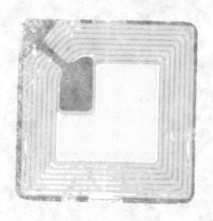

CASTLE CONNOLLY
AMERICA'S
TOP DOCTORS®
FOR CANCER

7th Edition

*America's Trusted Source
For Identifying Top Doctors*

Text by

John J. Connolly, Ed.D.

&

Jean Morgan, M.D.

A CASTLE CONNOLLY GUIDE

For more information, please contact:

Castle Connolly Medical Ltd., 42 West 24th St, New York, New York 10010
212-367-8400x10
E-mail: info@castleconnolly.com
Web site: http://www.castleconnolly.com.
Library of Congress Catalog Card Number 2010940314

| ISBN | 0-9845670-6-2; | 978-0-9845670-6-5 | (paperback) |
| ISBN | 0-9845670-7-0; | 978-0-9845670-7-2 | (hardcover) |

Printed in the United States of America

Table of Contents

Table of Contents

Section III: Physician Listings by Medical Specialty

Table of Contents

Table of Contents

Table of Contents

Table of Contents

Table of Contents

Table of Contents

Section IV: Appendices

Section V: Indices

About the Publishers

John K. Castle, the Chairman of Castle Connolly Medical Ltd., has spent much of the last three decades involved with healthcare institutions and issues. Mr. Castle served as Chairman of the Board of New York Medical College for eleven years, an institution where he served on the Board of Trustees for twenty-two years.

Mr. Castle has been extensively involved in other healthcare and voluntary activities as well. He served for five years as a commissioner and officer of the Joint Commission formerly known as (JCAHO), the body which accredits most public and private hospitals throughout the United States. Mr. Castle has also served as a trustee of five different hospitals in the metropolitan New York region, including NewYork Presbyterian Hospital, where he continues to serve.

Mr. Castle has also served as the Chairman of the Columbia Presbyterian Science Advisory Council and as a Director of the Whitehead Institute for Biomedical Research. He is a Fellow of New York Academy of Medicine and has served as a Trustee of the Academy. He was Chairman of the United Hospital Fund of New York's Capital Campaign and continues as Director Emeritus of the United Hospital Fund. He is a Life Member of the MIT Corporation, the governing body of the Massachusetts Institute of Technology.

Mr. Castle received his bachelor's degree from the Massachusetts Institute of Technology, his MBA as a Baker Scholar with High Distinction from Harvard, and two Honorary Doctorate degrees.

Mr. Castle's goal, as is the goal of Dr. John Connolly and all the Castle Connolly team, is to publish *America's Top Doctors®, America's Top Doctors® for Cancer, Top Doctors: New York Metro Area*, and other materials as well as build websites to help the public identify the very best in healthcare resources.

John J. Connolly, Ed.D., - the nation's foremost expert on identifying top physicians, is the President & CEO of Castle Connolly Medical Ltd. publisher of America's Top Doctors® and other consumer guides to help people find the best healthcare. He is also Vice-Chairman of Castle Connolly Graduate Medical Ltd., which publishes review manuals to assist resident physicians and fellows in preparing for their board exams.

Dr. Connolly served as President of New York Medical College, the nation's second largest private medical college, for more than ten years. He is a Fellow of the New York Academy of Medicine, a Fellow of the New York Academy of Sciences, a Director of the Northeast Business Group on Health, a member of the President's Council of the United Hospital Fund, and a member of the Board of Advisors of the Whitehead Institute for Biomedical Research.

Dr. Connolly has served as trustee of two hospitals and as Chairman of the Board of one. He is extensively involved in healthcare and community activities and has served on a number of voluntary and corporate boards including the Board of the American Lyme Disease Foundation, of which he is a founder and past chairman, and the Culinary Institute of America for over 20 years where he is now Chairman Emeritus. He also served as a director and Chairman of the Professional Examination Service and is presently on the board of the American Swiss Foundation. His current corporate board service includes: Baker and Taylor; Morton's of Chicago; Dearborn Risk Management and Perkins & Marie Callender's. He holds a Bachelor of Science degree from Worcester State College, a Master's degree from the University of Connecticut, and a Doctor of Education degree in College and University Administration from Teacher's College, Columbia University and an honorary doctorate (LHD) from Mercy College.

Dr. Connolly has appeared on or been interviewed by over 100 television and radio stations nationwide including "Good Morning America" (ABC-TV), "The Today Show" (NBC-TV), "20/20" (ABC-TV), "48 Hours" (CBS-TV), Fox Cable News, "Morning News" (CNN) and "Weekend Today in New York" (WNBC-TV). *The New York Times, The Chicago Tribune, The Daily News* (New York), *The Boston Herald* and other newspapers, as well as many national and regional magazines, have featured Castle Connolly Guides and/or Dr. Connolly in stories. He is the author and/or editor of seven books.

Castle Connolly Medical Advisory Board

Castle Connolly Medical Ltd. is pleased to have associated with a distinguished group of medical leaders who offer invaluable advice and wisdom in our efforts to assist consumers in making good healthcare choices. We thank each member of the Medical Advisory Board for their valuable contributions.

The Best in American Medicine
www.CastleConnolly.com

Foreword

Vincent T. DeVita, Jr., MD

Director, National Cancer Institute

(1980-1988)

As a physician, I've spent my professional career valuing the ability to find the right information and resources I need - quickly, efficiently and with the confidence that my sources are reliable. Similarly, healthcare consumers need to be able to find reliable information about the very best medical and healthcare services is critical, especially when confronting a diagnosis of cancer. That's why I like Castle Connolly's consumer guide, *America's Top Doctors® for Cancer*.

In creating this guide to more than 2,000 of the nation's leading medical specialists involved in the prevention, diagnosis and treatment of various cancer in both adults and children, Castle Connolly has invested a tremendous amount of time, energy and money in its research, screening and evaluation processes. To illustrate some of the complexity of doing this kind work, let me share a story with you. In my capacity as Director of the NCI from 1980 to 1988, I was often deluged with phone call requests, frequently from members of Congress or other well-placed individuals, to help them with their own personal problem with cancer or that of a friend or relative - and "pretty damn quick". They were not satisfied with just going to any doctor when their life, or the life of a friend or loved one was at stake - they wanted to know "who was doing what and where" and they wanted suggestions about the top doctors for their particular type of cancer. I often felt guilty that only a privileged few had access to this type of information. (This lack of fundamental information for the average patient is exactly what motivated Castle Connolly to start their "Top Doctors" series in 1991.)

The National Cancer Act had been established in 1971 by an Act of the U.S. Congress as part of a national "War on Cancer." Among its mandates for National Cancer Institute (NCI) was the creation of a cancer information service to get relevant information rapidly to cancer patients. Two unique individuals deserve credit and recognition for the role that they played in creating this information service. This part of the Cancer Act mandate was actually the brainchild of the philanthropist Mary Lasker, who was also one of the main architects of the passage of the Cancer Act itself. She had her finger on the pulse of the American public and was concerned, and correctly so in my view, that researchers and organizations that supported them, like the NIH, had a tendency to ignore the practical applications of their work for the public, despite the fact that their research was paid for by tax dollars. From the time of the passage of the act, Mary Lasker pursued each subsequent National Cancer Institute Director to build this information service. In 1981, Mr. Richard Bloch, of H&R Block, then a member of the National Cancer Advisory Board, and himself a successfully treated lung cancer patient, approached the NCI Director about his dream that a patient could use computerized information services to enter their personal information and get, in return, the most up-to-date management recommendations, and names of doctors using them. He was motivated by his own experience. He had had to fight his way through the system, being told by several doctors that he was incurable before he found where to go, and the physicians to provide the treatment that ultimately cured him. It was his goal, a goal to which he dedicated the rest of his life; to see that cancer patients like him got the information they needed.

With the strong advocacy of Mary Lasker and Richard Bloch, in 1984 NCI launched the PDQ system at the National Library of Medicine. It was the first computerized database in the world, aimed at the general public, devoted to a single disease, cancer. PDQ included lists of institutions, treatment protocols, and physicians devoted to managing cancer patients, all geographically matrixed, to allow patients, regardless of their status, to find the most appropriate doctor, treatment, and or clinical trial for them anywhere in the country and in their locale as well. Ironically, this aspect of PDQ - a list of specialists that seemed so logical and necessary - was controversial. From cancer specialists themselves, we heard that since not all cancer specialists (for example Cancer Surgeons) are "certified" by boards that test their qualifications for the cancer part of their work, the PDQ lists did not include " board certification" as a selection criteria. The PDQ physician list was also constructed primarily by using input and lists from specialty organizations. By building our list with assistance from specialty organizations, we were told, we had abrogated peer review and would be including doctors who might be only marginally qualified as specialists. To identify all doctors who were capable of providing modern care for cancer patients, on an individual basis, was not within the capability of the NCI or any government or private institution at the time. And to identify who were among the most qualified to diagnosis and treat specific types of cancers was simply not within our purview. And yet we knew that finding the right doctor at the right time could be a matter of life and death.

Foreword

Fast-forward to 2005 - PDQ and the Cancer Information Service have played a big part in the decline in national mortality rates from cancer in the US that began in 1990 and has continued since then. PDQ has now become a more complex information system about cancer and NCI cancer programs. But regrettably, the one thing that patients appreciated the most - the list of cancer doctors - is no longer a part of the PDQ system.

Castle Connolly's *America's Top Doctors® for Cancer* represents the much-needed and long-overdue answer for consumers – and physicians - seeking the top cancer specialists. Their physician-led Research Team has tackled some of the tough issues and developed criteria for selection, built on the foundation of Castle Connolly's well-respected national survey process that has enabled them to identify the leading physicians in more than twenty medical specialties associated with the prevention, diagnosis and treatment of cancers. The breadth and depth of the information they offer on each profiled physician will enable readers to be empowered consumers, to make informed decisions about the right doctor for their particular type of cancer. The guide also includes valuable information on some of the nation's most outstanding medical centers and specialty hospitals that are involved in the treatment of cancers.

America's Top Doctors® for Cancer will be an invaluable resource – a user-friendly, trusted source of information from an independent nationally renowned healthcare research and information company. I believe that using Castle Connolly's *America's Top Doctors® for Cancer* as a key source of information will help cancer patients and their loved ones navigate the complexities of the American healthcare system to find – and receive – the highest quality medical care.

Vincent T. DeVita, Jr., MD
Amy and Joseph Perella Professor of Medicine
Yale Cancer Center, Yale School of Medicine
(New Haven, Connecticut)
Director, National Cancer Institute (1980-1988)

The Best in American Medicine
www.CastleConnolly.com

The Best in American Medicine
www.CastleConnolly.com

Section I
Introduction

The Best in American Medicine
www.CastleConnolly.com

• 1 •

Cancer in the U.S. Today

If you or someone you love has been diagnosed with cancer, this book is for you. Although one in four Americans will be told they have cancer at some point during their lives, it is important to emphasize this no longer automatically carries a grim prognosis. Due to advances in treatment and, more importantly, early detection, people with cancer are living longer as well as healthier and more productive lives. While the overall quality of medical care throughout the United States is generally of very high quality, and in many places is superb, there are still those rare, complex or extremely difficult problems that demand resources beyond the ordinary or that require talents that are exceptional.

There is no denying fear is the most common reaction to the word "cancer," at least initially. Cancer has recently emerged as the leading cause of death of Americans under age 85. Bernadine Healy, M.D., former Director of the *National Institutes of Health*, wrote in *U.S. News and World Report* that cancer is both "sneaky and inexplicably virulent in many of its forms." These characteristics go a long way toward making cancer even more formidable than heart disease, another major killer.

However, Dr. Healy also described how advances in identification and prevention have restrained cancer from "galloping" through our population. We are all familiar with PAP smears which can identify early forms of cervical cancer in women, or the Prostate-Specific Antigen (PSA) test for prostate cancer in men, as well as colonoscopies that permit doctors to remove potentially cancerous polyps from the colon.

Many cancers are potentially curable, provided they are detected in the early stages. Growing awareness of early warning signs and symptoms, together with advances in screening, have resulted in major improvements in cancer survival.

Many cancers are potentially curable, provided they are detected in the early stages.

Prevention is even more important. Jane E. Brody, one of the nation's leading health columnists, wrote in *The New York Times* about life-enhancing changes involving diet and exercise we can make that may enable us to live cancer-free beyond the age of 85.

At the same time that methods of diagnosis and prevention have advanced, so too has our ability to treat cancer. In fact, today, many people are completely cured or are able to cope with their cancer as a chronic disease. There are nearly 10 million cancer survivors in the U.S. alone.

Americans' risk of getting cancer and dying from cancer continues to decline and survival rates for many cancers continue to improve. *The 2009 Annual Report to the Nation on the Status of Cancer, 1975-2006*, which is a colaboration among the American Cancer Society (ACS), the Centers for Disease Control and Prevention (CDC), the National Cancer Institute (NCI), and the North American Association of Central Cancer Registries (NAACR), provides updated information on cancer rates and trends in the United States, *found that both incidence and death rates decreased by <.05.*

In keeping with the current hopeful climate for cancer patients, the purpose of this book is to help you approach your diagnosis and treatment in the most effective way possible.

Cancer can occur in any cell in the body when the mechanisms that regulate normal cell growth fail. As a result, the cell experiences uncontrolled and excessive growth. These rapidly multiplying cells may go on to invade local tissues or spread (metastasize) to other parts of the body.

The field of cancer research is growing in leaps and bounds. Research is essential, not only to improve current methods of treatment, but also to develop new ways of treating what had previously been considered intractable types of cancer. As medical research and technology advances, more treatments and drugs are being introduced to combat cancer. In fact, every day we can read of new developments which may give renewed hope to many cancer patients.

The huge amount of information now available about all aspects of cancer can be quite daunting. New tests, new drugs, new technology, all may present a bewildering choice for many patients. You need guidance, and also psychological support, as you navigate through this strange new world. That's why it's vital for you to consult and be treated by a physician highly experienced in and knowledgeable about your particular type of cancer.

In certain types of cancer, different specialists may combine their efforts to work together as a team. For example, in successful skull base tumor surgery, the otolaryngologist and neurological surgeon operate together.

Different major medical centers may concentrate on different types of cancer treatments, their physicians working together to provide the "team approach" as needed. In other words, you're not just selecting a single doctor, but an entire hospital for your treatment.

Research is essential, not only to improve on current methods of treatment, but also to develop new ways of treating what had previously been considered intractable types of cancer.

The Best in American Medicine
www.CastleConnolly.com

• 2 •

Why Top Doctors and Top Hospitals

Finding the best physicians and best hospitals for your care is a major factor in achieving the best possible outcome. The average person may not be familiar with the various medical specialties, or know what constitutes medical education and the specifics of doctor "training," that period of residencies and fellowships that follows medical school. As a result, it is difficult for most Americans to choose physicians or hospitals in a well-informed fashion. Most people still find a doctor by asking a friend for a recommendation, or picking a name from a health plan directory or even a phone book.

In addition to listing excellent physicians identified by the Castle Connolly research team through our surveys, this book will describe the process you can use to find a "top doctor" for any medical problem or need. It will also provide up-to-date information on leading hospitals, and list valuable resources for cancer patients and their families. These resources are found in the appendices.

At times, our healthcare system, while good, may seem less than consumer friendly. The United States (and Canada) has many thousands of exceptionally well-trained and dedicated professionals involved in providing the best healthcare possible. Managed care, despite its shortcomings, has brought some much-needed structure to the healthcare delivery system. Most plans require that you have a primary care physician as well as specify referrals to selected specialists and hospitals. The health plans have the ability to monitor and assess the care delivered to you at all times, regardless of provider or location, because the plan has all your medical records in order to affect appropriate payment.

Unfortunately, the advantages offered by managed care plans have too frequently been directed toward controlling costs rather than enhancing quality. The hospitals and doctors to which patients are referred for more services or complex care are often selected on the basis of cost rather than other, more medically relevant, criteria. Therefore, even though a health plan directory may list a number of "centers of excellence" and several specialists for a given problem, they may not be the best for your particular needs.

Asking your primary care physician for a referral to a specialist can be a good place to start. However, too many of us don't have a close relationship with that all important "quarterback" of our healthcare, and this type of referral also has its limitations. Is the recommendation being made on the basis of a personal or professional relationship? Is the specialist to whom you are being referred truly the best, or is he or she simply in your primary care physician's group or in the network of your health plan? Even if your primary care physician is making a referral free from outside considerations, how broad is his or her knowledge of this particular specialty? Most primary care physicians have a limited number of referral channels. They are busy caring for their own patients and rarely have the time to devote hours of research to identifying top doctors for referrals. Typically, their referral network is local rather than regional or national

If you are already under the care of an excellent specialist, and he or she refers you to another specialist or sub-specialist for a particular problem, you can be confident of a more "meaningful" referral. When physicians are continually dealing with a specific disease, such as cancer, they are usually more aware of advances in the field, as well as the names of the top practitioners.

As the patient, finding the best physicians and best hospitals for your care is your responsibility. "Get a second opinion" is a common refrain. Everyone has heard stories of patients who were told by one physician (even at a top hospital) that their case was hopeless and yet, when they continued their search, they found another doctor or hospital that provided a different plan of treatment and perhaps even a cure.

Even the best doctors and the best hospitals are not perfect. Cancer treatment, like other medical care, is a combination of art and science. Frequently, opinions on diagnosis and treatment may differ - even among top doctors. That's why it's so important for you to seek second or even third opinions when a diagnosis, even one not involving cancer, is serious or may necessitate major surgery.

Even the best doctors and the best hospitals are not perfect. Cancer treatment is a combination of art and science.

One of the best known and inspirational stories of a patient undertaking this kind of search is that of Lance Armstrong, the seven time Tour de France champion cyclist. When Armstrong was first diagnosed with testicular cancer he received a grim prognosis from a number of excellent physicians at some of the nation's leading cancer centers. The recommended courses of treatment would have destroyed his ability to continue competing professionally. Refusing to accept that limitation, he continued his search until he found a physician and institution that offered different treatment options. As most people know, the treatment was successful. Seven of Armstrong's cycling championships (1999-2005) have come since his recovery from cancer.

Of course, there is a difference between seeking additional medical opinions and simply bouncing around from doctor to doctor until you find one that tells you what you want to hear. You need to find a doctor, hospital and treatment plan in which you have confidence, and which you honestly believe, based on extensive research, will work for you. Depending on the circumstances, it may be possible to find another physician or hospital that can offer a superior plan, or it may be that no better treatment options currently exist.

"Hope springs eternal" is not just a trite saying. It is something that should drive every patient and every doctor, simply because there are always unexpected and sometimes unexplainable remissions or cures occurring with cancer, and new breakthroughs in treatment could be just around the corner.

There is a significant amount of evidence that patients who are optimistic and fight, rather than surrender to their disease, have generally better outcomes. A positive attitude and the support of family and friends, as well as physicians and nurses, can be an important factor in your recovery. Knowing as much as possible about your diagnosis and your treatment options is another.

Reaching an initial diagnosis usually involves a number of medical tests including x-rays, MRIs and analysis of tissue samples obtained by a biopsy. It may be necessary to repeat these tests, or perform more specialized ones, in order to gain more thorough information or firmly establish a questionable diagnosis.

In the case of breast cancer, the disease is first likely to be identified either through a mammogram or else the discovery of a lump during a routine self or physician exam. Any breast lumps need to be biopsied for confirmation of cancer. Once that occurs, you will be referred to a surgeon who has special expertise in this field. He or she will recommend one or more possible treatments, including a total mastectomy, a lumpectomy, radiation therapy and chemotherapy.

As the patient, finding the best physicians and best hospitals for your care is your responsibility.

A suspicion of prostate cancer usually occurs following evidence of an enlarged prostate or an elevated PSA test. A urologist will make a definitive diagnosis based on a biopsy and examination of that tissue by a pathologist. Once cancer is found, the urologist can treat it by removing the prostate or by radiation.

Both the breast cancer and prostate cancer patient face the same basic questions: Is the surgeon treating you the most qualified and, more importantly, is surgery the only or best solution to deal with your disease?

Just like a number of additional options exist for breast cancer, surgery is not the only way to deal with prostate cancer, and may have unwanted side effects. Other alternative treatments include radiation therapy. In addition, since prostate cancer usually develops very slowly, some patients, especially older ones, may choose "watchful waiting." However, because most patients initially see a surgeon at the time of their diagnosis, they may end up having surgery without fully exploring the other alternatives.

Knowledge is not just power; in some instances it can make all the difference in not only your long-term survival, but also the quality of your life. This is why it is essential for you to be an informed consumer and find the best possible healthcare for yourself. This book will help you find the very best doctors and hospitals to treat cancer.

Factors to Consider When Identifying a Top Doctor

1. Medical Education

2. Residency & Fellowships

3. Board Certification

4. Hospital Appointment

5. Academic and Other Professional titles

6. Insurance Accepted

7. Personality

• 3 •

How Castle Connolly Identified the Top Doctors for Cancer

Castle Connolly is best known for its series of consumer guides including *America's Top Doctors*®, and *Top Doctors: New York Metro Area*. These books list "top doctors" in their respective regions. The New York edition profiles primary care physicians as well as other specialists and sub-specialists. *America's Top Doctors*® does not include any primary care physicians, but it lists the nation's top referral specialists. The Castle Connolly Guides are trusted by consumers and physicians alike. In fact, over 50% of the physicians listed in the Guides use them to make referrals.

Doctors do not and cannot pay to be listed in any Castle Connolly Guides. They are selected based on their nomination by peers solicited through mail and phone surveys, and on an extensive review of their credentials by the Castle Connolly physician-led research team.

For *America's Top Doctors*® *for Cancer* 7th Edition, Castle Connolly sent nomination forms to all physicians listed in *America's Top Doctors*® (10th edition) and *America's Top Doctors*® *for Cancer* (6th edition). In addition, nominations were solicited from the presidents and vice presidents of over 1500 of the nation's leading medical centers and specialty hospitals.

The physcians we have identified and listed are clearly among the best as nominated by their peers and screened by our research team.

Thousands of different physicians were nominated by their peers for inclusion in this guide. Of course, most of them received multiple nominations. In addition to the thousands of mail surveys, the Castle Connolly research team made hundreds of phone calls to leading specialists and sought additional nominations as well as using these conversations to reinforce the nominations received through the mail nomination process.

The Castle Connolly physician-led research team reviewed and analyzed the nominations and narrowed the field to those being considered for inclusion in *America's Top Doctors® for Cancer*. They contacted these physicians and asked them to complete an extensive biographical form describing their medical education, residencies, fellowships, hospital appointments and more. Particularly, we were interested in the physicians' area of special expertise; that is, the particular type of cancer (e.g. lung, breast, brain tumors, etc.,) or procedures (e.g. radical prostatectomy) in which the physician had particular experience, interest and expertise.

Finally, the research team checked on the disciplinary histories of the physicians by screening those that may have been disciplined by a medical board or state agency. After this intensive review, the final list was created.

The goal in creating this list was to select physicians viewed by their peers as the best in preventing, diagnosing and treating cancer and its related ramifications. Castle Connolly does not claim these are the only excellent doctors treating cancer in this country. Our nation is fortunate in having a generally excellent cadre of well-trained, dedicated physicians. The physicians we have identified and listed, however, are clearly among the very best as nominated by their peers and screened by our research team. In addition, they practice, for the most part, at major medical centers and leading specialty hospitals where they, and their patients, can receive the support of other highly skilled doctors, nurses and technicians as well as having access to the sophisticated and expensive equipment, laboratories and other resources that advance the level of cancer treatment and care from good to excellent. Furthermore, many of these physicians are engaged in teaching or research, or both. While the academic nature of their practice can limit the amount of time available to see patients, it keeps them, their colleagues and their institutions on the "cutting edge" of cancer treatment.

One important factor in our selection was geographic coverage. Some patients may be unable to travel long distances to a major medical center or specialty hospital due to financial resources, overall health status or some other reason. For them, a hospital in the immediate region is the only possible alternative. Since this is a guide for consumers and as many physicians use our guide to make referrals, we felt it was important to have broad geographic coverage and attempted to identify the top doctors for cancer in every state.

How Castle Connolly Identified the Top Doctors for Cancer

The reality is that the critical resources, the very best doctors and hospitals, are not dispersed evenly throughout the nation. For good reason they are clustered in large metropolitan areas or at academic medical centers that are part of major universities. It is only in these settings where it is possible to gather the combination of resources necessary to mount and maintain a superior medical program. The laboratories, technicians, intensive care beds, research fellows, scientists, specially trained nursing staff, equipment and, especially, the volume of patients and research subjects so necessary to enable these professional teams to continually develop and hone their skills, typically exist only in metropolitan areas or at university-based medical centers.

Therefore, it may be necessary for many Americans, if they are motivated to seek out the very best doctors and hospitals, to travel many miles, if possible, to obtain their care. It is also this reality that has motivated many outstanding medical centers and specialty hospitals to reach out and establish relationships with community hospitals throughout the nation. While it is not always possible to bring the labs, scientists, equipment and leading physicians to these communities, it is possible to raise the overall level of cancer care through these relationships.

Information on outcomes, procedure volume and malpractice is becoming increasingly available, but the public disclosure varies from state to state. Castle Connolly uses its best efforts to gather the information that is available and use it effectively. Ultimately, however, it is the professional judgment of the Castle Connolly editors, the Chief Medical and Research Officer and the research staff, which determines Castle Connolly Top Doctor™ selection.

Physicians may also be removed from the Castle Connolly lists if, in the judgment of the selection team, that is warranted. Some of the reasons physicians are removed include retirement, change in practice (taking a full time administrative post, for example), unavailability to patients, malpractice or disciplinary issues, negative physician or patient feedback, professional demeanor or a change in the "mix" of specialists Castle Connolly will present for a given community. Being removed from a Castle Connolly list does not necessarily indicate something negative about the physician. At the same time, Castle Connolly does not claim to identify every excellent physician in the nation or a region. The physicians identified through the Castle Connolly research process are clearly among the very best, but there are always other very good physicians not identified by Castle Connolly and that is why our guides, websites and other distribution channels for this critical information describe a process whereby consumers can identify excellent physicians using their own efforts.

The Best in American Medicine
www.CastleConnolly.com

• 4 •

Judging the Qualifications of a Physician

The National Cancer Institute (NCI) has declared its intention to eliminate suffering and death due to cancer by the year 2015. While that is clearly an ambitious goal, and one many may feel is unrealistic, it nonetheless demonstrates the optimism physicians and scientists are beginning to feel about the battle against cancer. As Ellen V. Sigal, Ph.D, founder and chairperson of Friends of Cancer Research in Washington, D.C. and a member of the National Cancer Institute's Board of Scientific Advisors, stated: "The consensus among the science community is that for the first time we understand the genetic underpinnings of this disease."

"How do you identify a top doctor?" is an important question for all Americans, not just those diagnosed with cancer. As we mentioned earlier, too many Americans are incredibly casual in selecting physicians and hospitals. They may pick a name from their health plan directory, or even from a phone book, with the location of the doctor's office being the primary factor in their selection. Others may simply ask a friend or relative and the recommendation they receive may be based on how well the person "likes" the doctor rather than on any particular medical expertise or skill.

The specialists listed in *America's Top Doctors® for Cancer* are clearly among the best in the nation and have been identified through a rigorous research process and thorough screening by the Castle Connolly physician-led research team. Through our extensive surveys and research we have done much of the work in finding a top referral specialist, but they are not the only excellent physicians in the nation.

The goal in creating this guide was to select physicians viewed by their peers as the best in preventing, diagnosing and treating cancer and its consequences.

So, how does one judge the qualifications of a physician who may not be listed in this Guide? If someone was trying to find a specialist on their own, how should they go about it? How can someone tell when a physician has the appropriate training in a specialty and how does one distinguish what is meaningful and what is not from among all those plaques and certificates on a doctor's wall?

The reality is that few of us see only one doctor in our lifetime. Each of us may be cared for by a primary care physician, an ophthalmologist, an orthopaedist, a dermatologist, a surgeon or a number of other specialists. The choices can be many and they can be among the most important choices we make.

The following pages will outline the process for selecting a well-qualified physician. In fact, what is written here reflects much of the logic that underlies the selection of physicians for this book. This section will help not only in finding a top specialist in this Guide, but it also should be helpful in choosing among the many specialists, primary care doctors and other physicians, that a person will need to consult throughout his/her life.

Education

The review of a prospective doctor's education and training should begin with medical school. While some may feel that the institution at which a physician earned a bachelor's degree could be an indication of the doctor's quality, most people in the medical field do not believe it plays a major role. A degree from a highly selective undergraduate college or university will help an aspiring doctor gain admission to a medical school, but once there all students are peers. Furthermore, where a doctor trains (i.e. completes residency) is more important than medical school in judging quality. American medical schools are highly standardized, at least in terms of basic quality standards.

A group known as the Liaison Committee for Medical Education (LCME) accredits all U.S. medical schools that grant medical degrees (MDs) and osteopathic degrees (DOs). Most also are accredited by the appropriate state agency, if one exists, and by regional agencies that accredit colleges and universities of all kinds.

Fortunately, U.S. medical schools have universally high standards for admission, including success on the undergraduate level and on the Medical College Admissions Tests (MCATs). Although frequently criticized for being slow to change and for training too many specialists, the system of medical education in the United States has assured consistent high quality in medical practice. One recent positive change is a strong effort in most medical schools to diversify the composition of the student body. While these schools have been less successful in enrolling racial minorities, the number of women in U.S. medical schools has increased to the point that women now make up about 50 percent of most classes. In certain specialties preferred by women medical graduates (pediatrics, for example), it is possible that in coming years the majority of specialists will be female.

Most doctors practicing in the United States are graduates of U.S. medical schools, but there are two other groups of doctors who make up a significant portion (30+%) of the total physician population. They are (1) foreign nationals who graduated from foreign schools and (2) U.S. nationals who graduated from foreign schools. (Canadian medical schools are not considered foreign.)

Foreign Medical Graduates

Foreign medical schools vary greatly in quality. Even some of the oldest and finest European schools have become virtually "open door," with huge numbers of unscreened students making teaching and learning difficult. Others are excellent and provided the model for our system of medical education.

The fact that someone graduated from a foreign school does not mean that he or she is a poor doctor. Foreign schools, like those in the U.S., produce both good and poor doctors. Foreign medical graduates who wish to practice here must pass the same exam taken by U.S. graduates for licensure. *In the 1998-2008 period of using the new United States Medical Licensing Exam (USMLE), 97% of U.S. medical school graduates passed Step II, the Clinical Knowledge Exam, as compared with 72% of the foreign graduates.* It is clear that the quality of many foreign schools, if not individual doctors, is not the same as U.S. medical schools, at least as measured by our standards. Nonetheless, many communities and patients have been well served by foreign medical graduates practicing in this counrty - often in sreas where it has been difficult to atract graduates of American schools. About 25% of practicing physicians in the U.S. today are graduates of foreign medical schools.

In addition, many foreign medical schools and their teaching hospitals are world renowned for their leadership in medical care, research and teaching, and many of the technologies and techniques we utilize in the U.S. today have been developed and perfected in foreign countries.

"How do you identify a top doctor?" is an important question for all Americans, not just those diagnosed with cancer.

Residency

Most doctors practicing today have at least three years of postgraduate training (following the MD or DO) in an approved residency program. This not only is an important step in the process of becoming a competent doctor, but it is also a requirement for board (specialty) certification. Most people assume that a prospective doctor needs to complete a three-year residency program to obtain a medical license. That is not an accurate assumption! New York State, for example, requires only one postgraduate year. However, since all approved residencies last at least three years and some, such as those in neurosurgery, general surgery, orthopaedic surgery and urology, may extend for five or more years, it is important to know the details of a doctor's training. Licensure alone is not enough of a basis on which to choose a physician.

Without undertaking extensive and detailed research on every residency program, the best assessment you can make of a doctor's residency program is to see if it took place in a large medical center whose name you recognize. The more prestigious institutions tend to attract the best medical students, sometimes regardless of the quality of the individual residency program. If in doubt about a doctor's training, ask the doctor if the residency he or she completed was in the specialty of the practice; if not, ask why not.

It is also important to be certain that a doctor completed a residency that has been approved by the appropriate governing board of the specialty, such as the American Board of Surgery, the American Board of Radiology, or the American Osteopathic Board of Pediatrics. These board groups are listed in Appendix A. If you are really concerned about a doctor's training, you should call the hospital that offered the residency and ask if the residency program was approved by the appropriate specialty group. If still in doubt, consult the publication Directory of Graduate Medical Education Programs, often called the "green book," found in medical school or hospital libraries, which lists all approved residencies.

> If in doubt about a doctor's training, ask the doctor if the residency program he or she completed was in the specialty of the practice; if not, ask why not.

Board Certification

With an MD or DO degree and a license, an individual may practice in any medical specialty with or without additional specialized training. For example, doctors with a license, but no special training, may call themselves a surgeon, oncologist or radiologist. This is why board certification is such an important factor. It assures the physician has had specific training in that specialty and has passed the board exam. The American Board of Medical Specialties (ABMS) recognizes 25 specialties and more than 90 subspecialties. Visit www.abms.org or call 866-275-2267 for more information. Eighteen boards certify in 20 specialties under the aegis of the American Osteopathic Association (AOA). Visit www.osteopathic.org or call 800-621-1773 for more information. Doctors who have qualified for such specialization are called board certified; they have completed an approved residency and passed the board's exam.

(See Appendix A for an approved ABMS and AOA lists). While many doctors who are not board certified call themselves "specialists," board certification is the best standard by which to measure competence and training.

You can be confident that doctors who are board certified have, at a minimum, the proper training in their specialty and have demonstrated their proficiency through supervision and testing. While there are many non-board certified doctors who are highly competent, it is more difficult to assess the level of their training. While board certification alone does not guarantee competence, it is a standard that reflects successful completion of an appropriate training program. If it is impossible to find a doctor in your area who is board certified in a particular subspecialty, for example, Medical Oncology or Radiation Oncology, at least be certain the physician is board certified in a related specialty such as Internal Medicine or Radiology.

Board certified doctors are referred to as Diplomates of the Board. Some of the colleges of medical specialties (e.g., the American College of Radiology, the American College of Surgeons) have multiple levels of recognition. The first is basic membership and the second, more prestigious and difficult to obtain, is status as a Fellow. Fellowship status in the colleges is meaningful and is based on experience, professional achievement and recognition by one's peers, including extensive experience in patient care. It should be viewed as a significant professional qualification.

It is important to know the details of a doctor's training. Licensure alone is not enough of a basis on which to choose a physician.

Board Eligibility

Many doctors who have been more recently trained are waiting to take the boards. They are sometimes described as "board eligible," a common term that the ABMS advocates abandoning because of its ambiguity. Board eligible means that the doctor has completed an approved residency and is qualified to sit for the related board's exam. Another term that is used is "board qualified." Once again, the term has no official standing, but could mean the doctor has completed residency and is awaiting the board exam. It could also mean the doctor took and failed to pass the exam to become board certified.

Each member board of the ABMS has its own policy regarding the use and recognition of the board eligible term. Therefore, the description "board eligible" should not be viewed as a genuine qualification, especially if a doctor has been out of medical school long enough to have taken the certification exam. To the boards, a doctor is either board certified or not. Furthermore, most of the specialty boards permit unlimited attempts to pass the exam and, in some cases, doctors who have failed the exam twice or even ten times, continue to call themselves board eligible. In Osteopathic Medicine, the board eligible status is recognized only for the first six years after completion of a residency.

In addition to the approved lists of specialties and subspecialties of the ABMS and AOA, there are a wide variety of other doctors and groups of doctors who call themselves specialists. At present there are at least 100 such groups called "self-designated medical specialties." They range from doctors who are working to create a recognized body of knowledge and subspecialty training to less formal groups interested in a particular approach to the practice of medicine. These groups may or may not have standards for membership. It may be difficult to determine the true extent of their members' training, and neither the ABMS or the AOA recognizes them. While you should be cautious of doctors who claim they are specialists in these areas, many do have advanced training and the groups at least offer a listing of people interested in a particular approach to medical care. Rely on board certification to assure yourself of basic competence, and use membership in one of these groups to indicate strong interest and possible additional training in a particular aspect of medicine.

You can be confident that doctors who are board certified have, at a minimum, the proper training in their specialty and have demonstrated their proficiency through supervision and testing.

Recertification

A relatively new focus of the specialty boards is the area of recertification. Until recently, board certification lasted for an unlimited time. Now, almost all the boards have put time limits on the certification period. For example, in Internal Medicine and Radiology, the time limit is ten years. These more stringent standards reflect an increasing emphasis on recertification by both the medical boards and state agencies responsible for licensing doctors.

Since the policies of the boards vary widely, it is a good procedure to check a doctor's background to see when certification was awarded. If the date was seven to ten years ago, see if he or she has been recertified. Unfortunately, many boards permit "grandfathering," whereby already certified doctors do not have to be recertified, and recertification requirements apply only to newly certified doctors. Even if recertification is not required, it is good professional practice for doctors to undertake the process. It assures you, the patient, that they are attempting to stay current.

Many states have a continuing medical education requirement for doctors. These states typically require a minimum number of continuing medical education (CME) credits for a doctor to maintain a medical license. Seven states require 150 CME credits over a three-year period. Osteopathic doctors are required to take 120 hours of CME credits within three years to maintain certification.

Fellowships

The purpose of a fellowship is to provide advanced training in the clinical techniques and research of a particular specialty. Fellowships usually, but not always, are designed to lead to board certification in a subspecialty such as medical oncology which is a subspecialty of internal medicine. Many physicians listed in this Guide have had fellowship training. In the U.S. there are a variety of fellowship programs available to doctors, which fall into two broad categories: approved and unapproved. Approved fellowships are those that are approved by the appropriate medical specialty board (e.g., the American Board of Radiology) and lead to subspecialty certificates. Fellowship programs that are unapproved are often in the same areas of training as those that are approved, but they do not lead to subspecialty certificates.

Unfortunately, all too often, unapproved fellowships exist only to provide relatively inexpensive labor for the research and/or patient care activities of a clinical department in a medical school or hospital. In such cases, the learning that takes place is secondary and may be a good deal less than in an approved fellowship. On the other hand, any fellowship is better than none at all and some unapproved fellowships have status for a valid reason that should not reflect negatively on the program. For example, the fellowship may have been recently created, with approval being sought. There are also some areas of medicine not yet recognized for sub-specialty certification, such as Transplant Surgery.

Some physicians may have completed more than one fellowship and may be boarded in two or more subspecialties. In addition, some physicians may pursue fellowship training and subspecialty certification but then choose to practice in their primary field of certification. For example, a doctor who is board certified in internal medicine also may have obtained board certification in oncology, but may choose to practice primarily internal medicine. For the most part, the physicians in this guide practice in their sub-specialties.

Professional Reputation

There are practitioners who meet every professional standard on paper, but who are simply not good doctors. In all probability, the medical community has ascertained this and, while the individual may still practice medicine, his or her reputation will reflect that collective assessment. There are also doctors who are outstanding leaders in their fields because of research or professional activities but who are not particularly strong, or perhaps even active, in patient care. It is important to distinguish that kind of professional reputation from a reputation as a competent, caring doctor in delivering patient care or, in the case of this guide, as an outstanding practitioner in a given specialty.

Hospital Appointment

Most doctors are on the medical staff of one or more hospitals and are known as "attendings;" some, however, are not. If a doctor does not have admitting privileges or is not on the attending staff of a hospital, you may wish to consider choosing a different doctor. It can be very difficult to ascertain whether or not the lack of hospital appointment is for a good reason. For example, it is understandable that some doctors who are raising families or heading toward retirement choose not to meet the demands (meetings, committees, etc.) of being an attending. However, if you need care in a hospital, the lack of such an appointment means that another doctor will have to oversee that care. In some specialties, such as dermatology and psychiatry, doctors may conduct their entire practice in the office and a hospital appointment is not as essential, or as good a criterion for assessment, as in other specialties.

If a doctor does not have admitting privileges or is not on the attending staff of a hospital, you may wish to consider choosing a different doctor.

While mistakes are made, most hospitals are quite careful about admissions to their medical staffs. The best hospitals are highly selective, so a degree of screening (or "credentialing") has been done for you. In other words, the best doctors usually practice at the best hospitals. Since caring for a patient in a hospital is often a team effort involving a number of specialists, the reputation of the hospital to which the doctor admits patients carries special weight. Hospital medical staffs review their colleagues' credentials and authorize performance of specific procedures. In addition, they typically review and reappoint their medical staff every two or three years. In effect, this is an additional screening to protect patients. It is especially true of hospitals that have what are known as closed staffs, where it is impossible to obtain admitting privileges unless there is a vacancy that the administration and medical staff deem necessary to fill. If you are having a surgical procedure and are concerned about the doctor's skill or experience, it may be worthwhile to call the Medical Affairs Office at the doctor's hospital to see if he or she is authorized to perform that procedure in that hospital.

The reasons for a hospital's selectivity are easy to understand: no hospital wishes to expose itself to liability and every hospital wants to have the best reputation possible in order to attract patients. Obviously, the quality of the medical staff is immensely important in creating that reputation.

Physicians listed in this guide are primarily on the staffs of major medical centers, university teaching hospitals and leading specialty hospitals. Occasionally, some may be on staff at a community hospital for one or two days a week and spend the majority of their time at the teaching hospital. There are many excellent physicians on the staffs of community hospitals that call themselves "medical centers," but they are typically not physicians who attract complex cases and referrals regionally, nationally and even internationally.

To learn about a hospital, visit its website. It is also useful to review a hospital's accreditation status under the Joint Commission on the Accreditation of Healthcare Organizations at www.jointcommission.org. *Also, http://hospitalcompare.hhs.gov/ offers data on hospital procedure numbers and outcomeds for a number of specific procedures.*

A last and very important reason why a hospital appointment is an essential requirement in your choice of doctor is that some states permit doctors to practice without malpractice insurance. If you are injured as a result of a doctor's poor care, you could be without recourse. However, few hospitals permit doctors to practice in them unless they carry malpractice insurance. This not only protects the hospital, but the patient as well.

The best doctors usually practice at the best hospitals.

Medical School Faculty Appointment

Many doctors have appointments on the faculties of medical schools. There is a range of categories from "straight" appointments, meaning full-time appointment as professor, associate professor, assistant professor or instructor, to clinical ranks that may reflect lesser degrees of involvement in teaching or research. If someone carries what is known as a straight academic rank (e.g. "professor of surgery," without "clinical" in the title), this usually means that the individual is engaged full-time in medical school research, teaching activities and patient care. The title "clinical professor of surgery" usually identifies a part-time or adjunct appointment and less direct involvement in medical school activities such as teaching and research.

Doctors who are full-time academicians are more likely to be in the forefront of new techniques and research, especially when it comes to a disease like cancer. They also have the advantage of the support of other faculty, residents and medical students.

When you are seeking a subspecialist, a doctor's relationship to a medical school becomes more meaningful since medical school faculties tend to be made up of sub-specialists. You are less likely to find large numbers of general or primary care practitioners engaged full-time on a medical school faculty. The newest approaches and techniques in medicine, for the most part, are explored and developed by medical school faculties in their laboratories and clinical practice settings. This is where they practice their sub-specialties, as well as teach and conduct research.

Medical Society Membership

Most medical society memberships sound very prestigious and some are; however, there are many societies that are not selective and virtually any doctor can join. In addition, membership in many of the more prestigious societies is based on research and publication or on leadership in the field and may have little to do with direct patient care. While it is clearly an honor to be invited to join these groups, membership may be less than helpful in discerning whether a doctor can meet your needs.

Physicians listed in this guide are primarily on the staffs of major medical centers, university teaching hospitals and leading specialty hospitals.

Experience

Experience is difficult to assess. Obviously, in most cases, an older doctor has more experience; on the other hand, a younger doctor has been more recently immersed in the challenge of medical school, residency, or even a fellowship, and may be the more up-to-date. If a doctor is board certified, you may assume that assures at least a minimal amount of experience, but since it could be as little as a year, check the date of graduation from medical school or completion of residency to know precisely how long a doctor has been in practice.

There is a good deal of evidence that there is a positive relationship between quantity of experience and quality of care. That is, the more a doctor performs a procedure, the better he or she becomes at it. That is why it is important to ask a doctor about his or her experience with the procedure that you need. Does the doctor see and treat similar cases every day, every week or only rarely? Of course, with some rare diseases, "rarely" is the only possible answer, but it is the relative frequency that is critical. In some states, data is available on volume or numbers of certain procedures performed at hospitals. For volume and outcome information in other states, visit the web site of Healthcare Choices at www.healthcarechoices.org. There is a good deal of controversy, however, on the validity and usefulness of such data. Opponents cite the fact that some of the data is produced from Medicare patient records only and, therefore, is based solely on an elderly population that does not represent the total activity of a hospital or doctor. Proponents of the use of such volume data agree that it is not perfect, but suggest it can be one useful criterion in selecting the best places to receive care for these specific problems. While recognizing the limitations of such data, the healthcare consumer may, nonetheless, find it of interest and use.

The one type of experience you should specifically want to know about is that dealing with any special procedure, particularly a surgical one, that has recently been developed and introduced into practice. For example, in the 1980's many doctors using laparoscopic cholecystectomy, a then new, minimally invasive surgical technique for removing gallbladders, experienced a high percentage of problems because they were not properly trained. This prompted the American Board of Surgery to promulgate new standards for the training of surgeons using this technique. Do not hesitate to ask about your doctor's training in a procedure and how frequently and with what degree of success he or she has performed it. Practice may not lead to perfection, but it does improve skills and enhance the probability of success.

Doctors who are full-time academicians are more likely to be in the forefront of new techniques and research, especially when it comes to a disease like cancer.

In some cases, relatively young doctors have recently completed residency or fellowship training under recognized leaders who have developed new approaches or techniques for dealing with a particular problem. They may have learned the new techniques from their mentors and may be far ahead of the field (and ahead of more senior and distinguished colleagues) in using those approaches. So age and experience must be considered and weighed along with other factors when choosing a physician.

Most doctors will be supportive if you request a second opinion and many will recommend it. In many cases, insurance companies will pay for second opinions, but check ahead of time to make sure your insurance plan does cover them. In an HMO you may have to be more assertive because one way health plans control costs is by limiting second opinions. Often, the opinion of a second doctor will confirm the opinion of the first, but the reassurance may be worth the time and extra cost. On the other hand, if the second opinion differs from the first, you have two alternatives: seek the opinion of a third doctor, or educate yourself as much as possible by talking to both doctors, reading up on the problem, and trusting your instincts about which diagnosis is correct. Sometimes obtaining a second opinion can be a major challenge. Occasionally, a physician may be offended. Nonetheless, you should not be dissuaded.

The simple logistics of getting a second opinion can be an obstacle. Tara Parker-Pope related in her column, *Health Journal* in *The Wall Street Journal*, the difficulty gathering her mother's records from five doctors, two radiology offices and the pathology lab. She also cited, in the same piece, a Northwestern University review of 340 breast cancer patients who sought second opinions. They reported that 20% of second opinions had no change in pathology or prognosis, but in the remaining 80% of patients some change did occur.

Office and Practice Arrangements

Some specialists will only see new patients who are referred to them by another doctor. Therefore, you may need to have your treating physician contact the specialist's office to arrange for your initial visit. Your health plan may also require that your primary care doctor provide a referral.

If English is not your first language, it may be advisable to determine whether someone in the specialist's office speaks your primary language or if a translator can be present during appointments or, perhaps take a bilingual person with you. This will ease communication and assure that all questions, responses and instructions are understood.

Research suggests that there is a positive relationship between
quantity of experience and
quality of care.

Accessibility of a physician's office may be a concern if you are wheelchair-bound, are elderly or cannot climb stairs or negotiate narrow corridors. Convenient parking may also be important to you.

When you are choosing a top specialist, these issues may be of lesser or greater importance, depending on the problem and type of care warranted. If you are traveling a great distance to have a specific procedure performed by a top specialist at a major medical center, continuing long-term monitoring or follow-up care by that physician may not be required or may not be feasible and such things as office practice arrangements are of less importance. On the other hand, if your disease needs to be monitored with follow-up care provided by the same top specialist, then such issues as accessibility of the doctor's office, appointment hours, waiting times and courtesy and professionalism of the staff become more significant.

Often, the opinion of a second doctor will confirm the opinion of the first, but the reassurance may be worth the time and extra cost.

Second Opinions

Second opinions are a valuable medical tool, too infrequently used in many instances and overused in others. Clearly, you do not want to seek another doctor's opinion on every ailment or problem that you face, but a second opinion should be pursued in the following situations:

- Before major surgery
- If a rare disease is diagnosed
- If a diagnosis is uncertain
- If the number of tests or procedures recommended might seem excessive
- If a test result has serious implications (e.g., a positive Pap smear)
- If the treatment suggested is risky or expensive
- If you are uncomfortable with the diagnosis and/or treatment
- If a course of treatment is not successful
- If you question your doctor's competence
- If your insurance company requires it

Personal Chemistry

One element of the doctor-patient relationship that we stress in our Guides is chemistry between doctor and patient, a part of which is often referred to as a doctor's "bedside manner." While this factor is of major importance in a long-term relationship such as you would have with your primary care physician, it is of less importance when you see a specialist only once or twice.

It is vital that there is a sense of mutual trust and respect between patient and doctor; this is a judgment that individuals must make for themselves. Among the many talented doctors listed in this Guide, there are very likely some to whom you would relate well and others with whom you may not feel as comfortable.

Patients prefer doctors who listen, demonstrate concern, are responsive to patient needs and spend sufficient time with them. The qualities of physicians in this regard, even the excellent ones in this Guide, vary widely.

You, the patient, are the only one who can assess these qualities because individuals react differently to various personalities. It is important for you to carefully judge your feelings towards a physician, especially if you are embarking on a long-term relationship. You should feel you can be open, trusting and responsive to your physician and that your relationship will be a positive one. Otherwise, find another doctor, since not doing so could adversely affect your care.

Once you have used this guide to identify the top specialist(s) best suited to treat your condition, there is much you can do to maximize the value of your first visit.

Patients prefer doctors who listen, demonstrate concern, are responsive to patient needs and spend sufficient time with them.

The Best in American Medicine
www.CastleConnolly.com

• 5 •

Maximizing Your First Appointment With a Top Doctor

After your research is done and you've secured an appointment for an initial consultation with a top doctor, known for his or her expertise in the diagnosis or treatment of your particular medical condition, what should you do?

Questions Concerning Payment

Other arrangements that may need to be made in advance of your first visit or discussed with the specialist's office staff concern payment. You may wish to ask the following:

- Is the specialist within your plan's network and will you need to make a co-payment? Or, is the specialist out-of-network and will you have to pay for your care out-of-pocket, meet a deductible or submit a form for reimbursement?

- Are credit cards an acceptable mode of payment?

- Does the specialist accept Medicare or Medicaid?

A specialist becoming newly involved in your care needs to learn as much as possible about the state of your health in a very limited time. Since top doctors are extremely busy people with many demands on their time, you should make certain that all relevant records and case summaries are obtained and sent to the specialist well in advance of your appointment.

Lastly, it may be advisable to take a relative or close friend with you for support.

Obtaining Your Records

All healthcare providers, including hospitals, doctors and their staffs, are under legal obligation to maintain the privacy of your medical records. In order to obtain release of those records, you must make a request in writing. If you need to obtain records from a number of providers, you should write one clear and concise letter authorizing release of your records and including your name, address, telephone number, date of birth, and hospital patient I.D. number. You then can make photocopies of this letter, but be sure to sign and date each copy as if it were an original. You also may want to specifically name those test results (e.g., pathology slides) or X-ray films (not just written reports or summaries) that must be included in addition to making a general request for your records. It's also a good idea to indicate the date of your appointment so the office staff can respond in a timely manner.

Although state laws require the timely release of medical records, hospital medical records departments and doctors' offices often take several weeks to pull and review patient charts and get them in the mail either to you or to another doctor. In addition to written authorization, you may be asked to pay the costs involved in copying your records, test results and X-ray films because many doctors' offices will not release the originals. Consider placing a call in advance to determine the procedure for releasing your records, how long you can expect it to take, and the costs involved so that you can save time by including payment with your release authorization letter. Be sure to allow sufficient time in advance of your consultation appointment for your request to be processed. Since you often must wait several weeks for an appointment with a specialist, allow at least that amount of time to obtain your records.

Even after making your written requests, you should follow up each letter with a telephone call to be sure that your records actually are sent. You should not assume that your request for records will be promptly fulfilled by an often overburdened, although well-intentioned, office staff.

It is vital that there is a sense of mutual trust and respect between patient and doctor; this is a judgment that individuals must make for themselves.

Remember, the more information the specialist has about your condition, the fewer repeat or additional tests or procedures you will need to undergo. This will lower the costs of your consultation and enable the specialist to more easily assess your condition.

The Facts and Only the Facts

Be thorough and organized in documenting your personal and familial medical histories, the medications you take and in relaying information about your condition. Even seemingly minor bits of information may provide subtle clues to the nature of your medical problem and the optimal way in which to treat it. It's also advisable to bring a list with you of names, addresses and telephone numbers of all physicians who have cared for you, especially those you have seen regarding your current medical problem.

Even though thoroughness is essential to presenting a clear picture of your medical condition, bear in mind that the specialist needs to get to your core health concerns as quickly as possible. Therefore, if you have a complex medical history, you may want to ask your current doctors to provide treatment summaries in addition to copies of your medical records. Hospital records should include your admission history and physical exam, dictated consultation and operation notes and discharge summaries for all hospitalizations. You may also be able to get a cumulative lab and X-ray summary for your hospital stays.

Unlike X-rays, which can be copied at reasonable cost, original pathology slides must be transported by mail or hand-carried. Your specialist may wish to have the pathologist with whom he or she works speak directly with the pathologist who initially interpreted your slides as part of the process of evaluating your case.

Being Prepared

To avoid leaving out important details of your condition or past treatment, prepare a concise, chronological summary before your consultation takes place. You may wish to type it and provide a copy to the specialist for inclusion in your chart. Highlight major medical results or significant events in the course of an illness or treatment if these will enlighten the doctor about your condition. Your personal perspective on the state of your health is vital to a full understanding of your medical problem.

You should make certain that all relevant records and case summaries are obtained and sent to the specialist well in advance of your appointment.

It is possible that the specialist will use terminology that you do not understand or may speak quickly assuming certain knowledge on your part about your condition or its treatment. Don't hesitate to ask for clarification as often or repeatedly as you may need to in order to fully comprehend what you are being told. If you are concerned that you may forget what the doctor tells you, ask the doctor's permission to take notes or ask if you might bring along a tape recorder so you can later replay what was said, especially any instructions you are given. You may prefer to bring along a relative or close friend to serve as a "second set of ears," but, again, seek the doctor's permission to do so in advance of your appointment.

Following this process will assure that you and the specialist you are consulting get the most from your appointment. After all, you both have the same goal: restoring you to optimal health and well being.

What To Do If You Can't Get an Appointment

At times it may be difficult, perhaps even impossible, to secure an appointment with the specific specialist you have identified. There are a number of reasons why this may occur. For example, the specialist may not be taking any new patients or may have such a busy schedule that it takes several weeks or months to get an appointment. He or she may only see patients during very limited hours because of teaching, research or other responsibilities or currently may have other limitations related to the acceptance of new patients.

However, bear in mind that the doctors in this guide are the leaders in their fields and therefore they work with and train the very best and brightest in their specialties. So, if you are unable to consult with a particular doctor, consider making an appointment with one of his or her outstanding colleagues. You can do this by asking a member of the doctor's office staff to refer you to an associate who is a member of the practice group or to another excellent physician who is specially trained to address your particular medical issue.

You can be comfortable knowing that you will receive high quality care from another specialist who practices in the same top setting.

Remember, the more information the specialist has about your condition, the fewer repeat or additional tests or procedures you will need to undergo.

Gathering The Facts

Have you done everything you can to prepare yourself and the specialist for the consultation? The following checklist will help you maximize the value of your visit to the specialist and will go a long way toward focusing you on the task at hand—getting the best advice or treatment for your health problem from one of the top doctors in the medical specialty related to your condition.

- Does the specialist have all the information needed to make a diagnosis of or treatment plan for your condition?

- Have your medical records, test results, and X-rays and MRIs been sent ahead of time to allow for their review by the specialist in advance of your first appointment?

- Have you written out your medical history, including that of your siblings, parents and grandparents, emphasizing the particular problem for which you are visiting this specialist?

- Are you prepared with a written list of questions?

- When you ask your questions, have you understood the answers?

The Best in American Medicine
www.CastleConnolly.com

• 6 •

Clinical Trials

The following information on special resources has been included to meet the needs of cancer patients and their families. These patients and their physicians may need to search for very new, cutting-edge, perhaps even experimental and not yet approved therapies. In such cases the search may lead to clinical trials, tests of new drugs and new medical devices, or innovative therapeutic approaches. Fortunately, these situations are rare, but when they do occur they are critical.

In addition to the outstanding private and public hospitals recognized in this guide, the U.S. government maintains its own unique, expert source of patient care and clinical research at the National Institutes of Health (NIH). In fact, the NIH operates its own hospital at which the care provided is usually related to clinical studies its researchers are undertaking.

In addition to those at the NIH, clinical trials also are conducted at leading medical centers and other organizations throughout the country. These facilities may be testing a new drug therapy, a new use for an existing medication or a medical device to deal with a problem that is not being resolved through the use of more traditional approaches.

This section will guide you in utilizing these special resources. These is also a listing of selected cancer resources in Appendix C.

If you are unable to consult with a particular doctor, consider making an appointment with one of his or her outstanding colleagues.

The Clinical Trial as a Treatment Option

For some patients the best medical treatment may only be available through clinical trials (also called treatment studies), which are designed to develop improved ways to use current medical treatments or to find new medical treatments by studying their effects on humans. Treatments are studied to determine if they are safe, effective and better treatments than conventional or standard therapies. Only if they meet all three of these criteria are they made available to the general public.

Many people are frightened by the term "clinical trial" because it conveys the notion of being a "guinea pig" in an experiment. Contrary to popular belief, however, new treatments are extensively studied by scientists in the laboratory before they are ever tested by physicians in clinical settings. Among the factors that keep patients from participating in clinical trials are: lack of awareness about clinical trials as a treatment option; fear of side effects or adverse reactions to treatment; refusal of insurance companies to pay for experimental treatments; failure of a physician to inform the patient about clinical trials; difficulty finding suitable clinical trials; unavailability of clinical trials for certain medical problems; distance of the patient from major medical centers conducting clinical trials; disruption of personal and family life; and the decision to stop medical treatment altogether.

Despite these and other obstacles, many people do seek out clinical trials. New medical treatments can offer participants hope for a cure, an extended lifespan, or an improvement in how they feel. Some participants also take comfort in knowing that others may benefit from their contribution to medical knowledge.

Deciding if a clinical trial is the right treatment option for you is no simple matter. Certainly, you will want to talk about it with your doctor(s) and other professionals involved in your care, as well as with family members and friends. But in order to fully benefit from what others have to say — based on either their professional knowledge or personal experience — you need to understand exactly what a clinical trial is and what your role as a volunteer will be.

Understanding Clinical Trials

Clinical trials are conducted for just about every medical condition, including life-threatening diseases such as AIDS or cancer; chronic illnesses such as diabetes and asthma; psychiatric disorders such as depression or anxiety; behavioral problems such as smoking and substance abuse; and even common ailments such as hair loss and acne. Chances are there is at least one trial (and probably more) that may be appropriate for you.

With more than 100 different types of cancer, it is understandable that a large number of clinical trials are cancer-related. Extensive information about clinical trials for cancer can be found on www.cancer.gov, the Web site of the National Cancer Institute (NCI). NCI is part of the National Institutes of Health (NIH). CenterWatch, an online clinical trials listing service, identifies over 14,000 clinical trials that are actively recruiting patients. Veritas Medicine, another useful online organization, allows individuals to perform personalized searches of its clinical trials database. See "Selected Cancer Resources" in Appendix C for more information on clinical trials.

Most clinical trials study new medical treatments, combinations of treatments, or improvements in conventional treatments using drugs, surgery and other medical procedures, medical devices, radiation or other therapies. Newer types of clinical trials, called screening or prevention trials, study how to prevent the incidence or recurrence of disease through the use of medicines, vitamins, minerals or other supplements; and how to screen for disease, especially in its early stages. Another type of trial studies how to improve the quality of life for patients, including both their physical and emotional well-being.

Clinical trials are sponsored both by the federal government (through the National Institutes of Health, the National Cancer Institute and many others) and by private industry through pharmaceutical and biotechnology companies, and through healthcare institutions (hospitals or health maintenance organizations) and community-based physician-investigators. The National Cancer Institute sponsors clinical trials at more than 1,000 sites in the United States. Trials are carried out in major medical research centers such as teaching hospitals as well as in community hospitals, specialized medical clinics and in doctors' offices.

Though clinical trials often involve hospitalized patients, a fair number of trials are conducted on an outpatient basis. Many trials are part of a cooperative network which may include as few as one or two sites or hundreds of locations, although one center generally assumes responsibility for overall coordination of the research. More than 45 research-oriented institutions, recognized for their scientific excellence, have been designated by the NCI as comprehensive or clinical cancer centers. See "Selected Cancer Resources" in Appendix C to find out how to locate these centers.

Clinical research is based on a protocol (established rules or procedures) describing who will be studied, how and when medications, procedures and/or treatments will be administered and how long the study will last. Trials that are conducted simultaneously at different sites use the same protocol to ensure that all patients are treated identically and all data are collected uniformly so that study findings can be compared.

The National Cancer Institute sponsors clinical trials at more than 1,000 sites in the United States.

Clinical trials generally are conducted in four phases. The first phase begins testing of the treatment on a small group of human subjects after rigorous and successful animal testing has been concluded. Phases Two and Three involve a broader test group and are designed to further evaluate the treatment's safety and more accurately determine appropriate dosage, application methods and side effects. The fourth phase, conducted after the treatment has been approved by the FDA for widespread use, monitors its long-term efficacy and is used to determine if any restrictions should be placed on the population of patients to whom the treatment is administered, or if any adverse effects result from interactions with other medications.

Some clinical trials test one treatment on one group of subjects, while others compare two or more groups of subjects. In such comparison studies participants are divided into two groups: the control group that receives the standard treatment and the experimental or treatment group which receives the new treatment. For example, the control group may undergo a surgical procedure while the experimental or treatment group undergoes a surgical procedure plus radiation to determine which treatment modality is more effective.

To ensure that patient characteristics do not unduly influence the study findings, patients may be randomly assigned to either the control or the experimental group, meaning that each patient's assignment is based purely on chance. In cases in which a standard treatment does not exist for a particular disease, the experimental group of patients receives the new treatment and the control group receives no treatment at all, or receives a placebo, an inactive medicine or procedure that has no treatment value. It is important to keep in mind that patients are never put into a control group without any treatment if there is a known treatment that could help them. Also, whether a patient is receiving an investigational drug or a placebo, he/she receives the same level and quality of medical care as those receiving the investigational treatment.

One of the most pressing reasons to participate in clinical trials is the opportunity to obtain treatment that might not be available otherwise.

Protecting the Rights of Participants

The safety of those who participate in clinical trials is a serious matter and is the number one priority of medical investigators. All clinical research, regardless of type of sponsorship results of long-term use and the occurrence of any serious side effect is guided by the same ethical and legal codes that govern the medical profession and the practice of medicine. Most clinical research is federally funded or federally regulated (at least in part) with built-in safeguards for patients. According to federal government regulations (and some state laws), every clinical trial in the United States must be approved and monitored by an Institutional Review Board (IRB), which is an independent committee of physicians, statisticians, community advocates and others (representing at least five distinct disciplines) to ensure that the protocol is being followed. Government regulations require researchers to fully inform participants about all aspects of a clinical trial before they agree to participate through a process called informed consent. To be sure that you understand your role in a clinical trial, you should jot down any questions beforehand so as not to forget them. You should also consider bringing along a friend or family member for support and additional input, and perhaps even tape recording the conversation (after asking permission to do so) to make sure you do not forget or misunderstand anything. Each participant in a clinical trial must be given a written consent form, which should be available in English and other languages. The consent form explains the issues listed in the box on page 46. Patients also are informed that they may leave the trial, or exclude themselves from any part of it, at any time. Informed consent means exactly what the term implies: you agree to join a clinical trial only after you completely understand exactly what your participation will involve for the duration of the study. By law, each patient must be provided with a copy of the signed consent form, which also must include the name and telephone number of a contact person for questions or additional information. Informed consent is a continuous process, so do not hesitate to ask questions before, during or after the trial.

The investigators must protect the privacy of each participant in a clinical trial by ensuring that all medical records are kept confidential except for inspection by the sponsoring agency, the Food and Drug Administration and other agencies involved in regulating the drug or treatment, and all data are collected anonymously by assigning a numeric code or initials to each individual.

During the course of the trial, participants are regularly seen by members of the research team to monitor their health and well-being. Participants also should be responsible for their own health by following the treatment plan (such as taking the proper dosage of medications on time), keeping all scheduled visits and informing members of the healthcare team about any symptoms that occur. If, during the course of the trial, the treatment proves to be ineffective or harmful, the patient is free to leave the study and still obtain conventional care. Conversely, as soon as there is evidence that one treatment modality is better than another, all patients in the trial are given the benefit of the new information.

Questions to Ask Your Doctor and the Trial's Research Team if You are Considering Participating in a Clinical Trial:

- Who is sponsoring the trial?

- How many patients will be involved?

- Will the trial be testing a single treatment or a combination of treatments?

- Will there be one treatment group or more than one treatment group?

- If more than one treatment group, how are patients assigned to each group?

- Has this treatment been studied in previous clinical trials? What were the findings?

- What are the requirements for patient eligibility?

Enrolling in Clinical Trials

Each clinical trial has its own guidelines, called eligibility criteria, for determining who can participate. Treatment studies recruit participants who have a disease or other medical condition, while screening and prevention studies generally recruit healthy volunteers. Inclusion criteria (those that allow you to participate in a study) and exclusion criteria (those that keep you from participating in a study) ensure that the study will answer the research questions posed in the research protocol while maintaining the safety of participants. The disease being studied is a primary factor in selecting suitable patients, but other factors such as the patient's gender, age, treatment history and other diagnosed medical conditions may also be important. Unfortunately, eligibility also may depend upon ability to pay. Many health plans do not cover all of the costs associated with clinical trials because they define these trials as experimental procedures. However, trials sometimes pay volunteers for their time and/or reimburse them for travel, childcare, meals and lodging.

To prevent people who qualify from being excluded from clinical trials for financial reasons, agencies such as the National Cancer Institute are working with health plans to find solutions and a growing number of states require insurance companies to pay for all routine patient care costs in cancer trials. To encourage more senior citizens to participate in cancer trials, Medicare plans to revise its payment policy to cover those trials.

When choosing a clinical trial you should determine the factors that are most important to you. For instance, patients generally prefer to participate in trials near their homes so that they can maintain their usual day-to-day activities, be surrounded by family and friends and avoid travel and lodging costs. If travel or temporary relocation becomes necessary, try to find a trial site that is near to some family member or friend or one that is in a locale similar to your own city or town. Many organizations, such as the National Cancer Institute, will work with patients and their families to identify support networks for them wherever they participate.

Participating in a Clinical Trial

Clinical trials are conducted by a research team led by a principal investigator (usually a physician) and are comprised of physicians, nurses and other health professionals such as social workers, psychologists and nutritionists. As a participant you may be required to commit a fair amount of time to a clinical trial, often within more than one geographic region or state.

Some participants also take comfort in knowing that others may benefit from their contribution to medical knowledge.

Participants in clinical trials should remain under the care of their regular physician(s) since clinical trials tend to provide short-term treatment for a specific medical condition and do not generally provide comprehensive primary care. In fact, some trials require that a patient's regular physician sign a consent form before the patient is enrolled. In addition, your regular physician can collaborate with the research team to make sure there are no adverse reactions between your other medications or treatments and the investigational treatment.

Weighing the Benefits and Risks of a Clinical Trial

If you are considering participation in a clinical trial, you need to consider the medical, emotional and financial ramifications of participation. Of course, the obvious benefit of a clinical trial is the chance that a new treatment may improve your health and prognosis. You will have access to drugs and other medical interventions before they are widely available to the public and you will obtain expert and specialized medical care at leading healthcare facilities. Many patients receive an added psychological benefit by taking an active role in their treatment.

It is important to bear in mind that some medical interventions used in clinical trials may carry potential risks depending upon the type of treatment and the patient's condition. While many side effects or adverse reactions are temporary (such as hair loss and nausea caused by some anti-cancer drugs), other more serious reactions can be permanent and even life-threatening (for example, heart, liver or kidney damage).

Deciding whether or not to participate in a clinical trial is often a matter of determining if the trial's potential benefits outweigh its possible risks. This is a highly personal decision that may be difficult to make in situations involving experimental treatment in which limited medical information may be available.

Getting Information on Clinical Trials

The more information you have about a clinical trial, the easier it will be to make a decision about whether or not it is right for you, and the more confident you will be that you made an appropriate decision. In addition to the "Selected Cancer Resources," Appendix C in this guide, the staff at your local public library, community hospital, or major medical center can assist you in locating the information you need from books, consumer organizations and on the Internet.

It is important to keep in mind that patients are never put into a control group without any treatment if there is a known treatment that could help them.

Questions to Ask the Sponsors About Your Rights as a Participant in a Clinical Trial:

- Who is responsible for approving and monitoring this research? Is there an IRB?

- Who informs me about the trial process? Do I sign a consent form? Will I receive a copy?

- May I leave the trial at any time? Have previous patients dropped out?

- Whom do I contact if I am experiencing any difficulty with this trial?

Learning about the National Institututes of Health (NIH)

The National Institutes of Health (NIH) comprise one the world's leading medical research centers and the Federal government's principal agency for biomedical research. An agency of the United States Department of Health, United States Public Health Service, NIH encompasses 25 separate institutions and centers with its main campus located in Bethesda, Maryland. Research is also conducted at several field units across the country and abroad.

Paitent Care at the NIH

The Warren Grant Magnuson Clinical Center, NIH's principal medical research center and hospital located in Bethesda, Maryland, provides medical care only to patients participating in clinical research programs. Two categories of patients participate in the Clinical Center studies: children and adults who wish to improve their own health, such as those with newly diagnosed medical problems, ongoing medical problems or family history of disease; and healthy volunteers wishing to advance knowledge about the causes, progress and treatment of disease. The patient's case must fit into an ongoing NIH research project for which the patient has the precise kind or stage of illness under investigation. General diagnostic and treatment services common to community hospitals are not available.

The Magnuson Clinical Center is the world's largest biomedical research hospital and ambulatory care facility, housing 1,600 laboratories conducting basic and clinical research. There are 1,200 tenured physicians, dentists and researchers on staff along with 660 nurses and 570 allied healthcare professionals (dieticians, imaging technologists, medical technologists, medical records and clerical staff, pharmacists and therapists).

The Center's hospital is specially designed for medical research and accommodates 540 carefully selected patients who are participating in clinical research programs. Its 350-bed facility has 24 inpatient care units to which 7,000 patients are admitted annually. The Center also has an Ambulatory Care Research Facility (ACRF) that serves 68,000 outpatient visits each year. A new facility, called the Mark O. Hatfield Clinical Research Center, which began accepting patients in early 2005, has 242 beds for inpatient care and 90 day-hospital stations for outpatient care. The Mark O. Hatfield Center carries out the latest biomedical research that results in new forms of disease diagnosis, prevention and treatment, which is then incorporated into improved methods of patient care.

The Consent Form Should Explain the Following:

- Why the research is being done.

- What the researchers hope to accomplish.

- What types of treatment interventions (and other test or procedures) will be performed?

- How long the study will continue.

- What the expected benefits and the possible risks are.

- What other treatments are available.

- What costs will be covered by the study, by the patient or by third-party payers such as Medicare, Medicaid or private insurance.

This is a fine example of Translational Medicine where excellent research discoveries are translated into new and improved methods of clinical treatment. In other words, the laboratory discoveries are brought to the bedside.

The Clinical Center also maintains a Children's Inn for pediatric outpatients and their families. This family-centered residence operates 24 hours a day, 7 days a week, 365 days a year.

In an effort to bring clinical research to the community, NIH supports approximately 80 General Clinical Research Centers (GCRCs) around the country, located within hospitals of major academic medical centers.

It is important to note that, as part of the federal government, the Warren Grant Magnuson Clinical Center provides treatment in clinical trials at no cost to its patients. In some cases, patients receive a stipend to help cover the costs of traveling to Bethesda for treatment and follow-up care. Travel costs for the initial screening visit, however, are not covered.

Areas of Clinical Study at the NIH

At the Magnuson Clinical Center alone, NIH physician-scientists conduct nearly 1,000 studies each year. Among the areas of study are cancer and related diseases.

Not all of these clinical areas are under investigation at any given time, however. The Patient Recruitment and Public Liaison Office (PRPL) at the NIH Clinical Center assists patients, their families and their physicians in obtaining information about participation in NIH clinical trials. Trained nurses are available to answer questions about the research programs and admission procedures.

Cancer Care at the Warren Grant Magnuson Clinical Center

The National Cancer Institute (NCI) is the largest of the biomedical research institutes and centers at NIH. There, clinical studies are designed to evaluate new and promising ways to prevent, detect, diagnose and treat cancer. The Warren Grant Magnuson Clinical Center provides a separate outpatient division for cancer patients and also has several designated inpatient units.

The investigators must protect the privacy of each participant in a clinical trial by ensuring that all medical records are kept confidential.

Questions to ask the trial's sponsor about eligibility criteria:

- What are the inclusion and exclusion criteria for the clinical trial(s) I am considering?

- How can I improve my chances of being accepted? Pre-existing conditions? Problems?

- If I am not eligible for one trial, what other trials being conducted for my condition?

- Will I be paid for my time or reimbursed for my out-of-pocket expenses?

If you are interested in entering a cancer study at the Magnuson Clinical Center (or at the General Clinical Research Centers), you should first discuss treatment options with a physician. As a general rule, patients interested in participating in clinical studies must be referred by a physician. However, in some instances, self-referral may be permitted.

Patients with medical problems other than cancer or healthy volunteers who wish to participate in a clinical study should contact the particular NIH institute responsible for the clinical area involved.

Cancer Care at the National Cancer Institute (NCI) Clinical Centers and Comprehensive Cancer Centers

You may also obtain clinical oncology services (education, screening, diagnosis or treatment) or participate in clinical trials at one of the 21 Cancer Centers or 39 Comprehensive Cancer Centers designated by the NCI for their scientific excellence and extensive resources devoted to cancer and cancer-related problems. Centers are located in 32 states, with the majority of sites in California, New York and Pennsylvania. You can find out about clinical trials at the NCI-designated centers by contacting NCI's Clinical Studies Support Center (CSSC) or by calling each center directly (See Appendix C for contact information). Information about other cancer-related services at these centers also may be obtained from the center itself. For more information, you can visit the National Cancer Institute's website at www.cancer.gov.

Questions to Ask the Research Team or Your Physician About Your Role in a Clinical Trial:

- Who are the members of the health team? Who will be in charge of my care?

- How long will the trial last?

- How does treatment in the trial compare with or differ from the standard treatment?

- Will I be hospitalized? How often? For how long a period of time?

- What will occur during each visit? What treatments or procedures will I be given?

- Will I still be able to see my regular physician(s)?

- Will my doctor and the research team collaborate?

- Can I be put in touch with other patients who have participated in this trial?

To encourage more senior citizens to participate in cancer trials, Medicare plans to revise its payment policy to cover those trials.

If Your Physician Concurs that a Clinical Study might be Appropriate for you, the NIH Recommends that the Following Steps be Taken:

- Contact National Cancer Institute's (NCI) Clinical Studies Support Center (CSSC), which is staffed by trained oncology (cancer) nurses who can identify appropriate clinical studies for you. Summaries of these trials and other pertinent information about the type of treatment being offered and the type of patients eligible for inclusion can be mailed or faxed to you and/or your physician.

- Review the clinical trials summaries and other information with your physician to decide which study or studies you should consider. Your physician also can contact the CSSC to communicate directly with the investigator in charge of the study.

- In cases in which you meet the initial eligibility requirements, it may be necessary for you to schedule a screening visit at the Clinical Center to learn more about the trial and possibly undergo some medical tests.

- If accepted for a clinical trial, make sure that you understand the details about the treatment and any possible risks and benefits.

Section II
Using this Guide to Find a Top Doctor

The Best in American Medicine
www.CastleConnolly.com

• 7 •

How to Use This Book

We assume most people who purchase this book have either received a diagnosis of cancer, or know someone who has. Although it would have been possible to arrange the listings by type of cancer, e.g. lung, breast, prostate, etc., that would not have been practical. For any particular type of cancer, a patient may be seeking one or more of a variety of different specialists. For example, any of the cancers mentioned could require, among other specialists, the involvement of pathologists, medical oncologists, surgeons, urologists, radiation oncologists and, possibly, psychiatrists.

Therefore, this guide and its list of physicians is organized first by specialty. Then, because many patients may prefer care as close to home as possible, we organized the lists by region. (See map on page 56)

The Special Expertise Index we include in the book, may also be of great help in locating the specialists a patient needs. We asked physicians making nominations to recommend individuals who were nationally recognized as leaders in the prevention, diagnosis and treatment of particular types of cancer, as well as leaders in various treatment modalities. When physicians selected for inclusion in *America's Top Doctors® for Cancer* completed and submitted their professional biographies, we also asked them to list their areas of special expertise. As a result, the Special Expertise Index lists hundreds of these areas.

The physicians are listed alphabetically within their specialties and then within their regions. A sample biography is presented and explained on the next page.

SAMPLE PHYSICIAN LISTING

Smith, John MD [Ped] - **Spec Exp:** Asthma Allergy; **Hospital:** Children's Hosp (page 120);

    Name [Specialty]   Special Expertise(s)   Admitting Hospital & Hospital Information Page

Address: 300 Ridge Road Boston, MA 12345; **Phone:** (617) 555-2343; **Board Cert:** Ped 75;

    Office Address   Office Phone   Board Certification(s)

Med School: Harvard Med Sch 70; **Resid:** Ped, Children's Hosp 73;

    Medical School   Residency(ies)

Fellow: AM, Children's Hosp 74; **Fac Appt:** Assoc Prof Ped, The Med Sch

    Fellowship(s)   Faculty Appointment

Step-by-Step Directions for Finding the Specialist you Need

1. Look for a doctor first by specialty. Turn to the Special Cancer Expertise Index on p. 609. Review the list which is organized alphabetically, and find the particular disease, organ, procedure or treatment of interest to you. Write down the page numbers of physicians with that expertise and turn to those pages.

2. Look in the area of the country closest to you. Each specialty lists doctors alphabetically within their geographical region. These regions start in New England (northeast) and go around the country in a consistent order to finish the West Coast and Pacific. Each state is grouped into one of these seven geographical regions. See map of the United States and the regions on page 56. If you don't find a doctor in that particular specialty in your first geographic preference, expand your search to other regions.

3. Check further in the special expertise index. If you don't find a doctor to meet your needs, the last chapter contains those specialties which include a small number of doctors. The Special Cancer Expertise index may include some diseases which are not related to cancer because a physician who treats cancer patients also may treat patients with these diseases.

Locating A Specialist

This guide is organized to make finding the right specialists for you or your loved ones as simple as possible. Physicians' biographies are presented by specialty and are organized by geographic region within each specialty or subspecialty. Thus, you may search for a particular type of specialist or subspecialist in one or more regions or throughout the nation.

A second way to locate the right specialist is to use the **Special Expertise Index** beginning on page 609. This index is organized according to diseases, conditions and procedures or techniques. If you already know a specialist's name, you can find his/her listing by using the **Alphabetical Listing of Doctors** beginning on page 653.

The information reported in each doctor's listing is, for the most part, provided by the doctor or his/her office staff. Castle Connolly attempts to verify the data through other sources but cannot guarantee that in all cases all data has been so verified or accurate. All such information is subject to change from time to time due to changes in physician practices.

Geographic Regions & States

To assist you in using *America's Top Doctors® for Cancer* in the most efficient and effective manner, the Guide is divided into seven geographic regions. This will help you to locate a specialist in your local or neighboring region. For example, if you live in Mississippi in the Southeast region and you are willing and able to travel to Louisiana in the Southwest region to consult with a specialist in medical oncology, you can review just those two regions, under the section headed "Medical Oncology." However, if you prefer to review the information on medical oncologists throughout the country, you can search the entire medical oncology section. Or, you can consult the "SPECIAL EXPERTISE INDEX" in the back of this Guide and choose a medical oncologist who has specific expertise to meet your particular needs.

The geographic regions are as follows:

New England	Great Plains and Mountains
Mid Atlantic	Southwest
Southeast	West Coast and Pacific
Midwest	

The states that are included in each region are listed on the following page and a map of the regions is also provided. Please note that not all regions are represented in all specialties. For example, in "Interventional Radiology" there are no listings in the Southwest region.

Section II

Geographic Regions and States

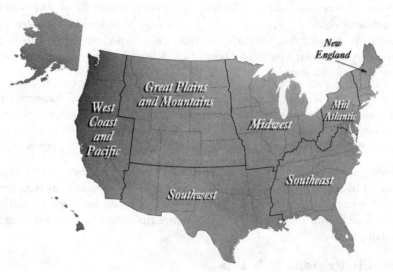

West Coast and Pacific:
Alaska
California
Hawaii
Nevada
Oregon
Washington

Great Plains and Mountains:
Colorado
Idaho
Kansas
Montana
Nebraska
North Dakota
South Dakota
Utah
Wyoming

Southwest:
Arizona
Arkansas
Louisiana
New Mexico
Oklahoma
Texas

Midwest:
Illinois
Indiana
Iowa
Michigan
Minnesota
Missouri
Ohio
Wisconsin

New England:
Connecticut
Maine
Massachusetts
New Hampshire
Rhode Island
Vermont

Mid Atlantic:
Delaware
Maryland
New Jersey
New York
Pennsylvania
Washington, DC
West Virginia

Southeast:
Alabama
Florida
Georgia
Kentucky
Mississippi
North Carolina
South Carolina
Tennessee
Virginia

• 8 •

Medical Specialties

In the pages that follow, each list of doctors in a medical specialty or subspecialty is preceded by a brief description of that specialty (or subspecialty) and the training required for board certification.

Critical Care Medicine has been excluded because in emergency situations there is neither time nor opportunity for choice. A number of other specialities not relevant to most patients (e.g., Forensic Psychiatry) have not been included as well.

The following descriptions of medical specialties and subspecialties were provided by the American Board of Medical Specialties (ABMS), an organization comprised of the 24 medical specialty boards that provide certification in 25 medical specialties. A complete listing of all specialists certified by the ABMS can be found in The Official ABMS Directory of Board Certified Medical Specialists, and is published by Marquis Who's Who. It is available (either in a multi-volume directory or on CD-ROM) in most public libraries, hospital libraries, university libraries and medical libraries. The ABMS also operates a toll-free phone line at 1-866-275-2267 and a website at www.abms.org to verify the certification status of individual doctors.

The following important policy statement, approved by the ABMS Assembly on March 19, 1987, remains valid.

The Purpose Of Certification

The intent of the certification process, as defined by the member boards of the American Board of Medical Specialties, is to provide assurance to the public that a certified medical specialist has successfully completed an approved educational program and an evaluation, including an examination process designed to assess the knowledge, experience and skills requisite to the provision of high quality patient care in that specialty.

Medical Specialty and Subspecialty Descriptions and Abbreviations

The following medical specialties and subspecialties are indicated in the doctors' listings by their abbreviations. Specialties are indicated in bold, subspecialties in italics, and the four primary care specialties in bold capitals. To review the official American Board of Medical Specialties (ABMS) organization of specialties, refer to Appendix A.

Addiction Psychiatry   AdP

Deals with habitual psychological and physiological dependence on a substance or practice which is beyond voluntary control.

Adolescent Medicine   AM

Involves the primary care treatment of adolescents and young adults.

Allergy & Immunology   **A&I**

Diagnosis and treatment of allergies, asthma, and skin problems such as hives and contact dermatitis.

Anesthesiology   **Anes**

Provides pain relief in maintenance or restoration of a stable condition during and following an operation. Anesthesiologists also diagnose and treat acute and long standing pain problems.

Cardiac Electrophysiology (Clinical)   CE

Involves complicated technical procedures to evaluate heart rhythms and determine appropriate treatment for them.

Cardiovascular Disease   Cv

Involves the diagnosis and treatment of disorders of the heart, lungs, and blood vessels.

Child & Adolescent Psychiatry   ChAP

Deals with the diagnosis and treatment of mental diseases in children and adolescents.

Child Neurology   ChiN

Diagnosis and medical treatment of disorders of the brain, spinal cord, and nervous system in children.

Clinical Genetics   **CG**

Deals with identifying the genetic causes of inherited diseases and ailments and preventing, when possible, their occurrence.

Colon and Rectal Surgery   **CRS**

Surgical treatment of diseases of the intestinal tract, colon and rectum, anal canal, and perianal area.

Critical Care Medicine   CCM

Involves diagnosing and taking immediate action to prevent death or further injury of a patient. Examples of critical injuries include shock, heart attack, drug overdose, and massive bleeding.

Dermatology **D**

Diagnosis and treatment of benign and malignant disorders of the skin, mouth, external genitalia, hair and nails, as well as a number of sexually transmitted diseases.

Diagnostic Radiology DR

Involves the study of all modalities of radiant energy in medical diagnoses and therapeutic procedures utilizing radiologic guidance.

Endocrinology, Diabetes & Metabolism EDM

Involves the study and treatment of patients suffering from hormonal and chemical disorders.

FAMILY MEDICINE **FP**

Deals with and oversees the total healthcare of individual patients and their family members. Family practitioners are more common in rural areas and may perform procedures more commonly performed by specialists (e.g., minor surgery).

Forensic Psychiatry FPsy

Concerns the evaluation of certain diagnostic groups of patients that include those with sexual disorders, antisocial personality disorders, paranoid disorders, and addictive disorders.

Gastroenterology Ge

The study, diagnosis and treatment of diseases of the digestive organs including the stomach, bowels, liver, and gallbladder.

Geriatric Medicine Ger

Deals with diseases of the elderly and the problems associated with aging.

Geriatric Psychiatry GerPsy

Involves the diagnosis, prevention, and treatment of mental illness in the elderly.

Gynecologic Oncology GO

Deals with cancers of the female genital tract and reproductive systems.

Hand Surgery HS

Involves the treatment of injury to the hand through surgical techniques.

Hematology Hem

Involves the diagnosis and treatment of diseases and disorders of the blood, bone marrow, spleen, and lymph glands.

Infectious Disease Inf

The study and treatment of diseases caused by a bacterium, virus, fungus, or animal parasite.

INTERNAL MEDICINE **IM**

Diagnosis and nonsurgical treatment of diseases, especially those of adults. Internists may act as primary care specialists, highly trained family doctors, or they may subspecialize in specialties such as cardiology or nephrology.

Maternal & Fetal Medicine MF

Involves the care of women with high-risk pregnancies and their unborn fetuses.

Medical Oncology   Onc

Refers to the study and treatment of tumors and other cancers.

Neonatal-Perinatal Medicine   NP

Involves the diagnosis and treatments of infants prior to, during, and one month beyond birth.

Nephrology   Nep

Concerned with disorders of the kidneys, high blood pressure, fluid and mineral balance, dialysis of body wastes when the kidneys do not function, and consultation with surgeons about kidney transplantation.

Neurological Surgery   **NS**

Involves surgery of the brain, spinal cord, and nervous system.

Neurology   **N**

Diagnosis and medical treatment of disorders of the brain, spinal cord, and nervous system.

Neuroradiology   NRad

Involves the utilization of imaging procedures during diagnosis as they relate to the brain, spine and spinal cord, head, neck, and organs of special sense in adults and children.

Nuclear Medicine   **NuM**

Evaluation of the functions of all the organs in the body and treatment of thyroid disease, benign and malignant tumors, and radiation exposure through the use of radioactive substances.

Nuclear Radiology   NR

Involves the use of radioactive substances to diagnose and treat certain functions and diseases of the body.

OBSTETRICS & GYNECOLOGY   **ObG**

Deals with the medical aspects of and intervention in pregnancy and labor and the overall health of the female reproductive system.

Occupational Medicine   OM

Concentrates on the effect of the work environment on the health of employees.

Ophthalmology   **Oph**

Diagnosis and treatment of diseases of and injuries to the eye.

Orthopaedic Surgery   **OrS**

Involves operations to correct injuries which interfere with the form and function of the extremities, spine, and associated structures.

Otolaryngology   **Oto**

Explores and treats diseases in the interrelated areas of the ears, nose and throat.

Otology/Neurotology   ON

Concentrates on the management, prevention, cure and care of patients with diseases of the ear and temporal bone, including disorders of hearing and balance.

Pain Medicine
PM

Involves providing a high level of care for patients experiencing problems with acute or chronic pain in both hospital and ambulatory settings.

Pediatric Cardiology
PCd

Involves the diagnosis and treatment of heart disease in children.

Pediatric Critical Care Medicine
PCCM

Involves the care of children who are victims of life threatening disorders such as severe accidents, shock, and diabetes acidosis.

Pediatric Dermatology
PD

Diagnosis and treatment of benign and malignant disorders of the skin, mouth, external genitalia, hair and nails in children.

Pediatric Endocrinology
PEn

Involves the study and treatment of children with hormonal and chemical disorders.

Pediatric Gastroenterology
PGe

The study, diagnosis, and treatment of diseases of the digestive tract in children.

Pediatric Hematology-Oncology
PHO

The study and treatment of cancers of the blood and blood-forming parts of the body in children.

Pediatric Infectious Disease
PInf

The study and treatment of diseases caused by a virus, bacterium, fungus, or animal parasite in children.

Pediatric Nephrology
PNep

Deals with the diagnosis and treatment of disorders of the kidneys in children.

Pediatric Otolaryngology
POto

Involves the diagnosis and treatment of disorders of the ear, nose, and throat which affect children.

Pediatric Pulmonology
PPul

Involves the diagnosis and treatment of diseases of the chest, lungs, and chest tissue in children.

Pediatric Radiology
PR

Involves diagnostic imaging as it pertains to the newborn, infant, child, and adolescent.

Pediatric Rheumatology
PRhu

Involves the treatment of diseases of the joints and connective tissues in children.

Pediatric Surgery
PS

Treatment of disease, injury, or deformity in children through surgical techniques.

PEDIATRICS
Ped

Diagnosis and treatment of diseases of childhood and monitoring of the growth, development, and well-being of preadolescents.

Physical Medicine & Rehabilitation   PMR

The use of physical therapy and physical agents such as water, heat, light electricity, and mechanical manipulations in the diagnosis, treatment, and prevention of disease and body disorders.

Plastic Surgery   PlS

Involves reconstructive and cosmetic surgery of the face and other body parts.

Preventive Medicine   PrM

A specialty focusing on the prevention of illness and on the health of groups rather than individuals.

Psychiatry   Psyc

Examination, treatment, and prevention of mental illness through the use of psychoanalysis and/or drugs.

Public Health & General Preventive Medicine   PHGPM

Involves the investigation of the causes of epidemic disease and the prevention of a wide variety of acute and chronic illness.

Pulmonary Disease   Pul

Involves the diagnosis and treatment of diseases of the chest, lungs, and airways.

Radiation Oncology   RadRo

Involves the use of radiant energy and isotopes in the study and treatment of disease, especially malignant cancer.

Reproductive Endocrinology   RE

Deals with the endocrine system (including the pituitary, thyroid, parathyroid, adrenal glands, placenta, ovaries, and testes) and how its failure relates to infertility.

Rheumatology   Rhu

Involves the treatment of diseases of the joints, muscles, bones and associated structures.

Sleep Medicine   Sleep Med

Involves the investigation and treatment of patients with sleep disorders.

Spinal Cord Injury Medicine   SpCdInj

Involves the prevention, diagnosis, treatment and management of traumatic spinal cord injuries.

Sports Medicine   SM

Refers to the practice of an orthopaedist or other physician who specializes in injuries to the bone or other soft tissues (muscles, tendons, ligaments) caused by participation in Athletic activity.

Surgery   S

Treatment of disease, injury, and deformity by surgical procedures.

Surgery of the Hand   SHd

Involves providing appropriate care for all structures in the upper extremity directly affecting the hand and wrist function.

Surgical Critical Care
SCC

Involves specialized care in the management of the critically ill patient, particularly **the trauma** victim and postoperative patient in the emergency department, intensive care unit, trauma unit, burn unit, and other similar settings.

Thoracic Surgery (includes open heart surgery)
TS

Involves surgery on the heart, lungs, and chest area.

Urology
U

Diagnosis and treatment of diseases of the genitals in men and disorders of the urinary tract and bladder in both men and women.

Vascular & Interventional Radiology
VIR

Involves diagnosing and treating diseases by percutaneous methods guided by various radiologic imaging modalities.

Vascular Surgery
VascS

Involves the operative treatment of disorders of the blood vessels excluding those to the heart, lungs, or brain.

The Training of a Specialist

Excerpted from "Which Medical Specialist For You?," American Board of Medical Specialties (ABMS), Evanston, IL, Revised 2000

Everyone knows that a "medical doctor" is a physician who has had years of training to understand the diagnosis, treatment and prevention of disease. The basic training for a physician specialist includes four years of premedical education in a college or university, four years of medical school, and after receiving the M.D. degree, at least three years of specialty training under supervision (called a "residency"). Training in subspecialties can take an additional one to three years.

Some specialists are primary care doctors such as family physicians, general internists and general pediatricians. Other specialists concentrate on certain body systems, specific age groups, or complex scientific techniques developed to diagnose or treat certain types of disorders. Specialties in medicine developed because of the rapidly expanding body of knowledge about health and illness and the constantly evolving new treatment techniques for disease.

A subspecialist is a physician who has completed training in a general medical specialty and then takes additional training in a more specific area of that specialty called a subspecialty. This training increases the depth of knowledge and expertise of the specialist in that particular field. For example, cardiology is a subspecialty of internal medicine and pediatrics, pediatric surgery is a subspecialty of surgery and child and adolescent psychiatry is a subspecialty of psychiatry. The training of a subspecialist within a specialty requires an additional one or more years of full-time education.

The training, or residency, of a specialist begins after the doctor has received the M.D. degree from a medical school. Resident physicians dedicate themselves for three to seven years to full-time experience in hospital and/or ambulatory care settings, caring for patients under the supervision of experienced specialists. Educational conferences and research experience are often part of that training. In years past, the first year of post-medical school training was called an internship, but is now called residency.

Licensure

The legal privilege to practice medicine is governed by state law and is not designed to recognize the knowledge and skills of a trained specialist. A physician is licensed to practice general medicine and surgery by a state board of medical examiners after passing a state or national licensure examination. Each state or territory has its own procedures to license physicians and sets the general standards for all physicians in that state or territory.

Who Credentials a Specialist and/or Subspecialist?

Specialty boards certify physicians as having met certain published standards. There are 24 specialty boards that are recognized by the American Board of Medical Specialties (ABMS) and the American Medical Association (AMA). All of the specialties and subspecialties recognized by the ABMS and the AMA are listed in the brief descriptions that follow. Remember, a subspecialist first must be trained and certified as a specialist.

In order to be certified as a medical specialist by one of these recognized boards a physician must complete certain requirements. See box on the next page.

All of the ABMS Member Boards now, or will soon, issue only time-limited certificates which are valid for six to ten years. In order to retain certification, diplomates must become "recertified," and must periodically go through an additional process involving continuing education in the specialty, review of credentials and further examination. Boards that may not yet require recertification have provided voluntary recertification with similar requirements.

How to Determine If a Physician is a Certified Specialist

Certified specialists are listed in The Official ABMS Directory of Board Certified Medical Specialists published by Marquis Who's Who. The ABMS Directory can be found in most public libraries, hospital libraries, university libraries and medical libraries, and is also available on CD-ROM. Alternatively, you could ask for that information from your county medical society, the American Board of Medical Specialties, or one of the specialty boards.

The ABMS operates a toll free number (1-866-275-2267) to verify the certification status of individual physicians. Additionally, information about the ABMS organization and links to an electronic directory of certified specialists can be accessed through the ABMS Web site at www.abms.org.

Almost all board certified specialists also are members of their medical specialty societies. These societies are dedicated to furthering standards, practice and professional and public education within individual medical specialties. Some, such as the American College of Surgeons and the American College of Obstetricians and Gynecologists, require board certification for full membership. A physician who has attained full membership is called a "Fellow" of the society and is entitled to use this designation in all formal communications such as certificates, publications, business cards, stationery and signage. Thus, "John Doe, M.D., F.A.C.S. (Fellow of the American College of Surgeons) is a board certified surgeon. Similarly, F.A.A.D. (Fellow of the American Academy of Dermatology) following the M.D. or D.O. in a physician's title would likely indicate board certification in that specialty.

To be Certified as a Medical Specialist by a Recognized Board, a Physician Must Complete Certain Requirements, these Include:

1 Completion of a course of study leading to the M.D. or D.O. (Doctor of Osteopathy) degree from a recognized school of medicine.

2 Completion of three to seven years of full-time training in an accredited residency program designed to train specialists in the field.

3 Many specialty boards require assessments and documentation of individual performance from the residency training director, or from the chief of service in the hospital where the specialist has practiced.

4 All of the ABMS Member Boards require that a person seeking certification have an unrestricted license to practice medicine in order to take the certification examination.

5 Finally, each candidate for certification must pass a written examination given by the specialty board. Fifteen of the 24 specialty boards also require an oral examination conducted by senior specialists in that field. Candidates who have passed the exams and other requirements are then given the status of "Diplomate" and are certified as specialists.

• 9 •

The Partnership for Excellence Program

Among the more than 6,000 acute care and specialty hospitals in the United States, many have extraordinary capabilities for superior patient care. These hospitals, renowned for their use of state-of-the-art equipment and up-to-the-minute technology, also attract outstanding physicians and other healthcare professionals. Many of their physicians are among those in the listings in this Guide.

To assist you in your search for top specialists and to supplement the information contained in the physician listings that follow, we invited a select group of these fine institutions to profile their services, special programs and centers of excellence in the Partnership for Excellence program. This special section contains pages sponsored by the included hospitals. This paid sponsorship program is totally separate from the physician selection process, which is based upon a completely independent review.

The Partnership for Excellence program provides an overview of the programs and services offered by the included hospitals with information related to their accreditation and sponsorship. Most also provide their physician referral numbers, should you wish to ask the hospitals for recommendations of doctors not listed in *America's Top Doctors® for Cancer* 7th edition.

In addition to the Partnership for Excellence program, profiled hospitals were also invited to highlight their special programs or services that focus on a particular disease or medical condition. These can be found in the "Centers of Excellence" sections that are interspersed throughout this book following the medical specialties and/or subspecialties to which they relate. Sponsored pages in the centers of excellence sections reflect the depth of commitment of these hospitals, which provide the staff, resources and financial support necessary to develop these special programs.

By visiting our website www.CastleConnolly.com, you may also link to the websites of these outstanding hospitals for even more detailed information on their cancer programs.

Participating Hospitals

- City of Hope National Medical Center

- Cleveland Clinic

- Continuum Health Partners

- Fox Chase Cancer Center

- Hackensack University Medical Center

- Maimonides Medical Center

- Memorial Sloan-Kettering Cancer Center

- Mount Sinai Medical Center

- New York Eye & Ear Infirmary

- NewYork-Presbyterian Hospital

- NYU Langone Medical Center

- Penn Medicine

- Thomas Jefferson University Hospital

- UHealth - University of Miami Health System

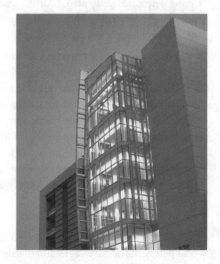

Cleveland Clinic

Every life deserves world class care.

Cleveland Clinic
Taussig Cancer Institute
9500 Euclid Avenue
Cleveland, OH 44195

Cancer Information and Support

Cancer Answer Line

The Cleveland Clinic Cancer Answer Line is here to help you understand your cancer diagnosis and available treatment options. The Cancer Answer Line is staffed by two clinical nurse specialists and their staff who can provide information and answer questions from patients and caregivers. If desired, they can also schedule appointments with expert physicians at Cleveland Clinic. The Cancer Answer Line hours are 8 a.m. – 5 p.m. ET, Monday – Friday.

The Scott Hamilton CARES Initiative

CARES was founded in 1999 as a partnership between Scott Hamilton, Olympic ice-skating champion and cancer survivor, and the Cleveland Clinic Taussig Cancer Center where he was treated. CARES was created to promote cancer awareness while raising significant funds for cancer research. Key components of CARES include:

- **4th Angel Mentoring Program** – a free phone-based program designed to match newly diagnosed patients with trained volunteers who are also cancer survivors. Emphasizing one-on-one contact, individuals are paired according to various demographics including age, cancer type and treatments. In addition, the 4th Angel Caregiver Mentoring program is designed to match a caregiver of a cancer survivor to a current cancer patient caregiver. A 4th Angel Caregiver Mentor uses her/his experience to help others cope with the difficult caregiver role. Call 866.520.3197

- **Chemocare.com** – a unique website designed to help patients better understand the chemotherapy experience. As the first website of its kind in the United States, Chemocare.com is written in easy-to-understand language, including both English and Spanish, and outlines everything patients and their families need to know about chemotherapy, side effects and their management.

clevelandclinic.org/scottcaresTCD

Appointments | Information: Call the Cancer Answer Line at 866.223.8100.

Cancer Treatment Guides

Cleveland Clinic has developed comprehensive treatment guides for many cancers. To download our free treatment guides, visit clevelandclinic.org/cancertreatmentguides.

Comprehensive Online Medical Second Opinion

Cleveland Clinic experts can review your medical records and render an opinion that includes treatment options and recommendations. Call 216.444.3223 or 800.223.2273 ext. 43223; email eclevelandclinic@ccf.org.

Special Assistance for Out-of-State Patients

Cleveland Clinic Global Patient Services offers a complimentary Medical Concierge service for patients who travel from outside of Ohio. Call 800.223.2273, ext. 55580, or email medicalconcierge@ccf.org.

Beth Israel | **Roosevelt Hospital** | **St. Luke's Hospital** | **NY Eye & Ear Infirmary**

Sponsorship: Voluntary Not-for-profit   **Beds:** 2,208 certified beds
Accreditation: Joint Commission of Accreditation of Healthcare Organizations (JCAHO), Accreditation Council for Graduate Medical Education, Medical Society of New York, in conjunction with the Accreditation Council for Continuing Medical Education

A STRONG PARTNERSHIP WITH A PROUD HERITAGE

Continuum Health Partners is a partnership of five venerable health care providers: Beth Israel Medical Center in Manhattan, Beth Israel Medical Center-Brooklyn, St. Luke's Hospital, Roosevelt Hospital, and The New York Eye and Ear Infirmary. Each of the five partner institutions was established more than a century ago by individuals committed to improving health and health care in their communities. Today, the system represents over 4,000 physicians and dentists and is superbly equipped to respond to the health care needs of the populations we serve. Our providers also see patients in group and private practice settings and in ambulatory centers in New York City and Westchester County.

LOCATIONS

Continuum Health Partners has campuses in Manhattan and Brooklyn. Beth Israel Medical Center has two divisions: the Milton and Caroll Petrie Division on the East Side, and the Brooklyn Division. The Phillips Ambulatory Care Center, a state-of-art outpatient center, is located at Union Square. St. Luke's Hospital is in Morningside Heights and Roosevelt Hospital is in the Columbus Circle and Lincoln Center neighborhoods on the West Side. The New York Eye and Ear Infirmary is located on Second Avenue and 14th street.

ACADEMIC AFFILIATIONS

Beth Israel Medical Center is the University Hospital and Manhattan Campus for the Albert Einstein College of Medicine. St. Luke's-Roosevelt Hospital Center is an Academic Affiliate of Columbia University College of Physicians and Surgeons. The New York Eye and Ear Infirmary is the primary teaching center of the New York Medical College and affiliated teaching hospitals in the areas of ophthalmology and otolaryngology.

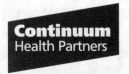

For a referral to a great doctor in your neighborhood, call (800) 420-4004.
Our Physician Referral Service can help you find a primary care physician or specialist affiliated with
Beth Israel, St. Luke's, Roosevelt or The New York Eye and Ear Infirmary.
Visit our Website at www.chpnyc.org

FOX CHASE
CANCER CENTER

333 Cottman Avenue
Philadelphia, PA 19111-2497
Phone: 1-888-FOX CHASE • Fax: 215-728-2702
www.foxchase.org

Sponsorship	Independent Nonprofit
Beds	100 licensed beds
Accreditation	The Joint Commission; American Hospital Association; American College of Surgeons Commission on Cancer with commendation; College of American Pathology; American College of Radiology; American Nurses Credentialing Center's Magnet designation

Overview

Fox Chase Cancer Center is one of the leading cancer research and treatment centers in the United States. Founded in 1904 in Philadelphia as one of the nation's first cancer hospitals, Fox Chase was also among the first institutions to be designated a National Cancer Institute Comprehensive Cancer Center in 1974. Fox Chase researchers have won the highest awards in their fields, including two Nobel Prizes. Fox Chase physicians are also routinely recognized in national rankings, and the Center's nursing program has received Magnet status for nursing excellence three consecutive times, having been the first hospital in Pennsylvania and the nation's first cancer hospital to earn this distinction from the American Nurses Credentialing Center. Today, Fox Chase conducts a broad array of nationally competitive basic, translational, and clinical research, with special programs in cancer prevention, detection, survivorship, and community outreach.

- Fox Chase's 100-bed hospital is one of the few in the country devoted entirely to adult cancer care.
- Fox Chase sees more than 7,900 new patients a year. Annual hospital admissions exceed 4,800, and outpatient visits to physicians total about 82,000 a year.
- Fox Chase's board-certified specialists are recognized nationally and internationally in medical, radiation and surgical oncology, diagnostic imaging, diagnostic pathology, pain management, oncology nursing and oncology social work.
- The staff provides a coordinated approach to meet the treatment needs of each patient. Special multidisciplinary centers provide consultations and treatment recommendations for specific types of cancer.
- The nursing staff of specially trained oncology nurses maintains excellent nurse-to-patient ratios.
- Fox Chase investigators have received numerous awards and honors, including Nobel Prizes in medicine and chemistry, a Kyoto Prize, a Lasker Clinical Research Award, memberships in the National Academy of Sciences and General Motors Cancer Research Foundation Prizes.
- Fox Chase maintains the first known cancer affiliate network in the United States. Established in 1986, Fox Chase Cancer Center Partners is a select group of 21 community hospitals in Pennsylvania and New Jersey with Fox Chase-affiliated cancer programs.
- Fox Chase is a founding member of the National Comprehensive Cancer Network, an alliance of the nation's leading academic cancer centers that is dedicated to improving the quality and effectiveness of cancer care.

For more about Fox Chase physicians and services, visit our website, www.foxchase.org, or call 1-888-FOX CHASE.

HACKENSACK UNIVERSITY MEDICAL CENTER

30 Prospect Avenue
Hackensack, New Jersey 07601
phone 201-996-2000

www.humc.com

Sponsorship	A not-for-profit, teaching and research hospital affiliated with the University of Medicine and Dentistry of New Jersey – New Jersey Medical School.
Beds	A 775-bed, Level II Trauma Center, providing tertiary and regional services for the New York/New Jersey metropolitan area.
Accreditation	Joint Commission.

BACKGROUND

Hackensack University Medical Center (HUMC) is a 775-bed teaching and research hospital that provides the largest number of admissions in New Jersey. Founded in 1888 with 12 beds and as Bergen County's first hospital, HUMC has demonstrated more than a century of growth and progress. Today, this not-for-profit, tertiary-care, teaching and research hospital serves as the hub of healthcare for northern New Jersey and the New York metropolitan area. HUMC is Bergen County's largest employer with a work force of more than 7,200 employees and an annual budget of $1 billion.

MEDICAL AND DENTAL STAFF

There are nearly 1,600 members on the medical and dental staff. These physicians and dentists represent a full spectrum of medical and dental specialties and subspecialties.

ACCOMPLISHMENTS

One of America's 50 Best Hospitals – In 2011, HealthGrades® named HUMC one of America's 50 Best Hospitals for the fifth consecutive year. These hospitals have achieved better survival rates and lower complication rates across dozens of medical procedures and diagnoses, from cardiac care to orthopedic surgery, consistently ranking among the top five percent in the nation for overall clinical outcomes. HUMC is the only healthcare facility in New Jersey, New York, and New England to be named one of America's 50 Best Hospitals for five years in a row. Also in 2011, *Becker's Hospital Review* named HUMC to its list of 50 Best Hospitals in America. *Becker's Hospital Review* is a leading national source of cutting-edge business and legal information relating to hospitals and health systems.

Nursing Excellence – HUMC is a Magnet® recognized hospital for nursing excellence, the first in New Jersey, receiving its fourth designation in April 2009. The medical center became the second hospital in the country to receive redesignation of this prestigious award and continues to have this highly honored recognition.

CENTERS OF EXCELLENCE

The **John Theurer Cancer Center** provides multidisciplinary care, personalized treatment, and innovative research within 14 divisions.

The **Heart & Vascular Hospital** is a new "hospital within a hospital," providing cutting-edge invasive and non-invasive services.

The **Joseph M. Sanzari Children's Hospital** offers 24 hour access to leading physicians, nurses, staff and a pediatric emergency department.

A consistent recipient of various women's health awards, the **Donna A. Sanzari Women's Hospital** provides superior care to its patients.

The **Jeffrey M. Creamer Emergency/Trauma Department** is a state-designated Level II Trauma Center open 24/7, treating all ages.

U.S. NEWS AND WORLD REPORT

Hackensack University Medical Center has been ranked in two specialties including geriatrics and heart surgery in *U.S. News and World Report's* 2010-11 publication of "America's Best Hospitals." Also, HUMC's Joseph M. Sanzari Children's Hospital has been named to U.S. News Media Group's 2011-12 Best Children's Hospitals' list, ranked in the top 50 in the specialty of neurology and neurosurgery. What's more, the children's hospital is the only hospital in New Jersey ever to be ranked in any Best Children's Hospitals specialty.

Maimonides Medical Center

4802 Tenth Avenue • Brooklyn, New York 11219
Phone: 718.283.6000
Physician Referral: 888.MMC.DOCS (662.3627)
www.maimonidesmed.org

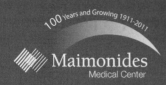

Sponsorship:	Voluntary, Not-for-Profit
Beds:	705 acute, 70 psychiatric
Accreditation:	The Joint Commission
	American College of Surgeons
	American Council of Graduate Medical Education (ACGME)

Maimonides Medical Center is among the largest independent teaching hospitals in the US, and trains more than 450 medical and surgical residents each year. Widely recognized for major achievements in medical technology and patient safety, Maimonides is a conductor of clinical trials for new treatments and therapies, and cited for clinical excellence by numerous health care evaluation services.

CENTERS OF EXCELLENCE

Cancer Center
Maimonides Cancer Center offers a fully integrated approach that includes prevention, screening, diagnostics, treatment, palliative care and clinical research. Staffed by leading physicians, nurses and social workers, the Center provides compassionate, patient-centered, state-of-the-art care.

Cardiac Institute
Maimonides is in the top 2% of hospitals in the nation for heart attack outcomes. Its renowned Cardiac Institute includes Catheterization Labs, state-of-the-art ORs, an electrophysiology lab, two ICUs, a Chest Pain Observation Unit, Advanced Cardiac Care Unit, Congestive Heart Failure Program, and Atrial Fibrillation Center.

Jaffe Stroke Center
The Jaffe Stroke Center at Maimonides received the *Gold Plus Quality Award* from the American Stroke Association. Currently the site of clinical trials for new stroke medications, medical devices and protocols, the Stroke Center offers interventional neuroradiology techniques and telemedicine.

Infants & Children's Hospital
The Maimonides Infants & Children's Hospital of Brooklyn, one of only five accredited children's hospitals in NYC, includes comprehensive inpatient services and more than 30 pediatric subspecialties. The Children's Hospital also has a Child Life Program, Pediatric ICU, Neonatal ICU, and Pediatric ER.

Vascular Institute
The Vascular Institute at Maimonides provides comprehensive diagnostic, clinical and vascular surgical services for patients with circulatory complications. The Vascular Institute is one of only five centers in New York certified to train vascular surgeons.

Stella & Joseph Payson Birthing Center
Maimonides delivers more babies than any other hospital in New York State. The Payson Birthing Center includes a Perinatal Testing Center, offers the services of doulas, and includes midwifery in a home-like setting – while utilizing the most advanced technology.

Geriatrics Program
Maimonides serves one of the oldest populations in New York City, with one in four patients over the age of 75. The Geriatrics Program is fully equipped to meet the special needs of seniors and encompasses inpatient and outpatient services.

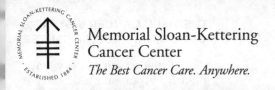

Memorial Sloan-Kettering Cancer Center
The Best Cancer Care. Anywhere.

1275 York Avenue
New York, NY 10065
Phone: (212) 639-2000
Make an Appointment: (800) 525-2225
www.mskcc.org

Sponsorship: Private, Non-Profit
Beds: 470
Accreditation: Awarded Accreditation from the Joint Commission on Accreditation of Healthcare Organizations (JCAHO)

At Memorial Sloan-Kettering Cancer Center, our sole focus is cancer. Our doctors are among the most skilled and experienced in the world in treating all kinds of cancer. The knowledge, talent, and expertise of our medical professionals lead to superb patient care, and often, a significant positive impact on the chances that their cancer will be cured or controlled.

SUB-SPECIALIZED MEDICAL EXPERTISE

Our patients benefit from individualized treatment plans developed by a team of specialists with unsurpassed depth and breadth of experience. The teams include surgeons, medical and radiation oncologists, radiologists, pathologists, nurses, and others who are specialists in a specific type of cancer. They develop treatment plans that reflect their combined expertise, so patients who need several different types of therapy will receive the best combination for them.

RESEARCH EXPANDS TREATMENT OPTIONS

One of Memorial Sloan-Kettering's great strengths is the close relationship between scientists and clinicians. Through the constant collaboration between our doctors and research scientists, new drugs and therapies developed in the laboratory can be quickly translated into improved treatment options for patients.

NURSING AND SUPPORTIVE CARE

Nurses are essential members of the healthcare team. Our specially trained oncology nurses care for patients throughout their treatment, help manage clinical trials, and educate patients about all aspects of their care.

Specialized psychiatrists and psychologists help patients deal with the stress, anxiety, and depression that sometimes accompany cancer and its treatment. Our social workers ensure that patients who need it receive assistance with needs such as housing and transportation. They offer individual and family counseling, as well as support groups for both inpatients and outpatients. After treatment, the Post-Treatment Resource Program offers patients seminars, lectures, support groups, and practical advice on various issues such as insurance and employment.

INTEGRATIVE MEDICINE

Our Integrative Medicine Service offers a full range of complementary therapies, including massage, reflexology, meditation, music therapy, and acupuncture. These do not replace medical care but are used along with clinical treatments to help patients relieve stress, reduce pain and anxiety, manage symptoms, and promote a feeling of well-being.

INSURANCE

Memorial Sloan-Kettering Cancer Center is in-network with most New York–area insurance plans.

A TRADITION OF EXCELLENCE

From its founding in 1884, Memorial Sloan-Kettering Cancer Center has been guided by a clear mission: to offer the best possible care for patients today, and to seek strategies to prevent, control, and ultimately cure cancer in the future. We are proud of our designation as one of the few select National Cancer Institute Comprehensive Cancer Centers and a member of the National Comprehensive Cancer Network.

To see one of our specialized cancer experts, call us at (800) 525-2225.

Make an Appointment: (800) 525-2225

MOUNT SINAI
SCHOOL OF
MEDICINE

THE TISCH CANCER INSTITUTE
AT THE MOUNT SINAI MEDICAL CENTER

One Gustave L. Levy Place
Fifth Avenue and 100th Street
New York, NY 10029-6574
Physician Referral: 1-800-MD-SINAI (637-4624)
www.tischcancerinstitute.org

THE TISCH CANCER INSTITUTE is embedded within a renowned medical center that has world-class research facilities, one of the nation's top-ranked hospitals, and an outstanding medical school. Patients have access to the best possible cancer care across a variety of disciplines, including medical, surgical, and radiation treatments; palliative care; behavioral medicine; physical therapy; psychosocial services—and cutting-edge cancer research. For fully integrated, multidisciplinary care, our patients are also treated by the best specialists in every field at Mount Sinai and can receive seamless referrals.

Services and Programs – The Tisch Cancer Institute employs a multidisciplinary treatment approach, providing access to clinical breakthroughs, innovative techniques, leading-edge technologies, and a wide range of diagnostic, therapeutic, and support services for all types of cancer. The Institute treats: breast cancer; hematological malignancies (including multiple myeloma, myelodysplastic syndrome, and myeloproliferative disorders); genitourinary cancers (including prostate, bladder, and kidney); head and neck cancers; thoracic cancer (including lung and esophagus); gynecologic cancers; brain tumors; and other diagnoses. In addition to surgical treatment, the Institute provides radiation and medical oncology therapies, as well as bone marrow transplantation. The Dubin Breast Center, consisting of 15,000 square feet, is a newly constructed facility that opened in April 2011 and significantly expands the treatment space for breast cancer patients.

THE RUTTENBERG TREATMENT CENTER
The Derald H. Ruttenberg Treatment Center houses the ambulatory cancer program of The Tisch Cancer Institute and is operated by the Mount Sinai Hospital.

THE DUBIN BREAST CARE CENTER
The Dubin Breast Care Center offers the latest, most innovative approaches available for breast health and the treatment of breast cancer.

The Tisch Cancer Institute encourages collaboration with colleagues across the Medical Center, drawing upon the knowledge of a vast network of specialists who are outstanding in their fields. These experts consist of award-winning physicians and surgeons specializing in cardiac care, neurology, urology, pediatrics, digestive diseases, obstetrics and gynecology, and other therapeutic areas. Oncologists, surgeons, radiation oncologists, and specialists from across the medical spectrum work together to provide the highest quality care to all cancer patients. Furthermore, Mount Sinai's nursing staff is an important part of the Medical Center's focus on delivering exceptional patient care, and it has received the prestigious Magnet Award for nursing excellence. Mount Sinai is also renowned for its palliative care program, which provides the highest level of care, focusing on the relief of pain, symptoms, and stress in cancer patients in both an inpatient and outpatient setting.

A Heritage of Breakthroughs – Teams of physicians and scientists at The Tisch Cancer Institute at Mount Sinai work together to rapidly translate laboratory research into new patient treatments. Among the advances pioneered at Mount Sinai are the first successful treatment of tumors of the bladder by transurethral electrocoagulation, the first demonstration of how asbestos can cause cancerous changes in the DNA of cells, and the first development of an ultrasound-guided technique to insert radioactive seeds into the prostate to treat prostate cancer.

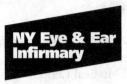

NY Eye & Ear Infirmary

Continuum Health Partners, Inc.

THE NEW YORK EYE AND EAR INFIRMARY

310 East 14th Street
New York, New York 10003
Tel. 212.979.4000   Fax. 212.228.0664
www.nyee.edu

OCULAR TUMOR SERVICE

The New York Eye and Ear Infirmary is a national referral center within the Collaborative Ocular Melanoma Study of the National Eye Institute/National Institutes of Health. New and innovative treatments for patients with eye cancer include radioactive plaques to treat intraocular tumors and chemotherapy for conjunctival neoplasia. Tumors of the eyelids, iris, retina, choroid and optic nerve are also treated by specialists in this service. A multidisciplinary Ocular Tumor Board meets monthly to discuss the most difficult cases and formulate therapeutic options

OTOLARYNGOLOGY/ HEAD & NECK SURGERY

Head & Neck Oncology: A team comprised of board-certified surgeons, medical & radiation oncologists, nutritionists and rehabilitation specialists ensure rapid recovery from complex, life saving surgical procedures and return to daily activities.

Thyroid Center: A unique center concentrates on streamlining the diagnosis and treatment of thyroid diseases and cancers with a highly skilled team of surgeons, endocrinologists and radiologists to manage the patient's care. An area of expertise is cancer resulting from radiation exposure such as that from Chernobyl.

Facial Plastics and Reconstructive Surgery: Treatment of facial tumors, both benign and cancerous, frequently requires expert reconstruction. Designed to restore the function and appearance of the face, these procedures may be required after appropriate treatment of skin cancers or deep tumors.

Otology–Neuro-otology: These rare cancers can be treated by our highly skilled team of surgeons which includes a neuro-otologist and a neurosurgeon.

Center for the Voice and Swallowing: Program cooperatively staffed by a team of specialists able to diagnose cancer of the vocal cords early and rehabilitate the voice after surgical and radiation treatment.

PATHOLOGY & LABORATORY MEDICINE

The Ocular Pathology Service is the leading laboratory in the Northeast and utilized by ophthalmologists throughout the region. The Infirmary is the site of some of the most promising studies into diseases and cancers of the eye, ear, nose and throat. Among them: cellular markers of oral cancer risk, non-invasive detection of thyroid cancer, basic cell biology of the growth of ocular melanoma cells, and persistence of biomaterials for repair in plastic and reconstructive surgery.

PLASTIC & RECONSTRUCTIVE SURGERY

The Department of Plastic & Reconstructive Surgery treats more than 1,500 patients a year who seek reconstructive surgery of the body as well as facial area as a result of accident, birth defect or cancer, and those who elect cosmetic surgery. It is one of the few hospitals in the region to perform breast reconstruction after mastectomy with microvascular surgery to harvest tissue from patients' lower body to create living, natural, and normal looking breasts, often preferred to artificial implants. State-of-the-art lymph node transfer to cure post-mastectomy lymphedema is also available.

About
The New York
Eye and Ear Infirmary

Established in 1820, The New York Eye and Ear Infirmary is nation's first specialty hospital and one of the most experienced in terms of the number of patients it treats and the complexity of its cases.

Each year the Ophthalmology Department performs more than 22,000 surgeries and sees more than 155,000 visits from outpatients. The Otolaryngology Department performs more than 6,000 surgeries and has some 70,000 outpatient visits. A third clinical department, Plastic & Reconstructive Surgery, is a natural complement to the Infirmary's other services with another 1,500 cases a year. Cutting-edge diagnostic tools and state-of-the-art surgical facilities with an experienced, caring staff assure high-tech treatment with a human touch for all.

The New York Eye and Ear Infirmay is a teaching affiliate of New York Medical College and a member of Continuum Health Partners, Inc.

**Physician Referral
1.800.449.HOPE (4673)**

⌐ NewYork-Presbyterian

⌐ The University Hospital of Columbia and Cornell

Affiliated with Columbia University College of Physicians and Surgeons and Weill Cornell Medical College

NewYork-Presbyterian Hospital	NewYork-Presbyterian Hospital
Columbia University Medical Center	Weill Cornell Medical Center
622 West 168th Street	525 East 68th Street
New York, NY 10032	New York, NY 10065

1-877-NYP-WELL (1-877-697-9355)   www.nyp.org

Sponsorship:	Voluntary Not-for-Profit
Beds:	2,409
Accreditation:	Joint Commission on Accreditation of Healthcare Organizations (JCAHO), Commission on Accreditation of Rehabilitation Facilities (CARF) and College of American Pathologists (CAP)

For 10 consecutive years, NewYork-Presbyterian Hospital has been listed on the prestigious "Honor Roll" of the *U.S. News & World Report* "Best Hospitals" survey and is ranked #1 in the New York metro area. NewYork-Presbyterian has the most physicians listed in *New York Magazine's* "Best Doctors" issue and is recognized for having more top doctors than any other hospital in the nation.

Overview

NewYork-Presbyterian Hospital is one of the foremost academic medical centers in the world and one of the most comprehensive healthcare institutions in the nation, with more than 6,100 physicians, some 117,00 discharges, and nearly 1.5 million outpatient visits annually. The Hospital enjoys a unique affiliation with two of the nation's leading Ivy League medical schools—the Joan and Sanford I. Weill Medical College of Cornell University and the Columbia University College of Physicians and Surgeons.

NewYork-Presbyterian Hospital Features Renowned CENTERS OF EXCELLENCE Including:

Morgan Stanley Children's Hospital and the Komansky Center for Children's Health— One of the largest, most comprehensive children's hospitals in the world, providing highly sophisticated pediatric medical, surgical, and intensive care services in a family-friendly, compassionate environment.

NewYork-Presbyterian Cancer Centers—Through a multidisciplinary team approach, we deliver seamless care and offer the latest therapeutic options and clinical trials for all cancer types.

NewYork-Presbyterian Digestive Disease Services—Our collaborative team manages and treats patients with digestive cancers and nonmalignant digestive diseases, such as inflammatory bowel disease and, pancreatic and biliary disorders, with compassionate care.

NewYork-Presbyterian Heart—Advances in cardiac care—from clinical cardiology, to interventional procedures, to surgical solutions—offer outstanding outcomes to adult and pediatric heart patients.

NewYork-Presbyterian Neuroscience Centers—Expert teams provide the most sophisticated diagnostic and treatment services for Alzheimer's disease, multiple sclerosis, Parkinson's disease, aneurysms, epilepsy, brain tumors, strokes, and other neurological disorders.

NewYork-Presbyterian Psychiatry—NewYork-Presbyterian Hospital's behavioral health and psychiatric services for adults, children, and adolescents offer a full continuum of programs at all levels of care.

NewYork-Presbyterian Transplant Institute—Our experts are internationally known for performing adult and pediatric heart, liver, kidney, pancreas, lung, bone marrow/stem cell, and intestinal and ex vivo transplantation.

NewYork-Presbyterian Vascular Care Center—We provide comprehensive, multidisciplinary preventive, diagnostic, and treatment services for aortic aneurysm, carotid artery disease, blood clots, and peripheral vascular diseases.

William Randolph Hearst Burn Center — NewYork-Presbyterian Hospital is home to the largest and busiest burn center in the nation, caring for more than 900 inpatients and 4,000 outpatients annually.

In addition, we offer extraordinary expertise, comprehensive programs, and specialized resources in the fields of AIDS, gene therapy, reproductive medicine and infertility, trauma care, and women's health.

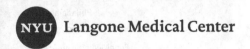
NYU Langone Medical Center

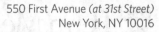

550 First Avenue *(at 31st Street)*
New York, NY 10016

www.NYULMC.org

Physician Referral: **(888)7-NYU-MED** *(888-769-8633)*

NYU Langone Medical Center is one of the nation's premier centers of excellence in health care, biomedical research, and medical education. For over 170 years, NYU physicians and researchers have made countless contributions to the practice and science of health care.

NYU Langone is comprised of three hospitals: Tisch Hospital, a 705-bed acute-care general hospital, Rusk Institute of Rehabilitation Medicine, the first and largest facility of its kind, and Hospital for Joint Diseases, a leader in musculoskeletal care; and NYU School of Medicine.

In a culture of humanism, where treating the whole person and not simply the disease is the norm, NYU Langone Medical Center is renowned for clinical excellence across a wide array of specialties, including: cardiology and cardiac and vascular surgery, cancer, musculoskeletal including orthopaedics and rehabilitation, neurosurgery, and children's services.

As an academic medical center, NYU Langone's clinical services are continually informed and enhanced by hundreds of basic and clinical research projects, as well as by major initiatives in translational research that promise to speed the transfer of laboratory discoveries to the patient's bedside.

We have brought together some of our most outstanding basic and translational scientists with clinicians to create six Centers of Excellence focusing on: addiction, brain aging, cancers of the skin, multiple sclerosis, musculoskeletal disease, and urologic disease. By applying the expertise and resources of multiple disciplines to focus on specific health problems, our Centers of Excellence are having a transformative effect, both on the productivity of our research and the quality of our patient care.

Additional Areas of Expertise:

Adult Cardiovascular Services	Otolaryngology
Internal Medicine	Pediatric Cardiology
Behavioral Health	Pediatric Critical Care
Cardiac Surgery	Pediatric Gastroenterology
Child and Adolescent Psychiatry	Pediatric Hematology
Clinical Genetics	Pediatric Rheumatology
Colon and Rectal Surgery	Pediatric Surgery
Dermatology	Program for IVF Reproductive
Gastroenterology	Psychiatry
Geriatric Medicine	Pulmonology
Hand Surgery	Radiology
Hematology/Oncology	Radiation Oncology
Infectious Diseases Pediatric Infectious Diseases	Reconstructive Plastic Surgery
Maternal and Fetal Medicine	Rheumatology
Pediatric Pulmonology	Thoracic Surgery
Minimally Invasive Surgery	Urology
Neonatal-Perinatal Medicine	Vascular Surgery
Nuclear Medicine	Wound Care
Obstetrics and Gynecology	Weight Management
Orthopaedic Services	

PENN CANCER SERVICES

Advancing Cancer Care

Penn Medicine is known for developing innovative approaches to the prevention, diagnosis and treatment of cancer. Through clinical excellence, advanced research and supportive care services, patients and their families are provided with outstanding comprehensive cancer care.

Abramson Cancer Center of the University of Pennsylvania

The Abramson Cancer Center is one of a select group of cancer centers in the country to be awarded the prestigious designation of *Comprehensive Cancer Center* by the National Cancer Institute (NCI).

The Cancer Center has established a variety of interdisciplinary centers dedicated to specific cancers. Each center offers patients a complete evaluation and treatment options by a team of doctors with subspecialty disease-specific expertise.

What Sets Abramson Apart?

- More than 400 full-time Penn faculty are actively involved in the diagnosis and treatment of patients with cancer.
- Clinical programs offering cutting-edge treatments such as robotic surgery for prostate, gynecologic cancer, and Transoral Robotic Surgery (TORS) for head and neck cancer.
- Developing immunotherapies that use the body's own immune system to fight cancer and reduce treatment-related side effects.
- One of the first cancer risk evaluation programs in the country for women concerned about their risk for breast and ovarian cancer.
- One of the foremost cancer research centers in the country and a leader in translational research, in which scientists translate discoveries from research laboratories into new treatments that benefit cancer patients.
- Comprehensive medical care for patients with other medical conditions such diabetes, pregnancy or heart disease.
- Utilizing personalized medicine which uses information about a person's genes, proteins, and environment to better prevent, diagnose, and treat cancer.
- Designated as a LIVESTRONG Center of Excellence™.
- Full range of support services to complement medical care including nutritional counseling, support groups, cancer rehabilitation, complementary and alternative therapies and pain and symptom management.

Joan Karnell Cancer Center at Pennsylvania Hospital

For patients and families facing cancer or blood-related illnesses, the Joan Karnell Cancer Center at Pennsylvania Hospital provides progressive, comprehensive and supportive cancer care through a wide range of services.
- A leader in the treatment of sarcoma and bloodless medicine.
- Committed to providing excellent cancer care in a supportive setting offering an interdisciplinary approach to diagnosis, treatment, research and education to help patients and their families achieve the best quality of life.

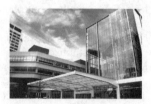

The Ruth and Raymond Perelman Center for Advanced Medicine

The Perelman Center is the home of the Abramson Cancer Center, which brings together outstanding cancer specialists with state-of-the-art technology to offer the most advanced cancer treatment options available.

The Roberts Proton Therapy Center

The Center, which is adjacent to the Perelman Center for Advanced Medicine, is the largest proton therapy treatment facility in the world and the first to be located on the campus of an academic medical center, facilitating scientific research to measure and improve this innovative therapy. Proton therapy is a treatment option for several types of cancer including prostate, lung, brain, head and neck, and sarcoma.

Additional Locations
Penn cancer services are also available at:

- Abramson Cancer Center at Penn Presbyterian Medical Center
- Hospital of the University of Pennsylvania
- Penn Medicine Radnor
- Penn Medicine Cherry Hill

For more information to schedule an appointment, call 800.789.PENN (7366) or visit PennMedicine.org/cancer.

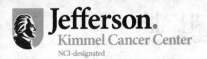

Jefferson®
Kimmel Cancer Center
NCI-designated

NCI·CC
A Cancer Center Designated by the
National Cancer Institute

111 S. 11th Street, Philadelphia, PA 19107-5098, 215-955-6000, *www.jeffersonhospital.org/cancer*

Designated Center of Excellence

Thomas Jefferson University Hospitals is an academic medical center comprised of Thomas Jefferson University Hospital, Jefferson Hospital for Neuroscience (JHN), Methodist Hospital and multiple outpatient sites. It is home to the Kimmel Cancer Center at Jefferson, a National Cancer Institute (NCI)-designated Center for Excellence in both cancer care and research, where world-famous cancer specialists provide breakthrough treatment with compassion, support and state-of-the-art technology. Jefferson doctors are ranked among the nation's best for cancer treatment on such prestigious lists as *Best Doctors in America®* database of experts. They also contribute to leading scientific and medical journals and hold leadership positions in national and local cancer organizations.

Recognized as Among the Best

- *U.S.News & World Report* recognizes Jefferson as one of the best hospitals in the nation for cancer care.
- Independence Blue Cross has designated Jefferson as a Blue Distinction Center for complex and rare cancers.
- Jefferson's Kimmel Cancer Center is one of only six cancer centers in the nation designated as a Center of Excellence by FertileHOPE, a non-profit organization providing reproductive information, support and hope to cancer patients and survivors.
- The Jefferson Breast Care Center has full accreditation from the National Accreditation Program for Breast Centers for achievement of the highest standards for breast cancer treatment.
- Jefferson's Center City Campus has been granted MAGNET® recognition for nursing excellence from the American Nurses Credentialing Center.

Jefferson's Approach to Cancer Care

- *Collaborative.* Specialists from our team of nationally renowned cancer experts will work with you and your referring physician to develop a personalized treatment plan. This is complemented by a support network for patients and their families, including specially trained nurses, educators, fellow patients and cancer survivors.
- *State-of-the-art.* Our experienced physicians utilize the most advanced technologies and pioneering therapies for diagnosis and treatment. Patients may have the opportunity to take part in one of the more than 120 clinical trials for promising new cancer treatments underway at Jefferson at any given time.
- *Personal.* We provide care for the whole person by addressing medical, emotional and spiritual needs. The Jefferson-Myrna Brind Center of Integrative Medicine's medical staff will work with your primary Kimmel Cancer Center provider to offer innovative natural therapies and counseling techniques, many of which can be applied during chemotherapy and radiation treatment, or at any time throughout survivorship.

Multidisciplinary Centers

Centers offer access to a team of specialists providing personalized care and leading-edge treatments:

- Brain Tumor
- Breast Care
- Colon and Rectal Cancer
- Genitourinary Oncology
- Gynecologic Cancer
- Head and Neck Cancer
- Liver Tumor
- Pancreatic, Biliary and Related Cancer
- Senior Adult Oncology
- Thoracic/Aerodigestive Cancer
- Uveal Melanoma

In addition, Jefferson offers innovative treatments for hematological malignancies, including new approaches to hematopoietic stem cell transplantation that make this option available to a greater number of patients.

Specialized Cancer Programs

- Bone Marrow Transplant
- Cancer Rehabilitation
- Musculoskeletal Oncology
- Hereditary Cancer
- Breast Cancer Risk Assessment
- Integrative Cancer Care

Physician Referral: Outpatient healthcare services are available throughout the Delaware Valley at the offices of 202 primary care physicians and 645 specialists affiliated with Thomas Jefferson University Hospitals. For an appointment with a Jefferson doctor, call **1-800-JEFF-NOW** or visit *www.jeffersonhospital.org*

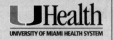
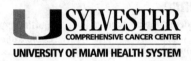

UNIVERSITY OF MIAMI HEALTH SYSTEM

DRIVEN TO BEAT CANCER

Sylvester Comprehensive Cancer Center serves as the cancer research diagnosis and treatment hub of UHealth – University of Miami Health System. Over the past decade and a half, Sylvester has grown with unstoppable momentum and singular focus – to develop and implement cancer breakthroughs and save lives.

Gaining the attention and respect of physicians and scientists from around the world, Sylvester has emerged as a magnet for today's leading cancer experts, attracting among the most innovative cancer professionals across a full spectrum of disciplines. Drawn to its entrepreneurial spirit, its unique international flair, and its awe-inspiring knowledge base, the team at Sylvester represents the future of university-based cancer care and research. It represents the real-world possibility to find the cure.

MORE CANCER SPECIALISTS. MORE SPECIALIZED CARE.

Patients who receive care from specialized hospitals often have better outcomes. At Sylvester we recognize the value of specialization, so we maintain a singular focus on cancer…only cancer. With more cancer experts than any other South Florida facility – more than 250 physicians and scientists, all faculty of the Miller School of Medicine – we have earned a reputation for delivering the most advanced treatment options available. This recognition has contributed to intense demand for care at Sylvester and more than a quarter million patient visits annually.

PHASE I CLINICAL TRIALS PROGRAM

Sylvester created South Florida's only academic phase I testing center dedicated to drug development for cancer patients. This novel program provides the necessary foundation to speed promising therapies from the laboratory to patients in need of care.

Phase I trials are the first studies in humans and, as a result, an important step to transition novel treatments from the bench to the bedside. The Phase I Clinical Trials Program assists physicians and scientists to establish important collaborative relationships that often translate into more treatment choices for patients.

Sylvester has assembled 15 multidisciplinary teams with focused expertise in specific types of cancers, including:

- Bone & Soft Tissue Cancers
- Breast Cancer
- Colorectal Cancer
- Eye Cancer
- Gynecologic Cancer
- Head & Neck Cancer
- Leukemia, Lymphoma & Myeloma
- Lung Cancer
- Melanoma & Related Skin Cancers
- Neurological Cancer
- Pancreatic, Liver & Related Cancers
- Pediatric Cancer
- Prostate, Bladder & Kidney Cancers
- Stomach & Esophageal Cancers
- Thyroid & Other Endocrine Cancers

As a leader in cancer research and treatment, Sylvester Comprehensive Cancer Center, with outpatient locations in Deerfield Beach and Kendall, is part of UHealth – University of Miami Health System, which includes more than 1,200 physicians, 30 outpatient locations, University of Miami Hospital, and the nation's top-ranked eye hospital, Bascom Palmer Eye Institute.

1475 N.W. 12th Avenue
Miami, Florida 33136
800-545-2292
www.sylvester.org

Section III
Physician Listings by Medical Specialty

The Best in American Medicine
www.CastleConnolly.com

Colon & Rectal Surgery

A colon and rectal surgeon is trained to diagnose and treat various diseases of the intestinal tract, colon, rectum, anal canal and perianal area by medical and surgical means. This specialist also deals with other organs and tissues (such as the liver, urinary and female reproductive system) involved with primary intestinal disease.

Colon and rectal surgeons have the expertise to diagnose and often manage anorectal conditions such as hemorrhoids, fissures (painful tears in the anal lining), abscesses and fistulae (infections located around the anus and rectum) in the office setting. They also treat problems of the intestine and colon and perform endoscopic procedures to evaluate and treat problems such as cancer, polyps (pre-cancerous growths) and inflammatory conditions.

Training Required: Five Years of General Surgery followed by one year in Colon & Rectal Surgery.

COLON & RECTAL SURGERY

New England

Bleday, Ronald MD [CRS] - **Spec Exp:** Colon & Rectal Cancer; **Hospital:** Brigham & Women's Hosp, Dana-Farber Cancer Inst; **Address:** Brigham & Women's Hosp, Dept Surgery, 75 Francis St, ASB II, Boston, MA 02115; **Phone:** 617-732-8460; **Board Cert:** Surgery 2009; Colon & Rectal Surgery 2003; **Med School:** McGill Univ 1982; **Resid:** Surgery, Rhode Island Hosp 1989; Surgical Oncology, Brigham & Womens Hosp 1986; **Fellow:** Endoscopy, Mass Genl Hosp 1990; Colon & Rectal Surgery, Univ Minn 1991; **Fac Appt:** Assoc Prof S, Harvard Med Sch

Harnsberger, Jeffrey R MD [CRS] - **Spec Exp:** Colon & Rectal Cancer; **Hospital:** Dartmouth - Hitchcock Med Ctr, Elliot Hosp; **Address:** Dartmouth-Hitchcock Manchester, 100 Hitchcock Way, Manchester, NH 03104; **Phone:** 603-695-2840; **Board Cert:** Surgery 2001; Colon & Rectal Surgery 2005; **Med School:** Med Coll OH 1987; **Resid:** Surgery, Dartamouth-Hitchkock Med Ctr 1992; **Fellow:** Colon & Rectal Surgery, St Louis Univ Med Ctr 1993; **Fac Appt:** Asst Prof S, Dartmouth Med Sch

Hyman, Neil H MD [CRS] - **Spec Exp:** Colon & Rectal Cancer; **Hospital:** Fletcher Allen Health Care- Med Ctr Campus; **Address:** FAHC 111 Colchester Ave, Burlington, VT 05401; **Phone:** 802-847-3339; **Board Cert:** Surgery 2008; Colon & Rectal Surgery 2003; **Med School:** Univ VT Coll Med 1984; **Resid:** Surgery, Mt Sinai Med Ctr 1989; **Fellow:** Colon & Rectal Surgery, Cleveland Clinic 1990; **Fac Appt:** Prof S, Univ VT Coll Med

Longo, Walter E MD [CRS] - **Spec Exp:** Colon & Rectal Cancer; Gastrointestinal Surgery; **Hospital:** Yale-New Haven Hosp, Yale Med Group; **Address:** Dept Surgery/Gastroenterology, 330 Cedar St, rm LH118, Box 208062, New Haven, CT 06520-8062; **Phone:** 203-785-2616; **Board Cert:** Surgery 2001; Colon & Rectal Surgery 2006; **Med School:** NY Med Coll 1984; **Resid:** Surgery, Yale-New Haven Hosp 1990; **Fellow:** Research, Yale-New Haven Hosp 1988; Colon & Rectal Surgery, Cleveland Clinic 1991; **Fac Appt:** Prof S, Yale Univ

Nagle, Deborah A MD [CRS] - **Spec Exp:** Colon & Rectal Cancer; Anal Cancer; Laparoscopic Surgery; **Hospital:** Beth Israel Deaconess Med Ctr - Boston; **Address:** Beth Israel Deaconess Med Ctr, 330 Brookline Ave Stoneman Bldg - rm 932, Boston, MA 02215; **Phone:** 617-667-4159; **Board Cert:** Colon & Rectal Surgery 2006; Surgery 2004; **Med School:** Univ Pennsylvania 1988; **Resid:** Surgery, Graduate Hosp 1993; Colon & Rectal Surgery, Thos Jefferson Univ Hosp 1994; **Fac Appt:** Prof CRS, Univ Pennsylvania

Orkin, Bruce A MD [CRS] - **Spec Exp:** Colon & Rectal Cancer; Laparoscopic Surgery; **Hospital:** Tufts Med Ctr; **Address:** Tufts Med Ctr, Div Colon & Rectal Surg, 860 Washington St, Box 6190, Boston, MA 02111; **Phone:** 617-636-6190; **Board Cert:** Colon & Rectal Surgery 2001; Surgery 2008; **Med School:** Univ Minn 1981; **Resid:** Surgery, Mayo Clinic 1986; **Fellow:** Surgical Research, Mayo Clinic 1988; Colon & Rectal Surgery, Cleveland Clinic 1989; **Fac Appt:** Prof S, Tufts Univ

Read, Thomas E MD [CRS] - **Spec Exp:** Colon & Rectal Cancer; Laparoscopic Surgery; Anorectal Disorders; **Hospital:** Lahey Clin; **Address:** Department of Colon and Rectal Surgery, Lahey Clinic Medical Center, 41 Mall Road, Burlington, MA 01805; **Phone:** 781-744-8971; **Board Cert:** Surgery 2005; Colon & Rectal Surgery 2008; **Med School:** UCSF 1988; **Resid:** Surgery, UCSF Med Ctr 1995; **Fellow:** Colon & Rectal Surgery, Lahey Clinic 1996; **Fac Appt:** Prof S, Tufts Univ

Roberts, Patricia L MD [CRS] - **Spec Exp:** Colon & Rectal Cancer; **Hospital:** Lahey Clin; **Address:** 41 Mall Rd, Burlington, MA 01805; **Phone:** 781-744-8243; **Board Cert:** Colon & Rectal Surgery 2003; **Med School:** Boston Univ 1981; **Resid:** Surgery, Boston City Hosp 1986; **Fellow:** Colon & Rectal Surgery, Lahey Clinic 1988; **Fac Appt:** Prof S, Tufts Univ

Schoetz Jr, David J MD [CRS] - **Spec Exp:** Colon & Rectal Cancer; Incontinence-Fecal; **Hospital:** Lahey Clin; **Address:** Lahey Clin Med Ctr, Dept Colon & Rectal Surg, 41 Mall Rd, Burlington, MA 01805-0001; **Phone:** 781-744-8889; **Board Cert:** Surgery 2001; Colon & Rectal Surgery 1983; **Med School:** Med Coll Wisc 1974; **Resid:** Surgery, Boston Univ Med Ctr 1981; Surgery, Boston Univ Med Ctr 1978; **Fellow:** Colon & Rectal Surgery, Lahey Clin 1982; **Fac Appt:** Prof S, Tufts Univ

Shah, Nishit S MD [CRS] - **Spec Exp:** Colon & Rectal Cancer; **Hospital:** Rhode Island Hosp; **Address:** University Surgical Associates Inc., 2 Dudley St, Ste 370, Providence, RI 02905; **Phone:** 401-553-8322; **Board Cert:** Surgery 2001; Colon & Rectal Surgery 2004; **Med School:** England, UK 1989; **Resid:** Surgery, Univ Pittsburgh Med Ctr 1995; **Fellow:** Colon & Rectal Surgery, Cleveland Clinic 1996

Shellito, Paul C MD [CRS] - **Spec Exp:** Colon & Rectal Cancer; Anorectal Disorders; **Hospital:** Mass Genl Hosp; **Address:** 15 Parkman St, Ste Wang 460, Mass General, Boston, MA 02114-3117; **Phone:** 617-724-0365; **Board Cert:** Surgery 2002; Colon & Rectal Surgery 1994; **Med School:** Harvard Med Sch 1977; **Resid:** Surgery, Mass Genl Hosp 1983; Surgery, Auckland Univ Med Sch 1981; **Fellow:** Colon & Rectal Surgery, Univ Minn 1985; **Fac Appt:** Asst Prof S, Harvard Med Sch

Mid Atlantic

Efron, Jonathan E MD [CRS] - **Spec Exp:** Colon & Rectal Cancer; Incontinence-Fecal; Anorectal Disorders; **Hospital:** Johns Hopkins Hosp, Johns Hopkins Bayview Med Ctr; **Address:** Johns Hopkins Hosp, 600 N Wolfe St, Baltimore, MD 21287; **Phone:** 410-933-1233; **Board Cert:** Surgery 2008; Colon & Rectal Surgery 2009; **Med School:** Univ MD Sch Med 1993; **Resid:** Surgery, LIJ Medical Ctr 1999; **Fellow:** Colon & Rectal Surgery, Cleveland Clinic 2000; Research, Cleveland Clinic 2001; **Fac Appt:** Assoc Prof S, Johns Hopkins Univ

Eisenstat, Theodore E MD [CRS] - **Spec Exp:** Colon Cancer; Anorectal Disorders; **Hospital:** Robert Wood Johnson Univ Hosp - New Brunswick, JFK Med Ctr - Edison; **Address:** 3900 Park Ave, Ste 101, Edison, NJ 08820-3032; **Phone:** 732-494-6640; **Board Cert:** Surgery 1974; Colon & Rectal Surgery 1994; **Med School:** NY Med Coll 1968; **Resid:** Surgery, Thomas Jefferson Univ Hosp 1971; Surgery, Pennsylvania Hosp 1973; **Fellow:** Colon & Rectal Surgery, Muhlenberg Med Ctr 1978; **Fac Appt:** Clin Prof S, UMDNJ-RW Johnson Med Sch

Fry, Robert D MD [CRS] - **Spec Exp:** Colon & Rectal Cancer; Anal Cancer; Anorectal Disorders; **Hospital:** Pennsylvania Hosp (page 80), Hosp Univ Penn - UPHS (page 80); **Address:** Pennsylvania Hospital, Div Colon & Rectal Surgery, 700 Spruce St, Ste 305, Philadelphia, PA 19106-4023; **Phone:** 215-662-2078; **Board Cert:** Surgery 2006; Colon & Rectal Surgery 1998; **Med School:** Washington Univ, St Louis 1972; **Resid:** Surgery, Barnes Jewish Hosp 1977; **Fellow:** Colon & Rectal Surgery, Cleveland Clinic 1978; **Fac Appt:** Prof S, Univ Pennsylvania

Gearhart, Susan L MD [CRS] - **Spec Exp:** Colon & Rectal Cancer-Hereditary; Incontinence-Fecal; **Hospital:** Johns Hopkins Hosp; **Address:** Johns Hopkins Hosp, Dept of Surgery, 600 N Wolfe St, Blalock 658, Baltimore, MD 21287; **Phone:** 410-955-7323; **Board Cert:** Surgery 2002; Colon & Rectal Surgery 2003; **Med School:** Loyola Univ-Stritch Sch Med 1993; **Resid:** Surgery, John Hopkins Hospital 2000; **Fellow:** Colon & Rectal Surgery, Cleveland Clin 2002; **Fac Appt:** Asst Prof S, Johns Hopkins Univ

Colon & Rectal Surgery

Geisler, Daniel P MD [CRS] - **Spec Exp:** Colon & Rectal Cancer & Surgery; Minimally Invasive Surgery; Rectal Cancer/Sphincter Preservation; Anal Cancer; **Hospital:** Allegheny General Hosp; **Address:** Allegheny Cancer Center, 320 East North Ave, Ste 261, Pittsburgh, PA 15212; **Phone:** 412-359-3901; **Board Cert:** Surgery 2003; Colon & Rectal Surgery 2005; **Med School:** St Louis Univ 1996; **Resid:** Surgery, Univ Oklahoma Hlth Sci Ctr 2001; **Fellow:** Colon & Rectal Surgery, Lankenau Hosp 2002; Minimally Invasive Surgery, Saint Vincent Hlth Ctr 2003; **Fac Appt:** Assoc Prof S, Cleveland Cl Coll Med/Case West Res

Goldstein, Scott D MD [CRS] - **Spec Exp:** Colon & Rectal Cancer; Laparoscopic Surgery; **Hospital:** Thomas Jefferson Univ Hosp (page 81); **Address:** 1100 Walnut St Fl 5 - Ste 500, Philadelphia, PA 19107; **Phone:** 215-955-5869; **Board Cert:** Surgery 1984; Colon & Rectal Surgery 1985; **Med School:** SUNY Buffalo 1978; **Resid:** Surgery, Lenox Hill Hosp 1983; Colon & Rectal Surgery, UMDNJ Med Ctr 1984; **Fac Appt:** Assoc Prof S, Thomas Jefferson Univ

Gorfine, Stephen R MD [CRS] - **Spec Exp:** Rectal Cancer; Anal Cancer; **Hospital:** Mount Sinai Med Ctr (page 76), Lenox Hill Hosp; **Address:** 25 E 69th St, New York, NY 10021-4925; **Phone:** 212-517-8600; **Board Cert:** Internal Medicine 1981; Surgery 2007; Colon & Rectal Surgery 1988; **Med School:** Univ Mass Sch Med 1978; **Resid:** Internal Medicine, Mt Sinai Hosp 1981; Surgery, Mt Sinai Hosp 1985; **Fellow:** Colon & Rectal Surgery, Ferguson Hosp 1987; **Fac Appt:** Clin Prof S, Mount Sinai Sch Med

Guillem, Jose MD [CRS] - **Spec Exp:** Colon & Rectal Cancer; Rectal Cancer/Sphincter Preservation; Colon & Rectal Cancer-Hereditary; Peritoneal Mucinous Carcinomatosis; **Hospital:** Meml Sloan-Kettering Cancer Ctr (page 75); **Address:** 1275 York Avenue, New York, NY 10065; **Phone:** 212-639-8278; **Board Cert:** Colon & Rectal Surgery 2005; Surgery 2004; **Med School:** Yale Univ 1983; **Resid:** Surgery, Columbia-Presby Med Ctr 1990; **Fellow:** Colon & Rectal Surgery, Lahey Clinic 1991; **Fac Appt:** Prof CRS, Cornell Univ-Weill Med Coll

Medich, David MD [CRS] - **Spec Exp:** Colon & Rectal Cancer; **Hospital:** UPMC Passavant-McCandless; **Address:** UPMC Cancer Ctr at UPMC Pasavant, Ground FL, South Pavilion, 9100 Babcock Blvd, Pittsburgh, PA 15237; **Phone:** 877-684-7189; **Board Cert:** Surgery 2004; Colon & Rectal Surgery 2006; **Med School:** Ohio State Univ 1987; **Resid:** Surgery, Univ Pittsburgh 1990; **Fellow:** Research, Univ Pittsburgh 1993; Colon & Rectal Surgery, Cleveland Clinic 1994; **Fac Appt:** Assoc Prof CRS, Drexel Univ Coll Med

Milsom, Jeffrey W MD [CRS] - **Spec Exp:** Laparoscopic Surgery; Colon & Rectal Cancer; **Hospital:** NY-Presby Hosp/Weill Cornell (page 78); **Address:** NY Cornell Med Ctr, Div Colorectal Surgery, 1315 York Ave Fl 2, New York, NY 10065-5304; **Phone:** 212-746-6030; **Board Cert:** Colon & Rectal Surgery 1986; **Med School:** Univ Pittsburgh 1979; **Resid:** Surgery, Roosevelt Hosp 1981; Surgery, Univ Virginia Med Ctr 1984; **Fellow:** Colon & Rectal Surgery, Ferguson Hosp 1985; **Fac Appt:** Prof S, Cornell Univ-Weill Med Coll

Pello, Mark J MD [CRS] - **Spec Exp:** Colon & Rectal Cancer; Laparoscopic Surgery; **Hospital:** Cooper Univ Hosp; **Address:** 3 Cooper Plaza, Ste 411, Camden, NJ 08103; **Phone:** 856-342-2270; **Board Cert:** Surgery 1997; Colon & Rectal Surgery 1980; **Med School:** Jefferson Med Coll 1975; **Resid:** Surgery, Cooper Med Ctr 1979; Colon & Rectal Surgery, Wm Beaumont Hosp 1980; **Fac Appt:** Assoc Prof S, UMDNJ-RW Johnson Med Sch

Rombeau, John L MD [CRS] - **Spec Exp:** Colon & Rectal Cancer; Rectal Cancer/Sphincter Preservation; **Hospital:** Temple Univ Hosp; **Address:** Dept Surg, 3401 N Broad St, Parkinson Pavilion Fl 4, Philadelphia, PA 19104-5103; **Phone:** 215-707-3133; **Board Cert:** Colon & Rectal Surgery 1977; **Med School:** Loma Linda Univ 1967; **Resid:** Surgery, Good Samaritan Hosp 1971; Surgery, LAC-USC Med Ctr 1975; **Fellow:** Colon & Rectal Surgery, Cleveland Clinic 1976; Nutrition & Metabolism, Brigham & Women's Hosp 1984; **Fac Appt:** Prof S, Temple Univ

Stein, David E MD [CRS] - **Spec Exp:** Colon & Rectal Cancer & Surgery; Laparoscopic Surgery; Anorectal Disorders; **Hospital:** Hahnemann Univ Hosp, St. Francis Hosp; **Address:** 245 N 15th St, Ste 413, Philadelphia, PA 19102; **Phone:** 215-762-1545; **Board Cert:** Surgery 2004; Colon & Rectal Surgery 2004; **Med School:** SUNY Downstate 1997; **Resid:** Surgery, T Jefferson Univ Hosp 2002; **Fellow:** Colon & Rectal Surgery, Cleveland Clinic 2003; **Fac Appt:** Asst Prof S, Drexel Univ Coll Med

Steinhagen, Randolph MD [CRS] - **Spec Exp:** Colon & Rectal Cancer; **Hospital:** Mount Sinai Med Ctr (page 76), St. John's Riverside Hosp-Andrus Pavil; **Address:** Div Colon & Rectal Surgery, 5 E 98th St Fl 14, Box 1259, New York, NY 10029-6501; **Phone:** 212-241-3547; **Board Cert:** Surgery 2002; Colon & Rectal Surgery 1985; **Med School:** Wayne State Univ 1977; **Resid:** Surgery, Mount Sinai Hosp 1982; **Fellow:** Colon & Rectal Surgery, Cleveland Clinic 1983; **Fac Appt:** Prof S, Mount Sinai Sch Med

Whelan, Richard L MD [CRS] - **Spec Exp:** Laparoscopic Surgery; Colon & Rectal Cancer; **Hospital:** St. Luke's - Roosevelt Hosp Ctr - Roosevelt Div (page 71); **Address:** 425 W 59th St, Ste 7B, New York, NY 10019; **Phone:** 212-523-8172; **Board Cert:** Surgery 1997; Colon & Rectal Surgery 1989; **Med School:** Columbia P&S 1982; **Resid:** Surgery, Columbia Presby Hosp 1987; **Fellow:** Colon & Rectal Surgery, Univ Minn Med Ctr 1988; **Fac Appt:** Assoc Clin Prof S, Columbia P&S

Southeast

Galandiuk, Susan MD [CRS] - **Spec Exp:** Colon & Rectal Cancer; **Hospital:** Univ of Louisville Hosp, Norton Hosp; **Address:** 401 E Chestnut St, Ste 710, Louisville, KY 40202; **Phone:** 502-583-8303; **Board Cert:** Surgery 2008; Colon & Rectal Surgery 2002; **Med School:** Germany 1982; **Resid:** Surgery, Cleveland Clinic Fdtn 1988; **Fellow:** Research, Univ Louisville Hosp 1989; Colon & Rectal Surgery, Mayo Clin 1990; **Fac Appt:** Prof CRS, Univ Louisville Sch Med

Golub, Richard W MD [CRS] - **Spec Exp:** Colon & Rectal Cancer; Laparoscopic Surgery; **Hospital:** Sarasota Meml Hosp, Doctors Hosp - Sarasota; **Address:** Surgical Specialists, 3333 Cattlemen Rd, Ste 206, Sarasota, FL 34232; **Phone:** 941-341-0042; **Board Cert:** Surgery 2000; Colon & Rectal Surgery 2003; **Med School:** Albert Einstein Coll Med 1984; **Resid:** Surgery, Univ Hosp 1990; **Fellow:** Colon & Rectal Surgery, Grant Medical Center 1991

Mantyh, Christopher R MD [CRS] - **Spec Exp:** Colon & Rectal Cancer & Surgery; Rectal Cancer/Sphincter Preservation; Incontinence-Fecal; Colon & Rectal Cancer-Familial Polyposis; **Hospital:** Duke Univ Hosp; **Address:** DUMC, Box 3117, Durham, NC 27710; **Phone:** 919-681-3977; **Board Cert:** Surgery 2010; Colon & Rectal Surgery 2000; **Med School:** Univ Wisc 1991; **Resid:** Surgery, Duke Univ Med Ctr 1998; **Fellow:** Colon & Rectal Surgery, Cleveland Clinic 1999; **Fac Appt:** Assoc Prof CRS, Univ Wisc

Marcet, Jorge E MD [CRS] - **Spec Exp:** Colon & Rectal Cancer; Anal Disorders & Reconstruction; **Hospital:** Tampa Genl Hosp; **Address:** USF Dept Surgery, 1 Tample General Circle, Ste F-145, Tampa, FL 33606; **Phone:** 813-844-4545; **Board Cert:** Surgery 2001; Colon & Rectal Surgery 2003; **Med School:** Cornell Univ-Weill Med Coll 1985; **Resid:** Surgery, St Luke's-Roosevelt Med Ctr 1990; **Fellow:** Colon & Rectal Surgery, Columbia Presby Hosp 1990; Colon & Rectal Surgery, St Luke's-Roosevelt Hosp 1991; **Fac Appt:** Assoc Prof S, Univ S Fla Coll Med

Nogueras, Juan J MD [CRS] - **Spec Exp:** Colon & Rectal Cancer; Incontinence-Fecal; Laparoscopic Surgery; **Hospital:** Cleveland Clin - Weston (page 70); **Address:** Cleveland Clinic, Dept Colorectal Surgery, 2950 Cleveland Clinic Blvd, Weston, FL 33331; **Phone:** 954-659-5251; **Board Cert:** Surgery 2007; Colon & Rectal Surgery 2003; **Med School:** Jefferson Med Coll 1982; **Resid:** Surgery, Columbia Presby Med Ctr 1987; **Fellow:** Colon & Rectal Surgery, Univ Minn 1991

Colon & Rectal Surgery

Vernava III, Anthony M MD [CRS] - **Spec Exp:** Colon & Rectal Cancer; Colon & Rectal Cancer-Familial Polyposis; Incontinence-Fecal; **Hospital:** Physicians Regl Hlthcare Med Ctr-Pine Ridge; **Address:** Physicians Regl Med Grp, 6101 Pine Ridge Rd, Naples, FL 34119; **Phone:** 239-348-4531; **Board Cert:** Surgery 2007; Colon & Rectal Surgery 1989; **Med School:** St Louis Univ 1982; **Resid:** Surgery, St Louis Univ Med Ctr 1988; Colon & Rectal Surgery, Univ Minnesota Med Ctr 1989; **Fellow:** Colon & Rectal Surgery, St Marks Hosp 1990; Colon & Rectal Surgery, Natl Cancer Ctr 1989

Wexner, Steven D MD [CRS] - **Spec Exp:** Colon & Rectal Cancer; Laparoscopic Surgery; Incontinence-Fecal; Anal Sphincter Repair; **Hospital:** Cleveland Clin - Weston (page 70); **Address:** 2950 Cleveland Clinic Blvd, Weston, FL 33331-3609; **Phone:** 954-659-5278; **Board Cert:** Surgery 2005; Colon & Rectal Surgery 2006; **Med School:** Cornell Univ-Weill Med Coll 1982; **Resid:** Surgery, Roosevelt Hosp 1987; **Fellow:** Colon & Rectal Surgery, Univ Minn 1988; **Fac Appt:** Prof S, Cleveland Cl Coll Med/Case West Res

Wise, Paul E MD [CRS] - **Spec Exp:** Colon & Rectal Cancer & Surgery; Minimally Invasive Surgery; Colon & Rectal Cancer-Hereditary; Anorectal Disorders; **Hospital:** Vanderbilt Univ Med Ctr; **Address:** Vanderbilt Univ Med Ctr, Dept of General Surgery, D-5248 Medical Center N, Nashville, TN 37232; **Phone:** 615-343-4612; **Board Cert:** Surgery 2004; Colon & Rectal Surgery 2005; **Med School:** Johns Hopkins Univ 1996; **Resid:** Surgery, Vanderbilt Univ Med Ctr 2003; **Fellow:** Colon & Rectal Surgery, Barnes-Jewish Hosp 2004; **Fac Appt:** Asst Prof S, Vanderbilt Univ

Midwest

Abcarian, Herand MD [CRS] - **Spec Exp:** Rectal Cancer/Sphincter Preservation; Incontinence-Fecal; **Hospital:** Univ of IL Med Ctr at Chicago, Gottlieb Meml Hosp; **Address:** University of Illinois, Dept of Colorectal Surgery, 840 S Wood St Fl 5, Chicago, IL 60612; **Phone:** 312-413-2708; **Board Cert:** Surgery 1972; Colon & Rectal Surgery 1972; **Med School:** Iran 1965; **Resid:** Surgery, Cook County Hosp 1971; Colon & Rectal Surgery, Cook County Hosp 1972; **Fac Appt:** Prof S, Univ IL Coll Med

Birnbaum, Elisa H MD [CRS] - **Spec Exp:** Colon & Rectal Cancer; **Hospital:** Barnes-Jewish Hosp; **Address:** Washington Univ Sch Med, Div Colorectal Surgery, 660 S Euclid, Box 8109, St Louis, MO 63110; **Phone:** 314-454-7177; **Board Cert:** Surgery 2009; Colon & Rectal Surgery 2003; **Med School:** Univ IL Coll Med 1985; **Resid:** Surgery, LIJ Med Ctr 1990; **Fellow:** Colon & Rectal Surgery, Barnes Jewish Hosp 1991; **Fac Appt:** Prof S, Washington Univ, St Louis

Church, James MD [CRS] - **Spec Exp:** Colon & Rectal Cancer-Familial Polyposis; Anorectal Disorders; Incontinence-Fecal; **Hospital:** Cleveland Clin (page 70); **Address:** Cleveland Clinic, 9500 Euclid Ave, MC A-30, Cleveland, OH 44195; **Phone:** 216-444-7000; **Med School:** New Zealand 1974; **Resid:** Surgery, Aukland Hosps 1980; **Fellow:** Research, Aukland Hosps 1983; Colon & Rectal Surgery, Cleveland Clinic 1984; **Fac Appt:** Prof CRS, Cleveland Cl Coll Med/Case West Res

Delaney, Conor P MD/PhD [CRS] - **Spec Exp:** Laparoscopic Surgery; Colon & Rectal Cancer; Rectal Cancer/Sphincter Preservation; **Hospital:** Univ Hosps Case Med Ctr; **Address:** 11100 Euclid Ave, Cleveland, OH 44106-5047; **Phone:** 216-844-8087; **Board Cert:** Surgery 1998; Colon & Rectal Surgery 1998; **Med School:** Ireland 1989; **Resid:** Surgery, Univ Hosp 1993; Surgery, Univ Hosp 1999; **Fellow:** Research, Univ of Pittsburgh 1995; Colon & Rectal Surgery, Cleveland Clinic 2000; **Fac Appt:** Prof S, Cleveland Cl Coll Med/Case West Res

Dietz, David W MD [CRS] - **Spec Exp:** Colon & Rectal Cancer; Anal Cancer; **Hospital:** Cleveland Clin (page 70); **Address:** Cleveland Clinic, Colorectal Surgery, 9500 Euclid Ave, Desk A30, Cleveland, OH 44195; **Phone:** 216-445-6597; **Board Cert:** Surgery 2001; Colon & Rectal Surgery 2002; **Med School:** Jefferson Med Coll 1993; **Resid:** Surgery, Cleveland Clinic 1999; Colon & Rectal Surgery, Cleveland Clinic 2001

America's Top Doctors® for Cancer 7th Edition

Fleshman Jr, James W MD [CRS] - **Spec Exp:** Colon & Rectal Cancer; Laparoscopic Surgery; **Hospital:** Barnes-Jewish Hosp, Barnes-Jewish West County Hosp; **Address:** Wash Univ Sch Med, Div Colorectal Surgery, 660 S Euclid Ave, Box 8109, St Louis, MO 63110; **Phone:** 314-454-7177; **Board Cert:** Colon & Rectal Surgery 1988; Surgery 2002; **Med School:** Washington Univ, St Louis 1980; **Resid:** Surgery, Jewish Hospital 1986; **Fellow:** Colon & Rectal Surgery, Univ Toronto 1987; **Fac Appt:** Prof S, Washington Univ, St Louis

Foley, Eugene F MD [CRS] - **Spec Exp:** Colon & Rectal Cancer; **Hospital:** Univ WI Hosp & Clins; **Address:** Univ WI Hosp & Clins, 600 Highland Ave, Madison, WI 53792-7375; **Phone:** 608-263-2521; **Board Cert:** Surgery 2003; Colon & Rectal Surgery 2005; **Med School:** Harvard Med Sch 1985; **Resid:** Surgery, New England Deaconess Hosp 1991; **Fellow:** Colon & Rectal Surgery, Lahey Clinic 1993; **Fac Appt:** Prof S, Univ Wisc

Kodner, Ira J MD [CRS] - **Spec Exp:** Colon & Rectal Cancer; Laparoscopic Surgery; **Hospital:** Barnes-Jewish Hosp; **Address:** Wash Univ Sch Med, Div Colorectal Surgery, 660 S Euclid Ave, Box 8109, St Louis, MO 63110; **Phone:** 314-454-7177; **Board Cert:** Surgery 1975; Colon & Rectal Surgery 1975; **Med School:** Washington Univ, St Louis 1967; **Resid:** Surgery, Barnes-Jewish Hosp 1974; **Fellow:** Colon & Rectal Surgery, Cleveland Clinic 1975; Medical Ethics, Univ Chicago Hosps & Hlth Sys 2004; **Fac Appt:** Prof S, Washington Univ, St Louis

Lavery, Ian C MD [CRS] - **Spec Exp:** Colon & Rectal Cancer; **Hospital:** Cleveland Clin (page 70); **Address:** 9500 Euclid Ave, Desk A30, Cleveland, OH 44195; **Phone:** 216-444-6930; **Board Cert:** Colon & Rectal Surgery 1998; **Med School:** Australia 1967; **Resid:** Surgery, Princess Alexandra Hosp 1974; Colon & Rectal Surgery, Cleveland Clinic 1977; **Fac Appt:** Prof S, Case West Res Univ

Ludwig, Kirk A MD [CRS] - **Spec Exp:** Colon & Rectal Cancer & Surgery; Rectal Cancer/Sphincter Preservation; Incontinence-Fecal; Colon & Rectal Cancer-Familial Polyposis; **Hospital:** Froedtert and Med Ctr of WI; **Address:** 9200 W Wisconsin Ave, Dept Surgery, Milwaukee, WI 53226; **Phone:** 414-805-5783; **Board Cert:** Surgery 2005; Colon & Rectal Surgery 2007; **Med School:** Univ Cincinnati 1988; **Resid:** Surgery, Med Coll Wisc 1994; **Fellow:** Colon & Rectal Surgery, Cleveland Clinic 1996; **Fac Appt:** Assoc Prof S, Med Coll Wisc

Madoff, Robert D MD [CRS] - **Spec Exp:** Colon & Rectal Cancer; **Address:** 420 Delaware St SE, MC MMC88, Minneapolis, MN 55455; **Phone:** 612-624-9708; **Board Cert:** Colon & Rectal Surgery 2002; **Med School:** Columbia P&S 1979; **Resid:** Surgery, Univ Minn Hosps 1987; **Fellow:** Colon & Rectal Surgery, Univ Minn Hosps 1988; **Fac Appt:** Prof S, Univ Minn

Mutch, Matthew G MD [CRS] - **Spec Exp:** Colon & Rectal Cancer; Laparoscopic Surgery; **Hospital:** Barnes-Jewish Hosp; **Address:** Washington U Med Sch, Dept Surgery, 660 S Euclid Ave, Ste 14102, Box 8109, St Louis, MO 63110-1010; **Phone:** 314-454-7177; **Board Cert:** Surgery 2002; Colon & Rectal Surgery 2003; **Med School:** Washington Univ, St Louis 1994; **Resid:** Surgery, Barnes Jewish Hosp 2001; **Fellow:** Research, Barnes Jewish Hosp 1998; Colon & Rectal Surgery, Lahey Clinic 2002; **Fac Appt:** Assoc Prof S, Washington Univ, St Louis

Nelson, Heidi MD [CRS] - **Spec Exp:** Colon & Rectal Cancer; Gastrointestinal Cancer; **Hospital:** Mayo Med Ctr & Clin - Rochester, Rochester Methodist Hosp; **Address:** Mayo Clinic, Gonda 9 South, 200 First St SW, Rochester, MN 55905; **Phone:** 507-284-3329; **Board Cert:** Surgery 2007; Colon & Rectal Surgery 1989; **Med School:** Univ Wash 1981; **Resid:** Surgery, Oregon Hlth Sci Univ Hosp 1987; Colon & Rectal Surgery, Oregon Hlth Sci Univ Hosp 1985; **Fellow:** Colon & Rectal Surgery, Mayo Clin 1988; **Fac Appt:** Prof S, Mayo Med Sch

Colon & Rectal Surgery

Pemberton, John H MD [CRS] - **Spec Exp:** Colon & Rectal Cancer; **Hospital:** St. Mary's Hosp - Rochester MN (Mayo), Rochester Methodist Hosp; **Address:** Mayo Clinic, Div Colon & Rectal Surg, 200 First St SW, Gonda 9-S, Rochester, MN 55905; **Phone:** 507-284-2359; **Board Cert:** Surgery 2001; Colon & Rectal Surgery 1985; **Med School:** Tulane Univ 1976; **Resid:** Surgery, Mayo Clinic 1983; **Fellow:** Colon & Rectal Surgery, Mayo Clinic 1984; **Fac Appt:** Prof S, Mayo Med Sch

Rafferty, Janice F MD [CRS] - **Spec Exp:** Colon & Rectal Cancer; Anal Disorders & Reconstruction; **Hospital:** Univ Hosp - Cincinnati, Christ Hosp, The - Cincinnati; **Address:** Univ Cincinnati, Colon & Rectal Surgery, 2123 Auburn Ave, Ste 524, Cincinnati, OH 45219; **Phone:** 513-929-0104; **Board Cert:** Surgery 2004; Colon & Rectal Surgery 2008; **Med School:** Ohio State Univ 1988; **Resid:** Surgery, Univ CincinnatiHosp 1995; Colon & Rectal Surgery, Barnes Jewish Hosp 1996; **Fac Appt:** Assoc Prof S, Univ Cincinnati

Remzi, Feza H MD [CRS] - **Spec Exp:** Colon & Rectal Cancer & Surgery; Laparoscopic Surgery; **Hospital:** Cleveland Clin (page 70); **Address:** Cleveland Clinic, 9500 Euclid Ave, Dept A30, Cleveland, OH 44195; **Phone:** 216-445-5020; **Board Cert:** Surgery 2006; Colon & Rectal Surgery 2007; **Med School:** Turkey 1989; **Resid:** Colon & Rectal Surgery, Cleveland Clinic 1996; Colon & Rectal Surgery, Cleveland Clinic 1997

Rothenberger, David A MD [CRS] - **Spec Exp:** Colon & Rectal Cancer; **Address:** Univ Minnesota Med Ctr, Dept Surg, 420 Delaware St SE MMC 88, Minneapolis, MN 55455; **Phone:** 612-624-9708; **Board Cert:** Colon & Rectal Surgery 2006; **Med School:** Tufts Univ 1973; **Resid:** Surgery, St Paul-Ramsey Med Ctr 1978; **Fellow:** Colon & Rectal Surgery, Univ Minnesota Hosps 1979; **Fac Appt:** Prof S, Univ Minn

Saclarides, Theodore J MD [CRS] - **Spec Exp:** Rectal Cancer/Sphincter Preservation; Laparoscopic Surgery; **Hospital:** Rush Univ Med Ctr, Skokie/North Shore Univ Htlh Syst; **Address:** University Surgeons, 1725 W Harrison St, Ste 810, Chicago, IL 60612-3832; **Phone:** 312-942-6500; **Board Cert:** Surgery 2007; Colon & Rectal Surgery 1989; **Med School:** Univ Miami Sch Med 1982; **Resid:** Surgery, Rush Univ Med Ctr 1987; **Fellow:** Colon & Rectal Surgery, Mayo Clinic 1988; **Fac Appt:** Prof S, Rush Med Coll

Stryker, Steven J MD [CRS] - **Spec Exp:** Colon & Rectal Cancer; Laparoscopic Surgery; **Hospital:** Northwestern Meml Hosp; **Address:** 676 N Saint Clair St, Ste 1525A, Chicago, IL 60611-2862; **Phone:** 312-943-5427; **Board Cert:** Surgery 2004; Colon & Rectal Surgery 1986; **Med School:** Northwestern Univ 1978; **Resid:** Surgery, Northwestern Meml Hosp 1983; **Fellow:** Colon & Rectal Surgery, Mayo Clinic 1985; **Fac Appt:** Clin Prof S, Northwestern Univ

Wolff, Bruce G MD [CRS] - **Spec Exp:** Colon & Rectal Cancer; **Hospital:** Mayo Med Ctr & Clin - Rochester; **Address:** Mayo Clinic, Gonda 9 South, 200 First St SW, Rochester, MN 55905; **Phone:** 507-284-3329; **Board Cert:** Surgery 2000; Colon & Rectal Surgery 2001; **Med School:** Duke Univ 1973; **Resid:** Surgery, NY Hosp-Cornell Med Ctr 1981; **Fellow:** Colon & Rectal Surgery, Mayo Clinic 1982; **Fac Appt:** Prof S, Mayo Med Sch

Great Plains and Mountains

Blatchford, Garnet J MD [CRS] - **Spec Exp:** Colon Cancer; Anal Disorders & Reconstruction; **Hospital:** Alegent Hlth - Immanuel Med Ctr; **Address:** Colon & Rectal Surgery Inc, 9850 Nicholas St, Ste 100, Omaha, NE 68114; **Phone:** 402-343-1122; **Board Cert:** Colon & Rectal Surgery 2009; **Med School:** Univ Nebr Coll Med 1983; **Resid:** Surgery, Univ Nebraska Med Ctr 1988; Colon & Rectal Surgery, Creighton Univ 1990; **Fac Appt:** Assoc Prof S, Creighton Univ

Thorson, Alan G MD [CRS] - **Spec Exp:** Colon & Rectal Cancer; Rectal Cancer/Sphincter Preservation; Incontinence-Fecal; Laparoscopic Surgery; **Hospital:** Nebraska Meth Hosp, Bergan Mercy Med Ctr-Alegant Hlth; **Address:** 9850 Nicholas St, Ste 100, Omaha, NE 68114-2191; **Phone:** 402-343-1122; **Board Cert:** Colon & Rectal Surgery 1999; **Med School:** Univ Nebr Coll Med 1979; **Resid:** Surgery, Univ Nebraska Affil Hosp 1984; Colon & Rectal Surgery, Univ Minn Affil Hosp 1985; **Fac Appt:** Clin Prof S, Creighton Univ

Southwest

Adkins, Terrance P MD [CRS] - **Spec Exp:** Colon & Rectal Cancer; **Hospital:** Tucson Med Ctr; **Address:** Southwestern Surgery Assoc, 1951 N Wilmot Rd Bldg 2, Tucson, AZ 85712; **Phone:** 520-795-5845; **Board Cert:** Surgery 2001; Colon & Rectal Surgery 2004; **Med School:** Univ Tex SW, Dallas 1985; **Resid:** Surgery, Univ Utah Med Ctr 1991; **Fellow:** Colon & Rectal Surgery, Univ Texas Med Ctr 1992; **Fac Appt:** Asst Clin Prof S, Univ Ariz Coll Med

Bailey, H Randolph MD [CRS] - **Spec Exp:** Rectal Cancer/Sphincter Preservation; Incontinence-Fecal; **Hospital:** Methodist Hosp - Houston, St. Luke's Episcopal Hosp-Houston; **Address:** Colon & Rectal Clinic, Smith Twr, 6550 Fannin St, Ste 2307, Houston, TX 77030-2717; **Phone:** 713-790-9250; **Board Cert:** Surgery 1974; Colon & Rectal Surgery 2004; **Med School:** Univ Tex SW, Dallas 1968; **Resid:** Surgery, Hermann Hosp-Univ Tex Med Sch 1973; **Fellow:** Colon & Rectal Surgery, Ferguson-Droste Hosp 1974; **Fac Appt:** Clin Prof S, Univ Tex, Houston

Beck, David E MD [CRS] - **Spec Exp:** Colon & Rectal Cancer; Minimally Invasive Surgery; **Hospital:** Ochsner Med Ctr-New Orleans, Ochsner Med Ctr-Baton Rouge; **Address:** Ochsner Clinic Fdn, Colorectal Surgery, 1514 Jefferson Hwy, 4th Fl, rm 04 East, New Orleans, LA 70121-2429; **Phone:** 504-842-4060; **Board Cert:** Colon & Rectal Surgery 1987; **Med School:** Univ Miami Sch Med 1979; **Resid:** Surgery, Wilford Hall USAF Med Ctr 1984; **Fellow:** Colon & Rectal Surgery, Cleveland Clinic Fdn 1986; **Fac Appt:** Assoc Clin Prof S, Louisiana State U, New Orleans

Haas, Eric M MD [CRS] - **Spec Exp:** Laparoscopic Surgery; Colon & Rectal Cancer; Incontinence-Fecal; **Hospital:** Methodist Hosp - Houston, St. Luke's Episcopal Hosp-Houston; **Address:** Colorectal Surgical Assocs, 7900 Fannin St, Ste 2700, Houston, TX 77054; **Phone:** 713-790-0600; **Board Cert:** Surgery 2003; Colon & Rectal Surgery 2004; **Med School:** Univ Tex, Houston 1997; **Resid:** Surgery, St Joseph Hosp 2002; **Fellow:** Colon & Rectal Surgery, Texas affil Hosps 2003

Heppell, Jacques P MD [CRS] - **Spec Exp:** Colon & Rectal Cancer; Anorectal Disorders; **Hospital:** Mayo Clinic - Phoenix; **Address:** Mayo Clinic, GENS/CB/Distribution 13, 5777 E Mayo Blvd, Phoenix, AZ 85054; **Phone:** 480-342-2697; **Board Cert:** Surgery 2004; Colon & Rectal Surgery 1995; **Med School:** Univ Montreal 1974; **Resid:** Surgery, Univ Montreal Med Ctr 1979; **Fellow:** Colon & Rectal Surgery, Mayo Clinic 1983; **Fac Appt:** Prof S, Mayo Med Sch

Hicks, Terry C MD [CRS] - **Spec Exp:** Colon & Rectal Cancer; **Hospital:** Ochsner Med Ctr-New Orleans; **Address:** Ochsner Clinic, Div Colorectal Surgery, 1514 Jefferson Hwy, New Orleans, LA 70121; **Phone:** 504-842-5884; **Board Cert:** Colon & Rectal Surgery 2002; **Med School:** Univ Tex, San Antonio 1977; **Resid:** Surgery, Univ Louisville Med Ctr 1982; Colon & Rectal Surgery, Ochsner Clinic 1983; **Fac Appt:** Assoc Prof S, Louisiana State U, New Orleans

Huber Jr, Philip J MD [CRS] - **Spec Exp:** Colon & Rectal Cancer; **Hospital:** Med City Dallas Hosp, TX Hlth Presby Hosp Dallas; **Address:** 7777 Forest Lane, Ste C-204, Dallas, TX 75230; **Phone:** 972-566-6115; **Board Cert:** Colon & Rectal Surgery 1993; **Med School:** Columbia P&S 1972; **Resid:** Surgery, Parkland Hosp 1977; Colon & Rectal Surgery, Presby Hosp 1978

Colon & Rectal Surgery

West Coast and Pacific

Beart Jr, Robert W MD [CRS] - **Spec Exp:** Colon & Rectal Cancer; **Hospital:** Glendale Mem Hosp & Hlth Ctr; **Address:** Colorectal Surgery Inst, 222 W Eulalia St, Ste 100A, Glendale, CA 91204; **Phone:** 818-244-8161; **Board Cert:** Colon & Rectal Surgery 1995; **Med School:** Harvard Med Sch 1971; **Resid:** Surgery, Univ Colo Med Ctr 1976; Colon & Rectal Surgery, Mayo Clinic 1978; **Fellow:** Transplant Surgery, Univ Colo Med Ctr 1975; **Fac Appt:** Prof Emeritus S, USC Sch Med

Senagore, Anthony MD [CRS] - **Spec Exp:** Laparoscopic Surgery; Colon & Rectal Cancer; Anorectal Disorders; Incontinence-Fecal; **Hospital:** USC Norris Cancer Hosp; **Address:** USC North Cancer Hosp, 1441 Eastlake Ave, Ste 7418, Los Angeles, CA 90033; **Phone:** 323-865-3690; **Board Cert:** Surgery 2006; Colon & Rectal Surgery 2009; Surgical Critical Care 2006; **Med School:** Mich State Univ 1981; **Resid:** Surgery, Butterworth Hosp 1987; Colon & Rectal Surgery, Ferguson Hosp 1989; **Fac Appt:** Prof S

Sokol, Thomas P MD [CRS] - **Spec Exp:** Colon & Rectal Cancer & Surgery; Incontinence-Fecal; **Hospital:** Cedars-Sinai Med Ctr; **Address:** 8737 Beverly Blvd, Ste 402, Los Angeles, CA 90048-1828; **Phone:** 310-854-3580; **Board Cert:** Colon & Rectal Surgery 2008; **Med School:** Ros Franklin Univ/Chicago Med Sch 1980; **Resid:** Surgery, Habor UCLA Med Ctr 1985; **Fellow:** Colon & Rectal Surgery, Carle Fdn Hosp/Univ Ill 1986; **Fac Appt:** Assoc Clin Prof S, UCLA

Stamos, Michael J MD [CRS] - **Spec Exp:** Rectal Cancer/Sphincter Preservation; Laparoscopic Surgery; Colon & Rectal Cancer; Anorectal Disorders; **Hospital:** UC Irvine Med Ctr; **Address:** UC Irvine Med Ctr, Div Colon & Rectal Surg, 333 City Blvd W, Ste 700, Orange, CA 92868-2993; **Phone:** 714-456-6262; **Board Cert:** Surgery 2010; Colon & Rectal Surgery 2003; **Med School:** Case West Res Univ 1985; **Resid:** Surgery, Jackson Meml Hosp 1990; Colon & Rectal Surgery, Ochsner Clinic 1991; **Fac Appt:** Prof S, UC Irvine

Varma, Madhulika G MD [CRS] - **Spec Exp:** Colon & Rectal Cancer & Surgery; Laparoscopic Surgery; **Hospital:** UCSF - Mt Zion Med Ctr; **Address:** Center for Colorectal Surgery, 2330 Post St, Ste 260, San Francisco, CA 94115-1799; **Phone:** 415-885-3606; **Board Cert:** Colon & Rectal Surgery 2010; Surgery 2007; **Med School:** Brown Univ 1991; **Resid:** Surgery, UCSF Med Ctr 1998; **Fellow:** Colon & Rectal Surgery, Univ Minnesota Med Ctr 2000; Research, UCSF Med Ctr 2001; **Fac Appt:** Asst Prof S, UCSF

Welton, Mark L MD [CRS] - **Spec Exp:** Colon & Rectal Cancer; Anal Cancer; **Hospital:** Stanford Univ Hosp & Clinics; **Address:** The Cancer Ctr, 875 Blake Wilbur Drive, Stanford, CA 94305; **Phone:** 650-723-5461; **Board Cert:** Surgery 2000; Colon & Rectal Surgery 2005; **Med School:** UCLA 1984; **Resid:** Surgery, UCLA Med Ctr 1992; **Fellow:** Colon & Rectal Surgery, Barnes Jewish Hosp 1993; **Fac Appt:** Assoc Prof S, Stanford Univ

Cleveland Clinic

Every life deserves world class care.

Cleveland Clinic
Taussig Cancer Institute
9500 Euclid Avenue
Cleveland, OH 44195

National Leader in Colorectal Cancer

At Cleveland Clinic Taussig Cancer Institute, more than 250 top cancer specialists, researchers, nurses and technicians are dedicated to delivering the most effective medical treatments and offering access to the latest clinical trials for more than 13,000 new cancer patients every year. Our doctors are nationally and internationally known for their contributions to cancer breakthroughs and their ability to deliver superior outcomes for our patients. In recognition of these and other achievements, *U.S.News & World Report* has ranked Cleveland Clinic as one of the top cancer centers in the nation.

Digestive Disease Institute

Taussig Cancer Institute's leading oncologists work closely with a multidisciplinary team of specialists from the Digestive Disease Institute to provide patients with innovative diagnostic techniques, the latest chemotherapy or anticancer agents, surgical options, clinical trials, novel therapies and genetic counseling to treat colorectal cancer.

The Digestive Disease Institute became the first in the nation to integrate its departments of Colorectal Surgery; Gastroenterology & Hepatology; General Surgery, including Hepato-pancreato-biliary and Transplant Surgery; and Human Nutrition. This integration provides unprecedented patient care, multidisciplinary education and collaborative research.

As one of the largest centers in the nation, the Digestive Disease Institute performs up to 10 laparoscopic intestinal resections a week. In addition, it houses the largest registries in the U.S. for inherited forms of colorectal cancer, the David G. Jagelman Inherited Colorectal Cancer Registries.

The Cleveland Clinic's digestive disease program has been ranked #2 in the nation since 2003, by *U.S.News and World Report*.

clevelandclinic.org/colorectalTCD

Appointments | Information: Call the Cancer Answer Line at 866.223.8100.

Cancer Treatment Guides

Cleveland Clinic has developed comprehensive treatment guides for many cancers. To download our free treatment guides, visit clevelandclinic.org/cancertreatmentguides.

Comprehensive Online Medical Second Opinion

Cleveland Clinic experts can review your medical records and render an opinion that includes treatment options and recommendations. Call 216.444.3223 or 800.223.2273 ext. 43223; email eclevelandclinic@ccf.org.

Special Assistance for Out-of-State Patients

Cleveland Clinic Global Patient Services offers a complimentary Medical Concierge service for patients who travel from outside of Ohio. Call 800.223.2273, ext. 55580, or email medicalconcierge@ccf.org.

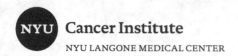

Cancer Institute
NYU LANGONE MEDICAL CENTER

NYU Langone Medical Center
550 First Avenue , New York, NY 10016
www.NYULMC.org

NYU Clinical Cancer Center
160 East 34th Street, New York, NY 10016
www.NYUCI.org

**The Stephen D. Hassenfeld Children's Center
for Cancer and Blood Disorders**
160 East 32nd Street, New York, NY 10016
www.NYUMC.org/Hassenfeld

The NYU Cancer Institute is an NCI-designated cancer center and provides personalized patient care that is both compassionate and state of the art. The doctors and researchers work together to develop innovative therapies for patients. The Cancer Institute is world-renowned for excellence in cancer-focused research, personalized care, education and community outreach. Its mission is to discover the origins of human cancer and to use that knowledge to eradicate the personal and societal burden of cancer in our community, the nation and the world. For more information about our expert physicians, call 212-731-5000. *We specialize in the following areas:*

Patient-Focused Setting
The NYU Clinical Cancer Center is the principal outpatient facility of The Cancer Institute and serves as home to our patients and their caregivers. The center and its multidisciplinary team of experts provide access to the latest treatment options and clinical trials along with a variety of programs in cancer risk reduction/prevention, screening, diagnostics, genetic counseling and supportive services. In addition the NYUCI emphasizes the importance of a holistic approach to management services in complementary medicine, psychosocial support, survivorship and palliative care.

Renowned Expertise
The NYU Cancer Institute brings together experts from a variety of disciplines to create collaborative research endeavors and clinical care teams. The Cancer Institute offers a full continuum of personalized care, from prevention through diagnosis, treatment and post-treatment support. The compassion and expertise of our team members helps patients better manage the symptoms of their diseases as well as meet their special needs. Additionally, we have created special emphasis programs in diseases such as breast cancer, melanoma, GI cancer, prostate cancer, hematologic malignancies and lung cancer among others, as well as, translational programs in cancer healthcare disparities, molecularly targeted therapy, and the cell signaling pathways involved in cancer.

A Translational Approach
NYU Langone Medical Center scientists and other researchers excel in uncovering how cancer develops at the molecular level, and how we can harness that knowledge to reduce the risk of cancer and treat the disease. The Medical Center constantly seeks to create new opportunities for collaboration between investigators within our own institution, those located elsewhere in the NYU network of campuses, and researchers at other institutions.

The Stephen D. Hassenfeld Children's Center for Cancer and Blood Disorders
The center is a leading pediatric outpatient facility for the treatment of childhood cancers and blood diseases. Its unique interdisciplinary and family-centered approach combines the most advanced medical treatments with psychosocial and emotional support services for young patients and their families.

Dermatology

A dermatologist is trained to diagnose and treat pediatric and adult patients with benign and malignant disorders of the skin, mouth, external genitalia, hair and nails, as well as a number of sexually transmitted diseases. The dermatologist has had additional training and experience in the diagnosis and treatment of skin cancers, melanomas, moles and other tumors of the skin, the management of contact dermatitis and other allergic and non-allergic skin disorders, and in the recognition of the skin manifestations of systemic (including internal malignancy) and infectious diseases.

Dermatologists may have special training in dermatopathology and in the surgical techniques used in dermatology. They also have expertise in the management of cosmetic disorders of the skin such as hair loss and scars, and the skin changes associated with aging.

Training Required: Four years

DERMATOLOGY

New England

Bolognia, Jean L MD [D] - **Spec Exp:** Melanoma; Skin Cancer; **Hospital:** Yale-New Haven Hosp, Yale Med Group; **Address:** 2 Church St S, Ste 305, New Haven, CT 06519; **Phone:** 203-789-1249; **Board Cert:** Dermatology 2005; **Med School:** Yale Univ 1980; **Resid:** Internal Medicine, Yale-New Haven Hosp 1982; Dermatology, Yale-New Haven Hosp 1985; **Fellow:** Dermatology, Yale-New Haven Hosp 1987; **Fac Appt:** Prof D, Yale Univ

Del Giudice, Stephen M MD [D] - **Spec Exp:** Skin Cancer; **Hospital:** Concord Hospital; **Address:** Dartmouth Hitchcock Concord Dermatology, 253 Pleasant St, Concord, NH 03301; **Phone:** 603-226-6119; **Board Cert:** Dermatology 1987; **Med School:** Tufts Univ 1981; **Resid:** Dermatology, Yale-New Haven Hosp 1987

Dufresne, Raymond G MD [D] - **Spec Exp:** Mohs' Surgery; **Hospital:** Rhode Island Hosp; **Address:** University Dermatology, 593 Eddy St, APC 10, Providence, RI 02903; **Phone:** 401-444-7024; **Board Cert:** Internal Medicine 1983; Dermatology 1986; **Med School:** Vanderbilt Univ 1980; **Resid:** Internal Medicine, Vanderbilt Univ Med Ctr 1983; Dermatology, Vanderbilt Univ Med Ctr 1986; **Fellow:** Mohs Surgery, Cleveland Clinic 1987; **Fac Appt:** Prof D, Brown Univ

Edelson, Richard L MD [D] - **Spec Exp:** Cutaneous Lymphoma; **Hospital:** Yale-New Haven Hosp, Yale Med Group; **Address:** 2 Church St S, Ste 305, New Haven, CT 06519; **Phone:** 203-789-1249; **Board Cert:** Dermatology 1977; **Med School:** Yale Univ 1970; **Resid:** Dermatology, Mass Genl Hosp 1972; Dermatology, Natl Inst Hlth 1975; **Fac Appt:** Prof D, Yale Univ

Fewkes, Jessica L MD [D] - **Spec Exp:** Mohs' Surgery; Skin Cancer-Head & Neck; Melanoma-Head & Neck; **Hospital:** Mass Eye & Ear Infirmary, Mass Genl Hosp; **Address:** Facial & Cosmetic Surgery Center, Mass Eye & Ear Infirmary, 243 Charles St, 9th Fl, Boston, MA 02114; **Phone:** 617-573-3789; **Board Cert:** Dermatology 1982; **Med School:** UCSF 1978; **Resid:** Dermatology, Mass Genl Hosp 1982; **Fellow:** Chemosurgery, Duke Univ Med Ctr 1983; **Fac Appt:** Asst Prof D, Harvard Med Sch

Gellis, Stephen MD [D] - **Spec Exp:** Melanoma; Pigmented Lesions; **Hospital:** Children's Hospital - Boston; **Address:** Chldn's Hosp-Boston, 300 Longwood Ave, Fegan-6, Boston, MA 02115-5737; **Phone:** 617-355-6117; **Board Cert:** Pediatrics 1978; Dermatology 1979; Pediatric Dermatology 2006; **Med School:** Harvard Med Sch 1973; **Resid:** Pediatrics, Chldn's Hosp 1976; Dermatology, Mass Genl Hosp 1978; **Fac Appt:** Asst Prof D, Harvard Med Sch

Gilchrest, Barbara MD [D] - **Spec Exp:** Melanoma; Skin Cancer; **Hospital:** Boston Med Ctr; **Address:** Boston Med Ctr- Dermatolgy Dept, 609 Albany St, Ste 8B, Doctor's Off Bldg, Boston, MA 02118; **Phone:** 617-638-7420; **Board Cert:** Internal Medicine 1975; Dermatology 1978; **Med School:** Harvard Med Sch 1971; **Resid:** Internal Medicine, Boston City Hosp 1973; Dermatology, Harvard Med Sch 1976; **Fellow:** Photo Biology, Harvard Med Sch 1975; **Fac Appt:** Prof D, Boston Univ

Kupper, Thomas S MD [D] - **Spec Exp:** Melanoma; Cutaneous Lymphoma; Skin Cancer; **Hospital:** Brigham & Women's Hosp, Dana-Farber Cancer Inst; **Address:** Brigham & Women's Hosp, Dept Dermatology, 77 Avenue Louis Pasteur, Ste 671, Boston, MA 02115; **Phone:** 617-525-5550; **Board Cert:** Dermatology 1989; **Med School:** Yale Univ 1981; **Resid:** Surgery, Yale-New Haven Hosp 1983; Dermatology, Yale-New Haven Hosp 1989; **Fac Appt:** Prof D, Harvard Med Sch

Leffell, David J MD [D] - **Spec Exp:** Mohs' Surgery; Melanoma; Skin Cancer; Skin Laser Surgery; **Hospital:** Yale-New Haven Hosp, Yale Med Group; **Address:** 40 Temple St, Ste 5a, New Haven, CT 06520; **Phone:** 203-785-3466; **Board Cert:** Internal Medicine 1984; Dermatology 2009; **Med School:** McGill Univ 1981; **Resid:** Internal Medicine, New York Hosp 1984; Dermatology, Yale-New Haven Hosp 1986; **Fellow:** Dermatology, Yale Sch Med 1987; Dermatologic Surgery, Univ Michigan Med Ctr 1988; **Fac Appt:** Prof D, Yale Univ

Maloney, Mary E MD [D] - **Spec Exp:** Mohs' Surgery; Skin Cancer; **Hospital:** UMass Memorial Med Ctr; **Address:** UMass Meml Med Ctr-Hahnemann Campus, 281 Lincoln St, Worcester, MA 01605; **Phone:** 508-334-5962; **Board Cert:** Dermatology 1982; **Med School:** Univ VT Coll Med 1977; **Resid:** Internal Medicine, Hartford Hospital 1979; Dermatology, Dartmouth-Hitchcock Med Ctr 1982; **Fellow:** Dermatologic Surgery, UCSF Med Ctr 1983; **Fac Appt:** Prof D, Univ Mass Sch Med

Mihm Jr, Martin C MD [D] - **Spec Exp:** Melanoma; Dermatopathology; **Hospital:** Brigham & Women's Hosp; **Address:** Skin Care & Dermatopathology Assocs, 1 Broadway Fl 14, Cambridge, MA 02142; **Phone:** 617-401-2231; **Board Cert:** Dermatology 1969; Dermatopathology 1974; Anatomic Pathology 1974; **Med School:** Univ Pittsburgh 1961; **Resid:** Internal Medicine, Mt Sinai Hosp 1964; Dermatology, Mass Genl Hosp 1967; **Fellow:** Anatomic Pathology, Mass Genl Hosp 1972; **Fac Appt:** Clin Prof Path, Harvard Med Sch

Neel, Victor A MD/PhD [D] - **Spec Exp:** Mohs' Surgery; Skin Cancer; **Hospital:** Mass Genl Hosp; **Address:** 50 Staniford St, Ste 270, Boston, MA 02114; **Phone:** 617-726-1869; **Board Cert:** Dermatology 2009; **Med School:** Cornell Univ-Weill Med Coll 1995; **Resid:** Pediatrics, Rhode Island Hosp 1997; Dermatology, Rhode Island Hosp 2000; **Fellow:** Mohs Surgery, UCLA Med Ctr 2001

Olbricht, Suzanne M MD [D] - **Spec Exp:** Skin Cancer; Mohs' Surgery; Muir-Torre Syndrome; **Hospital:** Lahey Clin; **Address:** Lahey Clinic, 41 Mall Rd, Burlington, MA 01805; **Phone:** 781-744-8348; **Board Cert:** Internal Medicine 1979; Dermatology 1983; **Med School:** Baylor Coll Med 1976; **Resid:** Internal Medicine, Mass General Hosp 1979; Dermatology, Mass General Hosp 1983; **Fellow:** Mohs Surgery, Mass General Hosp 1991; **Fac Appt:** Assoc Prof D, Harvard Med Sch

Sober, Arthur Joel MD [D] - **Spec Exp:** Melanoma; Skin Cancer; Merkel Cell Carcinoma; Mohs' Surgery; **Hospital:** Mass Genl Hosp; **Address:** 50 Staniford St, Ste 200, Boston, MA 02114; **Phone:** 617-726-2914; **Board Cert:** Internal Medicine 1974; Dermatology 1975; **Med School:** Geo Wash Univ 1968; **Resid:** Internal Medicine, Beth Israel Hosp 1970; Dermatology, Mass General Hosp 1974; **Fellow:** Immunology, Peter Bent Brigham Hosp 1976; **Fac Appt:** Prof D, Harvard Med Sch

Tsao, Hensin MD/PhD [D] - **Spec Exp:** Melanoma; Melanoma Genetics; Skin Cancer; **Hospital:** Mass Genl Hosp; **Address:** Mass Genl Hosp, Dept Dermatology, 55 Fruit St, Edwards Bldg, rm 211, Boston, MA 02114-2543; **Phone:** 617-726-2914; **Board Cert:** Dermatology 2006; **Med School:** Columbia P&S 1993; **Resid:** Dermatology, Brigham & Women's Hosp 1996; **Fellow:** Dermatology, Mass Genl Hosp 1997; **Fac Appt:** Assoc Prof D, Harvard Med Sch

Mid Atlantic

Bickers, David MD [D] - **Spec Exp:** Skin Cancer; Photodynamic Therapy; **Hospital:** NY-Presby Hosp/Columbia (page 78); **Address:** 16 E 60th St, Ste 300, New York, NY 10022-1002; **Phone:** 212-326-8465; **Board Cert:** Dermatology 1974; **Med School:** Univ VA Sch Med 1967; **Resid:** Dermatology, NYU Med Ctr 1973; **Fellow:** Pharmacology, Rockefeller Univ Hosp 1974; **Fac Appt:** Prof D, Columbia P&S

Dermatology

Braun III, Martin MD [D] - **Spec Exp:** Mohs' Surgery; Skin Cancer; **Hospital:** G Washington Univ Hosp, Washington Hosp Ctr; **Address:** 2112 F St NW, Ste 701, Washington, DC 20037; **Phone:** 202-293-7618; **Board Cert:** Dermatology 1977; Dermatopathology 1982; **Med School:** Univ MD Sch Med 1970; **Resid:** Dermatology, Univ Mich Med Ctr 1976; **Fellow:** Mohs Surgery, Precept w/ Dr Frederic Mohs 1975; **Fac Appt:** Clin Prof D, Geo Wash Univ

Brodland, David MD [D] - **Spec Exp:** Mohs' Surgery; Skin Cancer; Reconstructive Surgery-Skin; **Hospital:** UPMC Shadyside, Jefferson Reg Med Ctr - Pittsburgh; **Address:** South Hills Med Bldg, 575 Coal Valley Rd, Ste 360, Clairton, PA 15025; **Phone:** 412-466-9400; **Board Cert:** Dermatology 1989; **Med School:** Southern IL Univ 1985; **Resid:** Dermatology, Mayo Grad Sch Med 1989; **Fellow:** Mohs Surgery, John A Zitelli MD 1990; **Fac Appt:** Asst Clin Prof D, Univ Pittsburgh

Dzubow, Leonard M MD [D] - **Spec Exp:** Mohs' Surgery; Skin Cancer; **Address:** 101 Chesley Drive, Media, PA 19063; **Phone:** 484-621-0082; **Board Cert:** Internal Medicine 1978; Dermatology 2009; **Med School:** Univ Pennsylvania 1975; **Resid:** Internal Medicine, Hosp Univ Penn 1978; Dermatology, NYU-Skin Cancer Unit 1980; **Fellow:** Mohs Surgery, NYU-Skin Cancer Unit 1981; **Fac Appt:** Prof D, Univ Pennsylvania

Geronemus, Roy MD [D] - **Spec Exp:** Skin Laser Surgery; Mohs' Surgery; Skin Cancer; **Hospital:** NYU Langone Med Ctr (page 79), New York Eye & Ear Infirm (page 77); **Address:** 317 E 34 St, Ste 11N, New York, NY 10016-4974; **Phone:** 212-686-7306; **Board Cert:** Dermatology 1983; **Med School:** Univ Miami Sch Med 1979; **Resid:** Dermatology, NYU-Skin Cancer Unit 1983; **Fellow:** Mohs Surgery, NYU-Skin Cancer Unit 1984; **Fac Appt:** Clin Prof D, NYU Sch Med

Halpern, Allan C MD [D] - **Spec Exp:** Skin Cancer; Melanoma; Melanoma Early Detection/Prevention; **Hospital:** Meml Sloan-Kettering Cancer Ctr (page 75); **Address:** 160 E 53rd St Fl 2, Dermatology, New York, NY 10022; **Phone:** 212-610-0766; **Board Cert:** Internal Medicine 1984; Dermatology 1988; **Med School:** Albert Einstein Coll Med 1981; **Resid:** Internal Medicine, Montefiore Hosp 1985; Dermatology, Hosp Univ Penn 1989; **Fellow:** Epidemiology, Hosp Univ Penn 1989; **Fac Appt:** Assoc Prof Med, Cornell Univ-Weill Med Coll

Kriegel, David MD [D] - **Spec Exp:** Mohs' Surgery; Skin Laser Surgery; Mohs' Surgery; **Hospital:** Mount Sinai Med Ctr (page 76); **Address:** 250 W 57th St, Ste 825, New York, NY 10107-0809; **Phone:** 212-489-6669; **Board Cert:** Dermatology 2003; **Med School:** Boston Univ 1987; **Resid:** Dermatology, New England Med Ctr 1991; **Fellow:** Mohs Surgery, Stony Brook Univ Hosp 1993; **Fac Appt:** Assoc Prof D, Mount Sinai Sch Med

Lebwohl, Mark MD [D] - **Spec Exp:** Skin Cancer; Cutaneous Lymphoma; Melanoma; **Hospital:** Mount Sinai Med Ctr (page 76); **Address:** 5 E 98th St, Fl 5, New York, NY 10029-6501; **Phone:** 212-241-9728; **Board Cert:** Internal Medicine 1981; Dermatology 1983; **Med School:** Harvard Med Sch 1978; **Resid:** Internal Medicine, Mt Sinai Hosp 1981; Dermatology, Mt Sinai Hosp 1983; **Fellow:** Dermatology, Mt Sinai Hosp 1983; **Fac Appt:** Prof D, Mount Sinai Sch Med

Lessin, Stuart R MD [D] - **Spec Exp:** Cutaneous Lymphoma; Skin Cancer; Melanoma Risk Assessment; **Hospital:** Bryn Mawr Hosp; **Address:** Bryn Mawr Skin & Cancer Ctr, 919 Conestoga Rd, Rosemont, PA 19010; **Phone:** 610-525-5028; **Board Cert:** Dermatology 1986; **Med School:** Temple Univ 1982; **Resid:** Dermatology, Hosp Univ Penn 1986; **Fellow:** Molecular Biology, Wistar Inst 1987; **Fac Appt:** Prof D, Temple Univ

Lowitt, Mark H MD [D] - **Spec Exp:** Skin Cancer; Melanoma; **Hospital:** Greater Baltimore Med Ctr; **Address:** 6565 N Charles St, Ste 315, Baltimore, MD 21204; **Phone:** 410-321-1195; **Board Cert:** Dermatology 2003; **Med School:** Tulane Univ 1987; **Resid:** Internal Medicine, New England Deaconess Hosp 1990; **Fellow:** Dermatology, Univ Maryland 1993; **Fac Appt:** Assoc Clin Prof D, Univ MD Sch Med

Miller, Stanley J MD [D] - **Spec Exp:** Skin Cancer; Mohs' Surgery; Melanoma; **Hospital:** Johns Hopkins Hosp, Univ of MD Med Ctr; **Address:** Charles Towson Bldg, 1104 Kenilworth Drive, Ste 201, Towson, MD 21204; **Phone:** 443-279-0340; **Board Cert:** Dermatology 1989; **Med School:** Univ VT Coll Med 1984; **Resid:** Dermatology, UCSD Med Ctr 1989; **Fellow:** Dermatologic Surgery, Univ Penn 1991; **Fac Appt:** Assoc Prof D, Johns Hopkins Univ

Nigra, Thomas P MD [D] - **Spec Exp:** Skin Cancer; **Hospital:** Washington Hosp Ctr, Natl Rehab Hosp; **Address:** Dermatology Assocs, 110 Irving St NW, Ste 2B28, Washington, DC 20010; **Phone:** 202-877-6227; **Board Cert:** Dermatology 1973; **Med School:** Univ Pennsylvania 1967; **Resid:** Dermatology, Mass Genl Hosp 1973; Dermatology, Natl Inst of Health 1971; **Fac Appt:** Clin Prof D, Geo Wash Univ

Prioleau, Philip G MD [D] - **Spec Exp:** Melanoma; Skin Cancer; Mohs' Surgery; **Hospital:** NY-Presby Hosp/Weill Cornell (page 78); **Address:** 1035 Fifth Ave, Ste C, New York, NY 10028; **Phone:** 212-794-3548; **Board Cert:** Surgery 1973; Anatomic Pathology 1979; Dermatopathology 1980; Dermatology 1983; **Med School:** Med Univ SC 1967; **Resid:** Surgery, Univ Va Hosp 1972; Plastic Surgery, Duke Univ Hosp 1975; **Fellow:** Pathology, Barnes Jewish Hosp 1980; Dermatopathology, NYU Med Ctr 1981; **Fac Appt:** Assoc Prof D, Cornell Univ-Weill Med Coll

Ramsay, David L MD [D] - **Spec Exp:** Cutaneous Lymphoma; Skin Cancer; **Hospital:** NYU Langone Med Ctr (page 79); **Address:** 530 1st Ave, Ste 7G, New York, NY 10016-6402; **Phone:** 212-683-6283; **Board Cert:** Dermatology 1974; **Med School:** Indiana Univ 1969; **Resid:** Dermatology, NYU Med Ctr 1973; **Fellow:** Dermatology, Univ Ill Hosp 1973; **Fac Appt:** Clin Prof D, NYU Sch Med

Rigel, Darrell S MD [D] - **Spec Exp:** Melanoma; Skin Cancer; **Hospital:** NYU Langone Med Ctr (page 79), Mount Sinai Med Ctr (page 76); **Address:** 35 E 35th Street, Ste 208, New York, NY 10016-3823; **Phone:** 212-684-5964; **Board Cert:** Dermatology 1983; **Med School:** Geo Wash Univ 1978; **Resid:** Dermatology, NYU Med Ctr 1982; **Fellow:** Dermatologic Surgery, NYU Med Ctr 1983; **Fac Appt:** Clin Prof D, NYU Sch Med

Rook, Alain H MD [D] - **Spec Exp:** Cutaneous Lymphoma; **Hospital:** Hosp Univ Penn - UPHS (page 80); **Address:** Hosp Univ Penn, Dept Dermatology, Perelman Center Fl 1 - Ste 330-S, 3400 Civic Center Blvd, Philadelphia, PA 19104-4283; **Phone:** 215-662-2737; **Board Cert:** Internal Medicine 1979; Nephrology 1980; Dermatology 2001; **Med School:** Univ Mich Med Sch 1975; **Resid:** Internal Medicine, McGill Univ Med Ctr 1977; Dermatology, Hosp Univ Penn 1989; **Fellow:** Nephrology, McGill Univ Med Ctr 1979; Immunology, NIH 1986; **Fac Appt:** Prof D, Univ Pennsylvania

Zitelli, John MD [D] - **Spec Exp:** Mohs' Surgery; Skin Cancer; Melanoma; **Hospital:** UPMC Shadyside, Jefferson Reg Med Ctr - Pittsburgh; **Address:** South Hills Med Bldg, 575 Coal Valley Rd, Ste 360, Clairton, PA 15025; **Phone:** 412-466-9400; **Board Cert:** Dermatology 2009; **Med School:** Univ Pittsburgh 1976; **Resid:** Dermatology, Univ Hlth Ctr Hosp 1979; **Fellow:** Mohs Surgery, Univ Wisconsin 1980; **Fac Appt:** Assoc Clin Prof D, Univ Pittsburgh

Southeast

Amonette, Rex A MD [D] - **Spec Exp:** Skin Cancer; Mohs' Surgery; **Address:** Memphis Dermatology Clin, 1455 Union Ave, Memphis, TN 38104-6727; **Phone:** 901-726-6655; **Board Cert:** Dermatology 1974; **Med School:** Univ Ark 1966; **Resid:** Dermatology, Univ Tenn Med Ctr 1971; **Fellow:** Mohs Surgery, NYU Med Ctr 1972; **Fac Appt:** Clin Prof D, Univ Tenn Coll Med

Dermatology

Cook, Jonathan L MD [D] - **Spec Exp:** Skin Cancer; Mohs' Surgery; Reconstructive Surgery-Skin; **Hospital:** Duke Univ Hosp; **Address:** Duke Univ Med Ctr, 5324 McFarland Drive, Ste 400, Durham, NC 27707; **Phone:** 919-684-6805; **Board Cert:** Dermatology 2005; **Med School:** Med Univ SC 1992; **Resid:** Dermatology, Emory Univ Hosp 1996; **Fellow:** Dermatologic Surgery, Hosp Univ Penn 1997; **Fac Appt:** Prof D, Duke Univ

Eichler, Craig J MD [D] - **Spec Exp:** Skin Cancer; **Hospital:** Physicians Regl Hlthcare Med Ctr-Pine Ridge; **Address:** 6101 Pine Ridge Rd, Naples, FL 34119; **Phone:** 239-348-4335; **Board Cert:** Dermatology 2003; **Med School:** Univ Fla Coll Med 1989; **Resid:** Dermatology, Univ Texas Med Branch 1993

Elmets, Craig A MD [D] - **Spec Exp:** Skin Cancer; Photodynamic Therapy; Melanoma; **Hospital:** Univ of Ala Hosp at Birmingham, Birmingham, Alabama VA Med Ctr; **Address:** Univ of Alabama-Birmingham-Derm Dept, 1530 3rd Ave S EFH Bldg - rm 414, Birmingham, AL 35294; **Phone:** 205-996-7546; **Board Cert:** Internal Medicine 1978; Dermatology 2009; Clinical & Laboratory Dermatologic Immunology 1989; **Med School:** Univ Iowa Coll Med 1975; **Resid:** Internal Medicine, Kansas Med Ctr 1978; Dermatology, Univ Iowa Hosps 1980; **Fellow:** Immunological Dermatology, Univ Texas Hlth Sci Ctr 1982; **Fac Appt:** Prof D, Univ Alabama

Fenske, Neil A MD [D] - **Spec Exp:** Skin Cancer; Melanoma; **Hospital:** H Lee Moffitt Cancer Ctr & Research Inst, Tampa Genl Hosp; **Address:** 12901 Bruce B Downs Blvd, MDC-79, Tampa, FL 33612; **Phone:** 813-974-4744; **Board Cert:** Dermatology 1977; Dermatopathology 1984; **Med School:** St Louis Univ 1973; **Resid:** Dermatology, Wisc Hlth Sci Ctr 1977; **Fac Appt:** Prof Med, Univ S Fla Coll Med

Flowers, Franklin P MD [D] - **Spec Exp:** Mohs' Surgery; Dermatopathology; **Hospital:** Shands at Univ of FL; **Address:** Shands Healthcare, PO Box 100383, Gainesville, FL 32610-0383; **Phone:** 352-265-8001; **Board Cert:** Dermatology 1976; Dermatopathology 1981; **Med School:** Univ Fla Coll Med 1971; **Resid:** Dermatology, Ohio State Univ 1975; **Fellow:** Mohs Surgery, Univ Alabama 1993; **Fac Appt:** Prof Med, Univ Fla Coll Med

Garrett, Algin MD [D] - **Spec Exp:** Skin Cancer; Mohs' Surgery; **Hospital:** Med Coll of VA Hosp; **Address:** Stonypoint Medical Park, 9000 Stonypoint Pkwy Fl 2, Richmond, VA 23235; **Phone:** 804-560-8991; **Board Cert:** Dermatology 1983; **Med School:** Penn State Coll Med 1978; **Resid:** Internal Medicine, VA Med Ctr 1980; Dermatology, Med Col VA 1983; **Fellow:** Mohs Surgery, Cleveland Clin Fdn 1988; **Fac Appt:** Prof D, Va Commonwealth Univ Sch Med

Green, Howard A MD [D] - **Spec Exp:** Mohs' Surgery; Skin Cancer; **Hospital:** St. Mary's Med Ctr - W Palm Bch; **Address:** 120 Butler St, Ste A, West Palm Beach, FL 33407-6106; **Phone:** 561-659-1510; **Board Cert:** Internal Medicine 1988; Dermatology 2004; **Med School:** Boston Univ 1985; **Resid:** Internal Medicine, Jefferson Univ Hosp 1988; Dermatology, Harvard Affil Hosps 1992; **Fellow:** Mohs Surgery, Boston Univ Med Ctr 1993

Grichnik, James M MD/PhD [D] - **Spec Exp:** Melanoma; Skin Cancer; **Hospital:** Univ of Miami Hosp & Clins/Sylvester Comp Canc Ctr (page 82); **Address:** 1501 NW 10th Ave BRB Bldg - rm 912, Miami, FL 33136; **Phone:** 305-243-6045; **Board Cert:** Dermatology 2003; **Med School:** Harvard Med Sch 1990; **Resid:** Dermatology, Duke Univ Med Ctr 1994; **Fac Appt:** Prof D, Univ Miami Sch Med

Johr, Robert MD [D] - **Spec Exp:** Pigmented Lesions; Melanoma; **Hospital:** Boca Raton Regl Hosp, Univ of Miami Hosp & Clins/Sylvester Comp Canc Ctr (page 82); **Address:** 1050 NW 15th St, Ste 201A, Boca Raton, FL 33486-1341; **Phone:** 561-368-4545; **Board Cert:** Dermatology 1981; **Med School:** Mexico 1975; **Resid:** Dermatology, Roswell Park Cancer Ctr 1977; Dermatology, Metro Med Ctr 1979; **Fac Appt:** Clin Prof D, Univ Miami Sch Med

Leshin, Barry MD [D] - **Spec Exp:** Skin Cancer; Mohs' Surgery; **Address:** 125 Sunnynoll Ct, Ste 100, Winston-Salem, NC 27106; **Phone:** 336-724-2434; **Board Cert:** Dermatology 1985; **Med School:** Univ Tex, Houston 1981; **Resid:** Dermatology, Univ Iowa Hosp 1985; **Fellow:** Dermatologic Surgery, Univ Iowa Hosp 1986; **Fac Appt:** Clin Prof PlS, Wake Forest Univ

Nouri, Keyvan MD [D] - **Spec Exp:** Mohs' Surgery; Skin Cancer; **Hospital:** Univ of Miami Hosp & Clins/Sylvester Comp Canc Ctr (page 82); **Address:** 1475 NW 12th Ave, Miami, FL 33163; **Phone:** 305-243-4183; **Board Cert:** Dermatology 1997; **Med School:** Boston Univ 1993; **Resid:** Dermatology, Univ Miami 1997; **Fellow:** Dermatologic Surgery, NYU Med Ctr 1999; **Fac Appt:** Prof D, Univ Miami Sch Med

Olsen, Elise A MD [D] - **Spec Exp:** Cutaneous Lymphoma; **Hospital:** Duke Univ Hosp; **Address:** Trent and Erwin Road, Box 3294, Durham, NC 27710; **Phone:** 919-684-3432; **Board Cert:** Dermatology 1983; **Med School:** Baylor Coll Med 1978; **Resid:** Internal Medicine, Univ NC Meml Hosp 1980; Dermatology, Duke Univ Med Ctr 1983; **Fac Appt:** Prof D, Duke Univ

Sobel, Stuart A MD [D] - **Spec Exp:** Skin Cancer; **Hospital:** Meml Regl Hosp, Joe DiMaggio Chldns Hosp; **Address:** 4340 Sheridan St, Ste 101, Hollywood, FL 33021-3511; **Phone:** 954-983-5533; **Board Cert:** Dermatology 2009; **Med School:** Tufts Univ 1972; **Resid:** Dermatology, Mt Sinai Hosp 1976

Sokoloff, Daniel O MD [D] - **Spec Exp:** Skin Cancer; **Hospital:** Good Sam Med Ctr - W Palm Beach, St. Mary's Med Ctr - W Palm Bch; **Address:** Palm Beach Dermatology, 4475 Medical Center Way, Ste 2, West Palm Beach, FL 33407; **Phone:** 561-863-1000; **Board Cert:** Dermatology 1982; **Med School:** Geo Wash Univ 1977; **Resid:** Dermatology, Baylor Med Ctr 1982

Thiers, Bruce H MD [D] - **Spec Exp:** Cutaneous Lymphoma; Skin Cancer; **Hospital:** MUSC Med Ctr; **Address:** MUSC Dept Dermatology, 135 Rutledge Ave Fl 11, MS 578, Charleston, SC 29425; **Phone:** 843-792-9784; **Board Cert:** Dermatology 1978; **Med School:** SUNY Buffalo 1974; **Resid:** Dermatology, SUNY Buffalo Med Ctr 1978; **Fac Appt:** Prof D, Med Univ SC

Midwest

Arpey, Christopher J MD [D] - **Spec Exp:** Mohs' Surgery; Skin Cancer; Skin Laser Surgery; **Hospital:** Mayo Med Ctr & Clin - Rochester; **Address:** Mayo Clinic - Dept Dermatology, 200 First St SW, Rochester, MN 55905; **Phone:** 507-284-2536; **Board Cert:** Dermatology 2001; Internal Medicine 1989; **Med School:** Univ Rochester 1986; **Resid:** Internal Medicine, Univ Iowa Hosps & Clinics 1989; Dermatology, Univ Hosps 1992; **Fellow:** Mohs Surgery, Univ Iowa Hosps & Clinics 1994; **Fac Appt:** Prof D, Mayo Med Sch

Bailin, Philip L MD [D] - **Spec Exp:** Mohs' Surgery; Skin Laser Surgery; Skin Cancer; **Hospital:** Cleveland Clin (page 70); **Address:** 9500 Euclid Ave A Bldg Fl 6, MC A-61, Cleveland, OH 44195-5032; **Phone:** 216-444-2115; **Board Cert:** Dermatology 1975; **Med School:** Northwestern Univ 1968; **Resid:** Dermatology, Cleveland Clin Fdn 1974; **Fellow:** Dermatopathology, Armed Forces Inst Pathology 1975; Mohs Surgery, Univ Wisc Hosp & Clin

Cornelius, Lynn A MD [D] - **Spec Exp:** Melanoma; **Hospital:** Barnes-Jewish Hosp; **Address:** Washington Univ Dept Dermatology, 4921 Parkview Place, Campus Box 8123, St Louis, MO 63110; **Phone:** 314-362-2643; **Board Cert:** Dermatology 1989; **Med School:** Univ MO-Columbia Sch Med 1984; **Resid:** Dermatology, Barnes Jewish Hosp-Wash Univ 1989; **Fellow:** Immunological Dermatology, Emory Univ Med Ctr 1992; **Fac Appt:** Assoc Prof D, Washington Univ, St Louis

Dermatology

Fosko, Scott W MD [D] - **Spec Exp:** Mohs' Surgery; Skin Cancer; **Hospital:** St. Louis Univ Hosp; **Address:** 1755 S Grand Blvd, Ste 210, St Louis, MO 63104; **Phone:** 314-256-3420; **Board Cert:** Internal Medicine 1989; Dermatology 2001; **Med School:** Univ MD Sch Med 1986; **Resid:** Internal Medicine, Univ Va Med Ctr 1989; Dermatology, Yale-New Haven Hosp 1992; **Fellow:** Mohs Surgery, Hosp UPenn 1993; **Fac Appt:** Prof D, St Louis Univ

Hanke, C William MD [D] - **Spec Exp:** Mohs' Surgery; Skin Laser Surgery; Photodynamic Therapy; Melanoma; **Hospital:** St. Vincent Carmel Hosp; **Address:** Laser & Skin Surgery Ctr of Indiana, 13400 N Meridian St, Ste 290, Carmel, IN 46032-1486; **Phone:** 317-660-4900; **Board Cert:** Dermatology 2009; Dermatopathology 1982; **Med School:** Univ Iowa Coll Med 1971; **Resid:** Dermatology, Cleveland Clinic 1978; Dermatopathology, Indiana Univ 1982; **Fellow:** Cutaneous Oncology, Cleveland Clinic 1979; **Fac Appt:** Clin Prof D, Indiana Univ

Hruza, George J MD [D] - **Spec Exp:** Skin Laser Surgery; Mohs' Surgery; **Hospital:** St. Luke's Hosp - Chesterfield, MO, St. Louis Univ Hosp; **Address:** Laser & Derm Surg Ctr, 1001 Chesterfield Pkwy E, Ste 101, St Louis, MO 63017; **Phone:** 314-878-3839; **Board Cert:** Dermatology 1986; **Med School:** NYU Sch Med 1982; **Resid:** Dermatology, NYU Med Ctr-Skin Cancer Unit 1986; **Fellow:** Laser Surgery, Mass Genl Hosp-Harvard 1987; Mohs Surgery, Univ Wisc Affil Hosp 1988; **Fac Appt:** Clin Prof D, St Louis Univ

Johnson, Timothy M MD [D] - **Spec Exp:** Melanoma; Mohs' Surgery; **Hospital:** Univ of Michigan Hosp; **Address:** Univ Michigan Dermatology, 1910 Taubman Ctr, 1500 E Medical Center Drive, Ann Arbor, MI 48109-5314; **Phone:** 734-936-4190; **Board Cert:** Dermatology 1988; **Med School:** Univ Tex, Houston 1984; **Resid:** Dermatology, Univ Texas Med Ctr 1988; **Fellow:** Cutaneous Oncology, Univ Mich Med Ctr 1989; Mohs Surgery, Univ Oregon Hlth Sci Ctr 1990; **Fac Appt:** Prof D, Univ Mich Med Sch

Krunic, Aleksandar L MD [D] - **Spec Exp:** Mohs' Surgery; Skin Cancer; Melanoma; Skin Laser Surgery; **Hospital:** Univ of IL Med Ctr at Chicago; **Address:** 1801 W Taylor St, Ste 3E, Chicago, IL 60612; **Phone:** 312-996-8666; **Board Cert:** Dermatology 2003; **Med School:** Yugoslavia 1988; **Resid:** Dermatology, Univ Chicago Hosp 2003; **Fellow:** Mohs Surgery, Duke Univ Med Ctr 1997; Mohs Surgery, Univ Texas SW Med Ctr 2004; **Fac Appt:** Assoc Clin Prof D, Univ IL Coll Med

Lim, Henry W MD [D] - **Spec Exp:** Cutaneous Lymphoma; Skin Cancer; **Hospital:** Henry Ford Hosp; **Address:** Henry Ford Hosp, Dept Derm, 3031 W Grand Blvd, Ste 800, Detroit, MI 48202-3141; **Phone:** 313-916-4060; **Board Cert:** Dermatology 2005; Clinical & Laboratory Dematologic Immunology 1985; **Med School:** SUNY Downstate 1975; **Resid:** Dermatology, NYU Med Ctr 1979; **Fellow:** Immunological Dermatology, NYU Med Ctr 1980; **Fac Appt:** Prof Path, Wayne State Univ

Lowe, Lori MD [D] - **Spec Exp:** Dermatopathology; Skin Cancer; **Hospital:** Univ of Michigan Hosp; **Address:** Univ Michigan Dept Pathology, 1301 Catherine Rd, M3261-Med Sci 1, Ann Arbor, MI 48109-5602; **Phone:** 734-764-4460; **Board Cert:** Dermatology 1990; Dermatopathology 1991; **Med School:** Univ Tex, Houston 1985; **Resid:** Dermatology, Univ Tex Hlth Sci Ctr 1990; **Fellow:** Dermatopathology, Univ Colo Hlth Sci Ctr 1991; **Fac Appt:** Prof D, Univ Mich Med Sch

Neuburg, Marcelle MD [D] - **Spec Exp:** Mohs' Surgery; Skin Cancer; Pigmented Lesions; **Hospital:** Froedtert and Med Ctr of WI; **Address:** Dept Dermatology, 9200 W Wisconsin Ave, Milwaukee, WI 53226; **Phone:** 414-805-5300; **Board Cert:** Internal Medicine 1985; Dermatology 1988; **Med School:** Oregon Hlth & Sci Univ 1982; **Resid:** Internal Medicine, Georgetown Univ Hosp 1985; Dermatology, Boston Univ Sch Med Ctr 1988; **Fellow:** Mohs Surgery, Tufts New England Med Ctr 1990; **Fac Appt:** Prof D, Med Coll Wisc

Otley, Clark C MD [D] - **Spec Exp:** Mohs' Surgery; Skin Cancer; Skin Cancer in Transplant Patients; **Hospital:** Mayo Med Ctr & Clin - Rochester; **Address:** Mayo Clinic, 200 First St SW, Rochester, MN 55905; **Phone:** 507-284-3579; **Board Cert:** Dermatology 2004; **Med School:** Duke Univ 1991; **Resid:** Dermatology, Mass Genl Hosp 1995; **Fellow:** Dermatologic Surgery, Mayo Clinic 1996; **Fac Appt:** Assoc Prof D, Mayo Med Sch

Shea, Christopher R MD [D] - **Spec Exp:** Melanoma; Cutaneous Lymphoma; Pigmented Lesions; **Hospital:** Univ of IL Med Ctr at Chicago; **Address:** Univ Chicago Med Ctr, 5758 S Maryland Ave, MC 9815, Chicago, IL 60637; **Phone:** 773-702-6559; **Board Cert:** Anatomic Pathology 1998; Dermatology 2009; Dermatopathology 1991; **Med School:** Georgetown Univ 1983; **Resid:** Dermatology, Mass Genl Hosp 1986; Anatomic Pathology, Georgetown Univ Hosp 1981; **Fellow:** Dermatology, Mass Genl Hosp 1989; Dermatopathology, NY Presby Hosp/Weill Cornell 1991; **Fac Appt:** Prof Med, Univ IL Coll Med

Wheeland, Ronald G MD [D] - **Spec Exp:** Skin Laser Surgery; Mohs' Surgery; Cutaneous Lymphoma; **Hospital:** Univ of Missouri Hosp; **Address:** One Hospital Drive, One University Missouri Hospital Drive, Columbia, MO 65212; **Phone:** 573-882-4800 x2; **Board Cert:** Dermatology 2009; Dermatopathology 1978; **Med School:** Univ Ariz Coll Med 1973; **Resid:** Dermatology, Univ Ok Hlth Sci Ctr 1977; **Fellow:** Dermatopathology, Univ Ok Hlth Sci Ctr 1978; Mohs Surgery, Cleveland Clin Fnd 1984; **Fac Appt:** Prof D, Univ MO-Columbia Sch Med

Wood, Gary S MD [D] - **Spec Exp:** Cutaneous Lymphoma; Melanoma; Skin Cancer; **Hospital:** Univ WI Hosp & Clins, Wm S Middleton Mem Vet Hosp-Madison; **Address:** Univ Wisconsin Health, Dept Dermatology, 1 S Park St Fl 7, Madison, WI 53715-1375; **Phone:** 608-287-2620; **Board Cert:** Anatomic Pathology 1983; Dermatology 1986; Dermatopathology 1987; **Med School:** Univ IL Coll Med 1979; **Resid:** Anatomic Pathology, Stanford Univ Med Ctr 1983; Dermatology, Stanford Univ Med Ctr 1985; **Fellow:** Immunopathology, Stanford Univ Med Ctr 1981; **Fac Appt:** Prof D, Univ Wisc

Great Plains and Mountains

Bowen, Glen M MD [D] - **Spec Exp:** Melanoma; Cutaneous Lymphoma; Clinical Trials; Mohs' Surgery; **Hospital:** Univ Utah Hlth Care, Cottonwood Hosp & Med Ctr; **Address:** Huntsman Cancer Inst, 50 N Medical Drive, rm 4A330, Salt Lake City, UT 84132; **Phone:** 801-585-0197; **Board Cert:** Dermatology 2005; **Med School:** Univ Utah 1990; **Resid:** Dermatology, Univ Michigan Med Ctr 1993; **Fellow:** Immunological Dermatology, Univ Michigan Med Ctr 1995; Mohs Surgery, Univ Utah 2001; **Fac Appt:** Assoc Prof D, Univ Utah

Southwest

Butler, David F MD [D] - **Spec Exp:** Skin Cancer; **Hospital:** Scott & White Mem Hosp; **Address:** Scott White Meml Hosp, Dept Dermatology, 409 W Adams St, Temple, TX 76501; **Phone:** 254-742-3724; **Board Cert:** Dermatology 1985; **Med School:** Univ Tex Med Br, Galveston 1980; **Resid:** Dermatology, Walter Reed Army Med Ctr 1985; **Fac Appt:** Assoc Prof D, Texas Tech Univ

Carney, John M MD [D] - **Spec Exp:** Mohs' Surgery; Skin Cancer; **Hospital:** UAMS Med Ctr; **Address:** Southwest Med Arts Bldg, 11321 Interstate 30, Ste 201, Little Rock, AR 72209; **Phone:** 501-455-4700; **Board Cert:** Dermatology 1984; **Med School:** Northwestern Univ 1979; **Resid:** Dermatology, Univ Hosps 1984; **Fellow:** Physiology, Harvard Med Sch 1985; Dermatologic Surgery, Univ Tenn Med Ctr 1986

Dermatology

Curiel, Clara N MD [D] - **Spec Exp:** Skin Cancer; Cutaneous Lymphoma; **Hospital:** Univ Med Ctr - Tucson; **Address:** 3838 N Campbell Ave, Tucson, AZ 85719; **Phone:** 520-694-2873; **Board Cert:** Dermatology 2008; **Med School:** Venezuela 1992; **Resid:** Dermatology, Boston Univ Med Ctr 2000; **Fellow:** Dermatology, Boston Univ Med Ctr 2001; **Fac Appt:** Asst Prof D, Univ Ariz Coll Med

Duvic, Madeleine MD [D] - **Spec Exp:** Cutaneous Lymphoma; Skin Cancer; **Hospital:** UT MD Anderson Cancer Ctr, St. Luke's Episcopal Hosp-Houston; **Address:** UT MD Anderson Cancer Center, Dept of Dermatology, 1515 Holcombe Blvd, Unit 1452, Houston, TX 77030; **Phone:** 713-745-4615; **Board Cert:** Dermatology 1981; Internal Medicine 1982; **Med School:** Duke Univ 1977; **Resid:** Dermatology, Duke Univ Med Ctr 1980; Internal Medicine, Duke Univ Med Ctr 1982; **Fellow:** Geriatric Medicine, Duke Univ Med Ctr 1984; **Fac Appt:** Prof D, Univ Tex, Houston

Lim Quan, Katherine K MD [D] - **Spec Exp:** Mohs' Surgery; Skin Cancer; **Hospital:** Chandler Regional Med Ctr; **Address:** 1100 S Dobson Rd, Ste 223, Shea, Chandler, AZ 85286; **Phone:** 480-214-0388; **Board Cert:** Dermatology 2006; **Med School:** Northwestern Univ 1992; **Resid:** Dermatology, Mayo Clinic 1996; **Fellow:** Mohs Surgery, Mayo Clinic 1997

Orengo, Ida F MD [D] - **Spec Exp:** Melanoma; Mohs' Surgery; **Hospital:** St. Luke's Episcopal Hosp-Houston, DeBakey VA Med Ctr-Houston; **Address:** Baylor College of Medicine, 6620 Main St, Ste 1425, Houston, TX 77030; **Phone:** 713-798-6925; **Board Cert:** Dermatology 2009; **Med School:** Harvard Med Sch 1988; **Resid:** Dermatology, Baylor Coll Med 1991; **Fac Appt:** Assoc Prof D, Baylor Coll Med

Taylor, R Stan MD [D] - **Spec Exp:** Mohs' Surgery; Melanoma; Skin Cancer; **Hospital:** UT Southwestern Med Ctr at Dallas, Parkland Hlth & Hosp Sys; **Address:** Univ Tex SW Med Sch, Dept Derm, 5323 Harry Hines Blvd, MC 9192, Dallas, TX 75390-7208; **Phone:** 214-645-8950; **Board Cert:** Dermatology 1989; **Med School:** Univ Tex Med Br, Galveston 1985; **Resid:** Dermatology, Univ Mich Med Ctr 1989; **Fellow:** Immunological Dermatology, Univ Mich 1990; Mohs Surgery, Oregon Hlth Sci Univ 1991; **Fac Appt:** Prof D, Univ Tex SW, Dallas

West Coast and Pacific

Bennett, Richard G MD [D] - **Spec Exp:** Mohs' Surgery; Skin Cancer; Dermatofibrosarcoma Protruberans; **Hospital:** USC Univ Hosp, UCLA Ronald Reagan Med Ctr; **Address:** 1301 20th St, Ste 570, Santa Monica, CA 90404-2080; **Phone:** 310-315-0171; **Board Cert:** Dermatology 1975; **Med School:** Case West Res Univ 1970; **Resid:** Dermatology, Hosp Univ Penn 1974; **Fellow:** Mohs Surgery, NYU Med Ctr 1977; **Fac Appt:** Clin Prof D, UCLA

Berg, Daniel MD [D] - **Spec Exp:** Skin Cancer; Mohs' Surgery; Skin Laser Surgery; **Hospital:** Univ Wash Med Ctr; **Address:** 4225 Roosevelt Way NE, Box 354697, Seattle, WA 98105; **Phone:** 206-598-6647; **Board Cert:** Dermatology 2009; **Med School:** Univ Toronto 1985; **Resid:** Internal Medicine, Sunnybrook Med Ctr 1988; Dermatology, Duke Univ Med Ctr 1991; **Fellow:** Dermatologic Surgery, Univ Toronto 1992; Dermatologic Surgery, Univ British Columbia 1994; **Fac Appt:** Prof D, Univ Wash

Glogau, Richard G MD [D] - **Spec Exp:** Skin Laser Surgery; Mohs' Surgery; **Hospital:** UCSF Med Ctr; **Address:** 350 Parnassus Ave, Ste 400, San Francisco, CA 94117; **Phone:** 415-564-1261; **Board Cert:** Dermatology 2009; Dermatopathology 1982; **Med School:** Harvard Med Sch 1973; **Resid:** Dermatology, UCSF Med Ctr 1977; **Fellow:** Chemosurgery, UCSF Med Ctr 1978; **Fac Appt:** Clin Prof D, UCSF

Greenway, Hubert T MD [D] - **Spec Exp:** Skin Cancer; Mohs' Surgery; Melanoma; **Hospital:** Scripps Green Hosp; **Address:** Scripps Clinic, Div Mohs' Surgery, 10666 N Torrey Pines Rd, MS 112A, La Jolla, CA 92037; **Phone:** 858-554-8646; **Board Cert:** Dermatology 1982; **Med School:** Med Coll GA 1974; **Resid:** Dermatology, Naval Hosp 1982; **Fellow:** Mohs Surgery, Univ Wisconsin Med Ctr 1981

Kim, Youn-Hee MD [D] - **Spec Exp:** Cutaneous Lymphoma; Skin Cancer; **Hospital:** Stanford Univ Hosp & Clinics; **Address:** 875 Blake Wilbur Drive, Stanford, CA 94305; **Phone:** 650-723-6316; **Board Cert:** Dermatology 1989; **Med School:** Stanford Univ 1984; **Resid:** Dermatology, Metropolitan Hosp 1989

Nghiem, Paul T MD/PhD [D] - **Spec Exp:** Merkel Cell Carcinoma; Skin Cancer; **Hospital:** Univ Wash Med Ctr; **Address:** Seattle Cancer Care Alliance, 825 Eastlake Ave E, Seattle, WA 98109; **Phone:** 206-288-1024; **Board Cert:** Dermatology 2009; **Med School:** Stanford Univ 1994; **Resid:** Dermatology, Massachusetts General Hosp 1998; **Fellow:** Research, Harvard Univ 2002; **Fac Appt:** Assoc Prof D, Univ Wash

Swanson, Neil A MD [D] - **Spec Exp:** Skin Cancer; Mohs' Surgery; Reconstructive Surgery-Skin; **Hospital:** OR Hlth & Sci Univ, VA Medical Center - Portland; **Address:** 3303 SW Bond Ave, MC CH-5D, Portland, OR 97239; **Phone:** 503-418-3376; **Board Cert:** Dermatology 1980; **Med School:** Univ Rochester 1976; **Resid:** Dermatology, Univ Michigan Med Ctr 1979; **Fellow:** Dermatology, UCSF Med Ctr 1980; **Fac Appt:** Prof D, Oregon Hlth & Sci Univ

Swetter, Susan M MD [D] - **Spec Exp:** Melanoma; Melanoma Early Detection/Prevention; Skin Cancer; **Hospital:** Stanford Univ Hosp & Clinics, VA Hlth Care Sys - Palo Alto; **Address:** Stanford Univ Med Ctr, Dept Dermatology, 875 Blake Wilbur Dr, W0069, MC 5334, Stanford, CA 94305; **Phone:** 650-723-0119; **Board Cert:** Dermatology 2001; **Med School:** Univ Pennsylvania 1990; **Resid:** Dermatology, Stanford Univ Med Ctr 1994; **Fac Appt:** Assoc Prof D, Stanford Univ

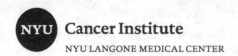

NYU Cancer Institute
NYU LANGONE MEDICAL CENTER

NYU Langone Medical Center
550 First Avenue , New York, NY 10016
www.NYULMC.org

NYU Clinical Cancer Center
160 East 34th Street, New York, NY 10016
www.NYUCI.org

**The Stephen D. Hassenfeld Children's Center
for Cancer and Blood Disorders**
160 East 32nd Street, New York, NY 10016
www.NYUMC.org/Hassenfeld

The NYU Cancer Institute is an NCI-designated cancer center and provides personalized patient care that is both compassionate and state of the art. The doctors and researchers work together to develop innovative therapies for patients. The Cancer Institute is world-renowned for excellence in cancer-focused research, personalized care, education and community outreach. Its mission is to discover the origins of human cancer and to use that knowledge to eradicate the personal and societal burden of cancer in our community, the nation and the world. For more information about our expert physicians, call 212-731-5000. *We specialize in the following areas:*

Patient-Focused Setting
The NYU Clinical Cancer Center is the principal outpatient facility of The Cancer Institute and serves as home to our patients and their caregivers. The center and its multidisciplinary team of experts provide access to the latest treatment options and clinical trials along with a variety of programs in cancer risk reduction/prevention, screening, diagnostics, genetic counseling and supportive services. In addition the NYUCI emphasizes the importance of a holistic approach to management services in complementary medicine, psychosocial support, survivorship and palliative care.

Renowned Expertise
The NYU Cancer Institute brings together experts from a variety of disciplines to create collaborative research endeavors and clinical care teams. The Cancer Institute offers a full continuum of personalized care, from prevention through diagnosis, treatment and post-treatment support. The compassion and expertise of our team members helps patients better manage the symptoms of their diseases as well as meet their special needs. Additionally, we have created special emphasis programs in diseases such as breast cancer, melanoma, GI cancer, prostate cancer, hematologic malignancies and lung cancer among others, as well as, translational programs in cancer healthcare disparities, molecularly targeted therapy, and the cell signaling pathways involved in cancer.

A Translational Approach
NYU Langone Medical Center scientists and other researchers excel in uncovering how cancer develops at the molecular level, and how we can harness that knowledge to reduce the risk of cancer and treat the disease. The Medical Center constantly seeks to create new opportunities for collaboration between investigators within our own institution, those located elsewhere in the NYU network of campuses, and researchers at other institutions.

The Stephen D. Hassenfeld Children's Center for Cancer and Blood Disorders
The center is a leading pediatric outpatient facility for the treatment of childhood cancers and blood diseases. Its unique interdisciplinary and family-centered approach combines the most advanced medical treatments with psychosocial and emotional support services for young patients and their families.

Endocrinology, Diabetes & Metabolism

a subspecialty of Internal Medicine

An internist who concentrates on disorders of the internal (endocrine) glands such as the thyroid and adrenal glands. This specialist also deals with disorders such as diabetes, metabolic and nutritional disorders, pituitary diseases, menstrual and sexual problems.

Training Required: Three years in internal medicine plus additional training and examination for certification in endocrinology, diabetes, and metabolism.

ENDOCRINOLOGY, DIABETES & METABOLISM

New England

Daniels, Gilbert H MD [EDM] - **Spec Exp:** Thyroid Disorders; Parathyroid Disease; Thyroid Cancer; Adrenal Cancer; **Hospital:** Mass Genl Hosp; **Address:** 15 Parkman St WACC Bldg - Ste 730, Boston, MA 02114; **Phone:** 617-726-8430; **Board Cert:** Internal Medicine 1972; Endocrinology, Diabetes & Metabolism 1975; **Med School:** Harvard Med Sch 1966; **Resid:** Internal Medicine, Mass Genl Hosp 1972; **Fellow:** Biochemistry, Natl Inst Hlth 1970; Endocrinology, Diabetes & Metabolism, UCSF Med Ctr 1971; **Fac Appt:** Prof Med, Harvard Med Sch

Levine, Robert A MD [EDM] - **Spec Exp:** Thyroid Cancer; Thyroid Disorders; Thyroid Ultrasound; **Hospital:** St. Joseph Hosp & Trauma Ctr; **Address:** Thyroid Center of New Hampshire, 5 Coliseum Ave, Ste 209, Nashua, NH 03063; **Phone:** 603-881-7141; **Board Cert:** Internal Medicine 1984; Endocrinology, Diabetes & Metabolism 1987; **Med School:** Univ Conn 1981; **Resid:** Internal Medicine, Mt Auburn Hosp 1984; **Fellow:** Endocrinology, Yale Univ 1987

Ross, Douglas S MD [EDM] - **Spec Exp:** Thyroid Disorders; Thyroid Cancer; **Hospital:** Mass Genl Hosp; **Address:** Mass General Thyroid Assocs, Thyroid Unit ACC-730, 55 Fruit St, Boston, MA 02114; **Phone:** 617-726-3872 x2; **Board Cert:** Internal Medicine 1980; Endocrinology, Diabetes & Metabolism 1983; **Med School:** Harvard Med Sch 1977; **Resid:** Internal Medicine, Mass General Hosp 1980; **Fellow:** Endocrinology, Mass General Hosp 1983; **Fac Appt:** Assoc Prof Med, Harvard Med Sch

Mid Atlantic

Ball, Douglas W MD [EDM] - **Spec Exp:** Thyroid Cancer; **Hospital:** Johns Hopkins Hosp; **Address:** Sidney Kimmel Cancer Ctr, 1830 E Monument St, Ste 333, Baltimore, MD 21287; **Phone:** 410-502-4926; **Board Cert:** Internal Medicine 1987; **Med School:** Geo Wash Univ 1984; **Resid:** Internal Medicine, Univ Pittsburgh 1987; **Fellow:** Endocrinology, Diabetes & Metabolism, Johns Hopkins Hosp 1991; **Fac Appt:** Assoc Prof Med, Johns Hopkins Univ

Burman, Kenneth D MD [EDM] - **Spec Exp:** Thyroid Disorders; Thyroid Cancer; **Hospital:** Washington Hosp Ctr; **Address:** Wash Hosp Ctr, Endocrinology Section, 110 Irving St NW, rm 2A72, Washington, DC 20010; **Phone:** 202-877-6563; **Board Cert:** Internal Medicine 1973; Endocrinology, Diabetes & Metabolism 1975; **Med School:** Univ MO-Columbia Sch Med 1970; **Resid:** Internal Medicine, Barnes Hosp 1972; **Fellow:** Endocrinology, Diabetes & Metabolism, Walter Reed Hosp 1974; **Fac Appt:** Prof Med, Georgetown Univ

Ladenson, Paul W MD [EDM] - **Spec Exp:** Thyroid Disorders; Thyroid Cancer; **Hospital:** Johns Hopkins Hosp; **Address:** Johns Hopkins Hosp, Div Endocrinology & Metabolism, 1830 E Monument St, rm 333, Baltimore, MD 21287; **Phone:** 410-955-3663; **Board Cert:** Internal Medicine 1978; Endocrinology, Diabetes & Metabolism 1981; **Med School:** Harvard Med Sch 1975; **Resid:** Internal Medicine, Mass Genl Hosp 1978; **Fellow:** Endocrinology, Diabetes & Metabolism, Mass Genl Hosp 1980; **Fac Appt:** Prof Med, Johns Hopkins Univ

Snyder, Peter J MD [EDM] - **Spec Exp:** Pituitary Tumors; **Hospital:** Hosp Univ Penn - UPHS (page 80); **Address:** Hosp Univ Pennsylvania, 3400 Civic Ctr Blvd, West Pavilion, Fl 4, Perelman Ctr, Philadelphia, PA 19104; **Phone:** 215-662-2300; **Board Cert:** Internal Medicine 1972; Endocrinology, Diabetes & Metabolism 1972; **Med School:** Harvard Med Sch 1965; **Resid:** Internal Medicine, Beth Israel Hosp 1967; Internal Medicine, Beth Israel Hosp 1970; **Fellow:** Endocrinology, Diabetes & Metabolism, Hosp Univ Penn 1971; **Fac Appt:** Prof Med, Univ Pennsylvania

Tuttle, R Michael MD [EDM] - **Spec Exp:** Thyroid Cancer; **Hospital:** Meml Sloan-Kettering Cancer Ctr (page 75); **Address:** 1275 York Avenue, New York, NY 10065; **Phone:** 800-525-2225; **Board Cert:** Endocrinology, Diabetes & Metabolism 2004; **Med School:** Univ Louisville Sch Med 1987; **Resid:** Internal Medicine, DD Eisenhower Army Med Ctr 1990; **Fellow:** Endocrinology, Diabetes & Metabolism, Madigan Army Med Ctr 1993; **Fac Appt:** Assoc Prof Med, Cornell Univ-Weill Med Coll

Wartofsky, Leonard MD [EDM] - **Spec Exp:** Thyroid Cancer; Thyroid Disorders; **Hospital:** Washington Hosp Ctr; **Address:** 110 Irving St NW, Ste 2A62, Washington, DC 20010-2975; **Phone:** 202-877-3109; **Board Cert:** Internal Medicine 1971; Endocrinology, Diabetes & Metabolism 1972; **Med School:** Geo Wash Univ 1964; **Resid:** Internal Medicine, Barnes Jewish Hosp 1966; Internal Medicine, Montefiore Med Ctr 1967; **Fellow:** Endocrinology, Diabetes & Metabolism, Boston City Hosp 1969; **Fac Appt:** Prof Med, Georgetown Univ

Southeast

Ain, Kenneth B MD [EDM] - **Spec Exp:** Thyroid Cancer; Thyroid Disorders; **Hospital:** Univ of Kentucky Albert B. Chandler Hosp, Lexington VA Med Ctr-Leestown Div; **Address:** Thyroid Oncology Program, rm MN524, 800 Rose St, Lexington, KY 40536-0298; **Phone:** 859-323-3778; **Board Cert:** Internal Medicine 1984; Endocrinology, Diabetes & Metabolism 1987; **Med School:** Brown Univ 1981; **Resid:** Internal Medicine, Hahnemann Univ Hosp 1984; **Fellow:** Endocrinology, Univ Chicago 1986; Thyroid Oncology, NIDDK, Natl Inst Hlth 1990; **Fac Appt:** Prof Med, Univ KY Coll Med

Earp III, H Shelton MD [EDM] - **Spec Exp:** Cancer-Hormonal Influences; **Hospital:** NC Memorial Hosp - UNC; **Address:** UNC Lineberger Comprehensive Cancer Center, 450 West Drive, Fl 1 - rm 10-012, Chapel Hill, NC 27599; **Phone:** 919-966-3036; **Board Cert:** Internal Medicine 1976; Endocrinology, Diabetes & Metabolism 1977; **Med School:** Univ NC Sch Med 1970; **Resid:** Internal Medicine, NC Memorial Hosp 1975; **Fellow:** Endocrinology, Diabetes & Metabolism, Univ North Carolina Hosp 1977; **Fac Appt:** Prof Pharm, Univ NC Sch Med

Koch, Christian A MD [EDM] - **Spec Exp:** Endocrine Cancers; Thyroid Cancer; **Hospital:** Univ Mississippi Med Ctr; **Address:** 2500 N State St, Dept Endocrinolgy, Jackson, MS 39216; **Phone:** 601-984-5525; **Board Cert:** Endocrinology, Diabetes & Metabolism 2000; **Med School:** Germany 1991; **Resid:** Internal Medicine, Ohio State Univ Hosp 1997; **Fellow:** Endocrinology, Natl Inst Hlth 2001; **Fac Appt:** Prof Med, Univ Miss

Midwest

Clutter, William E MD [EDM] - **Spec Exp:** Endocrine Cancers; **Hospital:** Barnes-Jewish Hosp, Washington Univ Med Ctr; **Address:** Washington Univ, Div Endo, Metabolism & Lipid Rsch, 660 S Euclid Ave, Campus Box 8121, St Louis, MO 63110; **Phone:** 314-362-3500; **Board Cert:** Internal Medicine 1978; Endocrinology, Diabetes & Metabolism 1981; **Med School:** Ohio State Univ 1975; **Resid:** Internal Medicine, Barnes Jewish Hosp 1978; **Fellow:** Endocrinology, Diabetes & Metabolism, Barnes Jewish Hosp 1980; **Fac Appt:** Assoc Prof Med, Washington Univ, St Louis

Hammer, Gary D MD [EDM] - **Spec Exp:** Adrenal Cancer; **Hospital:** Univ of Michigan Hosp; **Address:** Univ Michigan-Biomed Science Rsch Bldg, 109 Zina Pitcher Place, rm 1502, Ann Arbor, MI 48109-2200; **Phone:** 734-647-8906; **Board Cert:** Endocrinology, Diabetes & Metabolism 2007; **Med School:** Tufts Univ 1992; **Resid:** Internal Medicine, UCSF Med Ctr 1994; **Fellow:** Endocrinology, UCSF 1997; **Fac Appt:** Assoc Prof Med, Univ Mich Med Sch

Endocrinology, Diabetes & Metabolism

Kloos, Richard MD [EDM] - **Spec Exp:** Thyroid Cancer; **Hospital:** Ohio St Univ Med Ctr; **Address:** 1581 Dodd Drive, 4 Fl McCampbell Hall, Columbus, OH 43210; **Phone:** 614-292-3800; **Board Cert:** Internal Medicine 2002; Endocrinology, Diabetes & Metabolism 2005; Nuclear Medicine 2005; **Med School:** Case West Res Univ 1989; **Resid:** Internal Medicine, Metrohealth MC 1992; **Fellow:** Endocrinology, Diabetes & Metabolism, Univ Michigan 1995; Nuclear Medicine, Univ Michigan 1996; **Fac Appt:** Assoc Prof Med, Ohio State Univ

Kopp, Peter A MD [EDM] - **Spec Exp:** Thyroid Cancer; **Hospital:** Northwestern Meml Hosp; **Address:** Northwestern Medical Faculty Foundation, 675 N St Clair St, Ste 14-100, Galter Pavillion, Chicago, IL 60611; **Phone:** 312-695-7970; **Board Cert:** Internal Medicine 2003; Endocrinology, Diabetes & Metabolism 2004; **Med School:** Switzerland 1985; **Resid:** Internal Medicine, Regl Hosp 1992; Internal Medicine, Univ Bern 1992; **Fellow:** Endocrinology, Diabetes & Metabolism, Univ Bern 1992; Endocrinology, Diabetes & Metabolism, Northwestern Univ Hosp 1997; **Fac Appt:** Assoc Prof Med, Northwestern Univ-Feinberg Sch Med

Great Plains and Mountains

Ridgway, E Chester MD [EDM] - **Spec Exp:** Thyroid Cancer; **Hospital:** Univ of CO Hosp - Anschutz Inpatient Pav; **Address:** UCHSC at Fitzsimons, Div Endocrinology, 1635 Aurora Court, Box 6510, MS F732, Aurora, CO 80045; **Phone:** 720-848-2650; **Board Cert:** Internal Medicine 1972; Endocrinology 1973; **Med School:** Univ Colorado 1968; **Resid:** Internal Medicine, Mass Genl Hosp 1970; **Fellow:** Endocrinology, Mass Genl Hosp 1972; **Fac Appt:** Prof Med, Univ Colorado

Southwest

Robbins, Richard J MD [EDM] - **Spec Exp:** Thyroid Cancer; Pituitary Tumors; **Hospital:** Methodist Hosp - Houston; **Address:** The Methodist Hosp, 6550 Fannin St, Ste 1001, Houston, TX 77030; **Phone:** 713-441-6640; **Board Cert:** Internal Medicine 1978; Endocrinology, Diabetes & Metabolism 1983; **Med School:** Creighton Univ 1975; **Resid:** Internal Medicine, New York Hosp 1978; **Fellow:** Endocrinology, New England Med Ctr 1981; **Fac Appt:** Prof Med, Cornell Univ-Weill Med Coll

Rubenfeld, Sheldon MD [EDM] - **Spec Exp:** Thyroid Cancer; **Hospital:** St. Luke's Episcopal Hosp-Houston, Methodist Hosp - Houston; **Address:** 7515 S Main St, Ste 690, Houston, TX 77030; **Phone:** 713-795-5750; **Board Cert:** Internal Medicine 1976; Endocrinology, Diabetes & Metabolism 1979; **Med School:** Georgetown Univ 1971; **Resid:** Internal Medicine, Boston City Hosp 1972; Internal Medicine, Baylor Affil Hosps 1976; **Fellow:** Endocrinology, Baylor Affil Hosps 1978; **Fac Appt:** Clin Prof Med, Baylor Coll Med

Sherman, Steven I MD [EDM] - **Spec Exp:** Thyroid Cancer; Endocrine Cancers; **Hospital:** UT MD Anderson Cancer Ctr; **Address:** MD Anderson Cancer Ctr, 1515 Holcombe Blvd, Unit 1461, Houston, TX 77030; **Phone:** 713-792-2840; **Board Cert:** Internal Medicine 1988; Endocrinology, Diabetes & Metabolism 2007; **Med School:** Johns Hopkins Univ 1985; **Resid:** Internal Medicine, Johns Hopkins Hosp 1988; **Fellow:** Endocrinology, Diabetes & Metabolism, Johns Hopkins Hosp 1991; **Fac Appt:** Prof Med, Baylor Coll Med

Waguespack, Steven G MD [EDM] - **Spec Exp:** Thyroid Cancer; Pituitary Tumors; Hereditary Cancer; **Hospital:** UT MD Anderson Cancer Ctr; **Address:** MD Anderson Cancer Ctr, Dept Endocrine Neoplasia/Hormonal Disorders, 1515 Holcombe Blvd, Houston, TX 77030; **Phone:** 713-563-4400; **Board Cert:** Endocrinology, Diabetes & Metabolism 2002; Pediatric Endocrinology 2003; **Med School:** Univ Tex, Houston 1994; **Resid:** Internal Medicine & Pediatrics, Indiana Univ Hosps 1998; **Fellow:** Endocrinology, Diabetes & Metabolism, Indiana Univ Hosps 2001; Pediatric Endocrinology, Riley Chldns Hosp 2002; **Fac Appt:** Prof Med, Univ Tex, Houston

West Coast and Pacific

Fitzgerald, Paul A MD [EDM] - **Spec Exp:** Thyroid Disorders; Pituitary Tumors; **Hospital:** UCSF Med Ctr; **Address:** 350 Parnassus Ave, Ste 710, San Francisco, CA 94117-3685; **Phone:** 415-665-1136; **Board Cert:** Internal Medicine 1975; Endocrinology, Diabetes & Metabolism 1981; **Med School:** Jefferson Med Coll 1972; **Resid:** Internal Medicine, Presby Med Ctr-Univ Colo 1975; **Fellow:** Endocrinology, Diabetes & Metabolism, UCSF Med Ctr 1978; **Fac Appt:** Clin Prof Med, UCSF

Heber, David MD [EDM] - **Spec Exp:** Nutrition & Cancer Prevention; Nutrition & Disease Prevention/Control; **Hospital:** UCLA Ronald Reagan Med Ctr; **Address:** 900 Veteran Ave, Rm 12-217, UCLA Center for Human Nutrition, Los Angeles, CA 90095-1742; **Phone:** 310-206-1987; **Board Cert:** Internal Medicine 1976; Endocrinology, Diabetes & Metabolism 1977; **Med School:** Harvard Med Sch 1973; **Resid:** Internal Medicine, LAC Harbor Genl Hosp 1975; **Fellow:** Endocrinology, Diabetes & Metabolism, LAC Harbor Genl Hosp 1978; **Fac Appt:** Prof Med, UCLA

Hoffman, Andrew R MD [EDM] - **Spec Exp:** Pituitary Tumors; **Hospital:** Stanford Univ Hosp & Clinics, VA Hlth Care Sys - Palo Alto; **Address:** 300 Pasteur Drive, Div of Endocinology, Stanford, CA 94305-5103; **Phone:** 650-723-6961; **Board Cert:** Internal Medicine 1979; Endocrinology 1981; **Med School:** Stanford Univ 1976; **Resid:** Internal Medicine, Mass Genl Hosp 1978; **Fellow:** Endocrinology, Natl Inst Hlth 1980; Endocrinology, Mass Genl Hosp 1982; **Fac Appt:** Prof Med, Stanford Univ

Kandeel, Fouad MD/PhD [EDM] - **Spec Exp:** Thyroid Cancer; Endocrine Cancers; **Hospital:** City of Hope Natl Med Ctr (page 69); **Address:** City of Hope, Diabetes Dept, 1500 E Duarte Rd, Duarte, CA 91010; **Phone:** 626-256-4673 x62251; **Med School:** Egypt 1969; **Resid:** Internal Medicine, Birmingham & Midland Hosp for Women; Endocrinology, Diabetes & Metabolism, Queen Elizabeth Hosp; **Fac Appt:** Assoc Clin Prof Med, UCLA

Melmed, Shlomo MD [EDM] - **Spec Exp:** Pituitary Tumors; **Hospital:** Cedars-Sinai Med Ctr; **Address:** Cedars Sinai Med Ctr, 8700 Beverly Blvd, Ste 2015, Los Angeles, CA 90048; **Phone:** 310-423-4691; **Board Cert:** Internal Medicine 1979; Endocrinology, Diabetes & Metabolism 1983; **Med School:** South Africa 1970; **Resid:** Internal Medicine, Sheba Med Ctr 1976; **Fellow:** Endocrinology, Diabetes & Metabolism, Wadsworth VA Hosp 1980; **Fac Appt:** Prof Med, UCLA

The Best in American Medicine
www.CastleConnolly.com

Gastroenterology

a subspecialty of Internal Medicine

An internist who specializes in diagnosis and treatment of diseases of the digestive organs including the stomach, bowels, liver, and gallbladder. This specialist treats conditions such as abdominal pain, ulcers, diarrhea, cancer and jaundice and performs complex diagnostic and therapeutic procedures using endoscopes to see internal organs.

Training Required: Three years in internal medicine plus additional training and examination for certification in gastroenterology.

GASTROENTEROLOGY

New England

Aslanian, Harry R MD [Ge] - **Spec Exp:** Endoscopic Ultrasound; Esophageal Cancer; Pancre-atic Cancer; Rectal Cancer; **Hospital:** Yale-New Haven Hosp; **Address:** Yale Univ School of Med, Section of Digestive Diseases, 333 Cedar St, Box 208019, New Haven, CT 06520-8019; **Phone:** 203-200-5083; **Board Cert:** Gastroenterology 2002; **Med School:** Brown Univ 1996; **Resid:** Inter-nal Medicine, Mayo Clin 1999; **Fellow:** Gastroenterology, Yale Univ Affil Hosp 2002; Endoscopy, Yale Univ Affil Hosp 2003; **Fac Appt:** Assoc Prof Med, Yale Univ

Butterly, Lynn MD [Ge] - **Spec Exp:** Colonoscopy; Endoscopy; Colon & Rectal Cancer Detec-tion; Colon & Rectal Cancer-Familial Polyposis; **Hospital:** Dartmouth - Hitchcock Med Ctr; **Address:** Dartmouth-Hitchcock Med Ctr, Dept Gastro, 1 Med Ctr Drive, Lebanon, NH 03756; **Phone:** 603-650-5261; **Board Cert:** Internal Medicine 1983; Gastroenterology 1985; **Med School:** Harvard Med Sch 1979; **Resid:** Internal Medicine, Mass Genl Hosp 1983; **Fellow:** Gastroenterology, Mass Genl Hosp 1985; **Fac Appt:** Asst Prof Med, Dartmouth Med Sch

Chung, Daniel C MD [Ge] - **Spec Exp:** Colonoscopy; Colon & Rectal Cancer-Familial Polyposis; Pancreatic Cancer(Familial); Pancreatic Endocrine Tumors; **Hospital:** Mass Genl Hosp; **Address:** Gastroenterology Associates, 55 Fruit St, Blake 4, Boston, MA 02114; **Phone:** 617-726-3544; **Board Cert:** Internal Medicine 2001; Gastroenterology 2003; **Med School:** Harvard Med Sch 1988; **Resid:** Internal Medicine, Mass Genl Hosp 1991; **Fellow:** Gastroenterology, Mass Genl Hosp 1995; **Fac Appt:** Assoc Prof Med, Harvard Med Sch

Levine, Joel B MD [Ge] - **Spec Exp:** Colon & Rectal Cancer Detection; Colonoscopy; **Hospi-tal:** Univ of Conn Hlth Ctr, John Dempsey Hosp; **Address:** Univ Connecticut Hlth Ctr, Colon Cancer Prevention Prgm, 263 Farmington Ave, Farmington, CT 06030-2813; **Phone:** 860-679-4567; **Board Cert:** Internal Medicine 1973; Gastroenterology 1977; **Med School:** SUNY Downstate 1969; **Resid:** Internal Medicine, Univ Chicago Hosps 1971; Internal Medicine, Mass Genl Hosp 1974; **Fel-low:** Gastroenterology, Mass Genl Hosp 1977; **Fac Appt:** Prof Med, Univ Conn

Mason, Joel B MD [Ge] - **Spec Exp:** Nutrition & Cancer Prevention; **Hospital:** Tufts Med Ctr; **Address:** 800 Washington St, Box 239, Boston, MA 02111-1513; **Phone:** 617-636-5623; **Board Cert:** Internal Medicine 1984; Gastroenterology 1987; **Med School:** Univ Chicago-Pritzker Sch Med 1981; **Resid:** Internal Medicine, Univ Iowa Hosps 1984; **Fellow:** Gastroenterology, Univ Chicago Hosps 1986; Nutrition, Univ Chicago Hosps 1986; **Fac Appt:** Prof Med, Tufts Univ

Mid Atlantic

Canto, Marcia MD [Ge] - **Spec Exp:** Endoscopy; Endoscopic Ultrasound; Pancreatic Cancer-Early Detection; **Hospital:** Johns Hopkins Hosp; **Address:** Dept of Med, Gastroenterology, 1830 E Monument St, rm 426, Baltimore, MD 21205; **Phone:** 410-614-5388; **Board Cert:** Internal Medi-cine 1989; Gastroenterology 2008; **Med School:** Philippines 1985; **Resid:** Internal Medicine, SUNY Hlth Sci Ctr 1991; **Fellow:** Gastroenterology, SUNY Hlth Sci Ctr 1993; **Fac Appt:** Assoc Prof Med, Johns Hopkins Univ

Gerdes, Hans MD [Ge] - **Spec Exp:** Endoscopy; Endoscopic Ultrasound; Barrett's Esophagus; Gastrointestinal Cancer; **Hospital:** Meml Sloan-Kettering Cancer Ctr (page 75); **Address:** 1275 York Avenue, New York, NY 10065; **Phone:** 800-525-2225; **Board Cert:** Internal Medicine 1987; Gas-troenterology 1989; **Med School:** Cornell Univ-Weill Med Coll 1983; **Resid:** Internal Medicine, New York Hosp 1986; **Fellow:** Gastroenterology, Meml Sloan Kettering Cancer Ctr 1989

Giardiello, Francis MD [Ge] - **Spec Exp:** Colon Cancer; Colon & Rectal Cancer-Familial Polyposis; Cancer Risk Assessment; **Hospital:** Johns Hopkins Hosp; **Address:** 1830 E Mounument St, rm 431, Baltimore, MD 21205; **Phone:** 410-955-7495; **Board Cert:** Internal Medicine 1983; Gastroenterology 1985; **Med School:** Tufts Univ 1980; **Resid:** Internal Medicine, Univ Michigan 1983; **Fellow:** Gastroenterology, Johns Hopkins 1985; **Fac Appt:** Prof Med, Johns Hopkins Univ

Goggins, Michael MD [Ge] - **Spec Exp:** Pancreatic Cancer-Early Detection; **Hospital:** Johns Hopkins Hosp; **Address:** Johns Hopkins Univ Sch Med, 1550 Orleans St, St CRB-2 Bldg - rm 342, Baltimore, MD 21231; **Phone:** 410-933-7495; **Med School:** Ireland 1988; **Resid:** Internal Medicine, St Jame's Hosp 1990; **Fellow:** Gastroenterology, St Jame's Hosp 1992; **Fac Appt:** Assoc Prof Med, Johns Hopkins Univ

Greenwald, Bruce D MD [Ge] - **Spec Exp:** Endoscopic Ultrasound; Barrett's Esophagus; Esophageal Cancer; Clinical Trials; **Hospital:** Univ of MD Med Ctr; **Address:** Univ of Maryland Hosp, Gastroenterology, 22 S Greene St Fl 3 - rm N3W62, Baltimore, MD 21201; **Phone:** 410-328-8731; **Board Cert:** Internal Medicine 2000; Gastroenterology 2000; **Med School:** Univ MD Sch Med 1987; **Resid:** Internal Medicine, Univ Virginia Hosp 1990; **Fellow:** Gastroenterology, Univ Maryland Hosp 1992; **Fac Appt:** Assoc Prof Med, Univ MD Sch Med

Haluszka, Oleh MD [Ge] - **Spec Exp:** Pancreatic/Biliary Endoscopy (ERCP); Gastrointestinal Cancer; Endoscopic Ultrasound; Endoscopy; **Hospital:** Fox Chase Cancer Ctr (page 72); **Address:** 333 Cottman Ave, Ste EMB, Philadelphia, PA 19111; **Phone:** 215-214-1424; **Board Cert:** Internal Medicine 1987; Gastroenterology 2001; **Med School:** Uniformed Srvs Univ, Bethesda 1982; **Resid:** Internal Medicine, US Naval Hosp 1987; **Fellow:** Gastroenterology, US Naval Hosp 1990; Endoscopy, Med Coll Wisconsin 1993; **Fac Appt:** Assoc Clin Prof Med, Temple Univ

Itzkowitz, Steven H MD [Ge] - **Spec Exp:** Colon & Rectal Cancer; Colon & Rectal Cancer Detection; Hereditary Cancer; **Hospital:** Mount Sinai Med Ctr (page 76); **Address:** 5 E 98th St, Box 1625, New York, NY 10029-6501; **Phone:** 212-241-4299; **Board Cert:** Internal Medicine 1982; Gastroenterology 1985; **Med School:** Mount Sinai Sch Med 1979; **Resid:** Internal Medicine, Bellevue Hosp/NYU Med Ctr 1982; **Fellow:** Gastroenterology, UCSF Med Ctr 1984; **Fac Appt:** Prof Med, Mount Sinai Sch Med

Kastenberg, David M MD [Ge] - **Spec Exp:** Colon & Rectal Cancer Detection; Nutrition & Cancer Prevention; **Hospital:** Thomas Jefferson Univ Hosp (page 81); **Address:** 132 S 10th St Main Bldg - Ste 480, Dept Gastroenterology, Phildelphia, PA 19107; **Phone:** 215-955-8900; **Board Cert:** Internal Medicine 2000; Gastroenterology 2000; **Med School:** NYU Sch Med 1987; **Resid:** Internal Medicine, Temple Univ Hosp 1990; **Fellow:** Gastroenterology, Thomas Jefferson Univ Hosp 1992; **Fac Appt:** Assoc Prof Med, Jefferson Med Coll

Kochman, Michael L MD [Ge] - **Spec Exp:** Endoscopy; Pancreatic/Biliary Endoscopy (ERCP); Gastrointestinal Cancer; **Hospital:** Hosp Univ Penn - UPHS (page 80), Penn Presby Med Ctr - UPHS (page 80); **Address:** 3400 Spruce St Ravdin Bldg Fl 3 - Ste GI, Philadelphia, PA 19104-4206; **Phone:** 215-349-4279; **Board Cert:** Internal Medicine 1989; Gastroenterology 2003; **Med School:** Univ IL Coll Med 1986; **Resid:** Internal Medicine, Univ Illinois Med Ctr 1990; **Fellow:** Gastroenterology, Univ Michigan Med Ctr 1993; **Fac Appt:** Prof Med, Univ Pennsylvania

Kurtz, Robert C MD [Ge] - **Spec Exp:** Pancreatic Cancer(Familial); Gastrointestinal Cancer; Endoscopy; Nutrition & Cancer Prevention/Control; **Hospital:** Meml Sloan-Kettering Cancer Ctr (page 75); **Address:** 1275 York Avenue, New York, NY 10065; **Phone:** 212-639-7620; **Board Cert:** Internal Medicine 1971; Gastroenterology 1977; **Med School:** Jefferson Med Coll 1968; **Resid:** Internal Medicine, NY Hosp/Meml Sloan Kettering Cancer Ctr 1971; **Fellow:** Gastroenterology, Meml Sloan Kettering Cancer Ctr 1973; **Fac Appt:** Prof Med, Cornell Univ-Weill Med Coll

Gastroenterology

Lightdale, Charles J MD [Ge] - **Spec Exp:** Barrett's Esophagus; Gastrointestinal Cancer; Endoscopic Ultrasound; **Hospital:** NY-Presby Hosp/Columbia (page 78); **Address:** Columbia-Presby Med Ctr, Irving Pavilion, 161 Fort Washington Ave, rm 812, New York, NY 10032-3713; **Phone:** 212-305-3423; **Board Cert:** Internal Medicine 1972; Gastroenterology 1973; **Med School:** Columbia P&S 1966; **Resid:** Internal Medicine, Yale-New Haven Hosp 1968; Internal Medicine, NY Hosp-Cornell 1969; **Fellow:** Gastroenterology, NY Hosp-Cornell 1973; **Fac Appt:** Clin Prof Med, Columbia P&S

Okolo III, Patrick I MD [Ge] - **Spec Exp:** Liver Cancer; Pancreatic Cancer; Gastrointestinal Cancer; Clinical Trials; **Hospital:** Johns Hopkins Hosp; **Address:** The John Hopkins Hospital, 600 N Wolfe St, Baltimore, MD 21287; **Phone:** 410-933-7495; **Board Cert:** Internal Medicine 2004; Gastroenterology 2008; **Med School:** Nigeria 1988; **Resid:** Internal Medicine, Indiana Univ Med Ctr 1994; **Fellow:** Gastroenterology, John Hopkins Hosp 1997; **Fac Appt:** Assoc Prof Med, Johns Hopkins Univ

Pochapin, Mark B MD [Ge] - **Spec Exp:** Pancreatic Cancer; Endoscopic Ultrasound; Colon & Rectal Cancer Detection; Colon Cancer; **Hospital:** NY-Presby Hosp/Weill Cornell (page 78); **Address:** The Jay Monahan Ctr for GI Hlth, 1315 York Ave Fl Ground, New York, NY 10021; **Phone:** 212-746-4014; **Board Cert:** Gastroenterology 2004; **Med School:** Cornell Univ-Weill Med Coll 1988; **Resid:** Internal Medicine, NY Hosp-Cornell Med Ctr 1991; **Fellow:** Gastroenterology, Montefiore Med Ctr 1993; **Fac Appt:** Assoc Clin Prof Med, Cornell Univ-Weill Med Coll

Ravich, William J MD [Ge] - **Spec Exp:** Swallowing Disorders; Barrett's Esophagus; Eosinophilic Esophagitis; **Hospital:** Johns Hopkins Hosp, Greater Baltimore Med Ctr; **Address:** 10751 Falls Rd, Ste 401, Lutherville, MD 21093; **Phone:** 410-616-2840; **Board Cert:** Internal Medicine 1978; Gastroenterology 1981; **Med School:** Ros Franklin Univ/Chicago Med Sch 1975; **Resid:** Internal Medicine, Montefiore Hosp 1978; **Fellow:** Gastroenterology, Johns Hopkins Hosp 1981; **Fac Appt:** Assoc Prof Med, Johns Hopkins Univ

Shike, Moshe MD [Ge] - **Spec Exp:** Gastrointestinal Cancer; Nutrition & Cancer Prevention; Endoscopy; **Hospital:** Meml Sloan-Kettering Cancer Ctr (page 75); **Address:** 1275 York Ave, New York, NY 10065; **Phone:** 800-525-2225; **Board Cert:** Internal Medicine 1977; Gastroenterology 1981; **Med School:** Israel 1975; **Resid:** Internal Medicine, Mt Auburn Hosp 1977; **Fellow:** Gastroenterology, Toronto Genl Hosp 1981; **Fac Appt:** Prof Med, Cornell Univ-Weill Med Coll

Slivka, Adam MD/PhD [Ge] - **Spec Exp:** Pancreatic Cancer; **Hospital:** UPMC Presby, Pittsburgh; **Address:** Digestive Disorders Center, 200 Lothrop St, 3rd Fl-PUH, Pittsburgh, PA 15213; **Phone:** 412-647-8666; **Board Cert:** Internal Medicine 2002; Gastroenterology 1995; **Med School:** Mount Sinai Sch Med 1988; **Resid:** Internal Medicine, Brigham & Womens Hosp 1991; **Fellow:** Gastroenterology, Brigham & Womens Hosp 1994; **Fac Appt:** Assoc Prof Med, Univ Pittsburgh

Smoot, Duane T MD [Ge] - **Spec Exp:** Colon & Rectal Cancer Detection; Gastrointestinal Cancer; **Hospital:** Howard Univ Hosp; **Address:** Howard Univ Hosp, Med, Div Gastroenterology, Ste 5100, 2041 Georgia Ave NW Tower Bldg, Washington, DC 20060; **Phone:** 202-865-6620; **Board Cert:** Internal Medicine 1987; Gastroenterology 2003; **Med School:** Howard Univ 1983; **Resid:** Internal Medicine, Univ MD Hosp 1986; **Fellow:** Gastroenterology, Univ MD Hosp 1989; **Fac Appt:** Prof Med, Howard Univ

Waye, Jerome MD [Ge] - **Spec Exp:** Endoscopy; Colon Cancer; Colonoscopy; **Hospital:** Mount Sinai Med Ctr (page 76), Lenox Hill Hosp; **Address:** 650 Park Ave, New York, NY 10065; **Phone:** 212-439-7779; **Board Cert:** Internal Medicine 1965; Gastroenterology 1970; **Med School:** Boston Univ 1958; **Resid:** Internal Medicine, Mt Sinai Hosp 1961; **Fellow:** Gastroenterology, Mt Sinai Hosp 1962; **Fac Appt:** Clin Prof Med, Mount Sinai Sch Med

Weinberg, David Seth MD [Ge] - **Spec Exp:** Colonoscopy; Cancer Risk Assessment; Cancer Prevention; Endoscopy; **Hospital:** Fox Chase Cancer Ctr (page 72); **Address:** Fox Chase Cancer Ctr, Dept Medicine, 333 Cottman Ave, Ste P3047, Philadelphia, PA 19111; **Phone:** 215-214-1424; **Board Cert:** Gastroenterology 2006; **Med School:** Cornell Univ-Weill Med Coll 1989; **Resid:** Internal Medicine, Beth Israel Hosp 1992; **Fellow:** Gastroenterology, Hosp U Penn 1995; Epidemiology, Hosp U Penn 1995; **Fac Appt:** Prof Med, Temple Univ

Southeast

Barkin, Jamie S MD [Ge] - **Spec Exp:** Gastrointestinal Cancer; Endoscopy; **Hospital:** Mount Sinai Med Ctr - Miami, Univ of Miami Hosp & Clins/Sylvester Comp Canc Ctr (page 82); **Address:** Mount Sinai Medical Center, Gumenick Bldg, 4300 Alton Rd, Ste 2522, Miami Beach, FL 33140-2800; **Phone:** 305-674-2240; **Board Cert:** Internal Medicine 1973; Gastroenterology 1975; **Med School:** Univ Miami Sch Med 1970; **Resid:** Internal Medicine, Univ Miami Hosp 1973; **Fellow:** Gastroenterology, Univ Miami Hosp 1975; **Fac Appt:** Prof Med, Univ Miami Sch Med

Estores, David S MD [Ge] - **Spec Exp:** Barrett's Esophagus; **Hospital:** Tampa Genl Hosp; **Address:** Ctr for Swallowing Disorders, 12901 Bruce B Downs Blvd, MDC 72, Tampa, FL 33612-4742; **Phone:** 813-974-3374; **Board Cert:** Internal Medicine 1989; Gastroenterology 2001; **Med School:** Philippines 1985; **Resid:** Internal Medicine, St Lukes Hosp 1989; **Fellow:** Gastroenterology, Univ Pittsburgh-Presby Hosp 1992

Hoffman, Brenda J MD [Ge] - **Spec Exp:** Endoscopic Ultrasound; Gastrointestinal Cancer; Colon & Rectal Cancer-Familial Polyposis; **Hospital:** MUSC Med Ctr; **Address:** MUSC Digestive Disease Center, 25 Courteney Drive, ART7100A, MSC290, Charleston, SC 29425; **Phone:** 843-792-2301; **Board Cert:** Internal Medicine 1986; Gastroenterology 1989; **Med School:** Univ KY Coll Med 1983; **Resid:** Internal Medicine, Med Univ SC Med Ctr 1987; **Fellow:** Gastroenterology, Med Univ SC Med Ctr 1989; **Fac Appt:** Prof Med, Univ SC Sch Med

Porayko, Michael K MD [Ge] - **Spec Exp:** Transplant Medicine-Liver; Liver Cancer; **Hospital:** Vanderbilt Univ Med Ctr; **Address:** Digestive Disease Center, 1301 Medical Center Drive, Ste 1660, Nashville, TN 37232; **Phone:** 615-322-0128; **Board Cert:** Internal Medicine 1984; Gastroenterology 1987; Transplant Hepatology 2006; **Med School:** Univ IL Coll Med 1981; **Resid:** Internal Medicine, Michigan State Univ Affil Hosps 1984; **Fellow:** Gastroenterology, Lahey Clin & New England Deaconess Hosp 1987; Hepatology, Mayo Clinic 1988; **Fac Appt:** Prof Med, Vanderbilt Univ

Midwest

Brown, Kimberly A MD [Ge] - **Spec Exp:** Transplant Medicine-Liver; Liver Cancer; **Hospital:** Henry Ford Hosp; **Address:** Henry Ford Hosp, Dept Gastroenterology, 2799 W Grand Blvd K-747 Bldg Fl 7, Detroit, MI 48202-2608; **Phone:** 313-916-8865; **Board Cert:** Internal Medicine 1988; Gastroenterology 2002; Transplant Hepatology 2006; **Med School:** Wayne State Univ 1985; **Resid:** Internal Medicine, Univ Michigan Med Ctr 1989; **Fellow:** Gastroenterology, Univ Michigan Med Ctr 1992

Crippin, Jeffrey S MD [Ge] - **Spec Exp:** Transplant Medicine-Liver; Gastrointestinal Cancer; **Hospital:** Barnes-Jewish Hosp; **Address:** Barnes Jewish Hosp, Div Gastroenterology, 660 S Euclid Ave Campus Box 8124, St Louis, MO 63110; **Phone:** 314-454-8160; **Board Cert:** Internal Medicine 1987; Gastroenterology 2001; Transplant Hepatology 2006; **Med School:** Univ Kansas 1984; **Resid:** Internal Medicine, Kansas Univ Med Ctr 1988; **Fellow:** Gastroenterology, Mayo Clinic 1991; **Fac Appt:** Assoc Prof Med, Washington Univ, St Louis

Gastroenterology

Di Bisceglie, Adrian M MD [Ge] - **Spec Exp:** Liver Cancer; **Hospital:** St. Louis Univ Hosp; **Address:** St Louis Univ, Div Gastroenterology, 3635 Vista Ave, St Louis, MO 63110; **Phone:** 314-577-6000; **Board Cert:** Internal Medicine 2002; Gastroenterology 2002; **Med School:** South Africa 1977; **Resid:** Internal Medicine, Baragwanath Hosp 1984; **Fellow:** Hepatology, Natl Inst Hlth 1988; **Fac Appt:** Prof Med, St Louis Univ

Early, Dayna S MD [Ge] - **Spec Exp:** Colon & Rectal Cancer Detection; Endoscopic Ultrasound; Endoscopic Therapies; **Hospital:** Barnes-Jewish Hosp, Barnes-Jewish West County Hosp; **Address:** Center for Advanced Medicine, 4921 Parkview Pl Fl 8, Saint Louis, MO 63110; **Phone:** 314-747-2066; **Board Cert:** Internal Medicine 2003; Gastroenterology 2005; **Med School:** Univ MO-Columbia Sch Med 1990; **Resid:** Internal Medicine, Vanderbilt Univ Med Ctr 1993; **Fellow:** Gastroenterology, Vanderbilt Univ Med Ctr 1995; **Fac Appt:** Prof Med, Washington Univ, St Louis

Gholam, Pierre M MD [Ge] - **Spec Exp:** Transplant Medicine-Liver; **Hospital:** Univ Hosps Case Med Ctr; **Address:** UH Case Medical Center, 11100 Euclid Ave, WRN-5066, Cleveland, OH 44106; **Phone:** 216-844-5387; **Board Cert:** Gastroenterology 2002; Transplant Hepatology 2006; **Med School:** Lebanon 1996; **Resid:** Internal Medicine, St Lukes-Roosevelt Hosp 1999; **Fellow:** Gastroenterology, St Lukes-Roosevelt Hosp 2002; **Fac Appt:** Asst Prof Med, Case West Res Univ

Goldberg, Michael J MD [Ge] - **Spec Exp:** Colon Cancer; Pancreatic/Biliary Endoscopy (ERCP); Pancreatic Cancer; **Hospital:** Evanston/North Shore Univ Hlth Sys, Glenbrook Hosp-NorthShore Univ Hlth Syst; **Address:** 2650 Ridge Ave, Ste G-208, Evanston, IL 60201; **Phone:** 847-657-1900; **Board Cert:** Internal Medicine 1978; Gastroenterology 1981; **Med School:** Univ IL Coll Med 1975; **Resid:** Internal Medicine, Univ Illinois Hosp 1978; **Fellow:** Gastroenterology, Tufts-New England Med Ctr 1980; **Fac Appt:** Assoc Clin Prof Med, Northwestern Univ

Rex, Douglas K MD [Ge] - **Spec Exp:** Endoscopy; Endoscopic Ultrasound; Colon & Rectal Cancer Detection; **Hospital:** IU Health Methodist Hosp; **Address:** 550 N University Blvd, Ste 4100, Indianapolis, IN 46202; **Phone:** 317-948-9763; **Board Cert:** Internal Medicine 1985; Gastroenterology 1987; **Med School:** Indiana Univ 1980; **Resid:** Internal Medicine, Indiana Univ Med Ctr 1982; Internal Medicine, Indiana Univ Hosp 1985; **Fellow:** Gastroenterology, Indiana Univ Med Ctr 1984; **Fac Appt:** Prof Med, Indiana Univ

Waxman, Irving MD [Ge] - **Spec Exp:** Gastrointestinal Cancer; Pancreatic Cancer; Endoscopy; Endoscopic Ultrasound; **Hospital:** Univ of Chicago Med Ctr; **Address:** 5758 S Maryland Ave, MS MC 9028, Chicago, IL 60637; **Phone:** 773-702-1459; **Board Cert:** Internal Medicine 1988; Gastroenterology 2003; **Med School:** Mexico 1985; **Resid:** Internal Medicine, New Eng Deaconess Hosp 1988; **Fellow:** Gastroenterology, Georgetown Univ Med Ctr 1991; Endoscopy, Univ Academic Med Ctr 1991; **Fac Appt:** Prof Med, Univ Chicago-Pritzker Sch Med

Great Plains and Mountains

Burt, Randall W MD [Ge] - **Spec Exp:** Colon Cancer; Colon & Rectal Cancer-Familial Polyposis; **Hospital:** Univ Utah Hlth Care; **Address:** Huntsman Cancer Inst, 2000 Circle of Hope, Salt Lake City, UT 84112; **Phone:** 801-585-3281; **Board Cert:** Internal Medicine 1977; Gastroenterology 1979; **Med School:** Univ Utah 1974; **Resid:** Internal Medicine, Barnes Hosp 1977; **Fellow:** Gastroenterology, Univ Utah Med Ctr 1979; **Fac Appt:** Prof Med, Univ Utah

Southwest

Boland, C Richard MD [Ge] - **Spec Exp:** Colon & Rectal Cancer Detection; Cancer Genetics; **Hospital:** Baylor Univ Medical Ctr; **Address:** GI Cancer Rsch Lab H-250, 3500 Gaston Ave, Dallas, TX 75246; **Phone:** 214-820-2692; **Board Cert:** Internal Medicine 1978; Gastroenterology 1981; **Med School:** Yale Univ 1973; **Resid:** Internal Medicine, USPHS Hosp 1978; **Fellow:** Gastroenterology, UCSF Med Ctr 1981; **Fac Appt:** Clin Prof Med, Univ Tex SW, Dallas

Bresalier, Robert MD [Ge] - **Spec Exp:** Gastrointestinal Cancer; **Hospital:** UT MD Anderson Cancer Ctr; **Address:** MD Anderson Canc Ctr, GI Med & Nutrition, 1515 Holcombe Blvd - Unit 1466, Houston, TX 77030; **Phone:** 713-745-4340; **Board Cert:** Internal Medicine 1981; Gastroenterology 1983; **Med School:** Univ Chicago-Pritzker Sch Med 1978; **Resid:** Internal Medicine, Barnes Hosp-Washington Univ 1981; **Fellow:** Gastroenterology, UCSF Med Ctr 1983; **Fac Appt:** Prof Med, Univ Tex, Houston

Decker, Gustav Anton MD [Ge] - **Spec Exp:** Endoscopy; Pancreatic Cancer; **Hospital:** Mayo Clinic - Scottsdale; **Address:** Mayo Clinic, Div Gastroenterology, 13400 E Shea Blvd Fl 2, Scottsdale, AZ 85259; **Phone:** 480-301-6990; **Board Cert:** Internal Medicine 1999; Gastroenterology 2003; **Med School:** South Africa 1993; **Resid:** Internal Medicine, Mayo Clinic 1999; **Fellow:** Gastroenterology, Mayo Clinic 2002; **Fac Appt:** Asst Prof Med, Mayo Med Sch

Faigel, Douglas O MD [Ge] - **Spec Exp:** Endoscopic Ultrasound; Pancreatic/Biliary Endoscopy (ERCP); Gastrointestinal Cancer; **Hospital:** Mayo Clinic - Scottsdale; **Address:** Mayo Clinic, Dept Gastroenterology, 13400 E Shea Blvd Fl 2, Scottsdale, AZ 85259; **Phone:** 480-301-6990; **Board Cert:** Internal Medicine 2003; Gastroenterology 2005; **Med School:** Univ Pennsylvania 1990; **Resid:** Internal Medicine, UCSF Med Ctr 1993; **Fellow:** Gastroenterology, Hosp Univ Penn 1995

Fleischer, David MD [Ge] - **Spec Exp:** Barrett's Esophagus; Esophageal Cancer; **Hospital:** Mayo Clinic - Scottsdale; **Address:** Mayo Clinic - Scottsdale, 13400 E Shea Blvd, Div Gastroenterology 2A, Scottsdale, AZ 85259; **Phone:** 480-301-8484; **Board Cert:** Internal Medicine 1975; Gastroenterology 1977; **Med School:** Vanderbilt Univ 1970; **Resid:** Internal Medicine, Metro General Hosp 1975; **Fellow:** Gastroenterology, LA Co Harbor-UCLA Med Ctr 1977; **Fac Appt:** Prof Med, Mayo Med Sch

West Coast and Pacific

Gish, Robert MD [Ge] - **Spec Exp:** Liver Cancer; Transplant Medicine-Liver; Clinical Trials; **Hospital:** UCSD Med Ctr-Hillcrest; **Address:** UCSD Medical Center, 200 W Arbor Drive, Ste 342, MC 8413, San Diego, CA 92103; **Phone:** 619-543-3787; **Board Cert:** Internal Medicine 1984; Gastroenterology 1987; Transplant Hepatology 2006; **Med School:** Univ Kansas 1980; **Resid:** Internal Medicine, UCSD Med Ctr 1983; **Fellow:** Gastroenterology, UCLA Med Ctr 1988; **Fac Appt:** Assoc Clin Prof Med, UCSF

Lenz, Heinz Juergen MD [Ge] - **Spec Exp:** Gastrointestinal Cancer; Colon & Rectal Cancer; **Hospital:** USC Univ Hosp; **Address:** 1441 East Lake Ave, NOR 3456, Los Angeles, CA 90033; **Phone:** 323-865-3105; **Board Cert:** Internal Medicine 2000; Gastroenterology 2000; **Med School:** Germany 1981; **Resid:** Internal Medicine, Univ Hamburg Affil Hosp 1987; Internal Medicine, UC San Diego Med Ctr 1989; **Fellow:** Gastroenterology, UC San Diego Med Ctr 1990; **Fac Appt:** Prof Med, USC-Keck School of Medicine

Gastroenterology

Savides, Thomas MD [Ge] - **Spec Exp:** Gastrointestinal Cancer; Barrett's Esophagus; Colonoscopy; Endoscopic Ultrasound; **Hospital:** UCSD Med Ctr-Hillcrest; **Address:** UCSD Med Ctr, Div Gastroenterology, 200 W Arbor Drive, MC 8788, San Diego, CA 92103-8413; **Phone:** 619-543-2347; **Board Cert:** Internal Medicine 2003; Gastroenterology 2003; **Med School:** UCSD 1987; **Resid:** Internal Medicine, UCLA Med Ctr 1990; **Fellow:** Gastroenterology, UCLA Med Ctr 1993; Gastroenterology, Indiana Univ Med Ctr 1994; **Fac Appt:** Asst Clin Prof Med, UCSD

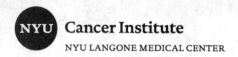

NYU **Cancer Institute**
NYU LANGONE MEDICAL CENTER

NYU Langone Medical Center
550 First Avenue , New York, NY 10016
www.NYULMC.org

NYU Clinical Cancer Center
160 East 34th Street, New York, NY 10016
www.NYUCI.org

**The Stephen D. Hassenfeld Children's Center
for Cancer and Blood Disorders**
160 East 32nd Street, New York, NY 10016
www.NYUMC.org/Hassenfeld

The NYU Cancer Institute is an NCI-designated cancer center and provides personalized patient care that is both compassionate and state of the art. The doctors and researchers work together to develop innovative therapies for patients. The Cancer Institute is world-renowned for excellence in cancer-focused research, personalized care, education and community outreach. Its mission is to discover the origins of human cancer and to use that knowledge to eradicate the personal and societal burden of cancer in our community, the nation and the world. For more information about our expert physicians, call 212-731-5000. *We specialize in the following areas:*

Patient-Focused Setting
The NYU Clinical Cancer Center is the principal outpatient facility of The Cancer Institute and serves as home to our patients and their caregivers. The center and its multidisciplinary team of experts provide access to the latest treatment options and clinical trials along with a variety of programs in cancer risk reduction/prevention, screening, diagnostics, genetic counseling and supportive services. In addition the NYUCI emphasizes the importance of a holistic approach to management services in complementary medicine, psychosocial support, survivorship and palliative care.

Renowned Expertise
The NYU Cancer Institute brings together experts from a variety of disciplines to create collaborative research endeavors and clinical care teams. The Cancer Institute offers a full continuum of personalized care, from prevention through diagnosis, treatment and post-treatment support. The compassion and expertise of our team members helps patients better manage the symptoms of their diseases as well as meet their special needs. Additionally, we have created special emphasis programs in diseases such as breast cancer, melanoma, GI cancer, prostate cancer, hematologic malignancies and lung cancer among others, as well as, translational programs in cancer healthcare disparities, molecularly targeted therapy, and the cell signaling pathways involved in cancer.

A Translational Approach
NYU Langone Medical Center scientists and other researchers excel in uncovering how cancer develops at the molecular level, and how we can harness that knowledge to reduce the risk of cancer and treat the disease. The Medical Center constantly seeks to create new opportunities for collaboration between investigators within our own institution, those located elsewhere in the NYU network of campuses, and researchers at other institutions.

The Stephen D. Hassenfeld Children's Center for Cancer and Blood Disorders
The center is a leading pediatric outpatient facility for the treatment of childhood cancers and blood diseases. Its unique interdisciplinary and family-centered approach combines the most advanced medical treatments with psychosocial and emotional support services for young patients and their families.

The Best in American Medicine
www.CastleConnolly.com

Hematology/Medical Oncology

a subspecialty of Internal Medicine

Hematology: An internist with additional training who specializes in diseases of the blood, spleen and lymph glands. This specialist treats conditions such as anemia, clotting disorders, sickle cell disease, hemophilia, leukemia and lymphoma.

Medical Oncology: An internist who specializes in the diagnosis and treatment of all types of cancer and other benign and malignant tumors. This specialist decides on and administers chemotherapy for malignancy, as well as consulting with surgeons and radiotherapists on other treatments for cancer.

Training Required: Three years in internal medicine plus additional training and examination for certification in hematology or medical oncology.

HEMATOLOGY

New England

Anderson, Kenneth C MD [Hem] - **Spec Exp:** Multiple Myeloma; Hematologic Malignancies; **Hospital:** Dana-Farber Cancer Inst, Brigham & Women's Hosp; **Address:** 450 Brookline Ave, Ste M557, Dana-Farber Cancer Inst, Div Hematology, Boston, MA 02215; **Phone:** 617-632-2144; **Board Cert:** Internal Medicine 1980; **Med School:** Johns Hopkins Univ 1977; **Resid:** Internal Medicine, Johns Hopkins Hosp 1980; **Fellow:** Hematology & Oncology, Dana Farber Cancer Inst 1983; **Fac Appt:** Prof Med, Harvard Med Sch

Ballen, Karen K MD [Hem] - **Spec Exp:** Leukemia; Bone Marrow Transplant; **Hospital:** Mass Genl Hosp; **Address:** Mass General Hospital, Hematology/Oncology, Zero Emerson Pl, Ste 118, Boston, MA 02114; **Phone:** 617-724-1124; **Board Cert:** Internal Medicine 1989; Medical Oncology 2003; Hematology 2004; **Med School:** Dartmouth Med Sch 1986; **Resid:** Internal Medicine, Beth Israel Deaconess Med Ctr 1989; **Fellow:** Hematology & Oncology, Brigham & Women's Hosp 1992; **Fac Appt:** Assoc Prof Med, Harvard Med Sch

Comenzo, Raymond MD [Hem] - **Spec Exp:** Plasma Cell Disorders; Stem Cell Transplant; **Hospital:** Tufts Med Ctr; **Address:** 800 Washington St, Box 826, Boston, MA 02111; **Phone:** 617-636-6454; **Board Cert:** Internal Medicine 1989; Hematology 2004; Blood Banking Transfusion Medicine 1992; **Med School:** Boston Univ 1986; **Resid:** Internal Medicine, Boston City Hosp 1989; **Fellow:** Hematology & Oncology, New Engl Med Ctr 1991

Duffy, Thomas P MD [Hem] - **Spec Exp:** Mast Cell Diseases; Leukemia; Lymphoma; Mast Cell Diseases; **Hospital:** Yale-New Haven Hosp, Yale Med Group; **Address:** Yale Univ, Sect Hematology, 333 Cedar St, rm 403-WWW, Box 208021, New Haven, CT 06520-8021; **Phone:** 203-785-4744; **Board Cert:** Internal Medicine 1972; Hematology 1974; **Med School:** Johns Hopkins Univ 1962; **Resid:** Internal Medicine, Johns Hopkins Hosp 1965; **Fellow:** Hematology, Johns Hopkins Hosp 1970; **Fac Appt:** Prof Med, Yale Univ

Klingemann, Hans-Georg MD/PhD [Hem] - **Spec Exp:** Bone Marrow Transplant; Stem Cell Transplant; **Hospital:** Tufts Med Ctr; **Address:** 800 Washington St, Box 245, Boston, MA 02111; **Phone:** 617-636-6227; **Med School:** Germany 1976; **Resid:** Internal Medicine, Univ Wurzburg Med Sch 1979; **Fellow:** Hematology & Oncology, Fred Hutchinson Cancer Rsch Ctr 1986; **Fac Appt:** Prof Med, Tufts Univ

Marks, Peter W MD/PhD [Hem] - **Spec Exp:** Leukemia; Platelet Disorders; Bleeding/Coagulation Disorders; **Hospital:** Yale-New Haven Hosp, Yale Med Group; **Address:** Yale Hematology, 333 Cedar St, Box 208302, New Haven, CT 06520; **Phone:** 203-200-4363; **Board Cert:** Internal Medicine 2004; Hematology 2007; Medical Oncology 2007; **Med School:** NYU Sch Med 1991; **Resid:** Internal Medicine, Brigham & Women's Hosp 1994; **Fellow:** Hematology & Oncology, Brigham & Women's Hosp 1996; **Fac Appt:** Assoc Prof Med, Yale Univ

Meehan, Kenneth MD [Hem] - **Spec Exp:** Bone Marrow Transplant; **Hospital:** Dartmouth - Hitchcock Med Ctr; **Address:** Norris Cotton Cancer Ctr, Dartmouth-Hitchcock Med Ctr, 1 Medical Center Drive, Lebanon, NH 03756; **Phone:** 603-650-4628; **Board Cert:** Internal Medicine 1989; Hematology 2004; **Med School:** Georgetown Univ 1986; **Resid:** Internal Medicine, Georgetown Univ 1989; **Fellow:** Hematology & Oncology, Dartmouth-Hitchcock Med Ctr 1992; **Fac Appt:** Assoc Prof Med, Dartmouth Med Sch

Miller, Kenneth B MD [Hem] - **Spec Exp:** Bone Marrow Transplant; Leukemia; Myelodysplastic Syndromes; **Hospital:** Tufts Med Ctr; **Address:** Tufts Med Ctr, Dept Medicine, 800 Washington St, Box 245, Boston, MA 02111; **Phone:** 617-636-2600; **Board Cert:** Internal Medicine 1976; Hematology 1980; **Med School:** NY Med Coll 1972; **Resid:** Internal Medicine, NYU Med Ctr/VA Hosp 1976; Internal Medicine, NYU Med Ctr 1976; **Fellow:** Hematology, New England Med Ctr 1979; **Fac Appt:** Prof Med, Tufts Univ

Richardson, Paul G MD [Hem] - **Spec Exp:** Multiple Myeloma; **Hospital:** Dana-Farber Cancer Inst, Brigham & Women's Hosp; **Address:** Dana Farber Cancer Inst, 44 Binney St, Boston, MA 02115; **Phone:** 617-632-2127; **Board Cert:** Hematology 1999; **Med School:** England, UK 1986; **Resid:** Internal Medicine, Baystate Med Ctr 1994; **Fellow:** Medical Oncology, Dana Farber Cancer Inst 1995; Hematology, Beth Israel Deaconess Med Ctr 1997; **Fac Appt:** Assoc Prof Med, Harvard Med Sch

Schiffman, Fred J MD [Hem] - **Spec Exp:** Hematologic Malignancies; Anemia-Cancer Related; Bleeding/Coagulation Disorders; **Hospital:** Miriam Hosp; **Address:** Comp Cancer Ctr at Miriam Hospital, 164 Summit Ave, Fain-3, Providence, RI 02906; **Phone:** 401-793-2920; **Board Cert:** Internal Medicine 1979; Hematology 1982; Medical Oncology 1987; **Med School:** NYU Sch Med 1973; **Resid:** Internal Medicine, Yale-New Haven Hosp 1975; Internal Medicine, Yale-New Haven Hosp 1979; **Fellow:** Hematology, Yale-New Haven Hosp 1981; **Fac Appt:** Prof Med, Brown Univ

Spitzer, Thomas R MD [Hem] - **Spec Exp:** Bone Marrow Transplant; Leukemia; **Hospital:** Mass Genl Hosp; **Address:** Mass Genl Hosp-Bone Marrow Tranplant Prog, 0 Emerson Pl, Ste 118, Boston, MA 02114; **Phone:** 617-724-1124; **Board Cert:** Internal Medicine 1977; Medical Oncology 1983; Hematology 1984; **Med School:** Univ Rochester 1974; **Resid:** Internal Medicine, NYew York Hosp-Cornell Med Ctr 1977; Internal Medicine, Mem Sloan Kettering Cancer Ctr 1977; **Fellow:** Hematology & Oncology, Case West Res Univ 1983; **Fac Appt:** Prof Med, Harvard Med Sch

Stone, Richard M MD [Hem] - **Spec Exp:** Leukemia; **Hospital:** Dana-Farber Cancer Inst, Brigham & Women's Hosp; **Address:** Dana Farber Cancer Inst, 44 Binney St, Mayer 1B-17, Boston, MA 02115-6084; **Phone:** 617-632-2214; **Board Cert:** Internal Medicine 1984; Medical Oncology 2008; Hematology 1988; **Med School:** Harvard Med Sch 1981; **Resid:** Internal Medicine, Brigham & Womens Hosp 1984; **Fellow:** Medical Oncology, Dana Farber Cancer Inst 1987; **Fac Appt:** Prof Med, Harvard Med Sch

Mid Atlantic

Allen, Steven Lee MD [Hem] - **Spec Exp:** Bleeding/Coagulation Disorders; Leukemia & Lymphoma; Multiple Myeloma; **Hospital:** N Shore Univ Hosp; **Address:** 450 Lakeville Rd, Lake Success, NY 11042; **Phone:** 516-734-8959; **Board Cert:** Internal Medicine 1980; Hematology 1982; Medical Oncology 1983; **Med School:** Johns Hopkins Univ 1977; **Resid:** Internal Medicine, NY Hosp-Cornell 1980; **Fellow:** Hematology & Oncology, NY Hosp-Cornell 1983; **Fac Appt:** Prof Med, Albert Einstein Coll Med

Baer, Maria R MD [Hem] - **Spec Exp:** Leukemia; Myelodysplastic Syndromes; Myeloproliferative Disorders; **Hospital:** Univ of MD Med Ctr; **Address:** Univ Maryland, Greenebaum Cancer Ctr, 22 S Greene St, rm S9D08, Baltimore, MD 21201; **Phone:** 410-328-7904; **Board Cert:** Internal Medicine 1983; Hematology 1984; **Med School:** Johns Hopkins Univ 1979; **Resid:** Internal Medicine, Vanderbilt Univ Hosp 1982; **Fellow:** Hematology, Vanderbilt Univ Hosp 1984; **Fac Appt:** Prof Med, Univ MD Sch Med

Hematology

Brodsky, Robert A MD [Hem] - **Spec Exp:** Hematologic Malignancies; Autoimmune Disease; Graft vs Host Disease; **Hospital:** Johns Hopkins Hosp; **Address:** 720 Rutland Ave, Ross Bldg - rm 1025, Baltimore, MD 21205; **Phone:** 410-955-3142; **Board Cert:** Internal Medicine 2002; Hematology 2006; **Med School:** Hahnemann Univ 1989; **Resid:** Internal Medicine, Vanderbilt Univ 1991; **Fellow:** Hematology, Vanderbilt Univ Hosp 1994; Medical Oncology, Johns Hopkins Hosp 1997; **Fac Appt:** Prof Med, Johns Hopkins Univ

Cheson, Bruce D MD [Hem] - **Spec Exp:** Leukemia; Hematologic Malignancies; **Hospital:** Georgetown Univ Hosp; **Address:** GUMC - Lombardi Cancer Ctr, 3800 Reservoir Rd NW, Podium B, Washington, DC 20007; **Phone:** 202-444-7932; **Board Cert:** Internal Medicine 1974; Hematology 1976; **Med School:** Tufts Univ 1971; **Resid:** Internal Medicine, Univ Virginia Hosp 1974; **Fellow:** Hematology, New England Med Ctr Hosp 1976

Dang, Chi V MD/PhD [Hem] - **Spec Exp:** Anaemia-Aplastic; Bone Marrow Failure Disorders; Myeloproliferative Disorders; **Hospital:** Johns Hopkins Hosp; **Address:** 1830 E Monument St, Ste 416, Baltimore, MD 21287; **Phone:** 410-614-0167; **Board Cert:** Internal Medicine 1985; Medical Oncology 1987; **Med School:** Johns Hopkins Univ 1982; **Resid:** Internal Medicine, Johns Hopkins Hosp 1985; **Fellow:** Medical Oncology, UCSF Med Ctr 1987; **Fac Appt:** Prof Med, Johns Hopkins Univ

Filicko-OHara, Joanne E MD [Hem] - **Spec Exp:** Hematologic Malignancies; Leukemia & Lymphoma; **Hospital:** Thomas Jefferson Univ Hosp (page 81); **Address:** 925 Chestnut St, Ste 320A, Phildelphia, PA 19107; **Phone:** 215-955-8874; **Board Cert:** Hematology 2009; Medical Oncology 2000; **Med School:** Hahnemann Univ 1992; **Resid:** Internal Medicine, Thomas Jefferson Univ Hosp 1995; **Fellow:** Hematology & Oncology, Thomas Jefferson Univ Hosp 1995

Goldberg, Jack MD [Hem] - **Spec Exp:** Leukemia; Lymphoma; Multiple Myeloma; Bone Marrow Transplant; **Hospital:** Penn Presby Med Ctr - UPHS (page 80), Hosp Univ Penn - UPHS (page 80); **Address:** 51 N 39th St MAB Bldg Fl 1 - Ste 103A, Philadelphia, PA 19104; **Phone:** 215-662-9801; **Board Cert:** Internal Medicine 1976; Hematology 1980; Medical Oncology 1989; **Med School:** SUNY Upstate Med Univ 1973; **Resid:** Internal Medicine, Boston Univ Hosp 1975; **Fellow:** Hematology & Oncology, SUNY Syracuse Med Ctr 1977; **Fac Appt:** Clin Prof Med, Univ Pennsylvania

Isola, Luis M MD [Hem] - **Spec Exp:** Bone Marrow Transplant; Stem Cell Transplant; Myelodysplastic Syndromes; **Hospital:** Mount Sinai Med Ctr (page 76); **Address:** Mount Sinai Med Ctr, 19 E 98th St, Ste 3D, New York, NY 10029; **Phone:** 212-241-6021; **Board Cert:** Internal Medicine 1986; Hematology 1988; **Med School:** Argentina 1979; **Resid:** Internal Medicine, Ctr for Med Education 1983; **Fellow:** Hematology, Mt Sinai Med Ctr 1985; **Fac Appt:** Assoc Prof Med, Mount Sinai Sch Med

Kempin, Sanford J MD [Hem] - **Spec Exp:** Bleeding/Coagulation Disorders; Leukemia; Lymphoma; **Hospital:** Beth Israel Med Ctr - Petrie Division (page 71); **Address:** Beth Israel Comprehensive Cancer Ctr, W Side Campus, Dept Med Oncology, 325 W 15th St, New York, NY 10011; **Phone:** 212-604-6010; **Board Cert:** Internal Medicine 1976; Medical Oncology 1977; Hematology 1978; **Med School:** Belgium 1971; **Resid:** Internal Medicine, Lemuel Shattuck Hosp 1972; **Fellow:** Hematology, St Jude Chldns Hosp 1975; Medical Oncology, Meml Sloan Kettering Cancer Ctr 1976; **Fac Appt:** Asst Prof Med, NY Med Coll

Kessler, Craig M MD [Hem] - **Spec Exp:** Bleeding/Coagulation Disorders; Hematologic Malignancies; **Hospital:** Georgetown Univ Hosp; **Address:** GUMC, Lombardi Cancer Ctr, 3800 Reservoir Rd NW, Washington, DC 20007; **Phone:** 202-444-8676; **Board Cert:** Internal Medicine 1976; Hematology 1980; **Med School:** Tulane Univ 1973; **Resid:** Internal Medicine, Ochsner Fdn Hosp 1976; **Fellow:** Hematology, Johns Hopkins Hosp 1978; **Fac Appt:** Prof Med, Georgetown Univ

Mangan, Kenneth F MD [Hem] - **Spec Exp:** Bone Marrow Transplant; Hematologic Malignancies; Anemia-Aplastic; **Hospital:** Temple Univ Hosp, Jeanes Hosp; **Address:** Temple BMT Program, Friends Hall Physicians Bldg, 7604 Central Ave, Lower Level, Philadelphia, PA 19111-2499; **Phone:** 215-214-3129; **Board Cert:** Internal Medicine 1976; Hematology 1978; **Med School:** Geo Wash Univ 1973; **Resid:** Internal Medicine, G Washington Univ Hosps 1976; **Fellow:** Hematology, Tufts-New England Med Ctr 1977; **Fac Appt:** Prof Med, Temple Univ

Marks, Stanley M MD [Hem] - **Spec Exp:** Leukemia; Lymphoma; Multiple Myeloma; **Hospital:** UPMC Shadyside; **Address:** UPMC- Hillman Cancer Ctr, 5115 Centre Ave Fl 3, Pittsburgh, PA 15232; **Phone:** 412-235-1020; **Board Cert:** Internal Medicine 1976; Hematology 1978; **Med School:** Univ Pittsburgh 1973; **Resid:** Internal Medicine, Presby Univ Hosp 1976; **Fellow:** Hematology & Oncology, Peter Bent Brigham Hosp 1978; **Fac Appt:** Clin Prof Med, Univ Pittsburgh

Maslak, Peter G MD [Hem] - **Spec Exp:** Leukemia; Stem Cell Transplant; Myelodysplastic Syndromes; Clinical Trials; **Hospital:** Meml Sloan-Kettering Cancer Ctr (page 75); **Address:** 1275 York Avenue, New York, NY 10065; **Phone:** 800-525-2225; **Board Cert:** Internal Medicine 1987; Hematology 2000; Medical Oncology 1989; **Med School:** Mount Sinai Sch Med 1984; **Resid:** Internal Medicine, Univ Michigan Med Ctr 1987; **Fellow:** Hematology & Oncology, Meml Sloan Kettering Cancer Ctr 1990

Mears, John Gregory MD [Hem] - **Spec Exp:** Lymphoma; Leukemia; Multiple Myeloma; Breast Cancer; **Hospital:** NY-Presby Hosp/Columbia (page 78); **Address:** 161 Ft Washington Ave, Ste 923, New York, NY 10032; **Phone:** 212-305-3506; **Board Cert:** Internal Medicine 1976; Hematology 1978; **Med School:** Columbia P&S 1973; **Resid:** Internal Medicine, Boston Univ Med Ctr 1975; **Fellow:** Hematology & Oncology, Columbia-Presby Med Ctr 1978; **Fac Appt:** Clin Prof Med, Columbia P&S

Millenson, Michael M MD [Hem] - **Spec Exp:** Leukemia & Lymphoma; Hematologic Malignancies; **Hospital:** Fox Chase Cancer Ctr (page 72); **Address:** Fox Chase Cancer Center, 333 Cottman Ave, Philadelphia, PA 19111; **Phone:** 215-728-2600; **Board Cert:** Internal Medicine 1987; Hematology 2000; Medical Oncology 2000; **Med School:** Temple Univ 1984; **Resid:** Internal Medicine, Temple Univ Hosp 1987; **Fellow:** Hematology & Oncology, Beth Israel Hosp 1991

Nimer, Stephen D MD [Hem] - **Spec Exp:** Bone Marrow Transplant; Myelodysplastic Syndromes; Leukemia; Stem Cell Transplant; **Hospital:** Meml Sloan-Kettering Cancer Ctr (page 75); **Address:** 1275 York Ave, New York, NY 10065; **Phone:** 800-525-2225; **Board Cert:** Internal Medicine 1982; Hematology 1986; Medical Oncology 1985; **Med School:** Univ Chicago-Pritzker Sch Med 1979; **Resid:** Internal Medicine, UCLA Med Ctr 1982; **Fellow:** Hematology & Oncology, UCLA Med Ctr 1986; **Fac Appt:** Prof Med, Cornell Univ-Weill Med Coll

Porter, David L MD [Hem] - **Spec Exp:** Leukemia; Bone Marrow Transplant; Lymphoma; **Hospital:** Hosp Univ Penn - UPHS (page 80); **Address:** Perelman Ctr for Advanced Med Fl 2, 3400 Civic Center Blvd, Philadelphia, PA 19104; **Phone:** 215-615-5858; **Board Cert:** Hematology 2006; **Med School:** Brown Univ 1987; **Resid:** Internal Medicine, Univ Hosp 1990; **Fellow:** Hematology & Oncology, Brigham & Womens Hosp 1992; **Fac Appt:** Assoc Prof Med, Univ Pennsylvania

Rai, Kanti R MD [Hem] - **Spec Exp:** Leukemia; Lymphoma; Multiple Myeloma; **Hospital:** Long Island Jewish Med Ctr; **Address:** 410 Lakeville Rd, Ste 212, Long Island Jewish Med Ctr, Div of Hem-Onc, New Hyde Park, NY 10042; **Phone:** 718-470-4050; **Board Cert:** Pediatrics 1960; **Med School:** India 1955; **Resid:** Pediatrics, Lincoln Hosp 1958; Pediatrics, North Shore Univ Hosp 1959; **Fellow:** Hematology, LI Jewish Med Ctr 1960; **Fac Appt:** Prof Med, Albert Einstein Coll Med

Hematology

Raphael, Bruce MD [Hem] - **Spec Exp:** Lymphoma; Leukemia; Multiple Myeloma; **Hospital:** NYU Langone Med Ctr (page 79), NY Downtown Hosp; **Address:** 160 E 34th Street Ave Fl 7, NYU Clinical Cancer Ctr, New York, NY 10016-6402; **Phone:** 212-731-5185; **Board Cert:** Internal Medicine 1978; Hematology 1980; Medical Oncology 1981; **Med School:** McGill Univ 1975; **Resid:** Internal Medicine, Jewish Genl Hosp 1977; **Fellow:** Medical Oncology, Meml Sloan Kettering Cancer Ctr 1978; Hematology, NYU Med Ctr 1980; **Fac Appt:** Assoc Prof Med, NYU Sch Med

Rapoport, Aaron P MD [Hem] - **Spec Exp:** Leukemia; Lymphoma; Myeloma; **Hospital:** Univ of MD Med Ctr; **Address:** University of MD Cancer Center, 22 S Greene St, Ste N9E12, Baltimore, MD 21201; **Phone:** 410-328-1230; **Board Cert:** Internal Medicine 1989; Hematology 2002; **Med School:** Harvard Med Sch 1986; **Resid:** Internal Medicine, Strong Meml Hosp 1989; **Fellow:** Hematology, Strong Meml Hosp 1989; **Fac Appt:** Prof Med, Univ MD Sch Med

Roodman, G David MD [Hem] - **Spec Exp:** Multiple Myeloma; **Hospital:** UPMC Shadyside, VA Pittsburgh Hlth Care Sys-Univ Dr; **Address:** VA Pittsburgh Healthcare System, R&D 151-U, rm 2E113, University Drive C, Pittsburgh, PA 15240; **Phone:** 412-692-4724; **Board Cert:** Internal Medicine 1978; Hematology 1980; **Med School:** Univ KY Coll Med 1973; **Resid:** Internal Medicine, Univ Minnesota Hosp 1978; **Fellow:** Hematology, Univ Minnesota Hosp 1980; **Fac Appt:** Prof Med, Univ Pittsburgh

Rowley, Scott D MD [Hem] - **Spec Exp:** Stem Cell Transplant; Bone Marrow Transplant; Graft vs Host Disease; **Hospital:** Hackensack Univ Med Ctr (page 73); **Address:** 360 Essex St, Ste 303, Hackensack, NJ 07601; **Phone:** 201-336-8297 x8291; **Board Cert:** Internal Medicine 1981; Medical Oncology 1983; Hematology 1984; **Med School:** Univ Mass Sch Med 1978; **Resid:** Internal Medicine, Rhode Island Hosp 1981; **Fellow:** Hematology & Oncology, Rhode Island Hosp 1984; **Fac Appt:** Assoc Prof Med, UMDNJ-NJ Med Sch, Newark

Savage, David G MD [Hem] - **Spec Exp:** Stem Cell Transplant; Multiple Myeloma; Lymphoma; **Hospital:** NY-Presby Hosp/Columbia (page 78); **Address:** 177 Fort Washington Ave, Millstein Bldg Fl 6 - rm 435, New York, NY 10032; **Phone:** 212-305-9783; **Board Cert:** Internal Medicine 1977; Hematology 1982; Medical Oncology 1985; **Med School:** Columbia P&S 1974; **Resid:** Internal Medicine, Harlem Hosp/Columbia Presby Med Ctr 1977; **Fellow:** Hematology & Oncology, Harlem Hosp/Columbia Presby Med Ctr 1979; **Fac Appt:** Assoc Prof Med, Columbia P&S

Schuster, Michael W MD [Hem] - **Spec Exp:** Bone Marrow Transplant; **Hospital:** Stony Brook Univ Med Ctr; **Address:** Stony Brook University, SUNY-7099, 100 Nichols Rd, Stony Brook, NY 11794-7909; **Phone:** 631-444-3577; **Board Cert:** Internal Medicine 1984; Hematology 1986; **Med School:** Dartmouth Med Sch 1980; **Resid:** Internal Medicine, New Eng Deaconess Hosp 1983; **Fellow:** Hematology & Oncology, Beth Israel Med Ctr 1987; **Fac Appt:** Assoc Prof Med, Cornell Univ-Weill Med Coll

Schuster, Stephen J MD [Hem] - **Spec Exp:** Lymphoma; Bone Marrow Transplant; **Hospital:** Hosp Univ Penn - UPHS (page 80); **Address:** Abramson Cancer Ctr, Perelman Ctr, West Pavilion Fl 2, 3400 Civic Ctr Blvd, Philadelphia, PA 19104; **Phone:** 215-614-1846; **Board Cert:** Internal Medicine 1984; Hematology 1986; Medical Oncology 1989; **Med School:** Jefferson Med Coll 1981; **Resid:** Internal Medicine, Pennsylvania Hosp 1984; **Fellow:** Hematology & Oncology, Thos Jefferson Univ Hosp 1986; **Fac Appt:** Assoc Prof Med, Univ Pennsylvania

Slease, Robert B MD [Hem] - **Spec Exp:** Hematologic Malignancies; Hodgkin's Disease; Stem Cell Transplant; Clinical Trials; **Hospital:** Wilmington Hosp; **Address:** Cristiana Care Hlth Svs, Div Hematology, Medical Pavilion, 4701 Ogletown-Stanton Rd, Ste 4200, Newark, DE 19713; **Phone:** 302-737-7700; **Board Cert:** Internal Medicine 1975; Hematology 1978; **Med School:** Univ Kansas 1972; **Resid:** Internal Medicine, Natl Naval Med Ctr 1975; **Fellow:** Hematology, Natl Naval Med Ctr 1977; **Fac Appt:** Clin Prof Med, Jefferson Med Coll

Spivak, Jerry L MD [Hem] - **Spec Exp:** Myeloproliferative Disorders; Leukemia; **Hospital:** Johns Hopkins Hosp; **Address:** 720 Rutland Ave Bldg Ross - Ste 1025, Baltimore, MD 21205; **Phone:** 410-955-3142; **Board Cert:** Internal Medicine 1971; Hematology 1974; **Med School:** Cornell Univ-Weill Med Coll 1964; **Resid:** Internal Medicine, Johns Hopkins Hosp 1966; Internal Medicine, Johns Hopkins Hosp 1972; **Fellow:** Hematology, Natl Cancer Inst 1968; Hematology, Johns Hopkins Hosp 1971; **Fac Appt:** Prof Med, Johns Hopkins Univ

Strair, Roger MD/PhD [Hem] - **Spec Exp:** Leukemia; Lymphoma; Bone Marrow Transplant; Multiple Myeloma; **Hospital:** Robert Wood Johnson Univ Hosp - New Brunswick; **Address:** Cancer Inst of NJ, 195 Little Albany St, New Brunswick, NJ 08903; **Phone:** 732-235-6044; **Board Cert:** Internal Medicine 1984; Hematology 1986; Medical Oncology 1987; **Med School:** Albert Einstein Coll Med 1981; **Resid:** Internal Medicine, Brigham & Women's Hosp 1984; **Fellow:** Hematology & Oncology, Brigham & Women's Hosp 1988; **Fac Appt:** Assoc Prof Med, UMDNJ-RW Johnson Med Sch

Streiff, Michael B MD [Hem] - **Spec Exp:** Bleeding Coagulation Disorders; Polycythemia Rubra Vera; Clinical Trials; **Hospital:** Johns Hopkins Hosp; **Address:** Division of Hematology, 1830 E Monument St, Ste 7300, Baltimore, MD 21205; **Phone:** 410-614-0727; **Board Cert:** Internal Medicine 2002; Hematology 2004; Medical Oncology 2005; **Med School:** Johns Hopkins Univ 1988; **Resid:** Internal Medicine, Shands Hosp-Univ Fla Coll Med 1991; **Fellow:** Hematology & Oncology, Johns Hopkins Univ Hosp 1994; **Fac Appt:** Assoc Prof Med, Johns Hopkins Univ

Tallman, Martin S MD [Hem] - **Spec Exp:** Bone Marrow Transplant; Leukemia; Hairy Cell Leukemia; **Hospital:** Meml Sloan-Kettering Cancer Ctr (page 75); **Address:** 1275 York Ave, Box 380, Ste 21-100, New York, NY 10065; **Phone:** 212-639-3842; **Board Cert:** Internal Medicine 1983; Medical Oncology 1987; Hematology 1988; **Med School:** Ros Franklin Univ/Chicago Med Sch 1980; **Resid:** Internal Medicine, Evanston Hosp 1983; **Fellow:** Medical Oncology, Fred Hutchinson Cancer Ctr 1987; **Fac Appt:** Prof Med, Cornell Univ-Weill Med Coll

Wisch, Nathaniel MD [Hem] - **Spec Exp:** Lymphoma; Breast Cancer; Leukemia; Anemia-Cancer Related; **Hospital:** Lenox Hill Hosp, Mount Sinai Med Ctr (page 76); **Address:** 12 E 86th St, New York, NY 10028-0506; **Phone:** 212-861-6660; **Board Cert:** Internal Medicine 1965; Hematology 1972; Medical Oncology 1977; **Med School:** Northwestern Univ 1958; **Resid:** Internal Medicine, VA Hosp 1960; Internal Medicine, Montefiore Hosp 1961; **Fellow:** Hematology, Mount Sinai Hosp 1962; **Fac Appt:** Clin Prof Med, Mount Sinai Sch Med

Yanovich, Saul MD [Hem] - **Spec Exp:** Bone Marrow Transplant; **Hospital:** Univ of MD Med Ctr; **Address:** Greenebaum Cancer Center, 22 S Greene St, Ste N9E12, Baltimore, MD 21201; **Phone:** 410-328-1230; **Board Cert:** Internal Medicine 1980; Medical Oncology 1981; Hematology 1976; **Med School:** Colombia 1970; **Resid:** Internal Medicine, Univ Miami-Jackson Meml Hosp 1974; Hematology, Univ Miami-Jackson Meml Hosp 1976; **Fellow:** Oncology, Dana Farber Canc Ctr 1978; **Fac Appt:** Prof Med, Univ MD Sch Med

Southeast

Bigelow, Carolyn L MD [Hem] - **Spec Exp:** Bone Marrow Transplant; Leukemia; **Hospital:** Univ Mississippi Med Ctr; **Address:** Univ Mississippi Med Ctr-Div Hematology, 2500 N State St, Jackson, MS 39216; **Phone:** 601-984-5615; **Board Cert:** Internal Medicine 1982; Hematology 1988; **Med School:** Univ Miss 1979; **Resid:** Internal Medicine, Univ Mississippi Med Ctr 1982; **Fellow:** Hematology & Oncology, Univ Washington Med Ctr 1987; **Fac Appt:** Prof Med, Univ Miss

Hematology

Djulbegovic, Benjamin MD/PhD [Hem] - **Spec Exp:** Multiple Myeloma; Lymphoma; Myelo-proliferative Disorders; Clinical Trials; **Hospital:** H Lee Moffitt Cancer Ctr & Research Inst, Tampa Genl Hosp; **Address:** 12901 Bruce B Downs Blvd, MDC 27, Tampa, FL 33612; **Phone:** 813-396-9178; **Board Cert:** Internal Medicine 2002; Hematology 2004; **Med School:** Bosnia 1976; **Resid:** Internal Medicine, Univ Med Ctr 1983; Internal Medicine, Univ Louisville Med Ctr 1988; **Fellow:** Univ Manchester 1985; Hematology & Oncology, Univ Louisville 1990; **Fac Appt:** Prof Med, Univ S Fla Coll Med

Files, Joe C MD [Hem] - **Spec Exp:** Bone Marrow Transplant; Stem Cell Transplant; Leukemia; **Hospital:** Univ Mississippi Med Ctr; **Address:** Univ Miss Med Ctr-Div Hematology, 2500 N State St, Jackson, MS 39216; **Phone:** 601-984-5615; **Board Cert:** Internal Medicine 1976; Hematology 1980; **Med School:** Univ Miss 1972; **Resid:** Internal Medicine, Univ Miss Med Ctr 1976; **Fellow:** Hematology, Univ Wash Sch Med 1979; **Fac Appt:** Prof Med, Univ Miss

Greer, John P MD [Hem] - **Spec Exp:** Leukemia & Lymphoma; Myelodysplastic Syndromes; Stem Cell Transplant; Clinical Trials; **Hospital:** Vanderbilt Univ Med Ctr; **Address:** 3927 The Vanderbilt Clinic, 1301 Medical Center Drive, Nashville, TN 37232; **Phone:** 615-936-8422; **Board Cert:** Pediatrics 1985; Internal Medicine 1979; Hematology 1984; Medical Oncology 1985; **Med School:** Vanderbilt Univ 1976; **Resid:** Internal Medicine, Tulane Univ Med Ctr 1979; Pediatrics, Med Coll Virginia 1981; **Fellow:** Hematology & Oncology, Vanderbilt Univ Med Ctr 1984; **Fac Appt:** Prof Med, Vanderbilt Univ

Komrokji, Rami S MD [Hem] - **Spec Exp:** Myelodysplastic Syndromes; Leukemia-Myeloid; Hodgkin's Disease; Clinical Trials; **Hospital:** H Lee Moffitt Cancer Ctr & Research Inst; **Address:** H Lee Moffitt Canc Ctr & Rsch Inst, 12902 Magnolia Drive, Tampa, FL 33612; **Phone:** 813-745-8986; **Board Cert:** Internal Medicine 2001; Hematology 2004; Medical Oncology 2004; **Med School:** Jordan 1996; **Resid:** Internal Medicine, Case Western Univ Affil Hosp 2001; **Fellow:** Hematology, Strong Meml Hosp 2004; **Fac Appt:** Assoc Prof

Laughlin, Mary J MD [Hem] - **Spec Exp:** Bone Marrow Transplant; Lymphoma; **Hospital:** Univ of Virginia Health Sys; **Address:** 1240 Lee St, Charlottesville, VA 22908; **Phone:** 434-982-6406; **Board Cert:** Internal Medicine 2003; Hematology 2004; **Med School:** SUNY Buffalo 1988; **Resid:** Internal Medicine, Duke Univ Med Ctr 1991; **Fellow:** Hematology & Oncology, Duke Univ Med Ctr 1992; Bone Marrow Transplant, Rosewell Park Cancer Inst 1994; **Fac Appt:** Assoc Prof Med, Case West Res Univ

Powell, Bayard L MD [Hem] - **Spec Exp:** Leukemia; Myelodysplastic Syndromes; **Hospital:** Wake Forest Univ Baptist Med Ctr; **Address:** Wake Forest Univ Baptist Med Ctr, Med Ctr Blvd-Cancer Center, Winston-Salem, NC 27157-1082; **Phone:** 336-716-7970; **Board Cert:** Internal Medicine 1983; Medical Oncology 1985; **Med School:** Univ NC Sch Med 1980; **Resid:** Internal Medicine, NC Baptist Hosp 1983; **Fellow:** Hematology & Oncology, Wake Forest Univ Sch Med 1986; **Fac Appt:** Prof Med, Wake Forest Univ

Rosenblatt, Joseph D MD [Hem] - **Spec Exp:** Lymphoma; Leukemia; Multiple Myeloma; Lymphomas-Rare; **Hospital:** Univ of Miami Hosp & Clins/Sylvester Comp Canc Ctr (page 82), Jackson Meml Hosp (page 82); **Address:** Sylvester Comprehensive Cancer Ctr, 1475 NW 12th Ave, D8-4, Ste 3300, Miami, FL 33136; **Phone:** 305-243-4909; **Board Cert:** Internal Medicine 1983; Medical Oncology 1985; **Med School:** UCLA 1980; **Resid:** Internal Medicine, UCLA Med Ctr 1983; **Fellow:** Hematology & Oncology, UCLA 1986; **Fac Appt:** Prof Med, Univ Miami Sch Med

Schwartzberg, Lee S MD [Hem] - **Spec Exp:** Breast Cancer; Lung Cancer; Stem Cell Transplant; **Hospital:** Baptist Memorial Hospital-Memphis; **Address:** The West Clinic, 100 N Humphreys Blvd, Memphis, TN 38120; **Phone:** 901-683-0055; **Board Cert:** Internal Medicine 1983; Medical Oncology 1985; Hematology 1986; **Med School:** NY Med Coll 1980; **Resid:** Internal Medicine, North Shore Univ Hosp 1983; Internal Medicine, Meml Sloan Kettering Cancer Ctr 1985; **Fellow:** Hematology & Oncology, Meml Sloan Kettering Cancer Ctr 1984; Hematology & Oncology, Meml Sloan Kettering Cancer Ctr 1987; **Fac Appt:** Assoc Prof Med, Univ Tenn Coll Med

Sokol, Lubomir MD/PhD [Hem] - **Spec Exp:** Lymphoma; Hematologic Malignancies; **Hospital:** H Lee Moffitt Cancer Ctr & Research Inst; **Address:** H Lee Moffitt Cancer Ctr & Rsch Inst, 12902 Magnolia Drive, MS FOB3, Tampa, FL 33612; **Phone:** 813-745-8212; **Board Cert:** Internal Medicine 2000; Medical Oncology 2002; Hematology 2003; **Med School:** Czech Republic 1981; **Resid:** Radiation Oncology, Charles Univ 1984; Internal Medicine, LSU Med Ctr 1999; **Fellow:** Radiation Oncology, Charles Univ 1990; Hematology & Oncology, USF Med Ctr 2002

Solberg, Lawrence Arthur MD/PhD [Hem] - **Spec Exp:** Leukemia & Lymphoma; Myelodysplastic Syndromes; Bone Marrow Transplant; Multiple Myeloma; **Hospital:** Mayo - Jacksonville; **Address:** 4500 San Pablo Rd Mayo Bldg Fl 8, Jacksonville, FL 32224; **Phone:** 904-953-7290; **Board Cert:** Internal Medicine 1978; Hematology 1980; **Med School:** St Louis Univ 1975; **Resid:** Internal Medicine, Mayo Clinic 1978; **Fellow:** Hematology, Mayo Clinic 1980; **Fac Appt:** Prof Med, Mayo Med Sch

Williams, Michael E MD [Hem] - **Spec Exp:** Lymphoma; Multiple Myeloma; Leukemia; Mantle Cell Lymphoma; **Hospital:** Univ of Virginia Health Sys; **Address:** UVA Hlth Sys, Div Hem/Oncology, PO Box 800716, Charlottesville, VA 22908-0716; **Phone:** 434-924-9637; **Board Cert:** Internal Medicine 1982; Medical Oncology 1987; Hematology 2009; **Med School:** Univ Cincinnati 1979; **Resid:** Internal Medicine, Univ Virginia Med Ctr 1983; **Fellow:** Hematology & Oncology, Univ Virginia Med Ctr 1986; **Fac Appt:** Prof Med, Univ VA Sch Med

Zuckerman, Kenneth S MD [Hem] - **Spec Exp:** Myeloproliferative Disorders; Leukemia; Myelodysplastic Syndromes; **Hospital:** H Lee Moffitt Cancer Ctr & Research Inst, Tampa Genl Hosp; **Address:** 12902 USF Magnolia Drive, Tampa, FL 33612-9416; **Phone:** 813-745-8090; **Board Cert:** Internal Medicine 1975; Hematology 1978; **Med School:** Ohio State Univ 1972; **Resid:** Internal Medicine, Ohio State Univ Hosps 1975; **Fellow:** Hematology, Peter Bent Brigham Hosp/Harvard Univ 1978; **Fac Appt:** Prof Med, Univ S Fla Coll Med

Midwest

Baron, Joseph M MD [Hem] - **Spec Exp:** Lymphoma; Myeloproliferative Disorders; **Hospital:** Univ of Chicago Med Ctr; **Address:** 5841 S Maryland Ave, MC 2115, Chicago, IL 60637-1463; **Phone:** 773-702-6149; **Board Cert:** Internal Medicine 1969; Hematology 1972; Medical Oncology 1975; **Med School:** Univ Chicago-Pritzker Sch Med 1962; **Resid:** Internal Medicine, Univ Chicago Hosps 1964; Internal Medicine, Univ Chicago Hosps 1968; **Fellow:** Hematology, Univ Chicago Hosps 1968; **Fac Appt:** Assoc Prof Med, Univ Chicago-Pritzker Sch Med

Bockenstedt, Paula MD [Hem] - **Spec Exp:** Bleeding/Coagulation Disorders; Leukemia; **Hospital:** Univ of Michigan Hosp; **Address:** Div Hematology, 1500 E Med Ctr Dr, MIB, rm C-344, Ann Arbor, MI 48109-8048; **Phone:** 734-936-6393; **Board Cert:** Internal Medicine 1981; Hematology 1984; **Med School:** Harvard Med Sch 1978; **Resid:** Internal Medicine, Brigham-Womens Hosp 1981; **Fellow:** Hematology, Brigham-Womens Hosp 1984; **Fac Appt:** Assoc Clin Prof Med, Univ Mich Med Sch

Hematology

Bricker, Leslie J MD [Hem] - **Spec Exp:** Palliative Care; **Hospital:** Henry Ford Hosp; **Address:** Henry Ford Hospital, 2799 W Grand Blvd, CFP 5, 13th Fl, Detroit, MI 48202; **Phone:** 313-916-1859; **Board Cert:** Internal Medicine 1980; Hematology 1982; Medical Oncology 1983; Hospice & Palliative Medicine 2008; **Med School:** Wayne State Univ 1977; **Resid:** Internal Medicine, Sinai Hosp 1980; **Fellow:** Hematology & Oncology, Univ Mich Hosp 1983; **Fac Appt:** Assoc Prof Med, Wayne State Univ

Byrd, John C MD [Hem] - **Spec Exp:** Leukemia-Chronic Lymphocytic; **Hospital:** Arthur G James Cancer Hosp & Research Inst; **Address:** 320 W 10th Ave, B302 Starling-Loving Hall, Columbus, OH 43210; **Phone:** 614-293-3196; **Board Cert:** Hematology 2007; **Med School:** Univ Ark 1991; **Resid:** Internal Medicine, Walter Reed AMC 1994; **Fellow:** Hematology & Oncology, Walter Reed AMC 1997; **Fac Appt:** Assoc Prof Med, Ohio State Univ

Copelan, Edward A MD [Hem] - **Spec Exp:** Leukemia; Myelodysplastic Syndromes; Bone Marrow Transplant; Multiple Myeloma; **Hospital:** Cleveland Clin (page 70); **Address:** Cleveland Clinic Fdn, 9500 Euclid Ave, Cleveland, OH 44195; **Phone:** 216-445-5647; **Board Cert:** Internal Medicine 1980; Hematology 1982; Medical Oncology 1983; **Med School:** Tufts Univ 1977; **Resid:** Internal Medicine, Ohio State Univ Hosp 1980; **Fellow:** Hematology & Oncology, Ohio State Univ Hosp 1983; Bone Marrow Transplant, UCLA Med Ctr; **Fac Appt:** Prof Med, Cleveland Cl Coll Med/Case West Res

Di Persio, John F MD/PhD [Hem] - **Spec Exp:** Bone Marrow Transplant; Hematologic Malignancies; Leukemia; **Hospital:** Barnes-Jewish Hosp; **Address:** Wash Univ Sch Med, Sect Bone Marrow Transplant & Leukemia, 660 S Euclid Ave, Box 8007, St Louis, MO 63110; **Phone:** 314-454-8306; **Board Cert:** Internal Medicine 1984; Medical Oncology 1987; Hematology 1988; **Med School:** Univ Rochester 1980; **Resid:** Internal Medicine, Parkland Meml Hosp 1984; **Fellow:** Hematology & Oncology, UCLA Med Ctr 1987; **Fac Appt:** Prof Med, Washington Univ, St Louis

Erba, Harry P MD/PhD [Hem] - **Spec Exp:** Leukemia; Myelodysplastic Syndromes; Lymphoma; **Hospital:** Univ of Michigan Hosp; **Address:** Univ Michigan Medical Ctr, 1500 E Medical Center Dr, C348MIB, MC 5PC5848, Ann Arbor, MI 48109-5848; **Phone:** 734-647-8901; **Board Cert:** Internal Medicine 2004; Hematology 2004; Medical Oncology 2005; **Med School:** Stanford Univ 1988; **Resid:** Internal Medicine, Brigham & Womens Hosp 1990; **Fellow:** Hematology & Oncology, Brigham & Womens Hosp 1993; **Fac Appt:** Assoc Prof Med, Univ Mich Med Sch

Farag, Sherif S MD/PhD [Hem] - **Spec Exp:** Multiple Myeloma; Leukemia & Lymphoma; Bone Marrow Transplant; Stem Cell Transplant; **Hospital:** IU Health Methodist Hosp; **Address:** Cancer Pavilion, 535 Barnhill Drive, rm 473, Indianapolis, IN 46202; **Phone:** 317-944-0920; **Med School:** Australia 1995; **Resid:** Internal Medicine, Univ Melbourne Med Ctr; **Fellow:** Hematology & Oncology, Roswell Park Cancer Inst; **Fac Appt:** Assoc Prof Med, Indiana Univ

Flynn, Patrick MD [Hem] - **Spec Exp:** Hematologic Malignancies; Colon & Rectal Cancer; Clinical Trials; Breast Cancer; **Hospital:** Abbott - Northwestern Hosp, Fairview Southdale Hosp; **Address:** 910 E 26th St, Ste 200, Minneapolis, MN 55404; **Phone:** 612-884-6300; **Board Cert:** Internal Medicine 1978; Medical Oncology 1981; Hematology 1982; **Med School:** Univ Minn 1975; **Resid:** Internal Medicine, Hennepin Co Med Ctr 1978; **Fellow:** Hematology & Oncology, Univ Minnesota Hosp 1981

Gertz, Morie MD [Hem] - **Spec Exp:** Multiple Myeloma; Waldenstrom's Macroglobulinemia; Plasma Cell Disorders; Bone Marrow Transplant; **Hospital:** Mayo Med Ctr & Clin - Rochester, Rochester Methodist Hosp; **Address:** 200 SW 1st St Fl W10, Rochester, MN 55905; **Phone:** 507-284-3725; **Board Cert:** Internal Medicine 1979; Hematology 1982; Medical Oncology 1983; **Med School:** Loyola Univ-Stritch Sch Med 1975; **Resid:** Internal Medicine, St Lukes Hosp 1979; **Fellow:** Hematology & Oncology, Mayo Clin 1982; **Fac Appt:** Prof Med, Mayo Med Sch

Godwin, John MD [Hem] - **Spec Exp:** Leukemia in Elderly; Head & Neck Cancer; Lymphoma; Lung Cancer; **Hospital:** St. John's Hosp - Springfield, Memorial Med Ctr-Springfield; **Address:** SIU School Medicine, Simmons Cooper Cancer Inst, PO Box 19678, Springfield, IL 62794; **Phone:** 217-545-5817; **Board Cert:** Internal Medicine 1981; Hematology 1986; **Med School:** Univ Alabama 1978; **Resid:** Internal Medicine, Baylor Coll Med 1981; Internal Medicine, Baylor Coll Med 1982; **Fellow:** Hematology, Baylor Coll Med 1983; Hematology, North Carolina Meml Hosp 1985; **Fac Appt:** Prof Med, Southern IL Univ

Gordon, Leo I MD [Hem] - **Spec Exp:** Lymphoma, Non-Hodgkin's; Hodgkin's Disease; Bone Marrow Transplant; **Hospital:** Northwestern Meml Hosp; **Address:** 676 N St Clair St, Ste 850, Chicago, IL 60611-3124; **Phone:** 312-695-4546; **Board Cert:** Internal Medicine 1976; Hematology 1978; Medical Oncology 1979; **Med School:** Univ Cincinnati 1973; **Resid:** Internal Medicine, Univ Chicago Hosps 1976; **Fellow:** Hematology, Univ Minnesota Hosps 1978; Hematology & Oncology, Univ Chicago Hosps 1979; **Fac Appt:** Prof Med, Univ Chicago-Pritzker Sch Med

Gregory, Stephanie A MD [Hem] - **Spec Exp:** Lymphoma; Leukemia; Plasma Cell Disorders; Multiple Myeloma; **Hospital:** Rush Univ Med Ctr; **Address:** Rush University Medical Center, 1725 W Harrison St, Ste 834, Chicago, IL 60612; **Phone:** 312-942-5982; **Board Cert:** Internal Medicine 1972; Hematology 1972; **Med School:** Med Coll PA Hahnemann 1965; **Resid:** Internal Medicine, Rush/Presby-St Luke's Med Ctr 1969; **Fellow:** Hematology, Rush/Presby-St Luke's Med Ctr 1972; **Fac Appt:** Prof Med, Rush Med Coll

Greipp, Philip R MD [Hem] - **Spec Exp:** Multiple Myeloma; **Hospital:** Mayo Med Ctr & Clin - Rochester; **Address:** Mayo Clinic, Div Hematology, 200 First St SW Mayo Bldg Fl W-10, Rochester, MN 55905-0001; **Phone:** 507-284-3159; **Board Cert:** Internal Medicine 1974; Hematology 1994; **Med School:** Georgetown Univ 1968; **Resid:** Internal Medicine, Mayo Clin 1973; **Fellow:** Hematology, Mayo Clin 1975; **Fac Appt:** Prof Med, Mayo Med Sch

Grever, Michael R MD [Hem] - **Spec Exp:** Hematologic Malignancies; Leukemia; Drug Development; Clinical Trials; **Hospital:** Ohio St Univ Med Ctr; **Address:** 395 W 12th Ave, Rm 392, Doan Tower, Columbus, OH 43210; **Phone:** 614-293-8724; **Board Cert:** Internal Medicine 1975; Medical Oncology 1979; Hematology 1988; **Med School:** Univ Pittsburgh 1971; **Resid:** Internal Medicine, Univ of Pittsburgh 1974; **Fellow:** Hematology & Oncology, Ohio State Univ 1978; **Fac Appt:** Prof Med, Ohio State Univ

Habermann, Thomas M MD [Hem] - **Spec Exp:** Lymphoma; Hodgkin's Disease; Leukemia; **Hospital:** Mayo Med Ctr & Clin - Rochester; **Address:** Mayo Clin, 200 1st St SW, Rochester, MN 55905; **Phone:** 507-284-3159; **Board Cert:** Internal Medicine 1982; Hematology 1984; **Med School:** Creighton Univ 1979; **Resid:** Internal Medicine, Mayo Clinic 1982; **Fellow:** Hematology, Mayo Clinic 1985; **Fac Appt:** Prof Med, Mayo Med Sch

Juckett, Mark B MD [Hem] - **Spec Exp:** Bone Marrow Transplant; **Hospital:** Univ WI Hosp & Clins; **Address:** 600 Highland Ave, Ste H4/534, Madison, WI 53792; **Phone:** 608-745-5660; **Board Cert:** Internal Medicine 2001; Hematology 2004; Medical Oncology 2005; **Med School:** Univ Louisville Sch Med 1987; **Resid:** Internal Medicine, Univ Minnesota 1990; **Fellow:** Hematology & Oncology, Univ Minnesota 1992; **Fac Appt:** Assoc Prof Med, Univ Wisc

Kraut, Eric H MD [Hem] - **Spec Exp:** Hematologic Malignancies; Leukemia; Drug Development; Clinical Trials; **Hospital:** Ohio St Univ Med Ctr; **Address:** 320 W 10th Ave, A358 SL, Columbus, OH 43210; **Phone:** 614-293-2887; **Board Cert:** Internal Medicine 1975; Medical Oncology 1977; Hematology 1978; **Med School:** Temple Univ 1972; **Resid:** Internal Medicine, Univ Pittsburgh 1975; **Fellow:** Hematology & Oncology, Ohio State Univ Hosp 1977; **Fac Appt:** Prof Med, Ohio State Univ

Hematology

Kuriakose, Philip MD [Hem] - **Spec Exp:** Leukemia; **Hospital:** Henry Ford Hosp; **Address:** Henry Ford Hosp, Hematology/Oncology, 2799 W Grand Blvd, K13, Detroit, MI 48202; **Phone:** 313-916-1841; **Board Cert:** Internal Medicine 1999; Medical Oncology 2002; Hematology 2002; **Med School:** India 1990; **Resid:** Internal Medicine, Christian Med Coll 1992; Internal Medicine, Henry Ford Hosp 1994; **Fellow:** Hematology & Oncology, Mayo Clinic 1995

Larson, Richard A MD [Hem] - **Spec Exp:** Leukemia & Lymphoma; Bone Marrow Transplant; Myelodysplastic Syndromes; **Hospital:** Univ of Chicago Med Ctr; **Address:** University of Chicago Medical Center, 5841 S Maryland Ave, MS 2115, Chicago, IL 60637; **Phone:** 773-702-6149; **Board Cert:** Internal Medicine 1980; Hematology 1982; Medical Oncology 1983; **Med School:** Stanford Univ 1977; **Resid:** Internal Medicine, Univ Chicago Hosps 1980; **Fellow:** Hematology & Oncology, Univ Chicago Hosps 1983; **Fac Appt:** Prof Hem & Onc, Univ Chicago-Pritzker Sch Med

Lazarus, Hillard M MD [Hem] - **Spec Exp:** Bone Marrow Transplant; Stem Cell Transplant; Leukemia; **Hospital:** Univ Hosps Case Med Ctr; **Address:** 11100 Euclid Ave, Wearn Bldg 351, Cleveland, OH 44106-5065; **Phone:** 216-844-3629; **Board Cert:** Internal Medicine 1977; Medical Oncology 1979; Hematology 1980; **Med School:** Univ Rochester 1974; **Resid:** Internal Medicine, Univ Hosps 1977; **Fellow:** Hematology & Oncology, Univ Hosps 1979; **Fac Appt:** Prof Med, Case West Res Univ

Litzow, Mark R MD [Hem] - **Spec Exp:** Bone Marrow Transplant; Leukemia; **Hospital:** Mayo Med Ctr & Clin - Rochester; **Address:** Mayo Clinic, Div Hematology, 200 First St SW, Rochester, MN 55905; **Phone:** 507-284-9448; **Board Cert:** Internal Medicine 1983; Hematology 1988; Medical Oncology 1989; **Med School:** Univ Chicago-Pritzker Sch Med 1980; **Resid:** Internal Medicine, Mayo Clinic 1984; **Fellow:** Medical Oncology, Mayo Clinic 1990; **Fac Appt:** Asst Prof Med, Mayo Med Sch

Maciejewski, Jaroslaw P MD/PhD [Hem] - **Spec Exp:** Anemia-Aplastic; Hematologic Malignancies; Stem Cell Transplant; **Hospital:** Cleveland Clin (page 70); **Address:** Cleveland Clinic, 9500 Euclid Ave, Desk R40, Cleveland, OH 44195; **Phone:** 216-445-5962; **Board Cert:** Internal Medicine 1999; Hematology 2001; **Med School:** Germany 1990; **Resid:** Internal Medicine, Univ Nevada Med Ctr 1997; **Fellow:** Hematology, Natl Inst Hlth 2000; **Fac Appt:** Prof Med, Case West Res Univ

McGlave, Philip B MD [Hem] - **Spec Exp:** Leukemia; Bone Marrow Transplant; **Address:** Univ Minn, Dept Med, Div Hem/Onc Transplanatation, 420 Delaware St SE, MMC 480, Minneapolis, MN 55455; **Phone:** 612-626-2446; **Board Cert:** Internal Medicine 1977; Hematology 1980; **Med School:** Univ IL Coll Med 1974; **Resid:** Internal Medicine, Univ Minnesota Med Ctr 1977; **Fellow:** Hematology & Oncology, Univ Minnesota Med Ctr 1980; **Fac Appt:** Prof Med, Univ Minn

Milhem, Mohammed M MD [Hem] - **Spec Exp:** Bone Cancer; Bone Marrow Transplant; Sarcoma; Melanoma; **Hospital:** Univ Iowa Hosp & Clinics; **Address:** UIHC, 200 Hawkins Drive, C32 GH, Iowa City, IA 52242; **Phone:** 319-356-4200; **Board Cert:** Internal Medicine 2000; Hematology 2003; Medical Oncology 2003; **Med School:** Jordan 1995; **Resid:** Internal Medicine, Univ IL Med Ctr 2000; **Fellow:** Hematology & Oncology, Univ IL Med Ctr 2003; Bone Marrow Transplant, Univ IL Med Ctr 2004; **Fac Appt:** Asst Clin Prof Hem & Onc, Univ Iowa Coll Med

Nand, Sucha MD [Hem] - **Spec Exp:** Myelodysplastic Syndromes; Myeloproliferative Disorders; Leukemia; Lymphoma, Non-Hodgkin's; **Hospital:** Loyola Univ Med Ctr; **Address:** Cardinal Bernardin Cancer Ctr, 2160 S First Ave Bldg 112 - rm 345, Maywood, IL 60153-3304; **Phone:** 708-327-3217; **Board Cert:** Internal Medicine 1979; Medical Oncology 1981; Hematology 1982; **Med School:** India 1971; **Resid:** Physical Medicine & Rehabilitation, Northwestern Meml Hosp 1976; Internal Medicine, North Chicago VA Hosp 1978; **Fellow:** Hematology & Oncology, Northwestern Meml Hosp 1981; **Fac Appt:** Prof Med, Loyola Univ-Stritch Sch Med

Porcu, Pierluigi MD [Hem] - **Spec Exp:** Lymphoma; Lymphoma, Non-Hodgkin's; Immunotherapy; **Hospital:** Ohio St Univ Med Ctr; **Address:** 320 W 10th Ave, B320 Starling Loving Hall, Columbus, OH 43210; **Phone:** 614-293-9273; **Board Cert:** Hematology 1999; Medical Oncology 1999; **Med School:** Italy 1987; **Resid:** Internal Medicine, Indiana Univ Hosp 1996; **Fellow:** Hematology & Oncology, Indiana Univ Hosp 1999; **Fac Appt:** Asst Prof Med, Ohio State Univ

Singhal, Seema MD [Hem] - **Spec Exp:** Multiple Myeloma; **Hospital:** Northwestern Meml Hosp; **Address:** Northwestern Div Hematology/Oncology, 676 N St Clair St, Ste 850, Chicago, IL 60611; **Phone:** 312-695-0990; **Board Cert:** Internal Medicine 2005; **Med School:** India 1989; **Resid:** Internal Medicine, King Edward Meml Hosp 1991; Hematology, King Edward Meml Hosp 1991; **Fellow:** Bone Marrow Transplant, Hadassah Univ Hosp 1992; **Fac Appt:** Prof Med, Northwestern Univ

Stiff, Patrick J MD [Hem] - **Spec Exp:** Bone Marrow Transplant; Leukemia; Lymphoma, Non-Hodgkin's; Vaccine Therapy; **Hospital:** Loyola Univ Med Ctr; **Address:** Cardinal Bernadin Cancer Ctr, 2160 S First Ave, Bldg 112, rm 255, Maywood, IL 60153; **Phone:** 708-327-3304; **Board Cert:** Internal Medicine 1978; Medical Oncology 1981; Hematology 1982; **Med School:** Loyola Univ-Stritch Sch Med 1975; **Resid:** Internal Medicine, Cleveland Clinic Fdn 1978; **Fellow:** Hematology & Oncology, Meml Sloan Kettering Cancer Ctr 1981; **Fac Appt:** Prof Med, Loyola Univ-Stritch Sch Med

Uberti, Joseph P MD/PhD [Hem] - **Spec Exp:** Bone Marrow Transplant; Stem Cell Transplant; **Hospital:** Barbara Ann Karmanos Cancer Inst; **Address:** Barbara Ann Karmanos Cancer Inst, 4100 John R St, MC HW04H0, Detroit, MI 48201; **Phone:** 313-576-8760; **Board Cert:** Internal Medicine 1986; Medical Oncology 1989; **Med School:** Wayne State Univ 1983; **Resid:** Internal Medicine, Detroit Receiving Hosp 1986; **Fellow:** Hematology & Oncology, Wayne State Univ Hosps 1988; **Fac Appt:** Prof Med, Wayne State Univ

Van Besien, Koen W MD [Hem] - **Spec Exp:** Lymphoma; Stem Cell Transplant; **Hospital:** Univ of Chicago Med Ctr; **Address:** Stem Cell Transplant Program, 5841 S Maryland Ave, MC 2115, Chicago, IL 60637; **Phone:** 773-702-4400; **Board Cert:** Internal Medicine 2005; Medical Oncology 2005; Hematology 2006; **Med School:** Belgium 1984; **Resid:** Internal Medicine, Univ Leuven Med Ctr 1987; **Fellow:** Hematology & Oncology, Indiana Univ Med Ctr 1990; **Fac Appt:** Prof Med, Univ Chicago-Pritzker Sch Med

Winter, Jane N MD [Hem] - **Spec Exp:** Lymphoma, Non-Hodgkin's; Hodgkin's Disease; Bone Marrow Transplant; Langerhans Cell Histiocytosis (LCH); **Hospital:** Northwestern Meml Hosp; **Address:** Northwestern Univ - Div Hem/Oncology, 675 N St Clair St, Ste 21-100, Chicago, IL 60611; **Phone:** 312-695-0990; **Board Cert:** Internal Medicine 1980; Hematology 2008; Medical Oncology 1983; **Med School:** Univ Pennsylvania 1977; **Resid:** Internal Medicine, Univ Chicago Hosps 1980; **Fellow:** Hematology & Oncology, Columbia Presby Hosp 1981; Hematology & Oncology, Northwestern Univ 1983; **Fac Appt:** Prof Med, Northwestern Univ

Great Plains and Mountains

Rodgers III, George M MD/PhD [Hem] - **Spec Exp:** Hematopathology; Anemia-Cancer Related; **Hospital:** Univ Utah Hlth Care; **Address:** Univ Utah Med Ctr - Div Hematology, 30 N 1900 E, rm 5C402, Salt Lake City, UT 84132; **Phone:** 801-585-3229; **Board Cert:** Internal Medicine 1979; Hematology 1982; Pathology 1984; **Med School:** Tulane Univ 1976; **Resid:** Internal Medicine, Baylor Affil Hosps 1979; **Fellow:** Hematology, UCSF Med Ctr 1982; **Fac Appt:** Prof Med, Univ Utah

Hematology

Vose, Julie M MD [Hem] - **Spec Exp:** Lymphoma; **Hospital:** Nebraska Med Ctr; **Address:** 987630 Nebraska Med Ctr, Emile @ 42nd St, Omaha, NE 68198-7630; **Phone:** 402-559-5600; **Board Cert:** Internal Medicine 1987; Medical Oncology 2000; Hematology 2000; **Med School:** Univ Nebr Coll Med 1984; **Resid:** Internal Medicine, Univ Nebraska Med Ctr 1987; **Fellow:** Hematology & Oncology, Univ Nebraska Med Ctr 1990; **Fac Appt:** Prof Med, Univ Nebr Coll Med

Southwest

Barlogie, Bart MD/PhD [Hem] - **Spec Exp:** Bone Marrow Transplant; Plasma Cell Disorders; Multiple Myeloma; **Hospital:** UAMS Med Ctr; **Address:** UAMS-Myeloma Inst Rsch & Therapy, 4301 West Markham St, Slot 816, Little Rock, AR 72205; **Phone:** 501-526-2873; **Med School:** Germany 1969; **Resid:** Internal Medicine, Univ Muenster Med Sch; **Fellow:** Medical Oncology, MD Anderson Cancer Ctr-Tumor Inst 1976; **Fac Appt:** Prof Med, Univ Ark

Brenner, Malcolm K MD/PhD [Hem] - **Spec Exp:** Gene Therapy; Bone Marrow Transplant; **Hospital:** Methodist Hosp - Houston, Texas Chldns Hosp; **Address:** 1102 Bates Ave, Ste 1630, Houston, TX 77030; **Phone:** 832-824-4671; **Med School:** England, UK 1975; **Resid:** Internal Medicine, Cambridge Univ 1979; **Fellow:** Immunology, Clinical Rsch Ctr 1984; Hematology & Oncology, Royal Free Hosp 1986; **Fac Appt:** Prof Med, Baylor Coll Med

Champlin, Richard E MD [Hem] - **Spec Exp:** Bone Marrow Transplant; Stem Cell Transplant; Leukemia & Lymphoma; **Hospital:** UT MD Anderson Cancer Ctr; **Address:** MD Anderson Cancer Ctr, Stem Cell Transplantation Ctr, 1515 Holcombe Blvd, Unit 0423 Blvd, Houston, TX 77030; **Phone:** 713-792-6100; **Board Cert:** Internal Medicine 1978; Hematology 1980; Medical Oncology 1981; **Med School:** Univ Chicago-Pritzker Sch Med 1975; **Resid:** Internal Medicine, LA Co Harbor/UCLA Med Ctr 1978; **Fellow:** Hematology & Oncology, LA Co Harbor/UCLA Med Ctr 1980; **Fac Appt:** Prof Med, Univ Tex, Houston

Cobos, Everardo MD [Hem] - **Spec Exp:** Bone Marrow Transplant; **Hospital:** Univ Med Ctr-Lubbock; **Address:** 602 Indiana Ave, SCRTC Dept, Lubbock, TX 779 418; **Phone:** 806-775-8600; **Board Cert:** Internal Medicine 1985; Medical Oncology 1987; Hematology 1988; **Med School:** Univ Tex, San Antonio 1981; **Resid:** Internal Medicine, Letterman Army Med Ctr 1985; **Fellow:** Hematology & Oncology, Letterman Army Med Ctr 1988; **Fac Appt:** Prof Med, Texas Tech Univ

Cooper, Barry MD [Hem] - **Spec Exp:** Leukemia; Lymphoma; **Hospital:** Baylor Univ Medical Ctr; **Address:** 3410 Worth St, Dallas, TX 75246-2096; **Phone:** 214-370-1002; **Board Cert:** Internal Medicine 1974; Medical Oncology 1977; Hematology 1978; **Med School:** Johns Hopkins Univ 1971; **Resid:** Internal Medicine, Johns Hopkins Hosp 1973; **Fellow:** Metabolism, Natl Inst Health 1975; Hematology, Peter Bent Brigham Hosp 1977; **Fac Appt:** Clin Prof Med, Univ Tex SW, Dallas

Cortes, Jorge E MD [Hem] - **Spec Exp:** Leukemia; Myelodysplastic Syndromes; Myeloproliferative Disorders; **Hospital:** UT MD Anderson Cancer Ctr; **Address:** UT MD Anderson Cancer Center, Leukemia Center, 1515 Holcombe Blvd, Unit 357, Houston, TX 77030; **Phone:** 713-792-8760; **Med School:** Mexico 1986; **Resid:** Internal Medicine, Instituto Nacional de la Nutricion 1989; **Fellow:** Hematology, UT MD Anderson Cancer Ctr 1992; Hematology & Oncology, UT MD Anderson Cancer Ctr 1995; **Fac Appt:** Prof Med, Univ Tex, Houston

Emanuel, Peter D MD [Hem] - **Spec Exp:** Lymphoma; Leukemia; Hodgkin's Disease; Multiple Myeloma; **Hospital:** UAMS Med Ctr; **Address:** 4301 W Markham, Slot 623, Little Rock, AR 72205; **Phone:** 501-526-2272; **Board Cert:** Internal Medicine 1988; **Med School:** Univ Wisc 1985; **Resid:** Internal Medicine, Univ Alabama Hosp 1988; **Fellow:** Hematology & Oncology, Univ Alabama 1991; **Fac Appt:** Prof Med, Univ Ark

Fonseca, Rafael MD [Hem] - **Spec Exp:** Multiple Myeloma; **Hospital:** Mayo Clinic - Scottsdale; **Address:** 13400 E Shea Blvd, MCCRB 1-105, Scottsdale, AZ 85259; **Phone:** 480-301-4280; **Board Cert:** Hematology 2010; **Med School:** Mexico 1991; **Resid:** Internal Medicine, Jackson Meml Hosp 1994; **Fellow:** Hematology & Oncology, Mayo Clinic 1998; **Fac Appt:** Assoc Prof Med, Mayo Med Sch

Kantarjian, Hagop M MD [Hem] - **Spec Exp:** Leukemia; **Hospital:** UT MD Anderson Cancer Ctr; **Address:** 1400 Holcombe Blvd, Unit 428, Houston, TX 77030; **Phone:** 713-792-7026; **Board Cert:** Internal Medicine 1983; Medical Oncology 1985; **Med School:** Amer Univ Beirut 1979; **Resid:** Internal Medicine, Univ Tex MD Anderson Cancer Ctr 1983; **Fellow:** Hematology & Oncology, Univ Tex MD Anderson Cancer Ctr 1983; **Fac Appt:** Prof Med, Univ Tex, Houston

Keating, Michael MD [Hem] - **Spec Exp:** Leukemia; **Hospital:** UT MD Anderson Cancer Ctr; **Address:** MD Anderson Cancer Ctr, 1400 Holcombe Blvd, Unit 428, Houston, TX 77030-4000; **Phone:** 713-745-2376; **Med School:** Australia 1966; **Resid:** Internal Medicine, St Vincents Hosp 1973; **Fellow:** Hematology, MD Anderson Cancer Ctr 1975; **Fac Appt:** Prof Med, Univ Tex, Houston

Lin, Weei-Chin MD/PhD [Hem] - **Spec Exp:** Hematologic Malignancies; **Hospital:** Baylor Clinic & Hosp, Ben Taub Genl Hosp; **Address:** One Baylor Plaza, rm 410, Houston, TX 77030; **Phone:** 713-873-3500; **Med School:** Taiwan 1986; **Resid:** Internal Medicine, Duke Univ Med Ctr 1996; **Fellow:** Hematology & Oncology, Duke Univ Med Ctr 1999; **Fac Appt:** Assoc Prof Med, Baylor Coll Med

Lyons, Roger M MD [Hem] - **Spec Exp:** Leukemia & Lymphoma; Multiple Myeloma; Myelodysplastic Syndromes; **Hospital:** Methodist Hosp-San Antonio, Methodist Spec & Transpl Hosp; **Address:** 4411 Med Drive, Ste 100, San Antonio, TX 78229-3325; **Phone:** 210-595-5300; **Board Cert:** Internal Medicine 1981; Hematology 1982; **Med School:** Canada 1967; **Resid:** Internal Medicine, Winnipeg Genl Hosp 1969; Internal Medicine, Barnes-Wohl Hosps 1972; **Fellow:** Hematology, Washington Univ Hosps 1975; **Fac Appt:** Clin Prof Med, Univ Tex, San Antonio

Maddox, Anne Marie MD [Hem] - **Spec Exp:** Hematologic Malignancies; Lung Cancer; Head & Neck Cancer; Clinical Trials; **Hospital:** UAMS Med Ctr; **Address:** Univ Arkansas Med Ctr, 4301 W Markham St, Slot 74-5, Little Rock, AR 72205; **Phone:** 501-686-8530; **Board Cert:** Internal Medicine 1979; Medical Oncology 1985; Hematology 2004; **Med School:** Dalhousie Univ 1975; **Resid:** Internal Medicine, Univ Toronto 1978; **Fellow:** Medical Oncology, TX MD Anderson Cancer Ctr 1982; **Fac Appt:** Prof, Univ Ark

Munker, Reinhold MD [Hem] - **Spec Exp:** Leukemia & Lymphoma; Bone Marrow Transplant; Hematologic Malignancies; **Hospital:** Louisiana State Univ Hosp; **Address:** LSUHSC-Shreveport, Feist-Weiller Cancer Ctr, 1501 Kings Hwy, Shreveport, LA 71130; **Phone:** 318-813-1016; **Board Cert:** Internal Medicine 2004; Hematology 2006; **Med School:** Germany 1979; **Resid:** Internal Medicine, Universit%otsklinikum Gro?hadern 1989; **Fellow:** Hematology & Oncology, Universit%otsklinikum Gro?hadern 1993; Blood Banking, Universit%otsklinikum Gro?hadern 1997; **Fac Appt:** Assoc Prof Med, Louisiana State U, Shrevport

Strauss, James F MD [Hem] - **Spec Exp:** Bleeding/Coagulation Disorders; Leukemia; Lymphoma; **Hospital:** TX Hlth Presby Hosp Dallas; **Address:** Texas Oncology at Presbyterian, 8220 Walnut Hill Ln Bldg 2 - Ste 700, Dallas, TX 75231; **Phone:** 214-739-4175; **Board Cert:** Internal Medicine 1976; Hematology 1978; Medical Oncology 1981; **Med School:** NYU Sch Med 1972; **Resid:** Internal Medicine, Baylor Univ Medical Ctr 1976; **Fellow:** Hematology, Univ Texas SW Medical Ctr 1977

Hematology

Yeager, Andrew M MD [Hem] - **Spec Exp:** Bone Marrow & Stem Cell Transplant; Graft vs Host Disease; Leukemia; **Hospital:** Univ Med Ctr - Tucson; **Address:** Arizona Cancer Ctr, 1515 N Campbell Ave, Ste 2956, Tucson, AZ 85724-5024; **Phone:** 520-626-3191; **Board Cert:** Pediatrics 1979; Pediatric Hematology-Oncology 1980; **Med School:** Johns Hopkins Univ 1975; **Resid:** Pediatrics, Johns Hopkins Hosp 1978; Pediatrics, Johns Hopkins Hosp 1982; **Fellow:** Pediatric Hematology-Oncology, Johns Hopkins Hosp 1980; **Fac Appt:** Prof Med, Univ Ariz Coll Med

West Coast and Pacific

Damon, Lloyd E MD [Hem] - **Spec Exp:** Leukemia; Lymphoma; Stem Cell Transplant; **Hospital:** UCSF Med Ctr; **Address:** UCSF Comprehensive Cancer Ctr, 400 Parnassus Ave, Ste A502, Box 0324, San Francisco, CA 94143; **Phone:** 415-353-2421; **Board Cert:** Internal Medicine 1985; Medical Oncology 1987; Hematology 1988; **Med School:** Univ Mich Med Sch 1982; **Resid:** Internal Medicine, UCSF Med Ctr 1985; **Fellow:** Hematology & Oncology, UCSF Med Ctr 1988; **Fac Appt:** Prof Med, UCSF

Forman, Stephen J MD [Hem] - **Spec Exp:** Lymphoma; Leukemia; Bone Marrow Transplant; **Hospital:** City of Hope Natl Med Ctr (page 69); **Address:** City Hope Natl Med Ctr, Dept Hematology, 1500 E Duarte Rd, rm 3002, Duarte, CA 91010-3012; **Phone:** 626-256-4673 x62403; **Board Cert:** Internal Medicine 1977; **Med School:** USC Sch Med 1974; **Resid:** Internal Medicine, LAC-Harbor-UCLA Med Ctr 1976; **Fellow:** Hematology, LAC-USC Med Ctr 1978; Hematology, City of Hope Med Ctr 1979; **Fac Appt:** Clin Prof Med, USC Sch Med

Heinrich, Michael C MD [Hem] - **Spec Exp:** Hematologic Malignancies; Sarcoma; Gastrointestinal Stromal Tumors; **Hospital:** VA Medical Center - Portland, OR Hlth & Sci Univ; **Address:** 3710 SW US Veteran's Hospital Rd, MC P3RND19, Portland, OR 97239; **Phone:** 503-220-8262 x51169; **Board Cert:** Internal Medicine 1987; Hematology 2000; Medical Oncology 2001; **Med School:** Johns Hopkins Univ 1984; **Resid:** Internal Medicine, Oreg Hlth Scis Univ 1988; **Fellow:** Hematology & Oncology, Oreg Hlth Scis Univ 1991; **Fac Appt:** Prof Med, Oregon Hlth & Sci Univ

Kipps, Thomas J MD/PhD [Hem] - **Spec Exp:** Leukemia; Lymphoma, Non-Hodgkin's; **Hospital:** UCSD Med Ctr-Hillcrest; **Address:** Moores UCSD Cancer Ctr, 3855 Health Sciences Drive, MC 0820, La Jolla, CA 92093; **Phone:** 858-822-5635; **Board Cert:** Internal Medicine 1982; Hematology 1984; **Med School:** Harvard Med Sch 1979; **Resid:** Internal Medicine, Stanford Univ Med Ctr 1981; **Fellow:** Hematology & Oncology, Stanford Univ Med Ctr 1984; **Fac Appt:** Prof Med, UCSD

Levine, Alexandra M MD [Hem] - **Spec Exp:** Lymphoma; AIDS Related Cancers; **Hospital:** City of Hope Natl Med Ctr (page 69); **Address:** 1500 E Duarte Rd, Needleman 213, Duarte, CA 91010; **Phone:** 626-471-7213; **Med School:** USC Sch Med 1971; **Resid:** Internal Medicine, LAC-USC Med Ctr 1974; **Fellow:** Hematology & Oncology, Grady Meml Hosp-Emory Univ 1975; Hematology, LAC-USC Med Ctr 1978; **Fac Appt:** Prof Med, USC Sch Med

Lill, Michael MD [Hem] - **Spec Exp:** Stem Cell Transplant; Lymphoma; Hematologic Malignancies; **Hospital:** Cedars-Sinai Med Ctr; **Address:** Cedars-Sinai Med Ctr-Outpt Cancer Ctr, 8700 Beverly Blvd, Ste AC 1070, Los Angeles, CA 90048; **Phone:** 310-423-1160; **Med School:** Australia 1982; **Resid:** Internal Medicine, Sir Charles Gairdner Hospital 1985; **Fellow:** Hematology, Royal Perth Hospital 1989; Hematopathology, Sir Charles Gairdner Hosp 1989; **Fac Appt:** Prof Med, UCLA

Linenberger, Michael MD [Hem] - **Spec Exp:** Bone Marrow Transplant; Leukemia & Lymphoma; Multiple Myeloma; **Hospital:** Univ Wash Med Ctr; **Address:** 825 Eastlake Ave E, MS G6-800, Seattle, WA 98109-1023; **Phone:** 206-288-1260; **Board Cert:** Internal Medicine 1985; Hematology 1988; **Med School:** Univ Kansas 1982; **Resid:** Internal Medicine, Rhode Island Hosp 1985; **Fellow:** Hematology, Univ Wash Med Ctr 1989; **Fac Appt:** Assoc Prof Med, Univ Wash

Maziarz, Richard MD [Hem] - **Spec Exp:** Leukemia; Immunotherapy; Bone Marrow Transplant; Lymphoma; **Hospital:** OR Hlth & Sci Univ; **Address:** OHSU Ctr Hematologic Malignancies, 3181 SW Sam Jackson Park Rd, Multnomah Pavilion, Ste 2502, MC L592, Portland, OR 97239; **Phone:** 503-494-5058; **Board Cert:** Internal Medicine 1982; Hematology 1988; Medical Oncology 1989; **Med School:** Harvard Med Sch 1979; **Resid:** Internal Medicine, Univ Hosp 1982; **Fellow:** Hematology & Oncology, Brigham & Womens Hosp 1988; **Fac Appt:** Prof Med, Oregon Hlth & Sci Univ

Mitchell, Beverly S MD [Hem] - **Spec Exp:** Hematologic Malignancies; Leukemia; Lymphoma; **Hospital:** Stanford Univ Hosp & Clinics; **Address:** Stanford Cancer Institute, Lorry Lokey Bldg-SIM 1, 265 Campus Drive, Ste G2167, Stanford, CA 94305; **Phone:** 650-736-7716; **Board Cert:** Internal Medicine 1973; Hematology 1978; **Med School:** Harvard Med Sch 1969; **Resid:** Internal Medicine, Univ Washington Med Ctr 1972; **Fellow:** Metabolism, Univ Zurich 1975; Hematology & Oncology, Univ Michigan 1977; **Fac Appt:** Prof Med, Stanford Univ

Nademanee, Auayporn P MD [Hem] - **Spec Exp:** Lymphoma; Hematologic Malignancies; Clinical Trials; **Hospital:** City of Hope Natl Med Ctr (page 69); **Address:** City of Hope Med Ctr-Dept Hematology, 1500 Duarte Rd, Duarte, CA 91010; **Phone:** 626-256-4673 x62691; **Board Cert:** Hematology 1982; Medical Oncology 1983; Internal Medicine 1978; **Med School:** Thailand 1973; **Resid:** Internal Medicine, Touro Infirm-Tulane Univ 1978; **Fellow:** Hematology & Oncology, Sepulveda VA Hosp 1980; Hematology & Oncology, USC Med Ctr 1981; **Fac Appt:** Prof Med, UCLA

Negrin, Robert S MD [Hem] - **Spec Exp:** Bone Marrow Transplant; **Hospital:** Stanford Univ Hosp & Clinics; **Address:** BMT Program, 300 Pasteur Drive, rm H0101, MC 5623, Stanford, CA 94305; **Phone:** 650-723-0822; **Board Cert:** Internal Medicine 1987; Hematology 2007; **Med School:** Harvard Med Sch 1984; **Resid:** Internal Medicine, Stanford Univ Hosp 1987; **Fellow:** Hematology, Stanford Univ Hosp 1990; **Fac Appt:** Prof Med, Stanford Univ

O'Donnell, Margaret R MD [Hem] - **Spec Exp:** Leukemia; Clinical Trials; **Hospital:** City of Hope Natl Med Ctr (page 69); **Address:** City of Hope National Med Ctr, 1500 E Duarte Rd, MOB-rm 3001, Duarte, CA 91010; **Phone:** 626-359-8111 x62405; **Board Cert:** Internal Medicine 1978; Hematology 1980; Medical Oncology 1979; **Med School:** Med Coll PA 1974; **Resid:** Internal Medicine, Montreal Genl Hosp 1976; Hematology, Royal Victoria Hosp-Montreal 1977; **Fellow:** Hematology & Oncology, Fred Hutchinson Cancer Ctr 1979

Saven, Alan MD [Hem] - **Spec Exp:** Leukemia; Lymphoma; **Hospital:** Scripps Green Hosp; **Address:** Scripps Green Hosp, Hematology, 10666 N Torrey Pines Rd, MS 312, La Jolla, CA 92037; **Phone:** 858-554-9489; **Board Cert:** Internal Medicine 1987; Medical Oncology 1989; **Med School:** South Africa 1982; **Resid:** Internal Medicine, Albert Einstein Med Ctr 1986; **Fellow:** Hematology & Oncology, Scripps Clinic 1987

Schiller, Gary J MD [Hem] - **Spec Exp:** Leukemia; **Hospital:** UCLA Ronald Reagan Med Ctr; **Address:** 10833 Le Conte Ave, rm 42-121 CHS, Los Angeles, CA 90095; **Phone:** 310-825-5513; **Board Cert:** Internal Medicine 1987; Medical Oncology 1989; Hematology 2000; **Med School:** USC Sch Med 1984; **Resid:** Internal Medicine, UCLA Med Ctr 1987; **Fellow:** Hematology & Oncology, UCLA Med Ctr 1990; **Fac Appt:** Prof Med, UCLA

Snyder, David S MD [Hem] - **Spec Exp:** Leukemia; Bone Marrow Transplant; Myeloproliferative Disorders; **Hospital:** City of Hope Natl Med Ctr (page 69); **Address:** 1500 E Duarte Rd, rm 1003, Duarte, CA 91010-3012; **Phone:** 626-256-4673 x62691; **Board Cert:** Internal Medicine 1980; Hematology 1984; **Med School:** Harvard Med Sch 1977; **Resid:** Internal Medicine, Beth Israel Hosp 1980; **Fellow:** Immunology, Harvard Med Sch 1982; Hematology & Oncology, New England Med Ctr 1984

MEDICAL ONCOLOGY

New England

Antin, Joseph H MD [Onc] - **Spec Exp:** Bone Marrow Transplant; Stem Cell Transplant; Leukemia; **Hospital:** Brigham & Women's Hosp, Dana-Farber Cancer Inst; **Address:** The Yawkey Center, 450 Brookline Ave, Boston, MA 02215; **Phone:** 617-632-3667; **Board Cert:** Internal Medicine 1981; Medical Oncology 1983; Hematology 1984; **Med School:** Cornell Univ-Weill Med Coll 1978; **Resid:** Internal Medicine, Peter Bent Brigham Hosp 1981; **Fellow:** Hematology & Oncology, Brigham & Womens Hosp/Dana Farber 1984; **Fac Appt:** Prof Med, Harvard Med Sch

Atkins, Michael B MD [Onc] - **Spec Exp:** Melanoma; Kidney Cancer; Immunotherapy; **Hospital:** Beth Israel Deaconess Med Ctr - Boston; **Address:** Beth Israel Deaconess Med Ctr, Cancer Clinical Trials 375 Longwood Ave, Masco Bldg Fl 4 - Ste 412, Boston, MA 02215; **Phone:** 617-632-9250; **Board Cert:** Internal Medicine 1983; Medical Oncology 1987; **Med School:** Tufts Univ 1980; **Resid:** Internal Medicine, New England Med Ctr 1983; **Fellow:** Hematology & Oncology, New England Med Ctr 1987; **Fac Appt:** Prof Med, Harvard Med Sch

Birrer, Michael J MD/PhD [Onc] - **Spec Exp:** Ovarian Cancer; Clinical Trials; Gynecologic Cancer; **Hospital:** Mass Genl Hosp; **Address:** MGH Cancer Ctr, 55 Fruit St, Yawkey 9E, Boston, MA 02114; **Phone:** 617-724-4000; **Board Cert:** Internal Medicine 1985; Medical Oncology 1987; **Med School:** Albert Einstein Coll Med 1982; **Resid:** Internal Medicine, Mass GeneralHosp 1985; **Fellow:** Medical Oncology, NIH 1987; **Fac Appt:** Prof Med, Harvard Med Sch

Bubley, Glenn J MD [Onc] - **Spec Exp:** Prostate Cancer; **Hospital:** Beth Israel Deaconess Med Ctr - Boston; **Address:** Beth Israel Deaconess Med Ctr, 330 Brookline Ave, Shapiro Bldg Fl 9, Boston, MA 02215; **Phone:** 617-735-2062; **Board Cert:** Internal Medicine 1980; Medical Oncology 1983; **Med School:** Mich State Univ 1977; **Resid:** Internal Medicine, St Francis Hosp 1980; **Fellow:** Hematology & Oncology, Beth Israel Deaconess Med Ctr 1983; **Fac Appt:** Assoc Prof Med, Harvard Med Sch

Burstein, Harold J MD [Onc] - **Spec Exp:** Breast Cancer; **Hospital:** Dana-Farber Cancer Inst, Brigham & Women's Hosp; **Address:** 450 Brookline Ave Yawkey Bldg Fl 12, Boston, MA 02215; **Phone:** 617-632-4587; **Board Cert:** Medical Oncology 2000; **Med School:** Harvard Med Sch 1994; **Resid:** Internal Medicine, Mass Genl Hosp 1997; **Fellow:** Medical Oncology, Dana Farber Cancer Inst 2000; **Fac Appt:** Assoc Prof Med, Harvard Med Sch

Canellos, George P MD [Onc] - **Spec Exp:** Lymphoma-Second Opinion; Hodgkin's Disease-Second Opinion; **Hospital:** Dana-Farber Cancer Inst, Brigham & Women's Hosp; **Address:** Dana Farber Cancer Inst, 44 Binney St, Dana 1B14, Boston, MA 02115; **Phone:** 617-632-3470; **Board Cert:** Internal Medicine 1967; Hematology 1972; Medical Oncology 1973; **Med School:** Columbia P&S 1960; **Resid:** Internal Medicine, Mass Genl Hosp 1963; Internal Medicine, Mass Genl Hosp 1966; **Fellow:** Medical Oncology, Natl Cancer Inst 1965; Hematology, Royal Post Graduate Sch of Med 1967; **Fac Appt:** Prof Med, Harvard Med Sch

Cannistra, Stephen A MD [Onc] - **Spec Exp:** Gynecologic Cancer; **Hospital:** Beth Israel Deaconess Med Ctr - Boston, Dana-Farber Cancer Inst; **Address:** Beth Israel Deaconess Med Ctr, 330 Brookline Ave, KS 158, Boston, MA 02215; **Phone:** 617-667-1909; **Board Cert:** Internal Medicine 1982; Medical Oncology 1985; **Med School:** Brown Univ 1979; **Resid:** Internal Medicine, Johns Hopkins Hosp 1982; **Fellow:** Medical Oncology, Dana-Farber Cancer Inst 1985; **Fac Appt:** Prof Med, Harvard Med Sch

Chabner, Bruce A MD [Onc] - **Spec Exp:** Breast Cancer; Colon & Rectal Cancer; **Hospital:** Mass Genl Hosp; **Address:** Mass General Hospital, 55 Fruit St, Lawrence House 214, Boston, MA 02114; **Phone:** 617-724-3200; **Board Cert:** Internal Medicine 1971; Medical Oncology 1973; **Med School:** Harvard Med Sch 1965; **Resid:** Internal Medicine, Peter Bent Brigham Hosp 1967; Internal Medicine, Yale-New Haven Hosp 1970; **Fellow:** Medical Oncology, Natl Inst Hlth 1969; **Fac Appt:** Prof Med, Harvard Med Sch

Come, Steven E MD [Onc] - **Spec Exp:** Breast Cancer; Hodgkin's Disease; **Hospital:** Beth Israel Deaconess Med Ctr - Boston, Dana-Farber Cancer Inst; **Address:** Beth Israel Deaconess Hosp, 330 Brookline Ave, Ste CC913, Boston, MA 02215-5400; **Phone:** 617-667-4599; **Board Cert:** Internal Medicine 1975; Medical Oncology 1979; **Med School:** Harvard Med Sch 1972; **Resid:** Internal Medicine, Beth Israel Hosp 1977; **Fellow:** Medical Oncology, Natl Cancer Inst 1976; **Fac Appt:** Assoc Prof Med, Harvard Med Sch

Demetri, George D MD [Onc] - **Spec Exp:** Sarcoma; Bone Tumors; **Hospital:** Dana-Farber Cancer Inst; **Address:** Dana Farber Cancer Inst, 450 Brookline Ave, MS Dana 1212, Boston, MA 02215; **Phone:** 617-632-3985; **Board Cert:** Internal Medicine 1986; Medical Oncology 1989; **Med School:** Stanford Univ 1983; **Resid:** Internal Medicine, Univ Wash Med Ctr 1986; **Fellow:** Medical Oncology, Dana Farber Cancer Inst 1989; **Fac Appt:** Assoc Prof Med, Harvard Med Sch

DeVita Jr, Vincent T MD [Onc] - **Spec Exp:** Lymphoma Consultation; Hodgkin's Disease Consultation; **Hospital:** Yale-New Haven Hosp, Yale Med Group; **Address:** Yale Cancer Ctr, 333 Cedar St, rm FMP117, New Haven, CT 06520-8028; **Phone:** 203-737-1010; **Board Cert:** Internal Medicine 1974; Hematology 1972; Medical Oncology 1973; **Med School:** Geo Wash Univ 1961; **Resid:** Internal Medicine, Geo Wash Hosp 1963; Internal Medicine, Yale-New Haven Hosp 1966; **Fellow:** Medical Oncology, Natl Cancer Inst 1965; **Fac Appt:** Prof Med, Yale Univ

Dizon, Don S MD [Onc] - **Spec Exp:** Gynecologic Cancer; Breast Cancer; **Hospital:** Women & Infants Hosp of RI; **Address:** Women & Infants Hosp, Womens Oncology Program, 101 Dudley St, Providence, RI 02905; **Phone:** 401-453-7520; **Board Cert:** Internal Medicine 2008; Medical Oncology 2002; **Med School:** Univ Rochester 1995; **Resid:** Internal Medicine, Yale-New Haven Hosp 1998; **Fellow:** Oncology, Meml Sloan Kettering Cancer Ctr 2001; **Fac Appt:** Asst Prof Med, Brown Univ

Erban III, John K MD [Onc] - **Spec Exp:** Breast Cancer; Hematologic Malignancies; Stem Cell Transplant; **Hospital:** Tufts Med Ctr; **Address:** Tuffs Med Cancer Ctr, 800 Washington St, Mailbox 5609, Boston, MA 02111; **Phone:** 617-636-5782; **Board Cert:** Internal Medicine 1984; Medical Oncology 1989; Hematology 1999; **Med School:** Tufts Univ 1981; **Resid:** Internal Medicine, Hosp Univ Penn 1984; **Fellow:** Hematology & Oncology, New England Med Ctr 1990; **Fac Appt:** Assoc Prof Med, Tufts Univ

Ernstoff, Marc Stuart MD [Onc] - **Spec Exp:** Melanoma; Genitourinary Cancer; Skin Cancer; **Hospital:** Dartmouth - Hitchcock Med Ctr; **Address:** 1 Medical Center Drive, Lebanon, NH 03756; **Phone:** 603-650-5534; **Board Cert:** Internal Medicine 1981; Medical Oncology 1989; **Med School:** NYU Sch Med 1978; **Resid:** Internal Medicine, Albert Einstein Coll Med 1981; **Fellow:** Medical Oncology, Yale Univ Affil Hosp 1984; **Fac Appt:** Prof Med, Dartmouth Med Sch

Flaherty, Keith T MD [Onc] - **Spec Exp:** Melanoma-Advanced; Clinical Trials; **Hospital:** Mass Genl Hosp; **Address:** Massachusetts Genl Cancer Ctr, 32 Fruit St, Yawkey 9E, Boston, MA 02114; **Phone:** 617-724-4800; **Board Cert:** Internal Medicine 2000; Medical Oncology 2003; **Med School:** Johns Hopkins Univ 1997; **Resid:** Internal Medicine, Brigham & Women's Hosp 2000; **Fellow:** Hematology & Oncology, Hosp Univ Penn 2002

Medical Oncology

Foss, Francine M MD [Onc] - **Spec Exp:** Lymphoma, Cutaneous T Cell (CTCL); Stem Cell Transplant; Graft vs Host Disease; Multiple Myeloma; **Hospital:** Yale-New Haven Hosp, Yale Med Group; **Address:** Yale Cancer Ctr, 333 Cedar St, Box 208032, New Haven, CT 06520-8032; **Phone:** 203-737-5312; **Board Cert:** Internal Medicine 1985; Medical Oncology 1987; **Med School:** Univ Mass Sch Med 1982; **Resid:** Internal Medicine, Brigham & Womens Hosp 1985; **Fellow:** Medical Oncology, Natl Cancer Inst 1988; **Fac Appt:** Prof Med, Yale Univ

Freedman, Arnold S MD [Onc] - **Spec Exp:** Lymphoma; Bone Marrow Transplant; Stem Cell Transplant; **Hospital:** Brigham & Women's Hosp, Dana-Farber Cancer Inst; **Address:** Dana-Farber Cancer Inst, 44 Binney St, Ste Dana-1B, Boston, MA 02115; **Phone:** 617-632-3441; **Board Cert:** Internal Medicine 1982; Medical Oncology 1985; **Med School:** Univ Mass Sch Med 1979; **Resid:** Internal Medicine, Memorial Hosp 1982; **Fellow:** Medical Oncology, Dana Farber Cancer Inst 1985; **Fac Appt:** Assoc Prof Med, Harvard Med Sch

Fuchs, Charles S MD [Onc] - **Spec Exp:** Gastrointestinal Cancer; Esophageal Cancer; **Hospital:** Dana-Farber Cancer Inst, Brigham & Women's Hosp; **Address:** Dana Farber Cancer Inst, 450 Brookline Ave, Boston, MA 02215; **Phone:** 617-632-5840; **Board Cert:** Internal Medicine 1989; Medical Oncology 2002; **Med School:** Harvard Med Sch 1986; **Resid:** Internal Medicine, Brigham & Womens Hosp 1989; **Fellow:** Hematology & Oncology, Dana Farber Cancer Inst 1992; **Fac Appt:** Assoc Prof Med, Harvard Med Sch

Garber, Judy E MD [Onc] - **Spec Exp:** Breast Cancer; Breast Cancer Genetics; Cancer Risk Assessment; **Hospital:** Dana-Farber Cancer Inst, Brigham & Women's Hosp; **Address:** Dana Farber Cancer Inst, 44 Binney St, Mayer 2 Fl 9, Boston, MA 02115; **Phone:** 617-632-5961; **Board Cert:** Internal Medicine 1984; Medical Oncology 1987; Hematology 1988; **Med School:** Yale Univ 1981; **Resid:** Internal Medicine, Brigham & Womens Hosp 1984; **Fellow:** Hematology & Oncology, Brigham & Womens Hosp/Dana Farber Cancer Inst 1988; Cancer Epidemiology, Dana Farber Cancer Inst 1990; **Fac Appt:** Assoc Prof Med, Harvard Med Sch

Garnick, Marc B MD [Onc] - **Spec Exp:** Prostate Cancer; Urologic Cancer; **Hospital:** Beth Israel Deaconess Med Ctr - Boston; **Address:** Beth Israel Deaconess Med Ctr, SCC9, 330 Brookline Ave, Boston, MA 02215; **Phone:** 617-735-2062; **Board Cert:** Internal Medicine 1976; Medical Oncology 1979; **Med School:** Univ Pennsylvania 1972; **Resid:** Internal Medicine, Hosp Univ Penn 1974; **Fellow:** Research, Natl Inst Hlth 1976; Medical Oncology, Dana-Farber Cancer Inst 1978; **Fac Appt:** Clin Prof Med, Harvard Med Sch

Grunberg, Steven M MD [Onc] - **Spec Exp:** Lung Cancer; Head & Neck Cancer; Thyroid Cancer; Cancer Risk Assessment; **Hospital:** Fletcher Allen Health Care- Med Ctr Campus; **Address:** FAHC Division of Hematology/Oncology, 89 Beaumont Ave, Given Bldg, E214, Burlington, VT 05405; **Phone:** 802-847-8400; **Board Cert:** Internal Medicine 1978; Medical Oncology 1983; **Med School:** Cornell Univ-Weill Med Coll 1975; **Resid:** Internal Medicine, Mofitt Hosp-U Calif 1978; **Fellow:** Medical Oncology, Sidney Farber Cancer Ctr 1981; **Fac Appt:** Prof Hem & Onc, Univ VT Coll Med

Hammond, Denis B MD [Onc] - **Spec Exp:** Breast Cancer; Prostate Cancer; **Hospital:** Elliot Hosp, Catholic Med Ctr; **Address:** NH Oncology, 200 Technology Drive, Hooksett, NH 03106; **Phone:** 603-622-6484; **Board Cert:** Internal Medicine 1977; Hematology 1978; **Med School:** Tufts Univ 1973; **Resid:** Internal Medicine, SUNY Buffalo Affil Hosps 1976; **Fellow:** Hematology, Mass Genl Hosp 1977; Medical Oncology, Dartmouth Med Sch 1978

Herbst, Roy S MD/PhD [Onc] - **Spec Exp:** Lung Cancer; Head & Neck Cancer; Breast Cancer; Drug Development; **Hospital:** Yale-New Haven Hosp; **Address:** Yale Cancer Ctr, 333 Cedar St, rm WWW-221, New Haven, CT 06520; **Phone:** 203-785-6879; **Board Cert:** Medical Oncology 2007; **Med School:** Cornell Univ-Weill Med Coll 1991; **Resid:** Internal Medicine, Brigham & Women's Hosp 1994; **Fellow:** Medical Oncology, Dana Farber Cancer Inst 1996; **Fac Appt:** Assoc Prof Med, Univ Tex, Houston

Hochberg, Ephraim P MD [Onc] - **Spec Exp:** Lymphoma; Hodgkin's Disease; Lymphomatoid Granulomatosis; **Hospital:** Mass Genl Hosp; **Address:** 55 Fruit St, YAW 7B, Boston, MA 02114; **Phone:** 617-724-4000; **Board Cert:** Medical Oncology 2002; Hematology 2004; **Med School:** Case West Res Univ 1996; **Resid:** Internal Medicine, Brigham & Women's Hosp 1999; **Fellow:** Hematology & Oncology, Dana Farber Cancer Inst 2002

Hochster, Howard S MD [Onc] - **Spec Exp:** Gastrointestinal Cancer; Gynecologic Cancer; Colon & Rectal Cancer; **Hospital:** Yale-New Haven Hosp, Yale Med Group; **Address:** Smilow Cancer Center, 333 Cedar St, Box 208028, New Haven, CT 06520-8028; **Phone:** 203-785-4191; **Board Cert:** Internal Medicine 1983; Medical Oncology 1985; Hematology 1986; **Med School:** Yale Univ 1980; **Resid:** Internal Medicine, NYU Med Ctr 1983; **Fellow:** Hematology & Oncology, NYU Med Ctr 1985; Medical Oncology, Jules Bordet Inst 1986; **Fac Appt:** Prof Med, Yale Univ

Hollister Jr, Dickerman MD [Onc] - **Spec Exp:** Breast Cancer; Lung Cancer; Colon Cancer; Leukemia & Lymphoma; **Hospital:** Greenwich Hosp; **Address:** 77 Lafayette Pl, Ste 260, Greenwich, CT 06830; **Phone:** 203-863-3737; **Board Cert:** Internal Medicine 1978; Hematology 1980; Medical Oncology 1981; **Med School:** Univ VA Sch Med 1975; **Resid:** Internal Medicine, NY Hosp-Cornell Med Ctr 1978; **Fellow:** Hematology & Oncology, NY Hosp-Cornell Med Ctr 1981; **Fac Appt:** Asst Clin Prof Med, Yale Univ

Johnson, Bruce E MD [Onc] - **Spec Exp:** Lung Cancer; Thoracic Cancers; Merkel Cell Carcinoma; Mesothelioma; **Hospital:** Dana-Farber Cancer Inst, Brigham & Women's Hosp; **Address:** Dana Farber Cancer Inst, 450 Brookline Ave, Ste 1234, Boston, MA 02215; **Phone:** 617-632-4790; **Board Cert:** Internal Medicine 1982; Medical Oncology 1985; **Med School:** Univ Minn 1979; **Resid:** Internal Medicine, Univ Chicago Hosps 1982; **Fellow:** Medical Oncology, Natl Cancer Inst 1985; **Fac Appt:** Prof Med, Harvard Med Sch

Kantoff, Philip W MD [Onc] - **Spec Exp:** Genitourinary Cancer; Prostate Cancer; Testicular Cancer; **Hospital:** Dana-Farber Cancer Inst, Brigham & Women's Hosp; **Address:** Dana Farber Cancer Inst, 450 Brookline Ave, Boston, MA 02215; **Phone:** 617-632-1914; **Board Cert:** Internal Medicine 1982; Medical Oncology 1989; **Med School:** Brown Univ 1979; **Resid:** Internal Medicine, NYU/Bellevue Hosp 1982; **Fellow:** Gene Therapy Research, NIH 1986; Hematology & Oncology, NIH/Dana Farber 1986; **Fac Appt:** Prof Med, Harvard Med Sch

Kaufman, Peter A MD [Onc] - **Spec Exp:** Breast Cancer; Clinical Trials; **Hospital:** Dartmouth - Hitchcock Med Ctr; **Address:** DHMC, Dept Hem-Onc, One Medical Center Drive, Lebanon, NH 03756; **Phone:** 603-653-6181; **Board Cert:** Internal Medicine 1986; Medical Oncology 1989; **Med School:** NYU Sch Med 1983; **Resid:** Internal Medicine, Duke Univ Med Ctr 1986; **Fellow:** Hematology & Oncology, Duke Univ Med Ctr 1989; **Fac Appt:** Assoc Prof Med, Dartmouth Med Sch

Lacy, Jill MD [Onc] - **Spec Exp:** Colon & Rectal Cancer; Brain Tumors; Gastrointestinal Cancer; Pancreatic Cancer; **Hospital:** Yale-New Haven Hosp, Yale Med Group; **Address:** Yale Univ Sch Med-Div Medical Oncology, 333 Cedar St, PO Box 208032, New Haven, CT 06520-8032; **Phone:** 203-785-4191; **Board Cert:** Internal Medicine 1982; Medical Oncology 2005; **Med School:** Yale Univ 1978; **Resid:** Internal Medicine, Yale-New Haven Hosp 1981; **Fellow:** Medical Oncology, Yale-New Haven Hosp 1985; **Fac Appt:** Assoc Prof Med, Yale Univ

Medical Oncology

Legare, Robert D MD [Onc] - **Spec Exp:** Breast Cancer; Breast Cancer Risk Assessment; **Hospital:** Women & Infants Hosp of RI; **Address:** Women & Infants Hosp, 101 Dudeley St Fl 2, Providence, RI 02905; **Phone:** 401-453-7520; **Board Cert:** Internal Medicine 2005; Hematology 2006; Medical Oncology 2008; **Med School:** Tufts Univ 1990; **Resid:** Internal Medicine, Yale-New Haven Hosp 1992; **Fellow:** Hematology & Oncology, Brigham & Women's Hosp 1996; **Fac Appt:** Asst Prof Med, Brown Univ

Lynch Jr, Thomas J MD [Onc] - **Spec Exp:** Lung Cancer; Thoracic Cancers; **Hospital:** Yale-New Haven Hosp, Yale Med Group; **Address:** Smilow Cancer Hosp, 333 Cedar St, Office WWW 205, New Haven, CT 06510; **Phone:** 203-688-5864; **Board Cert:** Internal Medicine 1989; Medical Oncology 2003; **Med School:** Yale Univ 1986; **Resid:** Internal Medicine, Mass Genl Hosp 1989; **Fellow:** Medical Oncology, Dana-Farber Cancer Inst 1991; **Fac Appt:** Assoc Prof Med, Yale Univ

Mathew, Paul MD [Onc] - **Spec Exp:** Prostate Cancer; Genitourinary Cancer; **Hospital:** Tufts Med Ctr; **Address:** Tufts Med Ctr, Dept Medicine, 800 Washington St, Box 245, Boston, MA 02111; **Phone:** 617-636-8483; **Board Cert:** Internal Medicine 2000; Medical Oncology 2003; Hematology 2004; **Med School:** Nigeria 1985; **Resid:** Internal Medicine, Cook Co Hosp 1990; **Fellow:** Hematology & Oncology, Mayo Clinic 1994; **Fac Appt:** Assoc Prof Med, Boston Univ

Matulonis, Ursula A MD [Onc] - **Spec Exp:** Gynecologic Cancer; Ovarian Cancer; Breast Cancer; Fertility Preservation in Cancer; **Hospital:** Dana-Farber Cancer Inst; **Address:** Dana Farber Cancer Inst, 450 Brookline Ave, Boston, MA 02215; **Phone:** 617-632-2334; **Board Cert:** Internal Medicine 2000; Medical Oncology 2000; **Med School:** Albany Med Coll 1987; **Resid:** Internal Medicine, Univ Pittsburgh Med Ctr 1990; **Fellow:** Medical Oncology, Dana Farber Cancer Inst 1993; **Fac Appt:** Assoc Prof Med, Harvard Med Sch

Nadler, Lee M MD [Onc] - **Spec Exp:** Lymphoma; **Hospital:** Dana-Farber Cancer Inst, Brigham & Women's Hosp; **Address:** Dana Farber Cancer Inst, 450 Brookline Ave, MS Smith 339, Boston, MA 02215; **Phone:** 617-632-3331; **Board Cert:** Internal Medicine 1976; **Med School:** Harvard Med Sch 1973; **Resid:** Internal Medicine, Columbia-Presby Hosp 1975; **Fellow:** Tumor Immunology, Natl Cancer Inst 1977; Medical Oncology, Dana-Farber Cancer Inst 1978; **Fac Appt:** Prof Med, Harvard Med Sch

Ryan, David MD [Onc] - **Spec Exp:** Colon Cancer; Pancreatic Cancer; Gastrointestinal Cancer; **Hospital:** Mass Genl Hosp; **Address:** MGH Cancer Ctr, 55 Fruit St, YAW 7B, Boston, MA 02114; **Phone:** 617-724-4000; **Board Cert:** Medical Oncology 2009; **Med School:** Columbia P&S 1992; **Resid:** Internal Medicine, Columbia Presby Med Ctr 1996; **Fellow:** Hematology & Oncology, Mass Genl Hosp 1998; **Fac Appt:** Asst Prof Med, Harvard Med Sch

Schnipper, Lowell E MD [Onc] - **Spec Exp:** Breast Cancer; Lymphoma; **Hospital:** Beth Israel Deaconess Med Ctr - Boston; **Address:** Beth Israel Deaconess Med Ctr, 330 Brookline Ave, RABB 430, Boston, MA 02215; **Phone:** 617-667-1198; **Board Cert:** Internal Medicine 1973; Medical Oncology 1983; **Med School:** SUNY Downstate 1968; **Resid:** Internal Medicine, Yale-New Haven Hosp 1970; Medical Oncology, Natl Cancer Inst 1973; **Fellow:** Hematology & Oncology, Barnes Jewish Hosp 1974; **Fac Appt:** Prof Med, Harvard Med Sch

Selvaggi, Kathy J MD [Onc] - **Spec Exp:** Palliative Care; Pain-Cancer; **Hospital:** Dana-Farber Cancer Inst; **Address:** Dana Farber Cancer Inst, 450 Brookline Ave, MC SW 411, Boston, MA 02215; **Phone:** 617-632-6464; **Board Cert:** Internal Medicine 1989; Medical Oncology 2005; Hospice & Palliative Medicine 2008; **Med School:** Penn State Coll Med 1985; **Resid:** Internal Medicine, UPMC Shadyside Hosp 1989; **Fellow:** Medical Oncology, UPMC Shadyside Hosp 1992

Shulman, Lawrence N MD [Onc] - **Spec Exp:** Breast Cancer; **Hospital:** Dana-Farber Cancer Inst, Brigham & Women's Hosp; **Address:** Dana-Farber Cancer Inst, 450 Brookline Ave, MS Dana-1608, Boston, MA 02215; **Phone:** 617-632-2277; **Board Cert:** Internal Medicine 1978; Medical Oncology 1981; Hematology 1982; **Med School:** Harvard Med Sch 1975; **Resid:** Internal Medicine, Beth Israel Hosp 1977; **Fellow:** Hematology & Oncology, Beth Israel Hosp 1980; **Fac Appt:** Assoc Prof Med, Harvard Med Sch

Smith, Matthew R MD/PhD [Onc] - **Spec Exp:** Prostate Cancer; **Hospital:** Mass Genl Hosp; **Address:** Mass Genl Hosp, Hematology/Oncology, 55 Fruit St, Yawkey 7E, Boston, MA 02114; **Phone:** 617-724-5257; **Board Cert:** Medical Oncology 2007; **Med School:** Duke Univ 1992; **Resid:** Internal Medicine, Brigham & Women's Hosp 1994; **Fellow:** Medical Oncology, Dana Farber Cancer Inst 1997; **Fac Appt:** Assoc Prof Med, Harvard Med Sch

Soiffer, Robert J MD [Onc] - **Spec Exp:** Stem Cell Transplant; Bone Marrow Transplant; Leukemia; Lymphoma; **Hospital:** Dana-Farber Cancer Inst, Brigham & Women's Hosp; **Address:** Dana-Farber Cancer Inst, 450 Brookline Ave, rm D1B09, Boston, MA 02115; **Phone:** 617-632-4711; **Board Cert:** Internal Medicine 1986; Medical Oncology 1989; **Med School:** NYU Sch Med 1983; **Resid:** Internal Medicine, Brigham & Women's Hosp 1986; **Fellow:** Medical Oncology, Brigham & Women's Hosp 1989; **Fac Appt:** Prof Med, Harvard Med Sch

Strauss, Gary M MD [Onc] - **Spec Exp:** Lung Cancer; Thoracic Cancers; Melanoma; Breast Cancer; **Hospital:** Tufts Med Ctr; **Address:** Tufts Medical Ctr, Div of Hem/Onc, 800 Washington St, Box 245, Boston, MA 02111; **Phone:** 617-636-5627; **Board Cert:** Internal Medicine 1975; Medical Oncology 1979; Hematology 1980; **Med School:** Yale Univ 1972; **Resid:** Internal Medicine, Boston City Hosp 1974; Internal Medicine, Mass Genl Hosp 1977; **Fellow:** Medical Oncology, Natl Cancer Inst 1976; Hematology & Oncology, Mass General Hosp 1979; **Fac Appt:** Prof Med, Tufts Univ

Strenger, Rochelle MD [Onc] - **Spec Exp:** Breast Cancer; Hematologic Malignancies; Lymphoma; **Hospital:** Miriam Hosp; **Address:** University Medicine, Comprehensive Cancer Center, 164 Summit Ave Fain 3, Providence, RI 02906; **Phone:** 401-793-2920; **Board Cert:** Internal Medicine 1986; Medical Oncology 2009; **Med School:** Albert Einstein Coll Med 1982; **Resid:** Internal Medicine, Brigham & Women's Hosp 1985; **Fellow:** Hematology & Oncology, Brigham & Women's Hosp 1988

Sweeney, Christopher J MD [Onc] - **Spec Exp:** Genitourinary Cancer; Prostate Cancer; Testicular Cancer; **Hospital:** Dana-Farber Cancer Inst; **Address:** Dana Farber Cancer Inst, 450 Brookline Ave, Ste D-1230, Boston, MA 02215; **Phone:** 617-632-5929; **Board Cert:** Medical Oncology 2000; **Med School:** Australia 1993; **Resid:** Internal Medicine, Gundersen Lutheran Med Ctr 1997; **Fellow:** Hematology & Oncology, Indiana Univ Med Ctr 2000

Taplin, Mary-Ellen MD [Onc] - **Spec Exp:** Prostate Cancer; Genitourinary Cancer; **Hospital:** Dana-Farber Cancer Inst, Brigham & Women's Hosp; **Address:** Dana Farber Cancer Inst, 450 Brookline Ave, MS D1230, Boston, MA 02215; **Phone:** 617-632-3237; **Board Cert:** Internal Medicine 1989; Hematology 2006; Medical Oncology 2003; **Med School:** Univ Mass Sch Med 1986; **Resid:** Internal Medicine, Univ Mass Med Ctr 1990; **Fellow:** Hematology & Oncology, Beth Israel Deaconess Med Ctr 1993; **Fac Appt:** Assoc Prof Med

Treon, Steven P MD/PhD [Onc] - **Spec Exp:** Waldenstrom's Macroglobulinemia; Multiple Myeloma; **Hospital:** Dana-Farber Cancer Inst; **Address:** Dana-Farber Cancer Inst, 450 Brookline Ave, MS LG 102, Boston, MA 02115; **Phone:** 617-632-2681; **Med School:** Boston Univ 1993; **Resid:** Internal Medicine, Boston Univ Med Ctr 1995; **Fellow:** Hematology & Oncology, Mass Genl Hosp 1996; Research, Dana Farber Cancer Inst 1997; **Fac Appt:** Assoc Prof Med, Harvard Med Sch

Medical Oncology

Verschraegen, Claire F MD [Onc] - **Spec Exp:** Ovarian Cancer; Drug Discovery; Mesothelioma; **Hospital:** Fletcher Allen Health Care- Med Ctr Campus; **Address:** Univ Vermont, Hematology/Oncology, Gven E-214, UVM363, 89 Beaumont Ave, Burlington, VT 05405; **Phone:** 802-656-5487; **Board Cert:** Internal Medicine 2000; Medical Oncology 2000; **Med School:** Belgium 1982; **Resid:** Internal Medicine, Bordet 1985; Internal Medicine, Univ Texas 1991; **Fellow:** Cancer Research, Stehlin Fdn for Cancer Research 1988; Oncology, MD Anderson Cancer Ctr 1994; **Fac Appt:** Prof Med, Univ VT Coll Med

Weisberg, Tracey MD [Onc] - **Spec Exp:** Breast Cancer; **Hospital:** Maine Med Ctr; **Address:** 100 Campus Drive, Unit 108, Scarborough, ME 04074; **Phone:** 207-885-7600; **Board Cert:** Internal Medicine 1987; Medical Oncology 1989; **Med School:** SUNY Stony Brook 1983; **Resid:** Internal Medicine, Mount Sinai Hosp 1985; Internal Medicine, Hartford Hosp 1986; **Fellow:** Medical Oncology, Yale Univ Hosp 1988

Winer, Eric P MD [Onc] - **Spec Exp:** Breast Cancer; **Hospital:** Dana-Farber Cancer Inst, Brigham & Women's Hosp; **Address:** Dana Farber Cancer Inst, 450 Brookline Ave, MS Mayer 228, Boston, MA 02215; **Phone:** 617-632-3800; **Board Cert:** Internal Medicine 1987; Medical Oncology 1989; **Med School:** Yale Univ 1983; **Resid:** Internal Medicine, Yale-New Haven Hosp 1987; **Fellow:** Hematology & Oncology, Duke Univ Med Ctr 1989; **Fac Appt:** Prof Med, Harvard Med Sch

Mid Atlantic

Abraham, Jame MD [Onc] - **Spec Exp:** Breast Cancer; **Hospital:** Ruby Memorial - WVU Hosp; **Address:** WVU School of Med-Hem/Onc, PO Box 9162, Morgantown, WV 26506; **Phone:** 304-293-4229; **Board Cert:** Internal Medicine 2007; Medical Oncology 2000; **Med School:** India 1991; **Resid:** Internal Medicine, Univ Conn Sch Med 1997; **Fellow:** Medical Oncology, Natl Cancer Inst 1999

Aghajanian, Carol A MD [Onc] - **Spec Exp:** Ovarian Cancer; Gynecologic Cancer; Trophoblastic Tumors; **Hospital:** Meml Sloan-Kettering Cancer Ctr (page 75); **Address:** 1275 York Ave, Ste H905, New York, NY 10065; **Phone:** 212-639-2252; **Board Cert:** Internal Medicine 2002; Medical Oncology 2005; **Med School:** SUNY Downstate 1989; **Resid:** Internal Medicine, Mt Sinai Med Ctr 1993; **Fellow:** Medical Oncology, Meml Sloan Kettering Cancer Ctr 1995; **Fac Appt:** Assoc Prof Med, Cornell Univ-Weill Med Coll

Ahlgren, James D MD [Onc] - **Spec Exp:** Gastrointestinal Cancer; Carcinoid Tumors; **Hospital:** G Washington Univ Hosp; **Address:** Geo Wash Univ Med Ctr, Div Hem/Oncology, 2150 Pennsylvania Ave NW, rm 1-203, Washington, DC 20037-3201; **Phone:** 202-741-2478; **Board Cert:** Internal Medicine 1980; Medical Oncology 1989; **Med School:** Georgetown Univ 1977; **Resid:** Internal Medicine, Georgetown Univ Hosp 1979; **Fellow:** Medical Oncology, Georgetown Univ Hosp 1981; **Fac Appt:** Prof Med, Geo Wash Univ

Aisner, Joseph MD [Onc] - **Spec Exp:** Lung Cancer; Solid Tumors; Thymoma; Mesothelioma; **Hospital:** Robert Wood Johnson Univ Hosp - New Brunswick; **Address:** Cancer Inst of New Jersey, 195 Little Albany St, rm 2006, New Brunswick, NJ 08903-2681; **Phone:** 732-235-6777; **Board Cert:** Internal Medicine 1973; Medical Oncology 1975; **Med School:** Wayne State Univ 1970; **Resid:** Internal Medicine, Georgetown Univ Hosp 1972; **Fellow:** Medical Oncology, Natl Cancer Inst 1975; **Fac Appt:** Prof Med, UMDNJ-RW Johnson Med Sch

Algazy, Kenneth M MD [Onc] - **Spec Exp:** Lung Cancer; Mesothelioma; Hematologic Malignancies; Head & Neck Cancer; **Hospital:** Hosp Univ Penn - UPHS (page 80), VA Med Ctr - Philadelphia; **Address:** Hosp Univ Pennsylvania, 3400 Convention Ave, The Perelman Ctr Fl 2, Philadelphia, PA 19104; **Phone:** 215-615-5810; **Board Cert:** Internal Medicine 1972; Hematology 1974; Medical Oncology 1979; **Med School:** Temple Univ 1969; **Resid:** Internal Medicine, Univ Rochester-Strong Meml Hosp 1972; **Fellow:** Hematology & Oncology, Johns Hopkins Med Ctr 1974; **Fac Appt:** Clin Prof Med, Temple Univ

Ambinder, Richard F MD/PhD [Onc] - **Spec Exp:** Lymphoma; Hodgkin's Disease; AIDS Related Cancers; **Hospital:** Johns Hopkins Hosp; **Address:** Cancer Research Bldg, 1650 Orleans St, rm CRB 389, Baltimore, MD 21231; **Phone:** 410-955-8964; **Board Cert:** Internal Medicine 1982; Medical Oncology 1985; **Med School:** Johns Hopkins Univ 1979; **Resid:** Internal Medicine, Johns Hopkins Hosp 1981; **Fellow:** Internal Medicine, Johns Hopkins Hosp 1982; Medical Oncology, Johns Hopkins Hosp 1985; **Fac Appt:** Prof Med, Johns Hopkins Univ

Argiris, Athanassios MD [Onc] - **Spec Exp:** Lung Cancer; Head & Neck Cancer; **Hospital:** UPMC Presby, Pittsburgh, UPMC Shadyside; **Address:** UPMC Presbyterian Cancer Ctr, 5115 Centre Ave Fl 2, Pittsburgh, PA 15232; **Phone:** 412-692-4724; **Board Cert:** Medical Oncology 2000; **Med School:** Greece 1990; **Resid:** Internal Medicine, Beth Israel Med Ctr 1997; **Fellow:** Medical Oncology, Yale-New Haven Hosp 2000; **Fac Appt:** Prof Med, Univ Pittsburgh

Arlen, Philip M MD [Onc] - **Spec Exp:** Prostate Cancer-Vaccine Therapy; Vaccine Therapy-Clinical Trials Only; Clinical Trials Only; **Hospital:** Natl Inst of Hlth - Clin Ctr, Natl Naval Med Ctr; **Address:** National Cancer Inst, MSC 1750, 10 Center Drive Bldg 10 - rm 5B52, Bethesda, MD 20892-1750; **Phone:** 301-496-0629; **Board Cert:** Medical Oncology 1998; **Med School:** Med Coll GA 1991; **Resid:** Internal Medicine, Georgia Baptist Hlth Care Syst 1994; **Fellow:** Hematology & Oncology, Emory Univ Med Ctr 1994; NCI/NIH 1999

Astrow, Alan MD [Onc] - **Spec Exp:** Ovarian Cancer; Breast Cancer; Lymphoma; **Hospital:** Maimonides Med Ctr (page 74); **Address:** MMC Hematology/Oncology, 6300 8th Ave, Brooklyn, NY 11220; **Phone:** 718-765-2653; **Board Cert:** Internal Medicine 1983; Hematology 1986; Medical Oncology 1987; **Med School:** Yale Univ 1980; **Resid:** Internal Medicine, Boston City Hosp 1983; **Fellow:** Hematology & Oncology, NYU Med Ctr 1986; **Fac Appt:** Assoc Clin Prof Med, NY Med Coll

Attas, Lewis MD [Onc] - **Spec Exp:** Breast Cancer; Lymphoma; Bleeding/Coagulation Disorders; **Hospital:** Englewood Hosp & Med Ctr, Holy Name Med Ctr; **Address:** 350 Engle St, Englewood, NJ 07631; **Phone:** 201-568-5250; **Board Cert:** Internal Medicine 1985; Medical Oncology 1987; Hematology 1988; **Med School:** Mount Sinai Sch Med 1982; **Resid:** Internal Medicine, Montefiore Hosp Med Ctr 1985; **Fellow:** Hematology & Oncology, North Shore Univ Hosp 1988; **Fac Appt:** Assoc Clin Prof Med, Mount Sinai Sch Med

Axelrod, Rita S MD [Onc] - **Spec Exp:** Head & Neck Cancer; Lung Cancer; Complementary Medicine; **Hospital:** Thomas Jefferson Univ Hosp (page 81); **Address:** Thomas Jefferson Univ Hosp, 925 Chestnut St Fl 2, Philadelphia, PA 19107; **Phone:** 215-955-8874; **Board Cert:** Internal Medicine 1976; Medical Oncology 1977; Hematology 1978; **Med School:** NYU Sch Med 1970; **Resid:** Internal Medicine, Med Coll Georgia Hosps 1973; **Fellow:** Hematology & Oncology, Hosp Univ Penn 1975; **Fac Appt:** Assoc Prof Med, Thomas Jefferson Univ

Azzoli, Christopher MD [Onc] - **Spec Exp:** Lung Cancer; Lung Cancer (advanced); **Hospital:** Meml Sloan-Kettering Cancer Ctr (page 75); **Address:** 1275 York Ave, New York, NY 10065; **Phone:** 866-675-5864; **Board Cert:** Internal Medicine 2009; Medical Oncology 2001; **Med School:** Johns Hopkins Univ 1996; **Resid:** Internal Medicine, Johns Hopkins Hosp 1999; **Fellow:** Medical Oncology, Meml Sloan Kettering Cancer Ctr 2002; **Fac Appt:** Asst Prof Med, Cornell Univ-Weill Med Coll

Medical Oncology

Bajorin, Dean F MD [Onc] - **Spec Exp:** Genitourinary Cancer; Bladder Cancer; Testicular Cancer; **Hospital:** Meml Sloan-Kettering Cancer Ctr (page 75); **Address:** 1275 York Avenue, New York, NY 10065; **Phone:** 646-497-9068; **Board Cert:** Internal Medicine 1981; Medical Oncology 1985; **Med School:** NY Med Coll 1978; **Resid:** Internal Medicine, Hartford Hosp 1981; **Fellow:** Medical Oncology, Meml Sloan Kettering Ctr 1986; **Fac Appt:** Prof Med, Cornell Univ-Weill Med Coll

Bashevkin, Michael MD [Onc] - **Spec Exp:** Solid Tumors; Hematologic Malignancies; **Hospital:** Maimonides Med Ctr (page 74); **Address:** 1660 E 14st St, Ste 501, Brooklyn, NY 11229; **Phone:** 718-382-8500 x501; **Board Cert:** Internal Medicine 1976; Hematology 1978; Medical Oncology 1979; **Med School:** SUNY Downstate 1973; **Resid:** Internal Medicine, VA Med Ctr 1976; Hematology & Oncology, Maimonides Med Ctr 1979

Belani, Chandra P MD [Onc] - **Spec Exp:** Lung Cancer; Drug Discovery; **Hospital:** Penn State Milton S Hershey Med Ctr; **Address:** Penn State Hershey Cancer Inst, 500 University Drive, MC CH72, Hershey, PA 17033; **Phone:** 717-531-1078; **Board Cert:** Internal Medicine 1986; Medical Oncology 1987; **Med School:** India 1978; **Resid:** Internal Medicine, SMS Med Hosp 1981; Internal Medicine, Good Samaritan/Univ MD Hosps 1984; **Fellow:** Hematology & Oncology, Univ Maryland Hosp 1987; **Fac Appt:** Prof Med

Biggs, David D MD [Onc] - **Spec Exp:** Breast Cancer; Kidney Cancer; Melanoma; Skin Cancer; **Hospital:** Wilmington Hosp; **Address:** Med. Onc. Hem. Consultants, 4701 Ogletown-Stanton Rd, Ste 3400, Newark, DE 19713; **Phone:** 302-366-1200; **Board Cert:** Internal Medicine 1988; Hematology 2002; Medical Oncology 2001; **Med School:** Univ Kansas 1984; **Resid:** Internal Medicine, Med Coll Wisconsin 1989; **Fellow:** Hematology & Oncology, Hosp Univ Penn 1991; **Fac Appt:** Asst Clin Prof Med

Bosl, George MD [Onc] - **Spec Exp:** Testicular Cancer; **Hospital:** Meml Sloan-Kettering Cancer Ctr (page 75); **Address:** 1275 York Avenue, New York, NY 10065; **Phone:** 212-639-8473; **Board Cert:** Internal Medicine 1976; Medical Oncology 1979; **Med School:** Creighton Univ 1973; **Resid:** Internal Medicine, NY Hosp 1975; Internal Medicine, Meml Sloan-Kettering Cancer Ctr 1977; **Fellow:** Medical Oncology, Univ Minn Hosps 1979; **Fac Appt:** Prof Med, Cornell Univ-Weill Med Coll

Brufsky, Adam M MD/PhD [Onc] - **Spec Exp:** Breast Cancer; **Hospital:** Magee-Womens Hosp - UPMC, UPMC Presby, Pittsburgh; **Address:** Univ Pitt Cancer Inst/Magee-Women's Hosp, 300 Halket St, Ste 4628, MS 15213, Pittsburgh, PA 15213; **Phone:** 412-641-6500; **Board Cert:** Internal Medicine 2004; Medical Oncology 2005; **Med School:** Univ Conn 1990; **Resid:** Internal Medicine, Brigham & Womens Hosp 1992; **Fellow:** Medical Oncology, Dana Farber Cancer Inst 1995; Bone Marrow Transplant, Dana Farber Cancer Inst 1993; **Fac Appt:** Prof Med, Univ Pittsburgh

Carabasi, Matthew H MD [Onc] - **Spec Exp:** Bone Marrow Transplant; Stem Cell Transplant; **Hospital:** Thomas Jefferson Univ Hosp (page 81); **Address:** Dept Med Oncology, Thomas Jefferson Univ, 925 Chestnut St, Philadelphia, PA 19107; **Phone:** 215-955-8874; **Board Cert:** Internal Medicine 1983; Medical Oncology 1987; **Med School:** Jefferson Med Coll 1980; **Resid:** Internal Medicine, Hahnemann MC Hosp 1984; **Fellow:** Hematology & Oncology, Meml Sloan-Kettering Cancer Ctr 1988; Research, Meml Sloan-Kettering Cancer Ctr 1989; **Fac Appt:** Assoc Prof Med, Jefferson Med Coll

Carducci, Michael A MD [Onc] - **Spec Exp:** Urologic Cancer; Drug Discovery & Development; Vaccine Therapy; Clinical Trials; **Hospital:** Johns Hopkins Hosp; **Address:** Sidney Kimmel Cancer Ctr, 1650 Orleans St 1M59 BB Bldg, Baltimore, MD 21231; **Phone:** 410-614-3977; **Board Cert:** Internal Medicine 2001; Medical Oncology 2005; **Med School:** Wayne State Univ 1988; **Resid:** Internal Medicine, Univ Colorado Hlth Sci Ctr 1992; **Fellow:** Medical Oncology, Johns Hopkins Hosp 1995; **Fac Appt:** Prof Med, Johns Hopkins Univ

Celano, Paul MD [Onc] - **Spec Exp:** Gynecologic Cancer; Gastrointestinal Cancer; Breast Cancer; **Hospital:** Greater Baltimore Med Ctr; **Address:** GBMC Cancer Ctr, 6569 N Charles St, Ste 205, Baltimore, MD 21204; **Phone:** 443-849-3051; **Board Cert:** Internal Medicine 1984; Medical Oncology 1987; **Med School:** Mount Sinai Sch Med 1981; **Resid:** Internal Medicine, Thos Jefferson Univ Hosp 1984; **Fellow:** Medical Oncology, Thos Jefferson Univ Hosp 1985; **Fac Appt:** Asst Prof Med, Johns Hopkins Univ

Chachoua, Abraham MD [Onc] - **Spec Exp:** Lung Cancer; Thoracic Cancers; **Hospital:** NYU Langone Med Ctr (page 79); **Address:** NYU Clinical Cancer Ctr, 160 E 34th St Fl 8, New York, NY 10016; **Phone:** 212-731-5388; **Med School:** Australia 1978; **Resid:** Internal Medicine, Alfred Hosp 1982; **Fellow:** Hematology & Oncology, Alfred Hosp 1985; Hematology & Oncology, NYU Med Ctr 1988; **Fac Appt:** Assoc Prof Med, NYU Sch Med

Chanan-Khan, Asher A MD [Onc] - **Spec Exp:** Multiple Myeloma; Leukemia-Chronic Lymphocytic; **Hospital:** Roswell Park Cancer Inst; **Address:** Roswell Park Cancer Inst, Elm & Carlton Sts, Buffalo, NY 14263; **Phone:** 716-845-3221; **Board Cert:** Medical Oncology 2001; Hematology 2004; **Med School:** Pakistan 1993; **Resid:** Internal Medicine, Harlem Hosp Ctr 1997; **Fellow:** Hematology & Oncology, NYU Med Ctr 1999; **Fac Appt:** Asst Prof Med, SUNY Buffalo

Chapman, Paul B MD [Onc] - **Spec Exp:** Melanoma; Immunotherapy; Clinical Trials; Vaccine Therapy; **Hospital:** Meml Sloan-Kettering Cancer Ctr (page 75); **Address:** 1275 York Avenue, New York, NY 10065; **Phone:** 646-888-2378; **Board Cert:** Internal Medicine 1984; Medical Oncology 1987; **Med School:** Cornell Univ-Weill Med Coll 1981; **Resid:** Internal Medicine, Univ Chicago Hosps 1984; **Fellow:** Medical Oncology, Meml Sloan-Kettering Cancer Ctr 1987; **Fac Appt:** Prof Med, Cornell Univ-Weill Med Coll

Chu, Edward MD [Onc] - **Spec Exp:** Colon & Rectal Cancer; Gastrointestinal Cancer; Clinical Trials; **Hospital:** UPMC Shadyside, UPMC Presby, Pittsburgh; **Address:** Univ of Pittsburgh Cancer Institute, 5150 Centre Ave Fl 5 - rm 571, Pittsburgh, PA 15232; **Phone:** 412-648-6589; **Board Cert:** Internal Medicine 1986; Medical Oncology 1989; **Med School:** Brown Univ 1983; **Resid:** Internal Medicine, Roger Williams Hosp 1987; **Fellow:** Medical Oncology, Natl Cancer Inst 1992; **Fac Appt:** Prof Med, Univ Pittsburgh

Claxton, David F MD [Onc] - **Spec Exp:** Leukemia; Bone Marrow Transplant; Hematologic Malignancies; Anemia-Aplastic; **Hospital:** Penn State Milton S Hershey Med Ctr; **Address:** 500 University Drive, rm T4422, Hershey, PA 17033; **Phone:** 717-531-8678; **Board Cert:** Internal Medicine 1984; Medical Oncology 2004; **Med School:** McGill Univ 1978; **Resid:** Internal Medicine, Royal Victoria Hosp 1984; **Fellow:** Hematology, Royal Victoria Hosp 1986; Medical Oncology, UTMD Anderson Cancer Ctr 1989; **Fac Appt:** Prof Med

Cohen, Gary I MD [Onc] - **Spec Exp:** Hematologic Malignancies; Stem Cell Transplant; Melanoma; **Hospital:** Greater Baltimore Med Ctr; **Address:** GBMC Cancer Ctr, 6569 N Charles St, Ste 205, Baltimore, MD 21204; **Phone:** 443-849-3051; **Board Cert:** Internal Medicine 1978; Medical Oncology 1985; Hematology 1982; **Med School:** Univ MD Sch Med 1975; **Resid:** Internal Medicine, SUNY Health Sci Ctr 1978; **Fellow:** Hematology & Oncology, Dana Farber Cancer Ctr 1980

Cohen, Philip MD [Onc] - **Spec Exp:** Breast Cancer; **Hospital:** Georgetown Univ Hosp; **Address:** Georgetown Univ Hosp, Lombardi Cancer Ctr, 3800 Reservoir Rd NW, Washington, DC 20007; **Phone:** 202-444-2198; **Board Cert:** Internal Medicine 1973; Medical Oncology 1975; Hematology 1976; **Med School:** Harvard Med Sch 1970; **Resid:** Internal Medicine, Mass Genl Hosp 1972; **Fellow:** Medical Oncology, Natl Cancer Inst 1974; **Fac Appt:** Assoc Prof Med, Geo Wash Univ

Medical Oncology

Cohen, Roger B MD [Onc] - **Spec Exp:** Drug Discovery & Development; Clinical Trials; Thyroid Cancer; Lung Cancer; **Hospital:** Hosp Univ Penn - UPHS (page 80); **Address:** Hosp Univ Penn, 16 Penn Tower, 3400 Spruce St, Philadelphia, PA 19104; **Phone:** 215-662-4469; **Board Cert:** Internal Medicine 1984; Hematology 1986; Medical Oncology 2005; **Med School:** Harvard Med Sch 1980; **Resid:** Internal Medicine, Mt Sinai Hosp 1982; **Fellow:** Research, Sloan Kettering Cancer Inst 1985; Hematology, Mt Sinai Hosp 1986

Cohen, Seymour M MD [Onc] - **Spec Exp:** Breast Cancer; Melanoma; Lung Cancer; Lymphoma; **Hospital:** Mount Sinai Med Ctr (page 76); **Address:** 1150 5th Ave, New York, NY 10128; **Phone:** 212-249-9141; **Board Cert:** Internal Medicine 1971; Medical Oncology 1973; **Med School:** Univ Pittsburgh 1962; **Resid:** Internal Medicine, Montefiore Med Ctr 1964; Internal Medicine, Mount Sinai Med Ctr 1965; **Fellow:** Hematology, Mount Sinai Med Ctr 1966; Hematology & Oncology, LI Jewish Hosp 1969; **Fac Appt:** Assoc Clin Prof Med, Mount Sinai Sch Med

Coleman, Morton MD [Onc] - **Spec Exp:** Leukemia & Lymphoma; Hodgkin's Disease; Multiple Myeloma; Waldenstrom's Macroglobulinemia; **Hospital:** NY-Presby Hosp/Weill Cornell (page 78); **Address:** 407 E 70th St, FL 3, New York, NY 10021-5302; **Phone:** 212-517-5900; **Board Cert:** Internal Medicine 1971; Hematology 1972; Medical Oncology 1973; **Med School:** Med Coll VA 1963; **Resid:** Internal Medicine, Grady Meml Hosp-Emory 1965; Internal Medicine, NY Hosp-Cornell 1968; **Fellow:** Hematology & Oncology, NY Hosp-Cornell 1970; **Fac Appt:** Clin Prof Med, Cornell Univ-Weill Med Coll

Cullen, Kevin MD [Onc] - **Spec Exp:** Head & Neck Cancer; **Hospital:** Univ of MD Med Ctr; **Address:** Univ Md Greenbaum Cancer Ctr, 22 S Greene St, rm N9E22, Baltimore, MD 21201; **Phone:** 410-328-5506; **Board Cert:** Internal Medicine 1986; Medical Oncology 1989; **Med School:** Harvard Med Sch 1983; **Resid:** Internal Medicine, Beth Israel Hosp 1986; Internal Medicine, Hammersmith Hosp 1985; **Fellow:** Medical Oncology, Natl Cancer Inst 1988

Czuczman, Myron S MD [Onc] - **Spec Exp:** Hodgkin's Disease; Multiple Myeloma; Leukemia-Chronic Lymphocytic; Waldenstrom's Macroglobulinemia; **Hospital:** Roswell Park Cancer Inst, Buffalo General Hosp; **Address:** Roswell Park Cancer Inst, Elm & Carlton Sts, Buffalo, NY 14263; **Phone:** 716-845-7695; **Board Cert:** Internal Medicine 1988; **Med School:** Penn State Coll Med 1985; **Resid:** Internal Medicine, North Shore Univ Hosp 1988; **Fellow:** Hematology & Oncology, Meml Sloan-Kettering Cancer Ctr 1992; **Fac Appt:** Assoc Prof Med, SUNY Buffalo

Daly, Mary B MD/PhD [Onc] - **Spec Exp:** Breast Cancer; Breast Cancer Risk Assessment; Cancer Prevention; Ovarian Cancer Risk Assessment; **Hospital:** Fox Chase Cancer Ctr (page 72); **Address:** Fox Chase Cancer Ctr, 333 Cottman Ave, P1054, Philadelphia, PA 19111; **Phone:** 215-728-2791; **Board Cert:** Internal Medicine 1981; Medical Oncology 1983; **Med School:** Univ NC Sch Med 1978; **Resid:** Internal Medicine, Univ Texas Hlth Sci Ctr 1981; **Fellow:** Medical Oncology, Univ Texas Hlth Sci Ctr 1983; **Fac Appt:** Clin Prof Med, Temple Univ

Davidson, Nancy E MD [Onc] - **Spec Exp:** Breast Cancer; **Hospital:** UPMC Shadyside, Magee-Womens Hosp - UPMC; **Address:** Univ Pittsburgh Cancer Inst, 5150 Centre Ave, Ste 500, Pittsburgh, PA 15232; **Phone:** 412-623-3205; **Board Cert:** Internal Medicine 1982; Medical Oncology 1985; **Med School:** Harvard Med Sch 1979; **Resid:** Internal Medicine, Johns Hopkins Hosp 1982; **Fellow:** Medical Oncology, Natl Cancer Inst 1986; **Fac Appt:** Prof Med, Univ Pittsburgh

Dawson, Nancy MD [Onc] - **Spec Exp:** Prostate Cancer; Kidney Cancer; Bladder Cancer; **Hospital:** Georgetown Univ Hosp; **Address:** Lombardi Cancer Ctr, Georgetown Univ Hosp, 3800 Reservoir Rd NW, Washington, DC 20007; **Phone:** 202-444-9094; **Board Cert:** Internal Medicine 1982; Hematology 1984; Medical Oncology 1985; **Med School:** Georgetown Univ 1979; **Resid:** Internal Medicine, Walter Reed AMC 1982; **Fellow:** Hematology & Oncology, Walter Reed AMC 1985; **Fac Appt:** Prof Med, Georgetown Univ

Dickler, Maura MD [Onc] - **Spec Exp:** Breast Cancer; **Hospital:** Meml Sloan-Kettering Cancer Ctr (page 75); **Address:** 1275 York Ave, New York, NY 10065; **Phone:** 646-497-9064; **Board Cert:** Medical Oncology 2008; **Med School:** Univ Chicago-Pritzker Sch Med 1991; **Resid:** Internal Medicine, Univ Chicago Hosps 1994; **Fellow:** Medical Oncology, Meml Sloan Kettering Cancer Ctr 1998; **Fac Appt:** Assoc Prof Med, Cornell Univ-Weill Med Coll

DiPaola, Robert S MD [Onc] - **Spec Exp:** Genitourinary Cancer; Prostate Cancer; Urologic Cancer; **Hospital:** Robert Wood Johnson Univ Hosp - New Brunswick; **Address:** Cancer Inst of New Jersey, 195 Little Albany St, New Brunswick, NJ 08903-2681; **Phone:** 732-235-6777; **Board Cert:** Internal Medicine 2001; Medical Oncology 2005; **Med School:** Univ Utah 1988; **Resid:** Internal Medicine, Duke Univ Med Ctr 1991; **Fellow:** Hematology & Oncology, Univ Penn Hosp 1994; **Fac Appt:** Assoc Prof Med, UMDNJ-RW Johnson Med Sch

Domchek, Susan M MD [Onc] - **Spec Exp:** Breast Cancer Genetics; Breast Cancer Risk Assessment; Ovarian Cancer Genetics; **Hospital:** Hosp Univ Penn - UPHS (page 80); **Address:** 3 West Perelman Center, Abramson Cancer Ctr Univ Penn, 3400 Civic Center Blvd, Philadelphia, PA 19104; **Phone:** 215-615-3341; **Board Cert:** Medical Oncology 2001; **Med School:** Harvard Med Sch 1995; **Resid:** Internal Medicine, Mass Genl Hosp 1998; **Fellow:** Medical Oncology, Dana Farber Cancer Inst 2001; **Fac Appt:** Prof Med, Univ Pennsylvania

Donehower, Ross Carl MD [Onc] - **Spec Exp:** Pancreatic Cancer; Colon Cancer; Prostate Cancer; **Hospital:** Johns Hopkins Hosp; **Address:** Hopkins Kimmel Cancer Ctr, 1650 Orleans St, CRB-I, rm 187, Baltimore, MD 21231-1000; **Phone:** 410-955-8964; **Board Cert:** Internal Medicine 1977; Medical Oncology 1979; **Med School:** Univ Minn 1974; **Resid:** Internal Medicine, Johns Hopkins Hosp 1976; **Fellow:** Medical Oncology, Natl Inst Hlth 1980; **Fac Appt:** Prof Med, Johns Hopkins Univ

Doroshow, James H MD [Onc] - **Spec Exp:** Drug Discovery & Development; Colon Cancer; Breast Cancer; **Hospital:** Natl Inst of Hlth - Clin Ctr; **Address:** National Cancer Institute, Div Cancer Treatment & Diagnosis, 31 Center Dr, Bldg 31-rm 3A44, Bethesda, MD 20892-2440; **Phone:** 301-496-4291; **Board Cert:** Internal Medicine 1976; Medical Oncology 1977; **Med School:** Harvard Med Sch 1973; **Resid:** Internal Medicine, Mass Genl Hosp 1975; **Fellow:** Medical Oncology, Natl Cancer Inst 1978

Dutcher, Janice P MD [Onc] - **Spec Exp:** Kidney Cancer; Melanoma; Breast Cancer; Lymphoma; **Hospital:** St. Luke's - Roosevelt Hosp Ctr - Roosevelt Div (page 71); **Address:** Continuum Cancer Center of NY, 1000 Tenth Ave, Ste 11C-02, New York, NY 10019; **Phone:** 212-636-3334; **Board Cert:** Internal Medicine 1978; Medical Oncology 1983; **Med School:** UC Davis 1975; **Resid:** Internal Medicine, Rush Presbyterian Med Ctr 1978; **Fellow:** Medical Oncology, National Cancer Inst 1981; **Fac Appt:** Prof Med, NY Med Coll

Edelman, Martin J MD [Onc] - **Spec Exp:** Thoracic Cancers; Lung Cancer; Drug Discovery & Development; **Hospital:** Univ of MD Med Ctr; **Address:** Greenebaum Cancer Ctr-Univ MD, 22 S Greene St, rm N9E08, Baltimore, MD 21201; **Phone:** 410-328-2703; **Board Cert:** Internal Medicine 1986; Medical Oncology 1989; **Med School:** Albany Med Coll 1982; **Resid:** Internal Medicine, Naval Hosp 1986; **Fellow:** Hematology & Oncology, Naval Hosp 1990; **Fac Appt:** Prof Med, Univ MD Sch Med

Eisenberger, Mario MD [Onc] - **Spec Exp:** Prostate Cancer; **Hospital:** Johns Hopkins Hosp; **Address:** 1650 Orleans St, rm 1M51, Baltimore, MD 21231; **Phone:** 410-614-3511; **Board Cert:** Internal Medicine 1976; Medical Oncology 1979; **Med School:** Brazil 1972; **Resid:** Internal Medicine, Michael Reese Hosp 1975; **Fellow:** Hematology, Michael Reese Hosp 1976; Medical Oncology, Jackson Meml Hosp/Univ Miami 1979; **Fac Appt:** Prof Med, Johns Hopkins Univ

Emens, Leisha A MD/PhD [Onc] - **Spec Exp:** Breast Cancer; Immunotherapy; **Hospital:** Johns Hopkins Hosp; **Address:** 1650 Orleans St CRB1 Bldg - rm 409, Baltimore, MD 21231; **Phone:** 410-955-8964; **Board Cert:** Internal Medicine 2008; Medical Oncology 2001; Hematology 2002; **Med School:** Baylor Coll Med 1995; **Resid:** Internal Medicine, Univ TX SW Affil Hosps 1998; **Fellow:** Medical Oncology, Johns Hopkins Hosps 2001; Research, Lab of Bio Chem- NCI 1993; **Fac Appt:** Assoc Prof Med, Johns Hopkins Univ

Engstrom, Paul F MD [Onc] - **Spec Exp:** Neuroendocrine Tumors; Gastrointestinal Cancer; **Hospital:** Fox Chase Cancer Ctr (page 72); **Address:** Fox Chase Cancer Ctr, Dept Medical Oncology, 333 Cottman Ave, Philadelphia, PA 19111; **Phone:** 215-728-2986; **Board Cert:** Internal Medicine 1969; Medical Oncology 1973; **Med School:** Univ Minn 1962; **Resid:** Internal Medicine, Univ Minn Hosp 1965; **Fac Appt:** Prof Med, Temple Univ

Ettinger, David S MD [Onc] - **Spec Exp:** Lung Cancer; Sarcoma; Clinical Trials; **Hospital:** Johns Hopkins Hosp; **Address:** Bunting Blaustein Cancer Rsrch Bldg, 1650 Orleans St, rm G88, Baltimore, MD 21231-1000; **Phone:** 410-955-8847; **Board Cert:** Internal Medicine 1976; Medical Oncology 1977; **Med School:** Univ Louisville Sch Med 1967; **Resid:** Internal Medicine, Mayo Grad Schl 1971; **Fellow:** Medical Oncology, Johns Hopkins Hosp 1975; **Fac Appt:** Prof Med, Johns Hopkins Univ

Fine, Howard Alan MD [Onc] - **Spec Exp:** Brain Tumors; Neuro-Oncology; **Hospital:** Natl Inst of Hlth - Clin Ctr; **Address:** 9030 Old Georgetown Rd, Block Bldg 82, Rm 225, MSC 8202, Bethesda, MD 20892-0001; **Phone:** 301-402-6298; **Board Cert:** Internal Medicine 1987; Medical Oncology 1989; **Med School:** Mount Sinai Sch Med 1984; **Resid:** Internal Medicine, Hosp Univ Penn 1987; **Fellow:** Medical Oncology, Dana Farber Cancer Ctr 1990

Fine, Robert Lance MD [Onc] - **Spec Exp:** Pancreatic Cancer; Drug Development; Brain Tumors; Clinical Trials; **Hospital:** NY-Presby Hosp/Columbia (page 78); **Address:** 650 W 168th St Fl 20th - Ste BB20-05, New York, NY 10032; **Phone:** 212-305-1168; **Board Cert:** Internal Medicine 1983; Medical Oncology 1985; **Med School:** Univ Chicago-Pritzker Sch Med 1979; **Resid:** Internal Medicine, Stanford Univ Med Ctr 1982; **Fellow:** Medical Oncology, National Cancer Inst 1988; **Fac Appt:** Assoc Prof Med, Columbia P&S

Fisher, Richard I MD [Onc] - **Spec Exp:** Lymphoma; Hodgkin's Disease; **Hospital:** Univ of Rochester Strong Meml Hosp; **Address:** James P Wilmot Cancer Ctr, 601 Elmwood Ave, Box 704, Rochester, NY 14642; **Phone:** 585-275-5823; **Board Cert:** Internal Medicine 1973; Medical Oncology 1977; **Med School:** Harvard Med Sch 1970; **Resid:** Internal Medicine, Mass Genl Hosp 1972; **Fac Appt:** Prof Med, Univ Rochester

Flomenberg, Neal MD [Onc] - **Spec Exp:** Bone Marrow Transplant; Stem Cell Transplant; Leukemia & Lymphoma; **Hospital:** Thomas Jefferson Univ Hosp (page 81); **Address:** Thomas Jefferson Univ Hosp, 925 Chestnut St Fl 2, Philadelphia, PA 19107; **Phone:** 215-955-8874; **Board Cert:** Internal Medicine 1979; Medical Oncology 1981; Hematology 1982; **Med School:** Jefferson Med Coll 1976; **Resid:** Internal Medicine, Montefiore Med Ctr 1979; **Fellow:** Hematology & Oncology, Meml Sloan Kettering Cancer Ctr 1982; **Fac Appt:** Clin Prof Med, Thomas Jefferson Univ

Forastiere, Arlene A MD [Onc] - **Spec Exp:** Esophageal Cancer; Head & Neck Cancer; **Hospital:** Johns Hopkins Hosp; **Address:** Bunting Blaustein Cancer Research Bldg, 1650 Orleans St, rm G90, Baltimore, MD 21231; **Phone:** 410-955-8964; **Board Cert:** Internal Medicine 1978; Medical Oncology 1981; **Med School:** NY Med Coll 1975; **Resid:** Internal Medicine, Albert Einstein Med Ctr 1977; Internal Medicine, Univ Conn Health Ctr 1978; **Fellow:** Medical Oncology, Meml Sloan Kettering Cancer Ctr 1980; **Fac Appt:** Prof Med, NY Med Coll

Fox, Kevin R MD [Onc] - **Spec Exp:** Breast Cancer; **Hospital:** Hosp Univ Penn - UPHS (page 80); **Address:** 3400 Civic Ctr Blvd, 3W Perelman Ctr, Philadelphia, PA 19104; **Phone:** 215-662-7469; **Board Cert:** Internal Medicine 1985; Medical Oncology 1987; **Med School:** Johns Hopkins Univ 1981; **Resid:** Internal Medicine, Johns Hopkins Hosp 1984; **Fellow:** Hematology & Oncology, Hosp Univ Penn 1987; **Fac Appt:** Prof Med, Univ Pennsylvania

Friedberg, Jonathan MD [Onc] - **Spec Exp:** Lymphoma; Hodgkin's Disease; Clinical Trials; **Hospital:** Univ of Rochester Strong Meml Hosp; **Address:** James P Wilmot Cancer Ctr, 601 Elmwood Ave, Box 704, Rochester, NY 14642-8704; **Phone:** 585-275-4911; **Board Cert:** Medical Oncology 2000; Hematology 2000; **Med School:** Harvard Med Sch 1994; **Resid:** Internal Medicine, Mass Genl Hosp 1997; Hematology & Oncology, Dana-Farber/Partners Cancer Ctr 1999; **Fac Appt:** Prof Med, Univ Rochester

Gabrilove, Janice MD [Onc] - **Spec Exp:** Myelodysplastic Syndromes; Leukemia; Hematologic Malignancies; Myeloproliferative Disorders; **Hospital:** Mount Sinai Med Ctr (page 76); **Address:** Mount Sinai Med Ctr, One Gustave L Levy Pl, Box 1079, Dept Hem Onc, New York, NY 10029-6574; **Phone:** 212-241-9650; **Board Cert:** Internal Medicine 1980; Medical Oncology 1983; **Med School:** Mount Sinai Sch Med 1977; **Resid:** Internal Medicine, Columbia-Presby Med Ctr 1980; **Fellow:** Hematology & Oncology, Meml Sloan-Kettering Cancer Ctr 1983; **Fac Appt:** Prof Med, Mount Sinai Sch Med

Gelmann, Edward P MD [Onc] - **Spec Exp:** Prostate Cancer; Bladder Cancer; Kidney Cancer; **Hospital:** NY-Presby Hosp/Columbia (page 78); **Address:** Columbia Univ Med Ctr, Milstein Hosp Bldg 6-435, 177 Fort Washington Ave, New York, NY 10032; **Phone:** 212-305-8602; **Board Cert:** Internal Medicine 1979; Medical Oncology 1981; **Med School:** Stanford Univ 1976; **Resid:** Internal Medicine, Univ Chicago Hosps 1978; **Fellow:** Medical Oncology, National Cancer Inst 1981; **Fac Appt:** Prof Med, Columbia P&S

Geyer Jr, Charles E MD [Onc] - **Spec Exp:** Breast Cancer; **Hospital:** Allegheny General Hosp; **Address:** Allegheny Cancer Ctr, 320 E North Ave Fl ACC 3, Pittsburgh, PA 15212; **Phone:** 412-359-6147; **Board Cert:** Internal Medicine 1983; Medical Oncology 1987; **Med School:** Texas Tech Univ 1980; **Resid:** Internal Medicine, Baylor Affil Hosps 1983; **Fellow:** Medical Oncology, Baylor Affil Hosps 1985

Glick, John H MD [Onc] - **Spec Exp:** Breast Cancer; Hodgkin's Disease; Lymphoma, Non-Hodgkin's; **Hospital:** Hosp Univ Penn - UPHS (page 80); **Address:** Abramson Cancer Ctr of Univ Penn, 3400 Civic Ctr Blvd, PCAM Bldg Fl 3 - Ste 3-300S, Philadelphia, PA 19104; **Phone:** 215-662-6065; **Board Cert:** Internal Medicine 1973; Medical Oncology 1975; **Med School:** Columbia P&S 1969; **Resid:** Internal Medicine, Presbyterian Hosp 1971; **Fellow:** Medical Oncology, Natl Cancer Inst 1973; Medical Oncology, Stanford Univ 1974; **Fac Appt:** Prof Med, Univ Pennsylvania

Goldstein, Lori J MD [Onc] - **Spec Exp:** Breast Cancer; **Hospital:** Fox Chase Cancer Ctr (page 72); **Address:** Fox Chase Cancer Ctr, Dept Med Oncology, 333 Cottman Ave, Philadelphia, PA 19111; **Phone:** 215-728-2689; **Board Cert:** Internal Medicine 1985; Medical Oncology 2002; **Med School:** SUNY Upstate Med Univ 1982; **Resid:** Internal Medicine, Presby Univ Hosp 1985; **Fellow:** Medical Oncology, Natl Cancer Inst/NIH 1990; **Fac Appt:** Assoc Prof Hem & Onc, Temple Univ

Goy, Andre MD [Onc] - **Spec Exp:** Lymphoma; Hodgkin's Disease; **Hospital:** Hackensack Univ Med Ctr (page 73); **Address:** 92 2nd St, Hackensack, NJ 07601; **Phone:** 201-996-5900; **Med School:** France 1988; **Resid:** Internal Medicine, Grenoble Univ Med Ctr 1992; **Fellow:** Hematology & Oncology, Grenoble Univ Med Ctr 1993

Medical Oncology

Grana, Generosa MD [Onc] - **Spec Exp:** Breast Cancer; Cancer Genetics; Cancer Prevention; **Hospital:** Cooper Univ Hosp; **Address:** 900 Centennial Blvd, Ste M, Voorhees, NJ 08043; **Phone:** 856-325-6740; **Board Cert:** Internal Medicine 1988; Medical Oncology 2001; **Med School:** Northwestern Univ 1985; **Resid:** Internal Medicine, Temple Univ Hosp 1988; **Fellow:** Hematology & Oncology, Fox Chase Cancer Ctr 1992; **Fac Appt:** Assoc Prof Med, UMDNJ-RW Johnson Med Sch

Grossbard, Michael L MD [Onc] - **Spec Exp:** Lymphoma; Gastrointestinal Cancer; Breast Cancer; **Hospital:** St. Luke's - Roosevelt Hosp Ctr - Roosevelt Div (page 71), Beth Israel Med Ctr - Petrie Division (page 71); **Address:** 1000 10th Ave, Fl 11, Ste C02, New York, NY 10019; **Phone:** 212-523-5419; **Board Cert:** Internal Medicine 1989; Medical Oncology 2001; **Med School:** Yale Univ 1986; **Resid:** Internal Medicine, Mass Genl Hosp 1989; **Fellow:** Medical Oncology, Dana Farber Cancer Inst 1991; **Fac Appt:** Clin Prof Med, Columbia P&S

Grossman, Stuart MD [Onc] - **Spec Exp:** Brain Tumors; Neuro-Oncology; Pain-Cancer; **Hospital:** Johns Hopkins Hosp; **Address:** Cancer Research Bldg 2, rm 1M16, 1550 Orleans St, Ste 1M16, Baltimore, MD 21231; **Phone:** 410-955-8837; **Board Cert:** Internal Medicine 1976; Medical Oncology 1983; **Med School:** Univ Rochester 1973; **Resid:** Internal Medicine, Strong Meml Hosp 1976; **Fellow:** Medical Oncology, Johns Hopkins Hosp 1981; **Fac Appt:** Prof Med, Johns Hopkins Univ

Gulley, James L MD/PhD [Onc] - **Spec Exp:** Prostate Cancer-Vaccine Therapy; Vaccine Therapy-Clinical Trials Only; Clinical Trials Only; **Hospital:** Natl Inst of Hlth - Clin Ctr; **Address:** NIH Cancer Research Ctr, Bldg 10, rm 13N208, 10 Center Dr, MSC 1750, Bethesda, MD 20892; **Phone:** 301-435-2956; **Board Cert:** Internal Medicine 2009; Medical Oncology 2000; **Med School:** Loma Linda Univ 1995; **Resid:** Internal Medicine, Emory Univ Med Ctr 1998; **Fellow:** Medical Oncology, Natl Cancer Inst 2000

Haas, Naomi S Balzer MD [Onc] - **Spec Exp:** Genitourinary Cancer; Kidney Cancer; Clinical Trials; **Hospital:** Hosp Univ Penn - UPHS (page 80); **Address:** Abramson Cancer Ctr, Dept Hem/Onc, 16 Penn Tower, 3400 Spruce St, Philadelphia, PA 19104; **Phone:** 215-662-7402; **Board Cert:** Internal Medicine 1988; Medical Oncology 2005; **Med School:** NE Ohio Univ 1985; **Resid:** Internal Medicine, Abington Meml Hosp 1988; **Fellow:** Hematology & Oncology, Fox Chase Cancer Ctr 1989

Hageboutros, Alexandre MD [Onc] - **Spec Exp:** Gastrointestinal Cancer; Lung Cancer; Colon & Rectal Cancer; **Hospital:** Cooper Univ Hosp; **Address:** 900 Centennial Blvd, Ste M, Voorhees, NJ 08043-4689; **Phone:** 856-325-6740; **Board Cert:** Internal Medicine 2001; Hematology 2004; Medical Oncology 2005; **Med School:** Lebanon 1987; **Resid:** Internal Medicine, Cooper Hosp 1991; **Fellow:** Hematology & Oncology, Temple Univ Hosp 1992; Hematology & Oncology, Fox Chase Cancer Ctr 1994; **Fac Appt:** Assoc Prof Med, UMDNJ-NJ Med Sch, Newark

Henry, David H MD [Onc] - **Spec Exp:** AIDS Related Cancers; **Hospital:** Pennsylvania Hosp (page 80); **Address:** 230 W Washington Square Fl 2, Philadelphia, PA 19106; **Phone:** 215-829-6088; **Board Cert:** Internal Medicine 1978; Hematology 1980; Medical Oncology 1981; **Med School:** Univ Pennsylvania 1975; **Resid:** Internal Medicine, Hosp Univ Penn 1978; **Fellow:** Hematology & Oncology, Hosp Univ Penn 1978; **Fac Appt:** Clin Prof Med, Univ Pennsylvania

Himelstein, Andrew L MD [Onc] - **Spec Exp:** Leukemia & Lymphoma; Palliative Care; **Hospital:** Christiana Hospital; **Address:** Medical Onc/Hem Consultants, 4701 Ogletown-Stanton Rd, Ste West 3400, Helen Graham Cancer Ctr, Newark, DE 19713; **Phone:** 302-366-1200; **Board Cert:** Internal Medicine 1988; Hematology 2000; Medical Oncology 2000; **Med School:** Washington Univ, St Louis 1985; **Resid:** Internal Medicine, Mt Sinai Hosp 1988; **Fellow:** Hematology & Oncology, Colum-Presby Univ Hosp 1991

Hogan, Thomas F MD [Onc] - **Spec Exp:** Genitourinary Cancer; Kidney Cancer; Urologic Cancer; **Hospital:** Ruby Memorial - WVU Hosp; **Address:** MBR Cancer Ctr, Robert T Byrd Hlth Sci Ctr, 1 Medical Center Drive, Morgantown, WV 26506-8110; **Phone:** 304-293-4500; **Board Cert:** Internal Medicine 1975; Medical Oncology 1977; Anatomic Pathology 1997; **Med School:** Med Coll VA 1972; **Resid:** Internal Medicine, Thomas Jefferson Univ Hosp 1975; **Fellow:** Medical Oncology, Univ Wisconsin Affil Hosp 1977; **Fac Appt:** Prof Med, W VA Univ

Holland, James F MD [Onc] - **Spec Exp:** Breast Cancer; Colon Cancer; Lung Cancer; Pancreatic Cancer; **Hospital:** Mount Sinai Med Ctr (page 76); **Address:** Ruttenberg Cancer Ctr, 1190 5th Ave, Box 1129, New York, NY 10029; **Phone:** 212-241-6756; **Board Cert:** Internal Medicine 1955; **Med School:** Columbia P&S 1947; **Resid:** Internal Medicine, Columbia-Presby Hosp 1949; **Fellow:** Medical Oncology, Francis Delafield Hosp 1953; **Fac Appt:** Prof Med, Mount Sinai Sch Med

Horwitz, Steven MD [Onc] - **Spec Exp:** Lymphoma, Cutaneous T Cell (CTCL); **Hospital:** Meml Sloan-Kettering Cancer Ctr (page 75); **Address:** Meml Sloan-Kettering Cancer Ctr, 1275 York Ave, New York, NY 10065; **Phone:** 212-639-3045; **Board Cert:** Medical Oncology 2001; **Med School:** Case West Res Univ 1993; **Resid:** Internal Medicine, Strong Memorial Hosp 1996; **Fellow:** Medical Oncology, Stanford Univ Med Ctr 1999

Hudes, Gary R MD [Onc] - **Spec Exp:** Prostate Cancer; Genitourinary Cancer; Kidney Cancer; **Hospital:** Fox Chase Cancer Ctr (page 72); **Address:** 333 Cottman Ave, rm C307, Philadelphia, PA 19111; **Phone:** 215-728-3889; **Board Cert:** Internal Medicine 1982; Hematology 1984; Medical Oncology 1985; **Med School:** SUNY Downstate 1979; **Resid:** Internal Medicine, Graduate Hosp 1982; **Fellow:** Hematology & Oncology, Presby-Univ Penn Med Ctr 1985

Hudis, Clifford A MD [Onc] - **Spec Exp:** Breast Cancer; **Hospital:** Meml Sloan-Kettering Cancer Ctr (page 75); **Address:** 1275 York Avenue, New York, NY 10065; **Phone:** 800-525-2225; **Board Cert:** Internal Medicine 1986; Medical Oncology 2001; **Med School:** Med Coll PA Hahnemann 1983; **Resid:** Internal Medicine, Hosp Med Coll Penn 1987; **Fellow:** Medical Oncology, Meml Sloan Kettering Cancer Ctr 1991; **Fac Appt:** Prof Med, Cornell Univ-Weill Med Coll

Ilson, David H MD [Onc] - **Spec Exp:** Esophageal Cancer; Colon & Rectal Cancer; Mesothelioma; Unknown Primary Cancer; **Hospital:** Meml Sloan-Kettering Cancer Ctr (page 75); **Address:** 1275 York Avenue, New York, NY 10065; **Phone:** 212-639-8306; **Board Cert:** Internal Medicine 1989; Medical Oncology 2002; **Med School:** NYU Sch Med 1986; **Resid:** Internal Medicine, Bellevue-NYU Sch Med 1989; **Fellow:** Medical Oncology, Meml Sloan Kettering Hosp 1992; **Fac Appt:** Assoc Prof Med, Cornell Univ-Weill Med Coll

Isaacs, Claudine J MD [Onc] - **Spec Exp:** Breast Cancer; Breast Cancer Risk Assessment; **Hospital:** Georgetown Univ Hosp; **Address:** Lombardi Cancer Ctr, Podium A, 3800 Reservoir Rd NW, Washington, DC 20007; **Phone:** 202-444-3677; **Board Cert:** Internal Medicine 2002; Medical Oncology 2003; **Med School:** McGill Univ 1987; **Resid:** Internal Medicine, Montreal Genl Hosp 1990; Hematology & Oncology, McGill Univ Hosp 1992; **Fellow:** Medical Oncology, Georgetown Univ Med Ctr 1993; **Fac Appt:** Assoc Prof Med, Georgetown Univ

Jurcic, Joseph G MD [Onc] - **Spec Exp:** Leukemia; Myelodysplastic Syndromes; Clinical Trials; **Hospital:** Meml Sloan-Kettering Cancer Ctr (page 75); **Address:** 1275 York Avenue, New York, NY 10065; **Phone:** 800-525-2225; **Board Cert:** Internal Medicine 2001; Medical Oncology 2005; Hematology 2008; **Med School:** Univ Pennsylvania 1988; **Resid:** Internal Medicine, Barnes Hosp 1991; **Fellow:** Hematology & Oncology, Meml Sloan Kettering Cancer Ctr 1994; **Fac Appt:** Assoc Prof Med, Cornell Univ-Weill Med Coll

Medical Oncology

Karp, Judith MD [Onc] - **Spec Exp:** Leukemia; Clinical Trials; Myelodysplastic Syndromes; **Hospital:** Johns Hopkins Hosp; **Address:** 1650 Orleans St, CRB1 Bldg - rm 2M44, Baltimore, MD 21287; **Phone:** 410-955-8964; **Board Cert:** Internal Medicine 1976; **Med School:** Stanford Univ 1971; **Resid:** Internal Medicine, John Hopkins Hosp 1974; **Fellow:** Medical Oncology, John Hopkins Hosp 1977; **Fac Appt:** Prof Med, Johns Hopkins Univ

Kelly, William K DO [Onc] - **Spec Exp:** Prostate Cancer; Genitourinary Cancer; Urologic Cancer; Solid Tumors; **Hospital:** Thomas Jefferson Univ Hosp (page 81); **Address:** 834 Chestnut St, Ben Franklin House St, Ste 314, Philadelphia, PA 19107; **Phone:** 215-955-8874; **Board Cert:** Medical Oncology 2003; **Med School:** Philadelphia Coll Osteo Med 1986; **Resid:** Internal Medicine, Montefiore Med Ctr 1990; **Fellow:** Hematology & Oncology, Meml Sloan Kettering Cancer Ctr 1993; **Fac Appt:** Prof Med, Thomas Jefferson Univ

Kelsen, David Paul MD [Onc] - **Spec Exp:** Gastrointestinal Cancer; Neuroendocrine Tumors; Unknown Primary Cancer; Merkel Cell Carcinoma; **Hospital:** Meml Sloan-Kettering Cancer Ctr (page 75); **Address:** 1275 York Ave Howard Bldg - rm 918, New York, NY 10065; **Phone:** 212-639-8470; **Board Cert:** Internal Medicine 1976; Medical Oncology 1979; **Med School:** Hahnemann Univ 1972; **Resid:** Internal Medicine, Temple Univ Hosp 1976; **Fellow:** Medical Oncology, Meml Sloan Kettering Cancer Ctr 1978; **Fac Appt:** Prof Med, Cornell Univ-Weill Med Coll

Kemeny, Nancy MD [Onc] - **Spec Exp:** Colon Cancer; Rectal Cancer; Liver Cancer; **Hospital:** Meml Sloan-Kettering Cancer Ctr (page 75); **Address:** 1275 York Ave, rm H916, New York, NY 10065; **Phone:** 800-525-2225; **Board Cert:** Internal Medicine 1974; Medical Oncology 1981; **Med School:** UMDNJ-NJ Med Sch, Newark 1971; **Resid:** Internal Medicine, St Luke's Hosp 1974; **Fellow:** Medical Oncology, Mem Sloan Kettering Cancer Ctr 1976; **Fac Appt:** Prof Med, Cornell Univ-Weill Med Coll

Kirkwood, John M MD [Onc] - **Spec Exp:** Melanoma; Immunotherapy; **Hospital:** UPMC Shadyside, UPMC Presby, Pittsburgh; **Address:** Hillman Cancer Research Pavilion, 5115 Centre Ave, Pittsburgh, PA 15213-1862; **Phone:** 412-623-7707; **Board Cert:** Internal Medicine 1976; Medical Oncology 1981; **Med School:** Yale Univ 1973; **Resid:** Internal Medicine, Yale-New Haven Hosp 1976; **Fellow:** Medical Oncology, Dana Farber Cancer Inst 1979; **Fac Appt:** Prof Med, Univ Pittsburgh

Kris, Mark G MD [Onc] - **Spec Exp:** Lung Cancer; Mediastinal Tumors; Thymoma; Thoracic Cancers; **Hospital:** Meml Sloan-Kettering Cancer Ctr (page 75); **Address:** 1275 York Ave, New York, NY 10065; **Phone:** 212-639-7590; **Board Cert:** Internal Medicine 1980; Medical Oncology 1983; **Med School:** Cornell Univ-Weill Med Coll 1977; **Resid:** Internal Medicine, New York Hosp 1980; **Fellow:** Medical Oncology, Meml Sloan Kettering Cancer Ctr 1983; **Fac Appt:** Prof Med, Cornell Univ-Weill Med Coll

Laheru, Daniel A MD [Onc] - **Spec Exp:** Pancreatic Cancer; Gastrointestinal Cancer; Vaccine Therapy; **Hospital:** Johns Hopkins Hosp; **Address:** Bunting-Blaustein Cancer Rsch Bldg, 1650 Orleans St, rm 4M09, Baltimore, MD 21231; **Phone:** 410-955-8974; **Board Cert:** Internal Medicine 1998; Medical Oncology 2000; **Med School:** Baylor Coll Med 1995; **Resid:** Internal Medicine, Univ Utah Hosp & Clinics 1998; **Fellow:** Medical Oncology, Johns Hopkins Hosp 1998; **Fac Appt:** Assoc Prof Med, Johns Hopkins Univ

Langer, Corey J MD [Onc] - **Spec Exp:** Lung Cancer; Head & Neck Cancer; Mesothelioma; Thoracic Cancers; **Hospital:** Hosp Univ Penn - UPHS (page 80); **Address:** Hospital U Penn, Abramson Cancer Ctr, 2 PCAM, 3400 Civic Center Blvd, Philadelphia, PA 19104; **Phone:** 215-615-5121; **Board Cert:** Internal Medicine 1984; Hematology 1986; Medical Oncology 1987; **Med School:** Boston Univ 1981; **Resid:** Internal Medicine, Graduate Hosp 1984; Hematology & Oncology, Presby Hosp 1986; **Fellow:** Medical Oncology, Fox Chase Cancer Ctr 1987; **Fac Appt:** Prof Med, Univ Pennsylvania

Levine, Ellis G MD [Onc] - **Spec Exp:** Breast Cancer; Testicular Cancer; Bladder Cancer; Prostate Cancer; **Hospital:** Roswell Park Cancer Inst; **Address:** Roswell Park Cancer Inst, Elm & Carlton St, Buffalo, NY 14263-0001; **Phone:** 716-845-8547; **Board Cert:** Internal Medicine 1982; Medical Oncology 1985; **Med School:** Univ Pittsburgh 1979; **Resid:** Internal Medicine, Univ Minn Hosps 1982; **Fellow:** Medical Oncology, Univ Minn Hosps 1984; **Fac Appt:** Prof Hem & Onc, SUNY Buffalo

Levy, Michael H MD/PhD [Onc] - **Spec Exp:** Pain Management; Palliative Care; Pain-Cancer; Ethics; **Hospital:** Fox Chase Cancer Ctr (page 72); **Address:** Fox Chase Cancer Ctr, Dept Med Oncology, Div Pain & Palliative Med, 333 Cottman Ave, Ste C307, Philadelphia, PA 19111; **Phone:** 215-728-3637; **Board Cert:** Internal Medicine 1979; Medical Oncology 1981; Hospice & Palliative Medicine 2008; **Med School:** Jefferson Med Coll 1976; **Resid:** Internal Medicine, Mt Sinai Med Ctr 1978; Internal Medicine, Hosp Univ Penn 1979; **Fellow:** Hematology & Oncology, Hosp Univ Penn 1981

Maki, Robert G MD/PhD [Onc] - **Spec Exp:** Sarcoma; Sarcoma-Soft Tissue; **Hospital:** Mount Sinai Med Ctr (page 76); **Address:** Mt Sinai Med Ctr, 1 Gustave Levy Pl, Box 1208, New York, NY 10029; **Phone:** 212-241-7022; **Board Cert:** Internal Medicine 2005; Medical Oncology 2007; **Med School:** Cornell Univ-Weill Med Coll 1992; **Resid:** Internal Medicine, Brigham & Womens Hosp 1995; **Fellow:** Medical Oncology, Dana-Farber Cancer Inst 1995; **Fac Appt:** Assoc Prof Med, Cornell Univ-Weill Med Coll

Marshall, John L MD [Onc] - **Spec Exp:** Gastrointestinal Cancer; Drug Development; **Hospital:** Georgetown Univ Hosp; **Address:** Lombardi Cancer Ctr, Podium A, 3800 Reservoir Rd NW, Washington, DC 20007; **Phone:** 202-444-7064; **Board Cert:** Internal Medicine 2001; Medical Oncology 2003; **Med School:** Univ Louisville Sch Med 1988; **Resid:** Internal Medicine, Georgetown Univ Hosp 1991; **Fellow:** Medical Oncology, Georgetown Univ Hosp 1993; **Fac Appt:** Assoc Prof Med, Georgetown Univ

Masters, Gregory A MD [Onc] - **Spec Exp:** Lung Cancer; Esophageal Cancer; Thoracic Cancers; **Hospital:** Christiana Hospital; **Address:** Medical Oncology-Hematology Consultants, Graham Cancer Ctr, 4701 Ogletown-Stanton Rd, Ste 3400, Newark, DE 19713; **Phone:** 302-366-1200; **Board Cert:** Internal Medicine 2003; Medical Oncology 2005; **Med School:** Northwestern Univ 1990; **Resid:** Internal Medicine, Hosp Univ Penn 1993; **Fellow:** Medical Oncology, Univ Chicago Hosps 1995; **Fac Appt:** Assoc Prof Med, Thomas Jefferson Univ

McGuire III, William P MD [Onc] - **Spec Exp:** Gynecologic Cancer; Ovarian Cancer; Breast Cancer; **Hospital:** Franklin Square Hosp; **Address:** Harry & Jeanette Weinberg Cancer Inst, 9103 Franklin Square Drive, Ste 2200, Baltimore, MD 21287; **Phone:** 443-777-7826; **Board Cert:** Internal Medicine 1974; Medical Oncology 1981; **Med School:** Baylor Coll Med 1971; **Resid:** Internal Medicine, Yale-New Haven Hosp 1973; **Fac Appt:** Clin Prof Med, Univ MD Sch Med

Miller, Vincent A MD [Onc] - **Spec Exp:** Lung Cancer; Drug Development; **Hospital:** Meml Sloan-Kettering Cancer Ctr (page 75); **Address:** Memorial Sloan-Kettering Cancer Ctr, 1275 York Ave, New York, NY 10065; **Phone:** 800-525-2225; **Board Cert:** Internal Medicine 2002; Medical Oncology 2005; **Med School:** UMDNJ-NJ Med Sch, Newark 1987; **Resid:** Internal Medicine, Thos Jefferson Univ Hosp 1991; **Fellow:** Medical Oncology, Meml Sloan Kettering Cancer Ctr 1994; **Fac Appt:** Assoc Prof Med, Cornell Univ-Weill Med Coll

Medical Oncology

Mintzer, David M MD [Onc] - **Spec Exp:** Breast Cancer; Gastrointestinal Cancer; Head & Neck Cancer; Palliative Care; **Hospital:** Pennsylvania Hosp (page 80); **Address:** 230 W Washington Square Fl 2, Philadelphia, PA 19106; **Phone:** 215-829-6088; **Board Cert:** Internal Medicine 1980; Hematology 1982; Medical Oncology 1983; Hospice & Palliative Medicine 2004; **Med School:** Jefferson Med Coll 1977; **Resid:** Internal Medicine, Pennsylvania Hosp 1980; **Fellow:** Hematology, Jefferson Med Coll 1982; Medical Oncology, Meml Sloan Kettering Cancer Ctr 1984; **Fac Appt:** Assoc Clin Prof Med, Univ Pennsylvania

Moore, Anne MD [Onc] - **Spec Exp:** Breast Cancer; **Hospital:** NY-Presby Hosp/Weill Cornell (page 78); **Address:** Weill Cornell Breast Ctr, 425 E 61st St Fl 8, New York, NY 10065; **Phone:** 212-821-0550; **Board Cert:** Internal Medicine 1973; Hematology 1976; Medical Oncology 2008; **Med School:** Columbia P&S 1969; **Resid:** Internal Medicine, Cornell Univ Med Ctr 1973; **Fellow:** Medical Oncology, Rockefeller Univ 1973; **Fac Appt:** Prof Med, Cornell Univ-Weill Med Coll

Motzer, Robert J MD [Onc] - **Spec Exp:** Kidney Cancer; Testicular Cancer; Prostate Cancer; **Hospital:** Meml Sloan-Kettering Cancer Ctr (page 75); **Address:** 1275 York Avenue, New York, NY 10065; **Phone:** 800-525-2225; **Board Cert:** Internal Medicine 1984; Medical Oncology 1987; **Med School:** Univ Mich Med Sch 1981; **Resid:** Internal Medicine, Meml Sloan Kettering Cancer Ctr 1984; **Fellow:** Medical Oncology, Meml Sloan Kettering Cancer Ctr 1987; **Fac Appt:** Assoc Prof Med, Cornell Univ-Weill Med Coll

Muggia, Franco MD [Onc] - **Spec Exp:** Gynecologic Cancer; **Hospital:** NYU Langone Med Ctr (page 79); **Address:** NYU Clinical Cancer Ctr, 160 E 34th St Fl 4, New York, NY 10016; **Phone:** 212-731-5433; **Board Cert:** Internal Medicine 1968; Medical Oncology 1973; Hematology 1974; **Med School:** Cornell Univ-Weill Med Coll 1961; **Resid:** Internal Medicine, Hartford Hosp 1964; Internal Medicine, Francis A Delafield Hosp 1966; **Fac Appt:** Prof Med, NYU Sch Med

Nanus, David M MD [Onc] - **Spec Exp:** Prostate Cancer; Bladder Cancer; Testicular Cancer; Genitourinary Cancer; **Hospital:** NY-Presby Hosp/Weill Cornell (page 78); **Address:** NY Hosp-Cornell Med Ctr, Payson Pavilion, 525 E 68th St Fl 3 - Ste 341, New York, NY 10021; **Phone:** 646-962-2072; **Board Cert:** Internal Medicine 1985; Medical Oncology 1987; **Med School:** Univ Hlth Scis, Chicago Med Sch 1982; **Resid:** Internal Medicine, Bronx Muni Hosp 1985; **Fellow:** Medical Oncology, Meml Sloan Kettering Canc Ctr 1989; **Fac Appt:** Prof Med, Cornell Univ-Weill Med Coll

Nissenblatt, Michael MD [Onc] - **Spec Exp:** Breast Cancer; Colon Cancer; Hereditary Cancer; Lymphoma; **Hospital:** Robert Wood Johnson Univ Hosp - New Brunswick, St. Peter's Univ Hosp; **Address:** 205 Easton Ave, New Brunswick, NJ 08901-1722; **Phone:** 732-828-9570; **Board Cert:** Internal Medicine 1976; Medical Oncology 1979; **Med School:** Columbia P&S 1973; **Resid:** Internal Medicine, Johns Hopkins Hosp 1976; **Fellow:** Medical Oncology, Johns Hopkins Hosp 1978; **Fac Appt:** Clin Prof Med

Norton, Larry MD [Onc] - **Spec Exp:** Breast Cancer; **Hospital:** Meml Sloan-Kettering Cancer Ctr (page 75); **Address:** 300 E 66th St, BAIC Bldg Fl 9 - Ste 933, New York, NY 10065; **Phone:** 646-888-5319; **Board Cert:** Internal Medicine 1975; Medical Oncology 1977; **Med School:** Columbia P&S 1972; **Resid:** Internal Medicine, Bronx Muni Hosp 1974; **Fellow:** Medical Oncology, Natl Cancer Inst 1977; **Fac Appt:** Prof Med, Cornell Univ-Weill Med Coll

O'Connor, Owen A MD/PhD [Onc] - **Spec Exp:** Lymphoma-Hodgkins & Non-Hodgkins; Drug Development; Clinical Trials; **Hospital:** NYU Langone Med Ctr (page 79); **Address:** NYU Clin Canc Ctr, 160 E 34th St Fl 7, New York, NY 10016; **Phone:** 212-731-6541; **Board Cert:** Internal Medicine 2004; Medical Oncology 2005; **Med School:** UMDNJ-RW Johnson Med Sch 1994; **Resid:** Internal Medicine, NY Presby Hosp 1996; **Fellow:** Medical Oncology, Memorial Sloan-Kettering Cancer Center 2000; **Fac Appt:** Prof Med, NYU Sch Med

O'Reilly, Eileen M MD [Onc] - **Spec Exp:** Pancreatic Cancer; Liver Cancer; Biliary Cancer; Neuroendocrine Tumors; **Hospital:** Meml Sloan-Kettering Cancer Ctr (page 75); **Address:** 1275 York Avenue, Meml Sloan-Kettering Cancer Ctr, New York, NY 10065; **Phone:** 212-639-6672; **Med School:** Ireland 1990; **Resid:** Internal Medicine, St Vincent's Hosp 1994; **Fellow:** Hematology, St Vincent's Hosp 1995; Medical Oncology, Memorial-Sloan Kettering Cancer Ctr 1997; **Fac Appt:** Assoc Prof Med, Cornell Univ-Weill Med Coll

Offit, Kenneth MD [Onc] - **Spec Exp:** Cancer Genetics; Breast Cancer; Lymphoma; **Hospital:** Meml Sloan-Kettering Cancer Ctr (page 75); **Address:** 1275 York Avenue, New York, NY 10065; **Phone:** 646-888-4050; **Board Cert:** Internal Medicine 1985; Medical Oncology 1987; **Med School:** Harvard Med Sch 1982; **Resid:** Internal Medicine, Lenox Hill Hosp 1985; **Fellow:** Hematology & Oncology, Meml Sloan Kettering Cancer Ctr 1988; **Fac Appt:** Prof Med, Cornell Univ-Weill Med Coll

Oh, William K MD [Onc] - **Spec Exp:** Genitourinary Cancer; Prostate Cancer; Testicular Cancer; Adrenal Cancer; **Hospital:** Mount Sinai Med Ctr (page 76); **Address:** 1 Gustave L Levy Pl, Box 1128, New York, NY 10029; **Phone:** 212-659-5429; **Board Cert:** Medical Oncology 2009; **Med School:** NYU Sch Med 1992; **Resid:** Internal Medicine, Brigham & Womens Hosp 1995; **Fellow:** Medical Oncology, Dana-Farber Cancer Inst 1997; **Fac Appt:** Prof Med, Mount Sinai Sch Med

Oratz, Ruth MD [Onc] - **Spec Exp:** Breast Cancer; Ovarian Cancer; **Hospital:** NYU Langone Med Ctr (page 79); **Address:** 345 E 37th St, Ste 202, New York, NY 10016; **Phone:** 212-400-4904; **Board Cert:** Internal Medicine 1985; Medical Oncology 1989; **Med School:** Albert Einstein Coll Med 1982; **Resid:** Internal Medicine, NYU Med Ctr 1982; **Fellow:** Medical Oncology, NYU Med Ctr 1985; **Fac Appt:** Assoc Clin Prof Med, NYU Sch Med

Oster, Martin W MD [Onc] - **Spec Exp:** Breast Cancer; Gastrointestinal Cancer; Head & Neck Cancer; **Hospital:** NY-Presby Hosp/Columbia (page 78); **Address:** NY Presby Hosp-Columbia Presby Med Ctr, 161 Fort Washington Ave, New York, NY 10032-3713; **Phone:** 212-305-8231; **Board Cert:** Internal Medicine 1974; Medical Oncology 1975; **Med School:** Columbia P&S 1971; **Resid:** Internal Medicine, Mass Genl Hosp 1973; **Fellow:** Medical Oncology, Natl Cancer Inst/NIH 1976; **Fac Appt:** Assoc Clin Prof Med, Columbia P&S

Pasmantier, Mark W MD [Onc] - **Spec Exp:** Lung Cancer; Ovarian Cancer; Breast Cancer; Lymphoma; **Hospital:** NY-Presby Hosp/Weill Cornell (page 78); **Address:** 407 E 70th St Fl 3, New York, NY 10021-5302; **Phone:** 212-517-5900; **Board Cert:** Internal Medicine 1972; Hematology 1974; Medical Oncology 1975; **Med School:** NYU Sch Med 1966; **Resid:** Internal Medicine, Harlem Hosp 1970; **Fellow:** Hematology, Montefiore Med Ctr 1971; Medical Oncology, NY Hosp 1972; **Fac Appt:** Clin Prof Med, Cornell Univ-Weill Med Coll

Pavlick, Anna C MD [Onc] - **Spec Exp:** Melanoma; Skin Cancer; Merkel Cell Carcinoma; **Hospital:** NYU Langone Med Ctr (page 79); **Address:** 160 E 34th St Fl 9, MS 10016, NYU Cancer Institute, New York, NY 10016; **Phone:** 212-731-5431; **Board Cert:** Medical Oncology 2008; **Med School:** UMDNJ Sch Osteo Med 1990; **Resid:** Internal Medicine, Hackensack Med Ctr 1993; **Fellow:** Hematology & Oncology, Meml Sloan Kettering Cancer Ctr 1996; **Fac Appt:** Assoc Prof Med, NYU Sch Med

Pecora, Andrew L MD [Onc] - **Spec Exp:** Stem Cell Transplant; Myelodysplastic Syndromes; Melanoma; Immunotherapy; **Hospital:** Hackensack Univ Med Ctr (page 73); **Address:** The Cancer Ctr-Hackensack Univ Med Ctr, 92 2nd St, Hackensack, NJ 07601; **Phone:** 201-996-5900; **Board Cert:** Internal Medicine 1986; Hematology 1988; Medical Oncology 1989; **Med School:** UMDNJ-NJ Med Sch, Newark 1983; **Resid:** Internal Medicine, New York Hosp 1986; **Fellow:** Hematology & Oncology, Meml Sloan Kettering Cancer Ctr 1988; **Fac Appt:** Prof Med, UMDNJ-NJ Med Sch, Newark

Medical Oncology

Perry, David J MD [Onc] - **Spec Exp:** Gastrointestinal Cancer; Lung Cancer; Genitourinary Cancer; Clinical Trials; **Hospital:** Washington Hosp Ctr; **Address:** Washington Hosp Ctr-Dept Med Oncology, 110 Irving St NW, rm C-2151, Washington, DC 20010; **Phone:** 202-877-2843; **Board Cert:** Internal Medicine 1979; Medical Oncology 1981; Hematology 1982; **Med School:** Univ Pennsylvania 1974; **Resid:** Internal Medicine, Walter Reed AMC 1979; **Fellow:** Hematology & Oncology, Walter Reed AMC 1979; **Fac Appt:** Assoc Prof Med, Eastern VA Med Sch

Petrylak, Daniel P MD [Onc] - **Spec Exp:** Testicular Cancer; Prostate Cancer; Bladder Cancer; Kidney Cancer; **Hospital:** NY-Presby Hosp/Columbia (page 78); **Address:** 161 Fort Washington Ave Fl 9, New York, NY 10032-3729; **Phone:** 212-305-1731; **Board Cert:** Internal Medicine 2001; Medical Oncology 2003; **Med School:** Case West Res Univ 1985; **Resid:** Internal Medicine, Jacobi Med Ctr 1988; **Fellow:** Oncology, Meml-Sloan Kettering Cancer Ctr 1991; **Fac Appt:** Assoc Prof Med, Columbia P&S

Pfister, David G MD [Onc] - **Spec Exp:** Head & Neck Cancer; Laryngeal Cancer; Thyroid Cancer; Skin Cancer; **Hospital:** Meml Sloan-Kettering Cancer Ctr (page 75); **Address:** 1275 York Avenue, New York, NY 10065; **Phone:** 800-525-2225; **Board Cert:** Internal Medicine 1985; Medical Oncology 1989; **Med School:** Univ Pennsylvania 1982; **Resid:** Internal Medicine, Hosp Univ Penn 1985; **Fellow:** Epidemiology, Yale-New Haven Hosp 1987; Hematology & Oncology, Meml Sloan Kettering Cancer Ctr 1989; **Fac Appt:** Prof Med, Cornell Univ-Weill Med Coll

Posner, Marshall R MD [Onc] - **Spec Exp:** Head & Neck Cancer; Skin Cancer-Head & Neck; **Hospital:** Mount Sinai Med Ctr (page 76); **Address:** Mount Sinai Med Ctr, 1 Gustave L Levy Pl, Box 1128, New York, NY 10029; **Phone:** 212-241-6756; **Board Cert:** Internal Medicine 1978; Medical Oncology 1981; **Med School:** Tufts Univ 1975; **Resid:** Internal Medicine, Boston City Hosp 1978; **Fellow:** Oncology, Dana-Farber Cancer Inst 1981; **Fac Appt:** Assoc Prof Med, Mount Sinai Sch Med

Raptis, George MD [Onc] - **Spec Exp:** Breast Cancer; **Hospital:** Mount Sinai Med Ctr (page 76); **Address:** Ruttenberg Treatment Ctr, 1190 5th Ave, Box 1129, New York, NY 10029; **Phone:** 212-241-6756; **Board Cert:** Medical Oncology 2003; **Med School:** Mount Sinai Sch Med 1987; **Resid:** Internal Medicine, Mt Sinai Med Ctr 1990; **Fellow:** Hematology & Oncology, Meml Sloan-Kettering Canc Ctr 1993; **Fac Appt:** Assoc Prof Med, Mount Sinai Sch Med

Remick, Scot C MD [Onc] - **Spec Exp:** AIDS Related Cancers; Clinical Trials; Drug Development; Thyroid Cancer; **Hospital:** Ruby Memorial - WVU Hosp; **Address:** WVU Mary Babb Randolph Cancer Ctr, MS 0, 1801 RCB Health Sciences Center S, Box 9300, Morgantown, WV 26506-9300; **Phone:** 304-598-4552; **Board Cert:** Internal Medicine 1985; Medical Oncology 1987; **Med School:** NY Med Coll 1982; **Resid:** Internal Medicine, Johns Hopkins Hosp 1985; **Fellow:** Medical Oncology, Univ Wisconsin Clin Cancer Ctr 1988; **Fac Appt:** Prof Med, W VA Univ

Ruggiero, Joseph T MD [Onc] - **Spec Exp:** Gastrointestinal Cancer; **Hospital:** NY-Presby Hosp/Weill Cornell (page 78); **Address:** 428 E 72nd St, Ste 300, New York, NY 10021-4635; **Phone:** 212-746-2083; **Board Cert:** Internal Medicine 1980; Hematology 1982; Medical Oncology 1983; **Med School:** NYU Sch Med 1977; **Resid:** Internal Medicine, New York Hosp 1980; **Fellow:** Hematology & Oncology, New York Hosp/Cornell 1983; **Fac Appt:** Assoc Clin Prof Med, Cornell Univ-Weill Med Coll

Saltz, Leonard B MD [Onc] - **Spec Exp:** Colon & Rectal Cancer; Gastrointestinal Cancer & Rare Tumors; Neuroendocrine Tumors; **Hospital:** Meml Sloan-Kettering Cancer Ctr (page 75); **Address:** 1275 York Ave, rm H-917, New York, NY 10065; **Phone:** 646-497-9053; **Board Cert:** Internal Medicine 1986; Hematology 1988; Medical Oncology 1989; **Med School:** Yale Univ 1983; **Resid:** Internal Medicine, New Yor Hosp 1986; **Fellow:** Hematology & Oncology, New York Hosp-Cornell/Rockefeller Univ 1989; **Fac Appt:** Prof Med, Cornell Univ-Weill Med Coll

Scheinberg, David MD/PhD [Onc] - **Spec Exp:** Leukemia; Immunotherapy; Vaccine Therapy; **Hospital:** Meml Sloan-Kettering Cancer Ctr (page 75); **Address:** 1275 York Avenue, New York, NY 10065; **Phone:** 646-888-2190; **Board Cert:** Internal Medicine 1986; Medical Oncology 2005; **Med School:** Johns Hopkins Univ 1983; **Resid:** Internal Medicine, NY Hosp-Cornell Med Ctr 1985; **Fellow:** Medical Oncology, Meml Sloan Kettering Cancer Ctr 1987; **Fac Appt:** Prof Med, Cornell Univ-Weill Med Coll

Scher, Howard MD [Onc] - **Spec Exp:** Genitourinary Cancer; Prostate Cancer; Bladder Cancer; **Hospital:** Meml Sloan-Kettering Cancer Ctr (page 75); **Address:** 1275 York Avenue, New York, NY 10065; **Phone:** 800-525-2225; **Board Cert:** Internal Medicine 1979; Medical Oncology 1985; **Med School:** NYU Sch Med 1976; **Resid:** Internal Medicine, Bellevue Hosp 1980; **Fellow:** Medical Oncology, Meml Sloan Kettering Cancer Ctr 1983; **Fac Appt:** Prof Med, Cornell Univ-Weill Med Coll

Schilder, Russell J MD [Onc] - **Spec Exp:** Gynecologic Cancer; Hematologic Malignancies; Drug Development; Clinical Trials; **Hospital:** Fox Chase Cancer Ctr (page 72); **Address:** Fox Chase Cancer Ctr, 333 Cottman Ave, Philadelphia, PA 19111; **Phone:** 215-728-3545; **Board Cert:** Internal Medicine 1986; Hematology 1988; Medical Oncology 1989; **Med School:** Univ Miami Sch Med 1983; **Resid:** Internal Medicine, Temple Univ Hosp 1986; **Fellow:** Hematology & Oncology, Fox Chase Cancer Ctr 1989; **Fac Appt:** Prof Med, Temple Univ

Schuchter, Lynn M MD [Onc] - **Spec Exp:** Melanoma; Breast Cancer; Clinical Trials; **Hospital:** Hosp Univ Penn - UPHS (page 80); **Address:** Univ Penn/Abramson Cancer Ctr, 3400 Spruce St Penn Tower Bldg Fl 16, Philadelphia, PA 19104-4206; **Phone:** 215-662-7907; **Board Cert:** Internal Medicine 1985; Medical Oncology 1989; **Med School:** Ros Franklin Univ/Chicago Med Sch 1982; **Resid:** Internal Medicine, Michael Reese Hosp 1985; **Fellow:** Medical Oncology, Johns Hopkins Hosp 1989; **Fac Appt:** Prof Med, Univ Pennsylvania

Shields, Peter G MD [Onc] - **Spec Exp:** Hematologic Malignancies; **Hospital:** Georgetown Univ Hosp; **Address:** Lombardi Cancer Ctr, 3800 Reservoir Rd NW, First Floor, Washington, DC 20007; **Phone:** 202-444-2198; **Board Cert:** Medical Oncology 1989; **Med School:** Mount Sinai Sch Med 1983; **Resid:** Internal Medicine, George Washington Univ Hosp 1986; **Fellow:** Hematology & Oncology, George Washington Univ Hosp 1990; **Fac Appt:** Prof Med, Georgetown Univ

Sidransky, David MD [Onc] - **Spec Exp:** Head & Neck Cancer; **Hospital:** Johns Hopkins Hosp; **Address:** 1550 Orleans St, rm 5-N03, Baltimore, MD 21231; **Phone:** 410-502-5153; **Board Cert:** Internal Medicine 1988; **Med School:** Baylor Coll Med 1984; **Resid:** Internal Medicine, Baylor Coll Med 1988; **Fellow:** Medical Oncology, Johns Hopkins Hosp 1992; **Fac Appt:** Prof Oto, Johns Hopkins Univ

Silverman, Lewis R MD [Onc] - **Spec Exp:** Myelodysplastic Syndromes; Leukemia & Lymphoma; Multiple Myeloma; **Hospital:** Mount Sinai Med Ctr (page 76); **Address:** Ruttenberg Treatment Ctr, 1190 5th Ave, Box 1129, New York, NY 10029; **Phone:** 212-241-6756; **Board Cert:** Internal Medicine 1981; Medical Oncology 1987; **Med School:** Belgium 1978; **Resid:** Internal Medicine, Metro Hospital 1980; Internal Medicine, Montefiore Med Ctr 1981; **Fellow:** Hematology, Montefiore Med Ctr 1982; Neoplastic Diseases, Mt Sinai Med Ctr 1984; **Fac Appt:** Assoc Prof Med, Mount Sinai Sch Med

Smith, Mitchell R MD/PhD [Onc] - **Spec Exp:** Lymphoma; Leukemia; Hodgkin's Disease; Multiple Myeloma; **Hospital:** Fox Chase Cancer Ctr (page 72); **Address:** Fox Chase Cancer Ctr, 333 Cottman Ave, Ste C307, Philadelphia, PA 19111; **Phone:** 215-728-2674; **Board Cert:** Internal Medicine 1985; Medical Oncology 1987; Hematology 1988; **Med School:** Case West Res Univ 1979; **Resid:** Pathology, Barnes Jewish Hosp 1983; Internal Medicine, Barnes Jewish Hosp 1984; **Fellow:** Medical Oncology, Meml Sloan-Ketter Cancer Ctr 1988

Medical Oncology

Speyer, James MD [Onc] - **Spec Exp:** Ovarian Cancer; Breast Cancer; Cardiac Toxicity in Cancer Therapy; **Hospital:** NYU Langone Med Ctr (page 79); **Address:** NYU Clinical Cancer Center, 160 E 34th St Fl 8, New York, NY 10016-4750; **Phone:** 212-731-5432; **Board Cert:** Internal Medicine 1977; Hematology 1978; Medical Oncology 1979; **Med School:** Johns Hopkins Univ 1974; **Resid:** Internal Medicine, Columbia-Presby Med Ctr 1976; Hematology, Columbia-Presby Med Ctr 1977; **Fellow:** Medical Oncology, Natl Cancer Inst 1979; **Fac Appt:** Prof Med, NYU Sch Med

Spriggs, David R MD [Onc] - **Spec Exp:** Ovarian Cancer; Drug Development; Uterine Cancer; Gynecologic Cancer; **Hospital:** Meml Sloan-Kettering Cancer Ctr (page 75); **Address:** 1275 York Ave, H Bldg Fl 9 - Ste 901, New York, NY 10065; **Phone:** 800-525-2225; **Board Cert:** Internal Medicine 1981; Medical Oncology 2006; **Med School:** Univ Wisc 1977; **Resid:** Internal Medicine, Columbia-Presby Hosp 1981; **Fellow:** Medical Oncology, Dana-Farber Cancer Inst 1985; **Fac Appt:** Prof Med, Cornell Univ-Weill Med Coll

Stadtmauer, Edward A MD [Onc] - **Spec Exp:** Bone Marrow & Stem Cell Transplant; Leukemia; Multiple Myeloma; **Hospital:** Hosp Univ Penn - UPHS (page 80); **Address:** Abramson Cancer Ctr, Univ of Penn, 2 PCAM, 34th & Cancer Ctr Blvd, Philadelphia, PA 19104; **Phone:** 215-662-7910; **Board Cert:** Internal Medicine 1986; Hematology 1988; Medical Oncology 1989; **Med School:** Univ Pennsylvania 1983; **Resid:** Internal Medicine, Bronx Muni Hosp 1986; **Fellow:** Hematology & Oncology, Hosp Univ Penn 1989; **Fac Appt:** Prof Med, Univ Pennsylvania

Stoopler, Mark Benjamin MD [Onc] - **Spec Exp:** Lung Cancer; Esophageal Cancer; Unknown Primary Cancer; **Hospital:** NY-Presby Hosp/Columbia (page 78); **Address:** 161 Fort Washington Ave, Ste 936, New York, NY 10032-3713; **Phone:** 212-305-8230; **Board Cert:** Internal Medicine 1978; Medical Oncology 1981; **Med School:** Cornell Univ-Weill Med Coll 1975; **Resid:** Internal Medicine, North Shore Univ Hosp 1978; Internal Medicine, NY Meml Hosp 1978; **Fellow:** Medical Oncology, Meml-Sloan Kettering Cancer Ctr 1980; **Fac Appt:** Assoc Clin Prof Med, Columbia P&S

Straus, David J MD [Onc] - **Spec Exp:** Lymphoma; Multiple Myeloma; **Hospital:** Meml Sloan-Kettering Cancer Ctr (page 75); **Address:** 1275 York Avenue, New York, NY 10065; **Phone:** 212-639-8365; **Board Cert:** Internal Medicine 1972; Hematology 1976; Medical Oncology 1977; **Med School:** Marquette Sch Med 1969; **Resid:** Internal Medicine, Montefiore Med Ctr 1972; Medical Oncology, Meml Sloan Kettering Cancer Ctr 1977; **Fellow:** Hematology, Beth Israel Hosp 1973; **Fac Appt:** Prof Med, Cornell Univ-Weill Med Coll

Sun, Weijing MD [Onc] - **Spec Exp:** Gastrointestinal Cancer; Pancreatic Cancer; **Hospital:** Hosp Univ Penn - UPHS (page 80); **Address:** Hosp Univ Pennsylvania, Division of Hematology-Oncology, 3400 Civic Center Blvd, Ste 300W, Philadelphia, PA 19104; **Phone:** 215-662-6319; **Board Cert:** Medical Oncology 2001; **Med School:** China 1982; **Resid:** Internal Medicine, Loyola Univ Med Ctr 1998; **Fellow:** Hematology & Oncology, Hosp Univ Penn 2001; **Fac Appt:** Assoc Prof Med, Univ Pennsylvania

Swain, Sandra MD [Onc] - **Spec Exp:** Breast Cancer; **Hospital:** Washington Hosp Ctr; **Address:** Washington Cancer Inst, 110 Irving St NW, rm C-2149, Washington, DC 20010; **Phone:** 202-877-8112; **Board Cert:** Internal Medicine 1983; Medical Oncology 1985; **Med School:** Univ Fla Coll Med 1980; **Resid:** Internal Medicine, Vanderbilt Univ Affil Hosp 1983; **Fellow:** Medical Oncology, NIH- Natl Cancer Inst 1986; **Fac Appt:** Assoc Prof Med, Georgetown Univ

Tagawa, Scott T MD [Onc] - **Spec Exp:** Prostate Cancer; Bladder Cancer; Kidney Cancer; Urologic Cancer; **Hospital:** NY-Presby Hosp/Weill Cornell (page 78); **Address:** NY Presby-Weill Cornell Med Ctr, 525 E 68th St, Box 403, New York, NY 10065; **Phone:** 646-962-2072; **Board Cert:** Internal Medicine 2001; Medical Oncology 2005; Hematology 2006; **Med School:** USC-Keck School of Medicine 1998; **Resid:** Internal Medicine, USC Med Ctr 2001; **Fellow:** Hematology & Oncology, USC Med Ctr 2005; **Fac Appt:** Asst Prof Hem & Onc, Cornell Univ-Weill Med Coll

Tester, William MD [Onc] - **Spec Exp:** Lung Cancer; Prostate Cancer; **Hospital:** Albert Einstein Med Ctr; **Address:** AEMC Cancer Center Fl 1, 5501 Old York Rd, Philadelphia, PA 19141; **Phone:** 215-456-3880; **Board Cert:** Internal Medicine 1980; Medical Oncology 1983; Hematology 1986; **Med School:** Hahnemann Univ 1977; **Resid:** Internal Medicine, Albert Einstein Med Ctr 1980; **Fellow:** Medical Oncology, NIH-Natl Cancer Inst 1982; Hematology, Georgetown Univ Affil Hosp 1983

Tkaczuk, Katherine H MD [Onc] - **Spec Exp:** Breast Cancer; **Hospital:** Univ of MD Med Ctr; **Address:** Univ MD Cancer Ctr, 22 S Greene St, rm S9D12, Baltimore, MD 21201; **Phone:** 410-328-7904; **Board Cert:** Internal Medicine 1989; Medical Oncology 2001; **Med School:** Poland 1984; **Resid:** Internal Medicine, St Agnes Hosp 1989; **Fellow:** Hematology & Oncology, Univ Maryland Cancer Ctr 1992; **Fac Appt:** Assoc Prof Med, Univ MD Sch Med

Toppmeyer, Deborah L MD [Onc] - **Spec Exp:** Breast Cancer; Hereditary Cancer; **Hospital:** Robert Wood Johnson Univ Hosp - New Brunswick; **Address:** Cancer Inst of New Jersey, 195 Little Albany St, New Brunswick, NJ 08903; **Phone:** 732-235-9692; **Board Cert:** Internal Medicine 1988; Medical Oncology 2006; **Med School:** Albany Med Coll 1985; **Resid:** Internal Medicine, Univ Pittsburgh Hlth Ctr Hosp 1988; **Fellow:** Medical Oncology, Dana Farber Cancer Inst 1993; **Fac Appt:** Assoc Prof Med

Trump, Donald L MD [Onc] - **Spec Exp:** Prostate Cancer; Genitourinary Cancer; Drug Discovery & Development; **Hospital:** Roswell Park Cancer Inst; **Address:** Roswell Park Cancer Inst, Elm and Carlton Streets, Buffalo, NY 14263; **Phone:** 716-845-3159; **Board Cert:** Internal Medicine 1973; Medical Oncology 1977; **Med School:** Johns Hopkins Univ 1970; **Resid:** Internal Medicine, Johns Hopkins Hosp 1975; **Fellow:** Medical Oncology, Johns Hopkins Hosp 1974; **Fac Appt:** Prof Med, SUNY Buffalo

Vaughn, David J MD [Onc] - **Spec Exp:** Testicular Cancer; Bladder Cancer; Prostate Cancer; Genitourinary Cancer; **Hospital:** Hosp Univ Penn - UPHS (page 80); **Address:** Hosp Univ Pennsylvania, Division Hematology/Oncology, 3400 Civic Center Blvd, Ste 300W, Philadelphia, PA 19104; **Phone:** 215-349-8498; **Board Cert:** Medical Oncology 2003; **Med School:** Harvard Med Sch 1987; **Resid:** Internal Medicine, NY Hosp-Cornell Med Ctr 1990; **Fellow:** Hematology & Oncology, Hosp Univ Penn 1993; **Fac Appt:** Prof Med, Univ Pennsylvania

Vinciguerra, Vincent P MD [Onc] - **Spec Exp:** Breast Cancer; Gastrointestinal Cancer; Lung Cancer; Cancer Prevention; **Hospital:** N Shore Univ Hosp; **Address:** 450 Lakeville Rd, Montra Cancer Ctr, Lake Success, NY 11042; **Phone:** 516-734-8954; **Board Cert:** Internal Medicine 1971; Hematology 1974; Medical Oncology 1975; **Med School:** Georgetown Univ 1966; **Resid:** Internal Medicine, NY Hosp-Cornell 1969; Internal Medicine, N Shore Univ Hosp 1971; **Fellow:** Hematology & Oncology, NY Hosp-Cornell 1970; Hematology & Oncology, N Shore Univ Hosp 1974; **Fac Appt:** Prof Med, NYU Sch Med

von Mehren, Margaret MD [Onc] - **Spec Exp:** Sarcoma; Melanoma; Immunotherapy; Gastrointestinal Stromal Tumors; **Hospital:** Fox Chase Cancer Ctr (page 72); **Address:** Fox Chase Cancer Ctr, Dept Med Oncology, 333 Cottman Ave, Philadelphia, PA 19111-2434; **Phone:** 215-728-2814; **Board Cert:** Medical Oncology 2007; **Med School:** Albany Med Coll 1989; **Resid:** Internal Medicine, NYU Med Ctr 1993; **Fellow:** Hematology & Oncology, Fox Chase Cancer Ctr 1996; **Fac Appt:** Assoc Prof Med, Temple Univ

Waintraub, Stanley MD [Onc] - **Spec Exp:** Breast Cancer; Bleeding/Coagulation Disorders; **Hospital:** Hackensack Univ Med Ctr (page 73); **Address:** Northern NJ Cancer Associates, 92 2nd St, Hackensack, NJ 07601; **Phone:** 201-996-5900; **Board Cert:** Internal Medicine 1980; Hematology 1982; Medical Oncology 1983; **Med School:** NY Med Coll 1977; **Resid:** Internal Medicine, Metropolitan Hosp Ctr 1980; **Fellow:** Hematology, Montefiore Hosp Med Ctr 1982; Medical Oncology, Meml Sloan Kettering Cancer Ctr 1983

Medical Oncology

Weiner, Louis M MD [Onc] - **Spec Exp:** Gastrointestinal Cancer; Immunotherapy; Liver Cancer; **Hospital:** Georgetown Univ Hosp; **Address:** Lombardi Cancer Ctr, Georgetown Univ, Research Bldg, 3800 Reservoir Rd NW, Washington, DC 20007; **Phone:** 202-444-2198; **Board Cert:** Internal Medicine 1980; Medical Oncology 1985; **Med School:** Mount Sinai Sch Med 1977; **Resid:** Internal Medicine, Med Ctr Hosp Vermont 1981; **Fellow:** Hematology & Oncology, New England Med Ctr 1984; **Fac Appt:** Prof Med, Georgetown Univ

Wetzler, Meir MD [Onc] - **Spec Exp:** Leukemia; **Hospital:** Roswell Park Cancer Inst; **Address:** Roswell Park Cancer Inst, Elm and Carlton Streets, Buffalo, NY 14263; **Phone:** 716-845-8447; **Board Cert:** Internal Medicine 2001; Medical Oncology 2003; **Med School:** Israel 1980; **Resid:** Internal Medicine, Kaplan Hosp 1986; **Fellow:** Medical Oncology, MD Anderson Cancer Ctr 1992; Clinical Immunology, MD Anderson Cancer Ctr 1992; **Fac Appt:** Prof Med, SUNY Buffalo

Wilson, Wyndham MD [Onc] - **Spec Exp:** Lymphoma; **Hospital:** Natl Inst of Hlth - Clin Ctr; **Address:** National Cancer Inst, Bldg 10 - rm 4N-115, 9000 Rockville Pike, Bethesda, MD 20892; **Phone:** 301-435-2415; **Board Cert:** Internal Medicine 1985; Medical Oncology 1987; **Med School:** Stanford Univ 1981; **Resid:** Internal Medicine, Stanford Univ 1984; **Fellow:** Oncology, NCI-NIH 1987

Wolchok, Jedd D MD/PhD [Onc] - **Spec Exp:** Melanoma; Immunotherapy; Clinical Trials; Vaccine Therapy; **Hospital:** Meml Sloan-Kettering Cancer Ctr (page 75); **Address:** Meml Sloan-Kettering Cancer Ctr, 1275 York Ave, New York, NY 10065; **Phone:** 646-888-2395; **Board Cert:** Medical Oncology 2000; **Med School:** NYU Sch Med 1994; **Resid:** Internal Medicine, NYU Med Ctr 1996; **Fellow:** Medical Oncology, Meml Sloan-Kettering Canc Ctr 1997

Wolff, Antonio C MD [Onc] - **Spec Exp:** Breast Cancer; Drug Development; **Hospital:** Johns Hopkins Hosp; **Address:** 1650 Orleans St, rm 189, CRB-1 Bldg, Baltimore, MD 21231; **Phone:** 410-614-4192; **Board Cert:** Internal Medicine 2000; Medical Oncology 2000; **Med School:** Brazil 1986; **Resid:** Internal Medicine, Mt Sinai Med Ctr 1991; **Fellow:** Hematology & Oncology, Washington Univ Med Ctr 1992; Medical Oncology, Johns Hopkins Hosp 1995; **Fac Appt:** Assoc Prof Med, Johns Hopkins Univ

Zelenetz, Andrew D MD/PhD [Onc] - **Spec Exp:** Lymphoma; **Hospital:** Meml Sloan-Kettering Cancer Ctr (page 75); **Address:** 1275 York Avenue, New York, NY 10065; **Phone:** 800-525-2225; **Board Cert:** Medical Oncology 2009; **Med School:** Harvard Med Sch 1984; **Resid:** Internal Medicine, Stanford Univ Med Ctr 1986; **Fellow:** Medical Oncology, Stanford Univ Med Ctr 1991; **Fac Appt:** Asst Prof Med, Cornell Univ-Weill Med Coll

Southeast

Antonia, Scott J MD/PhD [Onc] - **Spec Exp:** Kidney Cancer; Lung Cancer; **Hospital:** H Lee Moffitt Cancer Ctr & Research Inst; **Address:** H Lee Moffitt Cancer Ctr, 12902 Magnolia Drive, Tampa, FL 33612; **Phone:** 813-979-3883; **Board Cert:** Internal Medicine 2002; Medical Oncology 2006; **Med School:** Univ Conn 1989; **Resid:** Internal Medicine, Yale-New Haven Hosp 1991; **Fellow:** Medical Oncology, Yale-New Haven Hosp 1994; **Fac Appt:** Assoc Prof Med, Univ S Fla Coll Med

Arteaga, Carlos L MD [Onc] - **Spec Exp:** Breast Cancer; **Hospital:** Vanderbilt Univ Med Ctr, TN Valley Healthcare Sys-Nashville; **Address:** Vanderbilt-Ingram Cancer Ctr, 2220 Pierce Ave, 777 Preston Rsch Bldg, Nashville, TN 37232-6838; **Phone:** 615-936-3524; **Board Cert:** Internal Medicine 1984; Medical Oncology 1989; **Med School:** Ecuador 1980; **Resid:** Internal Medicine, Grady Meml Hosp 1984; **Fellow:** Hematology & Oncology, Univ Texas Hlth Sci Ctr 1987; **Fac Appt:** Prof Med, Vanderbilt Univ

Balducci, Lodovico MD [Onc] - **Spec Exp:** Genitourinary Cancer; Breast Cancer; **Hospital:** H Lee Moffitt Cancer Ctr & Research Inst, Tampa Genl Hosp; **Address:** H Lee Moffitt Cancer Ctr, 12902 Magnolia Drive, Tampa, FL 33612; **Phone:** 813-745-8658; **Board Cert:** Internal Medicine 1987; Hematology 1978; Medical Oncology 1979; **Med School:** Italy 1968; **Resid:** Internal Medicine, Univ Miss Med Ctr 1976; Hematology & Oncology, Univ Miss Med Ctr 1979; **Fellow:** Internal Medicine, A Gemelli Genl Hosp 1970; **Fac Appt:** Prof Med, Univ S Fla Coll Med

Benedetto, Pasquale W MD [Onc] - **Spec Exp:** Genitourinary Cancer; Bone Tumors; Gastrointestinal Cancer; Pancreatic Cancer; **Hospital:** Univ of Miami Hosp & Clins/Sylvester Comp Canc Ctr (page 82), Jackson Meml Hosp (page 82); **Address:** Sylvester Comp Cancer Ctr, Med Oncology, 1475 NW 12th Ave, rm 3310, Miami, FL 33136; **Phone:** 305-243-1000; **Board Cert:** Internal Medicine 1979; Medical Oncology 1981; Hematology 1982; **Med School:** Cornell Univ-Weill Med Coll 1976; **Resid:** Internal Medicine, Johns Hopkins Hosp 1979; **Fellow:** Medical Oncology, Meml Sloan Kettering Cancer Ctr 1981; **Fac Appt:** Prof Med, Univ Miami Sch Med

Berlin, Jordan D MD [Onc] - **Spec Exp:** Gastrointestinal Cancer; Pancreatic Cancer; Liver Cancer; Clinical Trials; **Hospital:** Vanderbilt Univ Med Ctr; **Address:** Vanderbilt-Ingram Cancer Ctr, 777 Preston Rsch Bldg, Nashville, TN 37232-6307; **Phone:** 615-322-6053; **Board Cert:** Internal Medicine 2002; Medical Oncology 2005; **Med School:** Univ IL Coll Med 1989; **Resid:** Internal Medicine, Univ Cincinnati Med Ctr 1992; **Fellow:** Medical Oncology, Univ Wisconsin 1995; **Fac Appt:** Assoc Prof Med, Vanderbilt Univ

Bernard, Stephen A MD [Onc] - **Spec Exp:** Gastrointestinal Cancer; Palliative Care; Clinical Trials; **Hospital:** NC Memorial Hosp - UNC; **Address:** Univ North Carolina Sch Med, 170 Manning Drive, CB 7305, Chapel Hill, NC 27599; **Phone:** 919-966-0000; **Board Cert:** Internal Medicine 1987; Medical Oncology 1979; Hospice & Palliative Medicine 2008; **Med School:** Univ NC Sch Med 1973; **Resid:** Internal Medicine, Columbia-Presby Med Ctr 1976; **Fellow:** Hematology & Oncology, Wash Univ Hosps 1978; **Fac Appt:** Prof Med, Univ NC Sch Med

Blackwell, Kimberly L MD [Onc] - **Spec Exp:** Breast Cancer; Clinical Trials; **Hospital:** Duke Univ Hosp; **Address:** Duke Univ Medical Ctr, Box 3893, Durham, NC 27710; **Phone:** 919-668-6688; **Board Cert:** Medical Oncology 2000; **Med School:** Mayo Med Sch 1994; **Resid:** Internal Medicine, Duke Univ Med Ctr 1997; **Fellow:** Medical Oncology, Duke Univ Med Ctr 2000; **Fac Appt:** Assoc Prof Med, Duke Univ

Blobe, Gerard C MD/PhD [Onc] - **Spec Exp:** Pancreatic Cancer; Colon & Rectal Cancer; Clinical Trials; **Hospital:** Duke Univ Hosp; **Address:** Duke Univ Medical Ctr, Dept Hematology/Oncology, Box 91004, Durham, NC 27708; **Phone:** 919-668-6688; **Board Cert:** Internal Medicine 2009; Medical Oncology 2000; **Med School:** Duke Univ 1995; **Resid:** Internal Medicine, Brigham & Women's Hosp 1997; **Fellow:** Medical Oncology, Dana-Farber Cancer Inst 2000; **Fac Appt:** Assoc Prof Med, Duke Univ

Bolger, Graeme B MD [Onc] - **Spec Exp:** Prostate Cancer; Testicular Cancer; **Hospital:** Univ of Ala Hosp at Birmingham; **Address:** 1530 3rd Ave S, Ste FOT-1105, Birmingham, AL 35294; **Phone:** 205-934-2992; **Board Cert:** Internal Medicine 1984; Medical Oncology 2000; **Med School:** McGill Univ 1981; **Resid:** Internal Medicine, Johns Hopkins Hosp 1984; **Fellow:** Medical Oncology, Fred Hutchinson Cancer Rsch 1985; Oncology, Meml Sloan-Kettering Cancer Ctr 1992; **Fac Appt:** Assoc Prof Med, Univ Alabama

Medical Oncology

Boston, Barry MD [Onc] - **Spec Exp:** Gastrointestinal Cancer; Genitourinary Cancer; Prostate Cancer; **Hospital:** St. Francis Hosp - Memphis, Methodist Univ Hosp - Memphis; **Address:** Univ of Tennessee Cancer Inst, 7945 Wolf River Blvd, Ste 300, Germantown, TN 38138; **Phone:** 901-752-6131; **Board Cert:** Internal Medicine 1974; Medical Oncology 1977; **Med School:** Louisiana State U, New Orleans 1971; **Resid:** Internal Medicine, Univ Tenn Hosp-VA Hosp 1973; Hematology, Univ Tenn Hosp-VA Hosp 1973; **Fellow:** Medical Oncology, Yale-New Haven Hosp 1975; **Fac Appt:** Assoc Prof Med, Univ Tenn Coll Med

Brenin, Christiana M MD [Onc] - **Spec Exp:** Breast Cancer; Colon & Rectal Cancer; **Hospital:** Univ of Virginia Health Sys; **Address:** Univ Virginia Med Ctr, Division of Hematology/Oncology, PO Box 800716, Charlottesville, VA 22908; **Phone:** 434-924-8552; **Board Cert:** Internal Medicine 2003; Medical Oncology 2008; **Med School:** NY Med Coll 1990; **Resid:** Internal Medicine, Northwestern Meml Hosp 1993; **Fellow:** Hematology & Oncology, Northwestern Meml Hosp 1996; **Fac Appt:** Assoc Prof Med, Univ VA Sch Med

Burris III, Howard A MD [Onc] - **Spec Exp:** Drug Development; Drug Discovery; Breast Cancer; **Hospital:** Centennial Med Ctr, Baptist Hosp - Nashville; **Address:** Tennessee Oncology, 250 25th Ave N, Ste 100, Nashville, TN 37203; **Phone:** 615-986-4300; **Board Cert:** Internal Medicine 1988; Medical Oncology 2001; **Med School:** Univ S Ala Coll Med 1985; **Resid:** Internal Medicine, Brooke Army Med Ctr 1988; **Fellow:** Medical Oncology, Brooke Army Med Ctr 1991

Butler, William M MD [Onc] - **Spec Exp:** Breast Cancer; Prostate Cancer; Lung Cancer; Clinical Trials; **Hospital:** Palmetto Health Richland Mem Hosp; **Address:** SC Oncology Associates, 166 Stoneridge Drive, Columbia, SC 29210; **Phone:** 803-461-3000; **Board Cert:** Internal Medicine 1975; Medical Oncology 1979; Hematology 1980; **Med School:** Tulane Univ 1972; **Resid:** Internal Medicine, Charity Hosp 1975; **Fellow:** Hematology & Oncology, Walter Reed AMC 1980; **Fac Appt:** Clin Prof Med, Univ SC Sch Med

Carbone, David MD/PhD [Onc] - **Spec Exp:** Lung Cancer; **Hospital:** Vanderbilt Univ Med Ctr; **Address:** Vanderbilt-Ingram Cancer Ctr, 685 Preston Rsch Bldg, 2220 Pierce Ave, Nashville, TN 37232-6838; **Phone:** 615-936-1279; **Board Cert:** Internal Medicine 1988; Medical Oncology 2001; **Med School:** Johns Hopkins Univ 1985; **Resid:** Internal Medicine, Johns Hopkins Hosp 1988; **Fellow:** Oncology, Natl Cancer Inst 1991; **Fac Appt:** Prof Med, Vanderbilt Univ

Carey, Lisa A MD [Onc] - **Spec Exp:** Breast Cancer; **Hospital:** NC Memorial Hosp - UNC; **Address:** Univ North Carolina-Div Hem/Onc, 170 Manning Drive Fl 3rd, POB Campus Box 7305, Chapel Hill, NC 27599-7300; **Phone:** 919-966-4431; **Board Cert:** Internal Medicine 2003; Medical Oncology 2007; **Med School:** Johns Hopkins Univ 1990; **Resid:** Internal Medicine, Johns Hopkins Hosp 1993; **Fellow:** Oncology, Johns Hopkins Hosp 1996; **Fac Appt:** Asst Prof Med, Univ NC Sch Med

Carpenter Jr, John T MD [Onc] - **Spec Exp:** Breast Cancer; **Hospital:** Univ of Ala Hosp at Birmingham; **Address:** Univ Alabama Birmingham, 1530 3rd Ave S, Ste FOT-510, Birmingham, AL 35294-3300; **Phone:** 205-934-2084; **Board Cert:** Internal Medicine 1972; Hematology 1981; Medical Oncology 1975; **Med School:** Tulane Univ 1968; **Resid:** Internal Medicine, Grady Meml Hosp 1971; **Fellow:** Hematology & Oncology, Emory Univ 1973; **Fac Appt:** Prof Med, Univ Alabama

Chao, Nelson J MD [Onc] - **Spec Exp:** Bone Marrow Transplant; Lymphoma; Leukemia; **Hospital:** Duke Univ Hosp; **Address:** Duke Univ Med Ctr, Box 3961, Durham, NC 27710; **Phone:** 919-668-1002; **Board Cert:** Internal Medicine 1984; Medical Oncology 1987; **Med School:** Yale Univ 1981; **Resid:** Internal Medicine, Stanford Univ Med Ctr 1984; **Fellow:** Oncology, Stanford Univ Med Ctr 1987; **Fac Appt:** Prof Med, Duke Univ

Chung, Ki Young MD [Onc] - **Spec Exp:** Gastrointestinal Cancer; **Address:** Cancer Ctrs of the Carolinas-Spartanburg, 120 Dillon Drive, Spartanburg, SC 29307; **Phone:** 864-699-5700; **Board Cert:** Medical Oncology 2004; **Med School:** Univ NC Sch Med 1995; **Resid:** Internal Medicine, Johns Hopkins Hosp/Sinai Hosp; **Fellow:** Hematology & Oncology, Meml Sloan Kettering Cancer Ctr 2003

Colon-Otero, Gerardo MD [Onc] - **Spec Exp:** Ovarian Cancer; Breast Cancer; Hematologic Malignancies; Pancreatic Cancer-Acinar Cell; **Hospital:** Mayo - Jacksonville; **Address:** Mayo Clinic, 4500 San Pablo Rd S, Jacksonville, FL 32224-1865; **Phone:** 904-953-2000; **Board Cert:** Internal Medicine 1982; Hematology 1984; Medical Oncology 1985; **Med School:** Puerto Rico 1979; **Resid:** Internal Medicine, Mayo Clinic 1982; **Fellow:** Hematology, Mayo Clinic 1984; Medical Oncology, Univ Va Med Ctr 1986; **Fac Appt:** Assoc Prof Med, Mayo Med Sch

Conry, Robert M MD [Onc] - **Spec Exp:** Melanoma; Lung Cancer; Colon & Rectal Cancer; Sarcoma; **Hospital:** Univ of Ala Hosp at Birmingham; **Address:** The Kirklin Clinic At Acton Rd, 2145 Bonner Way, Birmingham, AL 35243; **Phone:** 205-978-0250; **Board Cert:** Hematology 2001; **Med School:** Univ Alabama 1987; **Resid:** Internal Medicine, Univ Alabama Hosp 1990; **Fellow:** Medical Oncology, Univ Alabama Hosp 1993; **Fac Appt:** Assoc Prof Med, Univ Alabama

Crawford, Jeffrey MD [Onc] - **Spec Exp:** Lung Cancer; **Hospital:** Duke Univ Hosp; **Address:** Duke Univ Med Ctr, Box 3476, Durham, NC 27710; **Phone:** 919-668-6688; **Board Cert:** Internal Medicine 1977; Hematology 1980; Medical Oncology 1981; **Med School:** Ohio State Univ 1974; **Resid:** Internal Medicine, Duke Univ Med Ctr 1977; **Fellow:** Hematology & Oncology, Duke Univ Med Ctr 1981; **Fac Appt:** Prof Med, Duke Univ

De Simone, Philip MD [Onc] - **Spec Exp:** Colon Cancer; Pancreatic Cancer; **Hospital:** Univ of Kentucky Albert B. Chandler Hosp; **Address:** UKMC Markey Cancer Ctr, 800 Rose St Fl 1, Whitney-Hendrickson bldg, Lexington, KY 40536; **Phone:** 859-323-8043; **Board Cert:** Internal Medicine 1972; Hematology 1974; **Med School:** Univ VT Coll Med 1967; **Resid:** Internal Medicine, Univ Kentucky Hosp 1972; **Fellow:** Hematology & Oncology, Univ Kentucky Hosp 1974; **Fac Appt:** Prof Med, Univ KY Coll Med

Dunphy II, Frank R MD [Onc] - **Spec Exp:** Lung Cancer; Head & Neck Cancer; **Hospital:** Duke Univ Hosp; **Address:** Duke Univ Med Ctr, Box 3685, Durham, NC 27710; **Phone:** 919-668-6688; **Board Cert:** Internal Medicine 1984; Hematology 1986; Medical Oncology 1989; **Med School:** Louisiana State U, New Orleans 1979; **Resid:** Internal Medicine, Lousiana St Univ Hosp 1983; **Fellow:** Hematology & Oncology, Louisiana St Univ Hosp 1985; **Fac Appt:** Assoc Prof Med, Duke Univ

Flinn, Ian W MD/PhD [Onc] - **Spec Exp:** Leukemia; Lymphoma; Bone Marrow Transplant; Multiple Myeloma; **Hospital:** Centennial Med Ctr; **Address:** Tennessee Oncology, 250 25th Ave N, Ste 412, Nashville, TN 37203; **Phone:** 615-986-7600; **Board Cert:** Hematology 2007; Medical Oncology 2008; **Med School:** Johns Hopkins Univ 1990; **Resid:** Internal Medicine, Univ Michigan Med Ctr 1993; **Fellow:** Hematology & Oncology, Johns Hopkins 1996

Forero, Andres MD [Onc] - **Spec Exp:** Lymphoma; **Hospital:** Univ of Ala Hosp at Birmingham; **Address:** 615 18th St S, Birmingham, AL 35233; **Phone:** 205-934-9999; **Med School:** Colombia 1982; **Resid:** Internal Medicine, Javeriana Univ 1987; **Fellow:** Medical Oncology, Javeriana Univ 1991; **Fac Appt:** Assoc Prof Med, Univ Alabama

Medical Oncology

Fracasso, Paula M MD/PhD [Onc] - **Spec Exp:** Gynecologic Cancer; Breast Cancer; **Hospital:** Univ of Virginia Health Sys; **Address:** Univ Virginia- Dept Medicine, PO Box 800716, Charlottesville, VA 22908; **Phone:** 434-243-6143; **Board Cert:** Internal Medicine 1987; Medical Oncology 2003; **Med School:** Yale Univ 1984; **Resid:** Internal Medicine, Beth Israel Hosp 1987; **Fellow:** Cancer Research, Mass Inst Tech 1989; Hematology & Oncology, Tufts-New England Med Ctr 1991; **Fac Appt:** Prof Med, Univ VA Sch Med

Friedman, Henry S MD [Onc] - **Spec Exp:** Neuro-Oncology; Brain & Spinal Cord Tumors; Gliomas; **Hospital:** Duke Univ Hosp; **Address:** Preston Robert Tisch, Brain Tumor Ctr at Duke, DUMC, Box 3624, Durham, NC 27710; **Phone:** 919-684-5301; **Board Cert:** Pediatrics 1982; Pediatric Hematology-Oncology 1982; **Med School:** SUNY Upstate Med Univ 1977; **Resid:** Pediatrics, SUNY Upstate Med Ctr 1980; **Fellow:** Pediatric Hematology-Oncology, Duke Univ Med Ctr 1983; **Fac Appt:** Prof Neuro-Onc, Duke Univ

Garst, Jennifer L MD [Onc] - **Spec Exp:** Lung Cancer; Thoracic Cancers; Cancer Survivors-Late Effects of Therapy; **Hospital:** Duke Univ Hosp; **Address:** Duke Univ Hosp, Div Medical Oncology, 2301 Erwin Rd, Box 3198, Durham, NC 27710; **Phone:** 919-681-6932; **Board Cert:** Internal Medicine 2008; **Med School:** Med Coll GA 1990; **Resid:** Internal Medicine, Univ SW Texas Hosp 1993; **Fellow:** Hematology & Oncology, Duke Univ Med Ctr 1996; **Fac Appt:** Assoc Prof Med, Duke Univ

George, Daniel J MD [Onc] - **Spec Exp:** Prostate Cancer; Kidney Cancer; **Hospital:** Duke Univ Hosp; **Address:** Duke Univ Med Ctr, Box 102002, Durham, NC 27710; **Phone:** 919-668-8108; **Board Cert:** Medical Oncology 2007; **Med School:** Duke Univ 1992; **Resid:** Internal Medicine, Johns Hopkins Hosp 1995; **Fellow:** Medical Oncology, Johns Hopkins Hosp 1998; **Fac Appt:** Assoc Prof S, Duke Univ

Gockerman, Jon Paul MD [Onc] - **Spec Exp:** Leukemia; Lymphoma; **Hospital:** Duke Univ Hosp; **Address:** Duke Univ Med Ctr, 1 Trent Drive, rm 25153, Box 3872, Morris Bldg, Durham, NC 27710; **Phone:** 919-684-8964; **Board Cert:** Internal Medicine 1972; Medical Oncology 1973; Hematology 1974; **Med School:** Univ Chicago-Pritzker Sch Med 1967; **Resid:** Internal Medicine, Duke Univ Med Ctr 1969; **Fellow:** Hematology & Oncology, Duke Univ Med Ctr 1971

Godley, Paul A MD/PhD [Onc] - **Spec Exp:** Prostate Cancer (advanced); Testicular Cancer; Penile Cancer; Bladder Cancer; **Hospital:** NC Memorial Hosp - UNC; **Address:** UNC Hematology/Oncology, POB, Campus Box 7305, 3rd Floor, 170 Manning Drive, Chapel Hill, NC 27599; **Phone:** 919-966-4431; **Board Cert:** Internal Medicine 1987; Medical Oncology 2002; **Med School:** Harvard Med Sch 1984; **Resid:** Internal Medicine, Univ Hosps 1987; **Fellow:** Epidemiology, Univ NC Sch of Public Hlth 1989; Hematology & Oncology, Univ NC Hosps 1991; **Fac Appt:** Assoc Prof Med, Univ NC Sch Med

Goldberg, Richard M MD [Onc] - **Spec Exp:** Stomach Cancer; Esophageal Cancer; Pancreatic Cancer; Neuroendocrine Tumors; **Hospital:** NC Memorial Hosp - UNC; **Address:** Division of Hematology/Oncology, CB 7305, 170 Manning Drive, Chapel Hill, NC 27599-0001; **Phone:** 919-843-7711; **Board Cert:** Internal Medicine 1982; Medical Oncology 1985; **Med School:** SUNY Upstate Med Univ 1979; **Resid:** Internal Medicine, Emory Univ Med Ctr 1982; **Fellow:** Medical Oncology, Georgetown Univ Med Ctr 1984; **Fac Appt:** Prof Med, Univ NC Sch Med

Graham II, Mark L MD [Onc] - **Spec Exp:** Breast Cancer; Breast Cancer Genetics; **Hospital:** WakeMed Cary; **Address:** Waverly Hematology/Oncology, 300 Ashville Ave, Ste 310, Cary, NC 27518; **Phone:** 919-233-8585; **Board Cert:** Internal Medicine 1989; **Med School:** Mayo Med Sch 1982; **Resid:** Internal Medicine, Duke Univ Med Ctr 1985; **Fellow:** Medical Oncology, Univ CO Hlth Sci Ctr 1990; Medical Oncology, Mayo Clinic 1991; **Fac Appt:** Assoc Clin Prof Med, Univ NC Sch Med

Greco, F Anthony MD [Onc] - **Spec Exp:** Lung Cancer; Unknown Primary Cancer; **Hospital:** Centennial Med Ctr; **Address:** Sarah Cannon Research Inst, 250 25th Ave N Atrium Bldg - Ste 100, Nashville, TN 37203; **Phone:** 615-320-5090; **Board Cert:** Internal Medicine 1975; Medical Oncology 1977; **Med School:** W VA Univ 1972; **Resid:** Internal Medicine, Univ West Virginia Hosp 1974; **Fellow:** Medical Oncology, Natl Cancer Inst 1976

Grosh, William W MD [Onc] - **Spec Exp:** Melanoma; Sarcoma; Neuroendocrine Tumors; **Hospital:** Univ of Virginia Health Sys; **Address:** UVA Health System, Div Hem/Oncology, PO Box 800716, Charlottesville, VA 22908; **Phone:** 434-924-1904; **Board Cert:** Internal Medicine 1978; Medical Oncology 1985; **Med School:** Columbia P&S 1974; **Resid:** Internal Medicine, Vanderbilt Univ Med Ctr 1977; **Fellow:** Medical Oncology, Vanderbilt Univ Med Ctr 1983; **Fac Appt:** Assoc Prof Med, Univ VA Sch Med

Hande, Kenneth R MD [Onc] - **Spec Exp:** Drug Discovery; Sarcoma; Carcinoid Tumors; **Hospital:** Vanderbilt Univ Med Ctr, TN Valley Healthcare Sys-Nashville; **Address:** Vanderbilt Univ Med Ctr, 2220 Pierce Ave, Div Hematology/Oncology, 777 Preston Rsch Bldg, Nashville, TN 37232-6307; **Phone:** 615-322-4967; **Board Cert:** Internal Medicine 1975; Medical Oncology 1977; **Med School:** Johns Hopkins Univ 1972; **Resid:** Internal Medicine, Barnes Hosp 1974; **Fellow:** Medical Oncology, Natl Cancer Inst 1977; **Fac Appt:** Prof Med, Vanderbilt Univ

Hurd, David MD [Onc] - **Spec Exp:** Lymphoma; Leukemia; Bone Marrow Transplant; **Hospital:** Wake Forest Univ Baptist Med Ctr; **Address:** Wake Forest Sch Med, Comp Cancer Ctr, Medical Center Boulevard, Winston-Salem, NC 27157-1082; **Phone:** 336-713-5440; **Board Cert:** Internal Medicine 1977; Medical Oncology 1981; **Med School:** Univ IL Coll Med 1974; **Resid:** Internal Medicine, Univ Minn Hosp 1977; **Fellow:** Medical Oncology, Univ Minn Hosp 1979; **Fac Appt:** Prof Med, Wake Forest Univ

Jahanzeb, Mohammad MD [Onc] - **Spec Exp:** Breast Cancer; Lung Cancer; **Hospital:** Boca Raton Regl Hosp; **Address:** 1192 E Newport Center Drive, Ste 200, Deerfield Beach, FL 33442; **Phone:** 954-698-3665; **Board Cert:** Medical Oncology 2003; Hematology 2005; **Med School:** Pakistan 1986; **Resid:** Internal Medicine, New Britain Genl Hosp 1990; **Fellow:** Hematology & Oncology, Washington Univ 1993; **Fac Appt:** Prof Med

Jillella, Anand MD [Onc] - **Spec Exp:** Bone Marrow Transplant; Leukemia; Lymphoma; Multiple Myeloma; **Hospital:** Med Coll of GA Hosp and Clin (MCG Health Inc); **Address:** Med Coll Ga - BMT Program, 1120 15th St, BAA 5407, Augusta, GA 30912-3125; **Phone:** 706-721-2505; **Board Cert:** Medical Oncology 2007; **Med School:** India 1985; **Resid:** Internal Medicine, Med Coll Georgia 1992; **Fellow:** Medical Oncology, Yale-New Haven Hosp 1996; **Fac Appt:** Prof Med, Med Coll GA

Khuri, Fadlo MD [Onc] - **Spec Exp:** Lung Cancer; Head & Neck Cancer; Thyroid Cancer; Mesothelioma; **Hospital:** Emory Univ Hosp, Grady Hlth Sys; **Address:** 1365 Clifton Road Rd NE, C Bldg Fl 3 - Ste C300, Atlanta, GA 30322; **Phone:** 404-778-1900; **Board Cert:** Medical Oncology 2008; **Med School:** Columbia P&S 1989; **Resid:** Internal Medicine, Boston City Hosp 1992; **Fellow:** Hematology & Oncology, New England Med Ctr-Tufts 1995; **Fac Appt:** Prof Hem & Onc, Emory Univ

Kraft, Andrew S MD [Onc] - **Spec Exp:** Prostate Cancer; Sarcoma; Drug Development; Clinical Trials; **Hospital:** MUSC Med Ctr; **Address:** 86 Jonathan Lucas St, PO BOX 250955, Charleston, SC 29425; **Phone:** 843-792-8284; **Board Cert:** Internal Medicine 1980; Medical Oncology 1985; **Med School:** Univ Pennsylvania 1975; **Resid:** Internal Medicine, Mt Sinai Hosp 1979; **Fellow:** Medical Oncology, Natl Cancer Inst 1983; **Fac Appt:** Prof Med, Med Univ SC

Medical Oncology

Kucuk, Omer MD [Onc] - **Spec Exp:** Genitourinary Cancer; Nutrition in Cancer Therapy; Prostate Cancer; Nutrition & Cancer Prevention/Control; **Hospital:** Emory Univ Hosp; **Address:** Emory Winship Cancer Inst, 1365C Clifton Rd, Ste 2110, Atlanta, GA 30322; **Phone:** 404-778-1900; **Board Cert:** Internal Medicine 1978; Hematology 1984; Medical Oncology 1989; **Med School:** Turkey 1975; **Resid:** Internal Medicine, St Francis Hosp 1978; **Fellow:** Hematology & Oncology, Northwestern Univ 1981; **Fac Appt:** Prof Hem & Onc, Emory Univ

Kvols, Larry K MD [Onc] - **Spec Exp:** Gastrointestinal Cancer; Carcinoid Tumors; Neuroendocrine Tumors; **Hospital:** H Lee Moffitt Cancer Ctr & Research Inst; **Address:** H Lee Moffitt Cancer Ctr & Research Inst, 12902 Magnolia Drive, FOB-2, Tampa, FL 33612; **Phone:** 813-745-7257; **Board Cert:** Internal Medicine 1976; Medical Oncology 1977; **Med School:** Baylor Coll Med 1970; **Resid:** Internal Medicine, Johns Hopkins Hosp 1972; **Fellow:** Hematology & Oncology, Johns Hopkins Hosp 1973; **Fac Appt:** Prof Med, Mayo Med Sch

Lawson, David H MD [Onc] - **Spec Exp:** Melanoma; **Hospital:** Emory Univ Hosp; **Address:** Emory Winship Cancer Institute, 1365 Clifton Rd NE C Bldg Fl 2, Atlanta, GA 30322; **Phone:** 404-778-1900; **Board Cert:** Internal Medicine 1977; Medical Oncology 1979; **Med School:** Emory Univ 1974; **Resid:** Internal Medicine, Emory Univ Hosps 1977; **Fellow:** Medical Oncology, Emory Univ 1979; **Fac Appt:** Assoc Prof Hem & Onc, Emory Univ

Lesser, Glenn J MD [Onc] - **Spec Exp:** Neuro-Oncology; Brain Tumors; **Hospital:** Wake Forest Univ Baptist Med Ctr; **Address:** Wake Forest Univ-Div Hematolgy/Oncology, Medical Center Blvd, Winston-Salem, NC 27157-1082; **Phone:** 336-713-5440; **Board Cert:** Medical Oncology 2007; **Med School:** Penn State Coll Med 1987; **Resid:** Internal Medicine, NC Baptist Hosp/Bowman Gray Sch Med 1991; **Fellow:** Medical Oncology, Johns Hopkins Hosp 1995; **Fac Appt:** Prof Hem & Onc, Wake Forest Univ

Lilenbaum, Rogerio MD [Onc] - **Spec Exp:** Lung Cancer; **Hospital:** Mount Sinai Med Ctr - Miami; **Address:** Mount Sinai Cancer Ctr, 4306 Alton Rd, Ste 3, Miami Beach, FL 33140-2840; **Phone:** 305-535-3310; **Board Cert:** Internal Medicine 2005; Hematology 2008; Medical Oncology 2007; **Med School:** Brazil 1986; **Resid:** Internal Medicine, Univ Hosp-Rio de Janeiro 1989; **Fellow:** Hematology & Oncology, Washington Univ Sch Med 1992; Oncology, UCSD 1994; **Fac Appt:** Assoc Clin Prof Med, Univ Miami Sch Med

Limentani, Steven A MD [Onc] - **Spec Exp:** Breast Cancer; Multiple Myeloma; Clinical Trials; **Hospital:** Carolinas Med Ctr; **Address:** 1100 S Tryon St, Ste 400, Charlotte, NC 28203; **Phone:** 704-446-9046; **Board Cert:** Internal Medicine 1989; Medical Oncology 2001; Hematology 2002; **Med School:** Tufts Univ 1986; **Resid:** Internal Medicine, New England Deaconess Hosp 1989; **Fellow:** Hematology & Oncology, New England Med Ctr 1992; **Fac Appt:** Clin Prof Med, Univ NC Sch Med

Lippman, Marc E MD [Onc] - **Spec Exp:** Breast Cancer; **Hospital:** Univ of Miami Hosp & Clins/Sylvester Comp Canc Ctr (page 82), Univ of Miami Hosp (page 82); **Address:** Leonard M Miller Sch Med, Dept Med, 1430 NW 11th Ave, rm 1001, Miami, FL 33136; **Phone:** 305-243-1000; **Board Cert:** Internal Medicine 1987; Endocrinology 1975; Medical Oncology 1977; **Med School:** Yale Univ 1968; **Resid:** Internal Medicine, Johns Hopkins Hosp 1970; **Fellow:** Medical Oncology, Natl Cancer Inst 1973; Endocrinology, Yale-New Haven Hosp 1974; **Fac Appt:** Prof Med, Univ Mich Med Sch

List, Alan F MD [Onc] - **Spec Exp:** Myelodysplastic Syndromes; Leukemia; **Hospital:** H Lee Moffitt Cancer Ctr & Research Inst; **Address:** 12902 Magnolia Drive, MCC-VP, Tampa, FL 33612-9497; **Phone:** 813-745-6086; **Board Cert:** Internal Medicine 1983; Medical Oncology 1985; Hematology 1986; **Med School:** Univ Pennsylvania 1980; **Resid:** Internal Medicine, Good Samaritan Hosp 1983; Oncology, Vanderbilt Univ Med Ctr 1985; **Fellow:** Hematology, Vanderbilt Univ Med Ctr 1986

Lossos, Izidore MD [Onc] - **Spec Exp:** Lymphoma; Hodgkin's Disease; Leukemia; Lymphomas-Rare; **Hospital:** Univ of Miami Hosp & Clins/Sylvester Comp Canc Ctr (page 82), Jackson Meml Hosp (page 82); **Address:** Univ Miami - Sylvester Comp Cancer Ctr, 1475 NW 12th Ave, D8-4, Miami, FL 33136; **Phone:** 305-243-4785; **Med School:** Israel 1987; **Resid:** Internal Medicine, Hadassah Univ Hosp 1995; **Fellow:** Hematology & Oncology, Hadassah Univ Hosp 1997; Medical Oncology, Stanford Univ 2001; **Fac Appt:** Prof Med, Univ Miami Sch Med

Lyckholm, Laurel J MD [Onc] - **Spec Exp:** Neuro-Oncology; **Hospital:** Med Coll of VA Hosp; **Address:** Med Coll of VA, Div Hem/Onc, PO Box 980292, Richmond, VA 23298; **Phone:** 804-828-7999; **Board Cert:** Internal Medicine 1989; Medical Oncology 2003; Hematology 2004; Hospice & Palliative Medicine 2008; **Med School:** Creighton Univ 1985; **Resid:** Internal Medicine, Creighton Univ 1989; **Fellow:** Hematology & Oncology, Univ IA Coll Med 1992; **Fac Appt:** Assoc Prof Med, Med Coll VA

Lyman, Gary H MD [Onc] - **Spec Exp:** Breast Cancer; **Hospital:** Duke Univ Hosp; **Address:** Duke Comprehensive Cancer Center, Hock Plaza, 2424 Erwin Rd, Ste 205, Durham, NC 27705; **Phone:** 919-668-6688; **Board Cert:** Internal Medicine 1987; Medical Oncology 1977; Hematology 1978; **Med School:** SUNY Buffalo 1972; **Resid:** Internal Medicine, Univ North Carolina Hosp 1974; **Fellow:** Medical Oncology, Roswell Park Meml Inst 1976; Biostatistics, Harvard Med Sch 1982; **Fac Appt:** Prof Med, Duke Univ

Lynch Jr, James W MD [Onc] - **Spec Exp:** Lymphoma; Immunotherapy; Lung Cancer; **Hospital:** Shands at Univ of FL; **Address:** Shands Hlthcare, Div Hematology/Oncology, PO Box 100383, Gainesville, FL 32610-0383; **Phone:** 352-265-0725; **Board Cert:** Internal Medicine 1987; Medical Oncology 2001; **Med School:** Eastern VA Med Sch 1984; **Resid:** Internal Medicine, Univ Florida 1987; **Fellow:** Medical Oncology, Natl Cancer Inst 1991; **Fac Appt:** Prof Med, Univ Fla Coll Med

Marcom, Paul K MD [Onc] - **Spec Exp:** Breast Cancer; Clinical Trials; Cancer Genetics; **Hospital:** Duke Univ Hosp; **Address:** Duke Univ Med Ctr, Box 3476, Durham, NC 27710; **Phone:** 919-668-6688; **Board Cert:** Internal Medicine 2003; Medical Oncology 2005; **Med School:** Baylor Coll Med 1989; **Resid:** Internal Medicine, Duke Univ Med Ctr 1992; Hematology & Oncology, Duke Univ Med Ctr 1995; **Fac Appt:** Assoc Prof Med, Duke Univ

Miller, Antonius A MD [Onc] - **Spec Exp:** Lung Cancer; **Hospital:** Wake Forest Univ Baptist Med Ctr; **Address:** Wake Forest University, Comprehensive Cancer Center, Medical Center Blvd, Winston-Salem, NC 27157; **Phone:** 336-713-4392; **Med School:** Germany 1977; **Resid:** Internal Medicine, Univ Essen Med Sch 1979; Internal Medicine, Univ TN Med Ctr 1987; **Fellow:** Hematology & Oncology, UT MD Anderson Cancer Ctr 1981; **Fac Appt:** Prof Med, Wake Forest Univ

Miller, Donald M MD/PhD [Onc] - **Spec Exp:** Melanoma; Lung Cancer; **Hospital:** Univ of Louisville Hosp; **Address:** 529 S Jackson St, Louisville, KY 40202; **Phone:** 502-562-4790; **Board Cert:** Internal Medicine 1979; **Med School:** Duke Univ 1973; **Resid:** Internal Medicine, Peter Bent Brigham Hosp 1975; **Fellow:** Internal Medicine, Peter Bent Brigham Hosp 1978; Medical Oncology, Natl Cancer Inst 1979; **Fac Appt:** Prof Med, Univ Louisville Sch Med

Moore, Joseph O MD [Onc] - **Spec Exp:** Leukemia; Hodgkin's Disease; Lymphoma, Non-Hodgkin's; Neuroendocrine Tumors; **Hospital:** Duke Univ Hosp; **Address:** Duke Univ Med Ctr, Box 3872, Durham, NC 27710; **Phone:** 919-684-8964; **Board Cert:** Internal Medicine 1975; Medical Oncology 1977; **Med School:** Johns Hopkins Univ 1970; **Resid:** Internal Medicine, Johns Hopkins Hosp 1975; **Fellow:** Hematology & Oncology, Duke Univ Med Ctr 1977; **Fac Appt:** Prof Med, Duke Univ

Medical Oncology

Morgan, David S MD [Onc] - **Spec Exp:** Lymphoma & Leukemia; Hodgkin's Disease; Bone Marrow Transplant; **Hospital:** Vanderbilt Univ Med Ctr; **Address:** Vanderbilt University Medical Center, 2220 Pierce Ave, 777 Preston Research Bldg, Nashville, TN 37232-6307; **Phone:** 615-936-8422; **Board Cert:** Internal Medicine 2003; Medical Oncology 2008; **Med School:** Vanderbilt Univ 1990; **Resid:** Internal Medicine, Yale-New Haven Hosp 1993; **Fellow:** Medical Oncology, Stanford Univ Med Ctr 1997; **Fac Appt:** Asst Prof Med, Vanderbilt Univ

Muss, Hyman B MD [Onc] - **Spec Exp:** Breast Cancer; **Hospital:** NC Memorial Hosp - UNC; **Address:** Div of Hem/Onc, Physicians Office Bldg, 170 Manning Drive Fl 3 - rm 3120, Box 7305, Chapel Hill, NC 27599-7305; **Phone:** 919-966-0840; **Board Cert:** Internal Medicine 1973; Hematology 1974; Medical Oncology 1975; **Med School:** SUNY Downstate 1968; **Resid:** Internal Medicine, Peter Bent Brigham Hosp 1970; **Fellow:** Hematology & Oncology, Peter Bent Brigham Hosp 1974; Hematology & Oncology, Dana-Farber Cancer Ctr 1974; **Fac Appt:** Prof Med, Univ NC Sch Med

Nabell, Lisle M MD [Onc] - **Spec Exp:** Breast Cancer; Head & Neck Cancer; **Hospital:** Univ of Ala Hosp at Birmingham; **Address:** Univ of Alabama, 1530 3rd Ave S, Ste NP2540B, Birmingham, AL 35294; **Phone:** 205-934-3061; **Board Cert:** Internal Medicine 2000; Medical Oncology 2000; **Med School:** Univ NC Sch Med 1987; **Resid:** Internal Medicine, Univ Alabama Hosp 1990; **Fellow:** Hematology & Oncology, Univ Alabama Hosp 1992; **Fac Appt:** Assoc Prof Med, Univ Alabama

O'Regan, Ruth M MD [Onc] - **Spec Exp:** Breast Cancer; Breast Cancer Risk Assessment; Cancer Prevention; Clinical Trials; **Hospital:** Emory Univ Hosp; **Address:** Emory Winship Cancer Inst, 1365C Clifton Rd NE Fl 2, Atlanta, GA 30322; **Phone:** 404-778-1900; **Board Cert:** Medical Oncology 2000; **Med School:** Ireland 1988; **Resid:** Internal Medicine, Med Coll Wisconsin 1995; Medical Oncology, Northwestern Univ Hosp 1999; **Fellow:** Medical Oncology, Northwestern Univ 1998; **Fac Appt:** Assoc Prof Hem & Onc, Emory Univ

Pao, William MD/PhD [Onc] - **Spec Exp:** Thoracic Cancers; Lung Cancer; **Hospital:** Vanderbilt Univ Med Ctr; **Address:** 2220 Pierce Ave, rm 777 PRB, Nashville, TN 37232-6307; **Phone:** 615-322-3524; **Board Cert:** Internal Medicine 2001; Medical Oncology 2003; **Med School:** Yale Univ 1998; **Resid:** Internal Medicine, New York Hosp 2000; **Fellow:** Medical Oncology, Meml Sloan Kettering Canc Ctr 2004; **Fac Appt:** Assoc Prof Med, Vanderbilt Univ

Pasche, Boris C MD/PhD [Onc] - **Spec Exp:** Colon Cancer; Gastrointestinal Cancer; **Hospital:** Univ of Ala Hosp at Birmingham; **Address:** 2000 Morris Ave, Ste 1610, Birmingham, AL 35203; **Phone:** 205-934-9591; **Board Cert:** Medical Oncology 2008; **Med School:** Sweden 1986; **Resid:** Internal Medicine, NY Hosp/Cornell Med Ctr 1994; **Fellow:** Hematology & Oncology, Meml Sloan Kettering Cancer Ctr 1996; **Fac Appt:** Prof Med, Univ Alabama

Pegram, Mark D MD [Onc] - **Spec Exp:** Breast Cancer; Breast Cancer-Novel Therapies; **Hospital:** Univ of Miami Hosp & Clins/Sylvester Comp Canc Ctr (page 82); **Address:** UMHC/Sylvester Comp Cancer Ctr, 1475 NW 12th Ave, Miami, FL 33136; **Phone:** 305-243-1000; **Board Cert:** Internal Medicine 1989; Medical Oncology 2003; **Med School:** Univ NC Sch Med 1986; **Resid:** Internal Medicine, Parkland Meml Hosp 1989; **Fellow:** Hematology & Oncology, UCLA Med Ctr 1993; **Fac Appt:** Prof Med, Univ Miami Sch Med

Perez, Edith A MD [Onc] - **Spec Exp:** Breast Cancer; Breast Cancer Risk Assessment; Clinical Trials; **Hospital:** Mayo - Jacksonville; **Address:** Mayo Clinic-Jacksonville, 4500 San Pablo Rd Davis Bldg Fl 8, Jacksonville, FL 32224; **Phone:** 904-953-7283; **Board Cert:** Internal Medicine 1983; Hematology 1986; Medical Oncology 1987; **Med School:** Univ Puerto Rico 1979; **Resid:** Internal Medicine, Loma Linda Univ Med Ctr 1982; **Fellow:** Hematology & Oncology, Martinez VA Hosp/UC Davis 1987; **Fac Appt:** Prof Med, Mayo Med Sch

Posey III, James A MD [Onc] - **Spec Exp:** Gastrointestinal Cancer; Colon Cancer; Liver Cancer; Biliary Cancer; **Hospital:** Univ of Ala Hosp at Birmingham; **Address:** 1882 6th Ave S, NP-2540U, Birmingham, AL 35294-3300; **Phone:** 205-934-0916; **Board Cert:** Medical Oncology 1997; **Med School:** Howard Univ 1991; **Resid:** Internal Medicine, Georgetown Univ Med Ctr 1994; **Fellow:** Hematology & Oncology, Georgetown Univ Med Ctr 1997; **Fac Appt:** Assoc Prof Med, Univ Alabama

Ready, Neal E MD/PhD [Onc] - **Spec Exp:** Lung Cancer; Head & Neck Cancer; Clinical Trials; **Hospital:** Duke Univ Hosp; **Address:** Duke Univ Medical Ctr, DUMC, Box 3198, Durham, NC 27710; **Phone:** 919-668-6688; **Board Cert:** Internal Medicine 1989; Hematology 2005; Medical Oncology 2005; **Med School:** Vanderbilt Univ 1986; **Resid:** Internal Medicine, Rhode Island Hosp 1989; **Fellow:** Hematology, Rhode Island Hosp 1992; Medical Oncology, New England Med Ctr 1994

Reed, Eddie MD [Onc] - **Spec Exp:** Ovarian Cancer; Prostate Cancer; **Hospital:** Univ of S AL Med Ctr; **Address:** USA Mitchell Cancer Institute, 1660 Springhill Ave, Mobile, AL 36604; **Phone:** 251-665-8000; **Board Cert:** Internal Medicine 1982; **Med School:** Yale Univ 1979; **Resid:** Internal Medicine, Stanford Univ Med Ctr 1982; **Fellow:** Medical Oncology, Natl Cancer Inst 1985; **Fac Appt:** Prof Med, Univ S Ala Coll Med

Robert, Nicholas J MD [Onc] - **Spec Exp:** Breast Cancer; **Hospital:** Inova Fairfax Hosp; **Address:** 8503 Arlington Blvd, Ste 400, Fairfax, VA 22031; **Phone:** 703-280-5390; **Board Cert:** Internal Medicine 1978; Anatomic Pathology 1979; Medical Oncology 1981; Hematology 1984; **Med School:** McGill Univ 1974; **Resid:** Internal Medicine, Royal Victoria Hosp 1976; Pathology, Mass Genl Hosp 1979; **Fellow:** Hematology, Peter Bent Brigham Hosp 1980; Medical Oncology, Dana Farber Cancer Inst 1981

Robert-Vizcarrondo, Francisco MD [Onc] - **Spec Exp:** Lung Cancer; Mesothelioma; Drug Development; Clinical Trials; **Hospital:** Univ of Ala Hosp at Birmingham; **Address:** 1802 6th Ave S, rm NP-2555D, Birmingham, AL 35294-3300; **Phone:** 205-934-5077; **Board Cert:** Internal Medicine 1973; Medical Oncology 1975; Hematology 1976; **Med School:** Puerto Rico 1969; **Resid:** Internal Medicine, Univ PR Hosp 1972; Hematology, Univ PR Hosp 1974; **Fellow:** Medical Oncology, Univ AL Hosp at Birmingham 1976; **Fac Appt:** Prof Med, Univ Alabama

Romond, Edward H MD [Onc] - **Spec Exp:** Breast Cancer; **Hospital:** Univ of Kentucky Albert B. Chandler Hosp; **Address:** Univ Kentucky Med Ctr, Div Hematology/Oncology, CC413 Markey Cancer Center, Lexington, KY 40536; **Phone:** 859-323-8043; **Board Cert:** Internal Medicine 1980; Hematology 1984; Medical Oncology 1983; **Med School:** Univ KY Coll Med 1977; **Resid:** Internal Medicine, Michigan State Univ Hosps 1980; **Fellow:** Hematology & Oncology, Michigan State Univ 1983; **Fac Appt:** Prof Med, Univ KY Coll Med

Schwartz, Michael A MD [Onc] - **Spec Exp:** Breast Cancer; Lymphoma; Colon Cancer; **Hospital:** Mount Sinai Med Ctr - Miami; **Address:** 4306 Alton Rd Fl 3, Miami Beach, FL 33140; **Phone:** 305-535-3310; **Board Cert:** Internal Medicine 1989; Medical Oncology 2004; Hematology 2004; **Med School:** UMDNJ-RW Johnson Med Sch 1986; **Resid:** Internal Medicine, Mt Sinai Medical Ctr 1989; **Fellow:** Hematology & Oncology, Meml Sloan Kettering Cancer Ctr 1992; **Fac Appt:** Asst Clin Prof Med, Univ Miami Sch Med

Serody, Jonathan S MD [Onc] - **Spec Exp:** Breast Cancer Vaccine Therapy; Clinical Trials; Lymphoma; **Hospital:** NC Memorial Hosp - UNC; **Address:** Lineberger Comprehensive Cancer Ctr, 450 West Drive, CB 7295, Chapel Hill, NC 27599-7295; **Phone:** 919-966-8644; **Board Cert:** Internal Medicine 1989; Hematology 2007; **Med School:** Univ VA Sch Med 1986; **Resid:** Internal Medicine, Univ NC Med Ctr 1989; **Fellow:** Hematology, Univ NC Med Ctr 1992; Bone Marrow Transplant, Fred Hutchinson Transplant Program 1993; **Fac Appt:** Assoc Prof Med, Univ NC Sch Med

Medical Oncology

Shea, Thomas MD [Onc] - **Spec Exp:** Bone Marrow Transplant; Lymphoma; Leukemia; **Hospital:** NC Memorial Hosp - UNC; **Address:** Univ N Carolina, Dept Medicine, 170 Manning Drive, CB 7305, Chapel Hill, NC 27599; **Phone:** 919-966-7746; **Board Cert:** Internal Medicine 1982; Hematology 1984; Medical Oncology 1985; **Med School:** Univ NC Sch Med 1978; **Resid:** Internal Medicine, Beth Israel Deaconess Med Ctr 1982; **Fellow:** Hematology & Oncology, Beth Israel Deaconess Med Ctr 1985; Bone Marrow Transplant, Dana Farber Cancer Inst 1988; **Fac Appt:** Prof Med, Univ NC Sch Med

Sherman, Carol A MD [Onc] - **Spec Exp:** Lung Cancer; Thoracic Cancers; **Hospital:** MUSC Med Ctr; **Address:** 96 Jonathan Lucas St, Ste CSB-903, Charleston, SC 29425; **Phone:** 843-792-9621; **Board Cert:** Internal Medicine 1987; Medical Oncology 1989; **Med School:** Univ Mass Sch Med 1984; **Resid:** Internal Medicine, Univ Mass Med Ctr 1987; **Fellow:** Hematology & Oncology, Univ Mass Med Ctr 1989; **Fac Appt:** Assoc Prof Med, Med Univ SC

Shin, Dong Moon MD [Onc] - **Spec Exp:** Head & Neck Cancer; Mesothelioma; Thymoma; Lung Cancer; **Hospital:** Emory Univ Hosp; **Address:** Emory Winship Cancer Inst, 1365 C Clifton Rd NE, Ste 3094, Atlanta, GA 30322; **Phone:** 404-778-5990; **Board Cert:** Internal Medicine 1985; Medical Oncology 1989; **Med School:** South Korea 1975; **Resid:** Internal Medicine, Cook Co Hosp 1985; **Fellow:** Medical Oncology, UT- MD Anderson Cancer Ctr 1988; **Fac Appt:** Prof Med, Emory Univ

Simon, George R MD [Onc] - **Spec Exp:** Mesothelioma; Lung Cancer; Thymoma; **Hospital:** MUSC Med Ctr; **Address:** 96 Jonathan Lucas St, CSB Bldg, Ste 903, Charleston, SC 29425-6350; **Phone:** 843-792-8584; **Board Cert:** Internal Medicine 2007; Medical Oncology 2007; **Med School:** India 1986; **Resid:** Internal Medicine, St Joseph's Hosp 1995; **Fellow:** Hematology & Oncology, Univ Colorado Hlth Sciences Ctr 1997; **Fac Appt:** Assoc Prof Med, Med Univ SC

Smith, Thomas Joseph MD [Onc] - **Spec Exp:** Breast Cancer; Palliative Care; **Hospital:** VCU Med Ctr; **Address:** Massey Cancer Ctr, 9000 Stony Point Pkwy, Richmond, VA 23235; **Phone:** 804-327-8806; **Board Cert:** Internal Medicine 1982; Medical Oncology 1987; Hospice & Palliative Medicine 2008; **Med School:** Yale Univ 1979; **Resid:** Internal Medicine, Hosp Univ Penn 1982; **Fellow:** Medical Oncology, Med Coll Virginia 1987; **Fac Appt:** Prof Med, Va Commonwealth Univ Sch Med

Socinski, Mark A MD [Onc] - **Spec Exp:** Lung Cancer; **Hospital:** NC Memorial Hosp - UNC; **Address:** UNC Chapel Hill, Div Hem/Onc, 170 Manning Drive, Physicians Bldg, CB 7305, Chapel Hill, NC 27599-7305; **Phone:** 919-966-0000; **Board Cert:** Internal Medicine 1988; Medical Oncology 2002; **Med School:** Univ VT Coll Med 1984; **Resid:** Internal Medicine, Beth Israel Hosp 1986; **Fellow:** Medical Oncology, Dana-Farber Cancer Inst 1989; **Fac Appt:** Assoc Prof Med, Univ NC Sch Med

Sosman, Jeffrey MD [Onc] - **Spec Exp:** Melanoma; Skin Cancer; Immunotherapy; Drug Discovery; **Hospital:** Vanderbilt Univ Med Ctr; **Address:** Vanderbilt-Ingram Cancer Ctr, 777 Preston Rsch Bldg, Nashville, TN 37232-6307; **Phone:** 615-322-6053; **Board Cert:** Anatomic Pathology 1985; Internal Medicine 1987; Medical Oncology 1989; **Med School:** Albert Einstein Coll Med 1981; **Resid:** Anatomic Pathology, Univ Chicago Hosps 1985; Internal Medicine, Univ Wisconsin Hosp 1986; **Fellow:** Medical Oncology, Univ Wisconsin 1989; **Fac Appt:** Prof Med, Vanderbilt Univ

Sotomayor, Eduardo M MD [Onc] - **Spec Exp:** Lymphoma; Gene Therapy; Vaccine Therapy; Clinical Trials; **Hospital:** H Lee Moffitt Cancer Ctr & Research Inst; **Address:** H Lee Moffitt Cancer Inst, 12902 Magnolia Drive, FOB 3, rm 5.3125, Tampa, FL 33612; **Phone:** 813-745-1387; **Board Cert:** Medical Oncology 2009; **Med School:** Peru 1988; **Resid:** Internal Medicine, Univ Miami Sch Med 1995; **Fellow:** Immunology, Univ Miami Sch Med 1989; Oncology, Johns Hopkins Hosp 1998; **Fac Appt:** Assoc Prof Med, Univ S Fla Coll Med

Stone, Joel A MD [Onc] - **Spec Exp:** Lung Cancer; Breast Cancer; **Hospital:** St. Vincent's Med Ctr - Jacksonville; **Address:** N Florida Hematology/Oncology Assocs, 2 Shircliff Way, Ste 800, Jacksonville, FL 32204; **Phone:** 904-388-2619; **Board Cert:** Internal Medicine 1977; Medical Oncology 1979; **Med School:** Univ VA Sch Med 1974; **Resid:** Internal Medicine, Univ KY Med Ctr 1977; **Fellow:** Hematology & Oncology, Emory Univ Hosp 1979

Sutton, Linda Marie MD [Onc] - **Spec Exp:** Breast Cancer; Palliative Care; **Hospital:** Duke Univ Hosp; **Address:** University Tower, 3100 Tower Blvd, Ste 600, Durham, NC 27707; **Phone:** 919-419-5005; **Board Cert:** Internal Medicine 2002; Medical Oncology 2003; **Med School:** Univ Mass Sch Med 1987; **Resid:** Internal Medicine, Montefiore Med Ctr 1990; **Fellow:** Hematology & Oncology, Duke Univ Med Ctr 1993

Thigpen, James T MD [Onc] - **Spec Exp:** Gynecologic Cancer; Breast Cancer; Lung Cancer; **Hospital:** Univ Mississippi Med Ctr; **Address:** Univ Mississippi Med Ctr, Div Med Onc, 2500 N State St, Jackson, MS 39216; **Phone:** 601-984-5590; **Board Cert:** Internal Medicine 1972; Hematology 1974; Medical Oncology 1975; **Med School:** Univ Miss 1969; **Resid:** Internal Medicine, Univ Miss Med Ctr 1971; **Fellow:** Hematology & Oncology, Univ Miss Med Ctr 1973; **Fac Appt:** Prof Med, Univ Miss

Torti, Frank M MD [Onc] - **Spec Exp:** Prostate Cancer; Urologic Cancer; **Hospital:** Wake Forest Univ Baptist Med Ctr; **Address:** Wake Forest Med Ctr-Comp Cancer Ctr, Medical Center Blvd, Winston-Salem, NC 27157-1082; **Phone:** 336-716-7971; **Board Cert:** Internal Medicine 1978; Medical Oncology 1979; **Med School:** Harvard Med Sch 1974; **Resid:** Internal Medicine, Beth Israel Hosp 1976; **Fellow:** Medical Oncology, Stanford Univ Med Ctr 1979; **Fac Appt:** Prof Med, Wake Forest Univ

Troner, Michael MD [Onc] - **Spec Exp:** Head & Neck Cancer; Urologic Cancer; **Hospital:** Baptist Hosp of Miami; **Address:** 8940 N Kendall Drive, Ste 300, East Tower, Miami, FL 33176; **Phone:** 305-595-2141; **Board Cert:** Internal Medicine 1972; Medical Oncology 1973; **Med School:** SUNY Downstate 1968; **Resid:** Internal Medicine, Univ Maryland Hosp 1971; **Fellow:** Medical Oncology, Univ Miami Med Ctr 1973; **Fac Appt:** Assoc Clin Prof Med, Univ Miami Sch Med

Vance, Ralph MD [Onc] - **Spec Exp:** Lung Cancer; **Hospital:** Univ Mississippi Med Ctr; **Address:** Univ Mississippi Med Ctr, Div Med Onc, 2500 N State St, Jackson, MS 39216; **Phone:** 601-984-5590; **Med School:** Univ Miss 1972; **Resid:** Internal Medicine, Univ Hosp; **Fellow:** Hematology & Oncology, Univ Hosp; **Fac Appt:** Prof Med, Univ Miss

Vaughan, William P MD [Onc] - **Spec Exp:** Bone Marrow Transplant; Breast Cancer; **Hospital:** Univ of Ala Hosp at Birmingham; **Address:** Tinsley Harrison Twr, 1530 3rd Ave S, Birmingham, AL 35294; **Phone:** 205-934-1908; **Board Cert:** Internal Medicine 1975; Medical Oncology 1979; **Med School:** Univ Conn 1972; **Resid:** Internal Medicine, Univ Chicago Hosps 1975; **Fellow:** Oncology, Johns Hopkins Hosp 1977; **Fac Appt:** Prof Med, Univ Alabama

Vredenburgh, James J MD [Onc] - **Spec Exp:** Brain Tumors; Gliomas; Brain Tumors-Metastatic; **Hospital:** Duke Univ Hosp; **Address:** Duke Univ Medical Ctr, Brain Tumor Ctr, Box 3624, Durham, NC 27710; **Phone:** 919-668-2993; **Board Cert:** Internal Medicine 1986; Hematology 1988; Medical Oncology 1989; **Med School:** Univ VT Coll Med 1983; **Resid:** Internal Medicine, St Francis Med Ctr 1986; **Fellow:** Hematology & Oncology, Dartmouth-Hitchcock Med Ctr 1989; **Fac Appt:** Prof Med, Duke Univ

Waller, Edmund K MD [Onc] - **Spec Exp:** Bone Marrow & Stem Cell Transplant; **Hospital:** Emory Univ Hosp; **Address:** 1365 Clifton Rd NE, C Bldg, Atlanta, GA 30322; **Phone:** 404-778-4342; **Board Cert:** Internal Medicine 1988; Medical Oncology 2006; **Med School:** Cornell Univ-Weill Med Coll 1985; **Resid:** Internal Medicine, Stanford Univ Med Ctr 1988; **Fellow:** Oncology, Stanford Univ Med Ctr 1992; **Fac Appt:** Prof Hem & Onc, Emory Univ

Medical Oncology

Weber, Jeffrey S MD/PhD [Onc] - **Spec Exp:** Melanoma; **Hospital:** H Lee Moffitt Cancer Ctr & Research Inst; **Address:** H Lee Moffitt Cancer Ctr, 12902 Magnolia Ave, MS SRB-2, Tampa, FL 33612; **Phone:** 813-745-2691; **Board Cert:** Internal Medicine 1983; Medical Oncology 1987; **Med School:** NYU Sch Med 1980; **Resid:** Internal Medicine, UCSD Med Ctr 1983; **Fellow:** Medical Oncology, Natl Cancer Inst 1990; **Fac Appt:** Assoc Prof Med, USC Sch Med

Weiss, Geoffrey R MD [Onc] - **Spec Exp:** Gastrointestinal Cancer; Genitourinary Cancer; Melanoma; **Hospital:** Univ of Virginia Health Sys; **Address:** Univ Virginia Hlth System, Div Hem/Onc, PO Box 800716, Charlottesville, VA 22908-0716; **Phone:** 434-243-0066; **Board Cert:** Internal Medicine 1977; Medical Oncology 1981; **Med School:** St Louis Univ 1974; **Resid:** Internal Medicine, Temple Univ Hosp 1978; **Fellow:** Medical Oncology, Dana Farber Cancer Inst 1982; **Fac Appt:** Prof Med, Univ VA Sch Med

Wingard, John R MD [Onc] - **Spec Exp:** Bone Marrow Transplant; Leukemia; Multiple Myeloma; Lymphoma; **Hospital:** Shands at Univ of FL; **Address:** Gainsville Clin, PO Box 100278, Gainesville, FL 32610; **Phone:** 352-265-0111 x29452; **Board Cert:** Internal Medicine 1977; Medical Oncology 1983; **Med School:** Johns Hopkins Univ 1973; **Resid:** Internal Medicine, Memphis City Hosps 1976; Internal Medicine, VA Hosp 1977; **Fellow:** Medical Oncology, Johns Hopkins Hosp 1979; **Fac Appt:** Prof Med, Univ Fla Coll Med

Yunus, Furhan MD [Onc] - **Spec Exp:** Multiple Myeloma; Lymphoma; **Hospital:** Methodist Univ Hosp - Memphis, Regional Med Ctr - Memphis; **Address:** Univ TN Cancer Inst, 1331 Union Ave, Ste 800, Memphis, TN 38104; **Phone:** 901-725-1785; **Board Cert:** Medical Oncology 2008; **Med School:** Pakistan 1986; **Resid:** Internal Medicine, Methodist Hosp 1993; **Fellow:** Hematology & Oncology, Univ Ariz Coll Med Affil Hosp 1995; **Fac Appt:** Asst Prof Med, Univ Tenn Coll Med

Midwest

Adelstein, David J MD [Onc] - **Spec Exp:** Head & Neck Cancer; Esophageal Cancer; Lung Cancer; **Hospital:** Cleveland Clin (page 70); **Address:** Cleveland Clinic, Taussig Cancer Inst, 9500 Euclid Ave, R35, Cleveland, OH 44195; **Phone:** 216-444-9310; **Board Cert:** Internal Medicine 1978; Medical Oncology 1981; Hematology 1982; **Med School:** NYU Sch Med 1975; **Resid:** Internal Medicine, Univ Hosps Cleveland 1978; **Fellow:** Hematology & Oncology, Univ Hosps Cleveland 1981; **Fac Appt:** Prof Med, Cleveland Cl Coll Med/Case West Res

Albain, Kathy S MD [Onc] - **Spec Exp:** Breast Cancer; Lung Cancer; Cancer Survivors-Late Effects of Therapy; **Hospital:** Loyola Univ Med Ctr; **Address:** Loyola-Bernardin Cancer Ctr, 2160 S First Ave, Bldg 112 - Ste 109, Maywood, IL 60153-5590; **Phone:** 708-327-3214; **Board Cert:** Internal Medicine 1981; Medical Oncology 1983; **Med School:** Univ Mich Med Sch 1978; **Resid:** Internal Medicine, Univ Illinois Med Ctr 1981; **Fellow:** Hematology & Oncology, Univ Chicago 1984; **Fac Appt:** Prof Med, Loyola Univ-Stritch Sch Med

Albertini, Mark R MD [Onc] - **Spec Exp:** Melanoma; Melanoma-Metastatic; **Hospital:** Univ WI Hosp & Clins; **Address:** Univ Wisconsin-Medical Oncology, 600 Highland Ave, Ste H4/534, Madison, WI 53792; **Phone:** 608-265-1700; **Board Cert:** Internal Medicine 1987; Medical Oncology 2002; **Med School:** Univ VT Coll Med 1984; **Resid:** Internal Medicine, Univ Wisc Hosps Clins 1987; **Fellow:** Medical Oncology, Univ Wisconsin 1991; **Fac Appt:** Assoc Prof Med, Univ Wisc

Anderson, Joseph M MD [Onc] - **Spec Exp:** Breast Cancer; Palliative Care; Neuro-Oncology; **Hospital:** Henry Ford Hosp; **Address:** 2799 W Grand Blvd, Ste K13, Detroit, MI 48202; **Phone:** 313-916-1854; **Board Cert:** Internal Medicine 1985; Medical Oncology 1989; **Med School:** Univ Mich Med Sch 1982; **Resid:** Internal Medicine, Henry Ford Hosp 1986; **Fellow:** Medical Oncology, Henry Ford Hosp 1988

Benson III, Al B MD [Onc] - **Spec Exp:** Colon Cancer; Gastrointestinal Cancer; Liver Cancer; Pancreatic Cancer; **Hospital:** Northwestern Meml Hosp, Jesse Brown VA Med Ctr; **Address:** Northwestern Div Hematology/Oncology, 676 N St Clair St, Ste 850, Chicago, IL 60611; **Phone:** 312-695-0990; **Board Cert:** Internal Medicine 1979; Medical Oncology 1983; **Med School:** SUNY Buffalo 1976; **Resid:** Internal Medicine, Univ Wisc Hosps 1979; **Fellow:** Medical Oncology, Univ Wisc Hosps 1984; **Fac Appt:** Prof Med, Northwestern Univ

Bitran, Jacob D MD [Onc] - **Spec Exp:** Breast Cancer; Bone Marrow Transplant; Lung Cancer; **Hospital:** Adv Luth Genl Hosp; **Address:** Lutheran Genl Cancer Care Specialists, 1700 Luther Lane, Park Ridge, IL 60068-1270; **Phone:** 866-611-1991; **Board Cert:** Internal Medicine 1974; Medical Oncology 1977; Hematology 1986; **Med School:** Univ IL Coll Med 1971; **Resid:** Pathology, Rush Presby St Lukes Hosp 1973; Internal Medicine, Michael Reese Hosp 1975; **Fellow:** Hematology & Oncology, Univ Chicago Hosps 1977; **Fac Appt:** Prof Med, Ros Franklin Univ/Chicago Med Sch

Bolwell, Brian J MD [Onc] - **Spec Exp:** Bone Marrow Transplant; Hematologic Malignancies; **Hospital:** Cleveland Clin (page 70); **Address:** 9500 Euclid Ave, Desk R32, Cleveland, OH 44195; **Phone:** 216-444-6922; **Board Cert:** Internal Medicine 1985; Medical Oncology 1987; **Med School:** Case West Res Univ 1981; **Resid:** Internal Medicine, Univ Hosp 1984; **Fellow:** Hematology & Oncology, Hosp Univ Penn 1987; **Fac Appt:** Prof Med, Cleveland Cl Coll Med/Case West Res

Bonomi, Philip D MD [Onc] - **Spec Exp:** Lung Cancer; Thymoma; Mesothelioma; **Hospital:** Rush Univ Med Ctr; **Address:** Rush University Medical Center, 1725 W Harrison St, Ste 824, Chicago, IL 60612; **Phone:** 312-942-5904; **Board Cert:** Internal Medicine 1975; Medical Oncology 1977; **Med School:** Univ IL Coll Med 1970; **Resid:** Internal Medicine, Geisinger Med Ctr 1972; Internal Medicine, Geisinger Med Ctr 1975; **Fellow:** Medical Oncology, Rush Presby-St Luke's Med Ctr 1977; **Fac Appt:** Prof Med, Rush Med Coll

Borden, Ernest C MD [Onc] - **Spec Exp:** Melanoma; Immunotherapy; Sarcoma; Vaccine Therapy; **Hospital:** Cleveland Clin (page 70); **Address:** 9500 Euclid Ave, Desk R40, Cleveland, OH 44195; **Phone:** 216-444-8183; **Board Cert:** Internal Medicine 1973; Medical Oncology 1975; **Med School:** Duke Univ 1966; **Resid:** Internal Medicine, Hosp Univ Penn 1968; **Fellow:** Medical Oncology, Johns Hopkins Hosp 1973; **Fac Appt:** Prof Med, Cleveland Cl Coll Med/Case West Res

Brockstein, Bruce E MD [Onc] - **Spec Exp:** Head & Neck Cancer; Sarcoma; Melanoma; **Hospital:** Evanston/North Shore Univ Hlth Sys, Highland Park/North Shore Univ Hlth Syst; **Address:** North Shore Univ Hlth Sys, Div Hematology/Oncology, 2650 Ridge Ave, rm 4816, Evanston, IL 60201; **Phone:** 847-570-2515; **Board Cert:** Internal Medicine 2003; Medical Oncology 2005; **Med School:** Univ Chicago-Pritzker Sch Med 1990; **Resid:** Internal Medicine, Hosp Univ Penn 1993; **Fellow:** Hematology & Oncology, Univ Chicago Hosps 1996; **Fac Appt:** Assoc Clin Prof Med, Northwestern Univ

Buckner, Jan Craig MD [Onc] - **Spec Exp:** Brain Tumors; Neuro-Oncology; **Hospital:** Mayo Med Ctr & Clin - Rochester; **Address:** Mayo Clinic, 200 First St SW, Rochester, MN 55905; **Phone:** 507-284-4320; **Board Cert:** Internal Medicine 1983; Medical Oncology 1985; **Med School:** Univ NC Sch Med 1980; **Resid:** Internal Medicine, Butterworth Hosp 1983; **Fellow:** Medical Oncology, Mayo Clinic 1985; **Fac Appt:** Prof Med, Mayo Med Sch

Budd, George T MD [Onc] - **Spec Exp:** Breast Cancer; **Hospital:** Cleveland Clin (page 70); **Address:** Cleveland Clinic, Taussig Cancer Ctr, 9500 Euclid Ave, Desk R35, Cleveland, OH 44195; **Phone:** 216-444-6480; **Board Cert:** Internal Medicine 1980; Medical Oncology 1983; **Med School:** Univ Kansas 1977; **Resid:** Internal Medicine, Cleveland Clinic 1980; **Fellow:** Hematology & Oncology, Cleveland Clinic 1982

Chapman, Robert A MD [Onc] - **Spec Exp:** Lung Cancer; **Hospital:** Henry Ford Hosp; **Address:** 2799 W Grand Blvd, K13, Detroit, MI 48202; **Phone:** 313-916-1841; **Board Cert:** Internal Medicine 1985; Medical Oncology 1989; **Med School:** Cornell Univ-Weill Med Coll 1976; **Resid:** Internal Medicine, Henry Ford Hosp 1979; **Fellow:** Medical Oncology, Meml Sloan Kettering Cancer Ctr 1981

Chitambar, Christopher R MD [Onc] - **Spec Exp:** Lymphoma; Leukemia; Breast Cancer; **Hospital:** Froedtert and Med Ctr of WI; **Address:** Div Neoplastic Disease, 9200 W Wisconsin Ave, Milwaukee, WI 53226-3522; **Phone:** 414-805-4600; **Board Cert:** Internal Medicine 1980; Hematology 1982; Medical Oncology 1983; **Med School:** India 1977; **Resid:** Internal Medicine, Brackenridge Hosp 1980; **Fellow:** Hematology & Oncology, Univ CO Hlth Sci Ctr 1983; **Fac Appt:** Prof Med, Med Coll Wisc

Clamon, Gerald H MD [Onc] - **Spec Exp:** Lung Cancer; Palliative Care; **Hospital:** Univ Iowa Hosp & Clinics; **Address:** Holden Comprehensive Cancer Ctr, 200 Hawkins Drive, Ste C32GH, Iowa City, IA 52242; **Phone:** 319-384-8442; **Board Cert:** Internal Medicine 1976; Medical Oncology 1979; **Med School:** Washington Univ, St Louis 1971; **Resid:** Internal Medicine, Barnes Hosp 1976; **Fellow:** Research, Natl Cancer Inst 1974; Medical Oncology, Univ Iowa Hosp & Clinics 1977; **Fac Appt:** Prof Med, Univ Iowa Coll Med

Clark, Joseph I MD [Onc] - **Spec Exp:** Kidney Cancer; Melanoma; Head & Neck Cancer; **Hospital:** Loyola Univ Med Ctr, Edward Hines, Jr. VA Hosp; **Address:** Cardinal Bernardin Cancer Ctr, Loyola Univ Med Ctr, 2160 S 1st Ave, rm 346, Maywood, IL 60153-5500; **Phone:** 708-327-3217; **Board Cert:** Internal Medicine 2002; Medical Oncology 2006; **Med School:** Loyola Univ-Stritch Sch Med 1989; **Resid:** Internal Medicine, Loyola Univ Med Ctr/Hines VA Hosp 1992; **Fellow:** Hematology & Oncology, Fox Chase Cancer Ctr/Temple Univ Hosp 1995; **Fac Appt:** Prof Med, Loyola Univ-Stritch Sch Med

Cleary, James F MD [Onc] - **Spec Exp:** Palliative Care; Head & Neck Cancer; **Hospital:** Univ WI Hosp & Clins; **Address:** 600 Highland Ave CSC Bldg - rm k6/546, Madison, WI 53792; **Phone:** 608-263-8624; **Board Cert:** Hospice & Palliative Medicine 2011; **Med School:** Australia 1984; **Resid:** Internal Medicine, Royal Adelaide Hosp 1987; **Fellow:** Medical Oncology, Royal Adelaide Hosp 1990; **Fac Appt:** Assoc Prof Med, Univ Wisc

Clinton, Steven K MD/PhD [Onc] - **Spec Exp:** Genitourinary Cancer; Prostate Cancer; Nutrition & Cancer Prevention/Control; **Hospital:** Ohio St Univ Med Ctr; **Address:** 320 W 10th Ave, rm 456 SL, Columbus, OH 43210; **Phone:** 614-293-7560; **Board Cert:** Internal Medicine 1987; **Med School:** Univ IL Coll Med 1984; **Resid:** Internal Medicine, Univ Chicago Hosps 1987; **Fellow:** Medical Oncology, Dana Farber Cancer Inst/Harvard 1991; **Fac Appt:** Assoc Prof Med, Ohio State Univ

Cobleigh, Melody A MD [Onc] - **Spec Exp:** Breast Cancer; **Hospital:** Rush Univ Med Ctr; **Address:** Rush Univ Med Ctr, 1725 W Harrison St, Ste 821, Chicago, IL 60612-3828; **Phone:** 312-942-5904; **Board Cert:** Internal Medicine 1979; Medical Oncology 1981; **Med School:** Rush Med Coll 1976; **Resid:** Internal Medicine, Rush Presby-St Lukes Med Ctr 1979; **Fellow:** Medical Oncology, Indiana Univ 1981; **Fac Appt:** Prof Med, Rush Med Coll

Davis, Mellar P MD [Onc] - **Spec Exp:** Palliative Care; Lung Cancer (advanced); **Hospital:** Cleveland Clin (page 70); **Address:** Cleveland Clin Fdn, 9500 Euclid Ave, Desk R35, Cleveland, OH 44195; **Phone:** 216-445-4622; **Board Cert:** Internal Medicine 1980; Hematology 1982; Medical Oncology 1983; Hospice & Palliative Medicine 2004; **Med School:** Ohio State Univ 1977; **Resid:** Internal Medicine, Riverside Methodist Hosp 1979; **Fellow:** Hematology, Mayo Clinic 1981; Medical Oncology, Mayo Clinic 1982; **Fac Appt:** Prof Med, Cleveland Cl Coll Med/Case West Res

Dowlati, Afshin MD [Onc] - **Spec Exp:** Lung Cancer; Thoracic Cancers; **Hospital:** Univ Hosps Case Med Ctr; **Address:** UH Seidman Cancer Center, 11100 Euclid Ave, Cleveland, OH 44106; **Phone:** 216-844-1228; **Board Cert:** Internal Medicine 2000; Medical Oncology 2001; **Med School:** Belgium 1992; **Resid:** Internal Medicine, U Liege 1996; **Fellow:** Hematology & Oncology, Case Western/Univ Hosps 1998; **Fac Appt:** Assoc Prof Med, Case West Res Univ

Dreicer, Robert MD [Onc] - **Spec Exp:** Prostate Cancer; Kidney Cancer; Bladder Cancer; Testicular Cancer; **Hospital:** Cleveland Clin (page 70); **Address:** 9500 Euclid Ave, Desk R35, Cleveland, OH 44195; **Phone:** 216-445-4623; **Board Cert:** Internal Medicine 1986; Medical Oncology 1989; **Med School:** Univ Tex, Houston 1983; **Resid:** Internal Medicine, Ind Univ Med Ctr 1986; **Fellow:** Medical Oncology, Univ Wisconsin Hosp 1989; **Fac Appt:** Prof Med, Cleveland Cl Coll Med/Case West Res

Einhorn, Lawrence H MD [Onc] - **Spec Exp:** Testicular Cancer; Lung Cancer; Urologic Cancer; **Hospital:** IU Health Methodist Hosp; **Address:** 535 Barnhill Drive, rm 473, Indianapolis, IN 46202; **Phone:** 317-944-0920; **Board Cert:** Internal Medicine 1972; Medical Oncology 1975; **Med School:** UCLA 1967; **Resid:** Internal Medicine, Indiana Univ Hosp 1969; **Fellow:** Medical Oncology, Indiana Univ Hosp 1972; **Fac Appt:** Prof Med, Indiana Univ

Ellis, Matthew J MD/PhD [Onc] - **Spec Exp:** Breast Cancer; **Hospital:** Barnes-Jewish Hosp; **Address:** Washington University, 660 S Euclid Ave, Box 8056, St Louis, MO 63110; **Phone:** 314-747-1171; **Board Cert:** Internal Medicine 2004; Medical Oncology 2005; **Med School:** England, UK 1984; **Resid:** Internal Medicine, Hammersmith Hosp 1988; **Fellow:** Research, Georgetown Univ Med Ctr 1992; Medical Oncology, Georgetwon Univ Med Ctr 1994; **Fac Appt:** Prof Med, Washington Univ, St Louis

Ensminger, William D MD/PhD [Onc] - **Spec Exp:** Gastrointestinal Cancer; Liver Cancer; Clinical Trials; **Hospital:** Univ of Michigan Hosp; **Address:** 1150 W Med Ctr Drive, Med Sci II Rm #4742, Ann Arbor, MI 48109-5633; **Phone:** 734-647-8902; **Board Cert:** Internal Medicine 1976; Medical Oncology 1979; **Med School:** Harvard Med Sch 1973; **Resid:** Internal Medicine, Beth Israel Hosp 1975; **Fellow:** Medical Oncology, Dana Farber Cancer Inst 1977; **Fac Appt:** Prof Med, Univ Mich Med Sch

Fleming, Gini F MD [Onc] - **Spec Exp:** Breast Cancer-Novel Therapies; Gynecologic Cancer; Ovarian Cancer; **Hospital:** Univ of Chicago Med Ctr; **Address:** Univ Chicago Hosps, 5841 S Maryland MC2115, Chicago, IL 60637-1470; **Phone:** 773-702-6149; **Board Cert:** Internal Medicine 1988; Medical Oncology 2001; Hematology 2002; **Med School:** Univ IL Coll Med 1985; **Resid:** Internal Medicine, Univ Chicago Hosps 1988; **Fellow:** Hematology & Oncology, Univ Chicago Hosps 1992; **Fac Appt:** Prof Med, Univ Chicago-Pritzker Sch Med

Gaynor, Ellen MD [Onc] - **Spec Exp:** Breast Cancer; Gastrointestinal Cancer; Prostate Cancer; **Hospital:** Loyola Univ Med Ctr; **Address:** Loyola Bernardin Cancer Center, 2160 S First Ave Bldg 112 - rm 108, Maywood, IL 60153-3328; **Phone:** 708-327-3214; **Board Cert:** Internal Medicine 1982; Hematology 1986; Medical Oncology 1985; **Med School:** Univ Wisc 1978; **Resid:** Internal Medicine, Loyola Univ Med Ctr 1982; **Fellow:** Medical Oncology, Loyola Univ Med Ctr 1981; Hematology & Oncology, Univ Chicago 1984; **Fac Appt:** Prof Med, Loyola Univ-Stritch Sch Med

Gerson, Stanton MD [Onc] - **Spec Exp:** Leukemia; Lymphoma, Non-Hodgkin's; Stem Cell Transplant; Multiple Myeloma; **Hospital:** Univ Hosps Case Med Ctr; **Address:** Ireland Cancer Ctr, 11000 Euclid Ave, 1 WEARN 151, Cleveland, OH 44106-5065; **Phone:** 216-844-1232; **Board Cert:** Internal Medicine 1980; Hematology 1982; Medical Oncology 1983; **Med School:** Harvard Med Sch 1977; **Resid:** Internal Medicine, Hosp Univ Penn 1980; **Fellow:** Hematology & Oncology, Hosp Univ Penn 1983; **Fac Appt:** Prof Med, Case West Res Univ

Medical Oncology

Golomb, Harvey M MD [Onc] - **Spec Exp:** Lung Cancer; Leukemia; Lymphoma; **Hospital:** Univ of Chicago Med Ctr; **Address:** Univ Chicago Medical Ctr, 5841 S Maryland Ave, MC 2115, Chicago, IL 60637-1463; **Phone:** 773-702-6149; **Board Cert:** Internal Medicine 1975; Medical Oncology 1979; **Med School:** Univ Pittsburgh 1968; **Resid:** Internal Medicine, Johns Hopkins Hosp 1972; Clinical Genetics, Johns Hopkins Hosp 1973; **Fellow:** Hematology & Oncology, Univ Chicago Hosps 1975; **Fac Appt:** Prof Med, Univ Chicago-Pritzker Sch Med

Gradishar, William J MD [Onc] - **Spec Exp:** Breast Cancer; **Hospital:** Northwestern Meml Hosp; **Address:** 250 E Superior St, Ste 420, Chicago, IL 60611; **Phone:** 312-695-4125; **Board Cert:** Internal Medicine 1985; Medical Oncology 1989; **Med School:** Univ IL Coll Med 1982; **Resid:** Internal Medicine, Michael Reese Hosp 1985; **Fellow:** Hematology & Oncology, Univ Chicago Hosps 1990; **Fac Appt:** Prof Med, Northwestern Univ

Gruber, Stephen B MD/PhD [Onc] - **Spec Exp:** Cancer Genetics; Colon & Rectal Cancer; Melanoma; **Hospital:** Univ of Michigan Hosp; **Address:** 109 Zina Pitcher Pl, Ann Arbor, MI 48109-2200; **Phone:** 734-615-9712; **Board Cert:** Medical Oncology 2009; **Med School:** Univ Pennsylvania 1992; **Resid:** Internal Medicine, Hosp Univ Penn 1994; **Fellow:** Medical Oncology, Johns Hopkins Hosp 1997; Clinical Genetics, Univ Michigan Hlth Sys 1999; **Fac Appt:** Assoc Prof Med, Univ Mich Med Sch

Hartmann, Lynn Carol MD [Onc] - **Spec Exp:** Ovarian Cancer; **Hospital:** Mayo Med Ctr & Clin - Rochester; **Address:** Mayo Clinic Gonda 10 South, 200 First St SW, Rochester, MN 55905; **Phone:** 507-284-3903; **Board Cert:** Internal Medicine 1986; Medical Oncology 1989; **Med School:** Northwestern Univ 1983; **Resid:** Internal Medicine, Univ Ia Hosps/Clinics 1986; **Fellow:** Medical Oncology, Mayo Clinic 1989; **Fac Appt:** Prof Med, Mayo Med Sch

Hayes, Daniel F MD [Onc] - **Spec Exp:** Breast Cancer; **Hospital:** Univ of Michigan Hosp; **Address:** Univ Michigan Comprehensive Cancer Ctr, 6312 CCC SPC, 5942, 1500 E Medical Center Drive, Ann Arbor, MI 48109-5942; **Phone:** 734-615-6725; **Board Cert:** Internal Medicine 1982; Medical Oncology 1985; **Med School:** Indiana Univ 1979; **Resid:** Internal Medicine, Parkland Meml Hosp 1982; **Fellow:** Medical Oncology, Dana Farber Cancer Inst 1985; **Fac Appt:** Prof Med, Univ Mich Med Sch

Hoffman, Philip C MD [Onc] - **Spec Exp:** Lung Cancer; Breast Cancer; **Hospital:** Univ of Chicago Med Ctr, Little Company of Mary Hosp & Hlth Care Ctrs; **Address:** 5841 S Maryland Ave, MC 2115, Chicago, IL 60637-1447; **Phone:** 773-834-7424; **Board Cert:** Internal Medicine 1975; Hematology 1980; Medical Oncology 1981; **Med School:** Jefferson Med Coll 1972; **Resid:** Internal Medicine, Hosp Univ Penn 1975; **Fellow:** Hematology & Oncology, Univ Chicago Hosps 1980; **Fac Appt:** Prof Med, Univ Chicago-Pritzker Sch Med

Hussain, Maha H MD [Onc] - **Spec Exp:** Prostate Cancer; Bladder Cancer; Testicular Cancer; Genitourinary Cancer; **Hospital:** Univ of Michigan Hosp; **Address:** Univ Michigan Cancer Ctr, 1500 E Medical Ctr Drive, rm 7310, Ann Arbor, MI 48109; **Phone:** 734-936-8906; **Board Cert:** Internal Medicine 1986; Medical Oncology 1989; **Med School:** Iraq 1980; **Resid:** Internal Medicine, Wayne State Univ Affil Hosps 1986; **Fellow:** Medical Oncology, Wayne State Univ Affil Hosps 1989; **Fac Appt:** Prof Med, Univ Mich Med Sch

Ingle, James N MD [Onc] - **Spec Exp:** Breast Cancer; **Hospital:** Rochester Methodist Hosp, Mayo Med Ctr & Clin - Rochester; **Address:** Mayo Clinic, 200 First St SW, Gonda Bldg Fl 10, Rochester, MN 55905-0001; **Phone:** 507-284-8432; **Board Cert:** Internal Medicine 1974; Medical Oncology 1975; **Med School:** Johns Hopkins Univ 1971; **Resid:** Internal Medicine, Johns Hopkins Hosp 1976; Medical Oncology, Natl Cancer Inst 1975; **Fac Appt:** Prof Hem & Onc, Mayo Med Sch

Kalaycio, Matt E MD [Onc] - **Spec Exp:** Leukemia; Bone Marrow Transplant; **Hospital:** Cleveland Clin (page 70); **Address:** Taussig Cancer Ctr, 9500 Euclid Ave, Desk R35, Cleveland, OH 44195; **Phone:** 216-444-3705; **Board Cert:** Internal Medicine 2002; Hematology 2004; Medical Oncology 2005; **Med School:** W VA Univ 1988; **Resid:** Internal Medicine, Mercy Hosp 1991; **Fellow:** Hematology & Oncology, Cleveland Clinic 1994; **Fac Appt:** Prof Med, Cleveland Cl Coll Med/Case West Res

Kalemkerian, Gregory P MD [Onc] - **Spec Exp:** Lung Cancer; Mesothelioma; Thymoma; **Hospital:** Univ of Michigan Hosp; **Address:** 1500 E Med Ctr Drive, C350 Med Inn-SPC 5848, MS 5848, Ann Arbor, MI 48109-0848; **Phone:** 734-232-6046; **Board Cert:** Internal Medicine 1988; Medical Oncology 2001; **Med School:** Northwestern Univ 1985; **Resid:** Internal Medicine, Northwestern Meml Hosp 1988; **Fellow:** Medical Oncology, Johns Hopkins Hosp 1993; **Fac Appt:** Prof Hem & Onc, Univ Mich Med Sch

Kaminski, Mark S MD [Onc] - **Spec Exp:** Lymphoma; Bone Marrow Transplant; Drug Development; Clinical Trials; **Hospital:** Univ of Michigan Hosp; **Address:** Univ Michigan Cancer Ctr, 1500 E Medical Ctr Drive, rm 4316, Ann Arbor, MI 48109; **Phone:** 734-647-8901; **Board Cert:** Internal Medicine 1981; Medical Oncology 1983; **Med School:** Stanford Univ 1978; **Resid:** Internal Medicine, Barnes Hosp 1981; **Fellow:** Medical Oncology, Stanford Univ Med Ctr 1985; **Fac Appt:** Prof Med, Univ Mich Med Sch

Kindler, Hedy Lee MD [Onc] - **Spec Exp:** Pancreatic Cancer; Mesothelioma; Colon & Rectal Cancer; **Hospital:** Univ of Chicago Med Ctr; **Address:** Univ of Chicago Medical Ctr, 5841 S Maryland Ave, MC 2115, Chicago, IL 60637-1470; **Phone:** 773-702-6149; **Board Cert:** Internal Medicine 2002; Medical Oncology 2005; **Med School:** SUNY Buffalo 1985; **Resid:** Internal Medicine, UCLA Med Ctr 1992; **Fellow:** Medical Oncology, Meml Sloan Kettering Cancer Ctr 1995; **Fac Appt:** Assoc Prof Med, Univ Chicago-Pritzker Sch Med

Krishnamurthi, Smitha S MD [Onc] - **Spec Exp:** Gastrointestinal Cancer; Colon & Rectal Cancer; **Hospital:** Univ Hosps Case Med Ctr; **Address:** UH Case Medical Center, Seidman Cancer Center, 11100 Euclid Ave, Cleveland, OH 44106; **Phone:** 216-844-1006; **Board Cert:** Internal Medicine 2006; Medical Oncology 2008; **Med School:** Univ Pennsylvania 1993; **Resid:** Internal Medicine, Univ Penn Affil Hosps 1996; **Fellow:** Medical Oncology, Johns Hopkins Hosp 1996; **Fac Appt:** Asst Prof Med, Case West Res Univ

Kuzel, Timothy M MD [Onc] - **Spec Exp:** Kidney Cancer; Melanoma; Cutaneous Lymphoma; **Hospital:** Northwestern Meml Hosp; **Address:** Northwestern Meml Hosp, 675 N St Clair, Ste 21-100, Chicago, IL 60611; **Phone:** 312-695-0990; **Board Cert:** Internal Medicine 1987; Hematology 2000; Medical Oncology 1989; **Med School:** Univ Mich Med Sch 1984; **Resid:** Internal Medicine, McGraw MC-Northwestern Univ 1987; **Fellow:** Hematology & Oncology, McGraw MC-Northwestern Univ 1990; **Fac Appt:** Prof Med, Northwestern Univ

Loehrer, Patrick J MD [Onc] - **Spec Exp:** Gastrointestinal Cancer; Thymoma; Genitourinary Cancer; **Hospital:** IU Health Methodist Hosp; **Address:** Indiana Cancer Pavilion, 535 Barnhill Drive, rm 473, Indianapolis, IN 46202-5112; **Phone:** 317-944-0920; **Board Cert:** Internal Medicine 1981; Medical Oncology 2006; **Med School:** Rush Med Coll 1978; **Resid:** Internal Medicine, Rush-Presby-St Lukes Hosp 1981; **Fellow:** Medical Oncology, Indiana Univ 1983; **Fac Appt:** Prof Med, Indiana Univ

Loprinzi, Charles L MD [Onc] - **Spec Exp:** Breast Cancer; **Hospital:** Mayo Med Ctr & Clin - Rochester; **Address:** Mayo Clinic, Dept Med Oncology, 200 First St SW, Rochester, MN 55905-0001; **Phone:** 507-284-4849; **Board Cert:** Internal Medicine 1982; Medical Oncology 1985; **Med School:** Oregon Hlth & Sci Univ 1979; **Resid:** Internal Medicine, Maricopa Co Hosp 1982; **Fellow:** Medical Oncology, Univ Wisconsin Med Ctr 1984; **Fac Appt:** Prof Med, Mayo Med Sch

Medical Oncology

Markowitz, Sanford D MD [Onc] - **Spec Exp:** Colon & Rectal Cancer; Hereditary Cancer; **Hospital:** Univ Hosps Case Med Ctr; **Address:** Ireland Cancer Ctr, 11100 Euclid Ave Fl 6, Cleveland, OH 44106; **Phone:** 216-844-3951; **Board Cert:** Internal Medicine 1984; Medical Oncology 1987; **Med School:** Yale Univ 1980; **Resid:** Internal Medicine, Univ Chicago Hosp 1984; **Fellow:** Medical Oncology, Natl Cancer Inst 1986; **Fac Appt:** Prof Med, Case West Res Univ

Meropol, Neal J MD [Onc] - **Spec Exp:** Gastrointestinal Cancer; Colon Cancer; Pancreatic Cancer; **Hospital:** Univ Hosps Case Med Ctr; **Address:** 11100 Euclid Ave, Cleveland, OH 44106; **Phone:** 216-844-5220; **Board Cert:** Internal Medicine 1988; Medical Oncology 2001; **Med School:** Vanderbilt Univ 1985; **Resid:** Internal Medicine, Univ Hosps/Case West Res 1988; **Fellow:** Hematology & Oncology, Hosp Univ Penn 1992; **Fac Appt:** Prof Med, Case West Res Univ

O'Brien, Timothy E MD [Onc] - **Spec Exp:** Gastrointestinal Cancer; Colon & Rectal Cancer; Multiple Myeloma; Lung Cancer; **Hospital:** MetroHealth Med Ctr; **Address:** MetroHealth Cancer Care Ctr, 2500 MetroHealth Drive, rm C-2100, Cleveland, OH 44109; **Phone:** 216-778-5802; **Board Cert:** Medical Oncology 1997; Hematology 1998; **Med School:** Univ Rochester 1989; **Resid:** Internal Medicine, Univ Hosps Cleveland 1992; **Fellow:** Hematology & Oncology, Univ Hosps Cleveland 1997; **Fac Appt:** Assoc Prof Med, Case West Res Univ

Olopade, Olufunmilayo I MD [Onc] - **Spec Exp:** Breast Cancer; Hereditary Cancer; Breast Cancer Genetics; Cancer Risk Assessment; **Hospital:** Univ of Chicago Med Ctr; **Address:** Univ Chicago Med Ctr, 5841 S Maryland Ave, MC 2115, Chicago, IL 60637-1470; **Phone:** 773-702-6149; **Board Cert:** Internal Medicine 1986; Hematology 2001; Medical Oncology 1989; **Med School:** Nigeria 1980; **Resid:** Internal Medicine, Cook Co Hosp 1986; **Fellow:** Hematology & Oncology, Univ Chicago Hosps 1991; **Fac Appt:** Prof Med, Univ Chicago-Pritzker Sch Med

Ozer, Howard MD [Onc] - **Spec Exp:** Lymphoma; **Hospital:** Univ of IL Med Ctr at Chicago; **Address:** UIC Hematology/Oncology, Clinical Sciences Bldg, 840 S Wood St, Ste 820E, Chicago, IL 60612; **Phone:** 312-355-1625; **Board Cert:** Internal Medicine 1979; **Med School:** Yale Univ 1975; **Resid:** Internal Medicine, Mass Genl Hosp 1977; **Fellow:** Hematology & Oncology, PB Brigham/Dana Farber Cancer Inst 1979; **Fac Appt:** Prof Med, Univ IL Coll Med

Peace, David J MD [Onc] - **Spec Exp:** Prostate Cancer; Vaccine Therapy; Leukemia & Lymphoma; Immunotherapy; **Hospital:** Univ of IL Med Ctr at Chicago, MacNeal Hosp; **Address:** 840 S Wood St CSB Bldg - Ste 820, MS 713, Chicago, IL 60607; **Phone:** 312-413-1507; **Board Cert:** Internal Medicine 1983; Medical Oncology 1987; **Med School:** Univ Pittsburgh 1980; **Resid:** Internal Medicine, Univ Pittsburgh Med Ctr 1983; **Fellow:** Hematology & Oncology, Univ Washington Med Ctr 1988

Perry, Michael C MD [Onc] - **Spec Exp:** Lung Cancer; Breast Cancer; **Hospital:** Univ of Missouri Hosp; **Address:** Ellis Fischel Cancer Ctr, 115 Business Loop 70 W, DC 116.71, rm 524, Columbia, MO 65203-3299; **Phone:** 573-882-4979; **Board Cert:** Internal Medicine 1987; Hematology 1974; Medical Oncology 1975; **Med School:** Wayne State Univ 1970; **Resid:** Internal Medicine, Mayo Grad Sch 1972; **Fellow:** Hematology, Mayo Grad Sch 1974; Medical Oncology, Mayo Grad Sch 1975; **Fac Appt:** Prof Med, Univ MO-Columbia Sch Med

Peterson, Bruce MD [Onc] - **Spec Exp:** Lymphoma; Leukemia; **Address:** Univ of Minnesota, 420 Delaware St SE, MMC 480, Minneapolis, MN 55455; **Phone:** 612-625-5411; **Board Cert:** Internal Medicine 1974; Medical Oncology 1977; **Med School:** Univ Minn 1971; **Resid:** Internal Medicine, Fletcher Allen Hlthcare 1973; Internal Medicine, Fairview-Univ Med Ctr 1974; **Fellow:** Medical Oncology, Fairview-Univ Med Ctr 1977; **Fac Appt:** Prof Med, Univ Minn

Petruska, Paul J MD [Onc] - **Spec Exp:** Leukemia & Lymphoma; Solid Tumors; **Hospital:** St. Louis Univ Hosp; **Address:** SLU, Dept Hem/Onc, 3655 Vista Ave, St Louis, MO 63110; **Phone:** 314-577-6057; **Board Cert:** Internal Medicine 1972; Hematology 1974; Medical Oncology 1979; **Med School:** St Louis Univ 1967; **Resid:** Internal Medicine, St. Louis Hosp 1969; Internal Medicine, St. Louis Hosp 1972; **Fellow:** Hematology & Oncology, St. Louis Hosp 1974; **Fac Appt:** Prof Med, St Louis Univ

Pienta, Kenneth J MD [Onc] - **Spec Exp:** Prostate Cancer; **Hospital:** Univ of Michigan Hosp; **Address:** 1500 E Med Ctr Drive, rm 7303 CCC, Ann Arbor, MI 48109-5946; **Phone:** 734-647-3421; **Board Cert:** Internal Medicine 2001; Medical Oncology 2001; **Med School:** Johns Hopkins Univ 1986; **Resid:** Internal Medicine, Univ Chicago Hosps 1988; **Fellow:** Medical Oncology, Johns Hopkins Hosp 1991; **Fac Appt:** Prof Med, Univ Mich Med Sch

Pohlman, Brad L MD [Onc] - **Spec Exp:** Lymphoma; Lymphoma, Non-Hodgkin's; Bone Marrow Transplant; **Hospital:** Cleveland Clin (page 70); **Address:** Cleveland Clinic Fdn, 9500 Euclid Ave, Desk R35, Cleveland, OH 44195; **Phone:** 216-444-6070; **Board Cert:** Internal Medicine 1988; **Med School:** Indiana Univ 1985; **Resid:** Internal Medicine, Univ Wisconsin Hosp 1988; **Fellow:** Hematology, Univ Minnesota Hosp 1992

Ratain, Mark J MD [Onc] - **Spec Exp:** Solid Tumors; Drug Discovery & Development; **Hospital:** Univ of Chicago Med Ctr; **Address:** Univ Chicago Med Ctr, 5841 S Maryland Ave, MC 2115, Chicago, IL 60637; **Phone:** 773-702-6149; **Board Cert:** Internal Medicine 1983; Hematology 1986; Medical Oncology 1985; **Med School:** Yale Univ 1980; **Resid:** Internal Medicine, Johns Hopkins Hosp 1983; **Fellow:** Hematology & Oncology, Univ Chicago 1986; **Fac Appt:** Prof Med, Univ Chicago-Pritzker Sch Med

Richards, Jon M MD/PhD [Onc] - **Spec Exp:** Melanoma; **Hospital:** Adv Luth Genl Hosp, Skokie/North Shore Univ Htlh Syst; **Address:** Center for Advanced Care, 1700 Luther Ln Fl 2, Park Ridge, IL 60068; **Phone:** 847-268-8200; **Board Cert:** Medical Oncology 2007; **Med School:** Cornell Univ 1983; **Resid:** Internal Medicine, Univ Chicago Hosps 1985; **Fellow:** Hematology & Oncology, Univ Chicago Hosps 1988; **Fac Appt:** Assoc Prof Med, Univ IL Coll Med

Rosen, Steven T MD [Onc] - **Spec Exp:** Hematologic Malignancies; Breast Cancer; Leukemia & Lymphoma; **Hospital:** Northwestern Meml Hosp; **Address:** Northwestern Univ, 303 E Chicago Ave, Lurie 3-125, Chicago, IL 60611-3013; **Phone:** 312-695-0990; **Board Cert:** Internal Medicine 1979; Medical Oncology 1981; Hematology 1984; **Med School:** Northwestern Univ 1976; **Resid:** Internal Medicine, Northwestern Univ Hosp 1979; **Fellow:** Medical Oncology, Natl Cancer Inst 1981; **Fac Appt:** Prof Med, Northwestern Univ

Roth, Bruce J MD [Onc] - **Spec Exp:** Prostate Cancer; Bladder Cancer; Testicular Cancer; **Hospital:** Barnes-Jewish Hosp; **Address:** Washington University, 660 S Euclid Ave, Campus Box 8056, St Louis, MO 63110; **Phone:** 314-747-1171; **Board Cert:** Internal Medicine 1983; Medical Oncology 1985; **Med School:** St Louis Univ 1980; **Resid:** Internal Medicine, Indiana Univ Med Ctr 1983; **Fellow:** Hematology & Oncology, Indiana Univ Med Ctr 1986; **Fac Appt:** Prof Med, Washington Univ, St Louis

Salgia, Ravi MD/PhD [Onc] - **Spec Exp:** Lung Cancer; Mesothelioma; Thoracic Cancers; **Hospital:** Univ of Chicago Med Ctr; **Address:** Univ Chicago Medical Ctr, 5841 S Maryland Ave, MC 2115, Chicago, IL 60637; **Phone:** 773-702-6149; **Board Cert:** Medical Oncology 2006; **Med School:** Loyola Univ-Stritch Sch Med 1987; **Resid:** Internal Medicine, Johns Hopkins Hosp 1990; **Fellow:** Medical Oncology, Dana-Farber Cancer Inst 1993; **Fac Appt:** Prof Med, Univ Chicago-Pritzker Sch Med

Medical Oncology

Schiffer, Charles A MD [Onc] - **Spec Exp:** Leukemia; Lymphoma; Multiple Myeloma; **Hospital:** Barbara Ann Karmanos Cancer Inst, Harper Univ Hosp; **Address:** Karmanos Cancer Inst, Cancer Research Ctr, 4100 John R, HW04HO, Detroit, MI 48201; **Phone:** 313-576-8737; **Board Cert:** Internal Medicine 1972; Medical Oncology 1973; **Med School:** NYU Sch Med 1968; **Resid:** Internal Medicine, Bellevue-NY VA Hosp-NYU 1972; **Fellow:** Medical Oncology, Natl Cancer Inst 1974; **Fac Appt:** Prof Med, Wayne State Univ

Schilsky, Richard L MD [Onc] - **Spec Exp:** Gastrointestinal Cancer; Pancreatic Cancer; Drug Development; **Hospital:** Univ of Chicago Med Ctr; **Address:** Univ Chicago- Bio Sciences Div, 5841 S Maryland Ave, Chicago, IL 60637; **Phone:** 773-834-3914; **Board Cert:** Internal Medicine 1978; Medical Oncology 1979; **Med School:** Univ Chicago-Pritzker Sch Med 1975; **Resid:** Internal Medicine, Univ Texas 1977; **Fellow:** Medical Oncology, Natl Cancer Inst 1980; **Fac Appt:** Prof Med, Univ Chicago-Pritzker Sch Med

Schwartz, Burton S MD [Onc] - **Spec Exp:** Lymphoma; Breast Cancer; **Hospital:** Abbott - Northwestern Hosp; **Address:** 910 E 26th St, Ste 200, Minneapolis, MN 55404; **Phone:** 612-884-6300; **Board Cert:** Internal Medicine 1980; Hematology 1976; Medical Oncology 1977; **Med School:** Meharry Med Coll 1968; **Resid:** Internal Medicine, Michael Reese Hosp 1971; **Fellow:** Hematology, Univ Minn Hosp 1976; **Fac Appt:** Clin Prof Med, Univ Minn

Shapiro, Charles L MD [Onc] - **Spec Exp:** Breast Cancer; **Hospital:** Arthur G James Cancer Hosp & Research Inst; **Address:** 320 W 10th Ave, Starling-Loving Hall, rm B405, Columbus, OH 43210; **Phone:** 614-293-0066; **Board Cert:** Internal Medicine 1987; Medical Oncology 2005; **Med School:** SUNY Buffalo 1984; **Resid:** Internal Medicine, Temple Univ Hosp 1987; **Fellow:** Medical Oncology, Dana Farber Cancer Inst 1991; **Fac Appt:** Assoc Prof Med, Ohio State Univ

Silver, Samuel M MD/PhD [Onc] - **Spec Exp:** Hematologic Malignancies; Myelodysplastic Syndromes; Myeloproliferative Disorders; Platelet Disorders; **Hospital:** Univ of Michigan Hosp; **Address:** Univ Michigan Med Ctr, 4101 Med Sci I C- Wing, 1301 Catherine St, Ann Arbor, MI 48109-5624; **Phone:** 734-615-1332; **Board Cert:** Internal Medicine 1982; Medical Oncology 1985; Hematology 1984; **Med School:** Cornell Univ-Weill Med Coll 1978; **Resid:** Internal Medicine, UCSF-Moffit Hosp 1982; **Fellow:** Hematology & Oncology, Hosp Univ Penn 1985; **Fac Appt:** Clin Prof Med, Univ Mich Med Sch

Silverman, Paula MD [Onc] - **Spec Exp:** Breast Cancer; **Hospital:** Univ Hosps Case Med Ctr; **Address:** Univ Hosp Cleveland, Ireland Cancer Ctr, 11100 Euclid Ave Bolwell Bldg Fl 6, Cleveland, OH 44106; **Phone:** 216-844-8510; **Board Cert:** Internal Medicine 1984; Medical Oncology 1989; **Med School:** Case West Res Univ 1981; **Resid:** Internal Medicine, Univ Hosps 1984; **Fellow:** Hematology & Oncology, Case Western Reserve Univ 1987; **Fac Appt:** Assoc Prof Med, Case West Res Univ

Sledge Jr, George W MD [Onc] - **Spec Exp:** Breast Cancer; **Hospital:** IU Health Methodist Hosp, IU Health North Hosp; **Address:** 535 Barnhill Drive, rm 473, Indianapolis, IN 46202; **Phone:** 317-274-0920; **Board Cert:** Internal Medicine 1980; Medical Oncology 1983; **Med School:** Tulane Univ 1977; **Resid:** Internal Medicine, St Louis Univ Med Ctr 1980; **Fellow:** Medical Oncology, Univ Texas 1983; **Fac Appt:** Prof Med, Indiana Univ

Stadler, Walter M MD [Onc] - **Spec Exp:** Kidney Cancer; Bladder Cancer; Prostate Cancer; Testicular Cancer; **Hospital:** Univ of Chicago Med Ctr; **Address:** Univ Chicago Medical Center, 5841 S Maryland Ave, MC 2115, Chicago, IL 60637; **Phone:** 773-834-7424; **Board Cert:** Internal Medicine 2002; Medical Oncology 2003; **Med School:** Yale Univ 1988; **Resid:** Internal Medicine, Michael Reese Hosp 1991; **Fellow:** Medical Oncology, Univ Chicago Hosps 1994; **Fac Appt:** Prof Med, Univ Chicago-Pritzker Sch Med

Sweetenham, John W MD [Onc] - **Spec Exp:** Lymphoma; Stem Cell Transplant; **Hospital:** Cleveland Clin (page 70); **Address:** Cleveland Clin, Taussig Cancer Inst, 9500 Euclid Ave, Cleveland, OH 44195; **Phone:** 216-445-6707; **Med School:** England, UK 1980; **Resid:** Internal Medicine, Royal United Hosp 1984; **Fellow:** Hematology & Oncology, Univ Southampton 1989; **Fac Appt:** Prof Med, Cleveland Cl Coll Med/Case West Res

Triozzi, Pierre L MD [Onc] - **Spec Exp:** Melanoma; Vaccine Therapy; Clinical Trials; **Hospital:** Cleveland Clin (page 70); **Address:** Cleveland Clinic Fdn, 9500 Euclid Ave, MC R40, Cleveland, OH 44195; **Phone:** 216-445-5141; **Board Cert:** Internal Medicine 1983; Medical Oncology 1987; Hematology 1988; **Med School:** Ohio State Univ 1980; **Resid:** Internal Medicine, Duke Univ Med Ctr 1983; **Fellow:** Hematology & Oncology, Duke Univ Med Ctr 1987; **Fac Appt:** Prof Med, Case West Res Univ

Urba, Susan G MD [Onc] - **Spec Exp:** Head & Neck Cancer; **Hospital:** Univ of Michigan Hosp; **Address:** Level B1363, Reception C, 1500 E Med Ctr Drive, Ann Arbor, MI 48109-0922; **Phone:** 734-647-8902; **Board Cert:** Internal Medicine 1986; Medical Oncology 2002; **Med School:** Univ Mich Med Sch 1983; **Resid:** Internal Medicine, Univ Mich Med Ctr 1986; **Fellow:** Hematology & Oncology, Univ Mich Med Ctr 1988; **Fac Appt:** Assoc Prof Med, Univ Mich Med Sch

Von Roenn, Jamie H MD [Onc] - **Spec Exp:** Palliative Care; AIDS Related Cancers; Breast Cancer; **Hospital:** Northwestern Meml Hosp; **Address:** Northwestern Medical Faculty Foundation, 676 N St Clair St, Ste 850, Chicago, IL 60611; **Phone:** 312-695-6180; **Board Cert:** Internal Medicine 1983; Medical Oncology 2009; Hospice & Palliative Medicine 2008; **Med School:** Rush Med Coll 1980; **Resid:** Internal Medicine, Rush-Presby-St Lukes Hosp 1983; **Fellow:** Medical Oncology, Rush-Presby-St Lukes Hosp 1985; **Fac Appt:** Prof Med, Northwestern Univ

Weiner, George J MD [Onc] - **Spec Exp:** Lymphoma; Leukemia; Immunotherapy; **Hospital:** Univ Iowa Hosp & Clinics; **Address:** Holden Comprehensive Cancer Center, 200 Hawkins Drive, Ste 5970HJPP, Iowa City, IA 52242; **Phone:** 319-356-4422; **Board Cert:** Internal Medicine 1985; Hematology 1988; Medical Oncology 1987; **Med School:** Ohio State Univ 1981; **Resid:** Medical Oncology, Med Coll Ohio Affil Hosp 1984; **Fellow:** Hematology & Oncology, Univ Mich Med Ctr 1987; **Fac Appt:** Prof Med, Univ Iowa Coll Med

Wicha, Max S MD [Onc] - **Spec Exp:** Breast Cancer; Stem Cell Transplant; **Hospital:** Univ of Michigan Hosp; **Address:** Comp Cancer Ctr & Geriatrics Ctr, 1500 E Med Ctr Dr, rm 6302 CC, SPC 5942, Ann Arbor, MI 48109-5942; **Phone:** 734-936-1831; **Board Cert:** Internal Medicine 1977; Medical Oncology 1983; **Med School:** Stanford Univ 1974; **Resid:** Internal Medicine, Univ Chicago Hosp 1977; **Fellow:** Medical Oncology, Natl Inst Hlth 1980; **Fac Appt:** Prof Med, Univ Mich Med Sch

Wilding, George MD [Onc] - **Spec Exp:** Prostate Cancer; Kidney Cancer; Genitourinary Cancer; Drug Discovery & Development; **Hospital:** Univ WI Hosp & Clins; **Address:** 1111 Highland Ave, Ste 7057WIMR, Madison, WI 53705; **Phone:** 608-263-8610; **Board Cert:** Internal Medicine 1983; Medical Oncology 1985; **Med School:** Univ Mass Sch Med 1980; **Resid:** Internal Medicine, Univ Mass Med Ctr 1983; **Fellow:** Medical Oncology, Natl Cancer Inst 1985; **Fac Appt:** Prof Med, Univ Wisc

Worden, Francis P MD [Onc] - **Spec Exp:** Head & Neck Cancer; Palliative Care; Clinical Trials; **Hospital:** Univ of Michigan Hosp; **Address:** Level B1363, Reception C, 1500 E Medical Center Drive, Ann Arbor, MI 48109; **Phone:** 734-647-8902; **Board Cert:** Medical Oncology 2000; **Med School:** Indiana Univ 1993; **Resid:** Internal Medicine & Pediatrics, Detroit Med Ctr 1997; **Fellow:** Medical Oncology, Detroit Med Ctr 2000; **Fac Appt:** Asst Clin Prof Med, Univ Mich Med Sch

Medical Oncology

Yee, Douglas MD [Onc] - **Spec Exp:** Breast Cancer; **Address:** Masonic Cancer Ctr-Breast Ctr, 420 Delaware St SE, MMC 160, Minneapolis, MN 55455; **Phone:** 612-273-9685; **Board Cert:** Internal Medicine 1984; Medical Oncology 1987; **Med School:** Univ Chicago-Pritzker Sch Med 1981; **Resid:** Internal Medicine, Univ NC Med Ctr 1984; **Fellow:** Medical Oncology, NIH-Clin Ctr 1987; **Fac Appt:** Prof Med, Univ Minn

Great Plains and Mountains

Akerley III, Wallace L MD [Onc] - **Spec Exp:** Lung Cancer; Clinical Trials; **Hospital:** Univ Utah Hlth Care; **Address:** Huntsman Cancer Inst, 2000 Circle of Hope, rm 2165, Salt Lake City, UT 84112; **Phone:** 801-585-0100; **Board Cert:** Internal Medicine 1984; Medical Oncology 1987; Hematology 1988; **Med School:** Brown Univ 1981; **Resid:** Internal Medicine, USC Medical Ctr 1985; **Fellow:** Medical Oncology, USC Medical Ctr 1986; Hematology, Norris Cotton Cancer Ctr/Dartmouth 1988; **Fac Appt:** Prof Med, Univ Utah

Armitage, James MD [Onc] - **Spec Exp:** Lymphoma; Bone Marrow Transplant; **Hospital:** Nebraska Med Ctr; **Address:** 987630 Nebraska Medical Center, Emile @ 42nd St, Omaha, NE 68198-7630; **Phone:** 402-559-5600; **Board Cert:** Internal Medicine 1976; Medical Oncology 1977; Hematology 1984; **Med School:** Univ Nebr Coll Med 1973; **Resid:** Internal Medicine, Univ Nebraska Med Ctr 1975; **Fellow:** Hematology & Oncology, Univ Iowa Hosp 1977; **Fac Appt:** Prof Med, Univ Nebr Coll Med

Beatty, Patrick G MD/PhD [Onc] - **Spec Exp:** Hematologic Malignancies; Lymphoma; **Hospital:** St. Patrick Hospital - Missoula; **Address:** 500 W Broadway, PO Box 7877, Missoula, MT 59807; **Phone:** 406-728-2539; **Board Cert:** Internal Medicine 1980; Medical Oncology 1985; **Med School:** Univ Chicago-Pritzker Sch Med 1976; **Resid:** Internal Medicine, Vanderbilt Univ Med Ctr 1979; **Fellow:** Oncology, Univ Washington Hosps 1982

Bierman, Philip J MD [Onc] - **Spec Exp:** Lymphoma; Bone Marrow Transplant; **Hospital:** Nebraska Med Ctr; **Address:** Nebraska Medical Ctr, Dept Hem/Oncology, 987630 Nebraska Medical Ctr, Emile @ 42nd St, Omaha, NE 68198-7630; **Phone:** 402-559-5600; **Board Cert:** Internal Medicine 1982; Medical Oncology 1985; Hematology 1986; **Med School:** Univ MO-Kansas City 1979; **Resid:** Internal Medicine, Univ Nebraska Med Ctr 1983; **Fellow:** Medical Oncology, Univ Nebraska Med Ctr 1985; Hematology, City of Hope Natl Med Ctr 1986; **Fac Appt:** Prof Med, Univ Nebr Coll Med

Bunn Jr, Paul A MD [Onc] - **Spec Exp:** Lung Cancer; Clinical Trials; Thymoma; Mesothelioma; **Hospital:** Univ of CO Hosp - Anschutz Inpatient Pav; **Address:** Univ Colorado Hosp Cancer Ctr, 128001 E 17th Ave, Box 8117, Aurora, CO 80045; **Phone:** 720-848-0300; **Board Cert:** Internal Medicine 1974; Medical Oncology 1975; **Med School:** Cornell Univ-Weill Med Coll 1971; **Resid:** Internal Medicine, Moffitt Hosp/ UCSF Med Ctr 1973; **Fellow:** Medical Oncology, Natl Cancer Inst 1976; **Fac Appt:** Prof Med, Univ Colorado

Buys, Saundra S MD [Onc] - **Spec Exp:** Breast Cancer; Breast Cancer Risk Assessment; Breast Cancer Genetics; **Hospital:** Univ Utah Hlth Care; **Address:** Huntsman Cancer Inst, 2000 Circle of Hope, Salt Lake City, UT 84112; **Phone:** 801-585-0100; **Board Cert:** Internal Medicine 1982; Medical Oncology 1985; Hematology 1984; **Med School:** Tufts Univ 1979; **Resid:** Internal Medicine, Univ Utah Hosps 1982; **Fellow:** Hematology & Oncology, Univ Utah Hosps 1985; **Fac Appt:** Prof Med, Univ Utah

Cowan, Kenneth H MD/PhD [Onc] - **Spec Exp:** Breast Cancer; **Hospital:** Nebraska Med Ctr; **Address:** Eppley Cancer Center, 987630 Nebraska Medical Ctr, Emile @ 42nd St, Omaha, NE 68198-7630; **Phone:** 402-559-5600; **Board Cert:** Internal Medicine 1978; Medical Oncology 1981; **Med School:** Case West Res Univ 1975; **Resid:** Internal Medicine, Parkland Meml Hosp 1977

Dakhil, Shaker MD [Onc] - **Spec Exp:** Leukemia; Mesothelioma; Lymphoma; **Hospital:** Univ of Kansas Hosp; **Address:** Cancer Center Kansas, 818 N Emporia, Ste 403, Wichita, KS 67214; **Phone:** 316-262-4467; **Board Cert:** Internal Medicine 1978; Medical Oncology 1981; **Med School:** Lebanon 1976; **Resid:** Internal Medicine, Wayne State Univ Hosp 1978; **Fellow:** Hematology & Oncology, Univ Michigan Sch Med 1981; **Fac Appt:** Assoc Clin Prof Med, Univ Kansas

Eckhardt, S Gail MD [Onc] - **Spec Exp:** Gastrointestinal Cancer; Drug Development; **Hospital:** Univ of CO Hosp - Anschutz Inpatient Pav; **Address:** Univ Colorado Hosp Cancer Ctr, PO Box 6510, MS F-704, 1665 Aurora Court, Aurora, CO 80045-0510; **Phone:** 720-848-0300; **Board Cert:** Internal Medicine 1988; Medical Oncology 2006; **Med School:** Univ Tex Med Br, Galveston 1985; **Resid:** Internal Medicine, Univ Virginia Med Ctr 1988; **Fellow:** Research, Scripps Clinic 1989; Medical Oncology, UCSD Med Ctr 1992; **Fac Appt:** Prof Med, Univ Colorado

Elias, Anthony D MD [Onc] - **Spec Exp:** Breast Cancer; **Hospital:** Univ of CO Hosp - Anschutz Inpatient Pav; **Address:** UCH Breast Ctr, Anschutz OPD Pavillion, 1635 Aurora Ct, MS F724, Aurora, CO 80045; **Phone:** 720-848-1030; **Board Cert:** Internal Medicine 1983; Medical Oncology 1985; **Med School:** NYU Sch Med 1980; **Resid:** Internal Medicine, Johns Hopkins Hsop 1983; **Fellow:** Medical Oncology, Dana-Farber Cancer Inst 1983; **Fac Appt:** Assoc Prof Med, Univ Colorado

Fabian, Carol J MD [Onc] - **Spec Exp:** Breast Cancer; Breast Cancer Risk Assessment; **Hospital:** Univ of Kansas Hosp; **Address:** Westwood Med Pavilion, 2330 Shawnee Mission Pkwy, Ste 1102, MS 5015, Westwood, KS 66205; **Phone:** 913-588-7791; **Board Cert:** Internal Medicine 1976; Medical Oncology 1977; **Med School:** Univ Kansas 1972; **Resid:** Internal Medicine, Wesley Med Ctr 1975; **Fellow:** Medical Oncology, Univ Kansas Med Ctr 1977; **Fac Appt:** Prof Med, Univ Kansas

Glode, L Michael MD [Onc] - **Spec Exp:** Prostate Cancer; Genitourinary Cancer; **Hospital:** Univ of CO Hosp - Anschutz Inpatient Pav; **Address:** Univ Colorado Anschutz Cancer Pavilion, 1665 Aurora Court, CP 1004, MS F-710, Aurora, CO 80045; **Phone:** 720-848-0170; **Board Cert:** Internal Medicine 1975; Medical Oncology 1981; **Med School:** Washington Univ, St Louis 1972; **Resid:** Internal Medicine, Univ Texas SW Med Ctr 1973; Immunology, Natl Inst Hlth 1976; **Fellow:** Medical Oncology, Dana Farber Cancer Inst 1978; **Fac Appt:** Prof Med, Univ Colorado

Grem, Jean L MD [Onc] - **Spec Exp:** Colon & Rectal Cancer; Pancreatic Cancer; Stomach Cancer; Esophageal Cancer; **Hospital:** Nebraska Med Ctr; **Address:** 987630 Nebraska Medical Ctr, Emile @ 42nd St, Omaha, NE 68198-7630; **Phone:** 402-559-6210; **Board Cert:** Internal Medicine 1983; Medical Oncology 1985; **Med School:** Jefferson Med Coll 1980; **Resid:** Internal Medicine, Univ Iowa Hosps & Clinics 1983; **Fellow:** Medical Oncology, Univ Wisc Clin Cancer Ctr 1986; **Fac Appt:** Prof Med, Univ Nebr Coll Med

Hauke, Ralph J MD [Onc] - **Spec Exp:** Urologic Cancer; Clinical Trials; Testicular Cancer; Prostate Cancer; **Hospital:** Methodist Hosp - Omaha, Alegent Hlth - Bergan Mercy Med Ctr; **Address:** 8303 Dodge St, Ste 250, Omaha, NE 68114; **Phone:** 402-354-8124; **Board Cert:** Medical Oncology 2001; **Med School:** Panama 1990; **Resid:** Internal Medicine, Univ Nebraska Med Ctr 1996; **Fellow:** Medical Oncology, Univ Nebraska Med Ctr 2001; **Fac Appt:** Assoc Prof Med, Univ Nebr Coll Med

Medical Oncology

Kane, Madeleine A MD/PhD [Onc] - **Spec Exp:** Head & Neck Cancer; Gastrointestinal Cancer; Neuroendocrine Tumors; **Hospital:** Univ of CO Hosp - Anschutz Inpatient Pav, VA Eastern CO Health Care Sys-Denver; **Address:** Univ Colorado Hosp Cancer Ctr, PO Box 6510, MS F-704, 1665 Aurora Court, Aurora, CO 80045; **Phone:** 720-848-0300; **Board Cert:** Internal Medicine 1981; Medical Oncology 1983; Hematology 1986; **Med School:** Univ Miami Sch Med 1978; **Resid:** Internal Medicine, Stanford Univ Med Ctr 1981; **Fellow:** Hematology & Oncology, Univ Colo Hlth Sci Ctr 1984; **Fac Appt:** Prof Med, Univ Colorado

Messersmith, Wells A MD [Onc] - **Spec Exp:** Gastrointestinal Cancer; Colon & Rectal Cancer; **Hospital:** Univ of CO Hosp - Anschutz Inpatient Pav; **Address:** University of Colorado Hosp, 12605 E 16th Ave, Aurora, CO 80045; **Phone:** 720-848-0300; **Board Cert:** Internal Medicine 2001; Medical Oncology 2003; **Med School:** Harvard Med Sch 1998; **Resid:** Medical Oncology, Mass Genl Hosp 2000; **Fellow:** Medical Oncology, Johns Hopkins Hosp 2004; **Fac Appt:** Asst Prof Med, Univ Colorado

Samuels, Brian L MD [Onc] - **Spec Exp:** Sarcoma; **Hospital:** Kootenai Med Ctr; **Address:** 1440 Mullan Ave, Post Falls, ID 83854; **Phone:** 208-619-4100; **Board Cert:** Internal Medicine 1984; Medical Oncology 1987; **Med School:** Zimbabwe 1976; **Resid:** Internal Medicine, Albert Einstein Med Ctr 1981; Internal Medicine, Albert Einstein Med Ctr 1984; **Fellow:** Hematology & Oncology, Univ Chicago Hosps 1988

Steen, Preston D MD [Onc] - **Spec Exp:** Lymphoma; Lung Cancer; Breast Cancer; Palliative Care; **Hospital:** Sanford Med Ctr Fargo; **Address:** Sanford Health Roger Maris Cancer Ctr, 820 4th St N, Fargo, ND 58102; **Phone:** 701-234-6161; **Board Cert:** Internal Medicine 1987; Medical Oncology 2001; Hospice & Palliative Medicine ; **Med School:** Univ Minn 1984; **Resid:** Internal Medicine, Maricopa Med Ctr 1987; **Fellow:** Hematology & Oncology, Univ Utah 1990; **Fac Appt:** Clin Prof Med, Univ ND Sch Med

Ward, John H MD [Onc] - **Spec Exp:** Breast Cancer; Gastrointestinal Cancer; Brain Tumors; Unknown Primary Cancer; **Hospital:** Univ Utah Hlth Care, St. John's Med Ctr; **Address:** 2000 Circle of Hope, Ste 2100, rm 2141, Salt Lake City, UT 84112-5550; **Phone:** 801-585-0255; **Board Cert:** Internal Medicine 1979; Medical Oncology 1981; Hematology 1982; **Med School:** Univ Utah 1976; **Resid:** Internal Medicine, Duke Univ Med Ctr 1979; **Fellow:** Hematology & Oncology, Univ Utah Med Ctr 1982; **Fac Appt:** Prof Med, Univ Utah

Southwest

Abbruzzese, James L MD [Onc] - **Spec Exp:** Gastrointestinal Cancer; Pancreatic Cancer; Clinical Trials; **Hospital:** UT MD Anderson Cancer Ctr; **Address:** Univ Tex MD Anderson Cancer Ctr, 1515 Holcombe Blvd, Unit 426, Houston, TX 77030; **Phone:** 713-792-2828; **Board Cert:** Internal Medicine 1981; Medical Oncology 1983; **Med School:** Univ Chicago-Pritzker Sch Med 1978; **Resid:** Internal Medicine, Johns Hopkins Hosp 1981; **Fellow:** Medical Oncology, Dana-Farber Cancer Inst 1983; **Fac Appt:** Prof Med, Univ Tex, Houston

Ahmann, Frederick R MD [Onc] - **Spec Exp:** Prostate Cancer; Testicular Cancer; Bladder Cancer; **Hospital:** Univ Med Ctr - Tucson; **Address:** Arizona Cancer Ctr, 3838 N Campbell Ave, Tucson, AZ 85719; **Phone:** 520-694-2873; **Board Cert:** Internal Medicine 1977; Medical Oncology 1981; **Med School:** Univ MO-Columbia Sch Med 1974; **Resid:** Internal Medicine, Georgetown Univ Med Ctr 1977; **Fellow:** Medical Oncology, Univ Med Ctr 1980; **Fac Appt:** Prof Med, Univ Ariz Coll Med

Ajani, Jaffer A MD [Onc] - **Spec Exp:** Gastrointestinal Cancer; Esophageal Cancer; Stomach Cancer; Neuroendocrine Tumors; **Hospital:** UT MD Anderson Cancer Ctr; **Address:** Univ Tex MD Anderson Cancer Ctr, 1515 Holcombe Blvd, Unit 426, Houston, TX 77230; **Phone:** 713-792-2828; **Board Cert:** Internal Medicine 1979; Medical Oncology 1983; **Med School:** India 1971; **Resid:** Family Medicine, Penn Stae Univ-Altoona 1977; Internal Medicine, Tulane Univ Sch Med 1980; **Fellow:** Medical Oncology, MD Anderson Cancer Ctr 1983; **Fac Appt:** Prof Med, Univ Tex, Houston

Alberts, David S MD [Onc] - **Spec Exp:** Cancer Prevention; Ovarian Cancer; **Hospital:** Univ Med Ctr - Tucson; **Address:** Arizona Cancer Center, 1515N Campbell Ave, PO Box 245024, Tucson, AZ 85724; **Phone:** 520-626-7685; **Board Cert:** Internal Medicine 1973; Medical Oncology 1973; **Med School:** Univ VA Sch Med 1966; **Resid:** Medical Oncology, Natl Cancer Inst-NIH 1969; Internal Medicine, Univ Minn Hosps 1971; **Fellow:** Clinical Pharmacology, UC San Francisco 1974; **Fac Appt:** Prof Med, Univ Ariz Coll Med

Anthony, Lowell B MD [Onc] - **Spec Exp:** Gastrointestinal Cancer; Carcinoid Tumors; Neuroendocrine Tumors; **Hospital:** LSU Interim Public Hosp; **Address:** 200 W Esplanade, Ste 200, Kenner, LA 70065; **Phone:** 504-464-8500; **Board Cert:** Internal Medicine 1983; Medical Oncology 1989; **Med School:** Vanderbilt Univ 1979; **Resid:** Internal Medicine, Vanderbilt Univ Med Ctr 1982; **Fellow:** Medical Oncology, Vanderbilt Univ Med Ctr 1985; **Fac Appt:** Assoc Prof Med, Louisiana State U, New Orleans

Arun, Banu K MD [Onc] - **Spec Exp:** Breast Cancer; Cancer Prevention; Clinical Trials; **Hospital:** UT MD Anderson Cancer Ctr; **Address:** 1515 Holcombe Blvd, Unit 1354, Houston, TX 77030; **Phone:** 713-792-2817; **Med School:** Turkey 1990; **Resid:** Internal Medicine, Univ Istanbul 1994; **Fellow:** Hematology & Oncology, Lombardi Cancer Ctr-Georgetown Univ 1997; **Fac Appt:** Assoc Prof Med, Univ Tex, Houston

Benjamin, Robert S MD [Onc] - **Spec Exp:** Sarcoma; **Hospital:** UT MD Anderson Cancer Ctr; **Address:** UT MD Anderson Cancer Ctr, 1515 Holcombe Blvd, Unit 450, Houston, TX 77030; **Phone:** 713-792-3626; **Board Cert:** Internal Medicine 1973; Medical Oncology 1973; **Med School:** NYU Sch Med 1968; **Resid:** Internal Medicine, Bellevue Hosp Ctr-NYU 1970; **Fellow:** Medical Oncology, Baltimore Cancer Rsch Ctr 1972; **Fac Appt:** Prof Med, Univ Tex, Houston

Bergsagel, Peter Leif MD [Onc] - **Spec Exp:** Multiple Myeloma; Hematologic Malignancies; **Hospital:** Mayo Clinic - Scottsdale; **Address:** 13400 E Shea Blvd Fl 3, Scottsdale, AZ 85259; **Phone:** 480-301-8335; **Board Cert:** Internal Medicine 1987; Medical Oncology 1989; **Med School:** Univ Toronto 1984; **Resid:** Internal Medicine, Stanford Univ Med Ctr 1986; Internal Medicine, Sunnybrook Med Ctr 1987; **Fellow:** Medical Oncology, NIH Natl Cancer Inst 1990; **Fac Appt:** Prof Med, Mayo Med Sch

Bruera, Eduardo MD [Onc] - **Spec Exp:** Palliative Care; **Hospital:** UT MD Anderson Cancer Ctr; **Address:** 1515 Holcombe Blvd, Unit 1414, Houston, TX 77030; **Phone:** 713-792-6085; **Med School:** Argentina 1979; **Resid:** Internal Medicine, Hospital Privado; **Fellow:** Medical Oncology, Cross Cancer Inst; **Fac Appt:** Prof Med, Univ Tex, Houston

Buzdar, Aman U MD [Onc] - **Spec Exp:** Breast Cancer; **Hospital:** UT MD Anderson Cancer Ctr; **Address:** UT MD Anderson Canc Ctr, 1515 Holcome Blvd, Unit 1354, Houston, TX 77030; **Phone:** 713-792-2817; **Board Cert:** Internal Medicine 1975; Medical Oncology 1979; **Med School:** Pakistan 1967; **Resid:** Internal Medicine, Norwalk Hosp 1973; Internal Medicine, Lakewood Hosp 1971; **Fellow:** Hematology, Norwalk Hosp 1974; Oncology, MD Anderson Cancer Ctr 1975; **Fac Appt:** Prof Med, Univ Tex, Houston

Medical Oncology

Camoriano, John MD [Onc] - **Spec Exp:** Lymphoma; Breast Cancer; Bone Marrow Transplant; Myeloproliferative Disorders; **Hospital:** Mayo Clinic - Scottsdale; **Address:** Mayo Clinic - Scottsdale, 13400 E Shea Blvd Fl 3, Scottsdale, AZ 85259; **Phone:** 480-301-8335; **Board Cert:** Internal Medicine 1985; Hematology 1988; Medical Oncology 1989; **Med School:** Univ Nebr Coll Med 1982; **Resid:** Internal Medicine, Univ OK 1985; **Fellow:** Hematology & Oncology, Mayo Grad Sch Med 1989; **Fac Appt:** Asst Prof Med, Mayo Med Sch

Chang, Jenny C N MD [Onc] - **Spec Exp:** Breast Cancer; Clinical Trials; **Hospital:** Methodist Hosp - Houston; **Address:** 6445 Main St Fl 21, Outpatient Ctr, Houston, TX 77030; **Phone:** 713-441-9948; **Board Cert:** Internal Medicine 2004; **Med School:** England, UK 1989; **Resid:** Internal Medicine 1993; **Fellow:** Medical Oncology, Royal Marsden Hosp 1997; **Fac Appt:** Assoc Prof Med, Baylor Coll Med

Fay, Joseph W MD [Onc] - **Spec Exp:** Bone Marrow Transplant; Melanoma; Leukemia & Lymphoma; **Hospital:** Baylor Univ Medical Ctr; **Address:** 3410 Worth St, Ste 300, Sammons Cancer Ctr, Dallas, TX 75246; **Phone:** 214-370-1500; **Board Cert:** Internal Medicine 1975; Medical Oncology 1977; Hematology 1978; **Med School:** Ohio State Univ 1972; **Resid:** Internal Medicine, Duke Med Ctr 1974; Oncology, Natl Cancer Institute 1976; **Fellow:** Hematology, Duke Med Ctr 1977; **Fac Appt:** Clin Prof Med, Univ Tex SW, Dallas

Fitch, Tom R MD [Onc] - **Spec Exp:** Breast Cancer; Sarcoma; Cancer Prevention; Palliative Care; **Hospital:** Mayo Clinic - Scottsdale; **Address:** Mayo Clinic - Scottsdale, 13400 E Shea Blvd Fl 3, Scottsdale, AZ 85259; **Phone:** 480-301-8335; **Board Cert:** Internal Medicine 1985; Medical Oncology 1987; Hematology 1988; **Med School:** Univ Kansas 1982; **Resid:** Internal Medicine, Univ Michigan Med Ctr 1985; **Fellow:** Hematology & Oncology, Mayo Clinic 1988; **Fac Appt:** Asst Prof Med, Mayo Med Sch

Fossella, Frank V MD [Onc] - **Spec Exp:** Lung Cancer; **Hospital:** UT MD Anderson Cancer Ctr; **Address:** Dept Thoracic Head/Neck Med Oncol, 1400 Holcombe Blvd, Unit 432, Houston, TX 77030; **Phone:** 713-792-6363; **Board Cert:** Internal Medicine 1985; Medical Oncology 1987; **Med School:** Baylor Coll Med 1982; **Resid:** Internal Medicine, Baylor Coll Med 1985; **Fellow:** Medical Oncology, Baylor Coll Med 1987; **Fac Appt:** Prof Med, Univ Tex, Houston

Glisson, Bonnie S MD [Onc] - **Spec Exp:** Head & Neck Cancer; Lung Cancer; **Hospital:** UT MD Anderson Cancer Ctr; **Address:** UTMDACC- Unit 432, PO Box 301402, Houston, TX 77230-1402; **Phone:** 713-792-6363; **Board Cert:** Internal Medicine 1982; Medical Oncology 1985; **Med School:** Ohio State Univ 1979; **Resid:** Internal Medicine, Univ VA Med Ctr 1982; **Fellow:** Medical Oncology, Univ Fla Health Sci Ctr 1985; **Fac Appt:** Prof Med, Univ Tex, Houston

Haley, Barbara MD [Onc] - **Spec Exp:** Breast Cancer; **Hospital:** UT Southwestern Med Ctr at Dallas; **Address:** 5323 Harry Hines Blvd, Suite-NB2102, Dallas, TX 75390-8852; **Phone:** 214-648-4180; **Board Cert:** Internal Medicine 1979; Hematology 1984; **Med School:** Univ Tex SW, Dallas 1976; **Resid:** Internal Medicine, Parkland Meml Hosp 1979; **Fellow:** Hematology & Oncology, Parkland Meml Hosp 1981; **Fac Appt:** Prof Med, Univ Tex SW, Dallas

Hong, Waun Ki MD [Onc] - **Spec Exp:** Lung Cancer; Head & Neck Cancer; Thoracic Cancers; **Hospital:** UT MD Anderson Cancer Ctr; **Address:** Dept Thoracic Head/Neck, 1400 Holcombe Blvd, Unit 421, Houston, TX 77030; **Phone:** 713-792-6363; **Board Cert:** Internal Medicine 1976; Medical Oncology 1979; **Med School:** South Korea 1967; **Resid:** Internal Medicine, Boston VA Hosp 1973; **Fellow:** Medical Oncology, Meml Sloan-Kettering Cancer Ctr 1975; **Fac Appt:** Prof Med, Univ Tex, Houston

Hortobagyi, Gabriel N MD [Onc] - **Spec Exp:** Breast Cancer-Male; Clinical Trials; Gene Therapy; **Hospital:** UT MD Anderson Cancer Ctr; **Address:** 1515 Holcombe Blvd, ACB Bldg - Fl 5th, MS 1354, Dept Breast Oncology, PO Box 301429, Unit 1354, Houston, TX 77030-1439; **Phone:** 713-792-2817; **Board Cert:** Internal Medicine 1975; Medical Oncology 1977; **Med School:** Colombia 1970; **Resid:** Internal Medicine, St Lukes Hosp 1974; **Fellow:** Medical Oncology, MD Anderson Cancer Ctr 1976; **Fac Appt:** Prof Med, Univ Tex, Houston

Hutchins, Laura F MD [Onc] - **Spec Exp:** Breast Cancer; Melanoma; **Hospital:** UAMS Med Ctr; **Address:** Univ Arkansas Med Scis, Dept Hem/Onc, 4301 W Markham St, Slot 508, Little Rock, AR 72205; **Phone:** 501-686-8511; **Board Cert:** Internal Medicine 1980; Hematology 1984; Medical Oncology 1987; **Med School:** Univ Ark 1977; **Resid:** Internal Medicine, Univ Ark Affil Hosp 1980; **Fellow:** Hematology & Oncology, Univ Arkansas 1983; **Fac Appt:** Prof Med, Univ Ark

Hwu, Patrick MD [Onc] - **Spec Exp:** Melanoma; Immunotherapy; Clinical Trials; **Hospital:** UT MD Anderson Cancer Ctr; **Address:** UT MD Anderson Cancer Center, Melanoma & Skin Center, 1515 Holcombe Blvd, Unit 347, Houston, TX 77030; **Phone:** 713-792-6800; **Board Cert:** Medical Oncology 2008; **Med School:** Med Coll PA 1987; **Resid:** Internal Medicine, Johns Hopkins Hosp 1989; **Fellow:** Medical Oncology, Natl Cancer Inst 1993

Johnson, David H MD [Onc] - **Spec Exp:** Lung Cancer; Drug Discovery & Development; **Hospital:** UT Southwestern Med Ctr at Dallas; **Address:** UT Southwestern Med Ctr, 5323 Harry Hines Blvd, Dallas, TX 75390-9030; **Phone:** 214-648-3486; **Board Cert:** Internal Medicine 1979; Medical Oncology 2008; **Med School:** Med Coll GA 1976; **Resid:** Internal Medicine, Univ South Alabama Med Ctr 1979; Internal Medicine, Med Coll Georgia Hosp 1980; **Fellow:** Medical Oncology, Vanderbilt Univ Med Ctr 1983; **Fac Appt:** Prof Med, Univ Tex SW, Dallas

Karp, Daniel D MD [Onc] - **Spec Exp:** Lung Cancer; **Hospital:** UT MD Anderson Cancer Ctr; **Address:** UTMDACC- Unit 432, PO Box 301402, Houston, TX 77230-1402; **Phone:** 713-792-6363; **Board Cert:** Internal Medicine 1976; Hematology 1980; Medical Oncology 1981; **Med School:** Duke Univ 1973; **Resid:** Internal Medicine, Dartmouth-Hitchcock Med Ctr 1976; **Fellow:** Hematology, Dartmouth-Hitchcock Med Ctr 1978; Medical Oncology, Dana Farber Cancer Inst 1979; **Fac Appt:** Prof Med, Univ Tex, Houston

Kies, Merrill S MD [Onc] - **Spec Exp:** Head & Neck Cancer; Lung Cancer; **Hospital:** UT MD Anderson Cancer Ctr; **Address:** Div Cancer Med, Thoracic/Head & Neck Med Oncology, 1515 Holcombe Blvd, Unit 421, Houston, TX 77030; **Phone:** 713-792-7770; **Board Cert:** Internal Medicine 1976; Medical Oncology 1979; **Med School:** Loyola Univ-Stritch Sch Med 1973; **Resid:** Internal Medicine, Walter Reed AMC 1976; **Fellow:** Medical Oncology, Brooke AMC 1978; **Fac Appt:** Prof Med, Univ Tex, Houston

Kwak, Larry W MD/PhD [Onc] - **Spec Exp:** Lymphoma; Multiple Myeloma; Vaccine Therapy; Immunotherapy; **Hospital:** UT MD Anderson Cancer Ctr; **Address:** MD Anderson Cancer Ctr, Dept Lymphoma/Myeloma, 1515 Holcombe Blvd, Unit 429, Houston, TX 77030; **Phone:** 713-792-2860; **Board Cert:** Internal Medicine 1987; Medical Oncology 1989; **Med School:** Northwestern Univ 1982; **Resid:** Internal Medicine, Stanford Univ Hosp 1987; **Fellow:** Oncology, Stanford Univ Hosp 1989

Lippman, Scott M MD [Onc] - **Spec Exp:** Cancer Prevention; Lung Cancer; Head & Neck Cancer; **Hospital:** UT MD Anderson Cancer Ctr; **Address:** UT MD Anderson Cancer Ctr, 1515 Holcombe Blvd, Unit 432, Houston, TX 77030; **Phone:** 713-745-5439; **Board Cert:** Internal Medicine 1987; Hematology 1988; Medical Oncology 1989; **Med School:** Johns Hopkins Univ 1981; **Resid:** Internal Medicine, Harbor-UCLA Med Ctr 1983; **Fellow:** Hematology, Stanford Univ Med Ctr 1985; Hematology & Oncology, Univ Ariz Hlth Scis Ctr 1987; **Fac Appt:** Prof Med, Univ Tex, Houston

Medical Oncology

Livingston, Robert B MD [Onc] - **Spec Exp:** Bone Marrow Transplant; Breast Cancer; Lung Cancer; **Hospital:** Univ Med Ctr - Tucson; **Address:** Arizona Cancer Ctr, 3838 N Campbell Ave, Tucson, AZ 85719; **Phone:** 520-694-2873; **Board Cert:** Internal Medicine 1972; Medical Oncology 1973; **Med School:** Univ Okla Coll Med 1965; **Resid:** Internal Medicine, Univ Oklahoma Med Ctr 1971; **Fellow:** Medical Oncology, Univ Texas Cancer Ctr 1973; **Fac Appt:** Prof Med, Univ Wash

Logothetis, Christopher J MD [Onc] - **Spec Exp:** Prostate Cancer; Bladder Cancer; **Hospital:** UT MD Anderson Cancer Ctr; **Address:** UT MD Anderson Cancer Ctr, Dept GU Onc, Unit 1274, Box 301439, Houston, TX 77230; **Phone:** 713-563-7210; **Board Cert:** Internal Medicine 1978; Medical Oncology 1981; **Med School:** Greece 1974; **Resid:** Internal Medicine, Univ Texas 1979; **Fellow:** Hematology & Oncology, Univ Tex-MD Anderson Cancer Ctr 1981; **Fac Appt:** Prof Med, Univ Tex, Houston

Makhoul, Issam MD [Onc] - **Spec Exp:** Gastrointestinal Cancer; Breast Cancer; Colon Cancer; **Hospital:** UAMS Med Ctr; **Address:** 4301 W Markham St, Slot# 721-5, Little Rock, AR 72205; **Phone:** 501-686-8530; **Board Cert:** Medical Oncology 2002; Hematology 2003; **Med School:** Syria 1980; **Resid:** Internal Medicine, Genl Hosp 1984; Internal Medicine, Penn State Affil Hosp 1999; **Fellow:** Hematology & Oncology, Hershey Med Ctr 2002; **Fac Appt:** Asst Prof Med, Univ Ark

Miller, Thomas P MD [Onc] - **Spec Exp:** Lymphoma; **Hospital:** Univ Med Ctr - Tucson; **Address:** Arizona Cancer Ctr, 3838 N Campbell Ave, Tucson, AZ 85719; **Phone:** 520-694-2873; **Board Cert:** Internal Medicine 1977; Medical Oncology 1981; **Med School:** Univ IL Coll Med 1972; **Resid:** Internal Medicine, Univ Illinois Hosps 1977; **Fellow:** Hematology & Oncology, Univ Med Ctr 1980; **Fac Appt:** Prof Med, Univ Ariz Coll Med

Northfelt, Donald W MD [Onc] - **Spec Exp:** Breast Cancer; Colon & Rectal Cancer; Lung Cancer; **Hospital:** Mayo Clinic - Scottsdale; **Address:** Mayo Clinic Scottsdale, 13400 E Shea Blvd Fl 3, Scottsdale, AZ 85259; **Phone:** 480-301-8335; **Board Cert:** Internal Medicine 1988; Medical Oncology 2001; **Med School:** Univ Minn 1985; **Resid:** Internal Medicine, UCLA Med Ctr 1988; **Fellow:** Hematology & Oncology, UCSF Med Ctr 1991; **Fac Appt:** Assoc Prof Med, Mayo Med Sch

O'Brien, Susan M MD [Onc] - **Spec Exp:** Leukemia; Lymphoma; **Hospital:** UT MD Anderson Cancer Ctr; **Address:** Univ Texas MD Anderson Cancer Ctr, Dept Leukemia, Unit 428, PO Box 301402, Houston, TX 77230; **Phone:** 713-792-7305; **Board Cert:** Internal Medicine 1983; Medical Oncology 1987; **Med School:** UMDNJ-NJ Med Sch, Newark 1980; **Resid:** Internal Medicine, UMDNJ Med Ctr 1983; **Fellow:** Medical Oncology, Univ TX MD Anderson Med Ctr 1987; **Fac Appt:** Prof Med, Univ Tex, Houston

O'Shaughnessy, Joyce A MD [Onc] - **Spec Exp:** Breast Cancer; **Hospital:** Baylor Univ Medical Ctr; **Address:** Texas Oncology, 3410 Worth St, Dallas, TX 75246; **Phone:** 214-370-1000; **Board Cert:** Internal Medicine 1985; Medical Oncology 1987; **Med School:** Yale Univ 1982; **Resid:** Internal Medicine, Mass Genl Hosp 1985; **Fellow:** Medical Oncology, National Cancer Inst 1988

Orlowski, Robert Z MD/PhD [Onc] - **Spec Exp:** Multiple Myeloma; Lymphoma, Non-Hodgkin's; Leukemia; Clinical Trials; **Hospital:** UT MD Anderson Cancer Ctr; **Address:** MD Anderson Cancer Ctr, Lymphoma & Myeloma Clinic, 1515 Holcombe Blvd, Box 429, Houston, TX 77030; **Phone:** 713-792-3510; **Med School:** Yale Univ 1991; **Resid:** Internal Medicine, Barnes Hosp/Wash Univ 1994; **Fellow:** Hematology & Oncology, Johns Hopkins Hosp 1998; **Fac Appt:** Assoc Prof Med, Univ Tex, Houston

Osborne, C Kent MD [Onc] - **Spec Exp:** Breast Cancer; **Hospital:** Methodist Hosp - Houston; **Address:** 1 Baylor Plaza, MS BCM600, Houston, TX 77030; **Phone:** 713-798-1641; **Board Cert:** Internal Medicine 1975; Medical Oncology 1977; **Med School:** Univ MO-Columbia Sch Med 1972; **Resid:** Internal Medicine, Johns Hopkins Hosp 1974; **Fellow:** Medical Oncology, Natl Cancer Inst 1977; **Fac Appt:** Prof Med, Baylor Coll Med

Papadopoulos, Nicholas E MD [Onc] - **Spec Exp:** Melanoma; **Hospital:** UT MD Anderson Cancer Ctr; **Address:** 1515 Holcombe Blvd, Unit 430, Houston, TX 77030; **Phone:** 713-792-2921; **Med School:** Greece 1966; **Resid:** Internal Medicine, Baylor Coll Med 1976; **Fellow:** Medical Oncology, MD Anderson Cancer Ctr 1978; **Fac Appt:** Assoc Prof Med, Univ Tex, Houston

Patel, Shreyaskumar MD [Onc] - **Spec Exp:** Sarcoma; **Hospital:** UT MD Anderson Cancer Ctr; **Address:** 1515 Holcombe Blvd, Box 450, Houston, TX 77030; **Phone:** 713-792-3626; **Board Cert:** Internal Medicine 1987; Medical Oncology 2000; **Med School:** India 1983; **Resid:** Internal Medicine, Wayne State Univ 1987; **Fellow:** Medical Oncology, Mayo Clinic 1990

Patt, Yehuda Z MD [Onc] - **Spec Exp:** Liver Cancer; Biliary Cancer; Colon & Rectal Cancer; Gastrointestinal Cancer; **Hospital:** Univ Hosp - New Mexico; **Address:** Univ New Mexico CRTC, Div Hem/Onc, 1201 Camino de Salud NE, Albuquerque, NM 87131; **Phone:** 505-272-4946; **Board Cert:** Internal Medicine 1982; Medical Oncology 1987; **Med School:** Israel 1967; **Resid:** Internal Medicine, Tel Aviv-Sheba Med Ctr 1974; **Fellow:** Medical Oncology, UT MD Anderson Cancer Ctr 1977; **Fac Appt:** Prof Med, Univ New Mexico

Pisters, Katherine M W MD [Onc] - **Spec Exp:** Lung Cancer; **Hospital:** UT MD Anderson Cancer Ctr; **Address:** UT MD Anderson Cancer Ctr, PO Box 301402, Unit 432, Houston, TX 77230-1402; **Phone:** 713-792-6363; **Board Cert:** Internal Medicine 1988; Medical Oncology 2002; **Med School:** Univ Western Ontario 1985; **Resid:** Internal Medicine, N Shore Univ Hosp 1988; **Fellow:** Medical Oncology, Meml Sloan Kettering Cancer Ctr 1991; **Fac Appt:** Prof Med, Univ Tex, Houston

Romaguera, Jorge MD [Onc] - **Spec Exp:** Lymphoma; **Hospital:** UT MD Anderson Cancer Ctr; **Address:** 1515 Holcombe Blvd, Box 429, Lymphoma & Myeloma Clinic, Houston, TX 77030; **Phone:** 713-792-3510; **Board Cert:** Internal Medicine 1988; Medical Oncology 1989; **Med School:** Univ Puerto Rico 1982; **Resid:** Internal Medicine, Univ Hosp 1985; **Fellow:** Hematology & Oncology, Univ Hosp 1987

Ross, Helen J MD [Onc] - **Spec Exp:** Lung Cancer; Mesothelioma; Esophageal Cancer; **Hospital:** Mayo Clinic - Scottsdale; **Address:** Mayo Clinic, 13400 E Shea Blvd, Scottsdale, AZ 85259; **Phone:** 480-301-8335; **Board Cert:** Internal Medicine 1987; Medical Oncology 1989; **Med School:** UCLA 1984; **Resid:** Internal Medicine, Cedars Sinai Med Ctr 1987; **Fellow:** Medical Oncology, UCLA Med Ctr 1989; **Fac Appt:** Assoc Prof Med, Mayo Med Sch

Saiki, John H MD [Onc] - **Hospital:** Univ Hosp - New Mexico; **Address:** University of New Mexico Cancer Center, 1201 Camino de Salud NE, Albuquerque, NM 87106; **Phone:** 505-925-0423; **Board Cert:** Internal Medicine 1970; Medical Oncology 1973; **Med School:** McGill Univ 1961; **Resid:** Internal Medicine, Univ New Mexico 1968; Hematology, Univ New Mexico 1969; **Fellow:** Medical Oncology, MD Anderson Hosp 1970; **Fac Appt:** Prof Emeritus Med, Univ New Mexico

Schiller, Joan H MD [Onc] - **Spec Exp:** Lung Cancer; **Hospital:** UT Southwestern Med Ctr at Dallas; **Address:** Univ Texas Southwestern, 5323 Harry Hines Blvd, Dallas, TX 75390-8852; **Phone:** 214-648-4180; **Board Cert:** Internal Medicine 1983; Medical Oncology 1987; **Med School:** Univ IL Coll Med 1980; **Resid:** Internal Medicine, Northwestern Meml Hosp 1983; **Fellow:** Medical Oncology, Univ Wisconsin Hosp 1985; **Fac Appt:** Prof Med, Univ Wisc

Medical Oncology

Taetle, Raymond MD [Onc] - **Hospital:** St. Joseph's Hosp - Tucson; **Address:** Arizona Oncology Assoc, 6565 Carondolet St, Ste 155, Tucson, AZ 85710; **Phone:** 520-886-0206; **Board Cert:** Internal Medicine 1976; Hematology 1978; Medical Oncology 1979; **Med School:** Northwestern Univ 1973; **Resid:** Internal Medicine, Univ California Med Ctr 1976; **Fellow:** Hematology & Oncology, Univ California Med Ctr 1978; **Fac Appt:** Clin Prof Med, Univ Ariz Coll Med

Valero, Vicente MD [Onc] - **Spec Exp:** Breast Cancer; **Hospital:** UT MD Anderson Cancer Ctr; **Address:** Univ Texas MD Anderson Cancer Ctr, 1515 Holcombe Blvd, Unit 1354, Houston, TX 77030; **Phone:** 713-792-2817; **Board Cert:** Internal Medicine 1985; Medical Oncology 1987; Hematology 1988; **Med School:** Mexico 1980; **Resid:** Internal Medicine, Univ Cincinnati Med Ctr 1985; Hematology & Oncology, Univ Cincinnati Med Ctr 1987; **Fellow:** Hematology & Oncology, Univ Texas Med Br 1988; **Fac Appt:** Prof Med, Univ Tex, Houston

Varadhachary, Gauri MD [Onc] - **Spec Exp:** Unknown Primary Cancer; Pancreatic Cancer; **Hospital:** UT MD Anderson Cancer Ctr; **Address:** 1515 Holcombe Blvd, Box 426, Houston, TX 77030; **Phone:** 713-792-2828; **Board Cert:** Internal Medicine 2004; Medical Oncology 2008; **Med School:** India 1991; **Resid:** Internal Medicine, Greater Baltimore Med Ctr 1995; **Fellow:** Hematology & Oncology, Baylor Univ Affil Hosp 1998

Von Burton, Gary MD [Onc] - **Spec Exp:** Breast Cancer; Sarcoma; Brain Tumors; **Hospital:** Louisiana State Univ Hosp; **Address:** LSUHSC-Shreveport, Feist-Weiller Cancer Ctr, 1501 Kings Hwy, PO Box 33932, Shreveport, LA 71130; **Phone:** 318-675-5972; **Board Cert:** Internal Medicine 1981; Medical Oncology 1983; **Med School:** Univ Utah 1978; **Resid:** Internal Medicine, Duke Univ Med Ctr 1981; **Fellow:** Hematology & Oncology, Duke Univ Med Ctr 1983; **Fac Appt:** Prof Med, Louisiana State U, Shrevport

Von Hoff, Daniel D MD [Onc] - **Spec Exp:** Pancreatic Cancer; Breast Cancer; Drug Discovery; **Hospital:** Scottsdale Hlthcare - Shea; **Address:** Translational Genomics Rsch Inst, 445 N 5th St, Ste 600, Phoenix, AZ 85004; **Phone:** 602-343-8492; **Board Cert:** Internal Medicine 1976; Medical Oncology 1979; **Med School:** Columbia P&S 1973; **Resid:** Internal Medicine, UCSF Med Ctr 1975; **Fac Appt:** Prof Med, Univ Ariz Coll Med

Willson, James KV MD [Onc] - **Spec Exp:** Gastrointestinal Cancer; Colon Cancer; Pancreatic Cancer; **Hospital:** UT Southwestern Med Ctr at Dallas; **Address:** 5323 Harry Hines Blvd, Dallas, TX 75390-8590; **Phone:** 214-645-4673; **Board Cert:** Internal Medicine 1980; Medical Oncology 1981; **Med School:** Univ Alabama 1976; **Resid:** Internal Medicine, Johns Hopkins Hosp 1978; **Fellow:** Medical Oncology, Natl Cancer Inst-NIH 1980; **Fac Appt:** Prof Med, Univ Tex SW, Dallas

Wolff, Robert A MD [Onc] - **Spec Exp:** Gastrointestinal Cancer; Pancreatic Cancer; Colon & Rectal Cancer; Clinical Trials; **Hospital:** UT MD Anderson Cancer Ctr; **Address:** 1515 Holcombe Blvd, Unit 421, Houston, TX 77030; **Phone:** 713-745-5476; **Board Cert:** Internal Medicine 1989; Medical Oncology 2008; **Med School:** Albany Med Coll 1986; **Resid:** Internal Medicine, Duke Univ Med Ctr 1989; **Fellow:** Hematology & Oncology, Duke Univ Med Ctr 1992

West Coast and Pacific

Aboulafia, David M MD [Onc] - **Spec Exp:** AIDS Related Cancers; Leukemia; Lymphoma; Multiple Myeloma; **Hospital:** Virginia Mason Med Ctr; **Address:** Virginia Mason Med Ctr, Sect of Hematology/Oncology, 1100 Ninth Ave, Seattle, WA 98101; **Phone:** 206-223-6193; **Board Cert:** Internal Medicine 1986; Medical Oncology 1989; Hematology 2003; **Med School:** Univ Mich Med Sch 1983; **Resid:** Internal Medicine, UCLA Med Ctr 1986; **Fellow:** Hematology & Oncology, UCLA Med Ctr 1989; **Fac Appt:** Clin Prof Med, Univ Wash

Abrams, Donald I MD [Onc] - **Spec Exp:** AIDS Related Cancers; Complementary Medicine; **Hospital:** San Francisco Genl Hosp; **Address:** Positive Hlth Program-SF Genl Hosp, 995 Potrero Ave, Bldg 80, Ward 84, San Francisco, CA 94110; **Phone:** 415-476-4082 x444; **Board Cert:** Internal Medicine 1980; Medical Oncology 1983; **Med School:** Stanford Univ 1977; **Resid:** Internal Medicine, Kaiser Fdn Hosp 1980; **Fellow:** Medical Oncology, UCSF Cancer Rsch 1982; **Fac Appt:** Clin Prof Med, UCSF

Advani, Ranjana H MD [Onc] - **Spec Exp:** Lymphoma; Hematologic Malignancies; Clinical Trials; **Hospital:** Stanford Univ Hosp & Clinics; **Address:** Lymphoma Clinic, 875 Blake Wilbur Drive, Clinic C, Stanford, CA 94305; **Phone:** 650-498-6000; **Board Cert:** Internal Medicine 2001; Medical Oncology 2009; **Med School:** India 1982; **Resid:** Internal Medicine, Santa Clara Vly Med Ctr 1987; Internal Medicine, Stanford Univ 1991; **Fellow:** Hematology, Stanford Univ Med Ctr 1990; **Fac Appt:** Asst Prof Med, Stanford Univ

Appelbaum, Frederick R MD [Onc] - **Spec Exp:** Bone Marrow Transplant; Leukemia-Myeloid; Graft vs Host Disease; **Hospital:** Univ Wash Med Ctr; **Address:** 1100 Fairview Ave N, rm D5-310, PO Box 19024, Seattle, WA 98109; **Phone:** 206-288-1024; **Board Cert:** Internal Medicine 1975; Medical Oncology 1977; **Med School:** Tufts Univ 1972; **Resid:** Internal Medicine, Univ Michigan Med Ctr 1974; **Fellow:** Medical Oncology, Natl Cancer Inst 1976; **Fac Appt:** Prof Med, Univ Wash

Back, Anthony MD [Onc] - **Spec Exp:** Palliative Care; Gastrointestinal Cancer; **Hospital:** Univ Wash Med Ctr; **Address:** Seattle Cancer Care Alliance, 825 Eastlake Ave E, Box G4100, Seattle, WA 98109; **Phone:** 206-288-6478; **Board Cert:** Internal Medicine 1987; Medical Oncology 2001; Hospice & Palliative Medicine 2008; **Med School:** Harvard Med Sch 1984; **Resid:** Internal Medicine, Univ Washington Med Ctr 1988; **Fellow:** Oncology, Univ Washington Med Ctr 1991; **Fac Appt:** Prof Med, Univ Wash

Ball, Edward D MD [Onc] - **Spec Exp:** Bone Marrow & Stem Cell Transplant; Leukemia & Lymphoma; Multiple Myeloma; Immunotherapy; **Hospital:** UCSD Med Ctr-Hillcrest; **Address:** 3855 Health Sciences Dr, #0960, La Jolla, CA 92093-0960; **Phone:** 858-822-6600; **Board Cert:** Internal Medicine 1979; Medical Oncology 1983; Hematology 2011; **Med School:** Case West Res Univ 1976; **Resid:** Internal Medicine, Hartford Hosp 1979; **Fellow:** Hematology & Oncology, Univ Hosps Cleveland 1981; Hematology & Oncology, Dartmouth-Hitchcock Hosp 1982; **Fac Appt:** Prof Med, UCSD

Beer, Tomasz M MD [Onc] - **Spec Exp:** Prostate Cancer; **Hospital:** OR Hlth & Sci Univ, VA Medical Center - Portland; **Address:** 3303 SW Bond Ave, CH14R, Portland, OR 97239; **Phone:** 503-494-6594; **Board Cert:** Medical Oncology 2000; **Med School:** Johns Hopkins Univ 1991; **Resid:** Internal Medicine, Oreg Hlth Scis Univ 1994; Internal Medicine, Oreg Hlth Scis Univ 1996; **Fellow:** Hematology & Oncology, Oreg Hlth Scis Univ 1999; **Fac Appt:** Prof Med, Oregon Hlth & Sci Univ

Bensinger, William I MD [Onc] - **Spec Exp:** Multiple Myeloma; Stem Cell Transplant; **Hospital:** Univ Wash Med Ctr; **Address:** Fred Hutchinson Cancer Research Ctr, 1100 Fairview Ave N, MS DS-390, PO BOX 19024, Seattle, WA 98109-1024; **Phone:** 206-288-1024; **Board Cert:** Internal Medicine 1978; Medical Oncology 1979; **Med School:** Northwestern Univ 1973; **Resid:** Internal Medicine, Univ Wash Hosps 1978; **Fellow:** Medical Oncology, Univ Wash Hosps 1979; **Fac Appt:** Assoc Prof Med, Univ Wash

Berry, J Michael MD [Onc] - **Spec Exp:** Anal Cancer; HPV-Human Papilloma Virus; **Hospital:** UCSF - Mt Zion Med Ctr; **Address:** UCSF, Dysplasia Clinic, 1600 Divisadero St Fl 4th, Box 1705, San Francisco, CA 94143; **Phone:** 415-353-7100; **Board Cert:** Internal Medicine 1985; Medical Oncology 1989; **Med School:** Univ Miami Sch Med 1982; **Resid:** Internal Medicine, UCSF Med Ctr 1985; **Fellow:** Medical Oncology, Stanford Univ 1989; **Fac Appt:** Asst Clin Prof Med, UCSF

Medical Oncology

Carlson, Robert W MD [Onc] - **Spec Exp:** Breast Cancer; **Hospital:** Stanford Univ Hosp & Clinics; **Address:** Stanford Comprehensive Cancer Ctr, 875 Blake Wilbur Drive, rm CC-2236, Stanford, CA 94305; **Phone:** 650-498-6000; **Board Cert:** Internal Medicine 1981; Medical Oncology 1983; **Med School:** Stanford Univ 1978; **Resid:** Internal Medicine, Barnes Hosp 1980; Internal Medicine, Stanford Univ Hosp 1981; **Fellow:** Medical Oncology, Stanford Univ Hosp 1983; **Fac Appt:** Prof Med, Stanford Univ

Chang, Susan M MD [Onc] - **Spec Exp:** Brain Tumors; Spinal Cord Tumors; Pituitary Tumors; **Hospital:** UCSF Med Ctr; **Address:** UCSF, Dept Neurological Surgery, 400 Parnassus Ave Fl 8 - rm A808, San Francisco, CA 94143; **Phone:** 415-353-2966; **Med School:** Univ British Columbia Fac Med 1985; **Resid:** Internal Medicine, Plains Hlth Ctr 1987; Internal Medicine, Toronto Genl Hosp 1989; **Fellow:** Medical Oncology, Princess Margaret Hosp 1991; Neuro-Oncology, UCSF Med Ctr 1995; **Fac Appt:** Prof Med, UCSF

Chap, Linnea MD [Onc] - **Spec Exp:** Breast Cancer; **Hospital:** St. John's Hlth Ctr, Santa Monica; **Address:** Beverly Hills Cancer Center, 8900 Wilshire Blvd Fl 2, Beverly Hills, CA 90211; **Phone:** 310-432-8900; **Board Cert:** Medical Oncology 2005; **Med School:** Univ Chicago-Pritzker Sch Med 1988; **Resid:** Internal Medicine, Northwestern Meml Hosp 1991; **Fellow:** Hematology & Oncology, UCLA Med Ctr 1992

Chew, Helen MD [Onc] - **Spec Exp:** Breast Cancer; **Hospital:** UC Davis Med Ctr; **Address:** UC Davis Cancer Ctr, 4501 X St Fl 3, Sacramento, CA 95817; **Phone:** 916-734-3700; **Board Cert:** Medical Oncology 2007; **Med School:** Univ Tex, San Antonio 1991; **Resid:** Internal Medicine, UT Hlth Sci Ctr 1994; **Fellow:** Medical Oncology, UT Hlth Sci Ctr 1997

Chlebowski, Rowan T MD/PhD [Onc] - **Spec Exp:** Breast Cancer; **Hospital:** LAC - Harbor - UCLA Med Ctr; **Address:** 1124 W Carson St J3 Bldg, Torrance, CA 90502; **Phone:** 310-222-2218; **Board Cert:** Internal Medicine 1980; Medical Oncology 1981; **Med School:** Case West Res Univ 1974; **Resid:** Internal Medicine, MetroHealth Med Ctr 1976; Medical Oncology, LAC-USC Med Ctr 1979; **Fac Appt:** Prof Med, UCLA

Chow, Warren A MD [Onc] - **Spec Exp:** Sarcoma-Soft Tissue; Sarcoma; Melanoma; **Hospital:** City of Hope Natl Med Ctr (page 69); **Address:** 1500 E Duarte Rd, Duarte, CA 91010; **Phone:** 626-256-4673 x63712; **Board Cert:** Internal Medicine 1989; Medical Oncology 2003; Hematology 2004; **Med School:** Ros Franklin Univ/Chicago Med Sch 1986; **Resid:** Internal Medicine, Cedars-Sinai Med Ctr 1990; **Fellow:** Hematology & Oncology, City of Hope Med Ctr 1992; Molecular Genetics, City of Hope Med Ctr 1994; **Fac Appt:** Assoc Prof Med

Crocenzi, Todd MD [Onc] - **Spec Exp:** Gastrointestinal Cancer; **Hospital:** Providence Portland Med Ctr; **Address:** Providence Cancer Ctr, 4805 NE Glisan St, Ste 6N40, Portland, OR 97213; **Phone:** 503-215-5696; **Board Cert:** Medical Oncology 2004; **Med School:** Jefferson Med Coll 1994; **Resid:** Internal Medicine, Univ MD Med Ctr 1997; **Fellow:** Hematology & Oncology, Dartmouth Hitchcock Med Ctr 2004; Immunology, Dartmouth Hitchcock Med Ctr 2005

Daud, Adil I MD [Onc] - **Spec Exp:** Melanoma; Skin Cancer; Drug Development; **Hospital:** UCSF Med Ctr; **Address:** 1600 Divisadero St Fl 4, Box 1706, San Francisco, CA 94115; **Phone:** 415-353-9900; **Board Cert:** Hematology 2000; Medical Oncology 2000; **Med School:** India 1987; **Resid:** Internal Medicine, Indiana Univ Affil Hosp; **Fellow:** Hematology & Oncology, Meml Sloan Kettering Cancer Ctr

Deeg, H Joachim MD [Onc] - **Spec Exp:** Myelodysplastic Syndromes; Bone Marrow Failure Disorders; Hematologic Malignancies; Graft vs Host Disease; **Hospital:** Univ Wash Med Ctr; **Address:** Fred Hutchinson Cancer Research Center, 1100 Fairview Avenue N, D1-100, Box 19024, Seattle, WA 98109-1024; **Phone:** 206-667-5985; **Board Cert:** Internal Medicine 1976; Medical Oncology 1979; **Med School:** Germany 1972; **Resid:** Internal Medicine, Gennessee Hosp 1976; **Fellow:** Medical Oncology, Univ Wash Med Ctr 1978; **Fac Appt:** Prof Med, Univ Wash

Disis, Mary Lenora MD [Onc] - **Spec Exp:** Breast Cancer; Ovarian Cancer; Clinical Trials; **Hospital:** Univ Wash Med Ctr; **Address:** Univ Washington, Tumor Vaccine Group, 815 Mercer St, Box 358050, Seattle, WA 98109; **Phone:** 206-543-8557; **Board Cert:** Internal Medicine 1989; Medical Oncology 2008; **Med School:** Univ Nebr Coll Med 1986; **Resid:** Internal Medicine, Univ Illinois Med Ctr 1990; **Fellow:** Medical Oncology, Fred Hutchinson Cancer Ctr 1993; **Fac Appt:** Assoc Prof Med, Univ Wash

Druker, Brian J MD [Onc] - **Spec Exp:** Leukemia; Leukemia-Chronic Myeloid; Hematologic Malignancies; **Hospital:** OR Hlth & Sci Univ; **Address:** OHSU Ctr Hematologic Malignancies, 3181 Sam Jackson Park Rd, Multnomah Pavilion, Ste 2502, MC L592, Portland, OR 97239-3098; **Phone:** 503-494-5058; **Board Cert:** Internal Medicine 1984; Medical Oncology 1987; **Med School:** UCSD 1981; **Resid:** Internal Medicine, Barnes Jewish Hosp 1984; **Fellow:** Medical Oncology, Dana-Farber Cancer Inst 1987; **Fac Appt:** Prof Med, Oregon Hlth & Sci Univ

Ellis, Georgiana K MD [Onc] - **Spec Exp:** Breast Cancer; Clinical Trials; **Hospital:** Univ Wash Med Ctr; **Address:** Seattle Cancer Care Alliance, 825 Eastlake Ave E, Box 358081, MS G3-630, Seattle, WA 98109-1023; **Phone:** 206-288-1000; **Board Cert:** Internal Medicine 1985; Medical Oncology 1987; **Med School:** Univ Wash 1982; **Resid:** Internal Medicine, Univ Washington Med Ctr 1985; **Fellow:** Medical Oncology, Univ Washington Med Ctr 1988; **Fac Appt:** Assoc Prof Med, Univ Wash

Estey, Elihu H MD [Onc] - **Spec Exp:** Leukemia; Leukemia-Myeloid; Clinical Trials; Myelodysplastic Syndromes; **Hospital:** Univ Wash Med Ctr; **Address:** Seattle Cancer Care Alliance, 825 Eastlake Ave E, UW Box 3587710, Seattle, WA 98109; **Phone:** 206-288-7176; **Board Cert:** Internal Medicine 1975; Medical Oncology 1981; **Med School:** Johns Hopkins Univ 1972; **Resid:** Internal Medicine, Bellevue Hosp Ctr 1975; **Fellow:** Medical Oncology, MD Anderson Cancer Ctr 1978

Figlin, Robert A MD [Onc] - **Spec Exp:** Urologic Cancer; Kidney Cancer; Immunotherapy; **Hospital:** City of Hope Natl Med Ctr (page 69); **Address:** City of Hope, 1500 E Duarte Rd, Duarte, CA 91010; **Phone:** 626-256-4673; **Board Cert:** Internal Medicine 1979; Medical Oncology 1983; **Med School:** Med Coll PA Hahnemann 1976; **Resid:** Internal Medicine, Cedars Sinai Med Ctr 1980; **Fellow:** Hematology & Oncology, UCLA Ctr Hlth Sci 1982; **Fac Appt:** Prof Med, UCLA

Fisher Jr, George A MD/PhD [Onc] - **Spec Exp:** Gastrointestinal Cancer; Pancreatic Cancer; **Hospital:** Stanford Univ Hosp & Clinics; **Address:** Stanford Comp Cancer Ctr, GI Onc, 875 Blake Wilbur Drive, MC 5826, Stanford, CA 94305; **Phone:** 650-498-6000; **Board Cert:** Medical Oncology 1997; **Med School:** Stanford Univ 1987; **Resid:** Internal Medicine, Stanford Univ Med Ctr 1991; **Fellow:** Medical Oncology, Stanford Univ Med Ctr 1993; **Fac Appt:** Assoc Prof Med, Stanford Univ

Ford, James M MD [Onc] - **Spec Exp:** Gastrointestinal Cancer; Colon & Rectal Cancer; Cancer Genetics; **Hospital:** Stanford Univ Hosp & Clinics; **Address:** Stanford Comp Cancer Ctr, 875 Blake Wilbur Drive, Clinic A, Stanford, CA 94305; **Phone:** 650-723-7621; **Board Cert:** Medical Oncology 2005; **Med School:** Yale Univ 1989; **Resid:** Internal Medicine, Stanford Univ Med Ctr 1991; **Fellow:** Medical Oncology, Stanford Univ Med Ctr 1994; **Fac Appt:** Assoc Prof Med, Stanford Univ

Medical Oncology

Forscher, Charles A MD [Onc] - **Spec Exp:** Bone Tumors; Sarcoma-Soft Tissue; **Hospital:** Cedars-Sinai Med Ctr, UCLA Ronald Reagan Med Ctr; **Address:** Outpatient Cancer Ctr, Lower Level, 8700 Beverly Blvd, Ste AC1042D, Los Angeles, CA 90048; **Phone:** 310-423-8045; **Board Cert:** Internal Medicine 1981; Hematology 1986; Medical Oncology 1987; **Med School:** Albert Einstein Coll Med 1978; **Resid:** Internal Medicine, Montefiore Med Ctr 1981; **Fellow:** Hematology, Montefiore Med Ctr 1983; Neoplastic Diseases, Mt Sinai Med Ctr 1985; **Fac Appt:** Clin Prof Med, UCLA

Gandara, David R MD [Onc] - **Spec Exp:** Lung Cancer; **Hospital:** UC Davis Med Ctr; **Address:** UC Davis Cancer Ctr, 4501 X St Fl 2, Sacramento, CA 95817; **Phone:** 916-734-5959; **Board Cert:** Internal Medicine 1976; Medical Oncology 1979; **Med School:** Univ Tex Med Br, Galveston 1973; **Resid:** Internal Medicine, Madigan Med Ctr 1976; **Fellow:** Hematology & Oncology, Letterman AMC 1978; **Fac Appt:** Asst Prof Med, UC Davis

Ganz, Patricia A MD [Onc] - **Spec Exp:** Breast Cancer; Cancer Survivors-Late Effects of Therapy; **Hospital:** UCLA Ronald Reagan Med Ctr; **Address:** UCLA, Cancer Prev/Control Rsch, A2-125 CHS, 650 Charles Young Drive S, Box 956900, Los Angeles, CA 90095-6900; **Phone:** 310-206-1404; **Board Cert:** Internal Medicine 1976; Medical Oncology 1979; **Med School:** UCLA 1973; **Resid:** Internal Medicine, UCLA Med Ctr 1976; **Fellow:** Hematology, UCLA Med Ctr 1978; **Fac Appt:** Prof Med, UCLA

Glaspy, John A MD [Onc] - **Spec Exp:** Breast Cancer; Melanoma; Lymphoma; Gastrointestinal Cancer; **Hospital:** UCLA Ronald Reagan Med Ctr, Santa Monica - UCLA Med Ctr & Ortho Hosp; **Address:** 100 UCLA Medical Plaza, Ste 550, Los Angeles, CA 90095; **Phone:** 310-794-4955; **Board Cert:** Internal Medicine 1982; Medical Oncology 1985; Hematology 1986; **Med School:** UCLA 1979; **Resid:** Internal Medicine, UCLA Med Ctr 1982; **Fellow:** Hematology & Oncology, UCLA Med Ctr 1984; **Fac Appt:** Prof Med, UCLA

Gold, Philip J MD [Onc] - **Spec Exp:** Gastrointestinal Cancer; **Hospital:** Swedish Med Ctr-First Hill-Seattle; **Address:** Swedish Cancer Inst, 1221 Madison St Fl 2 - Ste 200, Seattle, WA 98104; **Phone:** 206-386-2121; **Board Cert:** Internal Medicine 2005; Medical Oncology 2007; **Med School:** Univ Miami Sch Med 1991; **Resid:** Internal Medicine, Univ of Washington Med Ctr 1994; **Fellow:** Medical Oncology, Fred Hutchinson Cancer Rsch Ctr 1997

Gralow, Julie MD [Onc] - **Spec Exp:** Breast Cancer; **Hospital:** Univ Wash Med Ctr; **Address:** Seattle Cancer Care Alliance, 825 Eastlake Ave E, MS G3-630, Seattle, WA 98109; **Phone:** 206-288-7222; **Board Cert:** Medical Oncology 2005; **Med School:** USC Sch Med 1988; **Resid:** Internal Medicine, Brigham & Women's Hosp 1991; **Fellow:** Oncology, Univ Wash Med Ctr 1994; **Fac Appt:** Assoc Prof Med, Univ Wash

Higano, Celestia MD [Onc] - **Spec Exp:** Genitourinary Cancer; Prostate Cancer; Testicular Cancer; **Hospital:** Univ Wash Med Ctr; **Address:** Seattle Cancer Care Alliance, 825 Eastlake Ave E, PO Box 19024, Seattle, WA 98109; **Phone:** 206-288-1152; **Board Cert:** Internal Medicine 1982; Medical Oncology 1985; **Med School:** Univ Mass Sch Med 1979; **Resid:** Internal Medicine, Mayo Clin 1982; **Fellow:** Oncology, Univ Washington Med Ctr 1985; **Fac Appt:** Prof Med, Univ Wash

Jacobs, Charlotte D MD [Onc] - **Spec Exp:** Sarcoma; Unknown Primary Cancer; **Hospital:** Stanford Univ Hosp & Clinics; **Address:** 875 Blake Wilbur Drive, Clinic B, Stanford, CA 94305; **Phone:** 650-498-6000; **Board Cert:** Internal Medicine 1975; Medical Oncology 1977; **Med School:** Washington Univ, St Louis 1972; **Resid:** Internal Medicine, Barnes Hosp 1974; Internal Medicine, UCSF Med Ctr 1975; **Fellow:** Medical Oncology, Stanford Univ 1977; **Fac Appt:** Prof Med, Stanford Univ

Kaplan, Lawrence D MD [Onc] - **Spec Exp:** AIDS Related Cancers; Lymphoma; **Hospital:** UCSF Med Ctr; **Address:** UCSF Medical Center, 400 Parnassus Ave, rm 502, Box 0324, San Francisco, CA 94143-0324; **Phone:** 415-353-2421; **Board Cert:** Internal Medicine 1983; Medical Oncology 1985; **Med School:** UCLA 1980; **Resid:** Internal Medicine, Boston City Hosp 1983; **Fellow:** Hematology & Oncology, UCSF Med Ctr 1985; **Fac Appt:** Clin Prof Med, UCSF

Kesari, Santosh MD/PhD [Onc] - **Spec Exp:** Neuro-Oncology; Stem Cell Therapy; Leukoencephalopathy; **Hospital:** John M & Sally B Thornton Hosp, UCSD Med Ctr-Hillcrest; **Address:** UCSD Moores Cancer Center, 3855 Health Sciences Drive, La Jolla, CA 92093; **Phone:** 858-822-7524; **Board Cert:** Neurology 2005; **Med School:** Univ Pennsylvania 1999; **Resid:** Neurology, Mass Genl Hosp 2003; **Fellow:** Neuro-Oncology, Dana Farber Cancer Inst 2004

Koczywas, Marianna MD [Onc] - **Spec Exp:** Lung Cancer; **Hospital:** City of Hope Natl Med Ctr (page 69); **Address:** City of Hope Med Ctr, Dept Med Onc, 1500 E Duarte Rd, Duarte, CA 91010; **Phone:** 626-471-9200; **Board Cert:** Hematology 2000; Medical Oncology 2001; **Med School:** Poland 1984; **Resid:** Internal Medicine, Troczewski City Hosp 1988; Internal Medicine, St Francis Med Ctr 1997; **Fellow:** Hematology & Oncology, City of Hope Natl Med Ctr 2000

Lim, Dean Wee MD [Onc] - **Hospital:** City of Hope Natl Med Ctr (page 69); **Address:** City of Hope Med Ctr, Dept Med Onc, 1500 E Duarte Rd, Duarte, CA 91010; **Phone:** 626-471-9200; **Board Cert:** Internal Medicine 1985; Medical Oncology 1989; **Med School:** Philippines 1980; **Resid:** Internal Medicine, Cabrini Med Ctr 1985; **Fellow:** Hematology & Oncology, St Lukes Roosevelt Hosp 1987; **Fac Appt:** Asst Clin Prof Med, USC-Keck School of Medicine

Maloney, David G MD/PhD [Onc] - **Spec Exp:** Lymphoma; Bone Marrow & Stem Cell Transplant; Vaccine Therapy; **Hospital:** Univ Wash Med Ctr; **Address:** Fred Hutchinson Cancer Rsch Ctr, 1100 Fairview Ave N, D1-100, Box 19024, Seattle, WA 98109-1024; **Phone:** 206-667-5616; **Board Cert:** Internal Medicine 1988; Medical Oncology 2005; **Med School:** Stanford Univ 1985; **Resid:** Internal Medicine, Brigham & Women's Hosp 1988; **Fellow:** Medical Oncology, Stanford Univ Med Ctr 1994; **Fac Appt:** Prof Med, Univ Wash

Margolin, Kim A MD [Onc] - **Spec Exp:** Melanoma; Kidney Cancer; Germ Cell Tumors; **Hospital:** Univ Wash Med Ctr; **Address:** 825 Eastlake Ave E, PO Box 19024, Seattle, WA 98109; **Phone:** 206-288-7222; **Board Cert:** Internal Medicine 1982; Medical Oncology 2006; Hematology 1986; **Med School:** Stanford Univ 1979; **Resid:** Internal Medicine, Yale-New Haven Hosp 1982; **Fellow:** Hematology & Oncology, UC San Diego Med Ctr 1983; Hematology & Oncology, City of Hope Med Ctr 1985; **Fac Appt:** Prof Med, Univ Wash

Martins, Renato G MD [Onc] - **Spec Exp:** Head & Neck Cancer; Lung Cancer; Mesothelioma; Salivary Gland Tumors; **Hospital:** Univ Wash Med Ctr; **Address:** Seattle Cancer Care Alliance, 825 Eastlake Ave E, MS G4-940, Seattle, WA 98109; **Phone:** 206-288-2048; **Board Cert:** Internal Medicine 2005; Medical Oncology 2008; **Med School:** Brazil 1992; **Resid:** Internal Medicine, Gunderson Clinic 1995; **Fellow:** Medical Oncology, Mass Genl Hosp 1998; **Fac Appt:** Assoc Prof Med, Univ Wash

Meyskens Jr, Frank MD [Onc] - **Spec Exp:** Cancer Prevention; Melanoma; Sarcoma; **Hospital:** UC Irvine Med Ctr; **Address:** UC Irvine Cancer Ctr, 101 The City Drive, Bldg 56, rm 215, Orange, CA 92868; **Phone:** 714-456-6310; **Board Cert:** Internal Medicine 1975; Medical Oncology 1981; **Med School:** UCSF 1972; **Resid:** Internal Medicine, Moffit-Calif Hosps 1974; **Fellow:** Hematology & Oncology, Natl Cancer Inst 1977; **Fac Appt:** Prof Med, UC Irvine

Medical Oncology

Mitsuyasu, Ronald T MD [Onc] - **Spec Exp:** AIDS Related Cancers; Hematologic Malignancies; **Hospital:** UCLA Ronald Reagan Med Ctr, Santa Monica - UCLA Med Ctr & Ortho Hosp; **Address:** 1399 S Roxbury Drive, Ste 100, 9911 W Pico Blvd, Ste 980, Los Angeles, CA 90035; **Phone:** 310-557-2273; **Board Cert:** Internal Medicine 1981; **Med School:** UCLA 1978; **Resid:** Internal Medicine, Rush Presby St Lukes Hosp 1981; **Fellow:** Hematology & Oncology, UCLA Med Ctr 1984; **Fac Appt:** Prof Hem & Onc, UCLA

Mortimer, Joanne MD [Onc] - **Spec Exp:** Breast Cancer; Clinical Trials; **Hospital:** City of Hope Natl Med Ctr (page 69); **Address:** 1500 E Duarte Rd, Duarte, CA 91010; **Phone:** 626-471-9200; **Board Cert:** Internal Medicine 1980; Medical Oncology 1983; **Med School:** Loyola Univ-Stritch Sch Med 1977; **Resid:** Internal Medicine, Cleveland Clinic 1980; **Fellow:** Medical Oncology, Cleveland Clinic 1982; **Fac Appt:** Prof Hem & Onc, Loyola Univ-Stritch Sch Med

Natale, Ronald B MD [Onc] - **Spec Exp:** Lung Cancer; **Hospital:** Cedars-Sinai Med Ctr; **Address:** Cedars-Sinai Outpatient Comp Cancer Ctr, 8700 Beverly Blvd, Ste MS-33, Los Angeles, CA. 90048; **Phone:** 310-423-1101; **Board Cert:** Internal Medicine 1977; Medical Oncology 1979; **Med School:** Wayne State Univ 1974; **Resid:** Internal Medicine, Wayne State Univ 1977; **Fellow:** Hematology & Oncology, Meml Sloan Kettering 1980; **Fac Appt:** Prof Med, Univ Mich Med Sch

O'Day, Steven J MD [Onc] - **Spec Exp:** Melanoma; Melanoma-Advanced; **Hospital:** St. John's Hlth Ctr, Santa Monica; **Address:** 11818 Wilshire Blvd, Ste 200, Los Angeles, CA 90025; **Phone:** 310-231-2121; **Med School:** Johns Hopkins Univ 1988; **Resid:** Internal Medicine, Johns Hopkins Hosp 1991; **Fellow:** Medical Oncology, Dana Farber Cancer Inst 1992; **Fac Appt:** Assoc Clin Prof Med, USC-Keck School of Medicine

Parker, Barbara A MD [Onc] - **Spec Exp:** Breast Cancer; Nutrition in Cancer Therapy; **Hospital:** UCSD Med Ctr-Hillcrest; **Address:** Moores UCSD Cancer Ctr, Hem/Onc Dept, 3855 Health Sciences Drive, MC 0987, La Jolla, CA 92093; **Phone:** 858-822-6195; **Board Cert:** Internal Medicine 1984; Medical Oncology 1987; **Med School:** Stanford Univ 1981; **Resid:** Internal Medicine, UCSD Med Ctr 1985; **Fellow:** Medical Oncology, UCSD Med Ctr 1987; **Fac Appt:** Prof Med, UCSD

Petersdorf, Stephen MD [Onc] - **Spec Exp:** Lymphoma; Myelodysplastic Syndromes; Leukemia; **Hospital:** Univ Wash Med Ctr; **Address:** Seattle Cancer Care Alliance, 825 Eastlake Ave E, MS E2102, Seattle, WA 98109-1023; **Phone:** 206-288-6202; **Board Cert:** Internal Medicine 1986; Hematology 2001; Medical Oncology 2001; **Med School:** Brown Univ 1983; **Resid:** Internal Medicine, Univ Washington Med Ctr 1986; **Fellow:** Hematology & Oncology, Univ Washington Med Ctr 1989; **Fac Appt:** Assoc Prof Med, Univ Wash

Picozzi Jr, Vincent J MD [Onc] - **Spec Exp:** Gastrointestinal Cancer; Pancreatic Cancer; Genitourinary Cancer; Myelodysplastic Syndromes; **Hospital:** Virginia Mason Med Ctr; **Address:** Virginia Mason Med Ctr, Div Hem/Onc, 1100 Nineth Ave, MS C2-Hem, Seattle, WA 98111; **Phone:** 206-223-6193; **Board Cert:** Internal Medicine 1981; Hematology 1986; Medical Oncology 1987; **Med School:** Stanford Univ 1978; **Resid:** Internal Medicine, Peter Bent Brigham Med Ctr 1981; **Fellow:** Hematology, Stanford Univ Med Ctr 1983; Medical Oncology, Stanford Univ MEd Ctr 1983; **Fac Appt:** Clin Prof Med, Univ Wash

Pinto, Harlan A MD [Onc] - **Spec Exp:** Head & Neck Cancer; Clinical Trials; **Hospital:** Stanford Univ Hosp & Clinics, VA Hlth Care Sys - Palo Alto; **Address:** Stanford Comp Cancer Ctr, 875 Blake Wilbur Drive, Clinic C, Stanford, CA 94305; **Phone:** 650-723-7621; **Board Cert:** Internal Medicine 1986; Medical Oncology 2002; **Med School:** Yale Univ 1983; **Resid:** Internal Medicine, Mass Genl Hosp 1986; **Fellow:** Medical Oncology, Stanford Univ Med Sch 1991; **Fac Appt:** Assoc Prof Med, Stanford Univ

Prados, Michael MD [Onc] - **Spec Exp:** Neuro-Oncology; Brain Tumors; **Hospital:** UCSF Med Ctr; **Address:** UCSF Med Ctr, Div Neuro-Oncology, 400 Parnassus Ave, rm A-808, San Francisco, CA 94143; **Phone:** 415-353-2966; **Board Cert:** Internal Medicine 1977; **Med School:** Louisiana State U, New Orleans 1974; **Resid:** Internal Medicine, Earl K Long Hosp 1977; **Fac Appt:** Prof NS, UCSF

Press, Oliver W MD/PhD [Onc] - **Spec Exp:** Lymphoma; Bone Marrow Transplant; **Hospital:** Univ Wash Med Ctr; **Address:** 1100 Fairview Ave N, MS D3-190, Seattle, WA 98109; **Phone:** 206-667-1864; **Board Cert:** Internal Medicine 1982; Medical Oncology 1985; **Med School:** Univ Wash 1979; **Resid:** Internal Medicine, Mass Genl Hosp 1982; Internal Medicine, Univ Washington Med Ctr 1983; **Fellow:** Medical Oncology, Univ Washington Med Ctr 1985; **Fac Appt:** Prof Med, Univ Wash

Quinn, David MD/PhD [Onc] - **Spec Exp:** Testicular Cancer; Kidney Cancer; Bladder Cancer; Adrenal Cancer; **Hospital:** USC Norris Cancer Hosp; **Address:** 1441 Eastlake Ave, Ste 3440, Los Angeles, CA 90033; **Phone:** 323-865-3956; **Med School:** Australia 1987; **Resid:** Internal Medicine, St Vincents Hosp 1992; **Fellow:** Medical Oncology, St Vincents Hosp 1995; **Fac Appt:** Assoc Prof Med, USC Sch Med

Reid, Tony R MD [Onc] - **Spec Exp:** Gastrointestinal Cancer; Pancreatic Cancer; Esophageal Cancer; Liver Cancer; **Hospital:** UCSD Med Ctr-Hillcrest; **Address:** 3855 Health Sciences Drive, Ste 1102, MC 0987, La Jolla, CA 92093; **Phone:** 858-822-6100; **Board Cert:** Medical Oncology 1999; **Med School:** Stanford Univ 1991; **Resid:** Internal Medicine, Stanford Univ Med Ctr 1997; **Fellow:** Oncology, Stanford Univ Med Ctr 1999; Cancer Research, Stanford Univ Med Ctr 2000; **Fac Appt:** Assoc Prof Med, UCSD

Rosove, Michael H MD [Onc] - **Spec Exp:** Bleeding/Coagulation Disorders; Myeloproliferative Disorders; Myelodysplastic Syndromes; Hematologic Malignancies; **Hospital:** UCLA Ronald Reagan Med Ctr; **Address:** 100 UCLA Med Plaza, Ste 550, Los Angeles, CA 90024-6970; **Phone:** 310-794-4955; **Board Cert:** Internal Medicine 1976; Hematology 1982; Medical Oncology 1981; **Med School:** UCLA 1973; **Resid:** Internal Medicine, UCLA Med Ctr 1976; **Fellow:** Hematology & Oncology, UCLA Med Ctr 1979; Hematology & Oncology, Columbia Presby Med Ctr 1978; **Fac Appt:** Clin Prof Med, UCLA-David Geffen Sch Med

Rugo, Hope S MD [Onc] - **Spec Exp:** Breast Cancer; Complementary Medicine; Breast Cancer-Novel Therapies; **Hospital:** UCSF Med Ctr; **Address:** UCSF Comp Cancer Ctr-Breast Care Ctr, 1600 Divisadero St Fl 2, San Francisco, CA 94115; **Phone:** 415-353-7070; **Board Cert:** Internal Medicine 1987; Medical Oncology 1989; **Med School:** Univ Pennsylvania 1984; **Resid:** Internal Medicine, UCSF Med Ctr 1987; **Fellow:** Hematology & Oncology, UCSF Med Ctr 1989; **Fac Appt:** Clin Prof Med, UCSF

Russell, Christy A MD [Onc] - **Spec Exp:** Breast Cancer; **Hospital:** USC Univ Hosp; **Address:** Norris Cancer Ctr, The Breast Ctr, 1441 Eastlake Ave, Los Angeles, CA 90033; **Phone:** 323-865-3371; **Board Cert:** Internal Medicine 1983; Medical Oncology 1985; **Med School:** Med Coll PA Hahnemann 1980; **Resid:** Internal Medicine, Good Sam Med Ctr 1983; **Fellow:** Hematology & Oncology, LAC-USC Med Ctr 1986; **Fac Appt:** Assoc Prof Med, USC Sch Med

Samlowski, Wolfram E MD [Onc] - **Spec Exp:** Kidney Cancer; Melanoma; Immunotherapy; **Hospital:** St. Rose Dom Hosp-San Martin; **Address:** Nevada Cancer Institute, One Breakthrough Way, Las Vegas, NV 89135; **Phone:** 702-822-5433; **Board Cert:** Internal Medicine 1981; Medical Oncology 1985; **Med School:** Ohio State Univ 1978; **Resid:** Internal Medicine, Wayne State Univ Affil Hosp 1981; **Fellow:** Hematology & Oncology, Univ Utah Affil Hosp 1984; **Fac Appt:** Prof Hem & Onc, Univ Nevada

Medical Oncology

Sandler, Alan MD [Onc] - **Spec Exp:** Lung Cancer; Sarcoma; **Hospital:** OR Hlth & Sci Univ; **Address:** 3181 SW Sam Jackson Park Rd, MC L586, Portland, OR 97239; **Phone:** 503-494-5586; **Board Cert:** Medical Oncology 2006; **Med School:** Rush Med Coll 1987; **Resid:** Internal Medicine, Yale-New Haven Hosp 1989; **Fellow:** Medical Oncology, Yale Univ 1993; **Fac Appt:** Prof Med, Oregon Hlth & Sci Univ

Scudder, Sidney MD [Onc] - **Spec Exp:** Ovarian Cancer; Cervical Cancer; **Hospital:** UC Davis Med Ctr; **Address:** 4501 X St, Ste 3016, Sacramento, CA 95817; **Phone:** 916-734-3700; **Board Cert:** Internal Medicine 1983; Medical Oncology 1985; **Med School:** Univ Fla Coll Med 1980; **Resid:** Internal Medicine, Barnes Hosp-Washington Univ 1983; **Fellow:** Medical Oncology, Stanford Univ 1985; **Fac Appt:** Prof Med, UC Davis

Shibata, Stephen I MD [Onc] - **Spec Exp:** Gastrointestinal Cancer; Clinical Trials; **Hospital:** City of Hope Natl Med Ctr (page 69); **Address:** City of Hope Cancer Ctr, 1500 E Duarte Rd, Duarte, CA 91010; **Phone:** 626-471-9200; **Board Cert:** Internal Medicine 1988; Medical Oncology 2004; **Med School:** UC Irvine 1985; **Resid:** Internal Medicine, St Mary Med Ctr 1988; **Fellow:** Medical Oncology, City of Hope Cancer Ctr 1990; Bone Marrow Transplant, City of Hope Cancer Ctr 1991; **Fac Appt:** Assoc Prof Med

Sikic, Branimir I MD [Onc] - **Spec Exp:** Unknown Primary Cancer; Clinical Trials; **Hospital:** Stanford Univ Hosp & Clinics; **Address:** Stanford Comp Cancer Ctr, 875 Blake Wilbur Drive, Clinic C, Palo Alto, CA 94305; **Phone:** 650-723-7621; **Board Cert:** Internal Medicine 1975; Medical Oncology 1979; **Med School:** Ros Franklin Univ/Chicago Med Sch 1972; **Resid:** Internal Medicine, Georgetown Univ Hosp 1975; **Fellow:** Medical Oncology, Natl Cancer Inst 1978; Medical Oncology, Georgetown Univ Hosp 1979; **Fac Appt:** Prof Med, Stanford Univ

Small, Eric J MD [Onc] - **Spec Exp:** Prostate Cancer; Vaccine Therapy; Genitourinary Cancer; **Hospital:** UCSF Med Ctr; **Address:** UCSF Urologic Oncology Practice, 1600 Divisadero St Fl 3, San Francisco, CA 94115; **Phone:** 415-353-7171; **Board Cert:** Internal Medicine 1988; Medical Oncology 2001; **Med School:** Case West Res Univ 1985; **Resid:** Internal Medicine, Beth Israel Hosp 1988; **Fellow:** Hematology & Oncology, Cancer Research Inst/UCSF 1991; **Fac Appt:** Prof Med, UCSF

Stewart, Forrest M MD [Onc] - **Spec Exp:** Unknown Primary Cancer; Sarcoma; **Hospital:** Univ Wash Med Ctr; **Address:** Seattle Cancer Care Alliance, 825 Eastlake Ave E, Box 19023, Seattle, WA 98109; **Phone:** 206-288-7222; **Board Cert:** Internal Medicine 1980; Hematology 1982; Medical Oncology 1985; **Med School:** Indiana Univ 1977; **Resid:** Internal Medicine, Indiana Univ Med Ctr 1980; Medical Oncology, Indiana Univ Med Ctr 1981; **Fellow:** Hematology, Univ Virginia Med Ctr 1983; **Fac Appt:** Prof Med, Univ Wash

Stockdale, Frank E MD/PhD [Onc] - **Spec Exp:** Breast Cancer; Tuberous Breasts; Sarcoma-Soft Tissue; **Hospital:** Stanford Univ Hosp & Clinics; **Address:** Stanford Univ Medical Ctr, 875 Blake Wilbur Drive, Stanford, CA 94305-5826; **Phone:** 650-498-6000; **Med School:** Univ Pennsylvania 1963; **Resid:** Internal Medicine, Stanford Univ Med Ctr 1967; Medical Oncology, Stanford Univ Med Ctr; **Fac Appt:** Prof Emeritus Med, Stanford Univ

Tempero, Margaret A MD [Onc] - **Spec Exp:** Pancreatic Cancer; Gastrointestinal Cancer; **Hospital:** UCSF Med Ctr, VA Med Ctr - San Francisco; **Address:** UCSF Medical Ctr, 1600 Divisadero St Fl 4, San Francisco, CA 94115; **Phone:** 415-353-9888; **Board Cert:** Internal Medicine 1980; Medical Oncology 1983; Hematology 1984; **Med School:** Univ Nebr Coll Med 1977; **Resid:** Internal Medicine, Univ Nebraska Hosp 1980; **Fellow:** Medical Oncology, Univ Nebraska Hosp 1982; **Fac Appt:** Prof Med, UCSF

Thompson, John Ainslie MD [Onc] - **Spec Exp:** Melanoma; Kidney Cancer; **Hospital:** Univ Wash Med Ctr; **Address:** Seattle Cancer Care Alliance, 825 Eastlake Ave E, MS G4-200, Seattle, WA 98109-1023; **Phone:** 206-288-2015; **Board Cert:** Internal Medicine 1982; Medical Oncology 1985; **Med School:** Univ Alabama 1979; **Resid:** Internal Medicine, Univ Wash Med Ctr 1982; **Fellow:** Medical Oncology, Univ Washington 1985

Tripathy, Debasish MD [Onc] - **Spec Exp:** Breast Cancer; Clinical Trials; **Hospital:** USC Norris Cancer Hosp; **Address:** USC Norris Cancer Ctr, 1441 Eastlake Ave, Ste 3447, Los Angeles, CA 90033; **Phone:** 323-865-3900; **Board Cert:** Internal Medicine 1988; Medical Oncology 2001; **Med School:** Duke Univ 1985; **Resid:** Internal Medicine, Duke Univ Med Ctr 1988; **Fellow:** Hematology & Oncology, USCF Med Ctr 1991; **Fac Appt:** Prof Med, Univ SC Sch Med

Twardowski, Przemyslaw W MD [Onc] - **Spec Exp:** Genitourinary Cancer; **Hospital:** City of Hope Natl Med Ctr (page 69); **Address:** 1500 E Duarte Rd, Duarte, CA 91010; **Phone:** 626-256-4673; **Board Cert:** Medical Oncology 2009; **Med School:** Univ MO-Columbia Sch Med 1990; **Resid:** Internal Medicine, Northwestern Meml Hosp 1994; **Fellow:** Hematology & Oncology, Northwestern Meml Hosp 1996; **Fac Appt:** Asst Prof Med, UCLA

Urba, Walter J MD/PhD [Onc] - **Spec Exp:** Breast Cancer; **Hospital:** Providence Portland Med Ctr; **Address:** Providence Oncology, 4805 NE Glisan Rd, Portland, OR 97213; **Phone:** 503-215-5696; **Board Cert:** Internal Medicine 1985; Medical Oncology 1987; **Med School:** Univ Miami Sch Med 1981; **Resid:** Internal Medicine, Morristown Meml Hosp 1983; **Fellow:** Medical Oncology, Natl Cancer Inst 1986; **Fac Appt:** Assoc Clin Prof Med, Oregon Hlth & Sci Univ

Venook, Alan P MD [Onc] - **Spec Exp:** Gastrointestinal Cancer; Colon & Rectal Cancer; Liver Cancer; **Hospital:** UCSF Med Ctr; **Address:** UCSF Comprehensive Cancer Ctr, Multi Disciplinary Practice, 1600 Divisadero St Fl 4 - rm 4202, San Francisco, CA 94115; **Phone:** 415-353-9888; **Board Cert:** Internal Medicine 1985; Medical Oncology 1987; Hematology 1988; **Med School:** UCSF 1980; **Resid:** Internal Medicine, UC Davis Med Ctr 1985; **Fellow:** Hematology & Oncology, UCSF Med Ctr 1987; **Fac Appt:** Prof Med

Vescio, Robert A MD [Onc] - **Spec Exp:** Multiple Myeloma; **Hospital:** Cedars-Sinai Med Ctr; **Address:** Cedars Sinai Med Ctr, Dept Hem/Oncology, 8700 Beverly Blvd, Ste AC1049, Los Angeles, CA 90048; **Phone:** 310-423-1825; **Board Cert:** Internal Medicine 1989; Hematology 2004; Medical Oncology 2003; **Med School:** UCSD 1986; **Resid:** Internal Medicine, UCSD Med Ctr 1989; **Fellow:** Hematology & Oncology, UCLA Med Ctr 1993; **Fac Appt:** Assoc Prof Med, UCLA

Volberding, Paul Arthur MD [Onc] - **Spec Exp:** AIDS Related Cancers; **Hospital:** UCSF Med Ctr, VA Med Ctr - San Francisco; **Address:** 4150 Clement St, VAMC 111, San Francisco, CA 94121; **Phone:** 415-750-2203; **Board Cert:** Internal Medicine 1978; Medical Oncology 1981; **Med School:** Univ Minn 1975; **Resid:** Internal Medicine, Univ Utah Med Ctr 1978; **Fellow:** Medical Oncology, UCSF Med Ctr 1981; **Fac Appt:** Prof Med, UCSF

von Gunten, Charles MD/PhD [Onc] - **Spec Exp:** Palliative Care; **Hospital:** San Diego Hospice; **Address:** San Diego Hospice, 4311 Third Ave, San Diego, CA 92103; **Phone:** 619-688-1600; **Board Cert:** Internal Medicine 2002; Medical Oncology 2003; Hospice & Palliative Medicine 2001; **Med School:** Univ Colorado 1988; **Resid:** Internal Medicine, Northwestern Univ 1991; **Fellow:** Medical Oncology, Northwestern Univ 1993; **Fac Appt:** Assoc Clin Prof Med, UCSD

Wierman, Ann MD [Onc] - **Spec Exp:** Breast Cancer; Lymphoma; Lung Cancer; **Hospital:** Mountainview Hosp - Las Vegas, Summerlin Hosp Med Ctr; **Address:** 7445 Peak Drive, Las Vegas, NV 89128; **Phone:** 702-952-2140; **Board Cert:** Internal Medicine 2002; Medical Oncology 2007; **Med School:** Baylor Coll Med 1989; **Resid:** Internal Medicine, Baylor Hosps 1992; Internal Medicine, Ben Taub Genl Hosp 1993; **Fellow:** Hematology & Oncology, Univ CO Hlth Sci Ctr 1996; **Fac Appt:** Assoc Clin Prof Med, Univ Nevada

Medical Oncology

Yen, Yun MD/PhD [Onc] - **Spec Exp:** Liver Cancer; Biliary Cancer; **Hospital:** City of Hope Natl Med Ctr (page 69); **Address:** City of Hope Comprehensive Cancer Ctr, 1500 E Duarte Rd, Duarte, CA 91010; **Phone:** 626-471-9200 x62307; **Board Cert:** Medical Oncology 2003; **Med School:** Taiwan 1982; **Resid:** Internal Medicine, St Luke's Hosp 1990; **Fellow:** Hematology & Oncology, Yale-New Haven Hosp 1993; **Fac Appt:** Prof Med, USC Sch Med

canswer.

Hematologic Oncology Experts

City of Hope was one of the first medical centers in the nation to successfully perform bone marrow transplantation for leukemia. Today, after more than 10,000 bone marrow and stem cell transplants, the Division of Hematology and Hematopoietic Cell Transplantation conducts one of the largest and most successful transplant programs in the world, with innovative protocols for patients with a variety of hematologic cancers and other diseases.

To learn more, call 800-826-HOPE
www.cityofhope.org/hct

1500 East Duarte Road, Duarte, California 91010

City of Hope is recognized as one of only 40 National Cancer Institute-designated Comprehensive Cancer Centers and is ranked by *U.S.News & World Report* as one of "America's Best Cancer Hospitals."

City of Hope's *Helford Clinical Research Hospital* integrates lifesaving research and superior clinical care. Multidisciplinary teams of medical professionals work together to deliver promising new therapies to patients quickly, safely and effectively. They care for the whole patient, including their emotional, psychological, spiritual and nutritional needs.

A recognized leader in compassionate patient care, innovative science and translational research, City of Hope collaborates with other top institutions around the globe, rapidly developing laboratory breakthroughs into revolutionary new treatments.

City of Hope welcomes patient referrals from physicians throughout the world. Please contact specialists directly or call **800-826-HOPE**.

City of Hope has answers to cancer.

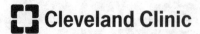
Cleveland Clinic

Every life deserves world class care.

Cleveland Clinic
Taussig Cancer Institute
9500 Euclid Avenue
Cleveland, OH 44195

Leukemia and Lymphoma Treatment Leader

At Cleveland Clinic Taussig Cancer Institute, more than 250 top cancer specialists, researchers, nurses and technicians are dedicated to delivering the most effective medical treatments and offering access to the latest clinical trials for more than 13,000 new cancer patients every year. Our doctors are nationally and internationally known for their contributions to cancer breakthroughs and their ability to deliver superior outcomes for our patients. In recognition of these and other achievements, *U.S.News & World Report* has ranked Cleveland Clinic as one of the top cancer centers in the nation.

National Treatment Leader in Blood Cancers

The Taussig Cancer Institute is a national leader in caring for and treating patients with leukemia, lymphoma, myeloma and myelodysplastic syndromes. For example, our Bone Marrow Transplant program has unsurpassed national outcomes. We have one of the most experienced teams in the nation, having performed more than 3,600 bone marrow transplant procedures since 1977.

Our teams of nurses, social workers, pharmacists and internationally recognized physicians work together to develop personalized treatment plans for every patient. We have a state-of-the-art, dedicated hospital floor with individual rooms for leukemia and BMT patients, and the most current treatments through clinical trials, many of which are developed at Cleveland Clinic. Our goal is to promote the highest quality of care for people who have hematologic cancers.

clevelandclinic.org/
bloodcancersTCD

**Appointments | Information:
Call the Cancer Answer Line at
866.223.8100.**

Cancer Treatment Guides

Cleveland Clinic has developed comprehensive treatment guides for many cancers. To download our free treatment guides, visit clevelandclinic.org/cancertreatmentguides.

**Comprehensive Online
Medical Second Opinion**

Cleveland Clinic experts can review your medical records and render an opinion that includes treatment options and recommendations. Call 216.444.3223 or 800.223.2273 ext. 43223; email eclevelandclinic@ccf.org.

**Special Assistance for
Out-of-State Patients**

Cleveland Clinic Global Patient Services offers a complimentary Medical Concierge service for patients who travel from outside of Ohio. Call 800.223.2273, ext. 55580, or email medicalconcierge@ccf.org.

☐ Cleveland Clinic

Every life deserves world class care.

Cleveland Clinic
Taussig Cancer Institute
9500 Euclid Avenue
Cleveland, OH 44195

clevelandclinic.org/cancerTCD

Committed to Patient Care, Transparency and Research

At Cleveland Clinic Taussig Cancer Institute, more than 250 top cancer specialists, researchers, nurses and technicians are dedicated to delivering the most effective medical treatments and offering access to the latest clinical trials for more than 13,000 new cancer patients every year. Our doctors are nationally and internationally known for their contributions to cancer breakthroughs and their ability to deliver superior outcomes for our patients. In recognition of these and other achievements, *U.S.News & World Report* has ranked Cleveland Clinic as one of the top cancer centers in the nation.

Compassionate Cancer Caregivers

The team in the Taussig Cancer Institute has extensive experience caring for patients with every kind of cancer. In our multidisciplinary clinics, medical, radiation and surgical oncologists work closely with pathologists, radiologists, oncology nurses and social workers to optimize the options for individual patients with complex conditions.

Outcomes Reporting

Cleveland Clinic is committed to transparency and strives to make data easily accessible for our patients. We were the first major medical center to publish annual outcomes and volume information for its medical specialties. Each Outcomes booklet includes comprehensive data on procedures, volumes, mortality, complications and innovations and is available online.

Center for Personalized Genetic Healthcare

Because some families are prone to developing cancer, advances in genetic research help us identify some of the risk factors. Cleveland Clinic's Center for Personalized Genetic Healthcare aims to prevent cancer by identifying high-risk individuals and by offering personalized medical management. For more information or to schedule an appointment, call 800.998.4785.

Appointments | Information: Call the Cancer Answer Line at 866.223.8100.

Clinical Trials Now Online

As part of a National Cancer Institute (NCI) Comprehensive Cancer Center, our cancer specialists consistently participate in more than 300 clinical trials, giving patients the chance to access new therapies and treatments first. Cleveland Clinic offers an online tool for patients, caregivers and physicians to search for open clinical trials. The site lists trials being managed by oncologists in the Taussig Cancer Institute that are accepting patients at Cleveland Clinic main campus and at some Cleveland Clinic regional facilities. Visit clevelandclinic.org/cancertrials.

Comprehensive Online Medical Second Opinion

Cleveland Clinic experts can review your medical records and render an opinion that includes treatment options and recommendations. Call 216.444.3223 or 800.223.2273 ext. 43223; email eclevelandclinic@ccf.org.

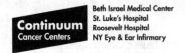

Beth Israel Medical Center
St. Luke's Hospital
Roosevelt Hospital
NY Eye & Ear Infirmary

Continuum Cancer Centers of New York

Continuum Cancer Centers
of New York
(212) 844-6027

The hospitals of Continuum – Beth Israel Medical Center, St. Luke's Hospital, Roosevelt Hospital and the New York Eye and Ear Infirmary – are leading providers of cancer care through Continuum Cancer Centers of New York (CCCNY). Last year as part of a major expansion of our cancer care services, Beth Israel Medical Center opened The Beth Israel Comprehensive Cancer Center-West Side Campus, a state-of-the-art facility comprising 88,000 square feet located in Manhattan.

We are dedicated to delivering care in ways that are more efficient, more attractive and more convenient for patients. Our cancer patients benefit from system-wide cancer expertise, facilities and resources. Continuum Cancer Centers feature world-renowned cancer specialists, including top-rated surgeons, medical oncologists, radiation oncologists, radiologists, pathologists, and oncology nurses.

Comprehensive diagnostic and treatment services are available for breast cancer, prostate cancer, head and neck and thyroid cancers, skin cancer, lung cancer, colorectal and other gastrointestinal cancers, lymphoma/Hodgkin's Disease, gynecological cancers, and cancers of the brain and central nervous system. Delivered efficiently in a friendly and supportive environment, our services include prevention programs – such as community education, screenings and early detection – expert diagnosis, outpatient treatment, inpatient services and home care. In addition, our Research Program offers patients access to investigational protocols through a wide number of clinical trials. Our physicians are leaders in both non-invasive and minimally invasive cancer treatments that focus on maximizing both the cure rate and the quality of life.

Support Services also play an important role at Continuum Cancer Centers. Our nurses, social workers, psychiatrists, chaplains, pharmacists, rehabilitation therapists and nutritionists all have specialized knowledge and expertise in the field of oncology.

In June 2011, CCCNY received a full three-year network accreditation from the American College of Surgeons Commission on Cancer (CoC), with commendation. Continuum first received a full, three-year accreditation in 2007, and was the only hospital system in New York State to receive such designation.

Continuum Health Partners, Inc.

Beth Israel   **Roosevelt Hospital**   **St. Luke's Hospital**   **NY Eye & Ear Infirmary**

www.chpnyc.org

FOX CHASE
CANCER CENTER

333 Cottman Avenue
Philadelphia, PA 19111-2497
Phone: 1-888-FOX CHASE • Fax: 215-728-2702
www.foxchase.org

MEDICAL ONCOLOGY

Medical oncologists at Fox Chase Cancer Center specialize in all major solid tumors in adults, rare tumors such as sarcomas, and cancers of the blood and bone marrow. Major clinical interests include breast, gastrointestinal, genitourinary, lung and ovarian cancers; adult lymphomas and leukemias; and phase I clinical trials.

New Drug Development

Fox Chase physicians and scientists are among the world's leaders in developing and testing new anticancer drugs, new methods of drug delivery and immunotherapy. A unique resource at Fox Chase, led by Anthony Olszanski, M.D., is the Center's Phase I Clinical Trials Program, which tests new drugs and treatments for the first time. Patients receive these state-of-the-art drugs under the close surveillance of dedicated nurses, physicians and scientists in the specialized clinical research unit.

Medical oncology research focuses on creating more effective anticancer drugs and investigating the molecular mechanisms that allow some tumor cells to acquire drug resistance. While new drug development focuses on testing new medications, it also develops important new biomarkers—tests which allow for better patient selection, helping to personalize the treatment strategy.

Targeted Therapy

Fox Chase medical oncologists are also leading the way in developing monoclonal antibody treatments that selectively target tumors or the microenvironment (such as tumor-related blood vessels) to disrupt cancer-related processes or activate the immune system to attack and eliminate cancer cells. The development of new, engineered antibodies has advanced the potential for immunotherapy to stimulate a patient's immune system and deliver activated immune cells directly to the cancer.

Monoclonal antibody therapies have become important tools in treating patients with various cancer types, including those with lymphoma, colorectal cancer, lung cancer and breast cancer, for example. Fox Chase medical oncologists continue to study combination therapies, pairing antibody treatments with other drugs or radioactive molecules that can be delivered directly to the tumor cells, leading the way to new discoveries aimed at treating cancer.

Clinical Trials Help Science and Medicine Work Together

Fox Chase translates new research findings into medical applications that may become models for improved comprehensive cancer care. Along with trials designed and offered only at Fox Chase, the Center participates in many national studies through the Eastern Cooperative Oncology Group, the Radiation Therapy Oncology Group, the Gynecologic Oncology Group and other national study groups. More than 200 clinical trials of new cancer prevention, diagnostic and treatment techniques are under way at any one time.

For healthy people who want to reduce their risk of cancer, Fox Chase conducts trials of agents that may prevent cancer in high-risk individuals. The Fox Chase advantage includes a leading role in national cancer prevention trials.

For more about Fox Chase physicians and services, visit our website, www.foxchase.org, or call 1-888-FOX CHASE.

THE JOHN THEURER CANCER CENTER
HACKENSACK UNIVERSITY MEDICAL CENTER

92 Second Street
Hackensack, New Jersey 07601
phone 201-996-5900 • fax 201-996-3452

jtcancercenter.org

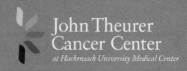

John Theurer Cancer Center – What does extraordinary cancer care mean? For us, extraordinary care is more than a catch phrase – it is an urgent call to action.

Cancer is hard enough for patients and their loved ones. At the John Theurer Cancer Center at Hackensack University Medical Center, we are committed to making the journey easier by delivering the complete spectrum of care.

Our five pillars of extraordinary care guide us as we strive to provide the best cancer care possible:
• Multidisciplinary care from teams of disease-specific experts;
• Personalized treatment that meets each patient's individual biologic, social, and emotional needs;
• Innovative research that brings tomorrow's novel research breakthroughs to patients today;
• Superior outcomes that improve survival rates through state-of-the-art treatments and prevention;
• Patient satisfaction that exceeds patients' needs and expectations.

Over the past 25 years, we have become one of the largest cancer centers in the United States. The John Theurer Cancer Center is transforming the cancer care experience one patient at a time by reaching for and delivering a new standard: extraordinary care.

Vision and Focus – The John Theurer Cancer Center's mission is to provide the highest quality cancer care, diagnosis, treatment, research, management, and preventive services. Fourteen specialized cancer-care teams provide advanced care that combines state-of-the-art technology, skilled medical expertise, research breakthroughs, and compassionate care giving. The Blood and Marrow Transplantation Program has been recognized with a Gold Seal of Approval™ for healthcare quality from the Joint Commission.

Bringing You Tomorrow's Breakthroughs Today™ – Most of today's cancer-care breakthroughs have come about from basic and clinical research into how cancer can be best detected, treated, or managed. Some of the most innovative cancer clinical trials are conducted at the cancer center, spearheaded by internationally renowned award-winning researchers. These trials give patients access to promising investigational medications, treatment protocols, and surgical techniques. This strong research component coupled with its patient care services elevates the John Theurer Cancer Center to a world-class academic medical center.

Finding Answers – The first step in cancer care is to define the illness, determine its location, and find out whether it has spread. At the cancer center, pathologists, radiologists, and other physicians use precise, sophisticated technology to gain answers to these questions. Among the equipment and tests used are a dedicated PET scanner, ultrasonography, nuclear medicine, computerized tomography, magnetic resonance imaging, mammography, and angiography.

Today's Treatment Innovations – Physicians at the cancer center have pioneered some of the most promising treatments for cancer – including peripheral stem cell transplantation. Through its specialized divisions, the cancer center offers patients the most advanced treatment options, including intensity modulated radiation therapy, image guided radiation therapy, brachytherapy, stereotactic radiosurgery; innovative adjuvant therapy approaches; and state-of-the-art surgical techniques, including video-assisted thoracic surgery, radioablation therapy, and minimally invasive procedures that reduce pain, lessen side effects, decrease recovery time, and increase patients' mobility.

To receive information on the John Theurer Cancer Center's services and its 14 specialized divisions, call 201-996-5900.

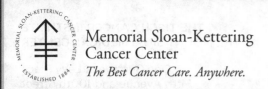

Memorial Sloan-Kettering Cancer Center
The Best Cancer Care. Anywhere.

1275 York Avenue
New York, NY 10065
Phone: (212) 639-2000
Make an Appointment: (800) 525-2225
www.mskcc.org

Sponsorship: Private, Non-Profit
Beds: 470
Accreditation: Awarded Accreditation from the Joint Commission on Accreditation of Healthcare Organizations (JCAHO)

At Memorial Sloan-Kettering Cancer Center, our sole focus is cancer. Our doctors are among the most skilled and experienced in the world in treating all kinds of cancer. The knowledge, talent, and expertise of our medical professionals lead to superb patient care, and often, a significant positive impact on the chances that their cancer will be cured or controlled.

SUB-SPECIALIZED MEDICAL EXPERTISE
Our patients benefit from individualized treatment plans developed by a team of specialists with unsurpassed depth and breadth of experience. The teams include surgeons, medical and radiation oncologists, radiologists, pathologists, nurses, and others who are specialists in a specific type of cancer. They develop treatment plans that reflect their combined expertise, so patients who need several different types of therapy will receive the best combination for them.

RESEARCH EXPANDS TREATMENT OPTIONS
One of Memorial Sloan-Kettering's great strengths is the close relationship between scientists and clinicians. Through the constant collaboration between our doctors and research scientists, new drugs and therapies developed in the laboratory can be quickly translated into improved treatment options for patients.

NURSING AND SUPPORTIVE CARE
Nurses are essential members of the healthcare team. Our specially trained oncology nurses care for patients throughout their treatment, help manage clinical trials, and educate patients about all aspects of their care.

Specialized psychiatrists and psychologists help patients deal with the stress, anxiety, and depression that sometimes accompany cancer and its treatment. Our social workers ensure that patients who need it receive assistance with needs such as housing and transportation. They offer individual and family counseling, as well as support groups for both inpatients and outpatients. After treatment, the Post-Treatment Resource Program offers patients seminars, lectures, support groups, and practical advice on various issues such as insurance and employment.

INTEGRATIVE MEDICINE
Our Integrative Medicine Service offers a full range of complementary therapies, including massage, reflexology, meditation, music therapy, and acupuncture. These do not replace medical care but are used along with clinical treatments to help patients relieve stress, reduce pain and anxiety, manage symptoms, and promote a feeling of well-being.

INSURANCE
Memorial Sloan-Kettering Cancer Center is in-network with most New York–area insurance plans.

A TRADITION OF EXCELLENCE

From its founding in 1884, Memorial Sloan-Kettering Cancer Center has been guided by a clear mission: to offer the best possible care for patients today, and to seek strategies to prevent, control, and ultimately cure cancer in the future. We are proud of our designation as one of the few select National Cancer Institute Comprehensive Cancer Centers and a member of the National Comprehensive Cancer Network.

To see one of our specialized cancer experts, call us at (800) 525-2225.

Make an Appointment: (800) 525-2225

MOUNT SINAI
SCHOOL OF
MEDICINE

THE TISCH CANCER INSTITUTE
AT THE MOUNT SINAI MEDICAL CENTER

One Gustave L. Levy Place
Fifth Avenue and 100th Street
New York, NY 10029-6574
Physician Referral: 1-800-MD-SINAI (637-4624)
www.tischcancerinstitute.org

THE TISCH CANCER INSTITUTE is embedded within a renowned medical center that has world-class research facilities, one of the nation's top-ranked hospitals, and an outstanding medical school. Patients have access to the best possible cancer care across a variety of disciplines, including medical, surgical, and radiation treatments; palliative care; behavioral medicine; physical therapy; psychosocial services—and cutting-edge cancer research. For fully integrated, multidisciplinary care, our patients are also treated by the best specialists in every field at Mount Sinai and can receive seamless referrals.

Services and Programs – The Tisch Cancer Institute employs a multidisciplinary treatment approach, providing access to clinical breakthroughs, innovative techniques, leading-edge technologies, and a wide range of diagnostic, therapeutic, and support services for all types of cancer. The Institute treats: breast cancer; hematological malignancies (including multiple myeloma, myelodysplastic syndrome, and myeloproliferative disorders); genitourinary cancers (including prostate, bladder, and kidney); head and neck cancers; thoracic cancer (including lung and esophagus); gynecologic cancers; brain tumors; and other diagnoses. In addition to surgical treatment, the Institute provides radiation and medical oncology therapies, as well as bone marrow transplantation. The Dubin Breast Center, consisting of 15,000 square feet, is a newly constructed facility that opened in April 2011 and significantly expands the treatment space for breast cancer patients.

THE RUTTENBERG TREATMENT CENTER
The Derald H. Ruttenberg Treatment Center houses the ambulatory cancer program of The Tisch Cancer Institute and is operated by the Mount Sinai Hospital.

THE DUBIN BREAST CARE CENTER
The Dubin Breast Care Center offers the latest, most innovative approaches available for breast health and the treatment of breast cancer.

The Tisch Cancer Institute encourages collaboration with colleagues across the Medical Center, drawing upon the knowledge of a vast network of specialists who are outstanding in their fields. These experts consist of award-winning physicians and surgeons specializing in cardiac care, neurology, urology, pediatrics, digestive diseases, obstetrics and gynecology, and other therapeutic areas. Oncologists, surgeons, radiation oncologists, and specialists from across the medical spectrum work together to provide the highest quality care to all cancer patients. Furthermore, Mount Sinai's nursing staff is an important part of the Medical Center's focus on delivering exceptional patient care, and it has received the prestigious Magnet Award for nursing excellence. Mount Sinai is also renowned for its palliative care program, which provides the highest level of care, focusing on the relief of pain, symptoms, and stress in cancer patients in both an inpatient and outpatient setting.

A Heritage of Breakthroughs – Teams of physicians and scientists at The Tisch Cancer Institute at Mount Sinai work together to rapidly translate laboratory research into new patient treatments. Among the advances pioneered at Mount Sinai are the first successful treatment of tumors of the bladder by transurethral electrocoagulation, the first demonstration of how asbestos can cause cancerous changes in the DNA of cells, and the first development of an ultrasound-guided technique to insert radioactive seeds into the prostate to treat prostate cancer.

NewYork-Presbyterian
The University Hospital of Columbia and Cornell

Affiliated with Columbia University College of Physicians and Surgeons and Weill Cornell Medical College

Herbert Irving Comprehensive Cancer Center	Weill Cornell Cancer Center
NewYork-Presbyterian Hospital	NewYork-Presbyterian Hospital
Columbia University Medical Center	Weill Cornell Medical Center
161 Fort Washington Avenue	525 East 68th Street
New York, NY 10032	New York, NY 10065

1-877-NYP-WELL (1-877-697-9355)   www.nyp.org/cancer

NewYork-Presbyterian Cancer Centers

Innovative cancer treatments. Personalized, compassionate care. Evidence-based medicine. These are the hallmarks of the cancer care available at NewYork-Presbyterian Hospital, where cutting-edge treatment goes beyond state-of-the-art. We treat more than 7,000 people who are newly diagnosed with cancer each year.

NewYork-Presbyterian features two of the country's top cancer centers: the National Cancer Institute-designated Herbert Irving Comprehensive Cancer Center (one of only three comprehensive NCI-designated cancer centers in New York State) and the Weill Cornell Cancer Center. Through a multidisciplinary team approach, we combine the expertise and talents of all of the individuals responsible for a patient's care—surgical, medical, and radiation oncologists, specialized oncology nurses, social workers, and nutritionists—to deliver seamless care in a supportive and healing environment.

Our team cares for patients with the following cancers:

- AIDS-related cancers
- Bladder cancer
- Brain and other nervous system cancers
- Breast cancer
- Colorectal, pancreatic, and other digestive cancers
- Eye cancer
- Gynecologic cancers (ovarian, cervical, endometrial)
- Head and neck cancers (oral, oropharyngeal, laryngeal)
- Kidney cancer
- Lymphomas (Hodgkin's and non-Hodgkin's)
- Leukemia and myelodysplastic syndromes
- Liver cancer
- Mesothelioma
- Myeloma
- Pediatric cancers
- Prostate cancer
- Sarcoma
- Thoracic cancers (lung, esophageal, chest wall)

Research underlies everything we do, and sets academic medical centers such as ours apart from other cancer treatment centers. Our scientists and clinical investigators are leading more than 500 clinical trials assessing new cancer management approaches in thousands of patients.

Specialized Cancer Care Includes:

- Surgical procedures for breast cancer that result in superior cosmetic outcomes, and evaluation of novel anticancer drugs for women with advanced disease

- Robotic surgery for prostate and gynecologic cancers

- Video-assisted thoracoscopy and lung-sparing surgery for some lung cancers

- Interventional endoscopy and laparoscopic surgery for colorectal and other cancers

- Targeted approaches to brain cancer treatment, including convection-enhanced chemotherapy and stereotactic radiosurgery

- Bone marrow and stem cell transplantation for hematologic cancers

- Renowned Mesothelioma Center

- Combination chemotherapy, targeted anticancer agents, novel drugs available through clinical trials, and highly targeted radiation therapy

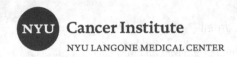

NYU Cancer Institute
NYU LANGONE MEDICAL CENTER

NYU Langone Medical Center
550 First Avenue , New York, NY 10016
www.NYULMC.org

NYU Clinical Cancer Center
160 East 34th Street, New York, NY 10016
www.NYUCI.org

**The Stephen D. Hassenfeld Children's Center
for Cancer and Blood Disorders**
160 East 32nd Street, New York, NY 10016
www.NYUMC.org/Hassenfeld

The NYU Cancer Institute is an NCI-designated cancer center and provides personalized patient care that is both compassionate and state of the art. The doctors and researchers work together to develop innovative therapies for patients. The Cancer Institute is world-renowned for excellence in cancer-focused research, personalized care, education and community outreach. Its mission is to discover the origins of human cancer and to use that knowledge to eradicate the personal and societal burden of cancer in our community, the nation and the world. For more information about our expert physicians, call 212-731-5000. *We specialize in the following areas:*

Patient-Focused Setting
The NYU Clinical Cancer Center is the principal outpatient facility of The Cancer Institute and serves as home to our patients and their caregivers. The center and its multidisciplinary team of experts provide access to the latest treatment options and clinical trials along with a variety of programs in cancer risk reduction/prevention, screening, diagnostics, genetic counseling and supportive services. In addition the NYUCI emphasizes the importance of a holistic approach to management services in complementary medicine, psychosocial support, survivorship and palliative care.

Renowned Expertise
The NYU Cancer Institute brings together experts from a variety of disciplines to create collaborative research endeavors and clinical care teams. The Cancer Institute offers a full continuum of personalized care, from prevention through diagnosis, treatment and post-treatment support. The compassion and expertise of our team members helps patients better manage the symptoms of their diseases as well as meet their special needs. Additionally, we have created special emphasis programs in diseases such as breast cancer, melanoma, GI cancer, prostate cancer, hematologic malignancies and lung cancer among others, as well as, translational programs in cancer healthcare disparities, molecularly targeted therapy, and the cell signaling pathways involved in cancer.

A Translational Approach
NYU Langone Medical Center scientists and other researchers excel in uncovering how cancer develops at the molecular level, and how we can harness that knowledge to reduce the risk of cancer and treat the disease. The Medical Center constantly seeks to create new opportunities for collaboration between investigators within our own institution, those located elsewhere in the NYU network of campuses, and researchers at other institutions.

The Stephen D. Hassenfeld Children's Center for Cancer and Blood Disorders
The center is a leading pediatric outpatient facility for the treatment of childhood cancers and blood diseases. Its unique interdisciplinary and family-centered approach combines the most advanced medical treatments with psychosocial and emotional support services for young patients and their families.

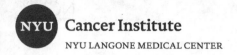

NYU **Cancer Institute**
NYU LANGONE MEDICAL CENTER

NYU Langone Medical Center
550 First Avenue , New York, NY 10016
www.NYULMC.org

NYU Clinical Cancer Center
160 East 34th Street, New York, NY 10016
www.NYUCI.org

**The Stephen D. Hassenfeld Children's Center
for Cancer and Blood Disorders**
160 East 32nd Street, New York, NY 10016
www.NYUMC.org/Hassenfeld

The NYU Cancer Institute is an NCI-designated cancer center and provides personalized patient care that is both compassionate and state of the art. The doctors and researchers work together to develop innovative therapies for patients. The Cancer Institute is world-renowned for excellence in cancer-focused research, personalized care, education and community outreach. Its mission is to discover the origins of human cancer and to use that knowledge to eradicate the personal and societal burden of cancer in our community, the nation and the world. For more information about our expert physicians, call 212-731-5000. *We specialize in the following areas:*

Patient-Focused Setting
The NYU Clinical Cancer Center is the principal outpatient facility of The Cancer Institute and serves as home to our patients and their caregivers. The center and its multidisciplinary team of experts provide access to the latest treatment options and clinical trials along with a variety of programs in cancer risk reduction/prevention, screening, diagnostics, genetic counseling and supportive services. In addition the NYUCI emphasizes the importance of a holistic approach to management services in complementary medicine, psychosocial support, survivorship and palliative care.

Renowned Expertise
The NYU Cancer Institute brings together experts from a variety of disciplines to create collaborative research endeavors and clinical care teams. The Cancer Institute offers a full continuum of personalized care, from prevention through diagnosis, treatment and post-treatment support. The compassion and expertise of our team members helps patients better manage the symptoms of their diseases as well as meet their special needs. Additionally, we have created special emphasis programs in diseases such as breast cancer, melanoma, GI cancer, prostate cancer, hematologic malignancies and lung cancer among others, as well as, translational programs in cancer healthcare disparities, molecularly targeted therapy, and the cell signaling pathways involved in cancer.

A Translational Approach
NYU Langone Medical Center scientists and other researchers excel in uncovering how cancer develops at the molecular level, and how we can harness that knowledge to reduce the risk of cancer and treat the disease. The Medical Center constantly seeks to create new opportunities for collaboration between investigators within our own institution, those located elsewhere in the NYU network of campuses, and researchers at other institutions.

The Stephen D. Hassenfeld Children's Center for Cancer and Blood Disorders
The center is a leading pediatric outpatient facility for the treatment of childhood cancers and blood diseases. Its unique interdisciplinary and family-centered approach combines the most advanced medical treatments with psychosocial and emotional support services for young patients and their families.

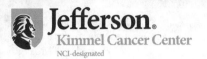

Jefferson.
Kimmel Cancer Center
NCI-designated

A Cancer Center Designated by the National Cancer Institute

111 S. 11th Street, Philadelphia, PA 19107-5098, 215-955-6000, *www.jeffersonhospital.org/cancer*

Designated Center of Excellence

Thomas Jefferson University Hospitals is an academic medical center comprised of Thomas Jefferson University Hospital, Jefferson Hospital for Neuroscience (JHN), Methodist Hospital and multiple outpatient sites. It is home to the Kimmel Cancer Center at Jefferson, a National Cancer Institute (NCI)-designated Center for Excellence in both cancer care and research, where world-famous cancer specialists provide breakthrough treatment with compassion, support and state-of-the-art technology. Jefferson doctors are ranked among the nation's best for cancer treatment on such prestigious lists as *Best Doctors in America*® database of experts. They also contribute to leading scientific and medical journals and hold leadership positions in national and local cancer organizations.

Recognized as Among the Best

- *U.S.News & World Report* recognizes Jefferson as one of the best hospitals in the nation for cancer care.
- Independence Blue Cross has designated Jefferson as a Blue Distinction Center for complex and rare cancers.
- Jefferson's Kimmel Cancer Center is one of only six cancer centers in the nation designated as a Center of Excellence by FertileHOPE, a non-profit organization providing reproductive information, support and hope to cancer patients and survivors.
- The Jefferson Breast Care Center has full accreditation from the National Accreditation Program for Breast Centers for achievement of the highest standards for breast cancer treatment.
- Jefferson's Center City Campus has been granted MAGNET® recognition for nursing excellence from the American Nurses Credentialing Center.

Jefferson's Approach to Cancer Care

- *Collaborative.* Specialists from our team of nationally renowned cancer experts will work with you and your referring physician to develop a personalized treatment plan. This is complemented by a support network for patients and their families, including specially trained nurses, educators, fellow patients and cancer survivors.
- *State-of-the-art.* Our experienced physicians utilize the most advanced technologies and pioneering therapies for diagnosis and treatment. Patients may have the opportunity to take part in one of the more than 120 clinical trials for promising new cancer treatments underway at Jefferson at any given time.
- *Personal.* We provide care for the whole person by addressing medical, emotional and spiritual needs. The Jefferson-Myrna Brind Center of Integrative Medicine's medical staff will work with your primary Kimmel Cancer Center provider to offer innovative natural therapies and counseling techniques, many of which can be applied during chemotherapy and radiation treatment, or at any time throughout survivorship.

Multidisciplinary Centers

Centers offer access to a team of specialists providing personalized care and leading-edge treatments:

- Brain Tumor
- Breast Care
- Colon and Rectal Cancer
- Genitourinary Oncology
- Gynecologic Cancer
- Head and Neck Cancer
- Liver Tumor
- Pancreatic, Biliary and Related Cancer
- Senior Adult Oncology
- Thoracic/Aerodigestive Cancer
- Uveal Melanoma

In addition, Jefferson offers innovative treatments for hematological malignancies, including new approaches to hematopoietic stem cell transplantation that make this option available to a greater number of patients.

Specialized Cancer Programs

- Bone Marrow Transplant
- Cancer Rehabilitation
- Musculoskeletal Oncology
- Hereditary Cancer
- Breast Cancer Risk Assessment
- Integrative Cancer Care

Physician Referral: Outpatient healthcare services are available throughout the Delaware Valley at the offices of 202 primary care physicians and 645 specialists affiliated with Thomas Jefferson University Hospitals. For an appointment with a Jefferson doctor, call **1-800-JEFF-NOW** or visit *www.jeffersonhospital.org*

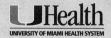
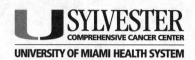

The Best in American Medicine
www.CastleConnolly.com

Neurological Surgery

A neurological surgeon provides the operative and non-operative management (i.e., prevention, diagnosis, evaluation, treatment, critical care and rehabilitation) of disorders of the central, peripheral and autonomic nervous systems, including their supporting structures and vascular supply; the evaluation and treatment of pathological processes which modify function or activity of the nervous system; and the operative and non-operative management of pain. A neurological surgeon treats patients with disorders of the nervous system; disorders of the brain, meninges, skull and their blood supply, including the extracranial carotid and vertebral arteries; disorders of the pituitary gland; disorders of the spinal cord, meninges and vertebral column, including those which may require treatment by spinal fusion or instrumentation; and disorders of the cranial and spinal nerves throughout their distribution.

Training Required: One year minimum of General Surgery followed by five years in Neurological Surgery.

Pediatric Neurological Surgery: The American Board of Pediatric Neurological Surgery (ABPNS) is not a recognized ABMS subspecialty. However, this designation has been included because the certification process is meaningful and rigorous. It is awarded to those doctors who hold a current ABMS certification in Neurological Surgery, have completed a fully accredited one year, post-graduate fellowship in pediatric neurological surgery, and have submitted surgical logs indicating a practice of pediatric neurological surgery for one year, followed by a written examination.

NEUROLOGICAL SURGERY

New England

Al-Mefty, Ossama MD [NS] - **Spec Exp:** Skull Base Surgery; Brain Tumors; Cerebrovascular Surgery; **Hospital:** Brigham & Women's Hosp; **Address:** Brigham & Women's Hosp, Dept Neurosurgery, 75 Francis St, Boston, MA 02115; **Phone:** 617-525-9451; **Board Cert:** Neurological Surgery 1980; **Med School:** Syria 1972; **Resid:** Surgery, Med Coll Ohio 1974; Neurological Surgery, West Va Med Ctr 1978; **Fac Appt:** Prof NS, Harvard Med Sch

Borges, Lawrence F MD [NS] - **Spec Exp:** Spinal Surgery; Spinal Tumors; **Hospital:** Mass Genl Hosp; **Address:** Mass General Hosp, 55 Fruit St, White 1205, Boston, MA 02114; **Phone:** 617-726-6156; **Board Cert:** Neurological Surgery 1986; **Med School:** Johns Hopkins Univ 1977; **Resid:** Neurological Surgery, Mass Genl Hosp 1983; **Fac Appt:** Assoc Prof S, Harvard Med Sch

Cosgrove, G Rees MD [NS] - **Spec Exp:** Brain Tumors; **Hospital:** Rhode Island Hosp, Miriam Hosp; **Address:** 55 Claverick St, Providence, RI 02903; **Phone:** 401-490-4176; **Board Cert:** Neurological Surgery 1989; **Med School:** Queens Univ 1980; **Resid:** Neurological Surgery, Montreal Neur Inst 1986; **Fac Appt:** Prof NS, Brown Univ

David, Carlos A MD [NS] - **Spec Exp:** Brain Tumors; Pituitary Tumors; **Hospital:** Lahey Clin, Emerson Hosp; **Address:** Lahey Clinic, Dept Neurosurgery, 41 Mall Rd, Burlington, MA 01805; **Phone:** 781-744-8643; **Board Cert:** Neurological Surgery 2001, **Med School:** Univ Miami Sch Med 1990; **Resid:** Neurological Surgery, Jackson Memorial Hosp 1995; **Fellow:** Cerebrovascular & Skull Base Surgery, Barrow Neuro Inst 1997; **Fac Appt:** Assoc Clin Prof NS, Tufts Univ

Duhaime, Ann Christine MD [NS] - **Spec Exp:** Pediatric Neurosurgery; Brain Tumors; **Hospital:** Mass Genl Hosp; **Address:** Mass Geneneral Hospital for Children, 15 Parkman St, WACC 331, Boston, MA 02114; **Phone:** 617-643-9175; **Board Cert:** Neurological Surgery 1990; Pediatric Neurological Surgery 2005; **Med School:** Univ Pennsylvania 1981; **Resid:** Neurological Surgery, Hosp Univ Penn 1987; **Fellow:** Pediatric Neurological Surgery, Chldns Hosp 1987

Goumnerova, Liliana MD [NS] - **Spec Exp:** Pediatric Neurosurgery; Brain Tumors; **Hospital:** Children's Hospital - Boston, Dana-Farber Cancer Inst; **Address:** 300 Longwood Ave Hunnewell Bldg Fl 2, Boston, MA 02115; **Phone:** 617-355-6364; **Board Cert:** Neurological Surgery 1992; Pediatric Neurological Surgery 2006; **Med School:** Canada 1980; **Resid:** Neurological Surgery, Univ Ottawa 1986; **Fellow:** Pediatric Neurological Surgery, Hosp for Sick Chldn 1988; Neurological Science, Univ Hosp Penn 1990; **Fac Appt:** Assoc Prof S, Harvard Med Sch

Martuza, Robert L MD [NS] - **Spec Exp:** Brain Tumors; Skull Base Surgery; **Hospital:** Mass Genl Hosp; **Address:** Mass General Hosp, Dept Neurosurgery, 55 Fruit St, White 502, Boston, MA 02114; **Phone:** 617-726-8581; **Board Cert:** Neurological Surgery 1983; **Med School:** Harvard Med Sch 1973; **Resid:** Neurological Surgery, Mass Genl Hosp 1980; **Fac Appt:** Prof NS, Harvard Med Sch

Penar, Paul L MD [NS] - **Spec Exp:** Brain & Spinal Tumors; Stereotactic Radiosurgery; Pain-Chronic; **Hospital:** Fletcher Allen Health Care- Med Ctr Campus; **Address:** Fletcher Allen Health Care, 111 Colchester Ave, Burlington, VT 05401; **Phone:** 802-847-4590; **Board Cert:** Neurological Surgery 1989; **Med School:** Univ Mich Med Sch 1981; **Resid:** Neurological Surgery, Yale-New Haven Hosp 1987

Piepmeier, Joseph MD [NS] - **Spec Exp:** Neuro-Oncology; Brain & Spinal Cord Tumors; **Hospital:** Yale-New Haven Hosp, Yale Med Group; **Address:** Yale Sch Med, Dept Neurosurgery, 333 Cedar St Fl TMP-410, New Haven, CT 06520; **Phone:** 203-785-2791; **Board Cert:** Neurological Surgery 1984; **Med School:** Univ Tenn Coll Med 1975; **Resid:** Neurological Surgery, Yale-New Haven Hosp 1982; **Fac Appt:** Prof NS, Yale Univ

Swearingen, Brooke MD [NS] - **Spec Exp:** Pituitary Tumors; Brain & Spinal Tumors; Neuroendocrine Tumors; Spinal Surgery; **Hospital:** Mass Genl Hosp; **Address:** 15 Parkman St, WACC 331, Boston, MA 02114-3117; **Phone:** 617-726-3910; **Board Cert:** Neurological Surgery 1993; **Med School:** Harvard Med Sch 1981; **Resid:** Neurological Surgery, Mass Genl Hosp 1987; **Fac Appt:** Assoc Prof NS, Harvard Med Sch

Mid Atlantic

Andrews, David MD [NS] - **Spec Exp:** Brain Tumors; Stereotactic Radiosurgery; **Hospital:** Thomas Jefferson Univ Hosp (page 81); **Address:** Thom Jefferson Univ Hosp, Dept Neurosurg, 909 Walnut St Fl 2, Philadelphia, PA 19107-5109; **Phone:** 215-503-7005; **Board Cert:** Neurological Surgery 1992; **Med School:** Univ Colorado 1983; **Resid:** Neurological Surgery, NY Presby Hosp-Cornell Med Ctr 1989; **Fellow:** Neuro-Oncology, Meml Sloan Kettering Cancer Ctr 1987; **Fac Appt:** Prof NS, Thomas Jefferson Univ

Bailes, Julian E MD [NS] - **Spec Exp:** Neuro-Oncology; Cancer Surgery; Spinal Surgery; Cerebrovascular Surgery; **Hospital:** Ruby Memorial - WVU Hosp; **Address:** W Virgina Univ Eye Inst, PO Box 9193, Morgantown, WV 26506; **Phone:** 304-598-6127; **Board Cert:** Neurological Surgery 1992; **Med School:** Louisiana State U, New Orleans 1982; **Resid:** Surgery, Northwestern Meml Hosp 1987; **Fellow:** Neurological Surgery, Barrow Neurological Inst 1988; **Fac Appt:** Prof NS

Bederson, Joshua B MD [NS] - **Spec Exp:** Brain & Spinal Cord Tumors; Pituitary Tumors; Skull Base Tumors; **Hospital:** Mount Sinai Med Ctr (page 76); **Address:** Mount Sinai Med Ctr, 1 Gustave Levy Pl, Box 1136, New York, NY 10029; **Phone:** 212-241-2377; **Board Cert:** Neurological Surgery 1993; **Med School:** UCSF 1984; **Resid:** Neurological Surgery, UCSF Med Ctr 1990; **Fellow:** Neurological Vascular Surgery, Barrow Neur Inst 1990; Neurological Vascular Surgery, Univ Hosp Zurich 1990; **Fac Appt:** Prof NS, Mount Sinai Sch Med

Bilsky, Mark H MD [NS] - **Spec Exp:** Brain & Spinal Tumors; Skull Base Tumors; Spinal Cord Tumors; Spinal Surgery; **Hospital:** Meml Sloan-Kettering Cancer Ctr (page 75), NY-Presby Hosp/Weill Cornell (page 78); **Address:** 1275 York Ave MSKCC Bldg Fl c705, New York, NY 10065; **Phone:** 212-639-8526; **Board Cert:** Neurological Surgery 2010; **Med School:** Emory Univ 1988; **Resid:** Neurological Surgery, NY Hosp-Cornell Med Ctr 1994; **Fellow:** Neuro-Oncology, Louisville Univ Med Ctr 1995; **Fac Appt:** Prof NS, Cornell Univ-Weill Med Coll

Brem, Henry MD [NS] - **Spec Exp:** Brain & Spinal Cord Tumors; Skull Base Tumors; Pituitary Tumors; **Hospital:** Johns Hopkins Hosp, Johns Hopkins Bayview Med Ctr; **Address:** Johns Hopkins Hosp, 600 N Wolfe St Meyer 7 Bldg - rm 113, Baltimore, MD 21287; **Phone:** 410-955-2248; **Board Cert:** Neurological Surgery 1986; **Med School:** Harvard Med Sch 1978; **Resid:** Neurological Surgery, Columbia-Presby Med Ctr 1984; **Fellow:** Neurological Surgery, Johns Hopkins Hosp 1980; **Fac Appt:** Prof NS, Johns Hopkins Univ

Bruce, Jeffrey MD [NS] - **Spec Exp:** Brain Tumors; Pituitary Tumors; Skull Base Surgery; Minimally Invasive Surgery; **Hospital:** NY-Presby Hosp/Columbia (page 78); **Address:** NY Presby Hosp, Dept Neurosurgery, 710 W 168th St N1 Bldg Fl 4 - rm 434, New York, NY 10032; **Phone:** 212-305-7346; **Board Cert:** Neurological Surgery 1993; **Med School:** UMDNJ-RW Johnson Med Sch 1983; **Resid:** Neurological Surgery, Columbia-Presby Med Ctr 1990; **Fellow:** Neurological Surgery, Nat Inst Hlth 1985; **Fac Appt:** Prof NS, Columbia P&S

Neurological Surgery

Carson, Benjamin S MD [NS] - **Spec Exp:** Brain & Spinal Cord Tumors; Pediatric Neurosurgery; **Hospital:** Johns Hopkins Hosp; **Address:** 600 N Wolfe St, Harvey 811, Baltimore, MD 21287-8811; **Phone:** 410-355-4259; **Board Cert:** Neurological Surgery 1988; Pediatric Neurological Surgery 1997; **Med School:** Univ Mich Med Sch 1977; **Resid:** Neurological Surgery, Johns Hopkins Hosp 1983; **Fellow:** Pediatric Neurological Surgery, Queen Elizabeth II Med Ctr 1984; **Fac Appt:** Assoc Prof NS, Johns Hopkins Univ

Chen, Chun Siang MD [NS] - **Spec Exp:** Skull Base Tumors; Skull Base Surgery; Microsurgery; Brain & Spinal Tumors; **Hospital:** Mount Sinai Med Ctr (page 76); **Address:** Mount Sinai Med Ctr, Annenberg Bldg, One Gustave L Levy Pl Fl 8 - rm 10, New York, NY 10029; **Phone:** 212-241-8480; **Med School:** Brazil 1978; **Resid:** Neurological Surgery, Santa Casa de Misericordia of Sao Paulo Med Sch 1983; Neurological Surgery, Mt Sinai Med Ctr 2005; **Fellow:** Skull Base Surgery, St Lukes Roosevelt Hosp 2006; **Fac Appt:** Asst Prof NS, Mount Sinai Sch Med

Di Giacinto, George V MD [NS] - **Spec Exp:** Spinal Surgery; Pain Management; **Hospital:** St. Luke's - Roosevelt Hosp Ctr - Roosevelt Div (page 71); **Address:** 425 W 59th St, Ste 4E, New York, NY 10019; **Phone:** 212-523-8500; **Board Cert:** Neurological Surgery 1981; **Med School:** Harvard Med Sch 1970; **Resid:** Neurological Surgery, Columbia-Presby Hosp 1978

Evans, James J MD [NS] - **Spec Exp:** Skull Base Surgery; Neuro-Oncology; Brain Tumors; **Hospital:** Thomas Jefferson Univ Hosp (page 81); **Address:** 909 Walnut St Fl 2, Philadelphia, PA 19107; **Phone:** 215-955-7000; **Board Cert:** Neurological Surgery 2006; **Med School:** Univ Mass Sch Med 1995; **Resid:** Neurological Surgery, Cleveland Clinic 1999; **Fellow:** Cranial Base Surgery, Inova Fairfax Hospital 2001; **Fac Appt:** Assoc Prof NS, Thomas Jefferson Univ

Feldstein, Neil A MD [NS] - **Spec Exp:** Pediatric Neurosurgery; Brain Tumors-Pediatric; Craniofacial Surgery-Pediatric; **Hospital:** NYPresby-Morgan Stanley Children's Hosp (page 78); **Address:** Neurological Inst, 710 W 168th St Fl 2 - rm 213, New York, NY 10032; **Phone:** 212-305-1396; **Board Cert:** Neurological Surgery 1995; Pediatric Neurological Surgery 2007; **Med School:** NYU Sch Med 1984; **Resid:** Neurological Surgery, Baylor Coll Med 1989; **Fellow:** Pediatric Neurological Surgery, NYU Med Ctr 1991; **Fac Appt:** Assoc Prof NS, Columbia P&S

Fenstermaker, Robert A MD [NS] - **Spec Exp:** Brain Tumors; Pituitary Tumors; Stereotactic Radiosurgery; Endoscopic Skull Base Surgery; **Hospital:** Roswell Park Cancer Inst; **Address:** Roswell Park Cancer Inst, Elm & Carlton Sts, Buffalo, NY 14263; **Phone:** 716-845-3154; **Board Cert:** Neurological Surgery 1991; **Med School:** NE Ohio Univ 1981; **Resid:** Neurological Surgery, Univ Hosps Cleveland 1987; **Fellow:** Pharmacology, Case Western Reserve 1989; **Fac Appt:** Prof NS, SUNY Buffalo

Golfinos, John G MD [NS] - **Spec Exp:** Brain Tumors; Stereotactic Radiosurgery; Skull Base Surgery; **Hospital:** NYU Langone Med Ctr (page 79), Bellevue Hosp Ctr; **Address:** 530 First Ave, Ste 8R, New York, NY 10016; **Phone:** 212-263-2950; **Board Cert:** Neurological Surgery 1998; **Med School:** Columbia P&S 1988; **Resid:** Neurological Surgery, Barrow Neuro Inst 1995; **Fac Appt:** Assoc Prof NS, NYU Sch Med

Gutin, Philip H MD [NS] - **Spec Exp:** Brain Tumors; **Hospital:** Meml Sloan-Kettering Cancer Ctr (page 75), NY-Presby Hosp/Weill Cornell (page 78); **Address:** 1275 York Ave, rm C 703, New York, NY 10065; **Phone:** 212-639-8556; **Board Cert:** Neurological Surgery 1981; **Med School:** Univ Pennsylvania 1971; **Resid:** Neurological Surgery, UCSF Med Ctr 1979; **Fellow:** Neurological Surgery, Natl Cancer Inst 1976; **Fac Appt:** Prof NS, Cornell Univ-Weill Med Coll

Jallo, George I MD [NS] - **Spec Exp:** Pediatric Neurosurgery; Brain & Spinal Cord Tumors; Minimally Invasive Neurosurgery; **Hospital:** Johns Hopkins Hosp, Johns Hopkins Bayview Med Ctr; **Address:** Johns Hopkins Hosp, Dept of Neurosurgery, 600 N Wolfe St, Ste Harvey 811, Baltimore, MD 21287; **Phone:** 410-955-7851; **Board Cert:** Neurological Surgery 2002; Pediatric Neurological Surgery 2004; **Med School:** Univ VA Sch Med 1991; **Resid:** Neurological Surgery, NYU Med Ctr 1998; **Fellow:** Pediatric Neurological Surgery, Beth Israel Med Ctr 1999; **Fac Appt:** Prof NS, Johns Hopkins Univ

Judy, Kevin MD [NS] - **Spec Exp:** Brain Tumors; Skull Base Tumors; **Hospital:** Thomas Jefferson Univ Hosp (page 81); **Address:** Jefferson Neurosurgical Assocs, 909 Walnut St, Philadelphia, PA 19107; **Phone:** 215-503-7005; **Board Cert:** Neurological Surgery 1997; **Med School:** Univ Pittsburgh 1984; **Resid:** Surgery, Mercy Hosp 1986; Neurological Surgery, Johns Hopkins Hosp 1992; **Fellow:** Neurological Surgery, Johns Hopkins Hosp 1991; **Fac Appt:** Prof NS, Jefferson Med Coll

Kobrine, Arthur MD/PhD [NS] - **Spec Exp:** Brain & Spinal Cord Tumors; Spinal Surgery; **Hospital:** Sibley Mem Hosp, Georgetown Univ Hosp; **Address:** 2440 M St NW, Ste 315, Washington, DC 20037-1404; **Phone:** 202-293-7136; **Board Cert:** Neurological Surgery 1976; **Med School:** Northwestern Univ 1968; **Resid:** Neurological Surgery, Northwestern Univ Hosp 1970; Neurological Surgery, Walter Reed Army Hosp 1973; **Fellow:** Physiology, Geo Wash Univ 1979; **Fac Appt:** Clin Prof NS, Georgetown Univ

Kondziolka, Douglas MD [NS] - **Spec Exp:** Brain Tumors-Adult & Pediatric; Brain Tumors-Metastatic; Stereotactic Radiosurgery; **Hospital:** UPMC Presby, Pittsburgh, Chldns Hosp of Pittsburgh - UPMC; **Address:** Univ Pittsburgh Med Ctr, Dept Neurological Surgery, 200 Lothrop St, Ste B400, Pittsburgh, PA 15213; **Phone:** 412-647-9990; **Board Cert:** Neurological Surgery 1994; **Med School:** Univ Toronto 1985; **Resid:** Neurological Surgery, Univ Toronto 1991; **Fellow:** Stereo Neurological Surgery, UPMC Presby Med Ctr 1991; **Fac Appt:** Prof NS, Univ Pittsburgh

Laske, Douglas W MD [NS] - **Spec Exp:** Brain & Spinal Cord Tumors; Stereotactic Radiosurgery; Brain Tumors-Metastatic; Pituitary Tumors; **Hospital:** Temple Univ Hosp, Fox Chase Cancer Ctr (page 72); **Address:** Temple University Hospital, 3401 N Broad St, Ste C540, Phildelphia, PA 19140; **Phone:** 215-707-7200; **Board Cert:** Neurological Surgery 1996; **Med School:** Columbia P&S 1985; **Resid:** Neurological Surgery, Med Coll Virginia 1991; **Fellow:** Neurosurgical Oncology, Natl Inst Hlth 1995; **Fac Appt:** Assoc Prof NS, Temple Univ

Lavyne, Michael H MD [NS] - **Spec Exp:** Spinal Tumors; **Hospital:** NY-Presby Hosp/Weill Cornell (page 78), Hosp For Special Surgery; **Address:** 110 E 55th St Fl 9, New York, NY 10022; **Phone:** 212-486-9100; **Board Cert:** Neurological Surgery 1982; **Med School:** Cornell Univ-Weill Med Coll 1972; **Resid:** Neurological Surgery, Mass Genl Hosp 1979; **Fellow:** Neurology, Beth Israel Hosp 1974; **Fac Appt:** Clin Prof NS, Cornell Univ-Weill Med Coll

Lunsford, L Dade MD [NS] - **Spec Exp:** Brain Tumors; Stereotactic Radiosurgery; **Hospital:** UPMC Presby, Pittsburgh, Chldns Hosp of Pittsburgh - UPMC; **Address:** UPMC Presbyterian Hosp; Dept Neuro Surg, 200 Lothrop St, Ste B-400, Pittsburgh, PA 15213-2536; **Phone:** 412-647-0953; **Board Cert:** Neurological Surgery 1983; **Med School:** Columbia P&S 1974; **Resid:** Neurological Surgery, Univ Pittsburgh Med Ctr 1980; **Fellow:** Stereo Neurological Surgery, Karolinska Hospital 1981; **Fac Appt:** Prof NS, Univ Pittsburgh

McCormick, Paul C MD [NS] - **Spec Exp:** Spinal Surgery; Spinal Tumors; **Hospital:** NY-Presby Hosp/Columbia (page 78); **Address:** 710 W 168th St, Ste 506, New York, NY 10032-2603; **Phone:** 212-305-7976; **Board Cert:** Neurological Surgery 1993; **Med School:** Columbia P&S 1982; **Resid:** Neurological Surgery, Columbia Presby Med Ctr 1989; **Fellow:** Neurological Surgery, Natl Inst Hlth 1984; Spinal Surgery, Med Coll Wisconsin 1990; **Fac Appt:** Prof NS, Columbia P&S

Neurological Surgery

Moore, Frank M MD [NS] - **Spec Exp:** Brain Tumors; Spinal Cord Tumors; Spinal Surgery; **Hospital:** Englewood Hosp & Med Ctr, Mount Sinai Med Ctr (page 76); **Address:** 1158 5th Ave, New York, NY 10029-6917; **Phone:** 212-410-6990; **Board Cert:** Neurological Surgery 1992; **Med School:** France 1983; **Resid:** Neurological Surgery, Mt Sinai Hosp 1988; **Fac Appt:** Assoc Prof NS, Mount Sinai Sch Med

Naff, Neal J MD [NS] - **Spec Exp:** Brain & Spinal Cord Tumors; Stereotactic Radiosurgery; Minimally Invasive Spinal Surgery; **Hospital:** St. Joseph Med Ctr; **Address:** Chesapeake Neurosurgery, 2700 Quarry Lake Drive, Ste 360, Baltimore, MD 21209; **Phone:** 410-486-0090; **Board Cert:** Neurological Surgery 2000; **Med School:** Johns Hopkins Univ 1991; **Resid:** Neurological Surgery, Johns Hopkins Hosp 1998

O'Rourke, Donald M MD [NS] - **Spec Exp:** Neuro-Oncology; Brain Tumors; **Hospital:** Hosp Univ Penn - UPHS (page 80); **Address:** Hosp Univ Penn-Dept Neurosurgery, 3400 Spruce St, 3 Silverstein, Philadelphia, PA 19104; **Phone:** 215-662-3490; **Board Cert:** Neurological Surgery 1998; **Med School:** Univ Pennsylvania 1987; **Resid:** Neurological Surgery, Hosp Univ Penn 1994; **Fac Appt:** Assoc Prof NS, Univ Pennsylvania

Olivi, Alessandro MD [NS] - **Spec Exp:** Brain & Spinal Cord Tumors; Skull Base Tumors; Brain Tumors-Metastatic; **Hospital:** Johns Hopkins Hosp; **Address:** 600 N Wolfe St, Phipps Bldg - Ste 1-100, Baltimore, MD 21287-0001; **Phone:** 410-955-0703; **Board Cert:** Neurological Surgery 1994; **Med School:** Italy 1979; **Resid:** Neurological Surgery, Univ of Padova; Neurological Surgery, Mayfield Neur Inst 1998; **Fellow:** Neuro-Oncology, Johns Hopkins Hosp 1991; **Fac Appt:** Prof NS, Johns Hopkins Univ

Pollack, Ian F MD [NS] - **Spec Exp:** Pediatric Neurosurgery; Brain Tumors; Craniofacial Surgery; Neuro-Oncology; **Hospital:** Chldns Hosp of Pittsburgh - UPMC, UPMC Presby, Pittsburgh; **Address:** Chldns Hosp Pittsburgh, Div Neurosurgery, 4401 Penn Ave, Ste FP4129, Pittsburgh, PA 15224; **Phone:** 412-692-5881; **Board Cert:** Neurological Surgery 1996; Pediatric Neurological Surgery 2006; **Med School:** Johns Hopkins Univ 1984; **Resid:** Neurological Surgery, Univ Pittsburgh Med Ctr 1991; **Fellow:** Pediatric Neurological Surgery, Hosp Sick Chldn 1992; **Fac Appt:** Prof NS, Univ Pittsburgh

Quigley, Matthew R MD [NS] - **Spec Exp:** Brain Tumors; Spinal Cord Tumors; Neuro-Oncology; **Hospital:** Allegheny General Hosp; **Address:** Allegeny General Hosp, Neurosurgery, 420 E North Ave, Ste 302, Pittsburgh, PA 15212; **Phone:** 412-359-4764; **Board Cert:** Neurological Surgery 1991; **Med School:** Northwestern Univ-Feinberg Sch Med 1981; **Resid:** Neurological Surgery, Northwestern Univ 1987; **Fac Appt:** Assoc Prof NS, Univ Pennsylvania

Schwartz, Theodore H MD [NS] - **Spec Exp:** Brain Tumors; Pituitary Tumors; Endoscopic Surgery; Pituitary Tumors; **Hospital:** NY-Presby Hosp/Weill Cornell (page 78); **Address:** Cornell Neurosurgery, 525 E 68th St, Starr Pavilion, rm 651, New York, NY 10021; **Phone:** 212-746-5620; **Board Cert:** Neurological Surgery 2002; **Med School:** Harvard Med Sch 1993; **Resid:** Neurological Surgery, Columbia-Presby Med Ctr 1999; **Fellow:** Neurological Surgery, Yale-New Haven Med Ctr 2000; **Fac Appt:** Prof NS, Cornell Univ-Weill Med Coll

Sen, Chandranath MD [NS] - **Spec Exp:** Brain Tumors; Skull Base Tumors; **Hospital:** NYU Langone Med Ctr (page 79); **Address:** NYU Langone Med Ctr, Dept Neurosurgery, 550 First Ave, Ste HCC-3F, New York, NY 10016; **Phone:** 212-263-5333; **Board Cert:** Neurological Surgery 1989; **Med School:** India 1976; **Resid:** Surgery, Univ Wisconsin Hosps 1980; Neurological Surgery, Univ Wisconsin Hosps 1985; **Fellow:** Microsurgery, Univ Pittsburgh Med Ctr 1986

Sisti, Michael B MD [NS] - **Spec Exp:** Brain Tumors; Stereotactic Radiosurgery; **Hospital:** NY-Presby Hosp/Columbia (page 78); **Address:** 710 W 168th St, New York, NY 10032-2603; **Phone:** 212-305-1728; **Board Cert:** Neurological Surgery 1991; **Med School:** Columbia P&S 1981; **Resid:** Neurological Surgery, Neuro Inst-Columbia-Presby Med Ctr 1988; **Fellow:** Neurological Surgery, Natl Inst Hlth 1983; **Fac Appt:** Assoc Prof NS, Columbia P&S

Souweidane, Mark M MD [NS] - **Spec Exp:** Pediatric Neurosurgery; Minimally Invasive Neurosurgery; Endoscopic Surgery; Brain Tumors-Pediatric; **Hospital:** NY-Presby Hosp/Weill Cornell (page 78), Meml Sloan-Kettering Cancer Ctr (page 75); **Address:** 525 E 68th St, Box 99, New York, NY 10065-4870; **Phone:** 212-746-2363; **Board Cert:** Neurological Surgery 1999; Pediatric Neurological Surgery 2000; **Med School:** Wayne State Univ 1988; **Resid:** Neurological Surgery, NYU Med Ctr 1994; **Fellow:** Pediatric Neurological Surgery, Hosp Sick Chldn 1995; **Fac Appt:** Prof NS, Cornell Univ-Weill Med Coll

Stieg, Philip E MD/PhD [NS] - **Spec Exp:** Skull Base Surgery; Brain Tumors; **Hospital:** NY-Presby Hosp/Weill Cornell (page 78), Hosp For Special Surgery; **Address:** 525 E 68th St, STARR 651, New York, NY 10021-9800; **Phone:** 212-746-4684; **Board Cert:** Neurological Surgery 1992; **Med School:** Med Coll Wisc 1983; **Resid:** Neurological Surgery, Dallas Chldns Hosp/Parkland Meml Hosp 1988; **Fellow:** Neurological Biology, Karolinska Inst 1988; **Fac Appt:** Prof NS, Cornell Univ-Weill Med Coll

Sutton, Leslie N MD [NS] - **Spec Exp:** Brain Tumors-Pediatric; **Hospital:** Chldns Hosp of Philadelphia; **Address:** Childrens Hosp of Philadelphia, Div, Neurosurgery, 34h & Civic Ctr Blvd Wood Bldg Fl 6, Philadelphia, PA 19104; **Phone:** 215-590-2780; **Board Cert:** Neurological Surgery 1984; Pediatric Neurological Surgery 1996; **Med School:** Univ Pennsylvania 1975; **Resid:** Neurological Surgery, Hosp Univ Penn 1981; **Fac Appt:** Prof NS, Univ Pennsylvania

Turtz, Alan R MD [NS] - **Spec Exp:** Brain Tumors; Pituitary Tumors; Spinal Surgery; **Hospital:** Cooper Univ Hosp; **Address:** 3 Cooper Plaza, Ste 104, Camden, NJ 08103; **Phone:** 856-968-7965; **Board Cert:** Neurological Surgery 1995; **Med School:** Med Coll PA 1986; **Resid:** Neurological Surgery, Med Coll Penn 1992; **Fac Appt:** Assoc Prof NS, UMDNJ-RW Johnson Med Sch

Weingart, Jon D MD [NS] - **Spec Exp:** Brain Tumors; Gliomas; **Hospital:** Johns Hopkins Hosp; **Address:** Johns Hopkins Hosp,Dept Neurosurgery, 600 N Wolfe St Phipps Bldg - rm 101, Baltimore, MD 21287; **Phone:** 410-614-3052; **Board Cert:** Neurological Surgery 1998; **Med School:** Duke Univ 1987; **Resid:** Neurological Surgery, John Hopkins Hosp 1993; **Fellow:** Neurosurgical Oncology, Johns Hopkins Hosp; **Fac Appt:** Prof NS, Johns Hopkins Univ

Wisoff, Jeffrey H MD [NS] - **Spec Exp:** Pediatric Neurosurgery; Brain Tumors-Pediatric; **Hospital:** NYU Langone Med Ctr (page 79), Maimonides Med Ctr (page 74); **Address:** 317 E 34th St, Ste 1002, New York, NY 10016-4974; **Phone:** 212-263-6419; **Board Cert:** Neurological Surgery 1990; Pediatric Neurological Surgery 2008; **Med School:** Geo Wash Univ 1978; **Resid:** Neurological Surgery, NYU/Bellevue Hosp 1984; **Fellow:** Pediatric Neurological Surgery, NYU Med Ctr 1985; **Fac Appt:** Assoc Prof NS, NYU Sch Med

Southeast

Asher, Anthony MD [NS] - **Spec Exp:** Brain Tumors; Stereotactic Radiosurgery; **Hospital:** Carolinas Med Ctr, Presby Hosp - Charlotte; **Address:** 225 Baldwin Ave, Charlotte, NC 28204; **Phone:** 704-376-1605; **Board Cert:** Neurological Surgery 1998; **Med School:** Wayne State Univ 1987; **Resid:** Neurological Surgery, Univ Mich Med Ctr 1995; **Fellow:** Surgical Oncology, Natl Cancer Inst 1991

Neurological Surgery

Boop, Frederick A MD [NS] - **Spec Exp:** Pediatric Neurosurgery; Brain Tumors; **Hospital:** Le Bonheur Chldns Med Ctr, Methodist Univ Hosp - Memphis; **Address:** 6325 Humphreys Blvd, Memphis, TN 38120; **Phone:** 901-259-5340; **Board Cert:** Neurological Surgery 1993; Pediatric Neurological Surgery 2005; **Med School:** Univ Ark 1983; **Resid:** Neurological Surgery, Univ Tex Hlth Sci Ctr 1989; Neurological Surgery, Inst Neur/Hosp Sick Chldn 1987; **Fellow:** Epilepsy, Univ Minn 1989; Pediatric Neurological Surgery, Ark Chldns Hosp 1990; **Fac Appt:** Assoc Prof NS, Univ Tenn Coll Med

Brem, Steven MD [NS] - **Spec Exp:** Brain Tumors; Pituitary Tumors; Clinical Trials; Neuro-Oncology; **Hospital:** H Lee Moffitt Cancer Ctr & Research Inst; **Address:** H Lee Moffitt Cancer Ctr/Neurosurgery, 12902 Magnolia Drive, Neuro Program, Tampa, FL 33612-9497; **Phone:** 813-745-3056; **Board Cert:** Neurological Surgery 1983; **Med School:** Harvard Med Sch 1972; **Resid:** Neurological Surgery, Massachusetts Genl Hosp 1981; **Fellow:** Oncology, Natl Cancer Inst 1976; **Fac Appt:** Prof NS, Univ S Fla Coll Med

Ewend, Matthew MD [NS] - **Spec Exp:** Brain Tumors; Pituitary Tumors; Pediatric Neurosurgery; **Hospital:** NC Memorial Hosp - UNC; **Address:** Univ North Carolina Neurosurgery, 170 Manning Drive, MC 7060, 2151 Physicians Office Bldg, Chapel Hill, NC 27599; **Phone:** 919-966-1374; **Board Cert:** Neurological Surgery 2001; **Med School:** Johns Hopkins Univ 1990; **Resid:** Neurological Surgery, Johns Hopkins Hospital 1994; **Fellow:** Neuro-Oncology, National Institutes of Health 1996; **Fac Appt:** Asst Prof NS, Univ NC Sch Med

Friedman, Allan H MD [NS] - **Spec Exp:** Brain Tumors; Skull Base Tumors; Gliomas; **Hospital:** Duke Univ Hosp; **Address:** Duke Univ Med Ctr, DUMC 3807, Dept of Neurosurgery, Durham, NC 27710; **Phone:** 919-681-6421; **Board Cert:** Neurological Surgery 1983; **Med School:** Univ IL Coll Med 1974; **Resid:** Neurological Surgery, Duke Univ Med Ctr 1980; **Fellow:** Vascular Surgery, Univ Western Ontario 1981; **Fac Appt:** Prof S, Duke Univ

Guthrie, Barton L MD [NS] - **Spec Exp:** Brain Tumors; Stereotactic Radiosurgery; **Hospital:** Univ of Ala Hosp at Birmingham; **Address:** Univ Alabama, Div Neurosurg, 510 20th St S, Ste FOT 1038, Birmingham, AL 35294-3410; **Phone:** 205-934-8136; **Board Cert:** Neurological Surgery 1992; **Med School:** Univ Alabama 1980; **Resid:** Neurological Surgery, Mayo Clinic 1988; **Fellow:** Neurological Surgery, Stanford Univ Med Ctr 1988; **Fac Appt:** Assoc Prof NS, Univ Alabama

Heros, Roberto MD [NS] - **Spec Exp:** Cerebrovascular Surgery; Skull Base Surgery; Brain Tumors; **Hospital:** Jackson Meml Hosp (page 82), Univ of Miami Hosp & Clins/Sylvester Comp Canc Ctr (page 82); **Address:** Univ Miami, Dept Neurosurgery, 1095 NW 14th Terrace, Miami, FL 33136; **Phone:** 305-243-4572; **Board Cert:** Neurological Surgery 1979; **Med School:** Univ Tenn Coll Med 1968; **Resid:** Surgery, Mass Genl Hosp 1970; Neurological Surgery, Mass Genl Hosp 1976; **Fac Appt:** Prof NS, Univ Miami Sch Med

Hodes, Jonathan MD [NS] - **Spec Exp:** Brain Tumors; **Hospital:** Frazier Rehab Inst, Univ of Louisville Hosp; **Address:** Univ Louisville Hlth Care Outpt Ctr, Dept Neurosurgery, 3900 Kresge Way, Ste 41, Louisville, KY 40202; **Phone:** 502-899-3623; **Board Cert:** Internal Medicine 1986; Neurological Surgery 1984; **Med School:** Indiana Univ 1980; **Resid:** Internal Medicine, Indiana Univ Hosp 1982; Neurological Surgery, UCSF Med Ctr 1989; **Fellow:** Geriatric Medicine, NIH 1984; Neurological Radiology, Lariboisiere Hosp 1991

Markert Jr, James M MD [NS] - **Spec Exp:** Brain Tumors; Stereotactic Radiosurgery; Clinical Trials; **Hospital:** Univ of Ala Hosp at Birmingham; **Address:** Univ Alabama, Div Neurosurgery, 510 20th St S, FOT, rm 1060, Birmingham, AL 35294; **Phone:** 205-975-6985; **Board Cert:** Neurological Surgery 1999; **Med School:** Columbia P&S 1988; **Resid:** Neurological Surgery, Univ Mich Med Ctr 1995; **Fellow:** Neuro-Oncology, Mass Genl Hosp; **Fac Appt:** Prof NS, Univ Alabama

Morcos, Jacques J MD [NS] - **Spec Exp:** Cerebrovascular Surgery; Brain Tumors; Skull Base Tumors & Surgery; **Hospital:** Jackson Meml Hosp (page 82); **Address:** University of Miami, Dept Neurosurgery, 1095 NW 14th Terr Fl 2, Miami, FL 33136; **Phone:** 305-243-4675; **Board Cert:** Neurological Surgery 1985; **Med School:** Lebanon 1985; **Resid:** Neurological Surgery, Natl Hosp for Nervous Diseases 1990; Neurological Surgery, Univ Minnesota 1993; **Fellow:** Cerebrovascular Neurosurgery, Univ Florida/Shands Med Ctr 1994; Skull Base Surgery, Barrow Neurolical Inst 1995; **Fac Appt:** Assoc Prof NS, Univ Miami Sch Med

Myseros, John S MD [NS] - **Spec Exp:** Pediatric Neurosurgery; Brain Tumors; **Hospital:** Inova Fairfax Hosp for Chldn; **Address:** 8501 Arlington Blvd, Ste 450, Fairfax, VA 22031; **Phone:** 571-226-8330; **Board Cert:** Neurological Surgery 2000; Pediatric Neurological Surgery 2000; **Med School:** Johns Hopkins Univ 1990; **Resid:** Neurological Surgery, Med Coll Virginia 1996; **Fellow:** Pediatric Neurological Surgery, Hosp for Sick Children 1997; **Fac Appt:** Assoc Prof NS, Geo Wash Univ

Olson, Jeffrey J MD [NS] - **Spec Exp:** Neuro-Oncology; Brain Tumors; Skull Base Tumors; Von Hippel-Lindau Disease; **Hospital:** Emory Univ Hosp, Emory Univ Hosp Midtown; **Address:** Emory Univ, Dept Neurosurgery, 1365B Clifton Rd NE, B Bldg - Fl 2 - Ste 2200, Atlanta, GA 30322; **Phone:** 404-778-5770; **Board Cert:** Neurological Surgery 1989; **Med School:** Univ Minn 1981; **Resid:** Neurological Surgery, Univ Iowa Hosps & Clinics 1987; **Fellow:** Neurological Surgery, Natl Inst Hlth 1990; **Fac Appt:** Prof NS, Emory Univ

Parent, Andrew D MD [NS] - **Spec Exp:** Pediatric Neurosurgery; Neuroendocrine Tumors; Pituitary Tumors; **Hospital:** Univ Mississippi Med Ctr; **Address:** Univ Miss Med Ctr-Dept Neurosurgery, 2500 N State St, Jackson, MS 39216-4500; **Phone:** 601-984-5702; **Board Cert:** Neurological Surgery 1981; Pediatric Neurological Surgery 2005; **Med School:** Univ VT Coll Med 1970; **Resid:** Neurological Surgery, Emory Univ 1978; **Fellow:** Neurological Surgery, Univ Tex Med Br 1974; **Fac Appt:** Prof NS, Univ Miss

Reid, William S MD [NS] - **Spec Exp:** Spinal Surgery; Brain & Spinal Cord Tumors; **Hospital:** Univ of Tennesee Med Ctr; **Address:** 1932 Alcoa Hwy, Bldg C, Ste 280, Knoxville, TN 37920; **Phone:** 865-329-4003; **Board Cert:** Neurological Surgery 1980; **Med School:** Univ Ariz Coll Med 1971; **Resid:** Neurological Surgery, Univ Texas Hlth Sci Ctr 1975; **Fac Appt:** Assoc Clin Prof NS, Univ Tex SW, Dallas

Sampson, John H MD/PhD [NS] - **Spec Exp:** Brain Tumors; Clinical Trials; **Hospital:** Duke Univ Hosp; **Address:** Duke Univ Med Ctr, Box 3050, Durham, NC 27710; **Phone:** 919-684-9041; **Board Cert:** Neurological Surgery 2002; **Med School:** Univ Manitoba 1990; **Resid:** Neurological Surgery, Duke Univ Med Ctr 1998; **Fellow:** Neurological Intensive Care, Duke Univ Med Ctr 1999; **Fac Appt:** Assoc Prof S, Duke Univ

Sandberg, David MD [NS] - **Spec Exp:** Pediatric Neurosurgery; Brain Tumors-Pediatric; Spinal Surgery; Minimally Invasive Spinal Surgery; **Hospital:** Miami Children's Hosp; **Address:** Miami Children's Hospital, Dept Neurosurgery, 3100 SW 62nd Ave, Ste 3109, Miami, FL 33135; **Phone:** 305-662-8386; **Board Cert:** Neurological Surgery 2007; **Med School:** Johns Hopkins Univ 1997; **Resid:** Surgery, NY Presby-Cornell Med Ctr 1998; Neurological Surgery, NY Presby-Cornell Med Ctr 2002; **Fellow:** Neurosurgical Oncology, Meml Sloan Kettering Cancer Ctr 2003; Pediatric Neurological Surgery, Children's Hosp 2004; **Fac Appt:** Assoc Prof NS, Univ Miami Sch Med

Sanford, Robert A MD [NS] - **Spec Exp:** Pediatric Neurosurgery; Brain Tumors-Pediatric; **Hospital:** Le Bonheur Chldns Med Ctr, St. Jude Children's Research Hosp; **Address:** 6325 Humphreys Blvd, Memphis, TN 38120; **Phone:** 901-259-5340; **Board Cert:** Neurological Surgery 1976; Pediatric Neurological Surgery 2005; **Med School:** Univ Ark 1967; **Resid:** Neurological Surgery, Univ Minneapolis Med Ctr 1973; **Fac Appt:** Prof NS, Univ Tenn Coll Med

Neurological Surgery

Shaffrey, Mark E MD [NS] - **Spec Exp:** Brain Tumors; Clinical Trials; Spinal Cord Tumors; Spinal Tumors; **Hospital:** Univ of Virginia Health Sys; **Address:** UVA Hlth Sys, Dept Neurosurgery, PO Box 800212, Charlottesville, VA 22908; **Phone:** 434-924-1843; **Board Cert:** Neurological Surgery 2000; **Med School:** Univ VA Sch Med 1987; **Resid:** Neurological Surgery, Univ Virginia Med Ctr 1991; **Fellow:** Microvascular Physiology, NIH 1992; Neurological Pathology, Univ Virginia Med Ctr 1993; **Fac Appt:** Prof NS, Univ VA Sch Med

Sills Jr, Allen MD [NS] - **Spec Exp:** Brain & Spinal Tumors; Stereotactic Radiosurgery; **Hospital:** Vanderbilt Univ Med Ctr; **Address:** 2009 Mallory Ln, Ste 230, Franklin, TN 37067; **Phone:** 615-778-2265; **Board Cert:** Neurological Surgery 2002; **Med School:** Johns Hopkins Univ 1990; **Resid:** Neurological Surgery, Johns Hopkins Hosp 1994; **Fellow:** Neuro-Oncology, Hunterian Neurosurg Lab/Johns Hopkins 1996; **Fac Appt:** Assoc Prof NS, Vanderbilt Univ

Tatter, Stephen MD/PhD [NS] - **Spec Exp:** Brain Tumors; Pituitary Tumors; Stereotactic Radiosurgery; **Hospital:** Wake Forest Univ Baptist Med Ctr; **Address:** Wake Forest Baptist Hlth, Dept Neurosurg, Medical Center Blvd, Winston-Salem, NC 27157-1029; **Phone:** 336-716-4047; **Board Cert:** Neurological Surgery 2004; **Med School:** Cornell Univ-Weill Med Coll 1990; **Resid:** Neurological Surgery, Mass Genl Hosp 1996; **Fellow:** Neurological Surgery, Mass Genl Hosp 1997; **Fac Appt:** Assoc Prof NS, Wake Forest Univ

Thompson, Reid C MD [NS] - **Spec Exp:** Neuro-Oncology; Brain & Spinal Cord Tumors; Skull Base Tumors; **Hospital:** Vanderbilt Univ Med Ctr; **Address:** Vanderbilt Univ Med Ctr, Dept Neurosurg, 1500 21st Ave S, Ste 1506, Nashville, TN 37212; **Phone:** 615-322-7417; **Board Cert:** Neurological Surgery 2001; **Med School:** Johns Hopkins Univ 1989; **Resid:** Neurological Surgery, Johns Hopkins Hosp 1995; **Fellow:** Neuro-Oncology, Rsch-Johns Hopkins Hosp 1996; Cerebrovascular Neurosurgery, Stanford Univ Med Ctr 1997; **Fac Appt:** Prof NS, Vanderbilt Univ

Wharen Jr, Robert E MD [NS] - **Spec Exp:** Brain Tumors; **Hospital:** Mayo - Jacksonville; **Address:** Mayo Clinic, Dept Neurosurgery, 4500 San Pablo Rd, Jacksonville, FL 32224-1865; **Phone:** 904-953-2103; **Board Cert:** Neurological Surgery 1988; **Med School:** Penn State Coll Med 1979; **Resid:** Neurological Surgery, Mayo Clinic 1985; **Fac Appt:** Prof NS, Mayo Med Sch

Midwest

Albright, A Leland MD [NS] - **Spec Exp:** Pediatric Neurosurgery; Brain Tumors; **Hospital:** Univ WI Hosp & Clins; **Address:** Dept Neurosurgery, 600 Highland Ave, rm K4/836, Madison, WI 53792; **Phone:** 608-263-9651; **Board Cert:** Neurological Surgery 1981; Pediatric Neurological Surgery 2005; **Med School:** Louisiana State U, New Orleans 1969; **Resid:** Surgery, Wash Hosps 1971; Neurological Surgery, Univ Pittsburgh Med Ctr 1978; **Fellow:** Neurological Surgery, Natl Inst Hlth 1974; Immunopathology, Univ Pittsburgh Med Ctr 1978; **Fac Appt:** Prof NS, Univ Wisc

Barnett, Gene H MD [NS] - **Spec Exp:** Brain Tumors; Stereotactic Radiosurgery; **Hospital:** Cleveland Clin (page 70); **Address:** Cleveland Clinic Brain Tumor Inst, 9500 Euclid Ave, MC S73, Cleveland, OH 44195; **Phone:** 216-444-5381; **Board Cert:** Neurological Surgery 1990; **Med School:** Case West Res Univ 1980; **Resid:** Neurological Surgery, Cleveland Clinic 1986; **Fellow:** Neurology, Cleveland Clinic 1982; Research, Mass Genl Hosp-Harvard 1987; **Fac Appt:** Prof NS, Cleveland Cl Coll Med/Case West Res

Chandler, William F MD [NS] - **Spec Exp:** Pituitary Surgery; Brain Tumors; **Hospital:** Univ of Michigan Hosp; **Address:** 1500 E Med Center Drive, Ste 3552, Tauban Center, Ann Arbor, MI 48109; **Phone:** 734-936-5020; **Board Cert:** Neurological Surgery 1980; **Med School:** Univ Mich Med Sch 1971; **Resid:** Neurological Surgery, Michigan Hosp 1977; **Fac Appt:** Prof NS, Univ Mich Med Sch

Chiocca, E Antonio MD [NS] - **Spec Exp:** Brain Tumors; Spinal Cord Tumors; **Hospital:** Arthur G James Cancer Hosp & Research Inst, Ohio St Univ Med Ctr; **Address:** OSU Med Ctr, Dept Neurosurgery, 410 W 10th Ave, 1021-N Doan Hall, Columbus, OH 43210; **Phone:** 614-293-9312; **Board Cert:** Neurological Surgery 2000; **Med School:** Univ Tex, Houston 1988; **Resid:** Neurological Surgery, Mass Genl Hosp 1995; **Fac Appt:** Prof NS, Ohio State Univ

Cohen, Alan R MD [NS] - **Spec Exp:** Pediatric Neurosurgery; Brain & Spinal Tumors-Pediatric; Minimally Invasive Surgery; **Hospital:** UH Rainbow Babies & Chldns Hosp, Univ Hosps Case Med Ctr; **Address:** 11100 Euclid Ave, Ste B501, Cleveland, OH 44106; **Phone:** 216-844-5741; **Board Cert:** Neurological Surgery 1991; Pediatric Neurological Surgery 2007; **Med School:** Cornell Univ-Weill Med Coll 1978; **Resid:** Surgery, NYU Medical Ctr 1980; Neurological Surgery, NYU Medical Ctr 1987; **Fellow:** Neurology, Natl Hosp Queen's Square 1982; **Fac Appt:** Prof NS, Case West Res Univ

Dacey Jr, Ralph G MD [NS] - **Spec Exp:** Cerebrovascular Surgery; Brain Tumors; **Hospital:** Barnes-Jewish Hosp, Barnes-Jewish West County Hosp; **Address:** Wash Univ Dept Neurosurgery, 660 S Euclid Ave, Box 8057, St Louis, MO 63110; **Phone:** 314-362-3577; **Board Cert:** Internal Medicine 1978; Neurological Surgery 1985; **Med School:** Univ VA Sch Med 1974; **Resid:** Internal Medicine, Strong Meml Hosp 1977; Neurological Surgery, Univ Virginia Med Ctr 1983; **Fac Appt:** Prof NS, Washington Univ, St Louis

Frim, David M MD/PhD [NS] - **Spec Exp:** Pediatric Neurosurgery; Brain & Spinal Tumors; **Hospital:** Univ of Chicago Med Ctr; **Address:** Univ of Chicago Medical Ctr, Pediatric Neurosurgery, 5841 S Maryland Ave, MC 3026, Chicago, IL 60637-1463; **Phone:** 773-702-2475; **Board Cert:** Neurological Surgery 1998; Pediatric Neurological Surgery 1998; **Med School:** Harvard Med Sch 1988; **Resid:** Neurological Surgery, Mass Genl Hosp 1995; **Fellow:** Pediatric Neurological Surgery, Chldns Hosp 1996; **Fac Appt:** Assoc Prof S, Univ Chicago-Pritzker Sch Med

Grubb Jr, Robert L MD [NS] - **Spec Exp:** Brain Tumors; Skull Base Tumors; **Hospital:** Barnes-Jewish Hosp, St. Louis Chldns Hosp; **Address:** Wash Univ Sch Med, Dept Neurosurgery, 660 S Euclid Ave, Box 8057, St Louis, MO 63110; **Phone:** 314-362-3577; **Board Cert:** Neurological Surgery 1976; **Med School:** Univ NC Sch Med 1965; **Resid:** Surgery, Barnes Jewish Hosp 1967; Neurological Surgery, Barnes Jewish Hosp 1973; **Fellow:** Neurological Surgery, National Inst Health 1969; **Fac Appt:** Prof NS, Washington Univ, St Louis

Guthikonda, Murali MD [NS] - **Spec Exp:** Skull Base Tumors; Pituitary Tumors; Spinal Tumors; **Hospital:** Harper Univ Hosp, Beaumont Hosp-Royal Oak; **Address:** Wayne St U Physicians Grp-Neurosurgery, 4160 John R, Ste 930, Detroit, MI 48201; **Phone:** 313-831-0777; **Board Cert:** Neurological Surgery 1982; **Med School:** India 1971; **Resid:** Surgery, St Elizabeth Hosp 1976; Neurological Surgery, Med Ctr Hosp VT 1980; **Fellow:** Skull Base Surgery, Univ Cincinnati 1993; **Fac Appt:** Assoc Prof NS, Wayne State Univ

Kaufman, Bruce A MD [NS] - **Spec Exp:** Pediatric Neurosurgery; Brain & Spinal Cord Tumors; **Hospital:** Chldns Hosp - Wisconsin; **Address:** Chldns Corporate Ctr, Dept Neurosurg, 999 N 92nd St, Ste 310, Milwaukee, WI 53226; **Phone:** 414-266-6435; **Board Cert:** Neurological Surgery 1992; Pediatric Neurological Surgery 2006; **Med School:** Case West Res Univ 1982; **Resid:** Neurological Surgery, Univ Hosp Cleveland/Case West Res 1988; **Fellow:** Pediatric Neurological Surgery, Chldns Meml Hosp/Northwestern Univ 1989; **Fac Appt:** Prof NS, Med Coll Wisc

Levy, Robert M MD/PhD [NS] - **Spec Exp:** Stereotactic Radiosurgery; Brain Tumors; Pain-Chronic; **Hospital:** Northwestern Meml Hosp; **Address:** 676 N Saint Clair St, Ste 2210, Chicago, IL 60611-2922; **Phone:** 312-695-8143; **Board Cert:** Neurological Surgery 1991; **Med School:** Stanford Univ 1981; **Resid:** Neurological Surgery, UCSF Med Ctr 1987; **Fellow:** Neurological Surgery, UCSF Med Ctr 1986; **Fac Appt:** Prof NS, Northwestern Univ

Neurological Surgery

Link, Michael J MD [NS] - **Spec Exp:** Skull Base Tumors; Brain Tumors; Cerebrovascular Surgery; **Hospital:** Mayo Med Ctr & Clin - Rochester; **Address:** Mayo Clinic, Dept Neurosurgery, 200 First St SW, Rochester, MN 55905; **Phone:** 507-284-8008; **Board Cert:** Neurological Surgery 2000; **Med School:** Mayo Med Sch 1990; **Resid:** Neurological Surgery, Mayo Clinic 1996; **Fellow:** Cerebrovascular & Skull Base Surgery, Univ Cincinnati/Mayfield Clinic 1998; **Fac Appt:** Assoc Prof NS, Mayo Med Sch

Malik, Ghaus M MD [NS] - **Spec Exp:** Cerebrovascular Surgery; Brain & Spinal Cord Tumors; **Hospital:** Henry Ford- W Bloomfield Hosp, Beaumont Hosp-Royal Oak; **Address:** Henry Ford Hosp, Dept Neurosurg, 6777 W Maple Rd, West Bloomfield, MI 48322; **Phone:** 248-661-6417; **Board Cert:** Neurological Surgery 1978; **Med School:** Pakistan 1968; **Resid:** Surgery, Henry Ford Hosp 1971; Neurological Surgery, Henry Ford Hosp 1975

Origitano, Thomas MD/PhD [NS] - **Spec Exp:** Skull Base Tumors & Surgery; Brain Tumors; Pituitary Tumors; Craniofacial Surgery; **Hospital:** Loyola Univ Med Ctr; **Address:** Loyola Univ Med Ctr, Dept Neurosurgery, 2160 S First Ave Bldg 105 - rm 1900, Maywood, IL 60153-3304; **Phone:** 708-216-8920; **Board Cert:** Neurological Surgery 1995; **Med School:** Loyola Univ-Stritch Sch Med 1984; **Resid:** Neurological Surgery, Loyola Univ Med Ctr 1990; **Fac Appt:** Prof NS, Loyola Univ-Stritch Sch Med

Park, Tae Sung MD [NS] - **Spec Exp:** Pediatric Neurosurgery; Neuro-Oncology; **Hospital:** St. Louis Chldns Hosp; **Address:** St Louis Children's Hospital, 1 Children's Place, Ste 4S20, St Louis, MO 63110; **Phone:** 314-454-2810; **Board Cert:** Neurological Surgery 1985; Pediatric Neurological Surgery 2006; **Med School:** Korea 1971; **Resid:** Neurological Surgery, Univ Virginia Hosp 1981; **Fellow:** Pediatric Neurological Surgery, Hosp for Sick Chldn 1983; **Fac Appt:** Prof NS, Washington Univ, St Louis

Raffel, Corey MD/PhD [NS] - **Spec Exp:** Pediatric Neurosurgery; Brain Tumors; Medulloblastoma; **Hospital:** Nationwide Chldn's Hosp; **Address:** Nationwide Chldn's Hosp, Dept Neurosurgery, 700 Children's Drive, Columbus, OH 43205; **Phone:** 614-722-2014; **Board Cert:** Neurological Surgery 1990; Pediatric Neurological Surgery 2006; **Med School:** UCSD 1980; **Resid:** Neurological Surgery, UCSF Med Ctr 1986; **Fellow:** Pediatric Neurological Surgery, Hosp Sick Chldn 1988

Rich, Keith M MD [NS] - **Spec Exp:** Brain Tumors; Stereotactic Radiosurgery; **Hospital:** Barnes-Jewish Hosp; **Address:** Wash Univ Dept Neurosurgery, 660 S Euclid Ave, Box 8057, St Louis, MO 63110; **Phone:** 314-362-3577; **Board Cert:** Neurological Surgery 1987; **Med School:** Indiana Univ 1977; **Resid:** Neurological Surgery, Barnes Jewish Hosp 1982; **Fellow:** Neurological Pharmacology, Barnes Jewish Hosp 1984; **Fac Appt:** Assoc Prof NS, Washington Univ, St Louis

Rock, Jack P MD [NS] - **Spec Exp:** Neuro-Oncology; Pituitary Surgery; Skull Base Surgery; Brain Tumors; **Hospital:** Henry Ford Hosp; **Address:** Henry Ford Hosp, Dept Neurosurg, 2799 W Grand Blvd, Detroit, MI 48202; **Phone:** 313-916-2241; **Board Cert:** Neurological Surgery 1989; **Med School:** Univ Miami Sch Med 1979; **Resid:** Neurological Surgery, New York Hosp-Cornell 1985; **Fellow:** Univ Maryland 1986

Rosenblum, Mark L MD [NS] - **Spec Exp:** Brain Tumors; Spinal Surgery; Neuro-Oncology; **Hospital:** Henry Ford Hosp; **Address:** Henry Ford Hospital, K11, 2799 W Grand Blvd, Detroit, MI 48202; **Phone:** 313-916-1340; **Board Cert:** Neurological Surgery 1982; **Med School:** NY Med Coll 1969; **Resid:** Surgery, UCLA Med Ctr 1973; Neurological Surgery, UCSF Med Ctr 1979; **Fellow:** Neuro-Oncology, NIH/Natl Cancer Inst 1972

Ruge, John R MD [NS] - **Spec Exp:** Pediatric Neurosurgery; Brain Tumors; **Hospital:** Adv Luth Genl Hosp; **Address:** Ctr Brain & Spine Surg-Parkside Ctr, 1875 Dempster St, Ste 605, Park Ridge, IL 60068; **Phone:** 847-698-1088; **Board Cert:** Neurological Surgery 1993; **Med School:** Northwestern Univ 1983; **Resid:** Neurological Surgery, Northwestern Meml Hosp 1989; **Fellow:** Pediatric Neurological Surgery, Childrens Hosp 1990; **Fac Appt:** Asst Prof S, Rush Med Coll

Ryken, Timothy C MD [NS] - **Spec Exp:** Brain Tumors; Spinal Surgery; **Hospital:** Covenant Med Ctr; **Address:** Iowa Spine & Brain Institute, 2710 St Francis Drive, Ste 110, Waterloo, IA 50702; **Phone:** 319-272-6700; **Board Cert:** Neurological Surgery 1998; **Med School:** Univ Iowa Coll Med 1988; **Resid:** Neurological Surgery, Univ Iowa 1995; **Fellow:** Research, Cambridge Univ 1996; **Fac Appt:** Assoc Prof NS, Univ Iowa Coll Med

Shapiro, Scott A MD [NS] - **Spec Exp:** Brain Tumors; Pituitary Tumors; **Hospital:** IU Health Methodist Hosp, Wishard Hlth Srvs; **Address:** Indiana Univ Health Methodist Hospital, 1801 N Senate Blvd, Ste 610, Indianapolis, IN 46202; **Phone:** 317-396-1300; **Board Cert:** Neurological Surgery 1990; **Med School:** Indiana Univ 1981; **Resid:** Neurological Surgery, Indiana Univ Med Ctr 1987; **Fac Appt:** Prof NS, Indiana Univ

Thompson, B Gregory MD [NS] - **Spec Exp:** Skull Base Tumors & Surgery; **Hospital:** Univ of Michigan Hosp; **Address:** Dept Neurosurgery, 3552 Taubman Ctr, 1500 E Medical Center Drive, Ann Arbor, MI 48109-5338; **Phone:** 734-936-7493; **Board Cert:** Neurological Surgery 1998; **Med School:** Univ Kansas 1986; **Resid:** Neurological Surgery, Univ Pittsburgh 1993; Research, Natl Inst Hlth 1992; **Fellow:** Neurological Surgery, Barrow Neuro Inst 1994; Interventional Radiology, Thomas Jefferson Univ 2005

Tomita, Tadanori MD [NS] - **Spec Exp:** Pediatric Neurosurgery; Brain Tumors-Pediatric; **Hospital:** Children's Mem Hosp -Chicago, Northwestern Meml Hosp; **Address:** Chldns Meml Hosp, Div Ped Neurosurg, 2300 Children's Plaza, Box 28, Chicago, IL 60614-3363; **Phone:** 773-880-4373; **Board Cert:** Neurological Surgery 1984; Pediatric Neurological Surgery 1996; **Med School:** Japan 1970; **Resid:** Neurological Surgery, Kobe Univ 1974; Neurological Surgery, Northwestern Meml Hosp 1980; **Fellow:** Surgery, Meml Sloan Kettering Canc Ctr 1981; **Fac Appt:** Prof NS, Northwestern Univ

Warnick, Ronald E MD [NS] - **Spec Exp:** Neuro-Oncology; Brain Tumors; **Hospital:** Univ Hosp - Cincinnati, Good Samaritan Hosp - Cincinnati; **Address:** 222 Piedmont Ave, Ste 3100, Cincinnati, OH 45219; **Phone:** 513-475-8629; **Board Cert:** Neurological Surgery 1995; **Med School:** Univ Rochester 1982; **Resid:** Neurological Surgery, NYU Med Ctr 1989; **Fellow:** Neuro-Oncology, UCSF Med Ctr 1991; **Fac Appt:** Prof NS, Univ Cincinnati

Great Plains and Mountains

Cherny, W Bruce MD [NS] - **Spec Exp:** Pediatric Neurosurgery; Brain Tumors; **Hospital:** St. Luke's Boise Med Ctr; **Address:** Childrens Specialty Ctr, 100 E Idaho St, Ste 202, Boise, ID 83712; **Phone:** 208-381-7360; **Board Cert:** Neurological Surgery 2000; **Med School:** Univ Ariz Coll Med 1987; **Resid:** Neurological Surgery, Barrow Neuro Inst/St Joseph's Med Ctr 1994; **Fellow:** Pediatric Neurological Surgery, Primary Chldns Hosp 1995

Couldwell, William T MD/PhD [NS] - **Spec Exp:** Brain Tumors; Skull Base Tumors; Pituitary Tumors; **Hospital:** Univ Utah Hlth Care; **Address:** Univ Utah, Dept Neurological Surgery, 175 N Medical Drive E, Salt Lake City, UT 84132-2303; **Phone:** 801-581-6908; **Board Cert:** Neurological Surgery 1994; **Med School:** McGill Univ 1984; **Resid:** Neurological Surgery, LAC/USC Med Ctr 1989; **Fellow:** Neurological Immunology, Montreal Neur Inst/McGill Univ 1990; Neurological Surgery, CHUV 1991; **Fac Appt:** Prof NS, Univ Utah

Neurological Surgery

Johnson, Stephen D MD [NS] - **Spec Exp:** Skull Base Tumors & Surgery; **Hospital:** Presby - St Luke's Med Ctr; **Address:** Western Neurological Group, 1601 E 19th Ave, Ste 4400, Denver, CO 80218; **Phone:** 303-861-2266; **Board Cert:** Neurological Surgery 1988; **Med School:** Univ Tenn Coll Med 1974; **Resid:** Neurological Surgery, Virginia Mason Med Ctr; Neurological Surgery, New York Hosp; **Fellow:** Neurological Surgery, Univ Tennessee; **Fac Appt:** Assoc Prof NS, Univ Colorado

Lillehei, Kevin O MD [NS] - **Spec Exp:** Neuro-Oncology; Pituitary Tumors; **Hospital:** Univ of CO Hosp - Anschutz Inpatient Pav; **Address:** Univ Colorado Hosp, Dept Neurosurgery, 12631 E 17th Ave, rm 501, MS C307, Aurora, CO 80045; **Phone:** 303-724-2280; **Board Cert:** Neurological Surgery 1989; **Med School:** Univ Minn 1979; **Resid:** Neurological Surgery, Univ Mich Med Ctr 1985; **Fac Appt:** Prof NS, Univ Colorado

Southwest

De Monte, Franco MD [NS] - **Spec Exp:** Skull Base Tumors & Surgery; Neuro-Oncology; **Hospital:** UT MD Anderson Cancer Ctr; **Address:** UT MD Anderson Cancer Ctr, Dept Neurosurgery, 1515 Holcombe Blvd, Unit 442, Houston, TX 77030; **Phone:** 713-792-2400; **Board Cert:** Neurological Surgery 1995; **Med School:** Canada 1985; **Resid:** Neurological Surgery, Univ Western Ontario 1991; **Fellow:** Skull Base Surgery, Loyola Univ-Stritch Sch Med 1992; **Fac Appt:** Prof NS, Baylor Coll Med

Greene Jr, Clarence S MD [NS] - **Spec Exp:** Pediatric Neurosurgery; Brain Tumors; **Hospital:** Children's Hospital - New Orleans; **Address:** 200 Henry Clay Ave, Ste 210, New Orleans, LA 70118; **Phone:** 504-896-9458; **Board Cert:** Neurological Surgery 1984; Pediatric Neurological Surgery 2007; **Med School:** Howard Univ 1974; **Resid:** Neurological Surgery, Chldns Hosp 1981; Neurological Surgery, Peter Bent Brigham Hosp 1981; **Fellow:** Pediatric Neurological Surgery, Chldns Hosp 1985; **Fac Appt:** Assoc Clin Prof NS, UC Irvine

Hankinson, Hal L MD [NS] - **Spec Exp:** Brain Tumors; **Hospital:** Christus St Vincent Reg Med Ctr-Santa Fe; **Address:** 465 St Michael's Drive, Ste 107, Sante Fe, NM 87505; **Phone:** 505-988-3233; **Board Cert:** Neurological Surgery 1977; **Med School:** Tulane Univ 1967; **Resid:** Neurological Surgery, UCSF Med Ctr 1975; **Fac Appt:** Clin Prof NS, Univ New Mexico

Lang Jr, Frederick F MD [NS] - **Spec Exp:** Brain & Spinal Tumors; Gliomas; Brain Tumors-Complex; Pediatric Neurosurgery; **Hospital:** UT MD Anderson Cancer Ctr; **Address:** Univ Texas MD Anderson Cancer Ctr, 1515 Holcombe Blvd, Unit 442, Houston, TX 77030; **Phone:** 713-792-6600; **Board Cert:** Neurological Surgery 2000; **Med School:** Yale Univ 1988; **Resid:** Neurological Surgery, NYU Med Ctr 1995; **Fellow:** Neurosurgical Oncology, MD Anderson Cancer Ctr 1996; **Fac Appt:** Prof NS, Univ Tex, Houston

Mapstone, Timothy B MD [NS] - **Spec Exp:** Brain Tumors-Adult & Pediatric; Pediatric Neurosurgery; **Hospital:** OU Med Ctr, Chldns Hosp OU Med Ctr; **Address:** Univ OK Hlth Sci Ctr, Dept Neurosurgery, 1000 N Lincoln Blvd, Ste 400, Oklahoma City, OK 73104; **Phone:** 405-271-4912; **Board Cert:** Neurological Surgery 1985; Pediatric Neurological Surgery 2005; **Med School:** Case West Res Univ 1977; **Resid:** Neurological Surgery, Univ Hosps 1983; **Fellow:** Research, Case West Reserve Univ; **Fac Appt:** Prof NS, Univ Okla Coll Med

Mickey, Bruce E MD [NS] - **Spec Exp:** Brain Tumors; Skull Base Surgery; Pituitary Tumors; **Hospital:** UT Southwestern Med Ctr at Dallas, Parkland Hlth & Hosp Sys; **Address:** UTSW Med Ctr, Dept Neurosurgery, 5323 Harry Hines Blvd, Dallas, TX 75390-8855; **Phone:** 214-645-2300; **Board Cert:** Neurological Surgery 1987; **Med School:** Univ Tex SW, Dallas 1978; **Resid:** Neurological Surgery, Parkland Meml Hosp 1984; **Fellow:** Research, Righospitalet 1983; **Fac Appt:** Prof NS, Univ Tex SW, Dallas

Sawaya, Raymond MD [NS] - **Spec Exp:** Brain Tumors; **Hospital:** UT MD Anderson Cancer Ctr, Baylor Univ Medical Ctr; **Address:** MD Anderson Cancer Ctr, 1515 Holcombe Blvd, Unit 442, Houston, TX 77030; **Phone:** 713-792-2400; **Board Cert:** Neurological Surgery 1985; **Med School:** Lebanon 1974; **Resid:** Neurological Surgery, Univ Cincinnati Med Ctr 1980; Neurological Surgery, Johns Hopkins Med Ctr 1981; **Fellow:** Neuro-Oncology, Natl Inst Hlth 1982; **Fac Appt:** Prof NS, Univ Tex, Houston

Spetzler, Robert F MD [NS] - **Spec Exp:** Skull Base Tumors & Surgery; Cerebrovascular Surgery; **Hospital:** St. Joseph's Hosp & Med Ctr - Phoenix; **Address:** Barrow Neurosurgical Assocs, 2910 N Third Ave, Phoenix, AZ 85013; **Phone:** 602-406-3489; **Board Cert:** Neurological Surgery 1979; **Med School:** Northwestern Univ 1971; **Resid:** Neurological Surgery, UCSF Med Ctr 1976; **Fac Appt:** Prof S, Univ Ariz Coll Med

West Coast and Pacific

Adler Jr, John R MD [NS] - **Spec Exp:** Stereotactic Radiosurgery; Brain Tumors; **Hospital:** Stanford Univ Hosp & Clinics; **Address:** Stanford Univ Med Ctr, Dept Neurosurg, 300 Pasteur Drive R Bldg - rm 205, Stanford, CA 94305-5327; **Phone:** 650-723-5573; **Board Cert:** Neurological Surgery 1990; **Med School:** Harvard Med Sch 1980; **Resid:** Neurological Surgery, Chldns Hosp 1987; Neurological Surgery, Mass Genl Hosp 1985; **Fellow:** Cerebrovascular Disease, Karolinska Inst 1986; **Fac Appt:** Prof NS, Stanford Univ

Ames, Christopher P MD [NS] - **Spec Exp:** Spinal Cord Tumors; **Hospital:** UCSF Med Ctr; **Address:** Spine Center, 400 Parnassus Ave, rm A311, San Francisco, CA 94143-0332; **Phone:** 866-817-7463; **Board Cert:** Neurological Surgery 2006; **Med School:** UCLA-David Geffen Sch Med 1994; **Resid:** Neurological Surgery, UCSD Med Ctr 2000; **Fellow:** Spinal Surgery, Barrow Neurological Inst 2002; **Fac Appt:** Assoc Clin Prof NS, UCLA-David Geffen Sch Med

Apuzzo, Michael L J MD [NS] - **Spec Exp:** Brain Tumors; Stereotactic Radiosurgery; **Hospital:** LAC & USC Med Ctr, USC Norris Cancer Hosp; **Address:** 1420 San Pablo Street, PMBA106, Los Angeles, CA 90033-1029; **Phone:** 323-226-7421; **Board Cert:** Neurological Surgery 1975; **Med School:** Boston Univ 1965; **Resid:** Neurological Surgery, Hartford Hosp 1970; Neurological Surgery, Hartford Hosp 1973; **Fellow:** Neurological Physiology, Yale Univ Hosp 1972; **Fac Appt:** Prof NS, USC Sch Med

Badie, Behnam MD [NS] - **Spec Exp:** Brain Tumors; **Hospital:** City of Hope Natl Med Ctr (page 69); **Address:** City of Hope Med Ctr, Dept Neurosurgery, 1500 E Duarte Rd, Duarte, CA 91010; **Phone:** 626-471-7100; **Board Cert:** Neurological Surgery 1998; **Med School:** UCLA 1989; **Resid:** Neurological Surgery, UCLA Med Ctr 1996; **Fac Appt:** Assoc Prof NS, UCLA

Berger, Mitchel S MD [NS] - **Spec Exp:** Brain & Spinal Cord Tumors; Pituitary Tumors; Neuro-Oncology; Pain Management; **Hospital:** UCSF Med Ctr; **Address:** UCSF Med Ctr, Dept Neurosurgery, 505 Parnassus Avenue, M-786, San Francisco, CA 94143-0112; **Phone:** 415-353-3933; **Board Cert:** Neurological Surgery 1991; **Med School:** Univ Miami Sch Med 1979; **Resid:** Neurological Surgery, UCSF Med Ctr 1984; **Fellow:** Neuro-Oncology, UCSF Med Ctr 1985; Pediatric Neurological Surgery, Hosp Sick Chldn 1986; **Fac Appt:** Prof NS, UCSF

Black, Keith L MD [NS] - **Spec Exp:** Brain Tumors; Pineal Tumors; Spinal Tumors; **Hospital:** Cedars-Sinai Med Ctr; **Address:** Cedars-Sinai Med Ctr, Dept Neurosugery, 8631 W Third St, Ste 800 East, Los Angeles, CA 90048; **Phone:** 310-423-7900; **Board Cert:** Neurological Surgery 1990; **Med School:** Univ Mich Med Sch 1981; **Resid:** Neurological Surgery, Univ Michigan Med Ctr 1987; **Fac Appt:** Prof NS, UCLA-David Geffen Sch Med

Boggan, James E MD [NS] - **Spec Exp:** Skull Base Tumors & Surgery; Pediatric Neurosurgery; **Hospital:** UC Davis Med Ctr; **Address:** Dept Neurological Surgery, 4860 Y St, Ste 3740, Sacramento, CA 95817-2307; **Phone:** 916-734-2371; **Board Cert:** Neurological Surgery 1985; **Med School:** Univ Chicago-Pritzker Sch Med 1976; **Resid:** Neurological Surgery, UCSF Med Ctr 1982; **Fac Appt:** Prof NS, UC Davis

Chen, Thomas C MD [NS] - **Spec Exp:** Brain & Spinal Tumors; Brain Tumors-Metastatic; Gliomas; **Hospital:** USC Norris Cancer Hosp, USC Univ Hosp; **Address:** USC Health Consultation Clinic 2, 1520 San Pablo St, rm 3800, MC 9197, Los Angeles, CA 90033; **Phone:** 323-442-5720; **Board Cert:** Neurological Surgery 2000; **Med School:** UCSF 1988; **Resid:** Neurological Surgery, USC Univ Hosp 1995; **Fellow:** Spinal Surgery, Med Coll Wisconsin 1997; **Fac Appt:** Assoc Prof NS, USC-Keck School of Medicine

Edwards, Michael S MD [NS] - **Spec Exp:** Brain Tumors-Pediatric; Pediatric Neurosurgery; Stereotactic Radiosurgery; **Hospital:** Lucile Packard Chldn's Hosp; **Address:** Pediatric Neurosurgery, 300 Pasteur Drive, Ste R211, MC 5327, Stanford, CA 94305; **Phone:** 650-497-8775; **Board Cert:** Neurological Surgery 1980; Pediatric Neurological Surgery 2006; **Med School:** Tulane Univ 1970; **Resid:** Neurological Surgery, Oschner Fdn Hosp/Charity Hosp 1977; **Fellow:** Pediatric Neuro-Oncology, UCSF Med Ctr 1978; **Fac Appt:** Prof NS, Stanford Univ

Ellenbogen, Richard MD [NS] - **Spec Exp:** Pediatric Neurosurgery; Brain Tumors; **Hospital:** Seattle Chldns Hosp, Univ Wash Med Ctr; **Address:** 4800 Sand Point Way NE, MS W-7729, Seattle, WA 98145; **Phone:** 206-987-2544; **Board Cert:** Neurological Surgery 1992; Pediatric Neurological Surgery 2009; **Med School:** Brown Univ 1983; **Resid:** Neurological Surgery, Brigham Womens Hosp/Childrens Hosp 1989; **Fac Appt:** Prof NS, Univ Wash

Giannotta, Steven L MD [NS] - **Spec Exp:** Skull Base Tumors; **Hospital:** USC Univ Hosp, LAC & USC Med Ctr; **Address:** 1520 San Pablo St, Ste 3800, Los Angeles, CA 90033; **Phone:** 323-442-5720; **Board Cert:** Neurological Surgery 1980; **Med School:** Univ Mich Med Sch 1972; **Resid:** Neurological Surgery, Univ Michigan Med Ctr 1978; **Fac Appt:** Prof NS, USC Sch Med

Harsh IV, Griffith R MD [NS] - **Spec Exp:** Brain & Spinal Cord Tumors; Skull Base Tumors; Pituitary Tumors; Endoscopic Surgery; **Hospital:** Stanford Univ Hosp & Clinics; **Address:** Stanford Center for Advanced Medicine, 875 Blake Wilbur Drive, MC 5826, Stanford, CA 94305; **Phone:** 650-723-7093; **Board Cert:** Neurological Surgery 1989; **Med School:** Harvard Med Sch 1980; **Resid:** Neurological Surgery, UCSF Med Ctr 1986; **Fellow:** Neuro-Oncology, UCSF Med Ctr 1987; **Fac Appt:** Prof NS, Stanford Univ

Kassam, Amin MD [NS] - **Spec Exp:** Skull Base Tumors & Surgery; Cerebrovascular Surgery; Endoscopic Surgery; Minimally Invasive Surgery; **Hospital:** St. John's Hlth Ctr, Santa Monica; **Address:** John Wayne Cancer Inst, 2200 Santa Monica Blvd, Santa Monica, CA 90404; **Phone:** 310-582-7450; **Med School:** Univ Toronto 1991; **Resid:** Neurological Surgery, Univ Ottawa Med Ctr 1997

Liau, Linda M MD/PhD [NS] - **Spec Exp:** Brain Tumors; Neuro-Oncology; **Hospital:** UCLA Ronald Reagan Med Ctr; **Address:** CHS 74-145, Box 956901, 10833 Le Conte Ave, Los Angeles, CA 90095-6901; **Phone:** 310-267-2621; **Board Cert:** Neurological Surgery 2002; **Med School:** Stanford Univ 1991; **Resid:** Neurological Surgery, UCLA Med Ctr 1998; **Fellow:** Neuro-Oncology, UCLA Med Ctr 1998; **Fac Appt:** Prof NS, UCLA

Linskey, Mark E MD [NS] - **Spec Exp:** Brain Tumors; Stereotactic Radiosurgery; Skull Base Surgery; Pituitary Tumors; **Hospital:** UC Irvine Med Ctr; **Address:** UCI Med Ctr, Dept Neurosurgery-Route 81, 101 The City Drive S Bldg 56 - Ste 400, Orange, CA 92868-3298; **Phone:** 714-456-6392; **Board Cert:** Neurological Surgery 1996; **Med School:** Columbia P&S 1986; **Resid:** Neurological Surgery, Univ Pittsburgh Hlth Ctrs 1993; **Fellow:** Neuro-Oncology, Ludwig Inst Cancer Rsch/Univ Coll London 1994; Neuro-Oncology, Pittsburgh Cancer Inst/Univ Pittsburgh 1992; **Fac Appt:** Assoc Prof NS, UC Irvine

Mamelak, Adam N MD [NS] - **Spec Exp:** Brain Tumors; Spinal Tumors; **Hospital:** Cedars-Sinai Med Ctr; **Address:** Maxine Dunitz Neurosurgical Institute, 8631 W Third St, Ste 800-East, Los Angeles, CA 90048; **Phone:** 310-423-7900; **Board Cert:** Neurological Surgery 2000; **Med School:** Harvard Med Sch 1990; **Resid:** Neurological Surgery, UCSF Med Ctr 1994; **Fellow:** Epilepsy, UCSF Epilepsy Research Lab 1996

Mayberg, Marc R MD [NS] - **Spec Exp:** Pituitary Surgery; Skull Base Tumors; **Hospital:** Swedish Med Ctr-First Hill-Seattle; **Address:** Seattle Neuroscience Inst, 550 17th Ave, Ste 500, James Tower, Seattle, WA 98122; **Phone:** 206-320-2800; **Board Cert:** Neurological Surgery 1988; **Med School:** Mayo Med Sch 1978; **Resid:** Neurological Surgery, Mass Genl Hosp 1984; **Fellow:** Neurological Surgery, Natl Hosp for Nervous Dis 1985

McDermott, Michael W MD [NS] - **Spec Exp:** Brain Tumors; Stereotactic Radiosurgery; Skull Base Tumors; **Hospital:** UCSF Med Ctr; **Address:** UCSF Dept Neurosurgery, 400 Parnassus Ave, rm A808, San Francisco, CA 94143; **Phone:** 415-353-7500; **Board Cert:** Neurological Surgery 2003; **Med School:** Univ Toronto 1982; **Resid:** Neurological Surgery, Univ British Columbia 1988; **Fellow:** Neuro-Oncology, UCSF Med Ctr 1990; **Fac Appt:** Prof NS, UCSF

Neuwelt, Edward A MD [NS] - **Spec Exp:** Neuro-Oncology; Brain Tumors; **Hospital:** OR Hlth & Sci Univ; **Address:** Oregon Hlth Sci Univ, Dept Neurosurgery, 3181 SW Sam Jackson Pk Rd, MC-L603, Portland, OR 97239; **Phone:** 503-494-5626; **Board Cert:** Neurological Surgery 1980; **Med School:** Univ Colorado 1972; **Resid:** Neurological Surgery, Univ Tex SW Med Sch 1978; **Fellow:** Neuro-Oncology, Natl Canc Inst/NIH 1976; **Fac Appt:** Prof NS, Oregon Hlth & Sci Univ

Ott, Kenneth H MD [NS] - **Spec Exp:** Brain Tumors; Stereotactic Radiosurgery; **Hospital:** Scripps Meml Hosp - La Jolla; **Address:** Neurosurgical Med Clin, 2100 Fifth Ave, Ste 200, San Diego, CA 92101; **Phone:** 619-297-4481 x102; **Board Cert:** Neurological Surgery 1980; **Med School:** UCSF 1970; **Resid:** Surgery, Mass Genl Hosp 1972; Neurological Surgery, Mass Genl Hosp 1976; **Fac Appt:** Assoc Clin Prof S, UCSD

Sekhar, Laligam N MD [NS] - **Spec Exp:** Brain Tumors; Skull Base Tumors; **Hospital:** Harborview Med Ctr, Univ Wash Med Ctr; **Address:** HMC-Neurosurgery, 9th & Jeff Bldg Fl 5, 908 Jefferson St, Seattle, WA 98104-2499; **Phone:** 206-744-9300; **Board Cert:** Neurological Surgery 1986; **Med School:** India 1973; **Resid:** Neurology, Univ Cincinnati Med Ctr 1977; Neurology, Univ Pittsburgh Med Ctr 1982; **Fellow:** Skull Base Surgery, Norstadt Krankenhaus 1983; Cerebrovascular Neurosurgery, Univ Zurich Hospital; **Fac Appt:** Prof NS, Univ Wash

Silbergeld, Daniel MD [NS] - **Spec Exp:** Brain Tumors; Brain Tumors-Metastatic; Brain Mapping; **Hospital:** Univ Wash Med Ctr; **Address:** Univ Wash Med Ctr, Dept Neurosurg, 1959 NE Pacific, Box 356470, Seattle, WA 98195; **Phone:** 206-598-5637; **Board Cert:** Neurological Surgery 1995; **Med School:** Univ Cincinnati 1984; **Resid:** Neurological Surgery, Univ Wash Med Ctr 1990; Research, Univ Wash Med Ctr 1988; **Fellow:** Neuro-Oncology, Univ Wash Med Ctr 1991; Epilepsy, Univ Wash Med Ctr 1991; **Fac Appt:** Assoc Prof NS, Univ Wash

Neurological Surgery

Sun, Peter P MD [NS] - **Spec Exp:** Pediatric Neurosurgery; Brain Tumors; **Hospital:** Chldns Hosp - Oakland; **Address:** 744 52nd St, Ste 5203, Oakland, CA 94609; **Phone:** 510-428-3319; **Board Cert:** Neurological Surgery 2002; Pediatric Neurological Surgery 2006; **Med School:** Columbia P&S 1991; **Resid:** Neurological Surgery, UC Davis Med Ctr 1994; Neurological Surgery, Yale-New Haven Hosp 1996; **Fellow:** Neurological Surgery, NYU Med Ctr 1997; Pediatric Neurological Surgery, Childrens Hosp 1998; **Fac Appt:** Asst Clin Prof NS, UCSF

Yu, John S MD [NS] - **Spec Exp:** Brain Tumors; Spinal Tumors; Clinical Trials; **Hospital:** Cedars-Sinai Med Ctr; **Address:** Maxine Dunitz Neurosurgical Institute, 8631 W 3rd St, Ste 800-East, Los Angeles, CA 90048; **Phone:** 310-423-7900; **Board Cert:** Neurological Surgery 2002; **Med School:** Harvard Med Sch 1990; **Resid:** Neurological Surgery, Mass General Hosp 1997

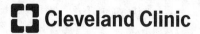
Cleveland Clinic

Every life deserves world class care.

Cleveland Clinic
Taussig Cancer Institute
9500 Euclid Avenue
Cleveland, OH 44195

Advanced Care for Brain and Spine Tumors

At Cleveland Clinic Taussig Cancer Institute, more than 250 top cancer specialists, researchers, nurses and technicians are dedicated to delivering the most effective medical treatments and offering access to the latest clinical trials for more than 13,000 new cancer patients every year. Our doctors are nationally and internationally known for their contributions to cancer breakthroughs and their ability to deliver superior outcomes for our patients. In recognition of these and other achievements, *U.S.News & World Report* has ranked Cleveland Clinic as one of the top cancer centers in the nation.

Multidisciplinary Treatment Approach

The Taussig Cancer Institute and the Rose Ella Burkhardt Brain Tumor and Neuro-Oncology Center collaborate on multidisciplinary teams to provide brain and spine cancer patients with comprehensive, individualized treatment strategies. The Burkhardt Brain Tumor Center is nationally recognized for its diagnosis and treatment of primary and metastatic tumors of the brain, spine and nerves. We offer both adult and pediatric patients the latest advances in diagnostic and treatment services including innovations such as laser interstitial thermal therapy (AutoLITT®), Gamma Knife® Perfexion™ radiosurgery, Novalis Tx™ stereotactic spine radiosurgery, advanced surgical navigation and intraoperative MRI.

Technology and Expertise in Treating Metastatic Disease

Stereotactic radiosurgery offers many patients an alternative to traditional treatment options, utilizing technology that precisely targets tumors which minimizes radiation exposure to nearby healthy tissue. Cleveland Clinic Gamma Knife Center® has performed more than 3,500 cranial radiosurgeries with expertise in treating brain metastases. Our Stereotactic Spine Radiosurgery Program has treated more than 400 patients providing effective pain and/or tumor control for metastatic spine tumors.

clevelandclinic.org/
braintumorTCD

**Appointments | Information:
Call the Cancer Answer Line at
866.223.8100.**

Cancer Treatment Guides

Cleveland Clinic has developed comprehensive treatment guides for many cancers. To download our free treatment guides, visit clevelandclinic.org/cancertreatmentguides.

**Comprehensive Online
Medical Second Opinion**

Cleveland Clinic experts can review your medical records and render an opinion that includes treatment options and recommendations. Call 216.444.3223 or 800.223.2273 ext. 43223; email eclevelandclinic@ccf.org.

**Special Assistance for
Out-of-State Patients**

Cleveland Clinic Global Patient Services offers a complimentary Medical Concierge service for patients who travel from outside of Ohio. Call 800.223.2273, ext. 55580, or email medicalconcierge@ccf.org.

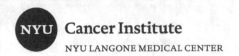

NYU **Cancer Institute**
NYU LANGONE MEDICAL CENTER

NYU Langone Medical Center
550 First Avenue , New York, NY 10016
www.NYULMC.org

NYU Clinical Cancer Center
160 East 34th Street, New York, NY 10016
www.NYUCI.org

**The Stephen D. Hassenfeld Children's Center
for Cancer and Blood Disorders**
160 East 32nd Street, New York, NY 10016
www.NYUMC.org/Hassenfeld

The NYU Cancer Institute is an NCI-designated cancer center and provides personalized patient care that is both compassionate and state of the art. The doctors and researchers work together to develop innovative therapies for patients. The Cancer Institute is world-renowned for excellence in cancer-focused research, personalized care, education and community outreach. Its mission is to discover the origins of human cancer and to use that knowledge to eradicate the personal and societal burden of cancer in our community, the nation and the world. For more information about our expert physicians, call 212-731-5000. *We specialize in the following areas:*

Patient-Focused Setting
The NYU Clinical Cancer Center is the principal outpatient facility of The Cancer Institute and serves as home to our patients and their caregivers. The center and its multidisciplinary team of experts provide access to the latest treatment options and clinical trials along with a variety of programs in cancer risk reduction/prevention, screening, diagnostics, genetic counseling and supportive services. In addition the NYUCI emphasizes the importance of a holistic approach to management services in complementary medicine, psychosocial support, survivorship and palliative care.

Renowned Expertise
The NYU Cancer Institute brings together experts from a variety of disciplines to create collaborative research endeavors and clinical care teams. The Cancer Institute offers a full continuum of personalized care, from prevention through diagnosis, treatment and post-treatment support. The compassion and expertise of our team members helps patients better manage the symptoms of their diseases as well as meet their special needs. Additionally, we have created special emphasis programs in diseases such as breast cancer, melanoma, GI cancer, prostate cancer, hematologic malignancies and lung cancer among others, as well as, translational programs in cancer healthcare disparities, molecularly targeted therapy, and the cell signaling pathways involved in cancer.

A Translational Approach
NYU Langone Medical Center scientists and other researchers excel in uncovering how cancer develops at the molecular level, and how we can harness that knowledge to reduce the risk of cancer and treat the disease. The Medical Center constantly seeks to create new opportunities for collaboration between investigators within our own institution, those located elsewhere in the NYU network of campuses, and researchers at other institutions.

The Stephen D. Hassenfeld Children's Center for Cancer and Blood Disorders
The center is a leading pediatric outpatient facility for the treatment of childhood cancers and blood diseases. Its unique interdisciplinary and family-centered approach combines the most advanced medical treatments with psychosocial and emotional support services for young patients and their families.

Neurology

A neurologist specializes in the diagnosis and treatment of all types of disease or impaired function of the brain, spinal cord, peripheral nerves, muscles and autonomic nervous system, as well as the blood vessels that relate to these structures.

Training Required: Four years

Certification in the following subspecialty requires additional training and examination.

Child Neurology: A neurologist with special qualifications in child neurology has special skills in the diagnosis and management of neurologic disorders of the neonatal period, infancy, early childhood and adolescence.

Training Required: Five years

Spinal Cord Injury Medicine: A physician who addresses the prevention, diagnosis, treatment and management of traumatic spinal cord injury and non-traumatic etiologies of spinal cord dysfunction by working in an interdisciplinary manner. Care is provided to patients of all ages on a lifelong basis and covers related medical, physical, psychological and vocational disabilities and complications.

Training Required: Five years

NEUROLOGY

New England

Batchelor, Tracy T MD [N] - **Spec Exp:** Brain Tumors; Gliomas; **Hospital:** Mass Genl Hosp; **Address:** Mass Genl Hosp Cancer Ctr - Neuro-Oncology, 55 Fruit St, Yawkey Ctr, Ste 9E, Boston, MA 02114; **Phone:** 617-724-8770; **Board Cert:** Neurology 2005; **Med School:** Emory Univ 1990; **Resid:** Neurology, Mass Genl Hosp 1994; **Fellow:** Neuro-Oncology, Meml Sloan Kettering Cancer Ctr 1995; **Fac Appt:** Prof N, Harvard Med Sch

Mid Atlantic

Dalmau, Josep O MD/PhD [N] - **Spec Exp:** Brain Tumors; **Hospital:** Hosp Univ Penn - UPHS (page 80); **Address:** Hosp Univ Penn, Dept Neuro-Oncology, 3 W Gates Bldg, 3400 Spruce St, Phildelphia, PA 19104; **Phone:** 215-746-4707; **Med School:** Spain 1971; **Resid:** Neurology, Univ Hosp de la Sta Cruz y San Pablo 1983; **Fellow:** Neurology, NY Hosp-Cornell Med Ctr 1992; Neuro-Oncology, Meml Sloan Kettering Cancer Ctr 1993; **Fac Appt:** Prof N, Univ Pennsylvania

De Angelis, Lisa M MD [N] - **Spec Exp:** Neuro-Oncology; **Hospital:** Meml Sloan-Kettering Cancer Ctr (page 75); **Address:** 1275 York Avenue, New York, NY 10065; **Phone:** 212-639-7123; **Board Cert:** Neurology 1986; **Med School:** Columbia P&S 1980; **Resid:** Neurology, Neuro Inst-Presby Hosp 1984; **Fellow:** Neuro-Oncology, Neuro Inst-Presby Hosp 1985; Neuro-Oncology, Meml Sloan-Kettering Cancer Ctr 1986; **Fac Appt:** Prof N, Cornell Univ-Weill Med Coll

Glass, Jon MD [N] - **Spec Exp:** Neuro-Oncology; Brain Tumors; Spinal Tumors; **Hospital:** Thomas Jefferson Univ Hosp (page 81); **Address:** 909 Walnut St Fl 2, Philadelphia, PA 19107; **Phone:** 215-503-7005; **Board Cert:** Neurology 1993; **Med School:** SUNY Downstate 1986; **Resid:** Neurology, Boston Univ 1990; **Fellow:** Neuro-Oncology, Mass Genl Hosp 1992; **Fac Appt:** Asst Prof N, NYU Sch Med

Hiesiger, Emile MD [N] - **Spec Exp:** Pain-Spine; Pain-Cancer, Spine; Pain-Back; **Hospital:** NYU Langone Med Ctr (page 79), VA NY Harbor Hlthcare Sys-Manhattan Campus; **Address:** 530 1st Ave, Ste 5A, New York, NY 10016-6402; **Phone:** 212-263-6123; **Board Cert:** Neurology 1983; **Med School:** NY Med Coll 1978; **Resid:** Neurology, NYU Med Ctr 1982; **Fellow:** Neurology, Meml Sloan-Kettering Cancer Ctr 1984; **Fac Appt:** Assoc Clin Prof N, NYU Sch Med

Kunschner, Lara MD [N] - **Spec Exp:** Neuro-Oncology; Brain Tumors; **Hospital:** Allegheny General Hosp; **Address:** 420 E North Ave, Ste 206, Ste 206, Pittsburgh, PA 15212; **Phone:** 412-359-8850; **Board Cert:** Neurology 1999; **Med School:** Univ Pittsburgh 1994; **Resid:** Neurology, Univ Michigan Hosps 1999; **Fellow:** Neuro-Oncology, MD Anderson Cancer Ctr 2000

Laterra, John J MD/PhD [N] - **Spec Exp:** Neuro-Oncology; Brain Tumors; **Hospital:** Johns Hopkins Hosp, Kennedy Krieger Inst; **Address:** Phipps 115, 600 N Wolfe St, Baltimore, MD 21287; **Phone:** 410-614-3853; **Board Cert:** Neurology 1990; **Med School:** Case West Res Univ 1984; **Resid:** Neurology, Univ Mich Hosps 1988; **Fellow:** Research, Johns Hopkins Hosp 1989; **Fac Appt:** Prof N, Johns Hopkins Univ

Posner, Jerome B MD [N] - **Spec Exp:** Neuro-Oncology; Brain Tumors; Paraneoplastic Syndromes; **Hospital:** Meml Sloan-Kettering Cancer Ctr (page 75); **Address:** 1275 York Ave, rm C731, New York, NY 10065; **Phone:** 212-639-7047; **Board Cert:** Neurology 1962; **Med School:** Univ Wash 1955; **Resid:** Neurology, Univ WA Affil Hosp 1959; **Fellow:** Biochemistry, Univ WA Affil Hosp 1963; **Fac Appt:** Prof N, Cornell Univ-Weill Med Coll

Rosenfeld, Myrna MD/PhD [N] - **Spec Exp:** Neuro-Oncology; Brain Tumors; **Hospital:** Hosp Univ Penn - UPHS (page 80); **Address:** Hosp Univ Penn, Dept Neurology, 3 West Gates Bldg, 3400 Spruce St, Philadelphia, PA 19104; **Phone:** 215-746-4707; **Board Cert:** Neurology 2004; **Med School:** Northwestern Univ 1985; **Resid:** Neurology, Northwestern Univ Hosp 1987; Neurology, Univ Hosp Cleveland 1989; **Fellow:** Neuro-Oncology, Meml Sloan Kettering Cancer Ctr; **Fac Appt:** Assoc Prof N, Univ Pennsylvania

Southeast

Janss, Anna J MD/PhD [N] - **Spec Exp:** Brain Tumors-Pediatric; Clinical Trials; Cancer Survivors-Late Effects of Therapy; **Hospital:** Chldns Hlthcare Atlanta @ Egleston, Chldns Hlthcare Atlanta @ Scottish Rite; **Address:** Aflac Cancer & Blood Disorders Ctr, Outpatient Clin, Tower 1 Fl 4, 1405 Clifton Rd NE, Atlanta, GA 30322; **Phone:** 404-785-1200; **Board Cert:** Neurology 1993; **Med School:** Univ Iowa Coll Med 1988; **Resid:** Neurology, Hosp Univ Penn 1992; **Fellow:** Pediatric Neuro-Oncology, Chldns Hosp 1996; **Fac Appt:** Assoc Prof N, Emory Univ

Moots, Paul L MD [N] - **Spec Exp:** Neuro-Oncology; Brain Tumors; Neurologic Complications of Cancer; Pain-Neuropathic; **Hospital:** Vanderbilt Univ Med Ctr, TN Valley Healthcare Sys-Nashville; **Address:** Vanderbilt Dept Neurology, 1161 21st Ave S, A-0118 Med Ctr North, Nashville, TN 37232; **Phone:** 615-322-6053; **Board Cert:** Neurology 1989; **Med School:** Ohio State Univ 1980; **Resid:** Neurology, Univ Va Med Ctr 1984; **Fellow:** Neuropathology, Univ Virginia 1986; Neuro-Oncology, Meml Sloan Kettering Canc 1989; **Fac Appt:** Assoc Prof N, Vanderbilt Univ

Nabors III, L Burt MD [N] - **Spec Exp:** Neuro-Oncology; Brain Tumors; **Hospital:** Univ of Ala Hosp at Birmingham; **Address:** UAB, FOT 1020, 510 20th St S, Birmingham, AL 35294-0001; **Phone:** 205-934-1432; **Board Cert:** Neurology 2009; **Med School:** Univ Tenn Coll Med 1991; **Resid:** Neurology, Univ Alabama Med Ctr; **Fellow:** Neuro-Oncology, Univ Alabama; **Fac Appt:** Prof N, Univ Alabama

Schiff, David MD [N] - **Spec Exp:** Brain Tumors; Spinal Cord Tumors; Neurologic Complications of Cancer; Neuro-Oncology; **Hospital:** Univ of Virginia Health Sys; **Address:** Univ VA, Div of Neuro-Oncology, PO Box 800432, Charlottesville, VA 22908; **Phone:** 434-982-4415; **Board Cert:** Neurology 1994; **Med School:** Harvard Med Sch 1988; **Resid:** Neurology, Harvard Longwood 1992; **Fellow:** Neuro-Oncology, Meml Sloan Kettering Cancer Ctr 1993; Mayo Clinic 1994; **Fac Appt:** Assoc Prof NS, Univ VA Sch Med

Midwest

Barger, Geoffrey R MD [N] - **Spec Exp:** Neuro-Oncology; Brain Tumors; **Hospital:** Harper Univ Hosp, Barbara Ann Karmanos Cancer Inst; **Address:** Wayne State Univ Hlth Ctr, 4201 St Antoine, Ste 8D-UHC, Detroit, MI 48201; **Phone:** 313-745-4275; **Board Cert:** Neurology 1981; **Med School:** Jefferson Med Coll 1975; **Resid:** Neurology, Penn Hosp 1979; **Fellow:** Neuro-Oncology, Moffitt Hosp & Brain Tumor Ctr/UCSF 1982; **Fac Appt:** Assoc Prof N, Wayne State Univ

Cascino, Terrence L MD [N] - **Spec Exp:** Neuro-Oncology; **Hospital:** Mayo Med Ctr & Clin - Rochester; **Address:** Mayo Clinic, Dept Neurology, 200 1st St SW, Rochester, MN 55905; **Phone:** 507-284-2576; **Board Cert:** Neurology 1984; **Med School:** Loyola Univ-Stritch Sch Med 1972; **Resid:** Neurology, Mayo Clinic 1980; **Fellow:** Neuro-Oncology, Meml Sloan Kettering Cancer Ctr; **Fac Appt:** Assoc Prof N, Mayo Med Sch

Neurology

Mikkelsen, Tommy MD [N] - **Spec Exp:** Brain Tumors; Gliomas; **Hospital:** Henry Ford Hosp; **Address:** Henry Ford Hospital, ER 3096, 2799 W Grand Blvd, Detroit, MI 48202; **Phone:** 313-916-8641; **Board Cert:** Neurology 2008; **Med School:** Univ Calgary 1983; **Resid:** Internal Medicine, Calgary General Hosp 1985; Neurology, Montreal Neuro Inst 1988; **Fellow:** Neuro-Oncology, Royal Victoria Hosp 1990; Neuro-Oncology, Ludwig Inst for Cancer Rsch 1992; **Fac Appt:** Assoc Prof N, Case West Res Univ

Newton, Herbert B MD [N] - **Spec Exp:** Neuro-Oncology; Brain & Spinal Tumors; Clinical Trials; **Hospital:** Ohio St Univ Med Ctr, Arthur G James Cancer Hosp & Research Inst; **Address:** 320 W 10th Ave, Starling Loving Bldg, rm M410, Columbus, OH 43210; **Phone:** 614-293-8930; **Board Cert:** Neurology 1989; **Med School:** SUNY Buffalo 1984; **Resid:** Neurology, Univ Michigan Med Ctr 1988; **Fellow:** Neuro-Oncology, Meml Sloan-Kettering Cancer Ctr 1990; **Fac Appt:** Prof N, Ohio State Univ

Rogers, Lisa R DO [N] - **Spec Exp:** Neuro-Oncology; Brain Tumors; Brain Radiation Toxicity; **Hospital:** Univ Hosps Case Med Ctr; **Address:** Univ Hosps-Case Med Ctr, Dept Neuro, Hanna House 506, MS HAN 5040, 11100 Euclid Ave, Cleveland, OH 44106-5040; **Phone:** 216-844-5160; **Board Cert:** Neurology 1982; **Med School:** Kirksville Coll Osteo Med 1976; **Resid:** Neurology, Cleveland Clin Fdn 1980; **Fellow:** Neuro-Oncology, Meml-Sloan Kettering Cancer Ctr 1982; **Fac Appt:** Prof N, Case West Res Univ

Rosenfeld, Steven S MD [N] - **Spec Exp:** Brain Tumors; Gliomas; Neuro-Oncology; **Hospital:** Cleveland Clin (page 70); **Address:** Cleveland Clinic, 9500 Euclid Ave, S-73, Cleveland, OH 44195; **Phone:** 216-444-4461; **Board Cert:** Neurology 1994; **Med School:** Northwestern Univ 1985; **Resid:** Neurology, Duke Univ Med Ctr 1989; **Fellow:** Neuro-Oncology, Duke Univ Med Ctr 1990; **Fac Appt:** Prof N, Cleveland Cl Coll Med/Case West Res

Vick, Nicholas A MD [N] - **Spec Exp:** Brain Tumors; Neuro-Oncology; **Hospital:** Evanston/North Shore Univ Hlth Sys; **Address:** Evanston Kellog Cancer Ctr, 2650 Ridge Ave, Evanston, IL 60201; **Phone:** 847-570-1808; **Board Cert:** Neurology 1971; **Med School:** Univ Chicago-Pritzker Sch Med 1965; **Resid:** Neurology, Univ Chicago Hosps 1968; **Fellow:** Neurology, Natl Inst Hlth 1970; **Fac Appt:** Prof N, Northwestern Univ

Southwest

Gilbert, Mark R MD [N] - **Spec Exp:** Brain Tumors; Neuro-Oncology; **Hospital:** UT MD Anderson Cancer Ctr; **Address:** Univ Tex MD Anderson Cancer Ctr, 1515 Holcombe Blvd, Unit 431, Houston, TX 77030; **Phone:** 713-792-4008; **Board Cert:** Internal Medicine 1985; Neurology 1990; **Med School:** Johns Hopkins Univ 1982; **Resid:** Internal Medicine, Johns Hopkins Hosp 1985; Neurology, Johns Hopkins Hosp 1988; **Fellow:** Neuro-Oncology, Johns Hopkins Hosp 1988; **Fac Appt:** Assoc Prof N, Univ Tex, Houston

Patchell, Roy Andrew MD [N] - **Spec Exp:** Neuro-Oncology; Brain Tumors; Spinal Tumors; **Hospital:** St. Joseph's Hosp & Med Ctr - Phoenix; **Address:** Barrow Neurological Institute, 350 W Thomas Rd, Ste 300, Phoenix, AZ 85013-4409; **Phone:** 602-406-2616; **Board Cert:** Neurology 1984; **Med School:** Univ KY Coll Med 1979; **Resid:** Neurology, Johns Hopkins Hosp 1983; **Fellow:** Neuro-Oncology, Meml Sloan-Kettering Canc Ctr 1985; **Fac Appt:** Prof N, Univ KY Coll Med

Shapiro, William R MD [N] - **Spec Exp:** Neuro-Oncology; **Hospital:** St. Joseph's Hosp & Med Ctr - Phoenix; **Address:** Barrow Neurology Clins, 500 W Thomas Rd, Ste 300, Phoenix, AZ 85013; **Phone:** 602-406-6262; **Board Cert:** Neurology 1969; **Med School:** UCSF 1961; **Resid:** Internal Medicine, Univ Wash Hosp 1963; Neurology, NY Hosp-Cornell Med Ctr 1966; **Fellow:** Neuro-Oncology, Natl Inst Hlth 1969; **Fac Appt:** Prof N, Univ Ariz Coll Med

Yung, WK Alfred MD [N] - **Spec Exp:** Neuro-Oncology; Brain Tumors; **Hospital:** UT MD Anderson Cancer Ctr; **Address:** 1515 Holcombe Blvd, Unit 431, Houston, TX 77030-4017; **Phone:** 713-794-1285; **Board Cert:** Neurology 1980; **Med School:** Univ Chicago-Pritzker Sch Med 1975; **Resid:** Neurology, UCSD Med Ctr 1978; **Fellow:** Neuro-Oncology, Meml Sloan Kettering Cancer Ctr 1981; **Fac Appt:** Prof N, Univ Tex, Houston

West Coast and Pacific

Chamberlain, Marc C MD [N] - **Spec Exp:** Brain Tumors; Neuro-Oncology; Clinical Trials; **Hospital:** Univ Wash Med Ctr; **Address:** Seattle Cancer Care Alliance, 825 Eastlake Ave E, POB 10923, MS G4940, Seattle, WA 98109-1023; **Phone:** 206-288-8280; **Board Cert:** Pediatrics 1985; Child Neurology 1989; **Med School:** Columbia P&S 1977; **Resid:** Pediatrics, Montefiore Med Ctr 1981; Neurology, UCLA Med Ctr 1983; **Fellow:** Neuro-Oncology, UCSF Med Ctr 1986; **Fac Appt:** Prof N, Univ Wash

Cloughesy, Timothy F MD [N] - **Spec Exp:** Neuro-Oncology; Brain Tumors; **Hospital:** UCLA Ronald Reagan Med Ctr; **Address:** UCLA Neurological Services, 710 Westwood Plaza, Ste 1230, Los Angeles, CA 90095; **Phone:** 310-825-5321; **Board Cert:** Neurology 1993; **Med School:** Tulane Univ 1987; **Resid:** Neurology, UCLA Med Ctr 1991; **Fellow:** Neuro-Oncology, Meml Sloan-Kettering Canc Ctr; **Fac Appt:** Clin Prof N, UCLA

Phuphanich, Surasak MD [N] - **Spec Exp:** Brain Tumors-Metastatic; Stem Cell Therapy; Spinal Tumors; Neurologic Complications of Cancer; **Hospital:** Cedars-Sinai Med Ctr; **Address:** 8631 W 3rd St, Ste 410E, Los Angeles, CA 90048; **Phone:** 310-423-4413; **Board Cert:** Neurology 1983; **Med School:** Thailand 1975; **Resid:** Neurology, Univ Illinois Med Ctr 1981; **Fellow:** Neuro-Oncology, UCSF Med Ctr 1984

Taylor, Lynne P MD [N] - **Spec Exp:** Brain Tumors; Gliomas; **Hospital:** Virginia Mason Med Ctr; **Address:** Virginia Mason Medical Ctr, Neurology, 1100 9th Ave, Fl 7, Seattle, WA 98101; **Phone:** 206-341-0420; **Board Cert:** Neurology 1987; Hospice & Palliative Medicine 2010; **Med School:** Washington Univ, St Louis 1982; **Resid:** Neurology, Hosp Univ Penn 1986; **Fellow:** Neuro-Oncology, Meml Sloan Kettering Cancer Ctr 1988; **Fac Appt:** Assoc Clin Prof N, Univ Wash

CHILD NEUROLOGY

New England

Pomeroy, Scott L MD/PhD [ChiN] - **Spec Exp:** Neuro-Oncology; Brain Tumors; **Hospital:** Children's Hospital - Boston, Dana-Farber Cancer Inst; **Address:** Chldns Hosp, Dept Neurology-Fegan 11, 300 Longwood Ave, Boston, MA 02115; **Phone:** 617-355-6386; **Board Cert:** Child Neurology 1988; **Med School:** Univ Cincinnati 1982; **Resid:** Pediatrics, Chldns Hosp 1984; Neurology, Barnes Hosp/Washington Univ 1985; **Fellow:** Pediatric Neurology, St Louis Chldns Hosp 1987; Neurological Biology, Washington Univ 1990; **Fac Appt:** Prof N, Harvard Med Sch

Mid Atlantic

Allen, Jeffrey MD [ChiN] - **Spec Exp:** Neuro-Oncology; Brain Tumors; **Hospital:** NYU Langone Med Ctr (page 79); **Address:** Hassenfeld Childrens Ctr, 160 E 32nd St Fl 2nd - Ste L3, New York, NY 10016; **Phone:** 212-263-9907; **Board Cert:** Child Neurology 1977; **Med School:** Harvard Med Sch 1969; **Resid:** Pediatrics, Montreal Chldns Hosp 1973; Pediatric Neurology, Montreal Neur Inst/McGill 1976; **Fac Appt:** Prof Ped, NYU Sch Med

Child Neurology

Duffner, Patricia K MD [ChiN] - **Spec Exp:** Brain Tumors; Cancer Survivors-Late Effects of Therapy; **Hospital:** Women's & Chldn's Hosp of Buffalo, The; **Address:** Women & Childrens Hosp, Dept Neurology, 219 Bryant St, Buffalo, NY 14222-2006; **Phone:** 716-878-7819; **Board Cert:** Pediatrics 1977; Child Neurology 1979; **Med School:** SUNY Buffalo 1972; **Resid:** Pediatrics, Buffalo Chldns Hosp 1975; **Fellow:** Child Neurology, SUNY Buffalo 1978; **Fac Appt:** Prof N, SUNY Buffalo

Packer, Roger J MD [ChiN] - **Spec Exp:** Brain Tumors; **Hospital:** Chldns Natl Med Ctr; **Address:** Chldns Natl Med Ctr, Dept Neurology, 111 Michigan Ave NW, Washington, DC 20010-2978; **Phone:** 202-476-6230; **Board Cert:** Child Neurology 1982; Pediatrics 1982; **Med School:** Northwestern Univ 1976; **Resid:** Pediatrics, Chldns Med Ctr 1978; Neurology, Chldns Hosp-Univ Penn 1981; **Fac Appt:** Prof N, Geo Wash Univ

Phillips, Peter C MD [ChiN] - **Spec Exp:** Brain Tumors; Neuro-Oncology; **Hospital:** Chldns Hosp of Philadelphia; **Address:** Chldns Hosp Philadelphia, 34th St & Civic Center Blvd, CTRB Bldg - Ste 4027, Philadelphia, PA 19104; **Phone:** 215-590-5188; **Board Cert:** Pediatrics 1985; Child Neurology 1986; **Med School:** Univ Conn 1978; **Resid:** Pediatrics, Chldns Hosp 1980; Pediatric Neurology, Neuro Inst 1983; **Fellow:** Neuro-Oncology, Meml Sloan Kettering Cancer Ctr 1986; **Fac Appt:** Prof N, Univ Pennsylvania

Midwest

Cohen, Bruce H MD [ChiN] - **Spec Exp:** Brain Tumors; **Hospital:** Akron Children's Hosp; **Address:** 215 W Bowery St, rm 400, Akron, OH 44308; **Phone:** 330-543-6048; **Board Cert:** Pediatrics 2004; Child Neurology 1990; **Med School:** Albert Einstein Coll Med 1982; **Resid:** Pediatrics, Chldns Hosp 1984; Child Neurology, Neurologic Inst-Columbia 1987; **Fellow:** Pediatric Neuro-Oncology, Chldns Hosp 1989; **Fac Appt:** Prof Ped, NE Ohio Univ

Keating, Gesina F MD [ChiN] - **Spec Exp:** Brain Tumors; Spinal Tumors; Cancer Survivors-Late Effects of Therapy; **Hospital:** Mayo Med Ctr & Clin - Rochester; **Address:** 200 First St SW, Mayo Clinic, Rochester, MN 55905; **Phone:** 507-284-2511; **Board Cert:** Child Neurology 2008; **Med School:** Mayo Med Sch 1991; **Resid:** Pediatric Neurology, Mayo Clinic 1996; Pediatrics, Vanderbilt Univ Med Ctr 1999; **Fellow:** Pediatric Neuro-Oncology, Beth Israel Med Ctr 2000

West Coast and Pacific

Fisher, Paul G MD [ChiN] - **Spec Exp:** Neuro-Oncology; Brain Tumors; **Hospital:** Lucile Packard Chldn's Hosp; **Address:** Stanford Cancer Ctr-Dept Neurology, 750 Welch Rd, Ste 317, MC 5, Palo Alto, CA 94304; **Phone:** 650-721-5889; **Board Cert:** Pediatrics 2003; Child Neurology 2008; **Med School:** UCSF 1989; **Resid:** Pediatrics, Johns Hopkins Univ Hosp 1991; Neurology, Johns Hopkins Univ Hosp 1994; **Fellow:** Neuro-Oncology, Children's Hosp 1994; **Fac Appt:** Assoc Prof Ped, Stanford Univ

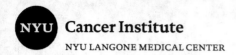

NYU **Cancer Institute**

NYU LANGONE MEDICAL CENTER

NYU Langone Medical Center
550 First Avenue , New York, NY 10016
www.NYULMC.org

NYU Clinical Cancer Center
160 East 34th Street, New York, NY 10016
www.NYUCI.org

The Stephen D. Hassenfeld Children's Center
for Cancer and Blood Disorders
160 East 32nd Street, New York, NY 10016
www.NYUMC.org/Hassenfeld

The NYU Cancer Institute is an NCI-designated cancer center and provides personalized patient care that is both compassionate and state of the art. The doctors and researchers work together to develop innovative therapies for patients. The Cancer Institute is world-renowned for excellence in cancer-focused research, personalized care, education and community outreach. Its mission is to discover the origins of human cancer and to use that knowledge to eradicate the personal and societal burden of cancer in our community, the nation and the world. For more information about our expert physicians, call 212-731-5000. *We specialize in the following areas:*

Patient-Focused Setting
The NYU Clinical Cancer Center is the principal outpatient facility of The Cancer Institute and serves as home to our patients and their caregivers. The center and its multidisciplinary team of experts provide access to the latest treatment options and clinical trials along with a variety of programs in cancer risk reduction/prevention, screening, diagnostics, genetic counseling and supportive services. In addition the NYUCI emphasizes the importance of a holistic approach to management services in complementary medicine, psychosocial support, survivorship and palliative care.

Renowned Expertise
The NYU Cancer Institute brings together experts from a variety of disciplines to create collaborative research endeavors and clinical care teams. The Cancer Institute offers a full continuum of personalized care, from prevention through diagnosis, treatment and post-treatment support. The compassion and expertise of our team members helps patients better manage the symptoms of their diseases as well as meet their special needs. Additionally, we have created special emphasis programs in diseases such as breast cancer, melanoma, GI cancer, prostate cancer, hematologic malignancies and lung cancer among others, as well as, translational programs in cancer healthcare disparities, molecularly targeted therapy, and the cell signaling pathways involved in cancer.

A Translational Approach
NYU Langone Medical Center scientists and other researchers excel in uncovering how cancer develops at the molecular level, and how we can harness that knowledge to reduce the risk of cancer and treat the disease. The Medical Center constantly seeks to create new opportunities for collaboration between investigators within our own institution, those located elsewhere in the NYU network of campuses, and researchers at other institutions.

The Stephen D. Hassenfeld Children's Center for Cancer and Blood Disorders
The center is a leading pediatric outpatient facility for the treatment of childhood cancers and blood diseases. Its unique interdisciplinary and family-centered approach combines the most advanced medical treatments with psychosocial and emotional support services for young patients and their families.

The Best in American Medicine
www.CastleConnolly.com

Obstetrics & Gynecology

An obstetrician/gynecologist possesses special knowledge, skills and professional capability in the medical and surgical care of the female reproductive system and associated disorders. This physician may serve as a consultant to other physicians, and may be a primary physician for some women.

Training Required: Four years plus two years in clinical practice before certification is complete.

Gynecolgic Oncology: An obstetrician/gynecologist who provides consultation and comprehensive management of patients with gynecologic cancer, including those diagnostic and therapeutic procedures necessary for the total care of the patient with gynecologic cancer and resulting complications.

Training Required: Four years plus two years in clinical practice before certification in obstetrics and gynecology is complete plus additional training and examination in gynecologic oncology.

Reproductive Endocrinology/Infertility: An obstetrician/gynecologist who is capable of managing complex problems relating to reproductive endocrinology and infertility.

Training Required: Four years plus two years in clinical practice before certification in obstetrics and gynecology is complete plus additional training and examination in reproductive endocrinology.

GYNECOLOGIC ONCOLOGY

New England

Azodi, Masoud MD [GO] - **Spec Exp:** Laparoscopic Surgery; Ovarian Cancer-Early Detection; Uterine Cancer; **Hospital:** Yale-New Haven Hosp, Yale Med Group; **Address:** Smilow Cancer Hosp, 35 Park St Fl 1, New Haven, CT 06519; **Phone:** 203-200-4176; **Board Cert:** Gynecologic Oncology 2009; Obstetrics & Gynecology 2009; **Med School:** Wright State Univ 1992; **Resid:** Obstetrics & Gynecology, Aultman Hospital 1996; **Fellow:** Obstetrics & Gynecology, Yale-New Haven Hosp 1999; **Fac Appt:** Assoc Prof ObG, Yale Univ

Berkowitz, Ross S MD [GO] - **Spec Exp:** Gynecologic Cancer; **Hospital:** Brigham & Women's Hosp, Dana-Farber Cancer Inst; **Address:** Div OB/GYN Oncology, 75 Francis St, Boston, MA 02115-6110; **Phone:** 617-732-8843; **Board Cert:** Obstetrics & Gynecology 1981; Gynecologic Oncology 1982; **Med School:** Boston Univ 1973; **Resid:** Surgery, Peter Bent Brigham Hosp 1975; Obstetrics & Gynecology, Boston Hosp for Women 1978; **Fellow:** Gynecologic Oncology, Boston Hosp for Women 1980; **Fac Appt:** Prof ObG, Harvard Med Sch

Brewer, Molly A MD [GO] - **Spec Exp:** Ovarian Cancer; Gynecologic Cancer; Gynecologic Cancer-Rare; **Hospital:** Univ of Conn Hlth Ctr, John Dempsey Hosp, Hartford Hosp; **Address:** Univ Conn Hlth Ctr, Div Gyn Oncology, 263 Farmington Ave, MC2875, Farmington, CT 06032-2875; **Phone:** 860-679-2100; **Board Cert:** Obstetrics & Gynecology 2009; Gynecologic Oncology 2009; **Med School:** SUNY Upstate Med Univ 1991; **Resid:** Obstetrics & Gynecology, Oregon Hlth Scis Ctr 1995; **Fellow:** Gynecologic Oncology, MD Anderson Cancer Ctr 1997; **Fac Appt:** Prof ObG, Univ Conn

Cain, Joanna M MD [GO] - **Spec Exp:** Ovarian Cancer; Breast Cancer Risk Assessment; Uterine Cancer; Ovarian Cancer-Early Detection; **Hospital:** Women & Infants Hosp of RI, Rhode Island Hosp; **Address:** Women & Infants Hospital, 101 Dudley St, Providence, RI 02905; **Phone:** 401-274-1122 x1575; **Board Cert:** Obstetrics & Gynecology 2009; Gynecologic Oncology 2009; **Med School:** Creighton Univ 1978; **Resid:** Obstetrics & Gynecology, Univ Washington Med Ctr 1981; **Fellow:** Gynecologic Oncology, Meml Sloan Kettering Cancer Ctr 1983; **Fac Appt:** Prof ObG, Brown Univ

DeMars, Leslie R MD [GO] - **Spec Exp:** Gynecologic Cancer; Laparoscopic Surgery; **Hospital:** Dartmouth - Hitchcock Med Ctr; **Address:** Dartmouth-Hitchcock Med Ctr, Gyn-Oncology, 1 Medical Center Drive, Lebanon, NH 03756; **Phone:** 603-653-3530; **Board Cert:** Obstetrics & Gynecology 2009; Gynecologic Oncology 2009; **Med School:** Univ VT Coll Med 1987; **Resid:** Obstetrics & Gynecology, Univ NC Hosp 1991; **Fellow:** Gynecologic Oncology, Univ NC Hosp 1994; **Fac Appt:** Assoc Prof ObG, Dartmouth Med Sch

Granai, Cornelius O MD [GO] - **Spec Exp:** Gynecologic Cancer; Complementary Medicine; **Hospital:** Women & Infants Hosp of RI, Rhode Island Hosp; **Address:** Womens & Infants Hosp, 101 Dudley St, GYN Oncology Department, Providence, RI 02905; **Phone:** 401-453-7520; **Board Cert:** Obstetrics & Gynecology 2009; Gynecologic Oncology 2009; **Med School:** Univ VT Coll Med 1977; **Resid:** Obstetrics & Gynecology, Hershey Med Ctr 1981; **Fellow:** Gynecologic Oncology, Tufts Univ 1984; **Fac Appt:** Prof ObG, Brown Univ

Muto, Michael G MD [GO] - **Spec Exp:** Ovarian Cancer; Cervical Cancer; Vulvar & Vaginal Cancer; Robotic Surgery; **Hospital:** Dana-Farber Cancer Inst, Brigham & Women's Hosp; **Address:** Brigham & Womens Hosp, Div Gynecologic Oncology, 75 Francis St, Boston, MA 02115; **Phone:** 617-732-8840; **Board Cert:** Obstetrics & Gynecology 2009; Gynecologic Oncology 2008; **Med School:** Univ Mass Sch Med 1983; **Resid:** Obstetrics & Gynecology, Brigham & Women's Hosp 1987; **Fellow:** Gynecologic Oncology, Brigham & Women's Hosp 1990; **Fac Appt:** Assoc Prof ObG, Harvard Med Sch

Rutherford, Thomas J MD [GO] - **Spec Exp:** Ovarian Cancer; Uterine Cancer; Ovarian Cancer-Early Detection; Cervical Cancer; **Hospital:** Yale-New Haven Hosp, Yale Med Group; **Address:** Smilow Cancer Hosp, 35 Park St Fl 1, New Haven, CT 06519; **Phone:** 203-200-4176; **Board Cert:** Obstetrics & Gynecology 2009; Gynecologic Oncology 2009; **Med School:** Med Coll OH 1989; **Resid:** Obstetrics & Gynecology, Cooper Hosp 1993; **Fellow:** Gynecologic Oncology, Yale-New Haven Hosp 1995; **Fac Appt:** Assoc Prof ObG, Yale Univ

Santin, Alessandro MD [GO] - **Spec Exp:** Immunotherapy; Ovarian Cancer; Vulvar & Vaginal Cancer; **Hospital:** Yale-New Haven Hosp, Yale Med Group; **Address:** Yale Gynecologic Oncology, 333 Cedar St, PO Box 208063, New Haven, CT 06510; **Phone:** 203-737-2280; **Med School:** Italy 1989; **Resid:** Obstetrics & Gynecology, Univ Brescia Sch Med 1993; **Fellow:** Gynecologic Oncology, UC Irvine 1995; Gynecologic Oncology, UAMS Med Ctr 2000; **Fac Appt:** Prof ObG, Yale Univ

Schorge, John O MD [GO] - **Spec Exp:** Ovarian Cancer; Uterine Cancer; Cervical Cancer; Minimally Invasive Surgery; **Hospital:** Mass Genl Hosp; **Address:** Gillette Ctr for Gynocological Oncology, 55 Fruit St, Yawkey Ctr 9E, Boston, MA 02114; **Phone:** 617-724-6899; **Board Cert:** Obstetrics & Gynecology 2009; Gynecologic Oncology 2009; **Med School:** Vanderbilt Univ 1993; **Resid:** Obstetrics & Gynecology, Brigham & Women's Hosp 1997; **Fellow:** Gynecologic Oncology, Brigham & Women's Hosp 2000; **Fac Appt:** Assoc Prof ObG, Harvard Med Sch

Schwartz, Peter E MD [GO] - **Spec Exp:** Ovarian Cancer; Uterine Cancer; Gynecologic Surgery-Complex; Cervical Cancer; **Hospital:** Yale-New Haven Hosp, Yale Med Group; **Address:** 333 Cedar St FMB Bldg Fl 3 - Ste 328, St, New Haven, CT 06510-3289; **Phone:** 203-785-4014; **Board Cert:** Obstetrics & Gynecology 1973; Gynecologic Oncology 1979; **Med School:** Albert Einstein Coll Med 1966; **Resid:** Obstetrics & Gynecology, Yale-New Haven Hosp 1970; **Fellow:** Gynecologic Oncology, MD Anderson Cancer Ctr 1975; **Fac Appt:** Prof ObG, Yale Univ

Tarraza, Hector M MD [GO] - **Spec Exp:** Gynecologic Cancer; **Hospital:** Maine Med Ctr; **Address:** 102 Campus Drive, rm 116, Scarborough, ME 04074; **Phone:** 207-883-0069; **Board Cert:** Obstetrics & Gynecology 2009; Gynecologic Oncology 2009; **Med School:** Harvard Med Sch 1981; **Resid:** Obstetrics & Gynecology, Mass Genl Hosp 1985; **Fellow:** Gynecologic Oncology, Mass Genl Hosp 1987; **Fac Appt:** Prof ObG, Univ VT Coll Med

Mid Atlantic

Abbas, Fouad M MD [GO] - **Spec Exp:** Gynecologic Cancer; Ovarian Cancer; Cervical Cancer; **Hospital:** Sinai Hosp - Baltimore; **Address:** Sinai Hosp Baltimore, 2411 W Belvedere Ave, Ste 206, Baltimore, MD 21215; **Phone:** 410-601-9030; **Board Cert:** Obstetrics & Gynecology 2008; Gynecologic Oncology 2008; **Med School:** Univ MD Sch Med 1986; **Resid:** Obstetrics & Gynecology, John Hopkins Hosp 1990; **Fellow:** Gynecologic Oncology, John Hopkins Hosp 1992; **Fac Appt:** Asst Prof ObG, Univ MD Sch Med

Gynecologic Oncology

Abu-Rustum, Nadeem R MD [GO] - **Spec Exp:** Ovarian Cancer; Uterine Cancer; Cervical Cancer; Vulvar Disease/Cancer; **Hospital:** Meml Sloan-Kettering Cancer Ctr (page 75); **Address:** 1275 York Ave, New York, NY 10065; **Phone:** 212-639-7051; **Board Cert:** Obstetrics & Gynecology 2009; Gynecologic Oncology 2009; **Med School:** Lebanon 1990; **Resid:** Obstetrics & Gynecology, Greater Baltimore Med Ctr 1994; **Fellow:** Gynecologic Oncology, Meml Sloan-Kettering Cancer Ctr 1997; **Fac Appt:** Assoc Prof ObG, Cornell Univ-Weill Med Coll

Barakat, Richard R MD [GO] - **Spec Exp:** Laparoscopic Surgery; Ovarian Cancer; Uterine Cancer; **Hospital:** Meml Sloan-Kettering Cancer Ctr (page 75); **Address:** 1275 York Ave, rm H1305, New York, NY 10065; **Phone:** 800-525-2225; **Board Cert:** Obstetrics & Gynecology 2006; Gynecologic Oncology 2006; **Med School:** SUNY Hlth Sci Ctr 1985; **Resid:** Obstetrics & Gynecology, Bellevue Hosp 1989; **Fellow:** Gynecologic Oncology, Meml Sloan Kettering Cancer Ctr 1991; **Fac Appt:** Assoc Prof ObG, Cornell Univ-Weill Med Coll

Barnes, Willard MD [GO] - **Spec Exp:** Pelvic Tumors; Gynecologic Cancer; **Hospital:** Georgetown Univ Hosp; **Address:** Georgetown Univ Hosp, Lombardi Cancer Ctr, Dept Gyn Oncology, 3800 Reservoir Rd NW, Washington, DC 20007-2194; **Phone:** 202-444-2114; **Board Cert:** Obstetrics & Gynecology 2009; Gynecologic Oncology 2009; **Med School:** Univ Miss 1979; **Resid:** Obstetrics & Gynecology, Univ Miss Med Ctr 1983; **Fellow:** Gynecologic Oncology, Georgetown Univ Med Ctr 1985; **Fac Appt:** Assoc Prof ObG, Georgetown Univ

Barter, James MD [GO] - **Spec Exp:** Laparoscopic Surgery; Ovarian Cancer; Gynecologic Cancer; **Hospital:** Holy Cross Hospital - Silver Spring, Suburban Hosp; **Address:** 6301 Executive Blvd, Rockville, MD 20852; **Phone:** 301-770-4967; **Board Cert:** Obstetrics & Gynecology 1997; Gynecologic Oncology 1997; **Med School:** Univ VA Sch Med 1977; **Resid:** Internal Medicine, Univ Kentucky Med Ctr 1979; Obstetrics & Gynecology, Duke Univ Med Ctr 1983; **Fellow:** Gynecologic Oncology, Univ Alabama 1985; **Fac Appt:** Clin Prof ObG, Georgetown Univ

Boice, Charles R MD [GO] - **Spec Exp:** Gynecologic Cancer; Ovarian Cancer; Cervical Cancer; **Hospital:** Washington Hosp Ctr; **Address:** 10301 Georgia Ave, Ste 205, Silver Springs, MD 20902; **Phone:** 301-592-1600; **Board Cert:** Obstetrics & Gynecology 1981; Gynecologic Oncology 1982; **Med School:** Loma Linda Univ 1973; **Resid:** Obstetrics & Gynecology, Los Angeles Med Ctr 1973; Surgery, City Hope Natl Med Ctr 1978; **Fellow:** Oncology, Univ Texas-MD Anderson Cancer Ctr 1980; **Fac Appt:** Assoc Clin Prof ObG, Univ Wash

Caputo, Thomas A MD [GO] - **Spec Exp:** Cervical Cancer; Ovarian Cancer; Uterine Cancer; Vulvar Disease/Cancer; **Hospital:** NY-Presby Hosp/Weill Cornell (page 78); **Address:** NY Presby Hosp-Weill Cornell, 525 E 68th St, Ste J130, New York, NY 10021; **Phone:** 212-746-3179; **Board Cert:** Obstetrics & Gynecology 1993; Gynecologic Oncology 1977; **Med School:** UMDNJ-NJ Med Sch, Newark 1965; **Resid:** Obstetrics & Gynecology, Martland Hosp 1969; **Fellow:** Gynecologic Oncology, Emory Univ Hosp 1974; **Fac Appt:** Clin Prof ObG, Cornell Univ-Weill Med Coll

Carlson, John A MD [GO] - **Spec Exp:** Gynecologic Cancer; Ovarian Cancer; Gynecologic Surgery-Complex; **Hospital:** St. Peter's Univ Hosp; **Address:** St Peter's Univ Hosp, 254 Easton Ave Cares Bldg, New Brunswick, NJ 08901; **Phone:** 732-937-6003; **Board Cert:** Obstetrics & Gynecology 1981; Gynecologic Oncology 1982; **Med School:** Georgetown Univ 1974; **Resid:** Obstetrics & Gynecology, Hosp Univ Penn 1978; **Fellow:** Gynecologic Oncology, MD Anderson Cancer Ctr 1980; **Fac Appt:** Prof ObG, Drexel Univ Coll Med

Cornelison, Terri L MD/PhD [GO] - **Spec Exp:** Gynecologic Cancer; Ovarian Cancer; Clinical Trials; **Hospital:** Johns Hopkins Hosp; **Address:** Kelly Gynecologic Oncology Service, 600 N Wolfe St Phipps Bldg - Ste 281, Baltimore, MD 21287; **Phone:** 410-502-4245; **Board Cert:** Obstetrics & Gynecology 2007; **Med School:** Yale Univ 1985; **Resid:** Obstetrics & Gynecology, Beth Israel Hosp 1989; **Fellow:** Gynecologic Oncology, Roswell Park Cancer Inst 1992; **Fac Appt:** Asst Prof ObG, Johns Hopkins Univ

Cosin, Jonathan A MD [GO] - **Spec Exp:** Gynecologic Cancer; **Hospital:** Washington Hosp Ctr; **Address:** Washington Hosp Ctr-Dept Gyn. Onc., 110 Irving St NW, rm 5B-33, Washington, DC 20010; **Phone:** 202-877-2391; **Board Cert:** Obstetrics & Gynecology 2009; Gynecologic Oncology 2009; **Med School:** Albany Med Coll 1991; **Resid:** Obstetrics & Gynecology, Baystate Med Ctr 1995; **Fellow:** Gynecology, Meml Sloan Kettering Cancer Ctr 1993; Gynecologic Oncology, Univ Minnesota Hosp 1998; **Fac Appt:** Asst Prof ObG, Georgetown Univ

Coukos, George MD/PhD [GO] - **Spec Exp:** Ovarian Cancer; Gynecologic Cancer; Vaccine Therapy; Clinical Trials; **Hospital:** Hosp Univ Penn - UPHS (page 80); **Address:** Hosp Univ Penn, 3400 Civic Center Blvd, Jordan Ctr Fl 3W, Philadelphia, PA 19104; **Phone:** 215-662-3318; **Board Cert:** Obstetrics & Gynecology 2004; Gynecologic Oncology 2004; **Med School:** Italy 1987; **Resid:** Obstetrics & Gynecology, Hosp Univ Penn 1997; **Fellow:** Gynecologic Oncology, Hosp Univ Penn 2000; **Fac Appt:** Assoc Prof ObG, Univ Pennsylvania

Curtin, John P MD [GO] - **Spec Exp:** Uterine Cancer; Ovarian Cancer; Laparoscopic Surgery; Gestational Trophoblastic Disease; **Hospital:** NYU Langone Med Ctr (page 79); **Address:** NYU Clin Cancer Ctr, 160 E 34th St Fl 4, New York, NY 10016-6402; **Phone:** 212-731-5345; **Board Cert:** Obstetrics & Gynecology 2008; Gynecologic Oncology 2009; **Med School:** Creighton Univ 1979; **Resid:** Obstetrics & Gynecology, Univ Minn Med Ctr 1984; **Fellow:** Gynecologic Oncology, Meml Sloan-Kettering Cancer Ctr 1988; **Fac Appt:** Prof ObG, NYU Sch Med

Dottino, Peter R MD [GO] - **Spec Exp:** Laparoscopic Surgery; Gynecologic Cancer; **Hospital:** Mount Sinai Med Ctr (page 76), Hackensack Univ Med Ctr (page 73); **Address:** 800-A 5th Ave, Ste 405, New York, NY 10065; **Phone:** 212-888-8439; **Board Cert:** Obstetrics & Gynecology 2007; Gynecologic Oncology 2007; **Med School:** Georgetown Univ 1979; **Resid:** Obstetrics & Gynecology, SUNY Downstate Med Ctr 1983; **Fellow:** Gynecologic Oncology, Mt Sinai Hosp 1985

Dunton, Charles J MD [GO] - **Spec Exp:** Ovarian Cancer; Uterine Cancer; Cervical Cancer; Pap Smear Abnormalities; **Hospital:** Lankenau Hosp; **Address:** 100 E Lancaster Ave, Med Office Bldg East, Ste 661, Wynnewood, PA 19096; **Phone:** 610-649-8085; **Board Cert:** Obstetrics & Gynecology 2009; Gynecologic Oncology 2009; **Med School:** Jefferson Med Coll 1980; **Resid:** Obstetrics & Gynecology, Lankenau Hosp 1984; **Fellow:** Gynecologic Oncology, Hosp Univ Penn 1989; **Fac Appt:** Prof ObG, Jefferson Med Coll

Edwards, Robert P MD [GO] - **Spec Exp:** Ovarian Cancer; Gynecologic Cancer; Cervical Cancer; Clinical Trials; **Hospital:** Magee-Womens Hosp - UPMC; **Address:** UPP-Dept Women's Health, 300 Halket St, Ste 2130, Pittsburgh, PA 15213; **Phone:** 412-641-1153; **Board Cert:** Obstetrics & Gynecology 2009; Gynecologic Oncology 2009; **Med School:** Univ Pittsburgh 1984; **Resid:** Obstetrics & Gynecology, Magee WomensHosp-UPMC 1989; **Fellow:** Gynecologic Oncology, Univ Alabama Med Ctr 1993; **Fac Appt:** Prof ObG, Univ Pittsburgh

Fields, Abbie L MD [GO] - **Spec Exp:** Fertility Preservation in Cancer; Robotic Surgery; Cancer Genetics; Pelvic Reconstruction; **Hospital:** Washington Hosp Ctr; **Address:** Washington Hospital Center, 110 Irving St NW, rm 5B-33B, Washington, DC 20010; **Phone:** 202-877-2391; **Board Cert:** Obstetrics & Gynecology 2009; Gynecologic Oncology 2009; **Med School:** Ohio State Univ 1987; **Resid:** Obstetrics & Gynecology, Northwestern Univ 1991; **Fellow:** Gynecologic Oncology, Johns Hopkins Hosp 1993

Fishman, David A MD [GO] - **Spec Exp:** Ovarian Cancer; Ovarian Cancer-Early Detection; Gynecologic Cancer; **Hospital:** Mount Sinai Med Ctr (page 76); **Address:** 5 E 98th St Fl 2, New York, NY 10029; **Phone:** 212-427-9898; **Board Cert:** Obstetrics & Gynecology 2009; Gynecologic Oncology 2009; **Med School:** Texas Tech Univ 1988; **Resid:** Obstetrics & Gynecology, Yale-New Haven Hosp 1992; **Fellow:** Gynecologic Oncology, Yale-New Haven Hosp 1994; **Fac Appt:** Prof ObG, Mount Sinai Sch Med

Gynecologic Oncology

Follen, Michele MD/PhD [GO] - **Spec Exp:** Gynecologic Cancer; Clinical Trials; Cervical Cancer; **Hospital:** Hahnemann Univ Hosp; **Address:** 245 N 15th St NCB Bldg Fl 17 - Ste 17113, Phildelphia, PA 19102; **Phone:** 215-762-1257; **Med School:** Univ Mich Med Sch 1980; **Resid:** Obstetrics & Gynecology, Columbia-Presby Med Ctr 1983; **Fellow:** Gynecologic Oncology, MD Anderson Cancer Ctr 1986; **Fac Appt:** Prof ObG, Drexel Univ Coll Med

Giuntoli II, Robert Lawrence MD [GO] - **Spec Exp:** Gynecologic Cancer; Ovarian Cancer; Gestational Trophoblastic Disease; Immunotherapy; **Hospital:** Johns Hopkins Hosp; **Address:** Johns Hopkins Hosp, Div Gyn Onc, 600 N Wolfe St, Phipps #281, Baltimore, MD 21287-1281; **Phone:** 410-502-4245; **Board Cert:** Obstetrics & Gynecology 2005; Gynecologic Oncology 2005; **Med School:** Univ Pennsylvania 1994; **Resid:** Obstetrics & Gynecology, Duke Univ Med Ctr 1998; **Fellow:** Gynecologic Oncology, Mayo Clin 2002; **Fac Appt:** Asst Prof ObG, Johns Hopkins Univ

Herzog, Thomas J MD [GO] - **Spec Exp:** Cervical Cancer; Gynecologic Cancer; Laparoscopic Surgery; Ovarian Cancer; **Hospital:** NY-Presby Hosp/Columbia (page 78); **Address:** Herbert Irving Pavilion, 161 Fort Washington Ave, 8-837, New York, NY 10032; **Phone:** 212-305-3410; **Board Cert:** Obstetrics & Gynecology 2008; Gynecologic Oncology 2008; **Med School:** Univ Cincinnati 1986; **Resid:** Obstetrics & Gynecology, Good Samaritan Hosp 1990; **Fellow:** Gynecologic Oncology, Barnes Jewish Hosp 1993; **Fac Appt:** Prof ObG, Columbia P&S

Kelley III, Joseph L MD [GO] - **Spec Exp:** Breast Cancer; Ovarian Cancer; Cervical Cancer; Gynecologic Cancer; **Hospital:** Magee-Womens Hosp - UPMC; **Address:** Magee-Womens Hosp-UPMC, 300 Halket St, Ste 1750, Pittsburgh, PA 15213; **Phone:** 412-641-5411; **Board Cert:** Obstetrics & Gynecology 2009; Gynecologic Oncology 2008; **Med School:** St Louis Univ 1985; **Resid:** Obstetrics & Gynecology, Magee-Womens Hosp 1989; **Fellow:** Gynecologic Oncology, MD Anderson Cancer Ctr 1991; **Fac Appt:** Assoc Prof ObG, Univ Pittsburgh

King, Stephanie A MD [GO] - **Spec Exp:** Ovarian Cancer; Uterine Cancer; Cervical Cancer; Trophoblastic Tumors; **Hospital:** Fox Chase Cancer Ctr (page 72); **Address:** Fox Chase Cancer Ctr, Dept Gynecologic Oncology, 333 Cottman Ave, Philadelphia, PA 19111; **Phone:** 215-728-5628; **Board Cert:** Obstetrics & Gynecology 2009; Gynecologic Oncology 2009; **Med School:** Univ Pennsylvania 1983; **Resid:** Obstetrics & Gynecology, Hosp Univ Penn 1988; **Fac Appt:** Assoc Prof S, Drexel Univ Coll Med

Koulos, John P MD [GO] - **Spec Exp:** Uterine Cancer; Ovarian Cancer; Cervical Cancer; **Hospital:** Beth Israel Med Ctr - Petrie Division (page 71); **Address:** Beth Israel Hosp Cancer Ctr, 10 Union Square E, Ste 4C, New York, NY 10003; **Phone:** 212-844-5729; **Board Cert:** Obstetrics & Gynecology 2010; Gynecologic Oncology 2010; **Med School:** Northwestern Univ 1978; **Resid:** Obstetrics & Gynecology, Northwestern Univ Med Sch 1982; **Fellow:** Gynecologic Oncology, Meml Sloan Kettering Cancer Ctr 1984; **Fac Appt:** Assoc Prof ObG, Albert Einstein Coll Med

Lele, Shashikant B MD [GO] - **Spec Exp:** Ovarian Cancer; Reconstructive Surgery; Pelvic Surgery-Complex; **Hospital:** Roswell Park Cancer Inst, Buffalo General Hosp; **Address:** Roswell Park Cancer Inst, Dept Gynecology, Elm & Carlton Sts, Buffalo, NY 14263; **Phone:** 716-845-5776; **Board Cert:** Obstetrics & Gynecology 1976; Gynecologic Oncology 1979; **Med School:** India 1968; **Resid:** Obstetrics & Gynecology, JJ Hosp-Grant Med Ctr 1970; Obstetrics & Gynecology, Mt Sinai Hosp 1973; **Fellow:** Gynecologic Oncology, Roswell Park Cancer Inst 1976; **Fac Appt:** Clin Prof ObG, SUNY Buffalo

Lin, Jeffrey Y MD [GO] - **Spec Exp:** Gynecologic Cancer; Gynecologic Surgery; Cervical Cancer; Ovarian Cancer; **Hospital:** Sibley Mem Hosp; **Address:** Sibley Ctr for GYN Oncology, 5255 Loughboro Rd NW, Washington, DC 20016; **Phone:** 202-741-2552; **Board Cert:** Obstetrics & Gynecology 2009; Gynecologic Oncology 2009; **Med School:** Albany Med Coll 1984; **Resid:** Obstetrics & Gynecology, George Washington Med Ctr 1988; Gynecologic Oncology, Univ Rochester Affil Hosp 1991; **Fac Appt:** Prof ObG, Geo Wash Univ

Morgan, Mark A MD [GO] - **Spec Exp:** Laparoscopic Surgery; Gynecologic Surgery-Complex; Gynecologic Cancer; Robotic Surgery; **Hospital:** Fox Chase Cancer Ctr (page 72); **Address:** Fox Chase Cancer Ctr-Department of Surgery, 333 Cottman Ave, Philadelphia, PA 19111; **Phone:** 215-214-1430; **Board Cert:** Obstetrics & Gynecology 2009; **Med School:** SUNY Downstate 1982; **Resid:** Obstetrics & Gynecology, Hosp Univ Penn 1986; **Fellow:** Gynecologic Oncology, Hosp Univ Penn 1988; **Fac Appt:** Prof Med, Univ Pennsylvania

Odunsi, Adekunle O MD/PhD [GO] - **Spec Exp:** Ovarian Cancer; Immunotherapy; Clinical Trials; **Hospital:** Roswell Park Cancer Inst; **Address:** Roswell Park Cancer Inst, Gyn Oncology, Elm and Carlton Streets, Buffalo, NY 14263; **Phone:** 716-845-2300; **Board Cert:** Obstetrics & Gynecology 2004; Gynecologic Oncology 2004; **Med School:** Nigeria 1984; **Resid:** Obstetrics & Gynecology, Rosie Maternity & Addenbrookes Hosps 1990; Obstetrics & Gynecology, Yale-New Haven Hosp 1999; **Fellow:** Gynecologic Oncology, Roswell Park Cancer Inst 2001; **Fac Appt:** Prof ObG, SUNY Buffalo

Randall, Thomas C MD [GO] - **Spec Exp:** Gynecologic Cancer; Robotic Surgery; **Hospital:** Pennsylvania Hosp (page 80); **Address:** Pennsylvania Hospital, Dept OB/GYN, 801 Spruce St Fl 7, Philadelphia, PA 19107; **Phone:** 215-829-2345; **Board Cert:** Obstetrics & Gynecology 2009; Gynecologic Oncology 2009; **Med School:** Johns Hopkins Univ 1987; **Resid:** Obstetrics & Gynecology, Johns Hopkins Hosp 1991; **Fellow:** Gynecologic Oncology, Hosp Univ Penn 1992; **Fac Appt:** Assoc Prof ObG, Univ Pennsylvania

Rosenblum, Norman G MD/PhD [GO] - **Spec Exp:** Ovarian Cancer; Uterine Cancer; Vulvar Disease/Cancer; **Hospital:** Thomas Jefferson Univ Hosp (page 81); **Address:** 834 Chesnut St, Ste 400, Philadelphia, PA 19107-5127; **Phone:** 215-955-6200; **Board Cert:** Obstetrics & Gynecology 2010; Gynecologic Oncology 2010; **Med School:** Jefferson Med Coll 1978; **Resid:** Obstetrics & Gynecology, Hosp Univ Penn 1982; **Fellow:** Gynecologic Oncology, Hosp Univ Penn 1984; **Fac Appt:** Prof ObG, Jefferson Med Coll

Rubin, Stephen C MD [GO] - **Spec Exp:** Ovarian Cancer; Uterine Cancer; Cervical Cancer; **Hospital:** Hosp Univ Penn - UPHS (page 80); **Address:** Perelman Center, Jordan Ctr for Gynecologic Cancer, 3400 Civic Center Blvd Fl 3 W, Philadelphia, PA 19104-4283; **Phone:** 215-662-3318; **Board Cert:** Obstetrics & Gynecology 2011; Gynecologic Oncology 2011; **Med School:** Univ Pennsylvania 1976; **Resid:** Obstetrics & Gynecology, Hosp Univ Penn 1980; **Fellow:** Gynecologic Oncology, Hosp Univ Penn 1982; **Fac Appt:** Prof ObG, Univ Pennsylvania

Southeast

Alvarez, Ronald D MD [GO] - **Spec Exp:** Gynecologic Cancer; Ovarian Cancer; **Hospital:** Univ of Ala Hosp at Birmingham, Brookwood Med Ctr; **Address:** Univ Alabama, Div Gyn Oncology, 619 19th St S, 176F, Ste 10250, Birmingham, AL 35249; **Phone:** 205-934-4986; **Board Cert:** Obstetrics & Gynecology 2007; Gynecologic Oncology 2007; **Med School:** Louisiana State U, New Orleans 1983; **Resid:** Obstetrics & Gynecology, Univ Alabama Hosp 1987; **Fellow:** Gynecologic Oncology, Univ Alabama Hosp 1990; **Fac Appt:** Assoc Prof ObG, Univ Alabama

Berchuck, Andrew MD [GO] - **Spec Exp:** Ovarian Cancer; Uterine Cancer; **Hospital:** Duke Univ Hosp; **Address:** Duke Univ Med Center, DUMC Box 3079, Durham, NC 27710; **Phone:** 919-684-3765; **Board Cert:** Obstetrics & Gynecology 2009; Gynecologic Oncology 2009; **Med School:** Case West Res Univ 1980; **Resid:** Obstetrics & Gynecology, Case Western Reserve Univ Hosp 1984; **Fellow:** Gynecology, UT Southwestern Affil Hosp 1985; Gynecologic Oncology, Meml Sloan-Kettering Cancer Ctr 1987; **Fac Appt:** Prof ObG, Duke Univ

Gynecologic Oncology

Bicher, Annette MD [GO] - **Spec Exp:** Ovarian Cancer; Laparoscopic Surgery; **Hospital:** Inova Fairfax Hosp; **Address:** 3289 Woodburn Rd, Ste 320, Annandale, VA 22003; **Phone:** 703-698-7100; **Board Cert:** Obstetrics & Gynecology 2009; Gynecologic Oncology 2009; **Med School:** Univ Mich Med Sch 1987; **Resid:** Obstetrics & Gynecology, George Washington Univ Med Ctr 1991; **Fellow:** Research, NCI-NIH 1992; Gynecologic Oncology, UT MD Anderson Cancer Ctr 1994

Clarke-Pearson, Daniel L MD [GO] - **Spec Exp:** Pelvic Reconstruction; Gynecologic Surgery-Complex; Gynecologic Cancer; **Hospital:** NC Memorial Hosp - UNC, Wesley Long Comm Hosp; **Address:** NC Women's Hospital, 101 Manning Drive, MS 27599, Chapel Hill, NC 27599; **Phone:** 919-966-5280; **Board Cert:** Obstetrics & Gynecology 2006; Gynecologic Oncology 2006; **Med School:** Case West Res Univ 1975; **Resid:** Obstetrics & Gynecology, Duke Univ Med Ctr 1979; **Fellow:** Gynecologic Oncology, Duke Univ Med Ctr 1981; **Fac Appt:** Prof ObG, Univ NC Sch Med

Creasman, William T MD [GO] - **Spec Exp:** Uterine Cancer; Ovarian Cancer; Cervical Cancer; Gynecologic Cancer-Rare; **Hospital:** MUSC Med Ctr; **Address:** Med Univ S Carolina-Dept ObGyn, Charleston, SC 29425; **Phone:** 843-792-4509; **Board Cert:** Obstetrics & Gynecology 1991; Gynecologic Oncology 1974; **Med School:** Baylor Coll Med 1960; **Resid:** Obstetrics & Gynecology, Rochester Med Ctr 1967; **Fellow:** Gynecologic Oncology, Anderson Hosp Tumor Inst 1969; **Fac Appt:** Prof ObG, Med Univ SC

Currie, John L MD [GO] - **Spec Exp:** Gynecologic Cancer; Pelvic Reconstruction; **Hospital:** Columbus Regl Med Ctr; **Address:** John B Amos Cancer Center, 1831 5th Ave, Columbus, GA 31904; **Phone:** 706-320-8700; **Board Cert:** Obstetrics & Gynecology 1991; Gynecologic Oncology 1982; **Med School:** Univ NC Sch Med 1967; **Resid:** Gynecologic Oncology, Hosp Univ Penn 1972; **Fellow:** Gynecologic Oncology, Duke Univ Med Ctr 1980

DePriest, Paul D MD [GO] - **Spec Exp:** Ovarian Cancer-Early Detection; Cervical Cancer; Pap Smear Abnormalities; **Hospital:** Univ of Kentucky Albert B. Chandler Hosp; **Address:** Univ Kentucky Gynecologic Oncology, Whiteney Hendrickson Bldg, 800 Rose St, rm 331E1, Lexington, KY 40536; **Phone:** 859-323-5277; **Board Cert:** Obstetrics & Gynecology 2009; Gynecologic Oncology 2009; **Med School:** Univ KY Coll Med 1985; **Resid:** Obstetrics & Gynecology, Univ Kentucky Med Ctr 1989; **Fellow:** Gynecologic Oncology, Univ Kentucky Med Ctr 1991; **Fac Appt:** Prof ObG, Univ KY Coll Med

Duska, Linda R MD [GO] - **Spec Exp:** Cervical Cancer; Gynecologic Cancer; Gynecologic Surgery-Complex; Ovarian Cancer; **Hospital:** Univ of Virginia Health Sys; **Address:** Dept of Obstetrics & Gynecology, Division of Gynecologic Oncology, P. O. Box 800712, Charlottesville, VA 22908; **Phone:** 434-924-1851; **Board Cert:** Obstetrics & Gynecology 2009; Gynecologic Oncology 2009; **Med School:** NYU Sch Med 1991; **Resid:** Obstetrics & Gynecology, John Hopkins Hosp 1995; **Fellow:** Gynecologic Oncology, MA Gen Hosp 1998; **Fac Appt:** Assoc Prof ObG, Univ VA Sch Med

Finan, Michael A MD [GO] - **Spec Exp:** Ovarian Cancer; Cervical Cancer; Uterine Cancer; **Hospital:** Univ of S AL Med Ctr, Univ of S Alabama Chil and Wom Hosp; **Address:** 1660 Springhill Ave, Mobile, AL 36604; **Phone:** 251-665-8000; **Board Cert:** Obstetrics & Gynecology 2008; Gynecologic Oncology 2008; **Med School:** Louisiana State U, New Orleans 1986; **Resid:** Obstetrics & Gynecology, Univ South Fla Affil Hosps 1990; **Fellow:** Gynecologic Oncology, H Lee Moffitt Cancer Ctr 1992; **Fac Appt:** Prof ObG, Univ S Ala Coll Med

Fiorica, James V MD [GO] - **Spec Exp:** Breast Cancer; Uterine Cancer; **Hospital:** Sarasota Meml Hosp; **Address:** 1888 Hillview St, Sarasota, FL 34239; **Phone:** 941-917-8383; **Board Cert:** Obstetrics & Gynecology 2009; Gynecologic Oncology 2009; **Med School:** Tufts Univ 1982; **Resid:** Obstetrics & Gynecology, Univ South Fla Affil Hosp 1986; **Fellow:** Gynecologic Oncology, Univ South Fla Affil Hosp 1989; Breast Disease, Tufts Univ 1990; **Fac Appt:** Clin Prof ObG, Univ S Fla Coll Med

Fowler Jr, Wesley C MD [GO] - **Spec Exp:** Vulvar Disease/Cancer; DES-Exposed Females; Cancer Prevention; Gynecologic Cancer; **Hospital:** NC Memorial Hosp - UNC; **Address:** UNC Chapel Hill, Div Ob/Gyn, Campus Box 7572, Chapel Hill, NC 27599-7572; **Phone:** 919-966-7822; **Board Cert:** Obstetrics & Gynecology 1991; Gynecologic Oncology 1979; **Med School:** Univ NC Sch Med 1966; **Resid:** Obstetrics & Gynecology, NC Memorial Hosp 1971; **Fellow:** Gynecologic Oncology, NC Memorial Hosp 1971; **Fac Appt:** Prof ObG, Univ NC Sch Med

Ghamande, Sharad A MD [GO] - **Spec Exp:** Ovarian Cancer; Gynecologic Surgery-Complex; Clinical Trials; **Hospital:** Med Coll of GA Hosp and Clin (MCG Health Inc), Univ HC Sys - Augusta; **Address:** MCG Health Cancer Centr, 1411 Laney Walker Blvd, Augusta, GA 30912; **Phone:** 706-721-6744; **Board Cert:** Obstetrics & Gynecology 2010; Gynecologic Oncology 2010; **Med School:** India 1990; **Resid:** Obstetrics & Gynecology, Boston Univ Hosp 1997; **Fellow:** Gynecologic Oncology, Roswell Park Cancer Inst 2000; **Fac Appt:** Assoc Prof ObG, Med Coll GA

Havrilesky, Laura J MD [GO] - **Spec Exp:** Ovarian Cancer; **Hospital:** Duke Univ Hosp; **Address:** Duke Univ Med Ctr, Gyno Oncology, Box 3079, Durham, NC 27710; **Phone:** 919-684-3765; **Board Cert:** Obstetrics & Gynecology 2005; Gynecologic Oncology 2005; **Med School:** Duke Univ 1995; **Resid:** Obstetrics & Gynecology, Duke Univ Med Ctr 1999; **Fellow:** Gynecologic Oncology, Duke Univ Med Ctr 2002; **Fac Appt:** Assoc Prof ObG, Duke Univ

Horowitz, Ira R MD [GO] - **Spec Exp:** Laparoscopic Surgery; Ovarian Cancer; Cervical Cancer; **Hospital:** Emory Univ Hosp, Emory Univ Hosp Midtown; **Address:** Emory Clinic, 1365A Clifton Rd NE, Fl 4, Atlanta, GA 30322; **Phone:** 404-778-3401; **Board Cert:** Obstetrics & Gynecology 2010; Gynecologic Oncology 2010; **Med School:** Baylor Coll Med 1980; **Resid:** Obstetrics & Gynecology, Baylor Affil Hosp 1984; **Fellow:** Gynecologic Oncology, Johns Hopkins Hosp 1987; **Fac Appt:** Prof ObG, Emory Univ

Kohler, Matthew F MD [GO] - **Spec Exp:** Gynecologic Surgery-Complex; **Hospital:** MUSC Med Ctr; **Address:** MUSC Med Ctr- Women's Hlth Ob/Gyn, 86 Jonathan Lucas St, MS 957, Charleston, SC 29425; **Phone:** 843-792-9300; **Board Cert:** Obstetrics & Gynecology 2009; Gynecologic Oncology 2009; **Med School:** Duke Univ 1987; **Resid:** Obstetrics & Gynecology, Duke Univ Med Ctr 1991; **Fellow:** Gynecologic Oncology, Duke Univ Med Ctr 1994; **Fac Appt:** Prof ObG, Med Univ SC

Lancaster, Johnathan M MD/PhD [GO] - **Spec Exp:** Ovarian Cancer; Cancer Genetics; Gene Therapy; **Hospital:** H Lee Moffitt Cancer Ctr & Research Inst; **Address:** H Lee Moffitt Cancer Ctr - Gyn Oncology, 12902 Magnolia Drive, The Ctr for Women's Oncology, Tampa, FL 33612; **Phone:** 888-860-2778; **Board Cert:** Obstetrics & Gynecology 2008; Gynecologic Oncology 2008; **Med School:** Wales, UK 1997; **Resid:** Obstetrics & Gynecology, Duke Univ Med Ctr 2000; **Fellow:** Gynecologic Oncology, Duke Univ Med Ctr 2003; **Fac Appt:** Asst Prof ObG, Univ S Fla Coll Med

Lentz, Samuel S MD [GO] - **Spec Exp:** Gynecologic Cancer; Pelvic Reconstruction; Incontinence-Fecal; **Hospital:** Wake Forest Univ Baptist Med Ctr, Forsyth Med Ctr; **Address:** Wake Forest Univ Sch Med, Div Gyn Oncology, Medical Center Blvd, Winston-Salem, NC 27157; **Phone:** 336-716-6673; **Board Cert:** Obstetrics & Gynecology 2008; Gynecologic Oncology 2010; **Med School:** Wake Forest Univ 1978; **Resid:** Obstetrics & Gynecology, NC Baptist Hosp 1982; **Fellow:** Gynecologic Oncology, Mayo Clinic 1989; **Fac Appt:** Prof ObG, Wake Forest Univ

Lucci, Joseph A MD [GO] - **Spec Exp:** Cervical Cancer; **Hospital:** Univ of Miami Hosp & Clins/Sylvester Comp Canc Ctr (page 82), Jackson Meml Hosp (page 82); **Address:** UMHC Sylvester Comp Cancer Ctr, 1475 NW 12th Ave, Ste 3500, Miami, FL 33136; **Phone:** 305-243-2233; **Board Cert:** Obstetrics & Gynecology 2007; Gynecologic Oncology 2007; **Med School:** Univ Tex, Houston 1984; **Resid:** Obstetrics & Gynecology, St Josephs Hosp 1988; **Fellow:** Gynecologic Oncology, UC Irvine 1992; **Fac Appt:** Clin Prof ObG, Univ Miami Sch Med

Gynecologic Oncology

Makhija, Sharmila K MD [GO] - **Spec Exp:** Ovarian Cancer; Cervical Cancer; Uterine Cancer; **Hospital:** Emory Univ Hosp; **Address:** The Emory Clinic Bldg A, 1365 Clifton Rd NE Fl 4, Atlanta, GA 30322; **Phone:** 404-778-3401; **Board Cert:** Obstetrics & Gynecology 2009; Gynecologic Oncology 2009; **Med School:** Univ Alabama 1992; **Resid:** Obstetrics & Gynecology, Univ Louisville Hosp 1996; **Fellow:** Gynecologic Oncology, Meml Sloan Kettering Cancer Ctr 1999; **Fac Appt:** Assoc Prof ObG, Emory Univ

Modesitt, Susan C MD [GO] - **Spec Exp:** Gynecologic Cancer; Ovarian Cancer; Vulvar Disease/Cancer; **Hospital:** Univ of Virginia Health Sys; **Address:** Div Gynecologic Oncology, P.O. Box 800712, Charlottesville, VA 22908-0712; **Phone:** 434-924-5197; **Board Cert:** Obstetrics & Gynecology 2005; Gynecologic Oncology 2005; **Med School:** Univ VA Sch Med 1995; **Resid:** Obstetrics & Gynecology, Univ NC Hlth Care System 1999; **Fellow:** Gynecologic Oncology, Univ TX- M.D. Anderson Cancer Ctr 2002; **Fac Appt:** Assoc Prof ObG, Univ VA Sch Med

Orr Jr, James W MD [GO] - **Spec Exp:** Gynecologic Cancer; **Hospital:** Lee Memorial Hlth Systems; **Address:** 8931 Colonial Ctr Drive, Ste 400, Fort Myers, FL 33905; **Phone:** 239-334-6626; **Board Cert:** Obstetrics & Gynecology 2008; Gynecologic Oncology 2008; **Med School:** Univ VA Sch Med 1976; **Resid:** Obstetrics & Gynecology, Univ Ala Med Ctr 1980; **Fellow:** Gynecologic Oncology, Univ Ala Med Ctr 1982; **Fac Appt:** Clin Prof ObG, Univ S Fla Coll Med

Penalver, Manuel A MD [GO] - **Spec Exp:** Gynecologic Cancer; Cervical Cancer; Pelvic Tumors; **Hospital:** Doctors' Hosp, Baptist Hosp of Miami; **Address:** South Florida Gyn Oncology, 5000 University Drive, Ste 3300, Coral Gables, FL 33146; **Phone:** 305-663-7001; **Board Cert:** Obstetrics & Gynecology 2009; Gynecologic Oncology 2009; **Med School:** Univ Miami Sch Med 1977; **Resid:** Obstetrics & Gynecology, Univ Miami/Jackson Meml Hosp 1982; **Fellow:** Gynecologic Oncology, Univ Miami/Jackson Meml Hosp 1984

Poliakoff, Steven R MD [GO] - **Spec Exp:** Ovarian Cancer; Minimally Invasive Surgery; Cancer Genetics; Robotic Surgery; **Hospital:** Mount Sinai Med Ctr - Miami, South Miami Hosp; **Address:** 6280 Sunset Dr, Ste 502, South Miami, FL 33143-4870; **Phone:** 305-596-0870; **Board Cert:** Obstetrics & Gynecology 1983; **Med School:** Univ NC Sch Med 1975; **Resid:** Obstetrics & Gynecology, Johns Hopkins Hosp 1979; **Fellow:** Gynecologic Oncology, Jackson Meml Hosp/Univ Miami 1981

Runowicz, Carolyn MD [GO] - **Spec Exp:** Ovarian Cancer; Cervical Cancer; Breast Cancer; **Hospital:** Jackson N Med Ctr (page 82); **Address:** 11200 S W 8th St SW, AHC2 Bldg Fl 6 - Ste 693, Miami, FL 33199; **Phone:** 305-348-0570; **Board Cert:** Obstetrics & Gynecology 2009; Gynecologic Oncology 2009; **Med School:** Jefferson Med Coll 1977; **Resid:** Obstetrics & Gynecology, Mount Sinai Med Ctr 1981; **Fellow:** Gynecologic Oncology, Mount Sinai Med Ctr 1983; **Fac Appt:** Prof ObG, Univ Conn

Soper, John T MD [GO] - **Spec Exp:** Gynecologic Cancer; Gynecologic Surgery-Complex; Gestational Trophoblastic Disease; **Hospital:** NC Memorial Hosp - UNC, Rex HlthCare; **Address:** Div Gyn-Onc, Dept OB/GYN, B110 Physicians Office Bldg, 170 Manning Drive, Chapel Hill, NC 27599-7572; **Phone:** 919-966-1195; **Board Cert:** Obstetrics & Gynecology 2009; Gynecologic Oncology 2009; **Med School:** Univ Iowa Coll Med 1978; **Resid:** Obstetrics & Gynecology, Univ Utah Med Ctr 1982; **Fellow:** Obstetrics & Gynecology, Duke Univ Med Ctr 1985; **Fac Appt:** Prof ObG, Univ NC Sch Med

Spann Jr, Cyril O MD [GO] - **Spec Exp:** Gynecologic Cancer; Ovarian Cancer; **Hospital:** Grady Hlth Sys, Emory Univ Hosp Midtown; **Address:** Dept Gynecology & Obstetrics, 69 Jesse Hill Jr Drive, Ste 400, Atlanta, GA 30303; **Phone:** 404-778-3401; **Board Cert:** Obstetrics & Gynecology 2005; Gynecologic Oncology 2005; **Med School:** Meharry Med Coll 1981; **Resid:** Obstetrics & Gynecology, Emory Univ Med Ctr 1985; **Fellow:** Gynecologic Oncology, Univ NC Meml Hosp 1989; **Fac Appt:** Prof ObG, Emory Univ

Taylor Jr, Peyton T MD [GO] - **Spec Exp:** Gynecologic Cancer; Gynecologic Surgery-Complex; **Hospital:** Univ of Virginia Health Sys; **Address:** Lee St, Cancer Cen Bldg, PO Box 800712, Charlottesville, VA 22908; **Phone:** 434-924-9933; **Board Cert:** Obstetrics & Gynecology 1994; Gynecologic Oncology 1981; **Med School:** Univ Alabama 1968; **Resid:** Obstetrics & Gynecology, Univ VA Hosp 1970; Obstetrics & Gynecology, Univ VA Hosp 1975; **Fellow:** Surgical Oncology, Natl Cancer Inst 1972; Gynecologic Oncology, Univ Va Hosp 1977; **Fac Appt:** Prof ObG, Univ VA Sch Med

Valea, Fidel A MD [GO] - **Spec Exp:** Cervical Cancer; Laparoscopic Surgery; **Hospital:** Duke Univ Hosp; **Address:** Duke Univ Med Ctr, Box 3079, Durham, NC 27710; **Phone:** 919-664-3725; **Board Cert:** Obstetrics & Gynecology 2007; Gynecologic Oncology 2007; **Med School:** SUNY Stony Brook 1985; **Resid:** Surgery, Univ NC Hosps 1987; Obstetrics & Gynecology, Univ NC Hosps 1990; **Fellow:** Gynecologic Oncology, Univ NC Hosps 1992; **Fac Appt:** Assoc Prof ObG, Duke Univ

Van Nagell Jr, John R MD [GO] - **Spec Exp:** Ovarian Cancer; Cervical Cancer; **Hospital:** Univ of Kentucky Albert B. Chandler Hosp; **Address:** 800 Rose St, Lexington, KY 40536-0001; **Phone:** 859-323-5553; **Board Cert:** Obstetrics & Gynecology 1973; Gynecologic Oncology 1976; **Med School:** Univ Pennsylvania 1967; **Resid:** Obstetrics & Gynecology, Univ Kentucky Med Ctr 1971; **Fellow:** Gynecologic Oncology, Univ Kentucky Med Ctr 1973; **Fac Appt:** Prof ObG, Univ KY Coll Med

Midwest

Cliby, William A MD [GO] - **Spec Exp:** Ovarian Cancer; **Hospital:** Mayo Med Ctr & Clin - Rochester; **Address:** Mayo Clinic, 200 First St SW, Rochester, MN 55905; **Phone:** 507-266-9323; **Board Cert:** Obstetrics & Gynecology 2009; Gynecologic Oncology 2009; **Med School:** Univ VT Coll Med 1987; **Resid:** Obstetrics & Gynecology, Duke Univ Med Ctr 1991; **Fellow:** Gynecologic Oncology, Mayo Clinic 1994; Research, Fred Hutchinson Cancer Rsch Ctr; **Fac Appt:** Prof ObG, Mayo Med Sch

Copeland, Larry J MD [GO] - **Spec Exp:** Ovarian Cancer; Uterine Cancer; Gynecologic Cancer; Gynecologic Cancer-Rare; **Hospital:** Arthur G James Cancer Hosp & Research Inst, Ohio St Univ Med Ctr; **Address:** 320 W 10th Ave, Starling L Bldg, Ste 210, Columbus, OH 43210; **Phone:** 614-293-7642; **Board Cert:** Obstetrics & Gynecology 1991; Gynecologic Oncology 1981; **Med School:** Univ Western Ontario 1973; **Resid:** Obstetrics & Gynecology, McMaster Univ Affil Hosps 1977; **Fellow:** Gynecologic Oncology, MD Anderson Cancer Ctr-Univ Tex 1979; **Fac Appt:** Prof ObG, Ohio State Univ

De Geest, Koen MD [GO] - **Spec Exp:** Ovarian Cancer; Uterine Cancer; Clinical Trials; **Hospital:** Univ Iowa Hosp & Clinics; **Address:** Univ Iowa, Div Gynecological Oncology, 200 Hawkins Drive, rm 4630 JCP, Iowa City, IA 52242; **Phone:** 319-356-2015; **Board Cert:** Obstetrics & Gynecology 2008; Gynecologic Oncology 2008; **Med School:** Belgium 1977; **Resid:** Obstetrics & Gynecology, Univ Ghent 1982; **Fellow:** Gynecologic Oncology, Penn State/Hershey Med Ctr 1990; **Fac Appt:** Prof ObG, Univ Iowa Coll Med

Del Priore, Giuseppe MD [GO] - **Spec Exp:** Fertility Preservation in Cancer; **Hospital:** IU Health University Hosp; **Address:** 535 Barnhill Drive, RT 433, Indianapolis, IN 46202; **Phone:** 317-944-2130; **Board Cert:** Obstetrics & Gynecology 2010; Gynecologic Oncology 2010; **Med School:** SUNY Downstate 1987; **Resid:** Obstetrics & Gynecology, Northwestern Meml Hosp 1991; **Fellow:** Gynecologic Oncology, Univ Rochester-Strong Meml 1995; **Fac Appt:** Prof ObG, Indiana Univ

Gynecologic Oncology

Fowler, Jeffrey M MD [GO] - **Spec Exp:** Laparoscopic Surgery; Gynecologic Cancer; Robotic Surgery; Pelvic Reconstruction; **Hospital:** Ohio St Univ Med Ctr; **Address:** Ohio State Univ, Div Gynecologic Oncology, 320 W Tenth Ave, M-210 SLH, Columbus, OH 43210; **Phone:** 614-293-3873; **Board Cert:** Obstetrics & Gynecology 2009; Gynecologic Oncology 2009; **Med School:** Northwestern Univ 1985; **Resid:** Obstetrics & Gynecology, Ohio State Univ Hosp 1989; **Fellow:** Gynecologic Oncology, Cedars-Sinai Med Ctr 1991; **Fac Appt:** Prof ObG, Ohio State Univ

Johnston, Carolyn M MD [GO] - **Spec Exp:** Gynecologic Surgery-Complex; Cervical Cancer; **Hospital:** Univ of Michigan Hosp; **Address:** Womens Hosp-Div Gyn Oncology, 1500 E Med Ctr Drive, rm L4510, Ann Arbor, MI 48109-0276; **Phone:** 734-647-8906; **Board Cert:** Obstetrics & Gynecology 2000; Gynecologic Oncology 2000; **Med School:** Yale Univ 1984; **Resid:** Obstetrics & Gynecology, Univ Chicago Hosp 1988; **Fellow:** Gynecologic Oncology, Mt Sinai Hosp 1990; **Fac Appt:** Assoc Clin Prof ObG, Univ Mich Med Sch

Lurain, John R MD [GO] - **Spec Exp:** Gestational Trophoblastic Disease; Uterine Cancer; Ovarian Cancer; Cervical Cancer; **Hospital:** Northwestern Meml Hosp; **Address:** Northwestern Medical Faculty Foundation, 250 E Superior St, Ste 04-420, Chicago, IL 60611-3056; **Phone:** 312-695-0990; **Board Cert:** Obstetrics & Gynecology 1977; Gynecologic Oncology 1981; **Med School:** Univ NC Sch Med 1972; **Resid:** Obstetrics & Gynecology, Univ Pittsburgh Magee-Womens Hosp 1975; **Fellow:** Gynecologic Oncology, Roswell Park Cancer Inst 1979; **Fac Appt:** Prof ObG, Northwestern Univ

Moore, David H MD [GO] - **Spec Exp:** Cervical Cancer; Ovarian Cancer; Laparoscopic Surgery; Robotic Surgery; **Hospital:** Franciscan St. Francis Hlth-Indianapolis, Franciscan St. Francis Hlth-Beech Grove; **Address:** Gynecologic Oncology of Indianapolis, 5255 E Stop 11 Rd, Ste 310, Indianapolis, IN 46237; **Phone:** 317-851-2555; **Board Cert:** Obstetrics & Gynecology 2009; Gynecologic Oncology 2009; **Med School:** Indiana Univ 1982; **Resid:** Obstetrics & Gynecology, Indiana Univ Hosp 1986; **Fellow:** Gynecologic Oncology, Univ N Carolina 1988

Mutch, David G MD [GO] - **Spec Exp:** Gynecologic Cancer; Pelvic Reconstruction; **Hospital:** Barnes-Jewish Hosp; **Address:** 4911 Barnes Jewish Hosp Plaza, CB 8064, St Louis, MO 63110; **Phone:** 314-362-3181; **Board Cert:** Obstetrics & Gynecology 2006; Gynecologic Oncology 2006; **Med School:** Washington Univ, St Louis 1980; **Resid:** Obstetrics & Gynecology, Barnes Hosp-Wash Univ 1984; **Fellow:** Gynecologic Oncology, Duke Univ Med Ctr 1987; **Fac Appt:** Prof ObG, Washington Univ, St Louis

Potkul, Ronald K MD [GO] - **Spec Exp:** Ovarian Cancer; Cervical Cancer; Robotic Surgery; Vulvar/Vaginal Cancer; **Hospital:** Loyola Univ Med Ctr; **Address:** Loyola Univ Med Ctr, 2160 S 1st Ave Bldg 112 - rm 267, Maywood, IL 60153; **Phone:** 708-327-3500; **Board Cert:** Obstetrics & Gynecology 2010; Gynecologic Oncology 2010; **Med School:** Univ Chicago-Pritzker Sch Med 1981; **Resid:** Obstetrics & Gynecology, Univ Chicago Hosps 1985; **Fellow:** Gynecologic Oncology, Georgetown Univ Hosp 1988; **Fac Appt:** Prof ObG, Loyola Univ-Stritch Sch Med

Rader, Janet S MD [GO] - **Spec Exp:** Cervical Cancer; Ovarian Cancer; Uterine Cancer; **Hospital:** Froedtert and Med Ctr of WI; **Address:** Med Coll of Wisconsin, Dept OB/GYN, 9200 W Wisconsin Ave, Milwaukee, WI 53226; **Phone:** 414-805-6606; **Board Cert:** Obstetrics & Gynecology 2009; Gynecologic Oncology 2009; **Med School:** Univ MO-Columbia Sch Med 1983; **Resid:** Obstetrics & Gynecology, Michael Reese Hosp 1987; **Fellow:** Gynecologic Oncology, Johns Hopkins Hosp 1990; **Fac Appt:** Prof ObG, Washington Univ, St Louis

Reynolds, R Kevin MD [GO] - **Hospital:** Univ of Michigan Hosp; **Address:** Women's Hosp, Div Gyn Onc, 1500 E Med Ctr Drive, rm L4510, Ann Arbor, MI 48109-0276; **Phone:** 734-764-9106; **Board Cert:** Obstetrics & Gynecology 2009; Gynecologic Oncology 2009; **Med School:** Univ New Mexico 1982; **Resid:** Obstetrics & Gynecology, Univ Vt Hosp 1986; **Fellow:** Gynecologic Oncology, Univ Mich Med Ctr 1991; **Fac Appt:** Asst Prof ObG, Univ Mich Med Sch

Rice, Laurel W MD [GO] - **Spec Exp:** Ovarian Cancer; Uterine Cancer; Cervical Cancer; **Hospital:** Univ WI Hosp & Clins; **Address:** 600 Highland Ave, Ste H4-636, Madison, WI 53792; **Phone:** 608-263-3194; **Board Cert:** Obstetrics & Gynecology 2006; Gynecologic Oncology 2006; **Med School:** Univ Colorado 1983; **Resid:** Obstetrics & Gynecology, Brigham-Womens Hosp 1987; **Fellow:** Obstetrics & Gynecology, Brigham-Womens Hosp 1989; **Fac Appt:** Assoc Prof ObG, Univ VA Sch Med

Rose, Peter G MD [GO] - **Spec Exp:** Cervical Cancer; Ovarian Cancer; Uterine Cancer; **Hospital:** Cleveland Clin (page 70), MetroHealth Med Ctr; **Address:** Cleveland Clin Fdn, 9500 Euclid Ave A-81, Cleveland, OH 44195; **Phone:** 216-444-1712; **Board Cert:** Obstetrics & Gynecology 2009; Gynecologic Oncology 2009; **Med School:** Boston Univ 1981; **Resid:** Surgery, Vanderbilt Univ Med Ctr 1983; Obstetrics & Gynecology, Ohio State Univ Med Ctr 1986; **Fellow:** Gynecologic Oncology, Roswell Park Cancer Inst 1988; **Fac Appt:** Prof ObG, Case West Res Univ

Rotmensch, Jacob MD [GO] - **Spec Exp:** Gynecologic Cancer; Ovarian Cancer; Cervical Cancer; Uterine Cancer; **Hospital:** Rush Univ Med Ctr; **Address:** Univ Gynecologic Oncology Assocs, 1725 W Harrison St, Professional Bldg, Ste 842, Chicago, IL 60612; **Phone:** 312-942-6300; **Board Cert:** Obstetrics & Gynecology 2009; Gynecologic Oncology 2008; **Med School:** Meharry Med Coll 1977; **Resid:** Obstetrics & Gynecology, Johns Hopkins Hosp 1981; **Fellow:** Gynecologic Oncology, Johns Hopkins Hosp 1984; **Fac Appt:** Prof ObG, Rush Med Coll

Schink, Julian C MD [GO] - **Spec Exp:** Ovarian Cancer; **Hospital:** Northwestern Meml Hosp; **Address:** Northwestern Medical Faculty Foundation, 250 E Superior St, Ste 04-420, Chicago, IL 60611; **Phone:** 312-695-0990; **Board Cert:** Obstetrics & Gynecology 2010; Gynecologic Oncology 2010; **Med School:** Univ Tex, San Antonio 1982; **Resid:** Obstetrics & Gynecology, Northwestern Univ Med Sch 1986; **Fellow:** Gynecologic Oncology, UCLA Med Ctr 1988; **Fac Appt:** Prof ObG, Northwestern Univ

Smith, Donna M MD [GO] - **Spec Exp:** Cervical Cancer; Ovarian Cancer; **Hospital:** Loyola Univ Med Ctr; **Address:** Loyola Univ Medical Ctr, 2160 S 1st Ave Bldg 112 - rm 267, Maywood, IL 60153; **Phone:** 708-327-3500; **Board Cert:** Obstetrics & Gynecology 2007; Gynecologic Oncology 2007; **Med School:** Univ MO-Kansas City 1980; **Resid:** Obstetrics & Gynecology, Emory Univ Hosp 1984; **Fellow:** Gynecologic Oncology, Georgetown Univ Med Ctr 1987; **Fac Appt:** Assoc Prof ObG, Loyola Univ-Stritch Sch Med

Stehman, Frederick B MD [GO] - **Spec Exp:** Clinical Trials; Gynecologic Cancer; **Hospital:** IU Health Methodist Hosp, Wishard Hlth Srvs; **Address:** Indiana Univ Cancer Pavilion, 535 Barnhill Drive, rm 436, Indianapolis, IN 46202; **Phone:** 317-278-7583; **Board Cert:** Obstetrics & Gynecology 2005; Gynecologic Oncology 2003; **Med School:** Univ Mich Med Sch 1972; **Resid:** Obstetrics & Gynecology, Univ Kansas Med Ctr 1975; Surgery, Univ Kansas Med Ctr 1977; **Fellow:** Gynecologic Oncology, UCLA Med Ctr 1979; **Fac Appt:** Prof ObG, Indiana Univ

Waggoner, Steven MD [GO] - **Spec Exp:** Ovarian Cancer; Cervical Cancer; Uterine Cancer; **Hospital:** Univ Hosps Case Med Ctr; **Address:** Dept Ob/Gyn & Gyn Oncology, 11100 Euclid Ave, rm 7128, UH MacDonald Women's Hospital, Cleveland, OH 44106; **Phone:** 216-844-3954; **Board Cert:** Obstetrics & Gynecology 2008; Gynecologic Oncology 2008; **Med School:** Univ Wash 1984; **Resid:** Obstetrics & Gynecology, Univ Chicago Hosps 1988; **Fellow:** Gynecologic Oncology, Georgetown Univ 1991; **Fac Appt:** Prof ObG, Case West Res Univ

Gynecologic Oncology

Great Plains and Mountains

Davidson, Susan MD [GO] - **Spec Exp:** Gynecologic Cancer; **Hospital:** Univ of CO Hosp - Anschutz Inpatient Pav; **Address:** Univ Colorado Hosp, Dept OB/GYN, PO Box 6510- F704, 1665 Aurora Ct, Denver, CO 80045; **Phone:** 720-848-0300; **Board Cert:** Obstetrics & Gynecology 2009; Gynecologic Oncology 2009; **Med School:** Univ Tex, San Antonio 1984; **Resid:** Obstetrics & Gynecology, Univ Texas Med Ctr 1988; **Fellow:** Gynecologic Oncology, Meml Sloan Kettering Cancer Ctr 1990; **Fac Appt:** Assoc Prof ObG, Univ Colorado

Remmenga, Steven W MD [GO] - **Spec Exp:** Ovarian Cancer; Cervical Cancer; Gynecologic Cancer; **Hospital:** Nebraska Med Ctr; **Address:** Department of Obsterics nd Gynecology, MS 0, 983255 Nebraska Med Ctr, Omaha, NE 68198-3255; **Phone:** 402-559-5068; **Board Cert:** Obstetrics & Gynecology 1998; Gynecologic Oncology 1998; **Med School:** Univ Nebr Coll Med 1981; **Resid:** Obstetrics & Gynecology, Naval Hospital 1986; **Fellow:** Gynecologic Oncology, Walter Reed Army Med Ctr 1990; **Fac Appt:** Prof ObG, Univ Nebr Coll Med

Soisson, Andrew P MD [GO] - **Spec Exp:** Cervical Cancer; HPV-Human Papilloma Virus; **Hospital:** LDS Hosp, Univ Utah Hlth Care; **Address:** Huntsman Cancer Hosp, 1950 Circle of Hope, Salt Lake City, UT 84112; **Phone:** 801-585-0100; **Board Cert:** Obstetrics & Gynecology 2006; Gynecologic Oncology 2006; **Med School:** Georgetown Univ 1981; **Resid:** Obstetrics & Gynecology, Madigan AMC 1985; **Fellow:** Gynecologic Oncology, Duke Univ Med Ctr 1990; **Fac Appt:** Assoc Prof ObG, Univ Utah

Southwest

Bodurka, Diane C MD [GO] - **Spec Exp:** Ovarian Cancer; Pelvic Surgery-Complex; **Hospital:** UT MD Anderson Cancer Ctr; **Address:** Univ Texas M.D. Anderson Cancer Center Dept of Gynecologic Oncology, 1155 Herman Pressler, Houston, TX 77030-4000; **Phone:** 713-745-3358; **Board Cert:** Gynecologic Oncology 2009; Obstetrics & Gynecology 2009; **Med School:** Georgetown Univ 1990; **Resid:** Obstetrics & Gynecology, Univ Alabama Hosp 1994; **Fellow:** Gynecologic Oncology, MD Anderson Cancer Ctr 1996; **Fac Appt:** Prof ObG, Univ Tex, Houston

Burke, Thomas W MD [GO] - **Spec Exp:** Uterine Cancer; Vulvar & Vaginal Cancer; **Hospital:** UT MD Anderson Cancer Ctr; **Address:** UT MD Anderson Cancer Ctr, 1515 Holcombe Blvd, Unit 43, Houston, TX 77030; **Phone:** 713-792-3825; **Board Cert:** Obstetrics & Gynecology 2009; Gynecologic Oncology 2009; **Med School:** Tulane Univ 1978; **Resid:** Obstetrics & Gynecology, Tripler Army Med Ctr 1982; **Fellow:** Gynecologic Oncology, Walter Reed Army Med Ctr 1986; **Fac Appt:** Prof ObG, Univ Tex, Houston

Burnett, Alexander F MD [GO] - **Spec Exp:** Laparoscopic Surgery; Fertility Preservation in Cancer; Gynecologic Cancer; **Hospital:** UAMS Med Ctr; **Address:** 4301 W Markham St, Slot 793, Little Rock, AR 72205; **Phone:** 501-686-8522; **Board Cert:** Obstetrics & Gynecology 2009; Gynecologic Oncology 2009; **Med School:** Georgetown Univ 1986; **Resid:** Obstetrics & Gynecology, Georgetown Univ Affil Hosp 1990; **Fellow:** Gynecologic Oncology, Georgetown Univ Affil Hosp 1993; **Fac Appt:** Assoc Prof ObG, Univ Ark

Chambers, Setsuko K MD [GO] - **Spec Exp:** Gynecologic Cancer; Breast Cancer; Ovarian Cancer; **Hospital:** Univ Med Ctr - Tucson; **Address:** 1515 N Campbell Ave, Arizona Cancer Center, Tucson, AZ 85724; **Phone:** 520-626-9285; **Board Cert:** Obstetrics & Gynecology 2008; Gynecologic Oncology 2008; **Med School:** Brown Univ 1980; **Resid:** Obstetrics & Gynecology, Yale-New Haven Hosp 1984; **Fellow:** Gynecologic Oncology, Yale-New Haven Hosp 1986; **Fac Appt:** Prof ObG, Univ Ariz Coll Med

Fromm, Geri-Lynn MD [GO] - **Spec Exp:** Cervical Cancer; Ovarian Cancer; Gestational Trophoblastic Disease; **Hospital:** St. Luke's Episcopal Hosp-Houston, Woman's Hosp TX; **Address:** 2223 Dorrington St, Houston, TX 77030; **Phone:** 713-665-0404; **Board Cert:** Obstetrics & Gynecology 2010; **Med School:** Northwestern Univ 1981; **Resid:** Obstetrics & Gynecology, Magee Womens Hosp 1985; **Fellow:** Gynecologic Oncology, MD Anderson Cancer Ctr 1987; **Fac Appt:** Assoc Clin Prof ObG, Baylor Coll Med

Gershenson, David M MD [GO] - **Spec Exp:** Ovarian Rare & Borderline Tumors; Uterine Cancer-Serous Carcinoma; Fertility Preservation in Cancer; Sex Cord-Stromal Tumors; **Hospital:** UT MD Anderson Cancer Ctr, St. Luke's Episcopal Hosp-Houston; **Address:** Univ Tex MD Anderson Cancer Ctr, PO Box 301439, Houston, TX 77030-1439; **Phone:** 713-745-2565; **Board Cert:** Obstetrics & Gynecology 1991; Gynecologic Oncology 1981; **Med School:** Vanderbilt Univ 1971; **Resid:** Obstetrics & Gynecology, Yale-New Haven Hosp 1975; **Fellow:** Gynecologic Oncology, MD Anderson Cancer Ctr 1979; **Fac Appt:** Prof ObG, Univ Tex, Houston

Hatch, Kenneth MD [GO] - **Spec Exp:** Cervical Cancer; **Hospital:** Univ Med Ctr - Tucson, NW Med Ctr; **Address:** Arizona Cancer Center, 1515 N Campbell Ave, Tucson, AZ 85724; **Phone:** 520-626-9285; **Board Cert:** Obstetrics & Gynecology 1993; Gynecologic Oncology 1981; **Med School:** Univ Nebr Coll Med 1971; **Resid:** Obstetrics & Gynecology, Univ AL Med Ctr Birmingham 1976; **Fellow:** Gynecologic Oncology, Univ AL Med Ctr Birmingham 1978; **Fac Appt:** Prof ObG, Univ Ariz Coll Med

Kline, Richard C MD [GO] - **Spec Exp:** Ovarian Cancer; Cervical Cancer; Uterine Cancer; Vulvar & Vaginal Cancer; **Hospital:** Ochsner Med Ctr-New Orleans; **Address:** Ochsner Clinic Foundation, 1514 Jefferson Hwy, New Orleans, LA 70121; **Phone:** 504-842-4165; **Board Cert:** Obstetrics & Gynecology 2009; Gynecologic Oncology 2009; **Med School:** Louisiana State U, New Orleans 1980; **Resid:** Obstetrics & Gynecology, Ochsner Fdn Hosp 1984; **Fellow:** Gynecologic Oncology, UT MD Anderson Cancer Ctr 1986

Levenback, Charles MD [GO] - **Spec Exp:** Vulvar Disease/Cancer; Cervical Cancer; Gynecologic Cancer; **Hospital:** UT MD Anderson Cancer Ctr; **Address:** 1515 Holcombe Blvd, PO Box 301439 - Unit 1362, Houston, TX 77230; **Phone:** 713-745-2563; **Board Cert:** Obstetrics & Gynecology 2009; Gynecologic Oncology 2009; **Med School:** Mount Sinai Sch Med 1983; **Resid:** Obstetrics & Gynecology, Albert Einstein Coll Med 1987; **Fellow:** Gynecologic Oncology, Meml Sloan Kettering Cancer Ctr 1989; **Fac Appt:** Prof ObG, Univ Tex, Houston

Lu, Karen Hsieh MD [GO] - **Spec Exp:** Ovarian Cancer; Ovarian Cancer-Early Detection; Uterine Cancer; Cancer Genetics; **Hospital:** UT MD Anderson Cancer Ctr; **Address:** Univ of Texas MD Anderson Cancer Ctr, 1515 Holcombe Blvd, Houston, TX 77030; **Phone:** 713-745-8902; **Board Cert:** Obstetrics & Gynecology 2003; Gynecologic Oncology 2003; **Med School:** Yale Univ 1991; **Resid:** Obstetrics & Gynecology, Brigham & Women's Hosp 1994; **Fellow:** Gynecologic Oncology, Brigham & Women's Hosp 1999; **Fac Appt:** Prof ObG, Univ Tex SW, Dallas

Magrina, Javier MD [GO] - **Spec Exp:** Gynecologic Cancer; Robotic Surgery; Minimally Invasive Surgery; **Hospital:** Mayo Clinic - Scottsdale; **Address:** Mayo Clinic, 5779 E Mayo Blvd, Phoenix, AZ 85054; **Phone:** 480-342-2668; **Board Cert:** Obstetrics & Gynecology 1994; Gynecologic Oncology 1982; **Med School:** Spain 1972; **Resid:** Obstetrics & Gynecology, Mayo Clinic 1977; **Fellow:** Gynecologic Oncology, Kansas Med Ctr 1980; **Fac Appt:** Prof ObG, Mayo Med Sch

Siller, Barry MD [GO] - **Spec Exp:** Cervical Cancer; **Hospital:** Meml Hermann Hosp - Texas Med Ctr; **Address:** 915 Gessner Rd, Ste 400, Medical Plaza 3, Houston, TX 77024; **Phone:** 713-242-2575; **Board Cert:** Obstetrics & Gynecology 2009; Gynecologic Oncology 2009; **Med School:** Baylor Coll Med 1988; **Resid:** Obstetrics & Gynecology, Univ Ala Med Ctr 1992; **Fellow:** Gynecologic Oncology, Univ Ala Med Ctr 1994

Gynecologic Oncology

Sood, Anil K MD [GO] - **Spec Exp:** Gynecologic Cancer; Ovarian Cancer; **Hospital:** UT MD Anderson Cancer Ctr; **Address:** Univ Texas MD Anderson Cancer Ctr, 1515 Holcombe Blvd Ste 440, Houston, TX 77030-4000; **Phone:** 713-745-5266; **Board Cert:** Obstetrics & Gynecology 2009; Gynecologic Oncology 2009; **Med School:** Univ NC Sch Med 1991; **Resid:** Obstetrics & Gynecology, Univ FL Med Ctr 1995; **Fellow:** Gynecologic Oncology, Univ Iowa Hosps & Clin 1998

Walker, Joan L MD [GO] - **Spec Exp:** Ovarian Cancer; Cervical Cancer; Uterine Cancer; **Hospital:** OU Med Ctr; **Address:** OU Physicians, 825 NE 10th St, Ste 5200, Oklahoma City, OK 73104; **Phone:** 405-271-7770; **Board Cert:** Obstetrics & Gynecology 2009; Gynecologic Oncology 2009; **Med School:** UCLA 1982; **Resid:** Obstetrics & Gynecology, Hosp Univ Penn 1986; **Fellow:** Gynecologic Oncology, UC-Irvine 1990; **Fac Appt:** Assoc Prof ObG, Univ Okla Coll Med

West Coast and Pacific

Berek, Jonathan S MD [GO] - **Spec Exp:** Ovarian Cancer; Uterine Cancer; Cervical Cancer; Vulvar & Vaginal Cancer; **Hospital:** Stanford Univ Hosp & Clinics; **Address:** Stanford Cancer Ctr, Stanford Univ Sch Med-Clin C, 875 Blake Wilbur Drive, Stanford, CA 94305; **Phone:** 650-498-6000; **Board Cert:** Obstetrics & Gynecology 2009; Gynecologic Oncology 2009; **Med School:** Johns Hopkins Univ 1975; **Resid:** Obstetrics & Gynecology, Brigham & Womens Hosp 1979; **Fellow:** Gynecologic Oncology, UCLA Sch Med 1981; **Fac Appt:** Prof ObG, Stanford Univ

Berman, Michael L MD [GO] - **Spec Exp:** Gynecologic Cancer; Cervical Cancer; **Hospital:** UC Irvine Med Ctr, Long Beach Meml Med Ctr; **Address:** Cho Family Comprehensive Cancer Ctr, 101 The City Drive S 23 rte81 Bldg - rm 800, Orange, CA 92868-3201; **Phone:** 714-456-8000; **Board Cert:** Obstetrics & Gynecology 2005; Gynecologic Oncology 2005; **Med School:** Geo Wash Univ 1967; **Resid:** Obstetrics & Gynecology, GW Univ Hosp 1969; Obstetrics & Gynecology, LAC-Harbor Hosp 1974; **Fellow:** Gynecologic Oncology, UCLA Med Ctr 1976; **Fac Appt:** Prof ObG, UC Irvine

Bristow, Robert E MD [GO] - **Spec Exp:** Ovarian Cancer; Gynecologic Cancer; **Hospital:** UC Irvine Med Ctr; **Address:** UC Irvine Med Ctr, 101 The City Drive, Route 81 Bldg 23 - rm 800, Orange, CA 92868; **Phone:** 714-456-8000; **Board Cert:** Obstetrics & Gynecology 2009; Gynecologic Oncology 2009; **Med School:** USC Sch Med 1991; **Resid:** Obstetrics & Gynecology, Johns Hopkins Hosp 1995; **Fellow:** Gynecologic Oncology, UCLA Med Ctr 1998; **Fac Appt:** Prof ObG, UC Irvine

Carney, Michael E MD [GO] - **Spec Exp:** Gynecologic Cancer; Pelvic Surgery-Complex; Minimally Invasive Surgery; **Hospital:** Kapiolani Med Ctr for Women & Chldn; **Address:** Womens Cancer Center, 1319 Punahou St, Ste 640, Honolulu, HI 96826; **Phone:** 808-983-6090; **Board Cert:** Obstetrics & Gynecology 2009; Gynecologic Oncology 2009; **Med School:** Loyola Univ-Stritch Sch Med 1990; **Resid:** Obstetrics & Gynecology, Duke Univ Med Ctr 1994; **Fellow:** Gynecologic Oncology, Duke Univ Med Ctr 1999; **Fac Appt:** Assoc Prof ObG, Univ Hawaii JA Burns Sch Med

Chan, John K MD [GO] - **Spec Exp:** Ovarian Cancer; Pelvic Surgery-Complex; Gene Therapy; Clinical Trials; **Hospital:** UCSF Med Ctr; **Address:** UCSF Medical Center, 1600 Divisadaro St, rm A747, Box 1702, San Francisco, CA 94143-1702; **Phone:** 415-353-9600; **Board Cert:** Obstetrics & Gynecology 2006; Gynecologic Oncology 2006; **Med School:** UCLA 1995; **Resid:** Obstetrics & Gynecology, UC Irvine Med Ctr 1999; **Fellow:** Gynecologic Oncology, MD Anderson Cancer Ctr 1999; Gynecologic Oncology, UC Irvine 2003; **Fac Appt:** Assoc Prof ObG, UCSF

Di Saia, Philip J MD [GO] - **Spec Exp:** Ovarian Cancer; Gynecologic Cancer; Cervical Cancer; **Hospital:** UC Irvine Med Ctr; **Address:** 101 The City Drive Bldg 56 - rm 800, Orange, CA 92668-3201; **Phone:** 714-456-5220; **Board Cert:** Obstetrics & Gynecology 1983; Gynecologic Oncology 1974; **Med School:** Tufts Univ 1963; **Resid:** Obstetrics & Gynecology, Yale-New Haven Hosp 1967; **Fellow:** Gynecologic Oncology, MD Anderson Hosp 1971; **Fac Appt:** Prof ObG, UC Irvine

Goff, Barbara A MD [GO] - **Spec Exp:** Ovarian Cancer; Uterine Cancer; Cervical Cancer; Gynecologic Surgery-Complex; **Hospital:** Univ Wash Med Ctr; **Address:** Univ Washington, Dept Gyn/Onc, 825 Eastlake Ave E, Seattle, WA 98109; **Phone:** 206-288-2273; **Board Cert:** Obstetrics & Gynecology 2009; Gynecologic Oncology 2009; **Med School:** Univ Pennsylvania 1986; **Resid:** Obstetrics & Gynecology, Mass Genl Hosp/Brigham & Womens Hosp 1990; **Fellow:** Gynecologic Oncology, Mass Genl Hosp 1993; **Fac Appt:** Prof ObG, Univ Wash

Greer, Benjamin E MD [GO] - **Spec Exp:** Gynecologic Cancer; **Hospital:** Univ Wash Med Ctr; **Address:** Seattle Cancer Care Alliance, 825 Eastlake Ave E, MS E2102, Seattle, WA 98109; **Phone:** 206-288-2273; **Board Cert:** Obstetrics & Gynecology 2002; Gynecologic Oncology 2002; **Med School:** Univ Pennsylvania 1966; **Resid:** Obstetrics & Gynecology, Univ Colorado Med Ctr 1970; **Fac Appt:** Prof ObG, Univ Wash

Husain, Amreen MD [GO] - **Spec Exp:** Cervical Cancer; **Hospital:** Stanford Univ Hosp & Clinics; **Address:** Stanford Comprehensive Cancer Center, 875 Blake Wilbur Drive, Clinic C, Gynecologic Oncology Clinic, Stanford, CA 94305; **Phone:** 650-498-8080; **Board Cert:** Obstetrics & Gynecology 2009; Gynecologic Oncology 2009; **Med School:** NY Med Coll 1991; **Resid:** Obstetrics & Gynecology, Cornell Univ Med Ctr/NY Hosp 1995; **Fellow:** Gynecologic Oncology, Meml Sloan-Kettering Cancer Ctr 2000; **Fac Appt:** Assoc Prof ObG, Stanford Univ

Karlan, Beth Y MD [GO] - **Spec Exp:** Ovarian Cancer; Gynecologic Cancer; **Hospital:** Cedars-Sinai Med Ctr; **Address:** 8700 Beverly Blvd, Ste 290W, Los Angeles, CA 90048; **Phone:** 310-423-3302; **Board Cert:** Obstetrics & Gynecology 1998; Gynecologic Oncology 1998; **Med School:** Harvard Med Sch 1982; **Resid:** Obstetrics & Gynecology, Yale-New Haven Hosp 1986; **Fellow:** Gynecologic Oncology, UCLA 1989; **Fac Appt:** Prof ObG, UCLA

Muntz, Howard G MD [GO] - **Spec Exp:** Robotic Surgery; Ovarian Cancer; Gynecologic Surgery-Complex; Gestational Trophoblastic Disease; **Hospital:** Northwest Hosp - Seattle; **Address:** Women's Cancer Care of Seattle, 1560 N 115th St, Ste 101, Seattle, WA 98133; **Phone:** 206-368-6806; **Board Cert:** Obstetrics & Gynecology 2009; Gynecologic Oncology 2009; **Med School:** Harvard Med Sch 1984; **Resid:** Obstetrics & Gynecology, Brigham & Womens Hosp 1988; **Fellow:** Gynecologic Oncology, Mass General Hosp 1991; **Fac Appt:** Assoc Clin Prof ObG, Univ Wash

Plaxe, Steven C MD [GO] - **Spec Exp:** Ovarian Cancer; Uterine Cancer; Gestational Trophoblastic Disease; **Hospital:** UCSD Med Ctr-Hillcrest; **Address:** Moores Cancer Center, 3855 Health Sciences Drive, MC 0987, La Jolla, CA 92093-0987; **Phone:** 858-822-6199; **Board Cert:** Obstetrics & Gynecology 2009; Gynecologic Oncology 2009; **Med School:** Mount Sinai Sch Med 1981; **Resid:** Obstetrics & Gynecology, Yale-New Haven Hosp 1985; **Fellow:** Gynecologic Oncology, Mt Sinai Med Ctr 1988; **Fac Appt:** Prof ObG, UCSD

Smith, Lloyd Herbert MD [GO] - **Spec Exp:** Ovarian Cancer; Uterine Cancer; Vulvar Disease/Cancer; Vaginal Cancer; **Hospital:** UC Davis Med Ctr, Sutter Mem Hospital-Sacramento; **Address:** UC Davis Med Ctr, Dept Ob/Gyn, 4860 Y St, Ste 2500, Sacramento, CA 95817-2307; **Phone:** 916-734-6946; **Board Cert:** Obstetrics & Gynecology 2009; Gynecologic Oncology 2009; **Med School:** UC Davis 1981; **Resid:** Obstetrics & Gynecology, UC Davis Med Ctr 1985; **Fellow:** Gynecologic Oncology, Stanford Univ Hosp 1988; **Fac Appt:** Prof ObG, UC Davis

Spirtos, Nicola Michael MD [GO] - **Spec Exp:** Gynecologic Cancer; Ovarian Cancer; **Hospital:** Sunrise Hosp & Med Ctr, Univ Med Ctr - Las Vegas; **Address:** 3131 La Canada St, Ste 241, Las Vegas, NV 89169; **Phone:** 702-693-6870; **Board Cert:** Obstetrics & Gynecology 2009; Gynecologic Oncology 2009; **Med School:** Northwestern Univ 1980; **Resid:** Obstetrics & Gynecology, Women's Hosp LAC-USC Med Ctr 1984; **Fellow:** Gynecologic Oncology, Stanford Univ Affil Hosp 1987; **Fac Appt:** Prof ObG

Stern, Jeffrey L MD [GO] - **Spec Exp:** Laparoscopic Surgery; Vulvar Disease/Cancer; **Hospital:** Alta Bates Summit Med Ctr-Alta Bates Campus; **Address:** Womens Cancer Ctr Northern Calif, 2001 Dwight Way, Berkley, CA 94704; **Phone:** 510-204-5770; **Board Cert:** Obstetrics & Gynecology 1983; Gynecologic Oncology 1984; **Med School:** SUNY Upstate Med Univ 1976; **Resid:** Obstetrics & Gynecology, Johns Hopkins Hosp 1980; **Fellow:** Gynecologic Oncology, USC Med Ctr 1982

Teng, Nelson NH MD/PhD [GO] - **Spec Exp:** Ovarian Cancer; Clinical Trials; **Hospital:** Stanford Univ Hosp & Clinics; **Address:** Dept Gyn Oncology, 300 Pasteur Drive, Stanford, CA 94305-5317; **Phone:** 650-498-8080; **Board Cert:** Obstetrics & Gynecology 2003; Gynecologic Oncology 2003; **Med School:** Univ Miami Sch Med 1977; **Resid:** Obstetrics & Gynecology, UCLA Med Ctr 1981; **Fellow:** Gynecologic Oncology, Stanford Univ Sch Med 1984; **Fac Appt:** Assoc Prof ObG, Stanford Univ

OBSTETRICS & GYNECOLOGY

New England

Cramer, Daniel W MD [ObG] - **Spec Exp:** Ovarian Cancer; Ovarian Cancer-High Risk; **Hospital:** Dana-Farber Cancer Inst, Brigham & Women's Hosp; **Address:** Brigham & Women's Hosp, Ob/Gyn Epidemiology Ctr, 221 Longwood Ave, RFB 366, Boston, MA 02115; **Phone:** 617-732-4895; **Board Cert:** Obstetrics & Gynecology 1979; **Med School:** Univ Colorado 1970; **Resid:** Obstetrics & Gynecology, Boston Womens Hosp 1976; **Fellow:** Public Health, Harvard Med Sch 1982; **Fac Appt:** Prof ObG, Harvard Med Sch

Southeast

Morgan, Linda S MD [ObG] - **Spec Exp:** Gynecologic Cancer; **Hospital:** Shands at Univ of FL; **Address:** 2000 SW Archer Rd, Gainesville, FL 32610; **Phone:** 352-265-8200; **Board Cert:** Obstetrics & Gynecology 2008; Gynecologic Oncology 2008; **Med School:** Med Coll PA Hahnemann 1975; **Resid:** Obstetrics & Gynecology, Shands Hosp 1979; **Fellow:** Gynecologic Oncology, Mass Genl Hosp 1981; **Fac Appt:** Prof ObG, Univ Fla Coll Med

Midwest

Argenta, Peter A MD [ObG] - **Spec Exp:** Laparoscopic Surgery; Cervical Cancer; Ovarian Cancer; Vulvar & Vaginal Cancer; **Address:** Womens Health Clin, 516 Delaware St SE, Clinic 1C Fl 1, Minneapolis, MN 55455; **Phone:** 612-626-3444; **Board Cert:** Obstetrics & Gynecology 2005; Gynecologic Oncology 2005; **Med School:** Duke Univ 1995; **Resid:** Obstetrics & Gynecology, Hosp U Penn 1999; **Fellow:** Gynecologic Oncology, Mt Sinai Med Ctr 2002; **Fac Appt:** Assoc Prof ObG, Univ Minn

Lengyel, Ernst MD/PhD [ObG] - **Spec Exp:** Ovarian Cancer; Cervical Cancer; **Hospital:** Univ of Chicago Med Ctr; **Address:** 5841 S Maryland Ave, rm L250, MC 2050, Chicago, IL 60637; **Phone:** 773-702-6722; **Board Cert:** Obstetrics & Gynecology 2010; **Med School:** Germany ; **Resid:** Obstetrics & Gynecology, Univ Munich; **Fellow:** Gynecologic Oncology, UCSF Med Ctr; **Fac Appt:** Prof ObG, Univ Chicago-Pritzker Sch Med

Shulman, Lee P MD [ObG] - **Spec Exp:** Breast Cancer Genetics; Ovarian Cancer Genetics; **Hospital:** Northwestern Meml Hosp, Rush Univ Med Ctr; **Address:** Northwestern Univ Dept Ob/Gyn, Division Clinical Genetics, 250 E Superior St, Ste 05-2168, Chicago, IL 60611; **Phone:** 312-472-4683; **Board Cert:** Obstetrics & Gynecology 1999; Clinical Genetics 1990; **Med School:** Cornell Univ 1983; **Resid:** Obstetrics & Gynecology, N Shore Univ Hosp 1987; **Fellow:** Reproductive Genetics, Univ Tenn Med Ctr 1989; **Fac Appt:** Prof ObG, Northwestern Univ

West Coast and Pacific

Goldman, Mindy E MD [ObG] - **Spec Exp:** Breast Cancer; **Hospital:** UCSF Med Ctr; **Address:** 2356 Sutter St, San Francisco, CA 94115; **Phone:** 415-885-7788; **Board Cert:** Obstetrics & Gynecology 2007; **Med School:** Univ VT Coll Med 1989; **Resid:** Obstetrics & Gynecology, UCSF Med Ctr 1993

REPRODUCTIVE ENDOCRINOLOGY

New England

Crowley, William F MD [RE] - **Spec Exp:** Fertility Preservation in Cancer; **Hospital:** Mass Genl Hosp; **Address:** Mass Genl Hosp, Reproductive Sci Ctr, 55 Fruit St, Bartlett Hall-Ext 511, Boston, MA 02114; **Phone:** 617-726-5390; **Board Cert:** Internal Medicine 1974; Endocrinology 1977; **Med School:** Tufts Univ 1969; **Resid:** Internal Medicine, Mass Genl Hosp 1971; Internal Medicine, Mass Genl Hosp 1974; **Fellow:** Endocrinology, Mass Genl Hosp 1976; **Fac Appt:** Prof Med, Harvard Med Sch

Ginsburg, Elizabeth S MD [RE] - **Spec Exp:** Fertility Preservation in Cancer; **Hospital:** Brigham & Women's Hosp, Dana-Farber Cancer Inst; **Address:** Brigham & Womens Hosp, Reproductive Med, 75 Francis St, ASB-1 3254, Boston, MA 02115; **Phone:** 617-732-4222; **Board Cert:** Obstetrics & Gynecology 2009; Reproductive Endocrinology 2009; **Med School:** Mount Sinai Sch Med 1985; **Resid:** Obstetrics & Gynecology, Brigham & Womens Hosp 1989; **Fellow:** Reproductive Endocrinology, Brigham & Womens Hosp 1991

Patrizio, Pasquale MD [RE] - **Spec Exp:** Fertility Preservation in Cancer; **Hospital:** Yale-New Haven Hosp, Yale Med Group; **Address:** Yale Fertility Ctr, Dept OB/GYN, 150 Sargent Drive, New Haven, CT 06511; **Phone:** 203-785-4708; **Board Cert:** Obstetrics & Gynecology 2007; Reproductive Endocrinology 2010; **Med School:** Italy 1983; **Resid:** Obstetrics & Gynecology, Univ Naples 1987; Reproductive Endocrinology, Univ Pisa 1990; **Fellow:** Infertility, UC Irvine 1995; **Fac Appt:** Prof ObG, Yale Univ

Reproductive Endocrinology

Mid Atlantic

Coutifaris, Christos MD/PhD [RE] - **Spec Exp:** Fertility Preservation in Cancer; **Hospital:** Hosp Univ Penn - UPHS (page 80); **Address:** Penn Fertility Care, 3701 Market St Fl 8 - Ste 800, Philadelphia, PA 19104; **Phone:** 215-662-6100; **Board Cert:** Obstetrics & Gynecology 2009; Reproductive Endocrinology 2009; **Med School:** Univ Pennsylvania 1982; **Resid:** Obstetrics & Gynecology, Hosp Univ Penn 1986; **Fellow:** Reproductive Endocrinology, Hosp Univ Penn 1987; **Fac Appt:** Prof ObG, Univ Pennsylvania

Gracia, Clarisa R MD [RE] - **Spec Exp:** Gynecology in Cancer Patients; Infertility in Cancer Patients; Fertility Preservation in Cancer; **Hospital:** Hosp Univ Penn - UPHS (page 80); **Address:** Penn Fertility Care, 3701 Market St, Ste 800, Philadelphia, PA 19104; **Phone:** 215-662-6100; **Board Cert:** Obstetrics & Gynecology 2007; Reproductive Endocrinology 2007; **Med School:** SUNY Buffalo 1997; **Resid:** Obstetrics & Gynecology, Hosp U Penn 2000; **Fellow:** Reproductive Endocrinology, Hosp U Penn; **Fac Appt:** Asst Prof ObG, Univ Pennsylvania

Licciardi, Frederick L MD [RE] - **Spec Exp:** Fertility Preservation in Cancer; **Hospital:** NYU Langone Med Ctr (page 79); **Address:** NYU Medical Ctr, 660 First Ave, 5th Fl, New York, NY 10016; **Phone:** 212-263-7754; **Board Cert:** Obstetrics & Gynecology 2007; Reproductive Endocrinology 2007; **Med School:** UMDNJ-Rutgers Med Sch 1986; **Resid:** Obstetrics & Gynecology, St Barnabas Med Ctr 1990; **Fellow:** Reproductive Endocrinology, NY Hosp-Cornell Med Ctr 1992; **Fac Appt:** Assoc Prof ObG, NYU Sch Med

Noyes, Nicole MD [RE] - **Spec Exp:** Fertility Preservation in Cancer; **Hospital:** NYU Langone Med Ctr (page 79); **Address:** NYU Med Ctr, 660 First Ave, 5th FL, New York, NY 10016; **Phone:** 212-263-7981; **Board Cert:** Obstetrics & Gynecology 2007; Reproductive Endocrinology 2007; **Med School:** Univ VT Coll Med 1986; **Resid:** Obstetrics & Gynecology, NY Hosp-Cornell Med Ctr 1990; **Fellow:** Reproductive Endocrinology, NY Hosp-Cornell Med Ctr 1992; **Fac Appt:** Assoc Prof ObG, NYU Sch Med

Rosenwaks, Zev MD [RE] - **Spec Exp:** Fertility Preservation in Cancer; **Hospital:** NY-Presby Hosp/Weill Cornell (page 78); **Address:** Ctr For Reproductive Medicine & Infertility, 1305 York Ave Fl 6, New York, NY 10021-4872; **Phone:** 646-962-3743; **Board Cert:** Obstetrics & Gynecology 1978; Reproductive Endocrinology 1981; **Med School:** SUNY Downstate 1972; **Resid:** Obstetrics & Gynecology, LI Jewish Med Ctr 1976; **Fellow:** Reproductive Endocrinology, Johns Hopkins Hosp 1978; **Fac Appt:** Prof ObG, Cornell Univ-Weill Med Coll

Midwest

Molo, Mary W MD [RE] - **Spec Exp:** Fertility Preservation in Cancer; **Hospital:** Rush Univ Med Ctr; **Address:** 1725 W Harrison St, Ste 408 East, Chicago, IL 60612; **Phone:** 312-997-2229; **Board Cert:** Obstetrics & Gynecology 2010; Reproductive Endocrinology 2010; **Med School:** Southern IL Univ 1982; **Resid:** Obstetrics & Gynecology, Southern Illinois Affil Hosps 1984; Obstetrics & Gynecology, Rush Presby St Lukes Hosp 1987; **Fellow:** Reproductive Endocrinology, Rush Presby St Lukes Hosp 1989; **Fac Appt:** Asst Prof ObG, Rush Med Coll

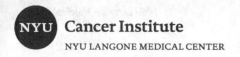

NYU **Cancer Institute**
NYU LANGONE MEDICAL CENTER

NYU Langone Medical Center
550 First Avenue , New York, NY 10016
www.NYULMC.org

NYU Clinical Cancer Center
160 East 34th Street, New York, NY 10016
www.NYUCI.org

**The Stephen D. Hassenfeld Children's Center
for Cancer and Blood Disorders**
160 East 32nd Street, New York, NY 10016
www.NYUMC.org/Hassenfeld

The NYU Cancer Institute is an NCI-designated cancer center and provides personalized patient care that is both compassionate and state of the art. The doctors and researchers work together to develop innovative therapies for patients. The Cancer Institute is world-renowned for excellence in cancer-focused research, personalized care, education and community outreach. Its mission is to discover the origins of human cancer and to use that knowledge to eradicate the personal and societal burden of cancer in our community, the nation and the world. For more information about our expert physicians, call 212-731-5000. *We specialize in the following areas:*

Patient-Focused Setting
The NYU Clinical Cancer Center is the principal outpatient facility of The Cancer Institute and serves as home to our patients and their caregivers. The center and its multidisciplinary team of experts provide access to the latest treatment options and clinical trials along with a variety of programs in cancer risk reduction/prevention, screening, diagnostics, genetic counseling and supportive services. In addition the NYUCI emphasizes the importance of a holistic approach to management services in complementary medicine, psychosocial support, survivorship and palliative care.

Renowned Expertise
The NYU Cancer Institute brings together experts from a variety of disciplines to create collaborative research endeavors and clinical care teams. The Cancer Institute offers a full continuum of personalized care, from prevention through diagnosis, treatment and post-treatment support. The compassion and expertise of our team members helps patients better manage the symptoms of their diseases as well as meet their special needs. Additionally, we have created special emphasis programs in diseases such as breast cancer, melanoma, GI cancer, prostate cancer, hematologic malignancies and lung cancer among others, as well as, translational programs in cancer healthcare disparities, molecularly targeted therapy, and the cell signaling pathways involved in cancer.

A Translational Approach
NYU Langone Medical Center scientists and other researchers excel in uncovering how cancer develops at the molecular level, and how we can harness that knowledge to reduce the risk of cancer and treat the disease. The Medical Center constantly seeks to create new opportunities for collaboration between investigators within our own institution, those located elsewhere in the NYU network of campuses, and researchers at other institutions.

The Stephen D. Hassenfeld Children's Center for Cancer and Blood Disorders
The center is a leading pediatric outpatient facility for the treatment of childhood cancers and blood diseases. Its unique interdisciplinary and family-centered approach combines the most advanced medical treatments with psychosocial and emotional support services for young patients and their families.

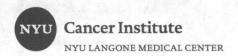
Cancer Institute

NYU LANGONE MEDICAL CENTER

NYU Langone Medical Center
550 First Avenue , New York, NY 10016
www.NYULMC.org

NYU Clinical Cancer Center
160 East 34th Street, New York, NY 10016
www.NYUCI.org

**The Stephen D. Hassenfeld Children's Center
for Cancer and Blood Disorders**
160 East 32nd Street, New York, NY 10016
www.NYUMC.org/Hassenfeld

The NYU Cancer Institute is an NCI-designated cancer center and provides personalized patient care that is both compassionate and state of the art. The doctors and researchers work together to develop innovative therapies for patients. The Cancer Institute is world-renowned for excellence in cancer-focused research, personalized care, education and community outreach. Its mission is to discover the origins of human cancer and to use that knowledge to eradicate the personal and societal burden of cancer in our community, the nation and the world. For more information about our expert physicians, call 212-731-5000. *We specialize in the following areas:*

Patient-Focused Setting
The NYU Clinical Cancer Center is the principal outpatient facility of The Cancer Institute and serves as home to our patients and their caregivers. The center and its multidisciplinary team of experts provide access to the latest treatment options and clinical trials along with a variety of programs in cancer risk reduction/prevention, screening, diagnostics, genetic counseling and supportive services. In addition the NYUCI emphasizes the importance of a holistic approach to management services in complementary medicine, psychosocial support, survivorship and palliative care.

Renowned Expertise
The NYU Cancer Institute brings together experts from a variety of disciplines to create collaborative research endeavors and clinical care teams. The Cancer Institute offers a full continuum of personalized care, from prevention through diagnosis, treatment and post-treatment support. The compassion and expertise of our team members helps patients better manage the symptoms of their diseases as well as meet their special needs. Additionally, we have created special emphasis programs in diseases such as breast cancer, melanoma, GI cancer, prostate cancer, hematologic malignancies and lung cancer among others, as well as, translational programs in cancer healthcare disparities, molecularly targeted therapy, and the cell signaling pathways involved in cancer.

A Translational Approach
NYU Langone Medical Center scientists and other researchers excel in uncovering how cancer develops at the molecular level, and how we can harness that knowledge to reduce the risk of cancer and treat the disease. The Medical Center constantly seeks to create new opportunities for collaboration between investigators within our own institution, those located elsewhere in the NYU network of campuses, and researchers at other institutions.

The Stephen D. Hassenfeld Children's Center for Cancer and Blood Disorders
The center is a leading pediatric outpatient facility for the treatment of childhood cancers and blood diseases. Its unique interdisciplinary and family-centered approach combines the most advanced medical treatments with psychosocial and emotional support services for young patients and their families.

Ophthalmology

An ophthalmologist has the knowledge and professional skills needed to provide eye and vision care. Ophthalmologists are medically trained to diagnose, monitor and medically or surgically treat all ocular and visual disorders. This includes problems affecting the eye and its component structures, the eyelids, the orbit and the visual pathways. In so doing, an ophthalmologist prescribes vision services, including glasses and contact lenses.

Training Required: Four years

OPHTHALMOLOGY

New England

Rubin, Peter A D MD [Oph] - **Spec Exp:** Oculoplastic Surgery; Orbital & Eyelid Tumors/Cancer; Eyelid Cancer & Reconstruction; **Hospital:** Beth Israel Deaconess Med Ctr - Boston; **Address:** 44 Washington St, Brookline, MA 02445; **Phone:** 617-232-9600; **Board Cert:** Ophthalmology 1991; **Med School:** Yale Univ 1985; **Resid:** Ophthalmology, Manhattan EET Hosp 1989; **Fellow:** Oculoplastic Surgery, Mass EE Infirmary 1990; **Fac Appt:** Assoc Clin Prof Oph, Univ Tenn Coll Med

Mid Atlantic

Abramson, David H MD [Oph] - **Spec Exp:** Eye Tumors/Cancer; Orbital Tumors/Cancer; Retinoblastoma; Melanoma-Choroidal (eye); **Hospital:** Meml Sloan-Kettering Cancer Ctr (page 75), NY-Presby Hosp/Weill Cornell (page 78); **Address:** 70 E 66th St, New York, NY 10065; **Phone:** 212-744-1700; **Board Cert:** Ophthalmology 1975; **Med School:** Albert Einstein Coll Med 1969; **Resid:** Ophthalmology, Harkness Eye Inst 1974; **Fellow:** Ocular Oncology, Columbia-Presby Med Ctr 1975; **Fac Appt:** Prof Oph, Cornell Univ-Weill Med Coll

Della Rocca, Robert C MD [Oph] - **Spec Exp:** Orbital Tumors/Cancer; Eyelid Tumors/Cancer; Oculoplastic Surgery; Eyelid Cancer & Reconstruction; **Hospital:** New York Eye & Ear Infirm (page 77), Sound Shore Med Ctr - Westchester; **Address:** 310 E 14th St, South Bldg, rm 319, New York, NY 10003; **Phone:** 212-979-4575; **Board Cert:** Ophthalmology 1975; **Med School:** Creighton Univ 1967; **Resid:** Ophthalmology, NY Eye & Ear Infirm 1973; **Fellow:** Oculoplastic Surgery, Albany Med Ctr

Finger, Paul T MD [Oph] - **Spec Exp:** Eye Tumors/Cancer; Melanoma-Choroidal (eye); Retinoblastoma; Orbital Tumors/Cancer; **Hospital:** New York Eye & Ear Infirm (page 77), NYU Langone Med Ctr (page 79); **Address:** 115 E 61 St Fl 5 - Ste B, New York, NY 10065; **Phone:** 212-832-8170; **Board Cert:** Ophthalmology 1990; **Med School:** Tulane Univ 1982; **Resid:** Ophthalmology, Manhattan EET Hosp 1986; **Fellow:** Ocular Oncology, N Shore Univ Hosp 1987; **Fac Appt:** Clin Prof Oph, NYU Sch Med

Handa, James T MD [Oph] - **Spec Exp:** Melanoma-Choroidal (eye); Retinoblastoma; **Hospital:** Johns Hopkins Hosp; **Address:** 600 N Wolfe St, Maumenee Building 710, Baltimore, MD 21287; **Phone:** 410-955-3518; **Board Cert:** Ophthalmology 1991; **Med School:** Univ Pennsylvania 1986; **Resid:** Ophthalmology, Wills Eye Hosp 1990; **Fellow:** Retina/Vitreous, Duke Eye Ctr 1992; Ophthalmic Oncololgy, USC Sch Med 1993; **Fac Appt:** Assoc Prof Oph, Johns Hopkins Univ

Iliff, Nicholas T MD [Oph] - **Spec Exp:** Oculoplastic Surgery; Orbital & Eyelid Tumors/Cancer; **Hospital:** Johns Hopkins Hosp; **Address:** Wilmer at Bayview Med Ctr, 4940 Eastern Ave, Baltimore, MD 21224; **Phone:** 410-550-2360; **Board Cert:** Ophthalmology 1978; **Med School:** Johns Hopkins Univ 1972; **Resid:** Ophthalmology, Johns Hopkins-Wilmer Inst 1977; **Fellow:** Retinal Surgery, Johns Hopkins-Wilmer Inst 1978; Oculoplastic & Reconstructive Surgery, Johns Hopkins-Wilmer Inst 1980; **Fac Appt:** Prof Oph, Johns Hopkins Univ

O'Brien, Joan M MD [Oph] - **Spec Exp:** Eye Tumors/Cancer; Retinoblastoma; **Hospital:** Hosp Univ Penn - UPHS (page 80); **Address:** Penn Presbyterian Med Ctr, Scheie Eye Inst, 51 N 39th St, Philadelphia, PA 19104; **Phone:** 215-662-8100; **Board Cert:** Ophthalmology 2007; **Med School:** Dartmouth Med Sch 1986; **Resid:** Ophthalmology, Mass Eye & Ear Infirm 1992; **Fellow:** Ophthalmic Pathology, Mass Eye & Ear Infirm 1989; Ophthalmological Pathology, UCSF Med Ctr 1993; **Fac Appt:** Prof Oph, Univ Pennsylvania

Shields, Carol L MD [Oph] - **Spec Exp:** Orbital Tumors/Cancer; Melanoma-Choroidal (eye); Retinoblastoma; Pediatric Ophthalmology; **Hospital:** Wills Eye Hosp, Jefferson Reg Med Ctr - Pittsburgh; **Address:** Wills Eye Inst, Ocular Oncology Service, 840 Walnut St, Ste 1440, Phildelphia, PA 19107; **Phone:** 215-928-3105; **Board Cert:** Ophthalmology 1989; **Med School:** Univ Pittsburgh 1983; **Resid:** Ophthalmology, Willis Eye Hosp 1988; **Fellow:** Ophthalmic Pathology, Willis Eye Hosp 1988; Ophthalmic Oncololgy, Willis Eye Hosp 1989; **Fac Appt:** Prof Oph, Jefferson Med Coll

Shields, Jerry MD [Oph] - **Spec Exp:** Eye Tumors/Cancer; Pediatric Ophthalmology; Retinoblastoma; Melanoma-Choroidal (eye); **Hospital:** Wills Eye Hosp, Thomas Jefferson Univ Hosp (page 81); **Address:** Wills Eye Hosp, Ocular Oncology Svce, 840 Walnut St, Ste 1440, Philadelphia, PA 19107; **Phone:** 215-928-3105; **Board Cert:** Ophthalmology 1972; **Med School:** Univ Mich Med Sch 1964; **Resid:** Ophthalmology, Wills Eye Hosp 1970; **Fellow:** Ophthalmology, Wills Eye Hosp 1972; **Fac Appt:** Prof Oph, Thomas Jefferson Univ

Southeast

Dutton, Jonathan J MD/PhD [Oph] - **Spec Exp:** Oculoplastic Surgery; Eye Tumors/Cancer; Melanoma-Choroidal (eye); **Hospital:** NC Memorial Hosp - UNC; **Address:** Univ North Carolina - Dept Ophthalmology, 130 Mason Farm Rd, 5156 Bioinformatics, CB 7040, Chapel Hill, NC 27599; **Phone:** 919-966-5296; **Board Cert:** Ophthalmology 1983; **Med School:** Washington Univ, St Louis 1977; **Resid:** Ophthalmology, Washington Univ Med Ctr 1982; **Fellow:** Oculoplastic Surgery, Univ Iowa Med Ctr 1983; **Fac Appt:** Prof Oph, Univ NC Sch Med

Grossniklaus, Hans E MD [Oph] - **Spec Exp:** Ophthalmic Pathology; Melanoma-Choroidal (eye); **Hospital:** Emory Univ Hosp; **Address:** Emory Clinic - LF Montgomery Lab, 1365-B Clifton Rd NE, rm BT428, Atlanta, GA 30322; **Phone:** 404-778-4611; **Board Cert:** Ophthalmology 1985; Anatomic Pathology 1987; **Med School:** Ohio State Univ 1980; **Resid:** Ophthalmology, Case West Res Univ Hosp 1984; Pathology, Case West Res Univ Hosp 1987; **Fellow:** Ophthalmological Pathology, Johns Hopkins Hosp 1985; **Fac Appt:** Prof Oph, Emory Univ

Haik, Barrett MD [Oph] - **Spec Exp:** Eye Tumors/Cancer; **Hospital:** St. Jude Children's Research Hosp; **Address:** Univ Tenn Med Group, Ophthamology, 930 Madison Ave, Ste 400, Memphis, TN 38103-3452; **Phone:** 901-448-6650; **Board Cert:** Ophthalmology 1981; **Med School:** Louisiana State U, New Orleans 1976; **Resid:** Ophthalmology, Columbia-Presby/Harkness Eye Inst 1980; **Fac Appt:** Prof Oph, Univ Tenn Coll Med

Murray, Timothy G MD [Oph] - **Spec Exp:** Eye Tumors/Cancer; **Hospital:** Bascom Palmer Eye Inst (page 82); **Address:** Bascom Palmer Eye Inst, 900 NW 17th St, rm 254, Miami, FL 33136-1119; **Phone:** 305-326-6166; **Board Cert:** Ophthalmology 1990; **Med School:** Johns Hopkins Univ 1985; **Resid:** Ophthalmology, UCSF Med Ctr 1989; **Fellow:** Ophthalmology, UCSF 1999; Ophthalmology, Med Coll Wisconsin 1991; **Fac Appt:** Prof Oph, Univ Miami Sch Med

Sternberg Jr, Paul MD [Oph] - **Spec Exp:** Eye Tumors/Cancer; **Hospital:** Vanderbilt Univ Med Ctr, Vanderbilt Monroe Carrell Jr. Chldn's Hosp; **Address:** Vanderbilt Eye Institute, 2311 Pierce Ave, Nashville, TN 37232-8808; **Phone:** 615-936-1453; **Board Cert:** Ophthalmology 1985; **Med School:** Univ Chicago-Pritzker Sch Med 1979; **Resid:** Ophthalmology, Johns Hopkins Hosp 1983; **Fellow:** Vitreoretinal Surgery, Duke Univ Med Ctr 1984; **Fac Appt:** Prof Oph, Vanderbilt Univ

Tse, David MD [Oph] - **Spec Exp:** Oculoplastic Surgery; Orbital Tumors/Cancer; Eyelid Tumors/Cancer; **Hospital:** Bascom Palmer Eye Inst (page 82), Jackson Meml Hosp (page 82); **Address:** Bascom Palmer Eye Inst, 900 NW 17th St, Miami, FL 33136; **Phone:** 305-326-6086; **Board Cert:** Ophthalmology 2002; **Med School:** Univ Miami Sch Med 1976; **Resid:** Ophthalmology, LAC/USC Med Ctr 1981; **Fellow:** Oculoplastic Surgery, Univ Iowa Hosps 1982; **Fac Appt:** Prof Oph, Univ Miami Sch Med

Ophthalmology

Wilson, Matthew W MD [Oph] - **Spec Exp:** Eye Tumors/Cancer; Retinoblastoma; Melanoma-Choroidal (eye); **Hospital:** St. Jude Children's Research Hosp, Methodist Univ Hosp - Memphis; **Address:** Univ Tenn Med Grp, Ophthalmology, 930 Madison Ave, Ste 200, Memphis, TN 38103; **Phone:** 901-448-6650; **Board Cert:** Ophthalmology 2007; **Med School:** Emory Univ 1990; **Resid:** Ophthalmology, Emory Univ Med Ctr 1994; Ophthalmic Pathology, Emory Univ Med Ctr 1995; **Fellow:** Ocular Oncology, Moorfields Eye Hosp 1996; Ophthalmic Plastic & Reconstructive Surgery, Casey Eye Inst 1998; **Fac Appt:** Assoc Prof Oph, Univ Tenn Coll Med

Yeatts, R Patrick MD [Oph] - **Spec Exp:** Oculoplastic Surgery; Orbital Tumors/Cancer; Eyelid Tumors/Cancer; **Hospital:** Wake Forest Univ Baptist Med Ctr; **Address:** Wake Forest Univ Eye Ctr, Janeway Clinical Sciences Bldg Fl 6, Medical Ctr Blvd, Winston-Salem, NC 27157; **Phone:** 336-716-4091; **Board Cert:** Ophthalmology 1983; **Med School:** Wake Forest Univ 1978; **Resid:** Ophthalmology, Mayo Clin 1982; **Fellow:** Oculoplastic & Reconstructive Surgery, Mass Eye & Ear Infirmary 1983; **Fac Appt:** Prof Oph, Wake Forest Univ

Midwest

Albert, Daniel M MD [Oph] - **Spec Exp:** Eye Tumors/Cancer; Ophthalmic Pathology; **Hospital:** Univ WI Hosp & Clins; **Address:** 600 Highland Ave CSC Bldg - rm K6/412, Madison, WI 53792-3284; **Phone:** 608-263-9798; **Board Cert:** Ophthalmology 1969; **Med School:** Univ Pennsylvania 1962; **Resid:** Ophthalmology, Hosp Univ Penn 1966; **Fellow:** Neuro-Ophthalmology, Natl Inst Hlth 1968; Pathology, Armed Forces Inst Path 1969; **Fac Appt:** Prof Oph, Univ Wisc

Augsburger, James MD [Oph] - **Spec Exp:** Eye Tumors/Cancer; Melanoma-Choroidal (eye); Retinoblastoma; **Hospital:** Univ Hosp - Cincinnati, Cincinnati Chldns Hosp Med Ctr; **Address:** Medical Arts Bldg, Ste 1500, 222 Piedmont Ave, ML 665-E, Cincinnati, OH 45267-0665; **Phone:** 513-475-7300; **Board Cert:** Ophthalmology 1979; **Med School:** Univ Cincinnati 1974; **Resid:** Ophthalmology, Univ Hosp-Cincinnati 1978; **Fellow:** Ocular Oncology, Wills Eye Hosp 1980; **Fac Appt:** Prof Oph, Univ Cincinnati

Elner, Victor H MD/PhD [Oph] - **Spec Exp:** Eyelid Tumors/Cancer; Orbital Tumors/Cancer; **Hospital:** Univ of Michigan Hosp; **Address:** Kellogg Eye Ctr, 1000 Wall St, Ann Arbor, MI 48105; **Phone:** 734-763-9142; **Board Cert:** Ophthalmology 1983; Pathology 1988; **Med School:** Univ Chicago-Pritzker Sch Med 1979; **Resid:** Ophthalmology, Univ Chicago 1982; Pathology, Univ Chicago 1984; **Fellow:** Ophthalmological Pathology, Armed Forces Inst 1985; Ophthalmic Plastic & Reconstructive Surgery, Univ Wisconsin 1987; **Fac Appt:** Prof Oph, Univ Mich Med Sch

Harbour, J William MD [Oph] - **Spec Exp:** Eye Tumors/Cancer; Melanoma-Choroidal (eye); Retinoblastoma; **Hospital:** Barnes-Jewish Hosp, St. Louis Chldns Hosp; **Address:** 1600 S Brentwood, Ste 800, St Louis, MO 63144; **Phone:** 314-367-1278 x2156; **Board Cert:** Ophthalmology 2007; **Med School:** Johns Hopkins Univ 1990; **Resid:** Ophthalmology, Wills Eye Hosp 1994; **Fellow:** Retina/Vitreous, Bascom Palmer Eye Inst 1995; Ocular Oncology, UCSF Med Ctr 1996; **Fac Appt:** Prof Oph, Washington Univ, St Louis

Lueder, Gregg T MD [Oph] - **Spec Exp:** Retinoblastoma; Eye Tumors-Pediatric; Pediatric Ophthalmology; **Hospital:** St. Louis Chldns Hosp; **Address:** St Louis Children's Hospital, One Children's Pl, Ste 2 South 89, St Louis, MO 63110; **Phone:** 314-454-6026; **Board Cert:** Ophthalmology 2003; **Med School:** Univ Iowa Coll Med 1985; **Resid:** Pediatrics, St Louis Children's Hosp 1988; Ophthalmology, Univ Iowa Med Ctr 1991; **Fellow:** Pediatric Ophthalmology, Hosp for Sick Children 1993; **Fac Appt:** Assoc Prof Oph, Washington Univ, St Louis

Mieler, William F MD [Oph] - **Spec Exp:** Eye Tumors/Cancer; **Hospital:** Univ of IL Med Ctr at Chicago, Weiss Meml Hosp; **Address:** Univ IL Chicago, Dept Ophthalmology, 1855 W Taylor St, MS 648, Chicago, IL 60637; **Phone:** 773-996-6660; **Board Cert:** Ophthalmology 1984; **Med School:** Univ Wisc 1979; **Resid:** Ophthalmology, Bascom-Palmer Eye Inst 1983; **Fellow:** Vitreoretinal Surgery & Disease, Med Ctr Wisconsin Eye Inst 1984; Oculoplastic Surgery, Wills Eye Hosp 1986; **Fac Appt:** Prof Oph, Univ IL Coll Med

Nerad, Jeffrey MD [Oph] - **Spec Exp:** Orbital Tumors/Cancer; Eyelid Cancer & Reconstruction; Oculoplastic Surgery; **Address:** Cincinnati Eye Institute, 1945 CEI Drive, Cincinnati, OH 45242; **Phone:** 513-984-5133; **Board Cert:** Ophthalmology 1984; **Med School:** St Louis Univ 1979; **Resid:** Ophthalmology, St Louis Univ Med Ctr 1983; **Fellow:** Oculoplastic & Reconstructive Surgery, Univ Iowa 1984; **Fac Appt:** Prof Oph, Univ Iowa Coll Med

Plager, David A MD [Oph] - **Spec Exp:** Pediatric Ophthalmology; Eye Tumors-Pediatric; Retinoblastoma; **Hospital:** Riley Hosp for Children; **Address:** Indiana University Medical Center, 702 Rotary Circle Fl 2, Indianapolis, IN 46202; **Phone:** 317-944-8103; **Board Cert:** Ophthalmology 2006; **Med School:** Indiana Univ 1983; **Resid:** Ophthalmology, Indiana Univ Hosps 1987; **Fellow:** Pediatric Ophthalmology, Chldns Hosp Natl Med Ctr 1988; **Fac Appt:** Prof Oph, Indiana Univ

Pulido, Jose S MD [Oph] - **Spec Exp:** Eye Tumors/Cancer; **Hospital:** Mayo Med Ctr & Clin - Rochester; **Address:** 200 1st St SW, Rochester, MN 55905; **Phone:** 507-284-3721; **Board Cert:** Ophthalmology 1986; **Med School:** Tulane Univ 1981; **Resid:** Ophthalmology, Illinois Eye & Ear Infirm 1986; **Fellow:** Vitreoretinal Surgery & Disease, Bascom-Palmer Eye Inst 1987; Ocular Oncology, Wills Eye Hosp; **Fac Appt:** Prof Oph, Mayo Med Sch

Great Plains and Mountains

Anderson, Richard L MD [Oph] - **Spec Exp:** Orbital & Eyelid Tumors/Cancer; **Hospital:** Salt Lake Regional Med Ctr, Intermountain Shriners Hosp; **Address:** 1002 E South Temple, Ste 308, Salt Lake City, UT 84102-1525; **Phone:** 801-363-3355; **Board Cert:** Ophthalmology 1976; **Med School:** Univ Iowa Coll Med 1971; **Resid:** Ophthalmology, Univ Iowa Hosps-Clins 1975; **Fellow:** Oculoplastic & Reconstructive Surgery, Albany Med Ctr 1975; Oculoplastic & Reconstructive Surgery, UCSF Med Ctr 1976; **Fac Appt:** Prof PlS, Univ Utah

Gigantelli, James W MD [Oph] - **Spec Exp:** Orbital Tumors/Cancer; Eyelid Cancer & Reconstruction; Lymphoma-Ocular (eye); **Hospital:** Nebraska Med Ctr; **Address:** 985540 Nebraska Medical Center, Omaha, NE 68198-5540; **Phone:** 402-559-4276; **Board Cert:** Ophthalmology 1991; **Med School:** Vanderbilt Univ 1985; **Resid:** Ophthalmology, Baylor Coll Med 1989; **Fellow:** Oculoplastic Surgery, Duke Unv Med Ctr 1990; **Fac Appt:** Prof Oph, Univ Nebr Coll Med

Southwest

Esmaeli-Azad, Bita MD [Oph] - **Spec Exp:** Orbital & Eyelid Tumors/Cancer; Eyelid Cancer & Reconstruction; Oculoplastic Surgery; **Hospital:** UT MD Anderson Cancer Ctr; **Address:** Dept of Head & Neck Surgery, Ophthalmology Section, 1515 Holcombe Blvd, Unit 1445, Houston, TX 77030; **Phone:** 713-792-6523; **Board Cert:** Ophthalmology 2006; **Med School:** Ros Franklin Univ/Chicago Med Sch 1990; **Resid:** Ophthalmology, Univ Michigan Affil Hosp 1994; **Fellow:** Ophthalmic Plastic & Reconstructive Surgery, Univ Toronto Affil Hosp 1996; **Fac Appt:** Assoc Prof Oph, Univ Tex, Houston

Ophthalmology

Lee, Andrew G MD [Oph] - **Spec Exp:** Neuro-Ophthalmology; Optic Nerve Tumors; **Hospital:** Methodist Hosp - Houston; **Address:** Methodist Hosp, Dept Ophthalmology, 6560 Fannin St, Ste 450, Houston, TX 77030; **Phone:** 713-441-8843; **Board Cert:** Ophthalmology 2006; **Med School:** Univ VA Sch Med 1989; **Resid:** Ophthalmology, Cullen Eye Inst-Baylor 1993; **Fellow:** Neuro-Ophthalmology, Wilmer Eye Inst-Johns Hopkins 1994; **Fac Appt:** Prof Oph, Univ Iowa Coll Med

Schiffman, Jade S MD [Oph] - **Spec Exp:** Neuro-Ophthalmology; **Hospital:** UT MD Anderson Cancer Ctr; **Address:** MD Anderson Cancer, 1515 Holcombe Blvd, Box 342, Houston, TX 77035; **Phone:** 713-792-3798; **Board Cert:** Neurology 1983; Ophthalmology 1991; **Med School:** SUNY Upstate Med Univ 1975; **Resid:** Neurology, Univ Miami Affil Hosp 1980; Ophthalmology, Univ California Affil Hosp 1989; **Fellow:** Neuro-Ophthalmology, Univ California Med Ctr 1981; **Fac Appt:** Prof Oph, Univ Tex, Houston

Soparkar, Charles MD [Oph] - **Spec Exp:** Eye Tumors/Cancer; Orbital & Eyelid Tumors/Cancer; Oculoplastic Surgery; **Hospital:** Methodist Hosp - Houston, Texas Chldns Hosp; **Address:** Plastic Eye Surg Assocs, 3730 Kirby Drive, Ste 900, Houston, TX 77098; **Phone:** 713-795-0705; **Board Cert:** Ophthalmology 2007; **Med School:** Univ Mass Sch Med 1990; **Resid:** Ophthalmology, Baylor Affil Hosps 1994; **Fellow:** Ophthalmic Oncololgy, Texas Med Ctr 1995; Ophthalmic Plastic Surgery, Texas Med Ctr 1995; **Fac Appt:** Asst Clin Prof Oph, Baylor Coll Med

West Coast and Pacific

Boxrud, Cynthia Ann MD [Oph] - **Spec Exp:** Oculoplastic Surgery; Eye Tumors/Cancer; **Hospital:** UCLA Ronald Reagan Med Ctr, St. John's Hlth Ctr, Santa Monica; **Address:** 2021 Santa Monica Blvd, Ste 700E, Santa Monica, CA 90404-2208; **Phone:** 310-829-9060; **Board Cert:** Ophthalmology 2008; **Med School:** Case West Res Univ 1986; **Resid:** Ophthalmology, NYU-Bellevue Hosp Ctr 1990; **Fellow:** Ophthalmic Oncololgy, New York Hosp-Cornell Med Ctr 1992; Ophthalmic Plastic Surgery, UCLA-Jules Stein Eye Inst 1993; **Fac Appt:** Asst Prof Oph, UCLA

Char, Devron H MD [Oph] - **Spec Exp:** Eye Tumors/Cancer; Oculoplastic Surgery; **Hospital:** CA Pacific Med Ctr-Pacific Campus, UCSF Med Ctr; **Address:** 45 Castro St, Ste 309, San Francisco, CA 94114; **Phone:** 415-522-0700; **Board Cert:** Ophthalmology 1978; **Med School:** Univ Minn 1970; **Resid:** Internal Medicine, Mass Genl Hosp 1972; Ophthalmology, UCSF Med Ctr 1977; **Fellow:** Medical Oncology, Natl Cancer Inst 1974; Ophthalmology, UCSF Med Ctr 1978; **Fac Appt:** Prof Oph, Stanford Univ

Cockerham, Kimberly P MD [Oph] - **Spec Exp:** Orbital Tumors/Cancer; Eyelid Cancer & Reconstruction; Neuro-Ophthalmology; **Hospital:** El Camino Hosp, Stanford Univ Hosp & Clinics; **Address:** 762 Altos Oaks Drive, Ste 2, Los Altos, CA 94024; **Phone:** 650-559-9150; **Board Cert:** Ophthalmology 2004; **Med School:** Geo Wash Univ 1987; **Resid:** Ophthalmology, Walter Reed Army Med Ctr 1992; **Fellow:** Neuro-Ophthalmology, Walter Reed Army Med Ctr 1993; Neuro-Ophthalmology, Allegheny General Hosp 1995

Kim, Jonathan W MD [Oph] - **Spec Exp:** Oculoplastic Surgery; Orbital Tumors/Cancer; **Hospital:** Stanford Univ Hosp & Clinics; **Address:** 900 Blake Wilbur Drive, rm W3002, MC 5353, Palo Alto, CA 94304; **Phone:** 650-723-6995; **Board Cert:** Ophthalmology 2000; **Med School:** Univ Iowa Coll Med 1994; **Resid:** Ophthalmology, CA Pacific Med Ctr 1998; **Fellow:** Oculoplastic Surgery, Jules Stein Eye Inst/UCLA Med Ctr 2000; Orbital Surgery, Mass Eye & Ear Infirm 2004

Murphree, A Linn MD [Oph] - **Spec Exp:** Retinoblastoma; Eye Tumors/Cancer; Ophthalmic Genetics; Pediatric Ophthalmology; **Hospital:** Chldns Hosp - Los Angeles, USC Norris Cancer Hosp; **Address:** Chldns Hosp, Div Oph, 4650 Sunset Blvd, MS 88, Los Angeles, CA 90027-6016; **Phone:** 323-361-2347; **Board Cert:** Ophthalmology 1978; **Med School:** Baylor Coll Med 1972; **Resid:** Ophthalmology, Baylor Coll Med 1973; Ophthalmology, Baylor Coll Med 1976; **Fellow:** Pediatric Ophthalmology, Wilmer Inst/Johns Hopkins 1977; **Fac Appt:** Prof Oph, USC Sch Med

Seiff, Stuart R MD [Oph] - **Spec Exp:** Oculoplastic Surgery; Orbital Tumors/Cancer; **Hospital:** UCSF Med Ctr, CA Pacific Med Ctr-Pacific Campus; **Address:** 2100 Webster St, Ste 214, San Francisco, CA 94115; **Phone:** 415-923-3007; **Board Cert:** Ophthalmology 1986; **Med School:** UCSF 1980; **Resid:** Ophthalmology, UCSF Med Ctr 1984; **Fellow:** Ophthalmic Plastic & Reconstructive Surgery, UCLA Med Ctr 1985; Oculoplastic Surgery, Moorfield's Eye Hosp 1986; **Fac Appt:** Prof Oph, UCSF

Stout, J Timothy MD/PhD [Oph] - **Spec Exp:** Retinoblastoma; **Hospital:** OR Hlth & Sci Univ, Providence St Vincent Med Ctr; **Address:** 3375 SW Terwilliger Blvd, Portland, OR 97239; **Phone:** 503-494-2435; **Board Cert:** Ophthalmology 2010; **Med School:** Baylor Coll Med 1989; **Resid:** Ophthalmology, Doheny Eye Inst 1993; **Fellow:** Ophthalmology, Moorfields Eye Hosp 1994; Retinal Surgery, Doheny Eye Inst 1995; **Fac Appt:** Assoc Prof Oph, Oregon Hlth & Sci Univ

Wilson, David Jean MD [Oph] - **Spec Exp:** Eye Tumors/Cancer; Ophthalmic Pathology; **Hospital:** OR Hlth & Sci Univ; **Address:** 3375 SW Terwilliger Blvd, Portland, OR 97239; **Phone:** 503-494-7881; **Board Cert:** Ophthalmology 2009; **Med School:** Baylor Coll Med 1981; **Resid:** Ophthalmology, Univ Oregon 1985; **Fellow:** Ophthalmic Pathology, John Hopkins Univ Hosp 1987; Retina/Vitreous, Mass Eye & Ear Infirm 1988; **Fac Appt:** Prof Oph, Oregon Hlth & Sci Univ

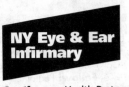

NY Eye & Ear Infirmary

Continuum Health Partners, Inc.

THE NEW YORK EYE AND EAR INFIRMARY

310 East 14th Street
New York, New York 10003
Tel. 212.979.4000   Fax. 212.228.0664
www.nyee.edu

OCULAR TUMOR SERVICE

The New York Eye and Ear Infirmary is a national referral center within the Collaborative Ocular Melanoma Study of the National Eye Institute/National Institutes of Health. New and innovative treatments for patients with eye cancer include radioactive plaques to treat intraocular tumors and chemotherapy for conjunctival neoplasia. Tumors of the eyelids, iris, retina, choroid and optic nerve are also treated by specialists in this service. A multidisciplinary Ocular Tumor Board meets monthly to discuss the most difficult cases and formulate therapeutic options

OTOLARYNGOLOGY/ HEAD & NECK SURGERY

Head & Neck Oncology: A team comprised of board-certified surgeons, medical & radiation oncologists, nutritionists and rehabilitation specialists ensure rapid recovery from complex, life saving surgical procedures and return to daily activities.

Thyroid Center: A unique center concentrates on streamlining the diagnosis and treatment of thyroid diseases and cancers with a highly skilled team of surgeons, endocrinologists and radiologists to manage the patient's care. An area of expertise is cancer resulting from radiation exposure such as that from Chernobyl.

Facial Plastics and Reconstructive Surgery. Treatment of facial tumors, both benign and cancerous, frequently requires expert reconstruction. Designed to restore the function and appearance of the face, these procedures may be required after appropriate treatment of skin cancers or deep tumors.

Otology–Neuro-otology: These rare cancers can be treated by our highly skilled team of surgeons which includes a neuro-otologist and a neurosurgeon.

Center for the Voice and Swallowing: Program cooperatively staffed by a team of specialists able to diagnose cancer of the vocal cords early and rehabilitate the voice after surgical and radiation treatment.

PATHOLOGY & LABORATORY MEDICINE

The Ocular Pathology Service is the leading laboratory in the Northeast and utilized by ophthalmologists throughout the region. The Infirmary is the site of some of the most promising studies into diseases and cancers of the eye, ear, nose and throat. Among them: cellular markers of oral cancer risk, non-invasive detection of thyroid cancer, basic cell biology of the growth of ocular melanoma cells, and persistence of biomaterials for repair in plastic and reconstructive surgery.

PLASTIC & RECONSTRUCTIVE SURGERY

The Department of Plastic & Reconstructive Surgery treats more than 1,500 patients a year who seek reconstructive surgery of the body as well as facial area as a result of accident, birth defect or cancer, and those who elect cosmetic surgery. It is one of the few hospitals in the region to perform breast reconstruction after mastectomy with microvascular surgery to harvest tissue from patients' lower body to create living, natural, and normal looking breasts, often preferred to artificial implants. State-of-the-art lymph node transfer to cure post-mastectomy lymphedema is also available.

Orthopaedic Surgery

An orthopaedic surgeon is trained in the preservation, investigation and restoration of the form and function of the extremities, spine and associated structures by medical, surgical and physical means. An orthopaedic surgeon is involved with the care of patients whose musculoskeletal problems include congenital deformities, trauma, infections, tumors, metabolic disturbances of the musculoskeletal system, deformities, injuries and degenerative diseases of the spine, hands, feet, knee, hip, shoulder and elbow in children and adults. An orthopaedic surgeon is also concerned with primary and secondary muscular problems and the effects of central or peripheral nervous system lesions of the musculoskeletal system.

Training Required: Five years (including general surgery training) plus two years in clinical practice before final certification is achieved.

Note: There are many Orthopaedic Surgeons who are trained in Sports Medicine and prefer to be listed under that heading; some trained in Sports Medicine prefer to be listed under Orthopaedics.

Hand Surgery: A specialist trained in the investigation, preservation and restoration by medical, surgical and rehabilitative means of all structures of the upper extremity directly affecting the form and function of the hand and wrist.

Training Required: Training required for Orthopaedic Surgery certification plus an additional year in hand surgery.

ORTHOPAEDIC SURGERY

New England

Friedlaender, Gary E MD [OrS] - **Spec Exp:** Bone & Soft Tissue Tumors; Tissue Banking; **Hospital:** Yale-New Haven Hosp, Yale Med Group; **Address:** 800 Howard Ave, Yale Physicians Fl 1, New Haven, CT 06519; **Phone:** 203-737-5660; **Board Cert:** Orthopaedic Surgery 1975; **Med School:** Univ Mich Med Sch 1969; **Resid:** Surgery, Michigan Med Ctr 1971; Orthopaedic Surgery, Yale-New Haven Hosp 1974; **Fellow:** Musculoskeletal Oncology, Mass Genl Hosp 1983; **Fac Appt:** Prof OrS, Yale Univ

Gebhardt, Mark MD [OrS] - **Spec Exp:** Musculoskeletal Tumors; Bone Tumors; **Hospital:** Beth Israel Deaconess Med Ctr - Boston, Children's Hospital - Boston; **Address:** 330 Brookline Ave, Stoneman 10, Boston, MA 02215; **Phone:** 617-667-9598; **Board Cert:** Orthopaedic Surgery 2007; **Med School:** Univ Cincinnati 1975; **Resid:** Surgery, Univ Pittsburg Med Ctr 1977; Orthopaedic Surgery, Harvard Affil Hosps 1982; **Fellow:** Pediatric Orthopaedic Surgery, Boston Chldns Hosp 1983; Orthopaedic Oncology, Mass Genl Hosp 1983; **Fac Appt:** Prof OrS, Harvard Med Sch

Hornicek, Francis J MD/PhD [OrS] - **Spec Exp:** Bone Tumors; Sarcoma; Bone Tumors-Metastatic; Soft Tissue Tumors; **Hospital:** Mass Genl Hosp; **Address:** MGH Orthpaedic Oncology, 55 Fruit St, Yawkey 3700, Boston, MA 02114; **Phone:** 617-724-3700; **Board Cert:** Orthopaedic Surgery 2010; **Med School:** Univ Pittsburgh 1991; **Resid:** Orthopaedic Surgery, Jackson Meml Hosp 1996; **Fellow:** Orthopaedic Oncology, Mass Genl Hosp/Chldns Hosp 1997; **Fac Appt:** Assoc Prof OrS, Harvard Med Sch

Ready, John E MD [OrS] - **Spec Exp:** Bone Cancer; Sarcoma-Soft Tissue; Hip & Knee Replacement in Bone Tumors; **Hospital:** Brigham & Women's Hosp, Dana-Farber Cancer Inst; **Address:** Brigham & Women's Hospital, Dept of Orthopedic Surgery, 75 Francis St, Boston, MA 02115; **Phone:** 617-732-5368; **Board Cert:** Orthopaedic Surgery 2002; **Med School:** Dalhousie Univ 1982; **Resid:** Orthopaedic Surgery, Dalhousie Univ Hosp 1987; **Fellow:** Orthopaedic Oncology, St Michael's Hosp 1988; Orthopaedic Oncology, Mass Genl Hosp/Childns Hosp 1989

Weinstein, James DO [OrS] - **Spec Exp:** Pain-Back; Spinal Tumors; **Hospital:** Dartmouth - Hitchcock Med Ctr; **Address:** DHMC, Dept Orthopaedic Surgery, One Medical Ctr Drive, Lebanon, NH 03756; **Phone:** 603-650-2225; **Board Cert:** Orthopaedic Surgery 2002; **Med School:** Chicago Coll Osteo Med 1973; **Resid:** Orthopaedic Surgery, Rush Presby-St Lukes Med Ctr 1983; **Fac Appt:** Prof OrS, Dartmouth Med Sch

Mid Atlantic

Aboulafia, Albert J MD [OrS] - **Spec Exp:** Bone Cancer; **Hospital:** Sinai Hosp - Baltimore; **Address:** Lapidus Cancer Inst, 2401 W Belvedere Ave, Baltimore, MD 21215; **Phone:** 410-601-9266; **Board Cert:** Orthopaedic Surgery 2004; **Med School:** Univ Mich Med Sch 1985; **Resid:** Orthopaedic Surgery, LAC/USC Sch Med 1990; **Fellow:** Orthopaedic Oncology, Chldn's Natl Med Ctr/NIH 1991; **Fac Appt:** Asst Clin Prof OrS, Univ MD Sch Med

Benevenia, Joseph MD [OrS] - **Spec Exp:** Limb Sparing Surgery; Bone Cancer; Sarcoma-Soft Tissue; **Hospital:** Univ Hosp-UMDNJ—Newark; **Address:** 140 Bergen St, Ste ACC1610, Newark, NJ 07103; **Phone:** 973-972-2153; **Board Cert:** Orthopaedic Surgery 2003; **Med School:** UMDNJ-NJ Med Sch, Newark 1984; **Resid:** Orthopaedic Surgery, UMDNJ-NJ Med Sch Hosp 1988; **Fellow:** Orthopaedic Oncology, Case Western Reserve Univ 1991; **Fac Appt:** Prof OrS, UMDNJ-NJ Med Sch, Newark

Dormans, John P MD [OrS] - **Spec Exp:** Bone Cancer; Pediatric Orthopaedic Surgery; **Hospital:** Chldns Hosp of Philadelphia; **Address:** 34th Street & Civic Center Blvd, Wood Bldg Fl 2 - rm 2315, Philadelphia, PA 19104-4399; **Phone:** 215-590-1534; **Board Cert:** Orthopaedic Surgery 2002; **Med School:** Indiana Univ 1983; **Resid:** Orthopaedic Surgery, Michigan State Univ Hosps 1988; **Fellow:** Pediatric Orthopaedic Surgery, Hosp for Sick Children 1989; **Fac Appt:** Prof OrS, Univ Pennsylvania

Frassica, Frank J MD [OrS] - **Spec Exp:** Bone Cancer; **Hospital:** Johns Hopkins Hosp, Univ of MD Med Ctr; **Address:** 601 N Caroline St, Ste 5215, Baltimore, MD 21287; **Phone:** 410-502-2698; **Board Cert:** Orthopaedic Surgery 2011; **Med School:** Univ SC Sch Med 1982; **Resid:** Orthopaedic Surgery, Mayo Clinic 1987; **Fellow:** Orthopaedic Oncology, Mayo Clinic 1988; **Fac Appt:** Prof OrS, Johns Hopkins Univ

Healey, John H MD [OrS] - **Spec Exp:** Bone Tumors; Hip & Knee Replacement in Bone Tumors; Sarcoma; Sarcoma-Soft Tissue; **Hospital:** Meml Sloan-Kettering Cancer Ctr (page 75), Hosp For Special Surgery; **Address:** 1275 York Ave, New York, NY 10065; **Phone:** 212-639-7610; **Board Cert:** Orthopaedic Surgery 2007; **Med School:** Univ VT Coll Med 1978; **Resid:** Orthopaedic Surgery, Hosp Special Surg 1983; **Fellow:** Musculoskeletal Oncology, Meml Sloan Kettering Cancer Ctr 1984; Orthopaedic Surgery, Hosp Special Surgery 1984; **Fac Appt:** Prof OrS, Cornell Univ-Weill Med Coll

Henshaw, Robert M MD [OrS] - **Spec Exp:** Musculoskeletal Tumors; Bone Tumors; Orthopaedic Oncology; **Hospital:** Washington Hosp Ctr, Chldns Natl Med Ctr; **Address:** 110 Irving St NW, Ste C2173, Washington, DC 20010; **Phone:** 202-877-3970; **Board Cert:** Orthopaedic Surgery 2010; **Med School:** Tufts Univ 1990; **Resid:** Orthopaedic Surgery, UCLA Med Ctr 1995; **Fellow:** Orthopaedic Surgery, Washington Hosp Ctr 1997; **Fac Appt:** Assoc Prof OrS, Georgetown Univ

Kenan, Samuel MD [OrS] - **Spec Exp:** Bone Tumors; **Hospital:** NYU Hosp For Joint Diseases (page 79), NYU Langone Med Ctr (page 79); **Address:** 300 Old Country Rd, Ste 221, Mineola, NY 11501; **Phone:** 516-280-3733; **Med School:** Israel 1976; **Resid:** Orthopaedic Surgery, Hadassah Univ Hosp 1984; **Fellow:** Orthopaedic Pathology, Hosp for Joint Diseases 1987; **Fac Appt:** Prof OrS, NYU Sch Med

Lackman, Richard D MD [OrS] - **Spec Exp:** Bone Cancer; Sarcoma; Limb Sparing Surgery; **Hospital:** Pennsylvania Hosp (page 80), Penn Presby Med Ctr - UPHS (page 80); **Address:** Penn Orthopaedics, 301 S 8th St, Garfield Duncan Bldg, Ste 2C, Philadelphia, PA 19106; **Phone:** 215-829-5022; **Board Cert:** Orthopaedic Surgery 1985; **Med School:** Univ Pennsylvania 1977; **Resid:** Orthopaedic Surgery, Hosp Univ Penn 1982; **Fellow:** Orthopaedic Oncology, Mayo Clin 1983; **Fac Appt:** Assoc Prof OrS, Univ Pennsylvania

Lane, Joseph MD [OrS] - **Spec Exp:** Bone Cancer; **Hospital:** Hosp For Special Surgery, NY-Presby Hosp/Weill Cornell (page 78); **Address:** Hosp for Special Surgery, 535 E 70th St, New York, NY 10021; **Phone:** 212-606-1172; **Board Cert:** Orthopaedic Surgery 1974; **Med School:** Harvard Med Sch 1965; **Resid:** Surgery, Hosp Univ Penn 1967; Orthopaedic Surgery, Hosp Univ Penn 1973; **Fac Appt:** Prof OrS, Cornell Univ-Weill Med Coll

Lee, Francis Y MD/PhD [OrS] - **Spec Exp:** Bone Tumors; Pediatric Orthopaedic Cancers; Pediatric Orthopaedic Surgery; **Hospital:** NYPresby-Morgan Stanley Children's Hosp (page 78), NYPresby Hosp/Columbia (page 78); **Address:** 3959 Broadway, Ste 800N, New York, NY 10032; **Phone:** 212-305-3293; **Board Cert:** Orthopaedic Surgery 2001; **Med School:** South Korea 1986; **Resid:** Orthopaedic Surgery, NJ Med Ctr 1997; **Fellow:** Orthopaedic Oncology, Harvard Med Sch 1998; Pediatric Orthopaedic Surgery, Hosp for Sick Chldn/Univ Toronto 1999; **Fac Appt:** Asst Prof OrS, Columbia P&S

Orthopaedic Surgery

Malawer, Martin M MD [OrS] - **Spec Exp:** Bone Tumors; Limb Sparing Surgery; Pediatric Orthopaedic Surgery; Sarcoma; **Hospital:** Georgetown Univ Hosp, G Washington Univ Hosp; **Address:** 7830 Old Georgetown Rd, Ste C15, Bethesda, MD 20814; **Phone:** 301-215-7940; **Board Cert:** Orthopaedic Surgery 1976; **Med School:** NYU Sch Med 1969; **Resid:** Surgery, Bronx Muni Hosp 1972; Orthopaedic Surgery, Bellevue Hosp Ctr 1975; **Fellow:** Orthopaedic Oncology, Shands Hosp-Univ Florida 1978; **Fac Appt:** Prof OrS, Geo Wash Univ

O'Keefe, Regis J MD/PhD [OrS] - **Spec Exp:** Bone & Soft Tissue Tumors; Reconstructive Surgery; **Hospital:** Univ of Rochester Strong Meml Hosp, Highland Hosp of Rochester; **Address:** Univ Rochester, Dept Orthopaedic Surgery, 601 Elmwood Ave, Box 665, Rochester, NY 14642; **Phone:** 585-275-3100; **Board Cert:** Orthopaedic Surgery 2007; **Med School:** Harvard Med Sch 1985; **Resid:** Surgery, New Eng Deaconess Hosp/Harvard 1986; Orthopaedic Surgery, Univ Rochester 1992; **Fellow:** Orthopaedic Oncology, Mass Genl Hosp 1993; **Fac Appt:** Prof S, Univ Rochester

Schmidt, Richard G MD [OrS] - **Spec Exp:** Bone Tumors; Sarcoma-Soft Tissue; Limb Sparing Surgery; Bone Tumors-Metastatic; **Hospital:** Lankenau Hosp, Fox Chase Cancer Ctr (page 72); **Address:** Musculoskeletal Tumor Ctr, 15 N Presidential Blvd, Ste 300, Bala Cynwyd, PA 19004; **Phone:** 610-667-2663; **Board Cert:** Orthopaedic Surgery 2009; **Med School:** Penn State Coll Med 1980; **Resid:** Orthopaedic Surgery, Hosp Univ Penn 1985; **Fellow:** Orthopaedic Oncology, Shands Hosp 1986

Wittig, James C MD [OrS] - **Spec Exp:** Bone Tumors; Sarcoma-Soft Tissue; Shoulder Tumors; Musculoskeletal Tumors; **Hospital:** Mount Sinai Med Ctr (page 76), Hackensack Univ Med Ctr (page 73); **Address:** 5 E 98th St, Fl 9, New York, NY 10029; **Phone:** 212-241-1807 x4817; **Board Cert:** Orthopaedic Surgery 2003; **Med School:** NYU Sch Med 1994; **Resid:** Orthopaedic Surgery, Columbia Presby Med Ctr 1999; **Fellow:** Orthopaedic Oncology, Washington Cancer Inst 2001; Orthopaedic Oncology, NIH 2001; **Fac Appt:** Assoc Prof OrS, Mount Sinai Sch Med

Southeast

Berrey, B Hudson MD [OrS] - **Spec Exp:** Musculoskeletal Tumors; Bone Cancer; Soft Tissue Tumors; Sarcoma; **Hospital:** Shands Jacksonville, Wolfson Chldns Hosp; **Address:** University of Florida Coll Med, Dept Orthopaedic Surgery, 655 W Eighth St ACC Bldg Fl 2, Jacksonville, FL 32209-6511; **Phone:** 904-244-5942; **Board Cert:** Orthopaedic Surgery 1982; **Med School:** Univ Tex Med Br, Galveston 1977; **Resid:** Orthopaedic Surgery, Tripler Army Med Ctr 1981; **Fellow:** Medical Oncology, Mass Genl Hosp/Harvard 1985; **Fac Appt:** Prof OrS, Univ Fla Coll Med

Kneisl, Jeffrey S MD [OrS] - **Spec Exp:** Bone Cancer; Musculoskeletal Tumors; **Hospital:** Carolinas Med Ctr; **Address:** 1025 Morhead Medical Drive, Ste 300, Charlotte, NC 28204; **Phone:** 704-355-5982; **Board Cert:** Orthopaedic Surgery 2010; **Med School:** Northwestern Univ 1980; **Resid:** Orthopaedic Surgery, Northwestern Univ 1987; **Fellow:** Orthopaedic Oncology, Univ Chicago 1990

Scarborough, Mark T MD [OrS] - **Spec Exp:** Bone Tumors; Sarcoma; **Hospital:** Shands at Univ of FL; **Address:** Shands Healthcare Univ FL, PO Box 112-733, Gainesville, FL 32611-2733; **Phone:** 352-273-7000; **Board Cert:** Orthopaedic Surgery 2004; **Med School:** Univ Fla Coll Med 1985; **Resid:** Orthopaedic Surgery, Univ Texas Med Ctr 1990; **Fellow:** Orthopaedic Surgery, Mass Genl Hosp 1991; **Fac Appt:** Prof OrS, Univ Fla Coll Med

Schwartz, Herbert S MD [OrS] - **Spec Exp:** Bone Tumors-Metastatic; Bone Tumors; Pelvic Surgery-Complex; Musculoskeletal Tumors; **Hospital:** Vanderbilt Univ Med Ctr, Baptist Hosp - Nashville; **Address:** Vanderbilt Orthopaedic Institute, Medical Center East, South Tower, Ste 4200, Nashville, TN 37232-8774; **Phone:** 615-322-0543; **Board Cert:** Orthopaedic Surgery 2007; **Med School:** Univ Chicago-Pritzker Sch Med 1981; **Resid:** Orthopaedic Surgery, Univ Chicago Hosps 1986; **Fellow:** Orthopaedic Oncology, Mayo Clinic 1987; **Fac Appt:** Prof OrS, Vanderbilt Univ

Siegel, Herrick J MD [OrS] - **Spec Exp:** Bone Cancer; Sarcoma; Bone Tumors-Metastatic; **Hospital:** Univ of Ala Hosp at Birmingham, UAB Highlands Hosp; **Address:** 1313 13th St S, Birmingham, AL 35205; **Phone:** 205-975-2310; **Board Cert:** Orthopaedic Surgery 2005; **Med School:** NYU Sch Med 1995; **Resid:** Orthopaedic Surgery, USC Univ Hosp 2000; **Fellow:** Orthopaedic Oncology, Mayo Clinic 2002; **Fac Appt:** Assoc Prof OrS, Univ Alabama

Walling, Arthur K MD [OrS] - **Spec Exp:** Bone Tumors; Soft Tissue Tumors; **Hospital:** Tampa Genl Hosp; **Address:** Florida Orthopaedic Inst, 13020 Telecom Pkwy N, Tampa, FL 33637; **Phone:** 813-978-9700; **Board Cert:** Orthopaedic Surgery 1982; **Med School:** Creighton Univ 1976; **Resid:** Orthopaedic Surgery, Univ South Florida Affil Hosps 1980; **Fellow:** Surgical Oncology, Univ Florida 1981; **Fac Appt:** Assoc Clin Prof OrS, Univ S Fla Coll Med

Ward Sr, William G MD [OrS] - **Spec Exp:** Bone Tumors; Soft Tissue Tumors; Reconstructive Surgery; Sarcoma; **Hospital:** Wake Forest Univ Baptist Med Ctr; **Address:** First Floor Comp Rehab, 131 Miller St, Winston-Salem, NC 27103; **Phone:** 336-716-8093; **Board Cert:** Orthopaedic Surgery 2004; **Med School:** Duke Univ 1975; **Resid:** Surgery, Duke Univ Med Ctr 1985; Orthopaedic Surgery, Duke Univ Med Ctr 1989; **Fellow:** Sports Medicine, Cleveland Clinic 1990; Orthopaedic Oncology, UCLA Med Ctr 1991; **Fac Appt:** Prof OrS, Wake Forest Univ

Midwest

Biermann, J Sybil MD [OrS] - **Spec Exp:** Sarcoma; Bone Cancer; Multiple Myeloma; Limb Sparing Surgery; **Hospital:** Univ of Michigan Hosp; **Address:** Univ Michigan Cancer Ctr, 1500 E Medical Ctr Drive, SPC 5912, Ann Arbor, MI 48109; **Phone:** 734-647-8902; **Board Cert:** Orthopaedic Surgery 2006; **Med School:** Stanford Univ 1987; **Resid:** Orthopaedic Surgery, Univ Iowa Hosp 1992; **Fellow:** Orthopaedic Oncology, Univ Chicago Hosps 1993; **Fac Appt:** Assoc Prof OrS, Univ Mich Med Sch

Buckwalter IV, Joseph A MD [OrS] - **Spec Exp:** Bone Cancer; Bone Tumors-Metastatic; **Hospital:** Univ Iowa Hosp & Clinics; **Address:** Univ Iowa Hosps, Dept Orthopaedics, 200 Hawkins Drive, Iowa City, IA 52242; **Phone:** 319-356-2595; **Board Cert:** Orthopaedic Surgery 1991; **Med School:** Univ Iowa Coll Med 1974; **Resid:** Orthopaedic Surgery, Iowa Hosp 1979; **Fac Appt:** Prof OrS, Univ Iowa Coll Med

Cheng, Edward Y MD [OrS] - **Spec Exp:** Bone & Soft Tissue Tumors; Reconstructive Surgery; **Address:** Univ Minnesota, Dept Orthopaedic Surgery, 2512 S Seventh St, Ste R-200, Minneapolis, MN 55454; **Phone:** 612-273-1177; **Board Cert:** Orthopaedic Surgery 2003; **Med School:** Northwestern Univ 1983; **Resid:** Surgery, Northwestern Univ 1985; Orthopaedic Surgery, Beth Israel Hosp 1989; **Fellow:** Surgical Oncology, Mass Genl Hosp 1990; **Fac Appt:** Prof OrS, Univ Minn

Clohisy, Denis MD [OrS] - **Spec Exp:** Bone Cancer; **Address:** Univ Minn, Dept Orthopaedic Surgery, 2512 S Seveth St, Ste R200, Minneapolis, MN 55454; **Phone:** 612-273-1177; **Board Cert:** Orthopaedic Surgery 2004; **Med School:** Northwestern Univ 1983; **Resid:** Orthopaedic Surgery, Univ Minn 1990; **Fellow:** Pathology, Wash Univ Med Ctr 1987; Musculoskeletal Oncology, Mass Genl Hosp 1991; **Fac Appt:** Prof OrS, Univ Minn

Orthopaedic Surgery

Gitelis, Steven MD [OrS] - **Spec Exp:** Bone Cancer; Soft Tissue Tumors; Limb Sparing Surgery; **Hospital:** Rush Univ Med Ctr; **Address:** 1611 W Harrison St, Ste 300, Chicago, IL 60612; **Phone:** 312-432-2397; **Board Cert:** Orthopaedic Surgery 1982; **Med School:** Rush Med Coll 1975; **Resid:** Orthopaedic Surgery, Rush Presby-St Lukes Med Ctr 1980; **Fellow:** Orthopaedic Oncology, Mayo Clinic 1982; **Fac Appt:** Prof OrS, Rush Med Coll

Irwin, Ronald B MD [OrS] - **Spec Exp:** Bone Cancer; Limb Sparing Surgery; Sarcoma-Soft Tissue; **Hospital:** Mount Clemens Regional Med Ctr; **Address:** Mount Clemens Regional Med Ctr, 1080 Harrington Blvd, Ste 201, Mount Clemens, MI 48043; **Phone:** 586-493-7575; **Board Cert:** Orthopaedic Surgery 1979; **Med School:** Univ Mich Med Sch 1971; **Resid:** Orthopaedic Surgery, William Beaumont Hosp 1978; **Fellow:** Orthopaedic Oncology, Mayo Clinic 1978

Joyce, Michael J MD [OrS] - **Spec Exp:** Bone & Soft Tissue Tumors; **Hospital:** Cleveland Clin (page 70); **Address:** 9500 Euclid Ave, Desk A41, Dept Orthopaedic Surgery, Cleveland, OH 44195; **Phone:** 216-444-4282; **Board Cert:** Orthopaedic Surgery 1985; **Med School:** Univ Louisville Sch Med 1976; **Resid:** Surgery, Johns Hopkins Hosp 1978; Orthopaedic Surgery, Harvard Combined Program 1981; **Fellow:** Orthopaedic Oncology, Mass General Hosp 1982; Trauma, Univ Toronto-Sunnybrook Hosp 1983; **Fac Appt:** Assoc Clin Prof OrS, Case West Res Univ

Les, Kimberly A MD [OrS] - **Spec Exp:** Bone Cancer; **Hospital:** Beaumont Hosp-Royal Oak; **Address:** Rose Cancer Treatment Ctr, 3577 W 13 Mile Rd, Ste 402, Royal Oak, MI 48073; **Phone:** 248-551-9910; **Board Cert:** Orthopaedic Surgery 2000; **Med School:** Geo Wash Univ 1992; **Resid:** Orthopaedic Surgery, Henry Ford Hosp 1997; **Fellow:** Orthopaedic Oncology, Univ Chicago Hosps 1978

Mayerson, Joel L MD [OrS] - **Spec Exp:** Bone Tumors; Sarcoma-Soft Tissue; Musculoskeletal Tumors; **Hospital:** Ohio St Univ Med Ctr; **Address:** Ohio State, Div of Musculoskeletal Onc, 410 W 10 Ave N Doan Hall Bldg - rm 1049, Columbus, OH 43210; **Phone:** 614-293-4420; **Board Cert:** Orthopaedic Surgery 2003; **Med School:** Johns Hopkins Univ 1994; **Resid:** Orthopaedic Surgery, Cleveland Clinic 1999; **Fellow:** Orthopaedic Oncology, Univ Wash Med Ctr 2000; **Fac Appt:** Assoc Prof OrS, Ohio State Univ

McDonald, Douglas J MD [OrS] - **Spec Exp:** Bone & Soft Tissue Tumors; Ewing's Sarcoma; Sarcoma; **Hospital:** Barnes-Jewish Hosp, St. Louis Chldns Hosp; **Address:** Ctr Advanced Med, Orthopaedic Surg Ctr, 4921 Parkview Pl Fl 6 - Ste A, Box 8605, St Louis, MO 63110; **Phone:** 314-747-2500; **Board Cert:** Orthopaedic Surgery 2011; **Med School:** Univ Minn 1982; **Resid:** Orthopaedic Surgery, Mayo Clinic 1987; **Fellow:** Orthopaedic Oncology, Mayo Clinic 1988; Orthopaedic Surgery, Rizzoli Inst 1989; **Fac Appt:** Prof OrS, Washington Univ, St Louis

Mott, Michael P MD [OrS] - **Spec Exp:** Soft Tissue Tumors; Musculoskeletal Tumors; Bone Cancer; **Hospital:** Henry Ford Hosp, Henry Ford- W Bloomfield Hosp; **Address:** Henry Ford Hosp, Dept Ortho Surg, 2799 W Grand Blvd Fl 12, Detroit, MI 48202; **Phone:** 313-916-1961; **Board Cert:** Orthopaedic Surgery 2007; **Med School:** Univ Mich Med Sch 1989; **Resid:** Orthopaedic Surgery, Wayne State Univ Affil Hosp 1994; **Fellow:** Musculoskeletal Oncology, Mass Genl Hosp 1995; Orthopaedic Oncology, Wayne State Univ 1996; **Fac Appt:** Assoc Prof OrS, Wayne State Univ

Parsons III, Theodore W MD [OrS] - **Spec Exp:** Bone & Soft Tissue Tumors; Reconstructive Surgery; **Hospital:** Henry Ford Hosp; **Address:** Henry Ford Hosp, Dept Orthopaedics, 2799 West Grand Blvd, CFP-6, Detroit, MI 48202; **Phone:** 313-916-1964; **Board Cert:** Orthopaedic Surgery 2005; **Med School:** Uniformed Srvs Univ, Bethesda 1986; **Resid:** Orthopaedic Surgery, Wilford Hall USAF Med Ctr 1991; **Fellow:** Pediatric Oncology, Boston Chldns Hosp 1992; Orthopaedic Oncology, Mass Genl Hosp 1992; **Fac Appt:** Prof OrS, Wayne State Univ

Peabody, Terrance D MD [OrS] - **Spec Exp:** Soft Tissue Tumors; Bone Tumors; Pediatric Orthopaedic Cancers; Limb Sparing Surgery; **Hospital:** Univ of Chicago Med Ctr; **Address:** Univ Chicago Medical Ctr, 5841 S Maryland Ave, MC 3079, Chicago, IL 60637; **Phone:** 773-702-3442; **Board Cert:** Orthopaedic Surgery 2004; **Med School:** UC Irvine 1985; **Resid:** Orthopaedic Surgery, UC Irvine Med Ctr 1990; **Fellow:** Orthopaedic Oncology, Univ Chicago Hosps 1991; **Fac Appt:** Prof OrS, Univ Chicago-Pritzker Sch Med

Sim, Franklin H MD [OrS] - **Spec Exp:** Sarcoma; Bone Cancer; **Hospital:** Mayo Med Ctr & Clin - Rochester; **Address:** Mayo Clinic, Orthopaedic Surg, Gonda 14, 200 1st St SW, Rochester, MN 55905; **Phone:** 507-284-2511; **Board Cert:** Orthopaedic Surgery 1971; **Med School:** Dalhousie Univ 1965; **Resid:** Orthopaedic Surgery, Mayo Clinic 1970; **Fac Appt:** Prof OrS, Mayo Med Sch

Wurtz, L Daniel MD [OrS] - **Spec Exp:** Bone & Soft Tissue Tumors; Limb Sparing Surgery; Sarcoma; Pediatric Orthopaedic Cancers; **Hospital:** IU Health Methodist Hosp; **Address:** University Orthopaedic Assocs, 541 Clinical Drive, Ste 2600, Indianapolis, IN 46202; **Phone:** 317-274-3227; **Board Cert:** Orthopaedic Surgery 2004; **Med School:** Univ S Ala Coll Med 1985; **Resid:** Orthopaedic Surgery, Wilford Hall USAF Med Ctr 1990; **Fellow:** Musculoskeletal Oncology, Univ Chicago; **Fac Appt:** Assoc Prof OrS, Indiana Univ

Great Plains and Mountains

Kelly, Cynthia M MD [OrS] - **Spec Exp:** Bone Tumors; Soft Tissue Tumors; Bone Cancer; **Hospital:** Presby - St Luke's Med Ctr; **Address:** 1601 E 19th Ave, Ste 3300, Denver, CO 80218; **Phone:** 303-837-0072; **Board Cert:** Orthopaedic Surgery 2000; **Med School:** UCLA 1989; **Resid:** Orthopaedic Surgery, Harbor-UCLA Med Ctr 1994; **Fellow:** Orthopaedic Oncology, UCLA Med Ctr 1995

Randall, R Lawrence L MD [OrS] - **Spec Exp:** Bone Tumors; Sarcoma-Soft Tissue; Pediatric Orthopaedic Surgery; **Hospital:** Univ Utah Hlth Care, Primary Children's Med Ctr; **Address:** Ped Ortho Surg, Primary Chlds Med Ctr, 100 N Mario Capecchi Drive, Ste 4550, Salt Lake City, UT 84113; **Phone:** 801-662-5600; **Board Cert:** Orthopaedic Surgery 2001; **Med School:** Yale Univ 1992; **Resid:** Orthopaedic Surgery, UCSF Med Ctr 1997; **Fellow:** Musculoskeletal Oncology, Univ WA Med Ctr 1998; **Fac Appt:** Assoc Prof OrS, Univ Utah

Wilkins, Ross M MD [OrS] - **Spec Exp:** Bone Cancer; **Hospital:** Presby - St Luke's Med Ctr; **Address:** 1601 E 19th Ave, Ste 3300, Denver, CO 80218; **Phone:** 303-837-0072; **Board Cert:** Orthopaedic Surgery 2007; **Med School:** Wayne State Univ 1978; **Resid:** Orthopaedic Surgery, Univ Colorado Med Ctr 1983; **Fellow:** Orthopaedic Oncology, Mayo Clinic 1984

Southwest

Williams, Ronald P MD [OrS] - **Spec Exp:** Bone Tumors; **Hospital:** Univ Hlth Syst-San Antonio; **Address:** Scarcoma Ctr at CTRC, 7979 Wurzbach Rd, Ste U219, MC 8226, San Antonio, TX 78229-3900; **Phone:** 210-450-1170; **Board Cert:** Orthopaedic Surgery 2003; **Med School:** Univ Tex, San Antonio 1984; **Resid:** Orthopaedic Surgery, Univ Kans Sch Med 1989; **Fellow:** Orthopaedic Oncology, Case West Res Univ 1990; **Fac Appt:** Prof OrS, Univ Tex, San Antonio

Orthopaedic Surgery

West Coast and Pacific

Bos, Gary D MD [OrS] - **Spec Exp:** Musculoskeletal Tumors; Sarcoma; Reconstructive Surgery; **Hospital:** Yakima Valley Mem Hosp; **Address:** 3003 TIETON Drive, Ste 350, Yakima, WA 98902; **Phone:** 509-573-3989; **Board Cert:** Orthopaedic Surgery 2008; **Med School:** Univ Chicago-Pritzker Sch Med 1978; **Resid:** Orthopaedic Surgery, Case West Reserve Univ 1984; **Fellow:** Orthopaedic Surgery, Case West Reserve Univ 1980; Orthopaedic Oncology, Mayo Clinic 1985; **Fac Appt:** Asst Clin Prof OrS

Brien, Earl Warren MD [OrS] - **Spec Exp:** Bone & Soft Tissue Tumors; **Hospital:** Cedars-Sinai Med Ctr; **Address:** 8700 Beverly Blvd, rm AC1058, Los Angeles, CA 90048; **Phone:** 310-423-9887; **Board Cert:** Orthopaedic Surgery 2006; **Med School:** Howard Univ 1986; **Resid:** Orthopaedic Surgery, LAC-King Drew Med Ctr 1992; **Fellow:** Musculoskeletal Disorders, Memorial Sloan Kettering 1993; Metabolic Bone Research, Hosp for Special Surgery 1994

Conrad, Ernest U MD [OrS] - **Spec Exp:** Pediatric Orthopaedic Surgery; Bone Tumors; Sarcoma; **Hospital:** Seattle Chldns Hosp, Univ Wash Med Ctr; **Address:** 4800 Sand Point Way NE, #W7706, Box 359300, Seattle, WA 98195-5371; **Phone:** 206-987-5678; **Board Cert:** Orthopaedic Surgery 2009; **Med School:** Univ VA Sch Med 1979; **Resid:** Orthopaedic Surgery, Hosp for Special Surgery 1984; **Fellow:** Orthopaedic Oncology, Univ Fla Coll Med 1985; Pediatric Orthopaedic Surgery, Hosp for Sick Chldn 1986; **Fac Appt:** Prof OrS, Univ Wash

Eckardt, Jeffrey J MD [OrS] - **Spec Exp:** Bone Tumors; Soft Tissue Tumors; Limb Sparing Surgery; **Hospital:** Santa Monica - UCLA Med Ctr & Ortho Hosp, UCLA Ronald Reagan Med Ctr; **Address:** UCLA Med Ctr, Dept Ortho Surg/Oncology, 1250 16th St Tower # 713, Santa Monica, CA 90404; **Phone:** 310-319-3816; **Board Cert:** Orthopaedic Surgery 1981; **Med School:** Cornell Univ-Weill Med Coll 1971; **Resid:** Orthopaedic Surgery, UCLA Med Ctr 1979; **Fellow:** Orthopaedic Oncology, Mayo Clinic 1980; **Fac Appt:** Prof OrS, UCLA

Luck Jr, James V MD [OrS] - **Spec Exp:** Musculoskeletal Tumors; **Hospital:** Santa Monica - UCLA Med Ctr & Ortho Hosp; **Address:** 2400 S Flower St, Fl 3, Los Angeles, CA 90007; **Phone:** 213-749-8255; **Board Cert:** Orthopaedic Surgery 2000; **Med School:** USC Sch Med 1967; **Resid:** Orthopaedic Surgery, Orthopaedic Hosp 1973; **Fellow:** Orthopaedic Oncology, Orthopaedic Hosp 1974; Reconstructive Surgery, Rancho Los Amigos 1974; **Fac Appt:** Prof OrS, UCLA

O'Donnell, Richard John MD [OrS] - **Spec Exp:** Bone Cancer; Sarcoma-Soft Tissue; Pediatric Orthopaedic Cancers; **Hospital:** UCSF Med Ctr; **Address:** UCSF Helen Diller Cancer Ctr, 1600 Divisadero St Fl 4, San Francisco, CA 94115; **Phone:** 415-885-3800; **Board Cert:** Orthopaedic Surgery 2010; **Med School:** Harvard Med Sch 1989; **Resid:** Orthopaedic Surgery, Mass Genl Hosp 1995; **Fellow:** Musculoskeletal Oncology, Univ WA Med Ctr 1996; **Fac Appt:** Assoc Prof OrS, UCSF

Singer, Daniel I MD [OrS] - **Spec Exp:** Bone Cancer; Hand & Upper Extremity Tumors; **Hospital:** Queen's Med Ctr - Honolulu; **Address:** Queen's Physicians' Office Blg 1, 1380 Lusitana St, Ste 615, Honolulu, HI 96813-2442; **Phone:** 808-521-8109; **Board Cert:** Orthopaedic Surgery 2010; Hand Surgery 2010; **Med School:** Boston Univ 1979; **Resid:** Surgery, Univ Conn Hlth Ctr 1981; Orthopaedic Surgery, Univ Hawaii Affil Hosp 1984; **Fellow:** Hand Surgery, Thomas Jefferson Univ Hosp 1985; Microvascular Surgery, St Vincent's Hosp 1986; **Fac Appt:** Assoc Prof OrS, Univ Hawaii JA Burns Sch Med

HAND SURGERY

Mid Atlantic

Athanasian, Edward MD [HS] - **Spec Exp:** Bone & Soft Tissue Tumors; Hand & Upper Extremity Tumors; **Hospital:** Hosp For Special Surgery, Meml Sloan-Kettering Cancer Ctr (page 75); **Address:** Hospital for Special Surgery, 535 E 70th St, New York, NY 10021; **Phone:** 212-606-1962; **Board Cert:** Orthopaedic Surgery 2008; Hand Surgery 2008; **Med School:** Columbia P&S 1988; **Resid:** Surgery, Beth Israel Hosp 1989; Orthopaedic Surgery, Hosp Special Surgery 1993; **Fellow:** Hand Surgery, Mayo Clinic 1994; Orthopaedic Oncology, Meml Sloan Kettering Cancer Ctr 1995; **Fac Appt:** Asst Prof OrS, Cornell Univ-Weill Med Coll

West Coast and Pacific

Szabo, Robert M MD [HS] - **Spec Exp:** Hand & Upper Extremity Tumors; **Hospital:** UC Davis Med Ctr, Mercy General Hosp - Sacramento; **Address:** UC Davis, Dept Orthopaedics, 4860 Y St, Ste 1700, Sacramento, CA 95817; **Phone:** 916-734-3678; **Board Cert:** Orthopaedic Surgery 2009; Hand Surgery 2009; **Med School:** SUNY Buffalo 1977; **Resid:** Surgery, Mt Sinai Hosp 1979; Orthopaedic Surgery, Mt Sinai Hosp 1982; **Fellow:** Hand Surgery, UCSD Med Ctr 1983; Epidemiology, UC Berkeley 1995; **Fac Appt:** Prof OrS, UC Davis

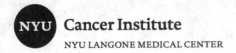

NYU Langone Medical Center
550 First Avenue , New York, NY 10016
www.NYULMC.org

NYU Clinical Cancer Center
160 East 34th Street, New York, NY 10016
www.NYUCI.org

**The Stephen D. Hassenfeld Children's Center
for Cancer and Blood Disorders**
160 East 32nd Street, New York, NY 10016
www.NYUMC.org/Hassenfeld

The NYU Cancer Institute is an NCI-designated cancer center and provides personalized patient care that is both compassionate and state of the art. The doctors and researchers work together to develop innovative therapies for patients. The Cancer Institute is world-renowned for excellence in cancer-focused research, personalized care, education and community outreach. Its mission is to discover the origins of human cancer and to use that knowledge to eradicate the personal and societal burden of cancer in our community, the nation and the world. For more information about our expert physicians, call 212-731-5000. *We specialize in the following areas:*

Patient-Focused Setting
The NYU Clinical Cancer Center is the principal outpatient facility of The Cancer Institute and serves as home to our patients and their caregivers. The center and its multidisciplinary team of experts provide access to the latest treatment options and clinical trials along with a variety of programs in cancer risk reduction/prevention, screening, diagnostics, genetic counseling and supportive services. In addition the NYUCI emphasizes the importance of a holistic approach to management services in complementary medicine, psychosocial support, survivorship and palliative care.

Renowned Expertise
The NYU Cancer Institute brings together experts from a variety of disciplines to create collaborative research endeavors and clinical care teams. The Cancer Institute offers a full continuum of personalized care, from prevention through diagnosis, treatment and post-treatment support. The compassion and expertise of our team members helps patients better manage the symptoms of their diseases as well as meet their special needs. Additionally, we have created special emphasis programs in diseases such as breast cancer, melanoma, GI cancer, prostate cancer, hematologic malignancies and lung cancer among others, as well as, translational programs in cancer healthcare disparities, molecularly targeted therapy, and the cell signaling pathways involved in cancer.

A Translational Approach
NYU Langone Medical Center scientists and other researchers excel in uncovering how cancer develops at the molecular level, and how we can harness that knowledge to reduce the risk of cancer and treat the disease. The Medical Center constantly seeks to create new opportunities for collaboration between investigators within our own institution, those located elsewhere in the NYU network of campuses, and researchers at other institutions.

The Stephen D. Hassenfeld Children's Center for Cancer and Blood Disorders
The center is a leading pediatric outpatient facility for the treatment of childhood cancers and blood diseases. Its unique interdisciplinary and family-centered approach combines the most advanced medical treatments with psychosocial and emotional support services for young patients and their families.

Otolaryngology

An otolaryngologist diagnoses and provides medical and/or surgical therapy prevention of diseases, allergies, neoplasms, deformities, disorders and/or injuries of the ears, nose, sinuses, throat, respiratory and upper alimentary systems, face, jaws and the other head and neck systems. Head and neck oncology, facial plastic and reconstructive surgery and the treatment of disorders of hearing and voice are fundamental areas of expertise.

An otolaraynogologist-head and neck surgeon provides comprehensive medical and surgical care for patients with diseases and disorders that affect the ears, nose, throat, the respiratory and upper alimentary systems and related structures of the head and neck.

Training Required: Five years. Certification in the following subspecialty requires additional training and examination.

Plastic Surgery within the Head and Neck: An otolaryngologist with additional training in plastic and reconstructive procedures within the head, face, neck and associated structures, including cutaneous head and neck oncology and reconstructioin, management of maxillofacial trauma, soft tissue repair and neural surgery.

This field is diverse and involves a wide range of patients, from the newborn to the aged. While both cosmetic and reconstructive surgeries are practiced, there are many additional procedures which interface with them.

Otolaryngology

New England

Couch, Marion E MD [Oto] - **Spec Exp:** Head & Neck Cancer; Thyroid & Parathyroid Cancer & Surgery; Microvascular Surgery; Airway Reconstruction; **Hospital:** Fletcher Allen Health Care- Med Ctr Campus; **Address:** 111 Colchester Ave, Div Otolaryngology, Burlington, VT 05401; **Phone:** 802-847-4537; **Board Cert:** Otolaryngology 1997; **Med School:** Rush Med Coll 1990; **Resid:** Surgery, Johns Hopkins Hosp 1991; Otolaryngology, Johns Hopkins Hosp 1995; **Fac Appt:** Assoc Prof Oto, Univ VT Coll Med

Deschler, Daniel G MD [Oto] - **Spec Exp:** Head & Neck Cancer; Head & Neck Reconstruction; Salivary Gland Tumors & Surgery; Voice after Laryngeal Cancer Surgery; **Hospital:** Mass Eye & Ear Infirmary, Mass Genl Hosp; **Address:** Mass Eye & Ear Infirmary, Head & Neck Surgery, 243 Charles St, Boston, MA 02114; **Phone:** 617-573-4100; **Board Cert:** Otolaryngology 1996; **Med School:** Harvard Med Sch 1990; **Resid:** Otolaryngology, UCSF Med Ctr 1995; **Fellow:** Head & Neck Surgical Oncology, Hahneman Univ Med Ctr 1996; **Fac Appt:** Assoc Prof Oto, Harvard Med Sch

Gosselin, Benoit J MD [Oto] - **Spec Exp:** Head & Neck Cancer; Facial Plastic & Reconstructive Surgery; Head & Neck Reconstruction; **Hospital:** Dartmouth - Hitchcock Med Ctr; **Address:** Dartmouth-Hitchcock Med Ctr, Dept Oto, 1 Med Ctr Drive, Lebanon, NH 03756; **Phone:** 603-650-8123; **Board Cert:** Otolaryngology 1994; **Med School:** Univ Ottawa 1988; **Resid:** Head and Neck Surgery, Univ Ottawa 1993; **Fellow:** Head and Neck Surgery, Univ Toronto 1994; Facial Plastic Surgery, Mercy Hosp 1995; **Fac Appt:** Assoc Clin Prof Oto, Dartmouth Med Sch

Grillone, Gregory A MD [Oto] - **Spec Exp:** Laryngeal Disorders; Laryngeal Cancer; Head & Neck Cancer; Voice Disorders; **Hospital:** Boston Med Ctr; **Address:** Boston Univ Med Ctr, Dept Otolaryngology, 830 Harrison Ave, Ste 1400, Boston, MA 02118; **Phone:** 617-414-4913; **Board Cert:** Otolaryngology 1988; **Med School:** Mount Sinai Sch Med 1983; **Resid:** Otolaryngology, Boston Univ Med Ctr 1988; **Fac Appt:** Assoc Prof Oto, Boston Univ

Randolph, Gregory W MD [Oto] - **Spec Exp:** Thyroid Disorders; Thyroid Cancer; Parathyroid Disease; **Hospital:** Mass Eye & Ear Infirmary; **Address:** Mass Eye & Ear Infirmary, 243 Charles St Fl 2, Boston, MA 02114; **Phone:** 617-573-4115; **Board Cert:** Otolaryngology 1993; **Med School:** Cornell Univ-Weill Med Coll 1987; **Resid:** Otolaryngology, Mass E&E Infirmary 1992; **Fellow:** Thyroid Oncology, Mass E&E Infirmary 1993; **Fac Appt:** Asst Prof Oto, Harvard Med Sch

Sasaki, Clarence T MD [Oto] - **Spec Exp:** Head & Neck Cancer; Skull Base Surgery; Voice Disorders; Swallowing Disorders; **Hospital:** Yale-New Haven Hosp, Yale Med Group; **Address:** Yale Sch Med, Dept Otolaryngology, 333 Cedar St, Box 208041, New Haven, CT 06520-8041; **Phone:** 203-785-2592; **Board Cert:** Otolaryngology 1973; **Med School:** Yale Univ 1966; **Resid:** Surgery, Mary Hitchcock Hosp 1968; Otolaryngology, Yale-New Haven Hosp 1973; **Fellow:** Head and Neck Surgery, Univ of Milan 1978; Skull Base Surgery, Univ Zurich 1982; **Fac Appt:** Prof Oto, Yale Univ

Zeitels, Steven MD [Oto] - **Spec Exp:** Laryngeal Disorders; Voice Disorders; Laryngeal Cancer; Head & Neck Cancer & Surgery; **Hospital:** Mass Genl Hosp; **Address:** MGH Center for Laryngeal Surgery, 1 Bowdoin Square Fl 11, Boston, MA 02114; **Phone:** 617-726-0218; **Board Cert:** Otolaryngology 1988; **Med School:** Boston Univ 1982; **Resid:** Surgery, Univ Hosp-Boston City Hosp 1983; Otolaryngology, Boston Univ-Tufts Univ Affil Hosps 1987; **Fellow:** Head and Neck Surgery, Boston VA Med Ctr 1988; **Fac Appt:** Prof Oto, Harvard Med Sch

Mid Atlantic

Califano III, Joseph A MD [Oto] - **Spec Exp:** Head & Neck Cancer; Thyroid Cancer; Skull Base Tumors; Melanoma; **Hospital:** Johns Hopkins Hosp, Greater Baltimore Med Ctr; **Address:** Johns Hopkins Hosp, 601 N Caroline St Fl 6th, Baltimore, MD 21287-0910; **Phone:** 410-502-2692; **Board Cert:** Otolaryngology 2000; **Med School:** Harvard Med Sch 1993; **Resid:** Otolaryngology, Johns Hopkins Hosp 1999; **Fellow:** Otolaryngology, Meml Sloan Kettering Cancer Ctr 2000; **Fac Appt:** Prof Oto, Johns Hopkins Univ

Chalian, Ara A MD [Oto] - **Spec Exp:** Head & Neck Cancer; Head & Neck Reconstruction; Thyroid Cancer; Reconstructive Surgery; **Hospital:** Hosp Univ Penn - UPHS (page 80); **Address:** Hosp Univ Penn, Dept Otolaryngology, 3400 Spruce St, 5 Silverstein Bldg, Philadelphia, PA 19104; **Phone:** 215-349-5559; **Board Cert:** Otolaryngology 1994; **Med School:** Indiana Univ 1988; **Resid:** Surgery, Indiana Univ Hosp 1990; Otolaryngology, Indiana Univ Hosp 1993; **Fellow:** Molecular Biology, Hosp U Penn 1994; Head and Neck Surgery, Hosp U Penn 1995; **Fac Appt:** Assoc Prof Oto, Univ Pennsylvania

Close, Lanny G MD [Oto] - **Spec Exp:** Skull Base Surgery; Head & Neck Cancer; **Hospital:** NY-Presby Hosp/Columbia (page 78); **Address:** 16 E 60th St, Ste 470, New York, NY 10022; **Phone:** 212-326-8475; **Board Cert:** Otolaryngology 1977; **Med School:** Baylor Coll Med 1972; **Resid:** Surgery, Johns Hopkins Hosp 1974; Otolaryngology, Baylor Affil Hosps 1977; **Fellow:** Head and Neck Surgery, MD Anderson Cancer Ctr 1979; **Fac Appt:** Prof Oto, Columbia P&S

Costantino, Peter D MD [Oto] - **Spec Exp:** Skull Base Tumors; Head & Neck Cancer; Craniofacial Surgery/Reconstruction; **Hospital:** Lenox Hill Hosp, NY-Presby Hosp/Columbia (page 78); **Address:** New York Head & Neck Inst, 110 E 59th St, Ste 10A, New York, NY 10022; **Phone:** 212-434-4500; **Board Cert:** Otolaryngology 1990; Facial Plastic & Reconstr Surgery 2000; **Med School:** Northwestern Univ 1984; **Resid:** Surgery, Northwestern Meml Hosp 1986; Otolaryngology, Northwestern Meml Hosp 1989; **Fellow:** Head and Neck Surgery, Northwestern Meml Hosp 1990; Skull Base Surgery, Univ Pittsburgh 1991; **Fac Appt:** Prof Oto, Columbia P&S

Davidson, Bruce J MD [Oto] - **Spec Exp:** Head & Neck Cancer; Thyroid Disorders; **Hospital:** Georgetown Univ Hosp; **Address:** Georgetown Univ Med Ctr, Dept Otolaryngology-Head & Neck Surgery, 3800 Reservoir Rd NW, Gorman Bldg - Fl 1, Washington, DC 20007; **Phone:** 202-444-1351; **Board Cert:** Otolaryngology 1993; **Med School:** W VA Univ 1987; **Resid:** Otolaryngology, Georgetown Univ Med Ctr 1992; **Fellow:** Head and Neck Surgery, Memorial Sloan-Kettering Cancer Ctr 1994; **Fac Appt:** Asst Prof Oto, Georgetown Univ

Ferris, Robert L MD/PhD [Oto] - **Spec Exp:** Head & Neck Cancer; Thyroid & Parathyroid Cancer & Surgery; **Hospital:** UPMC Presby, Pittsburgh; **Address:** 200 Lothrop St, Ste 500, Pittsburgh, PA 15213; **Phone:** 412-647-7110; **Board Cert:** Otolaryngology 2002; **Med School:** Johns Hopkins Univ 1995; **Resid:** Otolaryngology, Johns Hopkins Univ Hosp 2001; **Fac Appt:** Assoc Prof Oto, Univ Pittsburgh

Genden, Eric M MD [Oto] - **Spec Exp:** Head & Neck Cancer & Surgery; Head & Neck Cancer Reconstruction; Airway Reconstruction; Thyroid & Parathyroid Cancer & Surgery; **Hospital:** Mount Sinai Med Ctr (page 76); **Address:** Mt Sinai Dept Otolaryngology, 1 Gustave L Levy Pl, Box 1191, New York, NY 10029; **Phone:** 212-241-9410; **Board Cert:** Otolaryngology 1999; Facial Plastic & Reconstr Surgery 2000; **Med School:** Mount Sinai Sch Med 1992; **Resid:** Otolaryngology, Barnes Jewish Hosp 1998; **Fellow:** Head and Neck Surgery, Mt Sinai Med Ctr 1999; **Fac Appt:** Assoc Prof Oto, Mount Sinai Sch Med

Otolaryngology

Goldenberg, David MD [Oto] - **Spec Exp:** Head & Neck Cancer & Surgery; Thyroid & Parathyroid Cancer & Surgery; Salivary Gland Tumors & Surgery; **Hospital:** Penn State Milton S Hershey Med Ctr; **Address:** Otolaryngology-Head and Neck Surgery, 500 University Drive, MC H091, Hershey, PA 17033-0850; **Phone:** 717-531-8945; **Med School:** Israel 1995; **Resid:** Otolaryngology, Rambam Med Ctr; **Fellow:** Head & Neck Surgical Oncology, Johns Hopkins Med Ctr; **Fac Appt:** Assoc Prof S

Grandis, Jennifer R MD [Oto] - **Spec Exp:** Head & Neck Cancer; **Hospital:** UPMC Presby, Pittsburgh, Magee-Womens Hosp - UPMC; **Address:** Univ Pittsburgh Med Ctr EELB, 200 Lothrop St Fl 3, Ear, Nose & Throat Dept, Pittsburgh, PA 15213; **Phone:** 412-647-2100; **Board Cert:** Otolaryngology 1994; **Med School:** Univ Pittsburgh 1987; **Resid:** Otolaryngology, Univ Pittsburgh Med Ctr 1993; **Fac Appt:** Prof Oto, Univ Pittsburgh

Har-El, Gady MD [Oto] - **Spec Exp:** Head & Neck Cancer; Thyroid & Parathyroid Surgery; Sinus Tumors; Skull Base Tumors; **Hospital:** Lenox Hill Hosp, Lenox Hill Hosp (Manh Eye, Ear & Throat Hosp); **Address:** 186 E 76th St Fl 2, New York, NY 10021; **Phone:** 212-434-2323; **Board Cert:** Otolaryngology 1992; **Med School:** Israel 1982; **Resid:** Otolaryngology, SUNY Downstate Med Ctr 1991; **Fac Appt:** Prof Oto, SUNY Hlth Sci Ctr

Hicks Jr, Wesley L MD/DDS [Oto] - **Spec Exp:** Head & Neck Cancer & Surgery; Reconstructive Surgery; **Hospital:** Roswell Park Cancer Inst; **Address:** Roswell Park Cancer Inst, Dept Head & Neck Surgery, Elm & Carlton Sts, Buffalo, NY 14263; **Phone:** 716-845-3158; **Board Cert:** Otolaryngology 1993; **Med School:** SUNY Buffalo 1984; **Resid:** Otolaryngology, Manhattan Eye Ear & Throat Hosp 1988; Otolaryngology, New York Hosp/Meml Sloan Kettering Cancer Ctr 1989; **Fellow:** Head and Neck Surgery, Stanford Univ Med Ctr 1990; **Fac Appt:** Prof Oto, SUNY Buffalo

Hirsch, Barry MD [Oto] - **Spec Exp:** Ear Tumors; Skull Base Tumors; **Hospital:** UPMC Presby, Pittsburgh, UPMC St Margaret; **Address:** 200 Lothrop St Fl 3, Ear Nose Throat Inst, Dept Otolaryngology, Pittsburgh, PA 15213; **Phone:** 412-647-2100; **Board Cert:** Otolaryngology 1982; Neurotology 2005; **Med School:** Univ Pennsylvania 1977; **Resid:** Otolaryngology, Univ Pittsburgh Med Ctr 1982; **Fellow:** Neurotology, Univ Pittsburgh 1985; Neurotology, Univ Zurich 1986; **Fac Appt:** Prof Oto, Univ Pittsburgh

Holliday, Michael J MD [Oto] - **Spec Exp:** Neuro-Otology; Skull Base Surgery; **Hospital:** Johns Hopkins Hosp, Johns Hopkins Bayview Med Ctr; **Address:** Johns Hopkins Hosp-Otology Division, 601 N Caroline St Fl 6, Baltimore, MD 21287; **Phone:** 410-955-1686; **Board Cert:** Otolaryngology 1976; **Med School:** Marquette Sch Med 1969; **Resid:** Otolaryngology, Johns Hopkins Hosp 1976; **Fellow:** Neurotology, Univ Zurich 1979; **Fac Appt:** Assoc Prof Oto, Johns Hopkins Univ

Johnson, Jonas T MD [Oto] - **Spec Exp:** Head & Neck Surgery; Head & Neck Cancer; Parotid Gland Tumors; Thyroid Cancer; **Hospital:** UPMC Montefiore, Magee-Womens Hosp - UPMC; **Address:** Univ Physicians UPMC, Eye & Ear Inst, 200 Lothrop St, Ste 300, Pittsburgh, PA 15213; **Phone:** 412-647-2100; **Board Cert:** Otolaryngology 1977; **Med School:** SUNY Upstate Med Univ 1972; **Resid:** Surgery, Med Coll Virginia Hosps 1974; Otolaryngology, SUNY-Univ Hosp 1977; **Fac Appt:** Prof Oto, Univ Pittsburgh

Keane, William M MD [Oto] - **Spec Exp:** Head & Neck Cancer & Surgery; Thyroid Cancer; **Hospital:** Thomas Jefferson Univ Hosp (page 81); **Address:** Thomas Jefferson Hosp, 925 Chestnut St Fl 6, Philadelphia, PA 19107; **Phone:** 215-955-6760; **Board Cert:** Otolaryngology 1978; **Med School:** Harvard Med Sch 1970; **Resid:** Surgery, Strong Meml Hosp 1972; Otolaryngology, Univ Penn Hosp 1977; **Fac Appt:** Prof Oto, Thomas Jefferson Univ

Kennedy, David W MD [Oto] - **Spec Exp:** Sinus Disorders/Surgery; Skull Base Tumors & Surgery; Minimally Invasive Surgery; Esthesioneuroblastoma; **Hospital:** Hosp Univ Penn - UPHS (page 80), Pennsylvania Hosp (page 80); **Address:** 3400 Spruce St, Ravdin Bldg Fl 5, Philadelphia, PA 19104-4229; **Phone:** 215-662-6971; **Board Cert:** Otolaryngology 1978; **Med School:** Ireland 1972; **Resid:** Surgery, Johns Hopkins Hosp 1974; Otolaryngology, Johns Hopkins Hosp 1978; **Fac Appt:** Prof Oto, Univ Pennsylvania

Koch, Wayne Martin MD [Oto] - **Spec Exp:** Head & Neck Cancer; Sinus Tumors; **Hospital:** Johns Hopkins Hosp; **Address:** Johns Hopkins Hosp, Dept Otolaryngology, 601 N Caroline St, rm 6221, Baltimore, MD 21287; **Phone:** 410-955-1686; **Board Cert:** Otolaryngology 1987; **Med School:** Univ Pittsburgh 1982; **Resid:** Otolaryngology, Tufts-Boston Univ Hosps 1987; **Fellow:** Surgical Oncology, Johns Hopkins Hosp 1989; **Fac Appt:** Assoc Prof Oto, Johns Hopkins Univ

Kraus, Dennis H MD [Oto] - **Spec Exp:** Head & Neck Cancer; Skull Base Tumors; Thyroid & Parathyroid Surgery; **Hospital:** Meml Sloan-Kettering Cancer Ctr (page 75); **Address:** 1275 York Ave, Box 285, New York, NY 10065; **Phone:** 212-639-5621; **Board Cert:** Otolaryngology 1990; **Med School:** Univ Rochester 1985; **Resid:** Surgery, Cleveland Clinic 1987; Otolaryngology, Cleveland Clinic 1990; **Fellow:** Head and Neck Surgery, Meml Sloan Kettering Cancer Ctr 1991; **Fac Appt:** Prof Oto, Cornell Univ-Weill Med Coll

Krespi, Yosef P MD [Oto] - **Spec Exp:** Nasal & Sinus Cancer & Surgery; Head & Neck Cancer & Surgery; **Hospital:** Lenox Hill Hosp (Manh Eye, Ear & Throat Hosp), St. Luke's - Roosevelt Hosp Ctr - Roosevelt Div (page 71); **Address:** 425 W 59th St, Fl 10, New York, NY 10019-1128; **Phone:** 212-262-2929; **Board Cert:** Otolaryngology 1981; **Med School:** Israel 1973; **Resid:** Surgery, Mt Sinai Hosp 1976; Otolaryngology, Mt Sinai Hosp 1980; **Fellow:** Surgery, Northwestern Meml Hosp 1981; **Fac Appt:** Clin Prof Oto, Columbia P&S

Lawson, William MD [Oto] - **Spec Exp:** Nasal & Sinus Cancer & Surgery; Head & Neck Cancer; Skull Base Surgery; **Hospital:** Mount Sinai Med Ctr (page 76); **Address:** 5 E 98th St Fl 8, Box 1191, New York, NY 10029-6501; **Phone:** 212-241-9410; **Board Cert:** Otolaryngology 1974; **Med School:** NYU Sch Med 1965; **Resid:** Surgery, Bronx VA Hosp 1967; Otolaryngology, Mt Sinai Hosp 1973; **Fellow:** Otolaryngology, Mt Sinai Hosp 1970; **Fac Appt:** Prof Oto, Mount Sinai Sch Med

O'Malley Jr, Bert W MD [Oto] - **Spec Exp:** Head & Neck Cancer; Sinus Tumors; Skull Base Tumors; **Hospital:** Hosp Univ Penn - UPHS (page 80); **Address:** Hosp Univ Penn, Dept Otolaryngology, 3400 Spruce St, 5 Ravdin, Philadelphia, PA 19104; **Phone:** 215-615-4325; **Board Cert:** Otolaryngology 1995; **Med School:** Univ Tex SW, Dallas 1988; **Resid:** Surgery, UTSW Med Ctr/Parkland Meml Hosp 1989; Otolaryngology, Baylor Coll Med 1993; **Fellow:** Head & Neck Oncology, Univ Pittsburgh 1994; Skull Base Surgery, Univ Pittsburgh 1995; **Fac Appt:** Prof Oto, Univ Pennsylvania

Papel, Ira D MD [Oto] - **Spec Exp:** Reconstructive Surgery-Face; Skin Cancer/Facial Reconstruction; **Hospital:** Greater Baltimore Med Ctr, Johns Hopkins Hosp; **Address:** 1838 Greene Tree Rd, Ste 370, Baltimore, MD 21208; **Phone:** 410-486-3400; **Board Cert:** Otolaryngology 1986; Facial Plastic & Reconstr Surgery 1991; **Med School:** Boston Univ 1981; **Resid:** Otolaryngology, Johns Hopkins Hosp 1986; **Fellow:** Facial Plastic Surgery, UCSF Med Ctr 1987; **Fac Appt:** Assoc Prof Oto, Johns Hopkins Univ

Persky, Mark S MD [Oto] - **Spec Exp:** Head & Neck Cancer; Skull Base Tumors; Thyroid Cancer; **Hospital:** Beth Israel Med Ctr - Petrie Division (page 71), New York Eye & Ear Infirm (page 77); **Address:** 10 Union Square East, Ste 4J, New York, NY 10003; **Phone:** 212-844-8648; **Board Cert:** Otolaryngology 1976; **Med School:** SUNY Upstate Med Univ 1972; **Resid:** Otolaryngology, Bellevue Hosp 1976; **Fellow:** Head and Neck Surgery, Beth Israel Med Ctr 1977; **Fac Appt:** Clin Prof Oto, Albert Einstein Coll Med

Otolaryngology

Rassekh, Christopher MD [Oto] - **Spec Exp:** Laryngeal Cancer-Organ Preservation; Skull Base Tumors; Salivary Gland Tumors & Surgery; **Hospital:** Hosp Univ Penn - UPHS (page 80); **Address:** Hosp Univ Penn-Otorhinolaryngology, 5 Silverstein, Philadelphia, PA 19104; **Phone:** 215-662-2777; **Board Cert:** Otolaryngology 1993; **Med School:** Univ Iowa Coll Med 1986; **Resid:** Otolaryngology, Univ Iowa Med Ctr 1992; **Fellow:** Head and Neck Surgery, Univ Pittsburgh Med Ctr 1993; **Fac Appt:** Assoc Prof Oto, Univ Pennsylvania

Schantz, Stimson P MD [Oto] - **Spec Exp:** Head & Neck Surgery; Head & Neck Cancer; Thyroid Cancer; **Hospital:** New York Eye & Ear Infirm (page 77), Beth Israel Med Ctr - Petrie Division (page 71); **Address:** 310 E 14th St Fl 6N, New YorkNew York, NY 10003; **Phone:** 212-979-4535; **Board Cert:** Surgery 2005; **Med School:** Univ Cincinnati 1975; **Resid:** Surgery, Georgetown Univ Med CtrGeorgetown Univ Med Ctr 1982; Otolaryngology, Univ Illinois Eye & Ear Infirm 1980; **Fellow:** Surgical Oncology, MD Anderson Cancer Ctr 1984; **Fac Appt:** Prof Oto, NY Med Coll

Shapshay, Stanley M MD [Oto] - **Spec Exp:** Laryngeal Cancer; **Hospital:** Albany Med Ctr; **Address:** University Ear, Nose & Throat Ctr, 35 Hackett Blvd, Albany, NY 12208-3420; **Phone:** 518-262-5575; **Board Cert:** Otolaryngology 1975; **Med School:** Med Coll VA 1968; **Resid:** Surgery, New England Med Ctr 1971; Otolaryngology, Boston Med Ctr 1975; **Fellow:** Surgery, Serafimer Hosp/Karolinska Med Sch 1972; **Fac Appt:** Prof Oto, Albany Med Coll

Snyderman, Carl H MD [Oto] - **Spec Exp:** Skull Base Tumors & Surgery; Sinus Tumors; Head & Neck Cancer; Endoscopic Surgery; **Hospital:** UPMC Presby, Pittsburgh; **Address:** Eye Ear Inst, Dept of Otolaryngology, 200 Lothrop St, Ste 500, Pittsburgh, PA 15213; **Phone:** 412-647-8186; **Board Cert:** Otolaryngology 1987; **Med School:** Univ Chicago-Pritzker Sch Med 1982; **Resid:** Otolaryngology, Eye-Ear Hosp/Univ Pittsburgh 1987; **Fellow:** Skull Base Surgery, Eye-Ear Hosp/Univ Pittsburgh 1988; **Fac Appt:** Prof Oto, Univ Pittsburgh

Strome, Marshall MD [Oto] - **Spec Exp:** Voice Disorders; Head & Neck Cancer; Swallowing Disorders; Head & Neck Cancer Reconstruction; **Hospital:** St. Luke's - Roosevelt Hosp Ctr - St Luke's Hosp (page 71), Mount Sinai Med Ctr (page 76); **Address:** 110 E 59th St, Ste 10A, New York, NY 10022; **Phone:** 212-223-1333; **Board Cert:** Otolaryngology 1970; **Med School:** Univ Mich Med Sch 1964; **Resid:** Surgery, Harper Hosp 1966; Otolaryngology, Univ Michigan Hosp 1970; **Fac Appt:** Prof Oto

Strome, Scott E MD [Oto] - **Spec Exp:** Microsurgery; Head & Neck Cancer; Head & Neck Reconstruction; Laryngeal Cancer; **Hospital:** Univ of MD Med Ctr; **Address:** 16 S Eutaw St, Ste 500, Baltimore, MD 21201; **Phone:** 410-328-6467; **Board Cert:** Otolaryngology 1998; **Med School:** Harvard Med Sch 1991; **Resid:** Otolaryngology, Univ Michigan 1997; **Fellow:** Head and Neck Surgery, Allegheny Genl Hosp 1998; Microvascular Surgery, Allegheny Genl Hosp 1998; **Fac Appt:** Prof Oto, Univ MD Sch Med

Tufano, Ralph P MD [Oto] - **Spec Exp:** Thyroid Disorders; Parathyroid Disease; Head & Neck Cancer; **Hospital:** Johns Hopkins Hosp; **Address:** Johns Hopkins Hosp, Oto-Head & Neck Surg, 601 North Caroline St, Ste JHOC 6210, Baltimore, MD 21287; **Phone:** 410-955-3628; **Board Cert:** Otolaryngology 2001; **Med School:** SUNY Buffalo 1995; **Resid:** Otolaryngology, Univ Penn 2000; **Fellow:** Head and Neck Surgery, Johns Hopkins Hosp 2001; **Fac Appt:** Assoc Prof Oto, Johns Hopkins Univ

Urken, Mark MD [Oto] - **Spec Exp:** Head & Neck Cancer & Surgery; Head & Neck Cancer Reconstruction; Thyroid & Parathyroid Cancer & Surgery; Salivary Gland Tumors; **Hospital:** Beth Israel Med Ctr - Petrie Division (page 71); **Address:** Inst for Head, Neck & Thyroid Cancer, 10 Union Square E, Ste 5B, New York, NY 10003-3314; **Phone:** 212-844-8775; **Board Cert:** Otolaryngology 1986; **Med School:** Univ VA Sch Med 1981; **Resid:** Otolaryngology, Mt Sinai Hosp 1986; **Fellow:** Microvascular Surgery, Mercy Hosp 1987; **Fac Appt:** Prof Oto, Albert Einstein Coll Med

Weinstein, Gregory MD [Oto] - **Spec Exp:** Head & Neck Cancer; Laryngeal Cancer; **Hospital:** Hosp Univ Penn - UPHS (page 80); **Address:** Hosp Univ Penn, Dept Otolaryngology, 3400 Spruce St, 5 Ravdin, Philadelphia, PA 19104; **Phone:** 215-349-5390; **Board Cert:** Otolaryngology 1990; **Med School:** NY Med Coll 1985; **Resid:** Otolaryngology, Univ Iowa Hosp 1990; **Fellow:** Head & Neck Oncology, UC Davis Med Ctr 1991; **Fac Appt:** Assoc Prof Oto, Univ Pennsylvania

Woo, Peak MD [Oto] - **Spec Exp:** Voice Disorders; Laryngeal Cancer; **Hospital:** Mount Sinai Med Ctr (page 76); **Address:** 300 Central Park West, Ste 1-H, New York, NY 10024; **Phone:** 212-580-1004; **Board Cert:** Otolaryngology 1983; **Med School:** Boston Univ 1978; **Resid:** Otolaryngology, Boston Univ Med Ctr 1983; **Fac Appt:** Clin Prof Oto, Mount Sinai Sch Med

Southeast

Browne, J Dale MD [Oto] - **Spec Exp:** Head & Neck Cancer; Thyroid Cancer; Skull Base Surgery; Head & Neck Reconstruction; **Hospital:** Wake Forest Univ Baptist Med Ctr; **Address:** Wake Forest Baptist Med Ctr, Dept Otolaryngology, Medical Center Blvd, Winston Salem, NC 27103; **Phone:** 336-716-3854; **Board Cert:** Otolaryngology 1987; **Med School:** Med Coll GA 1982; **Resid:** Otolaryngology, NC Baptist Hosp 1987; **Fellow:** Otolaryngology, Univ Hosp 1991; **Fac Appt:** Prof Oto, Wake Forest Univ

Bumpous, Jeffrey MD [Oto] - **Spec Exp:** Head & Neck Cancer; Head & Neck Reconstruction; Thyroid & Parathyroid Cancer & Surgery; **Hospital:** Univ of Louisville Hosp, Norton Hosp; **Address:** 401 E Chestnut St, Ste 710, Louisville, KY 40202-1845; **Phone:** 502-583-8303; **Board Cert:** Otolaryngology 1994; **Med School:** Univ Louisville Sch Med 1988; **Resid:** Otolaryngology, Univ Louisville Hosp 1993; **Fellow:** Head and Neck Surgery, Univ Pittsburgh 1994; **Fac Appt:** Prof Oto, Univ Louisville Sch Med

Civantos, Francisco J MD [Oto] - **Spec Exp:** Head & Neck Cancer; Skull Base Surgery; **Hospital:** Univ of Miami Hosp & Clins/Sylvester Comp Canc Ctr (page 82); **Address:** Sylvester Cancer Ctr, Otolaryngology, 1475 NW 12th Ave, Miami, FL 33136; **Phone:** 305-243-5276; **Board Cert:** Otolaryngology 1992; **Med School:** Columbia P&S 1986; **Resid:** Otolaryngology, Univ Illinois Coll Med 1991; **Fellow:** Head & Neck Oncology, Vanderbilt Univ 1992; **Fac Appt:** Assoc Prof Oto, Univ Miami Sch Med

Day, Terrence A MD [Oto] - **Spec Exp:** Head & Neck Cancer; Reconstructive Microvascular Surgery; Skull Base Surgery; Facial Plastic & Reconstructive Surgery; **Hospital:** MUSC Med Ctr; **Address:** MUSC, Dept Otolaryngology, 135 Rutledge Ave, MSC550, Charleston, SC 29425; **Phone:** 843-792-0719; **Board Cert:** Otolaryngology 1996; **Med School:** Univ Okla Coll Med 1989; **Resid:** Otolaryngology, LSU Med Ctr 1995; **Fellow:** Head & Neck Surgical Oncology, UC Davis Med Ctr 1996; Maxillofacial Surgery, Univ Hosp 1994; **Fac Appt:** Assoc Prof Oto, Med Univ SC

DiNardo, Laurence J MD [Oto] - **Spec Exp:** Head & Neck Cancer; Sinus Disorders/Surgery; **Hospital:** Med Coll of VA Hosp; **Address:** VCU Dept Otolaryngology, 401 N 11th St, rm 7-100, Box 980146, Richmond, VA 23298-0146; **Phone:** 804-628-4368; **Board Cert:** Otolaryngology 1992; **Med School:** Stanford Univ 1986; **Resid:** Otolaryngology, Hosp Univ Penn 1991; **Fac Appt:** Prof Oto, Va Commonwealth Univ Sch Med

Goodwin, W Jarrard MD [Oto] - **Spec Exp:** Head & Neck Cancer; **Hospital:** Univ of Miami Hosp & Clins/Sylvester Comp Canc Ctr (page 82), Jackson Meml Hosp (page 82); **Address:** Sylvester Comp Cancer Ctr, Dept Otolaryngology, 1475 NW 12th Ave, rm 4037, Miami, FL 33136-1015; **Phone:** 305-243-3564; **Board Cert:** Otolaryngology 1978; **Med School:** Albany Med Coll 1972; **Resid:** Surgery, Jackson Meml Hosp 1974; Otolaryngology, Jackson Meml Hosp 1977; **Fellow:** Head & Neck Surgical Oncology, MD Anderson Hosp 1980; **Fac Appt:** Prof Oto, Univ Miami Sch Med

Otolaryngology

Lanza, Donald C MD [Oto] - **Spec Exp:** Skull Base Tumors; Sinus Disorders/Surgery; **Hospital:** St. Anthony's Hosp - St Petersburg, All Children's Hosp; **Address:** 900 Carillon Pkwy, Ste 200, St Petersburg, FL 33716; **Phone:** 727-573-0074; **Board Cert:** Otolaryngology 1990; **Med School:** SUNY Hlth Sci Ctr 1985; **Resid:** Surgery, Albany Med Ctr 1987; Otolaryngology, Albany Med Ctr 1990; **Fellow:** Rhinology, Johns Hopkins Univ 1990; Rhinology, Univ Penn 1991

Levine, Paul A MD [Oto] - **Spec Exp:** Head & Neck Cancer; Head & Neck Reconstruction; Skull Base Tumors; **Hospital:** Univ of Virginia Health Sys; **Address:** Dept Otolaryngology, PO Box 800713, Charlottesville, VA 22908; **Phone:** 434-924-5593; **Board Cert:** Otolaryngology 1978; **Med School:** Albany Med Coll 1973; **Resid:** Otolaryngology, Yale-New Haven Hosp 1977; **Fellow:** Head and Neck Surgery, Stanford Med Ctr 1978; **Fac Appt:** Prof Oto, Univ VA Sch Med

McCaffrey, Thomas V MD [Oto] - **Spec Exp:** Head & Neck Cancer; Thyroid Cancer; Tracheal Surgery; **Hospital:** H Lee Moffitt Cancer Ctr & Research Inst, Tampa Genl Hosp; **Address:** H Lee Moffitt Cancer Ctr, Dept Otolaryngology-HNS, 12902 Magnolia Drive, MS FOB2-HN, Tampa, FL 33612; **Phone:** 813-745-8463; **Board Cert:** Otolaryngology 1980; **Med School:** Loyola Univ-Stritch Sch Med 1974; **Resid:** Surgery, Mayo Affil Hosps 1976; Otolaryngology, Mayo Affil Hosps 1980; **Fac Appt:** Prof Oto, Univ S Fla Coll Med

Netterville, James L MD [Oto] - **Spec Exp:** Head & Neck Surgery; Head & Neck Cancer; Skull Base Tumors; **Hospital:** Vanderbilt Univ Med Ctr, Vanderbilt Monroe Carrell Jr. Chldn's Hosp; **Address:** Vanderbilt Univ Med Ctr, Dept Oto, 7209 Med Ctr East, South Twr, 1215 21st Ave S, Nashville, TN 37232-8605; **Phone:** 615-343-8840; **Board Cert:** Otolaryngology 1985; **Med School:** Univ Tenn Coll Med 1980; **Resid:** Surgery, Methodist Hosp 1982; Otolaryngology, Univ Tenn Med Ctr 1985; **Fellow:** Surgical Oncology, Univ Iowa 1986; **Fac Appt:** Prof Oto, Vanderbilt Univ

Osguthorpe, John D MD [Oto] - **Spec Exp:** Head & Neck Cancer; Thyroid & Parathyroid Cancer & Surgery; Salivary Gland Tumors & Surgery; Laryngeal Cancer; **Hospital:** MUSC Med Ctr, E Cooper Med Ctr; **Address:** MUSC Med Ctr-Dept Otolaryngology, 135 Rutledge Ave, PO Box 250550, Charleston, SC 29425; **Phone:** 843-792-3533; **Board Cert:** Otolaryngology 1978; **Med School:** Univ Utah 1973; **Resid:** Surgery, UCLA Med Ctr 1975; Otolaryngology, UCLA Med Ctr 1978; **Fellow:** Skull Base Surgery, Univ Zurich 1989; **Fac Appt:** Prof Oto, Med Univ SC

Peters, Glenn E MD [Oto] - **Spec Exp:** Thyroid & Parathyroid Cancer & Surgery; **Hospital:** Univ of Ala Hosp at Birmingham; **Address:** UAB Med Ctr, Div of Head & Neck Surgery, 1530 3rd Ave S, Ste BDB 563, Birmingham, AL 35294-0012; **Phone:** 205-934-9767; **Board Cert:** Otolaryngology 1985; **Med School:** Louisiana State U, New Orleans 1980; **Resid:** Surgery, Baptist Med Ctr 1982; Otolaryngology, Univ Alabama Hosp 1984; **Fellow:** Head & Neck Surgical Oncology, Johns Hopkins Hosp 1987; **Fac Appt:** Prof S, Univ Alabama

Pitman, Karen MD [Oto] - **Spec Exp:** Head & Neck Cancer & Surgery; Thyroid & Parathyroid Cancer & Surgery; Sentinel Node Surgery; **Hospital:** Univ Mississippi Med Ctr; **Address:** Univ Miss Med Ctr, Dept Otolaryngology, 2500 N State St, Jackson, MS 39216; **Phone:** 601-984-5160; **Board Cert:** Otolaryngology 1995; **Med School:** Uniformed Srvs Univ, Bethesda 1987; **Resid:** Otolaryngology, Naval Med Ctr 1994; **Fellow:** Head & Neck Oncology, Univ Pittsburgh 1996; **Fac Appt:** Prof Oto, Univ Miss

Rosenthal, Eben MD [Oto] - **Spec Exp:** Head & Neck Cancer; Microvascular Surgery; Reconstructive Surgery; Minimally Invasive Surgery; **Hospital:** Univ of Ala Hosp at Birmingham; **Address:** 2000 6th Ave S, Birmingham, AL 35233; **Phone:** 205-934-9766; **Board Cert:** Otolaryngology 2001; **Med School:** Univ Mich Med Sch 1994; **Resid:** Otolaryngology, Univ MI Med Ctr 2000; **Fellow:** Head and Neck Surgery, OR Hlth Sci Univ 2001; **Fac Appt:** Assoc Prof S, Univ Alabama

Samant, Sandeep MD [Oto] - **Spec Exp:** Head & Neck Cancer & Surgery; Skull Base Surgery; Endoscopic Surgery; Thyroid & Parathyroid Cancer & Surgery; **Hospital:** Methodist Univ Hosp - Memphis; **Address:** UT Med Grp-Oto-Head & Neck Surgery, 7945 Wolf River Blvd, Ste 220, Memphis, TN 38138; **Phone:** 901-347-8220; **Board Cert:** Otolaryngology 2009; **Med School:** India 1986; **Resid:** Otolaryngology, ALL-Indian Inst 1989; Otolaryngology, Royal Coll Surgeons 1994; **Fellow:** Head and Neck Surgery, Univ Miami/Sylvester Comprehensive Cancer Ctr 1995; Head & Neck Oncology, Univ TN Med Ctr 1996

Stringer, Scott P MD [Oto] - **Spec Exp:** Skull Base Surgery; **Hospital:** Univ Mississippi Med Ctr, G.V. (Sonny) Montgomery VA Med Ctr - Jackson; **Address:** Univ Miss Med Ctr, Dept Otolaryngology, 2500 N State St, Jackson, MS 39216-4505; **Phone:** 601-984-5160; **Board Cert:** Otolaryngology 1987; **Med School:** Univ Tex SW, Dallas 1982; **Resid:** Surgery, Univ Tex SW Med Ctr 1984; Otolaryngology, Univ Tex SW Med Ctr 1987; **Fac Appt:** Prof Oto, Univ Miss

Terris, David J MD [Oto] - **Spec Exp:** Thyroid Surgery; Thyroid Cancer; Parathyroid Disease; **Hospital:** Med Coll of GA Hosp and Clin (MCG Health Inc), Doctors Hosp; **Address:** MCG Health - Dept Otolaryngology, 1447 Harper St, Medical Office Bldg Fl 4, Augusta, GA 30912; **Phone:** 706-721-4400; **Board Cert:** Otolaryngology 1994; **Med School:** Duke Univ 1988; **Resid:** Surgery, Stanford Univ Med Ctr 1989; Otolaryngology, Stanford Univ Med Ctr 1993; **Fellow:** Head and Neck Surgery, Stanford Univ Med Ctr 1994; **Fac Appt:** Prof Oto, Med Coll GA

Valentino, Joseph MD [Oto] - **Spec Exp:** Head & Neck Cancer; Reconstructive Microvascular Surgery; Thyroid Cancer; **Hospital:** Univ of Kentucky Albert B. Chandler Hosp; **Address:** 800 Rose St, rm C236, Lexington, KY 40536; **Phone:** 859-257-5405; **Board Cert:** Otolaryngology 1993; **Med School:** UMDNJ-RW Johnson Med Sch 1987; **Resid:** Otolaryngology, Univ Minn 1992; **Fellow:** Otolaryngology, Univ Iowa Coll Med 1993; **Fac Appt:** Assoc Prof Oto, Univ KY Coll Med

Weissler, Mark C MD [Oto] - **Spec Exp:** Head & Neck Cancer; Salivary Gland Tumors; Thyroid Cancer; **Hospital:** NC Memorial Hosp - UNC; **Address:** 170 Manning Drive, G106 Physician's Office Bldg, CB#7070, Chapel Hill, NC 27599-7070; **Phone:** 919-843-4820; **Board Cert:** Otolaryngology 1985; **Med School:** Boston Univ 1980; **Resid:** Surgery, Mass Genl Hosp 1982; Otolaryngology, Mass Eye & Ear Infirm 1985; **Fellow:** Head & Neck Oncology, Univ Cincinnati 1986; **Fac Appt:** Prof Oto, Univ NC Sch Med

Yarbrough, Wendell G MD [Oto] - **Spec Exp:** Head & Neck Cancer; **Hospital:** Vanderbilt Univ Med Ctr; **Address:** Vanderbilt Otolaryngology, 1215 21st Ave S, Ste 7209, Nashville, TN 37232-8605; **Phone:** 615-322-6180; **Board Cert:** Otolaryngology 1995; **Med School:** Univ NC Sch Med 1989; **Resid:** Otolaryngology, Univ NC Hosps 1994; **Fellow:** Surgical Oncology, Univ NC Hosps 1996; **Fac Appt:** Assoc Prof Oto, Vanderbilt Univ

Midwest

Akervall, Jan A MD [Oto] - **Spec Exp:** Head & Neck Cancer; Head & Neck Reconstruction; Minimally Invasive Surgery; **Hospital:** Beaumont Hosp-Royal Oak, St. Joseph Mercy Hosp - Ann Arbor; **Address:** 28300 Orchard Lake Rd, Ste 100, Farmington Hills, MI 48334; **Phone:** 248-737-4030; **Med School:** Sweden 1990; **Resid:** Otolaryngology, Lund Univ Fac Med 1998; **Fellow:** Head & Neck Oncology, Univ MI Hosps 2002; **Fac Appt:** Clin Prof Oto, Oakland Univ-William Beaumont Med Sch

Alam, Daniel Syed MD [Oto] - **Spec Exp:** Nasal Reconstruction; Head & Neck Reconstruction; Parotid Gland Tumors; Cancer Reconstruction; **Hospital:** Cleveland Clin (page 70); **Address:** Cleveland Clin Main Campus, 9500 Euclid Ave, MC A71, Cleveland, OH 44195; **Phone:** 216-445-6594; **Board Cert:** Otolaryngology 2002; **Med School:** Johns Hopkins Univ 1996; **Resid:** Otolaryngology, Mass Genl Hosp 2001; **Fellow:** Facial Plastic & Reconstr Surgery, UCLA Med Ctr 2002

Otolaryngology

Arts, H Alexander MD [Oto] - **Spec Exp:** Skull Base Tumors & Surgery; Neuro-Otology; **Hospital:** Univ of Michigan Hosp; **Address:** Univ Michigan Health Systems, Dept Otolaryngology, 1500 E Medical Ctr Dr, 1904 Taubman Ctr, Ann Arbor, MI 48109; **Phone:** 734-936-8006; **Board Cert:** Otolaryngology 1992; Neurotology 2004; **Med School:** Baylor Coll Med 1983; **Resid:** Surgery, Univ Washington Med Ctr 1985; Otolaryngology, Univ Washington Med Ctr 1990; **Fellow:** Neurotology, Univ Virginia 1991; **Fac Appt:** Prof Oto, Univ Mich Med Sch

Blair, Elizabeth MD [Oto] - **Spec Exp:** Head & Neck Cancer & Surgery; Salivary Gland Tumors; Skull Base Tumors; **Hospital:** Univ of Chicago Med Ctr; **Address:** 5841 S Maryland Ave, MC 1035, Chicago, IL 60637; **Phone:** 773-702-4934; **Board Cert:** Otolaryngology 1994; **Med School:** Creighton Univ 1988; **Resid:** Otolaryngology, Univ Pittsburgh Med Ctr 1993; **Fellow:** Head & Neck Surgical Oncology, MD Anderson Cancer Ctr 1994; **Fac Appt:** Assoc Prof Oto, Univ Chicago-Pritzker Sch Med

Bojrab, Dennis I MD [Oto] - **Spec Exp:** Skull Base Tumors; **Hospital:** Providence Hosp - Southfield, Beaumont Hosp-Royal Oak; **Address:** Michigan Ear Inst, 30055 Northwestern Hwy, Ste 101, Farmington Hills, MI 48334; **Phone:** 248-865-4444; **Board Cert:** Otolaryngology 1985; Neurotology 2005; **Med School:** Indiana Univ 1979; **Resid:** Surgery, Butterworth Hosp 1981; Otolaryngology, Univ Indiana Sch Med 1984; **Fellow:** Skull Base Surgery, Vanderbilt Univ Med Ctr 1985; **Fac Appt:** Clin Prof Oto, Wayne State Univ

Bradford, Carol MD [Oto] - **Spec Exp:** Head & Neck Cancer; Melanoma-Head & Neck; Skin Cancer-Head & Neck; **Hospital:** Univ of Michigan Hosp; **Address:** University of Michigan Health System, 1500 E Medical Center Drive, rm 1904-TC, Ann Arbor, MI 48109-0312; **Phone:** 734-936-8029; **Board Cert:** Otolaryngology 1993; **Med School:** Univ Mich Med Sch 1986; **Resid:** Otolaryngology, Univ Michigan Med Ctr 1992; **Fellow:** Head and Neck Surgery, Univ Michigan Med Ctr 1988; **Fac Appt:** Prof Oto, Univ Mich Med Sch

Burkey, Brian MD [Oto] - **Spec Exp:** Parotid Gland Tumors; Head & Neck Cancer; Reconstructive Microvascular Surgery; **Hospital:** Cleveland Clin (page 70); **Address:** Head & Neck Inst, Desk A71, The Cleveland Clin, 9500 Euclid Ave, Cleveland, OH 44195; **Phone:** 216-445-8838; **Board Cert:** Otolaryngology 1992; **Med School:** Univ VA Sch Med 1986; **Resid:** Otolaryngology, Univ Mich Med Ctr 1991; **Fellow:** Microsurgery, Ohio State Univ 1991; **Fac Appt:** Assoc Prof Oto, Vanderbilt Univ

Campbell, Bruce H MD [Oto] - **Spec Exp:** Head & Neck Cancer; Thyroid Surgery; **Hospital:** Froedtert and Med Ctr of WI, Chldns Hosp - Wisconsin; **Address:** Med Coll Wisc-Dept Oto, 9200 W Wisconsin Ave, Milwaukee, WI 53226; **Phone:** 414-805-5583; **Board Cert:** Otolaryngology 1986; **Med School:** Rush Med Coll 1980; **Resid:** Otolaryngology, Med Coll Wisconsin 1985; **Fellow:** Head and Neck Surgery, MD Anderson Cancer Ctr 1987; **Fac Appt:** Prof Oto, Med Coll Wisc

Funk, Gerry F MD [Oto] - **Spec Exp:** Head & Neck Cancer; Head & Neck Reconstruction; **Hospital:** Univ Iowa Hosp & Clinics; **Address:** UIHC, Dept Otolaryngology, 200 Hawkins Drive, Iowa City, IA 52242-1007; **Phone:** 319-356-2165; **Board Cert:** Otolaryngology 1992; **Med School:** Univ Chicago-Pritzker Sch Med 1986; **Resid:** Surgery, LAC-USC Med Ctr 1987; Otolaryngology, LAC-USC Med Ctr 1991; **Fellow:** Head and Neck Surgery, Univ Iowa Hosp 1992; **Fac Appt:** Prof Oto, Univ Iowa Coll Med

Hartig, Gregory K MD [Oto] - **Spec Exp:** Head & Neck Cancer; Skull Base Tumors; **Hospital:** Univ WI Hosp & Clins; **Address:** 600 Highland Ave, rm K4/720, Madison, WI 53792-7375; **Phone:** 608-263-6190; **Board Cert:** Otolaryngology 1994; **Med School:** Univ Mich Med Sch 1988; **Resid:** Otolaryngology, Univ Mich Med Ctr 1993; **Fellow:** Otolaryngology, Univ Penn Med Ctr 1994; **Fac Appt:** Prof Oto, Univ Mich Med Sch

Haughey, Bruce H MD [Oto] - **Spec Exp:** Reconstructive Surgery-Face; Head & Neck Cancer; Head & Neck Reconstruction; **Hospital:** Barnes-Jewish Hosp, St. Louis Chldns Hosp; **Address:** Barnes Jewish Hosp South, 660 S Euclid Ave, Box 8115, St Louis, MO 63110; **Phone:** 314-362-7509; **Board Cert:** Otolaryngology 1984; **Med School:** New Zealand 1976; **Resid:** Surgery, Univ Auckland 1981; Otolaryngology, Univ Iowa Med Ctr 1984; **Fellow:** Otolaryngology, Univ Iowa Med Ctr 1985; **Fac Appt:** Prof Oto, Washington Univ, St Louis

Hoffman, Henry T MD [Oto] - **Spec Exp:** Voice Disorders; Head & Neck Cancer; Salivary Gland Tumors & Surgery; **Hospital:** Univ Iowa Hosp & Clinics; **Address:** Univ Iowa Hosp & Clins-Dept Oto, 200 Hawkins Drive, Iowa City, IA 52242; **Phone:** 319-356-2201; **Board Cert:** Otolaryngology 1985; **Med School:** UCSD 1980; **Resid:** Otolaryngology, Univ Iowa Hosp & Clinics 1985; **Fellow:** Head & Neck Oncology, Univ Michigan Hosp 1989; **Fac Appt:** Clin Prof Oto, Univ Iowa Coll Med

Lavertu, Pierre MD [Oto] - **Spec Exp:** Thyroid Cancer; Head & Neck Cancer; Skull Base Tumors; **Hospital:** Univ Hosps Case Med Ctr; **Address:** Univ Hosps, Dept Oto-Head & Neck Surg, 11100 Euclid Ave, Cleveland, OH 44106-5045; **Phone:** 216-844-4773; **Board Cert:** Otolaryngology 1981; **Med School:** Univ Montreal 1976; **Resid:** Otolaryngology, Univ Montreal Med Ctr 1981; **Fellow:** Head and Neck Surgery, Univ Montreal Med Ctr 1982; Head and Neck Surgery, Cleveland Clinic 1983; **Fac Appt:** Prof Oto, Case West Res Univ

Leonetti, John P MD [Oto] - **Spec Exp:** Skull Base Tumors & Surgery; Neuro-Otology; Head & Neck Cancer; **Hospital:** Loyola Univ Med Ctr; **Address:** Loyola University Medical Ctr, Dept Otolaryngology, 2160 S First Ave Bldg 105 - rm 1870, Maywood, IL 60153; **Phone:** 708-216-4804; **Board Cert:** Otolaryngology 1987; **Med School:** Loyola Univ-Stritch Sch Med 1982; **Resid:** Otolaryngology, Loyola Univ Med Ctr 1987; Research, House Ear Inst 1987; **Fellow:** Neurotology, Barnes Jewish Hosp 1988; **Fac Appt:** Prof Oto, Loyola Univ-Stritch Sch Med

Marentette, Lawrence J MD [Oto] - **Spec Exp:** Skull Base Tumors & Surgery; Facial Plastic & Reconstructive Surgery; **Hospital:** Univ of Michigan Hosp; **Address:** Univ Michigan Hlth Sys, Dept Oto, 1500 E Med Ctr Drive, 1904 Taubman Ctr, Ann Arbor, MI 48109; **Phone:** 734-936-8051; **Board Cert:** Otolaryngology 1981; Facial Plastic & Reconstr Surgery 1995; **Med School:** Wayne State Univ 1976; **Resid:** Otolaryngology, Wayne State Univ 1980; **Fellow:** Maxillofacial Surgery, Univ of Zurich 1985; **Fac Appt:** Prof Oto, Univ Mich Med Sch

Olsen, Kerry D MD [Oto] - **Spec Exp:** Head & Neck Cancer & Surgery; Esthesioneuroblastoma; Salivary Gland Tumors & Surgery; Skull Base Tumors; **Hospital:** Mayo Med Ctr & Clin - Rochester; **Address:** Mayo Clinic, Dept Otolaryngology, 200 1st St SW, Rochester, MN 55905-0001; **Phone:** 507-284-3542; **Board Cert:** Otolaryngology 1981; **Med School:** Mayo Med Sch 1976; **Resid:** Otolaryngology, Mayo Clinic 1981; **Fac Appt:** Prof Oto, Mayo Med Sch

Ozer, Enver MD [Oto] - **Spec Exp:** Head & Neck Cancer; Head & Neck Surgery; **Hospital:** Ohio St Univ Med Ctr; **Address:** 456 W 10th Ave, Ste 4A, Columbus, OH 43210; **Phone:** 614-293-8074; **Med School:** Turkey 1994; **Resid:** Otolaryngology, Marmara Univ Med Sch 1996; Head and Neck Surgery, Marmara Univ Med Sch 2000; **Fellow:** Head & Neck Oncology, Ohio St Univ Med Ctr 2005; **Fac Appt:** Asst Prof Oto, Ohio State Univ

Pelzer, Harold J MD/DDS [Oto] - **Spec Exp:** Head & Neck Cancer; **Hospital:** Northwestern Meml Hosp; **Address:** Northwestern Dept Otolaryngology, 675 N St Clair St, Ste 15-200, Chicago, IL 60611; **Phone:** 312-695-8182; **Board Cert:** Otolaryngology 1985; **Med School:** Northwestern Univ 1979; **Resid:** Surgery, Northwestern Meml Hosp 1983; **Fellow:** Head and Neck Surgery, Northwestern Meml Hosp 1985; **Fac Appt:** Assoc Prof Oto, Northwestern Univ

Pensak, Myles L MD [Oto] - **Spec Exp:** Skull Base Tumors; **Hospital:** Univ Hosp - Cincinnati, Good Samaritan Hosp - Cincinnati; **Address:** Univ Medical Arts Building, 222 Piedmont Ave, Ste 5200, Cincinnati, OH 45219; **Phone:** 513-475-8400; **Board Cert:** Otolaryngology 1983; Neurotology 2004; **Med School:** NY Med Coll 1978; **Resid:** Surgery, Upstate Med Ctr 1980; Otolaryngology, Yale Univ 1983; **Fellow:** Otology & Neurotology, The Otology Group 1984; **Fac Appt:** Prof Oto, Univ Cincinnati

Petruzzelli, Guy MD/PhD [Oto] - **Spec Exp:** Head & Neck Cancer & Surgery; Skull Base Tumors; Thyroid Cancer; Pituitary Tumors; **Hospital:** Rush Univ Med Ctr; **Address:** Rush Otolaryngology Head & Neck Surgery, 1611 W Harrison St, Ste 550, Chicago, IL 60612; **Phone:** 312-942-6100; **Board Cert:** Otolaryngology 1993; **Med School:** Rush Med Coll 1987; **Resid:** Otolaryngology, Univ Pittsburgh Med Ctr 1992; **Fellow:** Head & Neck Oncology, Univ Pittsburgh Med Ctr 1993; Skull Base Surgery, Univ Pittsburgh Ctr Cranial Base Surg 1993; **Fac Appt:** Prof Oto, Rush Med Coll

Siegel, Gordon J MD [Oto] - **Spec Exp:** Head & Neck Cancer; **Hospital:** Northwestern Meml Hosp; **Address:** 3 E Huron St Fl 1, Chicago, IL 60611-2705; **Phone:** 312-988-7777; **Board Cert:** Otolaryngology 1984; **Med School:** Ros Franklin Univ/Chicago Med Sch 1978; **Resid:** Otolaryngology, Northwestern Univ Affil Hosp 1982; **Fac Appt:** Asst Clin Prof Oto, Northwestern Univ

Stenson, Kerstin M MD [Oto] - **Spec Exp:** Head & Neck Cancer & Surgery; Head & Neck Cancer Reconstruction; **Hospital:** Univ of Chicago Med Ctr; **Address:** 5741 S Maryland Ave, MC 1035, Chicago, IL 60637-1463; **Phone:** 773-702-1865; **Board Cert:** Otolaryngology 1994; **Med School:** Ros Franklin Univ/Chicago Med Sch 1988; **Resid:** Otolaryngology, Univ Illinois Affil Hosp 1993; **Fellow:** Head & Neck Oncology, Univ Michigan Hosp 1994; Microvascular Surgery, Univ Michigan Hosp 1994; **Fac Appt:** Prof S, Univ Chicago-Pritzker Sch Med

Teknos, Theodoros N MD [Oto] - **Spec Exp:** Head & Neck Cancer; Thyroid Cancer; Facial Plastic & Reconstructive Surgery; Skull Base Tumors; **Hospital:** Ohio St Univ Med Ctr; **Address:** 456 W 10th Ave, Ste 4A, Columbus, OH 43210; **Phone:** 614-293-8074; **Board Cert:** Otolaryngology 1997; **Med School:** Harvard Med Sch 1991; **Resid:** Otolaryngology, Mass Eye & Ear Hosp 1996; **Fellow:** Head and Neck Surgery, Vanderbilt Univ Med Ctr 1997; Microvascular Surgery, Vanderbilt Univ Med Ctr 1997; **Fac Appt:** Prof Oto, Ohio State Univ

Wilson, Keith M MD [Oto] - **Spec Exp:** Head & Neck Cancer & Surgery; Voice Disorders; **Hospital:** Univ Hosp - Cincinnati; **Address:** Univ Cincinnati Medical Ctr, 222 Piedmont Ave, Ste 5200, Cincinnati, OH 45219-4222; **Phone:** 513-475-8400; **Board Cert:** Otolaryngology 1992; **Med School:** Cornell Univ-Weill Med Coll 1986; **Resid:** Otolaryngology, St Louis Univ Med Ctr 1991; **Fellow:** Head & Neck Surgical Oncology, Ohio State Med Ctr 1992; **Fac Appt:** Assoc Prof Oto, Univ Cincinnati

Wolf, Gregory T MD [Oto] - **Spec Exp:** Head & Neck Cancer; Laryngeal Cancer; **Hospital:** Univ of Michigan Hosp; **Address:** Univ Mich Med Ctr, Dept Oto-HNS, 1500 E Med Ctr, Taubman Ctr, rm 1904, Ann Arbor, MI 48109-0312; **Phone:** 734-936-8029; **Board Cert:** Otolaryngology 1978; **Med School:** Univ Mich Med Sch 1973; **Resid:** Surgery, Georgetown Univ Hosp 1975; Otolaryngology, SUNY Upstate Med Ctr 1977; **Fellow:** Immunology, NIH 1980; **Fac Appt:** Prof Oto, Univ Mich Med Sch

Yueh, Bevan MD [Oto] - **Spec Exp:** Head & Neck Cancer; **Address:** Univ Minn Med Ctr, Dept Otolaryngology/Head & Neck Surgery, 420 Delaware St SE, MMC 396, Minneapolis, MN 55455-0932; **Phone:** 612-625-2410; **Board Cert:** Otolaryngology 1995; **Med School:** Stanford Univ 1989; **Resid:** Otolaryngology, Johns Hopkins Hosp 1994; **Fellow:** Otolaryngology, Johns Hopkins Hosp 1995; **Fac Appt:** Assoc Prof Oto, Univ Minn

Great Plains and Mountains

Chowdhury, Khalid MD [Oto] - **Spec Exp:** Skull Base Tumors & Surgery; Craniofacial Surgery; Head & Neck Cancer; **Hospital:** Porter Adventist Hosp, Denver Health Med Ctr; **Address:** Center for Craniofacial Surgery, 1601 E 19th Ave, Ste 3000, Denver, CO 80218; **Phone:** 303-839-5155; **Board Cert:** Otolaryngology 1990; Facial Plastic & Reconstr Surgery 1995; **Med School:** Univ Saskatchewan 1982; **Resid:** Surgery, Univ Saskatchewan Hosp 1985; Otolaryngology, McGill Univ Hosps 1989; **Fellow:** Craniofacial Surgery, Univ Bern Hosp 1990; Facial Plastic & Reconstr Surgery, Univ Bern Hosp 1990; **Fac Appt:** Assoc Prof Oto, Univ Colorado

Lydiatt, Daniel D MD/DDS [Oto] - **Spec Exp:** Head & Neck Cancer; **Hospital:** Nebraska Med Ctr, Methodist Hosp - Omaha; **Address:** Nebraska Med Ctr, Dept Otolaryngology, 981225 Nebraska Medical Ctr, Omaha, NE 68198-1225; **Phone:** 402-559-6500; **Board Cert:** Otolaryngology 1992; **Med School:** Univ Nebr Coll Med 1983; **Resid:** Otolaryngology, Univ Nebraska Med Ctr 1990; **Fellow:** Head and Neck Surgery, MD Anderson Med Ctr 1991; **Fac Appt:** Assoc Prof Oto, Univ Nebr Coll Med

Lydiatt, William M MD [Oto] - **Spec Exp:** Head & Neck Cancer; Thyroid Cancer; Salivary Gland Tumors & Surgery; **Hospital:** Nebraska Med Ctr, Nebraska Meth Hosp; **Address:** 981225 Nebraska Medical Ctr, Omaha, NE 68198-7630; **Phone:** 402-559-6500; **Board Cert:** Otolaryngology 1994; **Med School:** Univ Nebr Coll Med 1988; **Resid:** Otolaryngology, Univ Nebraska Med Ctr 1993; **Fellow:** Head and Neck Surgery, Meml Sloan Kettering Cancer Ctr 1995; **Fac Appt:** Prof Oto, Univ Nebr Coll Med

Smith, Russell B MD [Oto] - **Spec Exp:** Head & Neck Cancer; Thyroid Cancer; Skull Base Tumors; **Hospital:** Nebraska Med Ctr, Nebraska Meth Hosp; **Address:** 981225 Nebraska Medical Center, Omaha, NE 68198-1225; **Phone:** 402-559-6500; **Board Cert:** Otolaryngology 2001; **Med School:** Univ MO-Columbia Sch Med 1995; **Resid:** Otolaryngology, Univ Missouri Med Ctr 2000; **Fellow:** Head & Neck Surgical Oncology, Univ Iowa Hosps & Clins 2001; **Fac Appt:** Assoc Prof Oto, Univ Nebr Coll Med

Song, John I MD [Oto] - **Spec Exp:** Head & Neck Cancer; Skull Base Tumors; Swallowing Disorders; **Hospital:** Univ of CO Hosp - Anschutz Inpatient Pav; **Address:** Univ Colorado Hosp, Otolaryngology, 1635 Aurora Ct, MS F737, Aurora, CO 80045; **Phone:** 720-848-2820; **Board Cert:** Otolaryngology 1998; **Med School:** NYU Sch Med 1991; **Resid:** Otolaryngology, UCLA Med Ctr 1997; **Fellow:** Head and Neck Surgery, Univ Pittsburgh Med Ctr 1998; **Fac Appt:** Asst Prof Oto, Univ Colorado

Southwest

Clayman, Gary Lee MD/DMD [Oto] - **Spec Exp:** Thyroid Cancer & Surgery; Salivary Gland Tumors & Surgery; Head & Neck Cancer; Thyroid & Parathyroid Surgery; **Hospital:** UT MD Anderson Cancer Ctr; **Address:** Univ TX/MD Anderson Cancer Center, 1515 Holcombe Blvd, Unit 1445, Houston, TX 77030-4009; **Phone:** 713-792-8837; **Board Cert:** Otolaryngology 1992; **Med School:** NE Ohio Univ 1986; **Resid:** Surgery, Hennepin Co Med Ctr 1987; Otolaryngology, Univ Minn Med Ctr 1991; **Fellow:** Head and Neck Surgery, MD Anderson Cancer Ctr 1993; **Fac Appt:** Prof Oto, Univ Tex, Houston

Otolaryngology

Diaz, Eduardo M MD [Oto] - **Spec Exp:** Head & Neck Cancer; Laryngeal Cancer; Laryngeal Cancer-Organ Preservation; Tongue Cancer; **Hospital:** UT MD Anderson Cancer Ctr; **Address:** UT MD Anderson Cancer Center, Head & Neck Center, 1515 Holcombe Blvd, Unit 460, Houston, TX 77030; **Phone:** 713-792-6920; **Board Cert:** Otolaryngology 1995; **Med School:** Baylor Coll Med 1989; **Resid:** Surgery, Univ Tex Hlth Sci Ctr 1991; Ophthalmology, Univ Tex Hlth Sci Ctr 1994; **Fellow:** Head & Neck Surgical Oncology, UT MD Anderson Cancer Ctr 1995; **Fac Appt:** Prof Oto, Univ Tex, Houston

Donovan, Donald T MD [Oto] - **Spec Exp:** Head & Neck Cancer; Voice Disorders; Thyroid Disorders; **Hospital:** Methodist Hosp - Houston, St. Luke's Episcopal Hosp-Houston; **Address:** 6550 Fannin St, Ste 1701, Smith Tower, Houston, TX 77030; **Phone:** 713-798-5900; **Board Cert:** Otolaryngology 1981; **Med School:** Baylor Coll Med 1976; **Resid:** Surgery, Baylor Affil Hosps 1978; Otolaryngology, Baylor Affil Hosps 1981; **Fellow:** Head and Neck Surgery, Columbia-Presby Med Ctr 1982; **Fac Appt:** Prof Oto, Baylor Coll Med

Hanna, Ehab YN MD [Oto] - **Spec Exp:** Skull Base Tumors & Surgery; Head & Neck Cancer & Surgery; **Hospital:** UT MD Anderson Cancer Ctr; **Address:** Univ Tex MD Anderson Cancer Ctr, 1515 Holcolmbe Blvd, Unit 1445, Houston, TX 77030; **Phone:** 713-745-1815; **Board Cert:** Otolaryngology 1994; **Med School:** Egypt 1982; **Resid:** Otolaryngology, Cleveland Clinic 1989; Otolaryngology, Cleveland Clinic 1993; **Fellow:** Otolaryngology, Univ Pittsburgh Med Ctr 1994; **Fac Appt:** Prof Oto, Univ Tex, Houston

Medina, Jesus E MD [Oto] - **Spec Exp:** Head & Neck Cancer & Surgery; **Hospital:** OU Med Ctr; **Address:** 825 NE 10th St Fl 4 - Ste 4200, Oklahoma City, OK 73104; **Phone:** 405-271-7559; **Board Cert:** Otolaryngology 1980; **Med School:** Peru 1974; **Resid:** Surgery, Wayne St Univ Affil Hosp 1977; Otolaryngology, Wayne St Univ Affil Hosp 1980; **Fellow:** Head and Neck Surgery, MD Anderson Hosp 1981; **Fac Appt:** Prof Oto, Univ Okla Coll Med

Myers, Jeffrey N MD/PhD [Oto] - **Spec Exp:** Head & Neck Cancer; Melanoma-Head & Neck; Tongue Cancer; **Hospital:** UT MD Anderson Cancer Ctr; **Address:** Univ Texas MD Anderson Cancer Ctr, 1515 Holcombe Blvd, Box 441, Houston, TX 77030; **Phone:** 713-745-2667; **Board Cert:** Otolaryngology 1997; **Med School:** Univ Pennsylvania 1991; **Resid:** Otolaryngology, Univ Pittsburgh Med Ctr 1996; **Fellow:** Head & Neck Surgical Oncology, MD Anderson Cancer Ctr 1997; **Fac Appt:** Assoc Prof Oto, Univ Tex, Houston

Nuss, Daniel W MD [Oto] - **Spec Exp:** Head & Neck Cancer; Skull Base Tumors & Surgery; **Hospital:** Our Lady of the Lake Regl Med Ctr; **Address:** Our Lady of the Lake Regl Med Ctr, 7777 Hennessy Blvd, Ste 409, Baton Rouge, LA 70808; **Phone:** 225-765-1765; **Board Cert:** Otolaryngology 1987; **Med School:** Louisiana State U, New Orleans 1981; **Resid:** Surgery, Charity Hosp 1983; Otolaryngology, LSU Med Ctr 1987; **Fellow:** Surgical Oncology, MD Anderson Hosp & Tumor Inst 1984; Head and Neck Surgery, Ctr Cranial Base Surg-Univ Pittsburgh 1991; **Fac Appt:** Prof Oto, Louisiana State U, New Orleans

Otto, Randal A MD [Oto] - **Spec Exp:** Head & Neck Cancer; Thyroid & Parathyroid Cancer & Surgery; **Hospital:** Univ Hlth Syst-San Antonio, Audie L Murphy Meml Vets Hosp - San Antonio; **Address:** 8300 Floyd Curl Drive, MSC 7777, San Antonio, TX 78229-3900; **Phone:** 210-450-0700; **Board Cert:** Otolaryngology 1987; **Med School:** Univ MO-Columbia Sch Med 1981; **Resid:** Pathology, Queens Med Ctr 1982; Otolaryngology, Univ of Missouri 1987; **Fac Appt:** Prof Oto, Univ Tex, San Antonio

Suen, James Y MD [Oto] - **Spec Exp:** Head & Neck Cancer; Thyroid Cancer; **Hospital:** UAMS Med Ctr, Arkansas Chldns Hosp; **Address:** Univ Hosp Arkansas Med Scis, 4301 W Markham St, Slot 543, Little Rock, AR 72205; **Phone:** 501-686-8224; **Board Cert:** Otolaryngology 1973; **Med School:** Univ Ark 1966; **Resid:** Surgery, Univ Arkansas Med Ctr 1970; Otolaryngology, Univ Arkansas Med Ctr 1973; **Fellow:** Head and Neck Surgery, MD Anderson Cancer Ctr 1974; **Fac Appt:** Prof Oto, Univ Ark

Weber, Randal S MD [Oto] - **Spec Exp:** Skin Cancer; Thyroid & Parathyroid Cancer & Surgery; Salivary Gland Tumors & Surgery; Head & Neck Cancer; **Hospital:** UT MD Anderson Cancer Ctr; **Address:** 1515 Holcombe Blvd, Unit 1445, Houston, TX 77030-4009; **Phone:** 713-745-0497; **Board Cert:** Otolaryngology 1985; **Med School:** Univ Tenn Coll Med 1976; **Resid:** Surgery, Baylor Coll Med 1982; Otolaryngology, Baylor Coll Med 1985; **Fellow:** Head and Neck Surgery, MD Anderson Cancer Ctr 1986; **Fac Appt:** Prof Oto, Univ Tex, Houston

Weber, Samuel C MD [Oto] - **Spec Exp:** Thyroid Cancer; Parathyroid Cancer; Head & Neck Surgery; **Hospital:** St. Luke's Episcopal Hosp-Houston, Methodist Hosp - Houston; **Address:** 6624 Fannin St, Ste 1480, Houston, TX 77030-2385; **Phone:** 713-795-5343; **Board Cert:** Otolaryngology 1972; **Med School:** Univ Tenn Coll Med 1965; **Resid:** Surgery, Baylor Coll Med 1971; Otolaryngology, Baylor Coll Med 1972; **Fac Appt:** Clin Prof Oto, Baylor Coll Med

West Coast and Pacific

Andersen, Peter MD [Oto] - **Spec Exp:** Laryngeal Cancer; Nasal & Sinus Cancer & Surgery; Head & Neck Cancer & Surgery; Neck Masses; **Hospital:** OR Hlth & Sci Univ; **Address:** Dept of Otolaryngology, 3181 SW Sam Jackson Park Rd, MC PV-01, Portland, OR 97239; **Phone:** 503-494-5355; **Board Cert:** Otolaryngology 1994; **Med School:** Washington Univ, St Louis 1988; **Resid:** Otolaryngology, Oregon Hlth & Science Univ 1993; **Fellow:** Head & Neck Surgical Oncology, Meml Sloan Kettering Cancer Ctr 1995; **Fac Appt:** Prof Oto, Oregon Hlth & Sci Univ

Berke, Gerald S MD [Oto] - **Spec Exp:** Head & Neck Surgery; Head & Neck Cancer; Voice Disorders; Laryngeal Disorders; **Hospital:** UCLA Ronald Reagan Med Ctr; **Address:** 200 UCLA Med Plaza, Ste 550, Los Angeles, CA 90095; **Phone:** 310-825-5179; **Board Cert:** Otolaryngology 1984; **Med School:** USC Sch Med 1978; **Resid:** Otolaryngology, LAC-USC Med Ctr 1979; **Fellow:** Head and Neck Surgery, UCLA Med Ctr 1984; **Fac Appt:** Prof Oto, UCLA

Blackwell, Keith Edward MD [Oto] - **Spec Exp:** Head & Neck Reconstruction; Head & Neck Cancer & Surgery; Microvascular Surgery; **Hospital:** UCLA Ronald Reagan Med Ctr; **Address:** UCLA Medical Center, Ste 550, Box 951624, Los Angeles, CA 90095; **Phone:** 310-206-6688; **Board Cert:** Otolaryngology 1995; **Med School:** Northwestern Univ 1988; **Resid:** Otolaryngology, UCLA Med Ctr1 1994; **Fellow:** Otolaryngology, Mt Sinai Med Ctr 1995; **Fac Appt:** Prof Oto, UCLA

Courey, Mark S MD [Oto] - **Spec Exp:** Laryngeal Cancer; **Hospital:** UCSF - Mt Zion Med Ctr, UCSF Med Ctr; **Address:** UCSF Voice & Swallowing Ctr, 2330 Post St Fl 5 - Ste 526, San Francisco, CA 94115; **Phone:** 415-885-7700; **Board Cert:** Otolaryngology 1993; **Med School:** SUNY Buffalo 1987; **Resid:** Otolaryngology, SUNY-Buffalo Med Ctr 1992; **Fellow:** Laryngology, Vanderbilt Univ 1993; **Fac Appt:** Prof Oto, UCSF

Donald, Paul J MD [Oto] - **Spec Exp:** Skull Base Tumors & Surgery; Head & Neck Cancer; **Hospital:** UC Davis Med Ctr; **Address:** 2521 Stockton Blvd, rm 7200, Sacramento, CA 95817; **Phone:** 916-734-2832; **Board Cert:** Otolaryngology 1973; **Med School:** Univ British Columbia Fac Med 1964; **Resid:** Surgery, St Pauls Hosp 1969; Otolaryngology, Univ Iowa Hosp 1973; **Fac Appt:** Prof Oto, UC Davis

Otolaryngology

Eisele, David W MD [Oto] - **Spec Exp:** Salivary Gland Tumors & Surgery; Head & Neck Cancer; Thyroid Cancer; Neck Masses; **Hospital:** UCSF Med Ctr; **Address:** UCSF, Dept Head & Neck Surgery, 2380 Sutter St Fl 2, Box 1703, San Francisco, CA 94115-1703; **Phone:** 415-885-7528; **Board Cert:** Otolaryngology 1988; **Med School:** Cornell Univ-Weill Med Coll 1982; **Resid:** Surgery, Univ Wash Med Ctr 1984; Otolaryngology, Univ Wash Med Ctr 1988; **Fac Appt:** Prof Oto, UCSF

Fee Jr, Willard E MD [Oto] - **Spec Exp:** Head & Neck Cancer; Parotid Gland Tumors; Thyroid Cancer; **Hospital:** Stanford Univ Hosp & Clinics; **Address:** Stanford Cancer Ctr, 875 Blake Lake Wilbur Dr, CC-2227, Stanford, CA 94305-5826; **Phone:** 650-498-6000; **Board Cert:** Otolaryngology 1974; **Med School:** Univ Colorado 1969; **Resid:** Surgery, Wadsworth VA Hosp 1971; Otolaryngology, UCLA Med Ctr 1974; **Fac Appt:** Prof Oto, Stanford Univ

Futran, Neal D MD/DMD [Oto] - **Spec Exp:** Head & Neck Cancer & Surgery; Head & Neck Cancer Reconstruction; Skull Base Tumors & Surgery; **Hospital:** Univ Wash Med Ctr, Harborview Med Ctr; **Address:** Univ Wash Med Ctr, Oto Office, 1959 NE Pacific St, Box 356161, Seattle, WA 98195-6515; **Phone:** 206-543-3060; **Board Cert:** Otolaryngology 1993; **Med School:** SUNY Downstate 1987; **Resid:** Surgery, Kings Co-SUNY Downstate 1985; Otolaryngology, Univ Rochester Med Ctr 1992; **Fellow:** Microvascular Surgery, Mt Sinai Hosp 1993; **Fac Appt:** Prof Oto, Univ Wash

Jackler, Robert K MD [Oto] - **Spec Exp:** Neuro-Otology; Skull Base Surgery; Ear Tumors; **Hospital:** Stanford Univ Hosp & Clinics; **Address:** Stanford Univ Med Ctr, Dept Head & Neck Surg, 801 Welch Rd Fl 2, Stanford, CA 94305-5739; **Phone:** 650-725-6500; **Board Cert:** Otolaryngology 1984; Neurotology 2004; **Med School:** Boston Univ 1979; **Resid:** Otolaryngology, UCSF Med Ctr 1984; **Fellow:** Otolaryngology, Oto Med Grp 1985; **Fac Appt:** Prof Oto, Stanford Univ

Kaplan, Michael J MD [Oto] - **Spec Exp:** Head & Neck Surgery; Skull Base Surgery; Head & Neck Cancer; **Hospital:** Stanford Univ Hosp & Clinics; **Address:** Stanford Cancer Ctr, Dept Otolaryngology, 801 Welch Rd Fl 2, Stanford, CA 94305-5739; **Phone:** 650-498-6000; **Board Cert:** Otolaryngology 1982; **Med School:** Harvard Med Sch 1977; **Resid:** Surgery, Beth Israel-Chldns Hosps 1979; Otolaryngology, Mass EE Infirm 1982; **Fellow:** Head and Neck Surgery, Univ Virginia 1984; **Fac Appt:** Prof Oto, Stanford Univ

McMenomey, Sean O MD [Oto] - **Spec Exp:** Skull Base Tumors & Surgery; Head & Neck Surgery; Stereotactic Radiosurgery; **Hospital:** OR Hlth & Sci Univ, Providence St Vincent Med Ctr; **Address:** Oregon Hlth & Sci Univ, Dept Otolaryngology, 3181 SW Sam Jackson Park Rd, MC PV-01, Portland, OR 97239; **Phone:** 503-494-8135; **Board Cert:** Otolaryngology 1993; Neurotology 2004; **Med School:** St Louis Univ 1987; **Resid:** Otolaryngology, Oregon Hlth Sci Ctr 1992; **Fellow:** Otology & Neurotology, Baptist Hosp 1993; **Fac Appt:** Assoc Prof Oto, Oregon Hlth & Sci Univ

Rice, Dale H MD [Oto] - **Spec Exp:** Head & Neck Cancer; Sinus Disorders/Surgery; **Hospital:** USC Univ Hosp, USC Norris Cancer Hosp; **Address:** 1520 San Pablo St, Ste 4600, Los Angeles, CA 90033-1029; **Phone:** 323-442-5790; **Board Cert:** Otolaryngology 1976; **Med School:** Univ Mich Med Sch 1968; **Resid:** Surgery, Univ Mich Med Ctr 1970; Otolaryngology, Univ Mich Med Ctr 1976; **Fac Appt:** Prof Oto, USC Sch Med

Shindo, Maisie L MD [Oto] - **Spec Exp:** Head & Neck Cancer & Surgery; Thyroid Cancer; Parathyroid Surgery; Parathyroid Cancer; **Hospital:** OR Hlth & Sci Univ; **Address:** Thyroid & Parathyroid Clinic, 3181 SW Sam Jackson Park Rd, MC PV-01, Portland, OR 97239-3098; **Phone:** 503-494-2544; **Board Cert:** Otolaryngology 1989; **Med School:** Univ Saskatchewan 1984; **Resid:** Otolaryngology, LAC-USC Med Ctr 1989; **Fellow:** Head and Neck Surgery, Northwestern Meml Hosp 1991; **Fac Appt:** Prof Oto, Oregon Hlth & Sci Univ

Singer, Mark I MD [Oto] - **Spec Exp:** Head & Neck Surgery; Head & Neck Cancer; Melanoma; **Hospital:** CA Pacific Med Ctr-Pacific Campus; **Address:** 2340 Clay St Fl 2, San Francisco, CA 94115; **Phone:** 415-600-3800; **Board Cert:** Otolaryngology 1976; **Med School:** Columbia P&S 1970; **Resid:** Surgery, Northwestern Meml Hosp 1973; Otolaryngology, Northwestern Meml Hosp 1976; **Fellow:** Oncology, Northwestern Meml Hosp 1976

Sinha, Uttam K MD [Oto] - **Spec Exp:** Head & Neck Cancer; Voice Disorders; Thyroid Cancer; Swallowing Disorders; **Hospital:** USC Univ Hosp, House Ear Inst; **Address:** 1200 N State St, rm 4136, Los Angeles, CA 90033; **Phone:** 323-226-7315; **Board Cert:** Otolaryngology 1998; **Med School:** India 1985; **Resid:** Otolaryngology, LAC-USC Med Ctr 1995; **Fellow:** Microvascular Surgery, Mount Sinai Med Ctr 1996; Laryngology 1997; **Fac Appt:** Assoc Prof Oto, USC Sch Med

Wang, Steven J MD [Oto] - **Spec Exp:** Head & Neck Cancer & Surgery; **Hospital:** UCSF Med Ctr; **Address:** 2380 Sutter St Fl Second, San Francisco, CA 94115; **Phone:** 415-885-7528; **Board Cert:** Otolaryngology 2002; **Med School:** Harvard Med Sch 1995; **Resid:** Otolaryngology, UCLA Med Ctr 2001; Head and Neck Surgery, UCLA Med Ctr 2001; **Fellow:** Head & Neck Surgical Oncology, Univ Michigan 2003; **Fac Appt:** Assoc Prof Oto, UCSF

Wax, Mark K MD [Oto] - **Spec Exp:** Skull Base Tumors & Surgery; Facial Plastic & Reconstructive Surgery; Head & Neck Cancer; **Hospital:** OR Hlth & Sci Univ; **Address:** Oregon Hlth Scis Univ, Dept Ototlaryngology, 3181 SW Sam Jackson Park Rd, MC PV-01, Portland, OR 97201; **Phone:** 503-494-5355; **Board Cert:** Otolaryngology 1985; Facial Plastic & Reconstr Surgery 2000; **Med School:** Univ Toronto 1980; **Resid:** Otolaryngology, Univ Toronto 1985; Surgery, Cedars-Sinai Med Ctr 1983; **Fellow:** Head and Neck Surgery, St Michaels Hosp 1991; **Fac Appt:** Prof Oto, Oregon Hlth & Sci Univ

Weisman, Robert A MD [Oto] - **Spec Exp:** Head & Neck Cancer; Clinical Trials; Thyroid & Parathyroid Cancer & Surgery; Head & Neck Cancer Reconstruction; **Hospital:** UCSD Med Ctr-Hillcrest; **Address:** Moores-UCSD Cancer Center, 3855 Hlth Sci Drive, MC 0987, La Jolla, CA 92093-0987; **Phone:** 858-822-6197; **Board Cert:** Otolaryngology 1978; **Med School:** Washington Univ, St Louis 1973; **Resid:** Head and Neck Surgery, UCLA Med Ctr 1978; **Fac Appt:** Prof S, UCSD

Weymuller Jr, Ernest MD [Oto] - **Spec Exp:** Head & Neck Cancer; Sinus Disorders/Surgery; **Hospital:** Univ Wash Med Ctr; **Address:** 1959 NE Pacific St, Box 356161, Seattle, WA 98159; **Phone:** 206-598-4022; **Board Cert:** Otolaryngology 1973; **Med School:** Harvard Med Sch 1966; **Resid:** Surgery, Vanderbilt Univ Hosp 1968; Otolaryngology, Mass Eye and Ear Infirm 1973; **Fac Appt:** Prof Oto, Univ Wash

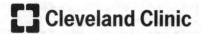 **Cleveland Clinic**

Every life deserves world class care.

Head and Neck Cancer Innovations

At Cleveland Clinic Taussig Cancer Institute, more than 250 top cancer specialists, researchers, nurses and technicians are dedicated to delivering the most effective medical treatments and offering access to the latest clinical trials for more than 13,000 new cancer patients every year. Our doctors are nationally and internationally known for their contributions to cancer breakthroughs and their ability to deliver superior outcomes for our patients. In recognition of these and other achievements, *U.S.News & World Report* has ranked Cleveland Clinic as one of the top cancer centers in the nation.

Unique Team Treatments

Cleveland Clinic Taussig Cancer Institute and the Head & Neck Institute bring together the expertise of world-renowned specialists to treat patients with cancer of the head and neck. Using the least invasive, most effective and innovative treatment approaches, Cleveland Clinic specialists strive to cure the patient's cancer, and also preserve the patient's normal function such as speech, taste, vision, hearing and swallowing.

Innovative Treatments

The treatment team uses innovative chemotherapy and combined chemotherapy-radiation therapy regimens for treating advanced head and neck cancers, including the newest molecularly targeted therapies available. Radiation oncologists have pioneered the use of the most advanced radiation therapy technique, such as intensity modulated radiation therapy, image-guided radiation therapy and adaptive radiation therapy planning. Surgeons in the Head and Neck Institute pioneered a flexible laser for throat surger and use new techniques to optimally treat cancers of the parotid gland, skull base and others which affect facial nerve function.

U.S.News & World Report ranks Cleveland Clinic's ear, nose and throat programs as #8 in the nation.

Cleveland Clinic
Taussig Cancer Institute
9500 Euclid Avenue
Cleveland, OH 44195

clevelandclinic.org/
headandneckcancersTCD

**Appointments | Information:
Call the Cancer Answer Line at
866.223.8100.**

Cancer Treatment Guides

Cleveland Clinic has developed comprehensive treatment guides for many cancers. To download our free treatment guides, visit clevelandclinic.org/cancertreatmentguides.

Comprehensive Online Medical Second Opinion

Cleveland Clinic experts can review your medical records and render an opinion that includes treatment options and recommendations. Call 216.444.3223 or 800.223.2273 ext. 43223; email eclevelandclinic@ccf.org.

Special Assistance for Out-of-State Patients

Cleveland Clinic Global Patient Services offers a complimentary Medical Concierge service for patients who travel from outside of Ohio. Call 800.223.2273, ext. 55580, or email medicalconcierge@ccf.org.

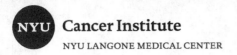

NYU Cancer Institute
NYU LANGONE MEDICAL CENTER

NYU Langone Medical Center
550 First Avenue , New York, NY 10016
www.NYULMC.org

NYU Clinical Cancer Center
160 East 34th Street, New York, NY 10016
www.NYUCI.org

The Stephen D. Hassenfeld Children's Center
for Cancer and Blood Disorders
160 East 32nd Street, New York, NY 10016
www.NYUMC.org/Hassenfeld

The NYU Cancer Institute is an NCI-designated cancer center and provides personalized patient care that is both compassionate and state of the art. The doctors and researchers work together to develop innovative therapies for patients. The Cancer Institute is world-renowned for excellence in cancer-focused research, personalized care, education and community outreach. Its mission is to discover the origins of human cancer and to use that knowledge to eradicate the personal and societal burden of cancer in our community, the nation and the world. For more information about our expert physicians, call 212-731-5000. *We specialize in the following areas:*

Patient-Focused Setting
The NYU Clinical Cancer Center is the principal outpatient facility of The Cancer Institute and serves as home to our patients and their caregivers. The center and its multidisciplinary team of experts provide access to the latest treatment options and clinical trials along with a variety of programs in cancer risk reduction/prevention, screening, diagnostics, genetic counseling and supportive services. In addition the NYUCI emphasizes the importance of a holistic approach to management services in complementary medicine, psychosocial support, survivorship and palliative care.

Renowned Expertise
The NYU Cancer Institute brings together experts from a variety of disciplines to create collaborative research endeavors and clinical care teams. The Cancer Institute offers a full continuum of personalized care, from prevention through diagnosis, treatment and post-treatment support. The compassion and expertise of our team members helps patients better manage the symptoms of their diseases as well as meet their special needs. Additionally, we have created special emphasis programs in diseases such as breast cancer, melanoma, GI cancer, prostate cancer, hematologic malignancies and lung cancer among others, as well as, translational programs in cancer healthcare disparities, molecularly targeted therapy, and the cell signaling pathways involved in cancer.

A Translational Approach
NYU Langone Medical Center scientists and other researchers excel in uncovering how cancer develops at the molecular level, and how we can harness that knowledge to reduce the risk of cancer and treat the disease. The Medical Center constantly seeks to create new opportunities for collaboration between investigators within our own institution, those located elsewhere in the NYU network of campuses, and researchers at other institutions.

The Stephen D. Hassenfeld Children's Center for Cancer and Blood Disorders
The center is a leading pediatric outpatient facility for the treatment of childhood cancers and blood diseases. Its unique interdisciplinary and family-centered approach combines the most advanced medical treatments with psychosocial and emotional support services for young patients and their families.

The Best in American Medicine
www.CastleConnolly.com

Pain Medicine

a subspecialty of Anesthesiology, Neurology, Physical Medicine & Rehabilitation or Psychiatry

Some physicians who have their primary board certification in anesthesiology, neurology, physical medicine and rehabilitation, or psychiatry have completed additional training and passed an examination in the subspecialty called pain management. These doctors provide a high level of care, either as a primary physcian or consultant, for patients experiencing problems with acute, chronic and/or cancer pain in both hospital and ambulatory settings.

For more information about the main specialties of these physicians, see Anesthesiology, Neurology, Physical Medicine and Rehabilitation or Psychiatry.

Training Required: Number of years required for primary specialty plus additional one year training and examination.

PAIN MEDICINE

New England

Abrahm, Janet L MD [PM] - **Spec Exp:** Palliative Care; Pain-Cancer; **Hospital:** Dana-Farber Cancer Inst, Brigham & Women's Hosp; **Address:** Dana-Farber Cancer Institute, 450 Brookline St, Shields-Warren 420, Boston, MA 02215; **Phone:** 617-632-6464; **Board Cert:** Internal Medicine 1976; Medical Oncology 1981; Hematology 1978; Hospice & Palliative Medicine 2008; **Med School:** UCSF 1973; **Resid:** Internal Medicine, Mass Genl Hosp 1975; Internal Medicine, Moffitt Hosp-UCSF 1977; **Fellow:** Hematology, Mass Genl Hosp 1976; Hematology & Oncology, Hosp Univ Penn 1980; **Fac Appt:** Assoc Prof Med, Harvard Med Sch

Mid Atlantic

Ballantyne, Jane C MD [PM] - **Spec Exp:** Pain-Chronic; Pain-Cancer; **Hospital:** Hosp Univ Penn - UPHS (page 80); **Address:** Penn Pain Medicine Ctr, 1840 South St, The Tuttleman Bldg Fl 2, Philadelphia, PA 19146; **Phone:** 215-893-7246; **Board Cert:** Anesthesiology 2007; **Med School:** England, UK 1978; **Resid:** Surgery, London & Oxford 1985; Anesthesiology, John Radcliffe Hosp 1990; **Fellow:** Anesthesiology, Mass Genl Hosp 1992; Pain Medicine, Mass Genl Hosp 1994; **Fac Appt:** Prof Anes, Univ Pennsylvania

DeLeon, Oscar A MD [PM] - **Spec Exp:** Pain-Acute; Pain-Chronic; Pain-Cancer; **Hospital:** Roswell Park Cancer Inst; **Address:** Roswell Park Cancer Inst, Dept Anesthesia/Pain Medicine, Elm & Carlton Sts, Buffalo, NY 14263; **Phone:** 716-845-4595; **Board Cert:** Anesthesiology 1991; Critical Care Medicine 1993; Pain Medicine 2005; **Med School:** Guatemala 1982; **Resid:** Surgery, SUNY-Downstate Med Ctr 1986; Anesthesiology, Univ Buffalo 1989; **Fac Appt:** Prof Anes, SUNY Buffalo

Jain, Subhash MD [PM] - **Spec Exp:** Pain-Cancer; Pain-Back; **Hospital:** Beth Israel Med Ctr - Petrie Division (page 71); **Address:** 360 E 72nd St, Ste C, New York, NY 10021; **Phone:** 212-439-6100; **Board Cert:** Anesthesiology 1994; Pain Medicine 1998; **Med School:** India 1968; **Resid:** Surgery, St Vincent Med Ctr 1977; Anesthesiology, New York Hosp 1979; **Fellow:** Pain Medicine, New York Hosp/Meml Sloan Kettering Cancer Ctr 1980; **Fac Appt:** Assoc Prof Anes, Cornell Univ-Weill Med Coll

Kreitzer, Joel MD [PM] - **Spec Exp:** Pain-Back; Pain-Cancer; Pain-Neuropathic; **Hospital:** Mount Sinai Med Ctr (page 76), Mount Sinai Hosp of Queens (page 76); **Address:** Upper East Side Pain Medicine, 1540 York Ave, New York, NY 10028; **Phone:** 212-288-2180; **Board Cert:** Anesthesiology 1990; Pain Medicine 2004; **Med School:** Albert Einstein Coll Med 1985; **Resid:** Anesthesiology, Mt Sinai Hosp 1989; **Fellow:** Pain Medicine, Mt Sinai Hosp 1989; **Fac Appt:** Assoc Clin Prof Anes, Mount Sinai Sch Med

Portenoy, Russell MD [PM] - **Spec Exp:** Pain-Cancer; Palliative Care; **Hospital:** Beth Israel Med Ctr - Petrie Division (page 71); **Address:** Beth Israel Med Ctr, Dept Pain Medicine/Palliative Care, First Ave at 16th St, New York, NY 10003; **Phone:** 212-844-1403; **Board Cert:** Neurology 1985; Hospice & Palliative Medicine 2008; **Med School:** Univ MD Sch Med 1980; **Resid:** Neurology, Montefiore Med Ctr 1984; **Fellow:** Pain Medicine, Meml Sloan-Kettering Cancer Ctr 1985; **Fac Appt:** Prof N, Albert Einstein Coll Med

Staats, Peter MD [PM] - **Spec Exp:** Pain-Cancer; **Hospital:** Riverview Med Ctr, CentraState Med Ctr; **Address:** Metzger Staats Pain Mgmt, 160 Avenue at the Commons, Ste 1, Shrewsbury, NJ 07702; **Phone:** 732-380-0200; **Board Cert:** Anesthesiology 1994; Pain Medicine 2005; **Med School:** Univ Mich Med Sch 1989; **Resid:** Anesthesiology, Johns Hopkins Hosp 1993; **Fellow:** Pain Medicine, Johns Hopkins Hosp 1994

Weinberger, Michael L MD [PM] - **Spec Exp:** Pain-Cancer; Pain-Back; Palliative Care; **Hospital:** NY-Presby Hosp/Columbia (page 78); **Address:** 630 W 168th St, PH5, rm 500, New York, NY 10032-3720; **Phone:** 212-305-7114; **Board Cert:** Internal Medicine 1986; Anesthesiology 1990; Pain Medicine 2004; Hospice & Palliative Medicine 2006; **Med School:** Columbia P&S 1983; **Resid:** Internal Medicine, St Vincent's Hosp 1986; Anesthesiology, Columbia-Presby Med Ctr 1989; **Fellow:** Pain Medicine, Meml Sloan Kettering Cancer Ctr 1990; **Fac Appt:** Assoc Prof Anes, Columbia P&S

Southeast

Anghelescu, Doralina L MD [PM] - **Spec Exp:** Pain Management-Pediatric; Pain-Cancer; **Hospital:** St. Jude Children's Research Hosp; **Address:** St Jude Chldn's Rsch Hosp, Anesthesiology, 262 Danny Thomas Pl, MS 130, Memphis, TN 38105; **Phone:** 901-595-4034; **Board Cert:** Anesthesiology 1998; Pain Medicine 2001; **Med School:** Romania 1985; **Resid:** Anesthesiology, Univ N Mex Hosp 1997; **Fellow:** Pain Medicine, Chldns Natl Med Ctr 1998; Pain Medicine, Univ NMex Hosp 1999

Rauck, Richard L MD [PM] - **Spec Exp:** Pain-Cancer; **Hospital:** Forsyth Med Ctr, Wake Forest Univ Baptist Med Ctr; **Address:** Carolinas Pain Institute, 145 Kimel Park Drive, Ste 330, Winston-Salem, NC 27103; **Phone:** 336-765-6181; **Board Cert:** Anesthesiology 1987; Pain Medicine 2005; **Med School:** Bowman Gray 1982; **Resid:** Anesthesiology, Univ Cincinnati Hosp 1985; **Fellow:** Pain Medicine, Univ Cincinnati Hosp 1986; **Fac Appt:** Assoc Prof Anes, Wake Forest Univ

Midwest

Amin, Sandeep D MD [PM] - **Spec Exp:** Pain-Cancer; Pain-after Spinal Intervention; **Hospital:** Rush Univ Med Ctr, Rush Oak Park Hosp; **Address:** Rush Pain Ctr, 1725 W Harrison St, Ste 550, Chicago, IL 60612; **Phone:** 312-942-6631; **Board Cert:** Anesthesiology 1998; Pain Medicine 2011; **Med School:** India 1991; **Resid:** Anesthesiology, Univ Illinois Hosps 1997; **Fellow:** Pain Medicine, Univ Illinois Hosps 1998; Pain Medicine, Johns Hopkins Hosp 1999; **Fac Appt:** Prof Anes, Rush Med Coll

Benedetti, Costantino MD [PM] - **Spec Exp:** Pain-Cancer; Palliative Care; Pain-Acute; Pain-Chronic; **Hospital:** Ohio St Univ Med Ctr, Arthur G James Cancer Hosp & Research Inst; **Address:** Ohio State Univ Med Ctr, 300 W 10th Ave, Ste 410, Columbus, OH 43210; **Phone:** 614-293-8487; **Board Cert:** Hospice & Palliative Medicine 1997; **Med School:** Italy 1972; **Resid:** Anesthesiology, Univ Colorado Hosp 1975; Anesthesiology, Univ Wash Med Ctr 1976; **Fellow:** Pain Medicine, Univ Wash Med Ctr 1978; **Fac Appt:** Clin Prof Anes, Ohio State Univ

Benzon, Honorio T MD [PM] - **Spec Exp:** Pain-Back; Pain-Neuropathic; Pain-Cancer; **Hospital:** Northwestern Meml Hosp; **Address:** 675 N Saint Clair St, Fl 20, Ste 100, Chicago, IL 60611-3015; **Phone:** 312-695-2500; **Board Cert:** Anesthesiology 2009; Pain Medicine 2004; **Med School:** Philippines 1971; **Resid:** Anesthesiology, Univ Cincinnati Med Ctr 1975; Anesthesiology, Northwestern Meml Hosp 1976; **Fellow:** Research, Brigham & Womens Hosp 1986; **Fac Appt:** Prof Anes, Northwestern Univ

Pain Medicine

Huntoon, Marc MD [PM] - **Spec Exp:** Pain-Cancer; Pain-after Spinal Intervention; Palliative Care; **Hospital:** Mayo Med Ctr & Clin - Rochester; **Address:** Mayo Clinic-Pain Medicine, 200 First St SW, Rochester, MN 55905; **Phone:** 507-266-9240; **Board Cert:** Anesthesiology 2003; Pain Medicine 2004; Hospice & Palliative Medicine 2004; **Med School:** Wayne State Univ 1985; **Resid:** Anesthesiology, Naval Hosp Med Ctr 1991; **Fellow:** Pain Medicine, Naval Hosp Med Ctr 1992

Swarm, Robert A MD [PM] - **Spec Exp:** Pain-Acute; Pain-Chronic; Pain-Cancer; **Hospital:** Barnes-Jewish Hosp; **Address:** Ctr for Advanced Med-Pain Mngmt Ctr, 4921 Parkview Pl, Ste 10A, MS 90-35-706, St Louis, MO 63110; **Phone:** 314-362-8820; **Board Cert:** Anesthesiology 1990; Pain Medicine 2004; **Med School:** Washington Univ, St Louis 1983; **Resid:** Surgery, Barnes Hosp 1986; Anesthesiology, Barnes Hosp 1989; **Fellow:** Pain Medicine, Univ Sydney 1991; **Fac Appt:** Assoc Prof Anes, Washington Univ, St Louis

Weisman, Steven J MD [PM] - **Spec Exp:** Pain Management-Pediatric; Palliative Care-Pediatric; Pain-Cancer; **Hospital:** Chldns Hosp - Wisconsin; **Address:** Chldns Hosp Wisconsin, Chldns Pain Clin, PO Box 1997, Milwaukee, WI 53201-1997; **Phone:** 414-266-2775; **Board Cert:** Pediatrics 1982; Pediatric Hematology-Oncology 1984; Anesthesiology 1996; **Med School:** Albert Einstein Coll Med 1978; **Resid:** Pediatrics, Chldns Hosp 1981; Anesthesiology, Univ Conn Hlth Ctr 1994; **Fellow:** Pediatric Hematology-Oncology, Indiana Univ Sch Med 1984; **Fac Appt:** Prof Anes, Med Coll Wisc

Great Plains and Mountains

Fine, Perry G MD [PM] - **Spec Exp:** Pain-Cancer; Palliative Care; Pain-Chronic; **Hospital:** Univ Utah Hlth Care; **Address:** 546 S Chipeta Way, Ste 220, Salt Lake City, UT 84108; **Phone:** 801-581-7246; **Board Cert:** Anesthesiology 1985; Pain Medicine 2004; **Med School:** Med Coll VA 1981; **Resid:** Anesthesiology, Univ Utah Hlth Sci Ctr 1984; **Fellow:** Pain Medicine, Univ Toronto Affil Hosp 1985; **Fac Appt:** Prof Anes, Univ Utah

Weinstein, Sharon M MD [PM] - **Spec Exp:** Pain-Cancer; Palliative Care; **Hospital:** Univ Utah Hlth Care; **Address:** Huntsman Cancer Institute, 2000 Circle of Hope, Salt Lake City, UT 84112; **Phone:** 801-585-0112; **Board Cert:** Neurology 1993; Pain Medicine 2000; Hospice & Palliative Medicine 2008; **Med School:** Albert Einstein Coll Med 1986; **Resid:** Neurology, Montefiore Med Ctr 1990; **Fellow:** Pain Medicine, Meml Sloan Kettering Cancer Ctr 1991; **Fac Appt:** Assoc Prof Anes, Univ Utah

Southwest

Burton, Allen W MD [PM] - **Spec Exp:** Pain-Cancer; Palliative Care; **Hospital:** St. Luke's Episcopal Hosp-Houston; **Address:** 7700 Main St, Ste 400, Houston, TX 77030; **Phone:** 832-553-1336; **Board Cert:** Anesthesiology 1996; Pain Medicine 1998; **Med School:** Baylor Coll Med 1991; **Resid:** Anesthesiology, Brigham & Women's Hosp 1995; **Fellow:** Pain Medicine, U Texas Med Branch Hosp 1998; **Fac Appt:** Assoc Prof Anes, Univ Tex Med Br, Galveston

Driver, Larry C MD [PM] - **Spec Exp:** Pain-Cancer; Palliative Care; **Hospital:** UT MD Anderson Cancer Ctr; **Address:** UT MD Anderson Cancer Ctr, Dept Pain Medicine, 1400 Holcombe Blvd, Unit 409, Houston, TX 77030; **Phone:** 713-745-7246; **Board Cert:** Anesthesiology 1992; Pain Medicine 2002; **Med School:** Univ Tex, San Antonio 1980; **Resid:** Anesthesiology, Univ Colorado Hlth Sci Ctr 1984; **Fellow:** Pain Medicine, MD Anderson Cancer Ctr 1999; **Fac Appt:** Assoc Prof Anes, Univ Tex, Houston

West Coast and Pacific

Audell, Laura G MD [PM] - **Spec Exp:** Pain-Cancer; **Hospital:** Cedars-Sinai Med Ctr; **Address:** 444 S San Vincente, Ste 1101, Los Angeles, CA 90048; **Phone:** 310-423-9600; **Board Cert:** Internal Medicine 1986; Anesthesiology 1988; Pain Medicine 2007; **Med School:** Univ Wash 1982; **Resid:** Internal Medicine, UCLA-Hosps 1985; Anesthesiology, UCLA-Hosps 1987; **Fellow:** Pain Medicine, UCLA-Hosps 1988

Fishman, Scott M MD [PM] - **Spec Exp:** Pain-Cancer; Pain-Chronic; **Hospital:** UC Davis Med Ctr; **Address:** UC Davis Med Ctr, Pain Management Clinic, 4860 Y St, Ste 2700, Sacramento, CA 95817; **Phone:** 916-734-7246; **Board Cert:** Psychiatry 1998; Pain Medicine 1995; **Med School:** Univ Mass Sch Med 1990; **Resid:** Internal Medicine, Greenwich Hosp 1993; Psychiatry, Mass Genl Hosp 1996; **Fellow:** Pain Medicine, Mass Genl Hosp 1995; **Fac Appt:** Prof Anes, UC Davis

Fitzgibbon, Dermot R MD [PM] - **Spec Exp:** Pain-Cancer; **Hospital:** Univ Wash Med Ctr; **Address:** Univ Wash Med Ctr, Dept Anesthesiology, 1959 NE Pacific St, Box 356540, Seattle, WA 98195; **Phone:** 206-598-4100; **Board Cert:** Anesthesiology 1996; Pain Medicine 2009; **Med School:** Ireland 1983; **Resid:** Anesthesiology, St Vincent's Hosp 1992; Anesthesiology, Univ Washington Med Ctr 1995; **Fellow:** Pain Medicine, Univ Wash-Pain Mngmt Clinic 1994; **Fac Appt:** Assoc Prof Anes, Univ Wash

Slatkin, Neal E MD [PM] - **Spec Exp:** Pain-Cancer; Palliative Care; **Hospital:** El Camino Hosp, Good Samaritan Hosp - San Jose; **Address:** 4850 Union Ave, San Jose, CA 95124-5156; **Phone:** 408-559-5600; **Board Cert:** Neurology 1982; Pain Medicine 2000; **Med School:** SUNY Stony Brook 1976; **Resid:** Neurology, Bellevue Hosp Ctr-NYU 1978; Neurology, Med Coll Va Hosps 1981; **Fellow:** Neurology, Med Coll Va 1982; Neuro-Oncology, Meml Sloan-Kettering Cancer Ctr 1984

Wallace, Mark Steven MD [PM] - **Spec Exp:** Pain-Chronic; Pain-Cancer; Palliative Care; **Hospital:** UCSD Med Ctr-Hillcrest; **Address:** 9350 Campus Point Drive, MC 7651, La Jolla, CA 92037; **Phone:** 858-657-6035; **Board Cert:** Anesthesiology 1992; Pain Medicine 2005; **Med School:** Creighton Univ 1987; **Resid:** Anesthesiology, Univ Maryland Hosp 1991; **Fellow:** Pain Medicine, UCSD Med Ctr 1994

The Best in American Medicine
www.CastleConnolly.com

Pathology

A pathologist deals with the causes and nature of disease and contributes to diagnosis, prognosis and treatment through knowledge gained by the laboratory application of the biologic, chemical and physical sciences.

A pathologist uses information gathered from the microscopic examination of tissue specimens, cells and body fluids, and from clinical laboratory tests on body fluids and secretions for the diagnosis, exclusion and monitoring of the disease.

Training Required: Three to four years. Certification in the following subspecialty requires additional training and examination.

Dermatopathology: A dermatopathologist has the expertise to diagnose and monitor diseases of the skin including infectious, immunologic, degenerative and neoplastic diseases. This entails the examination and interpretation of specially prepared tissue sections, cellular scrapings and smears of skin lesions by means of routine and special (electron and fluorescent) microscopes.

PATHOLOGY

New England

Bhan, Atul K MD [Path] - **Spec Exp:** Immunopathology; Liver Pathology; Liver Cancer; **Hospital:** Mass Genl Hosp; **Address:** Mass Genl Hosp, Dept Pathology, 55 Fruit St, Warren 501, Boston, MA 02114-2620; **Phone:** 617-726-2588; **Board Cert:** Anatomic Pathology 1976; Immunopathology 1985; **Med School:** India 1965; **Resid:** Pathology, Boston Univ Hosp 1971; Pathology, Chldns Univ Hosp 1974; **Fac Appt:** Prof Path, Harvard Med Sch

Connolly, James L MD [Path] - **Spec Exp:** Breast Pathology; Breast Cancer; **Hospital:** Beth Israel Deaconess Med Ctr - Boston, Brigham & Women's Hosp; **Address:** Beth Israel Deaconess Med Ctr, Dept Path, Dept Pathology, 330 Brookline Ave, rm ES 112, Boston, MA 02215-5400; **Phone:** 617-667-4344; **Board Cert:** Anatomic Pathology 1980; **Med School:** Vanderbilt Univ 1974; **Resid:** Anatomic Pathology, Beth Israel Hosp 1978; **Fac Appt:** Prof Path, Harvard Med Sch

DeLellis, Ronald A MD [Path] - **Spec Exp:** Thyroid Cancer; Endocrine Cancers; **Hospital:** Rhode Island Hosp, Miriam Hosp; **Address:** Rhode Island Hosp, Dept Pathology, 593 Eddy St, Providence, RI 02903-4923; **Phone:** 401-444-5154; **Board Cert:** Anatomic Pathology 1972; **Med School:** Tufts Univ 1966; **Resid:** Anatomic Pathology, Natl Inst Hlth 1971; **Fellow:** Pathology, Univ Hosp 1973; **Fac Appt:** Prof Path, Brown Univ

Fletcher, Christopher D M MD [Path] - **Spec Exp:** Soft Tissue Tumors; Sarcoma; Surgical Pathology; **Hospital:** Brigham & Women's Hosp, Dana-Farber Cancer Inst; **Address:** Brigham & Women's Hospital, Dept Pathology, 75 Francis St, Boston, MA 02115-6110; **Phone:** 617-732-8558; **Med School:** England, UK 1981; **Resid:** Pathology, St Thomas Hosp 1985; **Fellow:** Pathology, St Thomas Hosp 1986; **Fac Appt:** Prof Path, Harvard Med Sch

Harris, Nancy L MD [Path] - **Spec Exp:** Lymphoma; Hematopathology; **Hospital:** Mass Genl Hosp; **Address:** Mass Genl Hosp, Dept Pathology, 55 Fruit St, Warren 211, Boston, MA 02114; **Phone:** 617-726-5155; **Board Cert:** Anatomic Pathology 1978; Clinical Pathology 1978; **Med School:** Stanford Univ 1970; **Resid:** Pathology, Beth Israel Hosp 1978; **Fellow:** Immunopathology, Mass Genl Hosp 1980; **Fac Appt:** Prof Path, Harvard Med Sch

Mark, Eugene J MD [Path] - **Spec Exp:** Pulmonary Pathology; Occupational Lung Disease; Lung Pathology-Rare Tumors; **Hospital:** Mass Genl Hosp; **Address:** Mass Genl Hosp, Dept Path, 55 Fruit St, Warren 246, Boston, MA 02114; **Phone:** 617-726-8891; **Board Cert:** Anatomic & Clinical Pathology 1973; Dermatopathology 1975; **Med School:** Harvard Med Sch 1967; **Resid:** Pathology, Mass Genl Hosp 1972; **Fellow:** Pathology, Kantonspital 1966; **Fac Appt:** Prof Path, Harvard Med Sch

Morrow, Jon Stanley MD/PhD [Path] - **Spec Exp:** Kidney Cancer; Colon Cancer; Breast Cancer; Hematopathology; **Hospital:** Yale-New Haven Hosp; **Address:** Yale Pathology, Bady Memorial Laboratory, 310 Cedar St, BML 140, New Haven, CT 06510; **Phone:** 203-785-3624; **Board Cert:** Pathology 1980; **Med School:** Yale Univ 1976; **Resid:** Pathology, Yale-New Haven Hosp 1978; **Fellow:** Pathology, Yale-New Haven Hosp 1980; **Fac Appt:** Prof Path, Yale Univ

Odze, Robert D MD [Path] - **Spec Exp:** Gastrointestinal Pathology; Liver Pathology; Esophageal Cancer; **Hospital:** Brigham & Women's Hosp; **Address:** Brigham & Women's Hosp, Dept Pathology, 75 Francis St, Boston, MA 02115; **Phone:** 617-732-7549; **Board Cert:** Anatomic Pathology 1990; **Med School:** McGill Univ 1984; **Resid:** Surgery, McGill Univ 1987; Pathology, McGill Univ 1990; **Fellow:** Gastrointestinal Pathology, New England Deaconess Med Ctr 1991; **Fac Appt:** Assoc Prof Path, Harvard Med Sch

Schnitt, Stuart J MD [Path] - **Spec Exp:** Breast Pathology; Breast Cancer; **Hospital:** Beth Israel Deaconess Med Ctr - Boston; **Address:** Beth Israel Deaconess Med Ctr, Dept Pathology, 330 Brookline Ave, rm ES 112, Boston, MA 02215-5400; **Phone:** 617-667-4344; **Board Cert:** Anatomic & Clinical Pathology 1983; **Med School:** Albany Med Coll 1979; **Resid:** Anatomic Pathology, Beth Israel Deaconess Med Ctr 1983; **Fellow:** Surgical Pathology, Beth Israel Deaconess Med Ctr 1984; **Fac Appt:** Assoc Prof Path, Harvard Med Sch

Young, Robert H MD [Path] - **Spec Exp:** Ovarian Cancer; Gynecologic Cancer; **Hospital:** Mass Genl Hosp; **Address:** Mass General Hosp, 55 Fruit St, Dept Pathology, Warren 215, Boston, MA 02114; **Phone:** 617-726-8892; **Board Cert:** Anatomic Pathology 1980; **Med School:** Ireland 1974; **Resid:** Pathology, Mass Genl Hosp 1979; Pathology, Dublin Univ 1977; **Fac Appt:** Prof Path, Harvard Med Sch

Mid Atlantic

Bagg, Adam MD [Path] - **Spec Exp:** Hematopathology; Leukemia & Lymphoma; Myelodysplastic Syndromes; **Hospital:** Hosp Univ Penn - UPHS (page 80); **Address:** Hosp Univ Penn, Dept Pathology & Lab Med, 3400 Spruce St, Philadelphia, PA 19104; **Phone:** 215-662-4280; **Board Cert:** Clinical Pathology 1992; Hematology 1999; **Med School:** South Africa 1981; **Resid:** Internal Medicine, Univ Witwatersrand 1992; Clinical Pathology, Georgetown Univ 1992; **Fellow:** Hematopathology, Georgetown Univ 1993; **Fac Appt:** Prof Path, Univ Pennsylvania

Bastian, Boris C MD/PhD [Path] - **Spec Exp:** Melanoma; Skin Cancer; Dermatopathology; **Hospital:** Meml Sloan-Kettering Cancer Ctr (page 75); **Address:** Meml Sloan Kettering Cancer Ctr, 1275 York Ave, Dept Pathology, New York, NY 10065; **Phone:** 212-639-8410; **Med School:** Germany 1988; **Resid:** Dermatology, University of Wurzburg 1994; **Fellow:** Hematology, Ludwig-Maximilian-University 1989; UCSF Canc Ctr; **Fac Appt:** Asst Prof D, UCSF

Brooks, John S MD [Path] - **Spec Exp:** Tumor Pathology; Sarcoma; Bone & Soft Tissue Pathology; **Hospital:** Pennsylvania Hosp (page 80), Hosp Univ Penn - UPHS (page 80); **Address:** Pennsylvania Hospital, Preston 6 FL, 800 Spruce St, Philadelphia, PA 19107; **Phone:** 215-829-3541; **Board Cert:** Anatomic Pathology 1978; Immunopathology 1983; **Med School:** Thomas Jefferson Univ 1974; **Resid:** Pathology, Hosp Univ Penn 1978; **Fellow:** Immunopathology, Hosp Univ Penn 1978; **Fac Appt:** Prof Path, Univ Pennsylvania

Burger, Peter MD [Path] - **Spec Exp:** Brain Tumors; Neuro-Pathology; **Hospital:** Johns Hopkins Hosp; **Address:** Johns Hopkins Hosp-Dept Pathology, 600 N Wolfe St, Pathology 710, Baltimore, MD 21287; **Phone:** 410-955-8378; **Board Cert:** Anatomic Pathology 1976; Neuropathology 1976; **Med School:** Northwestern Univ 1966; **Resid:** Anatomic Pathology, Duke Univ Med Ctr 1973; **Fellow:** Neuropathology, Duke Univ Med Ctr 1973

Crawford, James M MD/PhD [Path] - **Spec Exp:** Liver Pathology; Gastrointestinal Pathology; Gastrointestinal Cancer; **Hospital:** N Shore Univ Hosp, Long Island Jewish Med Ctr; **Address:** N Shore-LI Jewish Laboratories, 10 Nevada Drive, Lake Success, NY 11042-1114; **Phone:** 516-719-1060; **Board Cert:** Anatomic Pathology 1987; **Med School:** Duke Univ 1982; **Resid:** Pathology, Brigham & Women's Hosp 1984; **Fellow:** Gastrointestinal Pathology, Brigham & Women's Hosp 1987; Pathology, Royal Free hosp 1989

Ehya, Hormoz MD [Path] - **Spec Exp:** Cytopathology; Breast Pathology; Lung Pathology; **Hospital:** Fox Chase Cancer Ctr (page 72); **Address:** Fox Chase Cancer Center, 333 Cottman Ave, rm C427, Philadelphia, PA 19111-2497; **Phone:** 215-728-5389; **Board Cert:** Anatomic Pathology 1979; Cytopathology 1989; **Med School:** Iran 1974; **Resid:** Pathology, Univ Miss Med Ctr 1979; **Fellow:** Cytopathology, Meml Sloan-Kettering Cancer Ctr 1980

Pathology

Epstein, Jonathan MD [Path] - **Spec Exp:** Bladder Cancer; Prostate Cancer; Urologic Pathology; **Hospital:** Johns Hopkins Hosp; **Address:** 401 N Broadway, Weinberg 2242, Baltimore, MD 21231; **Phone:** 410-955-5043; **Board Cert:** Anatomic Pathology 1986; **Med School:** Boston Univ 1981; **Resid:** Pathology, Johns Hopkins Hosp 1985; **Fellow:** Pathology, Meml Sloan Kettering Cancer Ctr 1984; **Fac Appt:** Prof Path, Johns Hopkins Univ

Fogt, Franz MD/PhD [Path] - **Spec Exp:** Gastrointestinal Pathology; **Hospital:** Penn Presby Med Ctr - UPHS (page 80); **Address:** Presbyterian Medical Ctr, Dept Pathology, 51 N 39th St, 551 Wright Saunders Bldg, Philadelphia, PA 19104; **Phone:** 215-662-8077; **Board Cert:** Anatomic & Clinical Pathology 1995; **Med School:** Germany 1988; **Resid:** Anatomic & Clinical Pathology, New England Deaconess Hosp 1995; **Fellow:** Gastrointestinal Pathology, New England Deaconess Hosp 1996; **Fac Appt:** Assoc Prof Path, Univ Pennsylvania

Gottlieb, Geoffrey J MD [Path] - **Spec Exp:** Dermatopathology; Melanoma; **Address:** Ackerman Academy Dermatopathology, 145 E 32nd St Fl 10, New York, NY 10016; **Phone:** 212-889-6225; **Board Cert:** Anatomic Pathology 1979; Dermatopathology 1982; **Med School:** Cornell Univ-Weill Med Coll 1976; **Resid:** Pathology, NY Hosp-Cornell Med Ctr 1979; **Fellow:** Dermatopathology, NYU Med Ctr 1982

Gupta, Prabodh K MD [Path] - **Spec Exp:** Lung Pathology; Cervical Cancer; Fine Needle Aspiration Biopsy; **Hospital:** Hosp Univ Penn - UPHS (page 80); **Address:** Hosp Univ Penn - Cytopathology, 3400 Spruce St, 6 Founders, Philadelphia, PA 19104; **Phone:** 215-662-3238; **Board Cert:** Anatomic Pathology 1975; Cytopathology 1989; **Med School:** India 1960; **Resid:** Pathology, All India Inst Med Scis 1967; **Fellow:** Pathology, Mass Genl Hosp 1968; Cytopathology, Johns Hopkins Hosp 1969; **Fac Appt:** Prof Path, Univ Pennsylvania

Heller, Debra S MD [Path] - **Spec Exp:** Gynecologic Pathology; Pediatric Pathology; **Hospital:** Univ Hosp-UMDNJ—Newark; **Address:** UMDNJ-NJ Med Sch Dept Pathology, 185 S Orange Ave, UH/E158, Newark, NJ 07101; **Phone:** 973-972-0751; **Board Cert:** Anatomic Pathology 1988; Obstetrics & Gynecology 2008; Pediatric Pathology 1999; **Med School:** NY Med Coll 1977; **Resid:** Obstetrics & Gynecology, Beth Israel Med Ctr 1981; Anatomic Pathology, Mt Sinai Med Ctr 1988; **Fellow:** Pediatric Pathology, Mt Sinai Med Ctr 1987; Gynecologic Pathology, Mt Sinai Med Ctr 1989; **Fac Appt:** Prof Path, UMDNJ-NJ Med Sch, Newark

Hoda, Syed A MD [Path] - **Spec Exp:** Breast Cancer; Surgical Pathology; **Hospital:** NY-Presby Hosp/Weill Cornell (page 78); **Address:** 525 E 68th St, 1028 Starr, New York, NY 10021-4870; **Phone:** 212-746-2700; **Board Cert:** Anatomic & Clinical Pathology 1990; Cytopathology 1991; Pathology 2001; **Med School:** Pakistan 1984; **Resid:** Anatomic & Clinical Pathology, Tulane Univ Affil Hosps 1990; **Fellow:** Cytopathology, Meml Sloan Kettering Cancer Ctr 1991; Pathology, Meml Sloan Kettering Cancer Ctr 1992; **Fac Appt:** Clin Prof Path, Cornell Univ-Weill Med Coll

Hruban, Ralph H MD [Path] - **Spec Exp:** Gastrointestinal Pathology; Pancreatic Cancer; **Hospital:** Johns Hopkins Hosp; **Address:** Johns Hopkins Hosp, Dept Pathology, 401 N Broadway Bldg Weinberg - rm 2242, Baltimore, MD 21231; **Phone:** 410-955-2660; **Board Cert:** Anatomic Pathology 1990; **Med School:** Johns Hopkins Univ 1985; **Resid:** Pathology, Johns Hopkins Hosp 1990; **Fellow:** Anatomic Pathology, Meml Sloan Kettering Cancer Ctr 1989; **Fac Appt:** Prof Path, Johns Hopkins Univ

Jones, Robert V MD [Path] - **Spec Exp:** Neuro-Pathology; Brain Tumors; **Hospital:** Georgetown Univ Hosp; **Address:** GWUMC, Dept Path, 2300 Eye St NW, Ross Hall, Ste 502, Washington, DC 20037; **Phone:** 202-994-3391; **Board Cert:** Anatomic & Clinical Pathology 1981; Neuropathology 1994; **Med School:** Univ VA Sch Med 1977; **Resid:** Anatomic & Clinical Pathology, Walter Reed AMC 1981; **Fellow:** Neurological Pathology, ARmed Forces Inst Path 1990; **Fac Appt:** Assoc Prof Path, Geo Wash Univ

Katzenstein, Anna-Luise A MD [Path] - **Spec Exp:** Lung Cancer; Pulmonary Pathology; **Hospital:** SUNY Upstate Med Univ Shos, Crouse Hosp; **Address:** SUNY Upstate Medical Univ, 750 E Adams St UH Bldg - rm 6709, Syracuse, NY 13210; **Phone:** 315-464-7125; **Board Cert:** Anatomic Pathology 1976; **Med School:** Johns Hopkins Univ 1971; **Resid:** Pathology, Univ Hosp 1975; **Fellow:** Surgical Pathology, Barnes Hosp-Wash Univ 1976; **Fac Appt:** Prof Path, SUNY Upstate Med Univ

Kurman, Robert J MD [Path] - **Spec Exp:** Gynecologic Pathology; Ovarian Cancer; Uterine Cancer; **Hospital:** Johns Hopkins Hosp; **Address:** Johns Hopkins Hosp, Dept Pathology, 401 N Broadway, Weinberg-2242, Baltimore, MD 21231; **Phone:** 410-955-0471; **Board Cert:** Anatomic Pathology 1972; Obstetrics & Gynecology 1980; **Med School:** SUNY Upstate Med Univ 1968; **Resid:** Pathology, Peter Bent Brigham Hosp/Mass Genl Hosp 1977; Obstetrics & Gynecology, LAC Hosp/USC 1978; **Fellow:** Obstetrics & Gynecology, Harvard Univ 1973; **Fac Appt:** Prof Path, Johns Hopkins Univ

Li Volsi, Virginia A MD [Path] - **Spec Exp:** Endocrine Cancers; Thyroid Cancer; Gynecologic Cancer; **Hospital:** Hosp Univ Penn - UPHS (page 80); **Address:** Hosp Univ Penn - Pathology, 3400 Spruce St, Founders Bldg Fl 6 - rm 6009, Philadelphia, PA 19104; **Phone:** 215-662-6545; **Board Cert:** Anatomic Pathology 1974; **Med School:** Columbia P&S 1969; **Resid:** Anatomic Pathology, Presbyterian Hosp 1974; **Fac Appt:** Prof Path, Univ Pennsylvania

Melamed, Jonathan MD [Path] - **Spec Exp:** Prostate Cancer; Tumor Banking-Prostate; **Hospital:** NYU Langone Med Ctr (page 79); **Address:** NYU Medical Ctr, Dept Pathology, TH-461, 560 First Ave, New York, NY 10016; **Phone:** 212-263-8927; **Board Cert:** Anatomic & Clinical Pathology 1992; **Med School:** South Africa 1985; **Resid:** Pathology, Lenox Hill Hosp 1991; **Fellow:** Pathology, Meml Sloan Kettering Cancer Ctr 1992; Urologic Pathology, Meml Sloan Kettering Cancer Ctr 1993; **Fac Appt:** Assoc Prof Path, NYU Sch Med

Mies, Carolyn MD [Path] - **Spec Exp:** Breast Cancer; **Hospital:** Hosp Univ Penn - UPHS (page 80); **Address:** Hosp Univ Penn-Surgical Pathology, 3400 Spruce St, Founders 6, Philadelphia, PA 19104; **Phone:** 215-662-6503; **Board Cert:** Anatomic Pathology 1984; **Med School:** Rush Med Coll 1980; **Resid:** Pathology, Tufts-New England Med Ctr 1982; Pathology, New England Deaconess Hosp 1984; **Fellow:** Surgical Pathology, Meml Sloan Kettering Cancer Ctr 1986; **Fac Appt:** Assoc Prof Path, Univ Pennsylvania

Montgomery, Elizabeth A MD [Path] - **Spec Exp:** Barrett's Esophagus; Esophageal Cancer; Gastrointestinal Pathology; **Hospital:** Johns Hopkins Hosp; **Address:** Johns Hopkins Univ, Dept Pathology, 401 N Broadway Weinberg Bldg - rm 2242, Baltimore, MD 21231; **Phone:** 410-614-2308; **Board Cert:** Anatomic Pathology 1988; Cytopathology 1994; **Med School:** Geo Wash Univ 1984; **Resid:** Pathology, Walter Reed AMC 1988; **Fac Appt:** Assoc Prof Path, Johns Hopkins Univ

Orazi, Attilio MD [Path] - **Spec Exp:** Hematopathology; Bone Marrow Pathology; Lymph Node Pathology; Spleen Pathology; **Hospital:** NY-Presby Hosp/Weill Cornell (page 78); **Address:** NY Presby-Cornell Medical Ctr, 525 E 68th St, Starr Pavilion, rm 715, New York, NY 10021; **Phone:** 212-746-2050; **Board Cert:** Anatomic Pathology 1997; Hematology 1998; **Med School:** Italy 1979; **Resid:** Internal Medicine, Leicester Royal Infirmary 1982; Histopathology, Northampton Genl Hosp 1983; **Fellow:** Anatomic Pathology, Natl Cancer Inst 1985; **Fac Appt:** Prof Path, Cornell Univ-Weill Med Coll

Patchefsky, Arthur S MD [Path] - **Spec Exp:** Breast Cancer; Pulmonary Pathology; Sarcoma; **Hospital:** Fox Chase Cancer Ctr (page 72); **Address:** Fox Chase Cancer Center, 333 Cottman Ave, rm C4333, Philadelphia, PA 19111; **Phone:** 215-728-5390; **Board Cert:** Anatomic Pathology 1969; **Med School:** Hahnemann Univ 1963; **Resid:** Pathology, John Hopkins Hosp 1966; Pathology, Hosp Univ Penn 1967; **Fellow:** Pathology, Meml Sloan Kettering Cancer Ctr 1968; **Fac Appt:** Prof Path, Thomas Jefferson Univ

Reuter, Victor E MD [Path] - **Spec Exp:** Prostate Cancer; Genitourinary Pathology; Bladder Cancer; Testicular Cancer; **Hospital:** Meml Sloan-Kettering Cancer Ctr (page 75); **Address:** Memorial Sloan Kettering Cancer Ctr, Dept Pathology, 1275 York Ave, New York, NY 10021; **Phone:** 212-639-8225; **Board Cert:** Anatomic & Clinical Pathology 1983; **Med School:** Dominican Republic 1978; **Resid:** Anatomic Pathology, Thos Jefferson Univ Hosp 1981; Clinical Pathology, Thos Jefferson Univ Hosp 1983; **Fellow:** Surgical Pathology, Meml Sloan Kettering Cancer Ctr 1985; **Fac Appt:** Prof Path, Cornell Univ-Weill Med Coll

Rosenblum, Marc K MD [Path] - **Spec Exp:** Neuropathology; Brain Tumors; **Hospital:** Meml Sloan-Kettering Cancer Ctr (page 75); **Address:** 1275 York Ave, Meml Sloan-Kettering Cancer Ctr, New York, NY 10065; **Phone:** 212-639-3844; **Board Cert:** Anatomic Pathology 1984; Neuropathology 1988; **Med School:** Univ Miami Sch Med 1979; **Resid:** Anatomic Pathology, Mt Sinai Med Ctr 1984; **Fellow:** Pathology, Meml Sloan-Kettering Cancer Ctr 1985; Neurological Pathology, Bellevue-NYU Med Ctr 1987; **Fac Appt:** Prof Path, Cornell Univ-Weill Med Coll

Ross, Jeffrey S MD [Path] - **Spec Exp:** Urologic Cancer; Prostate Cancer; Breast Cancer; **Hospital:** Albany Med Ctr; **Address:** Albany Med Coll, Dept Path, 47 New Scotland Ave, MC 81, Albany, NY 12208; **Phone:** 518-262-5471; **Board Cert:** Anatomic & Clinical Pathology 1974; **Med School:** SUNY Buffalo 1970; **Resid:** Pathology, Mass Genl Hosp 1974; **Fellow:** Pathology, Harvard Med Sch 1974; **Fac Appt:** Prof Path, Albany Med Coll

Sanchez, Miguel A MD [Path] - **Spec Exp:** Breast Cancer; Thyroid Cancer; **Hospital:** Englewood Hosp & Med Ctr; **Address:** 350 Engle St Dean Bldg Fl LL1, Englewood, NJ 07631-1898; **Phone:** 201-894-3423; **Board Cert:** Anatomic Pathology 1975; Clinical Pathology 1979; Cytopathology 1991; **Med School:** Spain 1969; **Resid:** Pathology, Englewood Hosp 1972; Pathology, Temple Univ 1973; **Fellow:** Pathology, Meml Sloan Kettering Cancer Ctr 1974; Clinical Pathology, St Vincents Hosp 1975; **Fac Appt:** Assoc Prof Path, Mount Sinai Sch Med

Schiller, Alan L MD [Path] - **Spec Exp:** Bone & Joint Pathology; Soft Tissue Pathology; Bone Tumors; **Hospital:** Mount Sinai Med Ctr (page 76); **Address:** Mt Sinai Sch Med, Dept Pathology, 1 Gustave Levy Pl, Box 1194, New York, NY 10029-6500; **Phone:** 212-241-8014; **Board Cert:** Anatomic Pathology 1973; **Med School:** Ros Franklin Univ/Chicago Med Sch 1967; **Resid:** Pathology, Mass Genl Hosp 1972; **Fac Appt:** Prof Path, Mount Sinai Sch Med

Silverman, Jan F MD [Path] - **Spec Exp:** Fine Needle Aspiration Biopsy; Surgical Pathology; Gastrointestinal Pathology; Cytopathology; **Hospital:** Allegheny General Hosp, West Penn Hosp-Forbes Campus; **Address:** Allegheny Gen Hosp-Dept Lab Medicine, 320 E North Ave, Pittsburgh, PA 15212; **Phone:** 412-359-6886; **Board Cert:** Anatomic & Clinical Pathology 1975; Cytopathology 1989; **Med School:** Med Coll VA 1970; **Resid:** Pathology, Med Coll Virginia 1975; **Fellow:** Surgical Pathology, Med Coll Virginia 1975; **Fac Appt:** Prof Path, Drexel Univ Coll Med

Soslow, Robert A MD [Path] - **Spec Exp:** Gynecologic Pathology; **Hospital:** Meml Sloan-Kettering Cancer Ctr (page 75); **Address:** 1275 York Avenue, Pathology Department, New York, NY 10065; **Phone:** 800-525-2225; **Board Cert:** Anatomic Pathology 1995; **Med School:** Univ Pennsylvania 1991; **Resid:** Anatomic Pathology, Stanford Univ Med Ctr 1994; **Fellow:** Immunopathology, Stanford Univ Med Ctr 1995; **Fac Appt:** Assoc Prof Path, Cornell Univ

Swerdlow, Steven H MD [Path] - **Spec Exp:** Lymphoma; Hematopathology; Transplant Pathology; **Hospital:** UPMC Presby, Pittsburgh; **Address:** Div Hematopathology, 200 Lothrop St, Ste G-300, Pittsburgh, PA 15213-2536; **Phone:** 412-647-5191; **Board Cert:** Anatomic & Clinical Pathology 2005; **Med School:** Harvard Med Sch 1975; **Resid:** Pathology, Beth Israel Hosp 1979; **Fellow:** Hematopathology, Vanderbilt Univ 1981; Hematopathology, St Bartholmew's Hosp 1983; **Fac Appt:** Prof Path, Univ Pittsburgh

Tomaszewski, John E MD [Path] - **Spec Exp:** Kidney Pathology; Lung Pathology; Uterine Cancer; Genitourinary Pathology; **Hospital:** Hosp Univ Penn - UPHS (page 80); **Address:** Hosp Univ Penn, Dept Pathology & Lab Med, 3400 Spruce St, 6 Founders Bldg, Ste 6042, Philadelphia, PA 19104; **Phone:** 215-662-6852; **Board Cert:** Anatomic Pathology 1982; Immunopathology 1983; **Med School:** Univ Pennsylvania 1977; **Resid:** Pathology, Hosp Univ Penn 1982; **Fellow:** Surgical Pathology, Hosp Univ Penn 1983; **Fac Appt:** Prof Path, Univ Pennsylvania

Tornos, Carmen MD [Path] - **Spec Exp:** Gynecologic Cancer; Breast Cancer; Ovarian Cancer; **Hospital:** Stony Brook Univ Med Ctr; **Address:** Stony Brook Univ Hosp, Dept Pathology, Level 2, rm 766, Stony Brook, NY 11794; **Phone:** 631-444-2222; **Board Cert:** Anatomic & Clinical Pathology 1989; **Med School:** Spain 1977; **Resid:** Hematology, Ciudad Sanitaria Valle de Hebron 1982; Anatomic & Clinical Pathology, Univ Texas HSC 1989; **Fellow:** Surgical Pathology, MD Anderson Cancer Ctr 1990; **Fac Appt:** Prof Path, SUNY Stony Brook

Travis, William MD [Path] - **Spec Exp:** Pulmonary Pathology; Lung Cancer; **Hospital:** Meml Sloan-Kettering Cancer Ctr (page 75); **Address:** 1275 York Ave, MSKCC Bldg, Pathology Dept, New York, NY 10065; **Phone:** 212-639-6364; **Board Cert:** Anatomic & Clinical Pathology 1985; **Med School:** Univ Fla Coll Med 1981; **Resid:** Anatomic Pathology, New England Deaconess Hosp 1983; Clinical Pathology, Mayo Clinic 1985; **Fellow:** Surgical Pathology, Mayo Clinic 1986

Wang, Beverly Y MD [Path] - **Spec Exp:** Head & Neck Pathology; **Hospital:** NYU Langone Med Ctr (page 79); **Address:** NYU Medical Ctr, Dept Pathology, 530 First Ave Fl 4 - rm 461, New York, NY 10016; **Phone:** 212-263-6032; **Board Cert:** Anatomic Pathology 1998; Cytopathology 1999; **Med School:** China 1982; **Resid:** Pathology, Mount Sinai Med Ctr 1999; **Fac Appt:** Prof Path, NYU Sch Med

Yousem, Samuel A MD [Path] - **Spec Exp:** Pulmonary Pathology; Transplant-Lung (Pathology); Lung Cancer; **Hospital:** UPMC Presby, Pittsburgh; **Address:** Dept Pathology, A-610, UPMC-Presbyterian Campus, 200 Lothrop St, Pittsburgh, PA 15213; **Phone:** 412-647-6193; **Board Cert:** Anatomic Pathology 1985; Cytopathology 1997; **Med School:** Univ MD Sch Med 1981; **Resid:** Pathology, Stanford Univ Med Ctr 1983; **Fellow:** Surgical Pathology, Stanford Univ Med Ctr 1984; **Fac Appt:** Prof Path, Univ Pittsburgh

Zagzag, David MD/PhD [Path] - **Spec Exp:** Neuropathology; Brain Tumors; Tumor Banking-Brain; **Hospital:** NYU Langone Med Ctr (page 79), Bellevue Hosp Ctr; **Address:** NYU Med Ctr, Dept Pathology, 550 First Ave, Div Neuropathology, NB-4N30, New York, NY 10016; **Phone:** 212-263-6449; **Board Cert:** Anatomic Pathology 1993; Neuropathology 1993; **Med School:** France 1984; **Resid:** Surgical Pathology, NYU Med Ctr 1990; **Fellow:** Neurological Pathology, NYU Med Ctr 1992; **Fac Appt:** Assoc Prof Path, NYU Sch Med

Southeast

Banks, Peter MD [Path] - **Spec Exp:** Hematopathology; Lymphoma; **Hospital:** Carolinas Med Ctr; **Address:** Dept Pathology, 1000 Blythe Blvd, 4th Fl Pathology Lab, Charlotte, NC 28203; **Phone:** 704-355-2251; **Board Cert:** Anatomic Pathology 2008; **Med School:** Harvard Med Sch 1971; **Resid:** Pathology, National Cancer Inst 1974; Pathology, Duke Univ Med Ctr 1975; **Fellow:** Surgical Pathology, Univ Minn Med Ctr 1976; **Fac Appt:** Prof Path, Univ NC Sch Med

Bostwick, David MD [Path] - **Spec Exp:** Urologic Pathology; Prostate Cancer; Bladder Cancer; Gastrointestinal Pathology; **Address:** 4355 Innslake Drive, Glen Allen, VA 23060; **Phone:** 804-967-9225; **Board Cert:** Anatomic Pathology 2003; **Med School:** Univ MD Sch Med 1979; **Resid:** Pathology, Stanford Univ Med Ctr 1981; **Fellow:** Surgical Pathology, Stanford Univ Med Ctr 1984

Pathology

Cote, Richard J. MD [Path] - **Spec Exp:** Lymph Node Pathology; Bladder Cancer; Breast Cancer; **Hospital:** Univ of Miami Hosp (page 82); **Address:** 1120 NW 14th St, CRB Bldg - Fl 14 - Ste 1416 (R5), Miami, FL 33136; **Phone:** 305-243-2683; **Board Cert:** Anatomic Pathology 1987; **Med School:** Univ Chicago-Pritzker Sch Med 1980; **Resid:** Pathology, New York Hosp 1987; **Fellow:** Pathology, Meml Sloan-Kettering Cancer Ctr 1990; **Fac Appt:** Prof Path, USC-Keck School of Medicine

Lage, Janice MD [Path] - **Spec Exp:** Gynecologic Pathology; Breast Pathology; **Hospital:** MUSC Med Ctr; **Address:** MUSC Med Ctr, Dept Path, 165 Ashley Ave, Ste 309, Box 250908, Charleston, SC 29425; **Phone:** 843-792-3121; **Board Cert:** Anatomic Pathology 2001; **Med School:** Washington Univ, St Louis 1980; **Resid:** Pathology, Barnes Hosp/Wash Univ 1982; Obstetrics & Gynecology, Barnes Hosp/Wash Univ 1983; **Fellow:** Surgical Pathology, Barnes Hosp/Wash Univ 1984; **Fac Appt:** Prof Path, Med Univ SC

Masood, Shahla MD [Path] - **Spec Exp:** Breast Cancer; Breast Pathology; **Hospital:** Shands Jacksonville; **Address:** Univ of Florida, Dept Pathology, 655 W 8th St, Jacksonville, FL 32209-6511; **Phone:** 904-244-4387; **Board Cert:** Anatomic & Clinical Pathology 1977; Cytopathology 1990; **Med School:** Iran 1973; **Resid:** Anatomic Pathology, Univ Hosp 1977; **Fac Appt:** Prof Path, Univ Fla Coll Med

McCurley, Thomas L MD [Path] - **Spec Exp:** Hematopathology; Immunopathology; **Hospital:** Vanderbilt Univ Med Ctr, TN Valley Healthcare Sys-Nashville; **Address:** Hematopathology Dept, 1301 Med Ctr Drive, 4601 TVC, Nashville, TN 37232-5310; **Phone:** 615-343-9167; **Board Cert:** Anatomic & Clinical Pathology 1981; Immunopathology 1986; Hematology 1999; **Med School:** Vanderbilt Univ 1974; **Resid:** Internal Medicine, UCSF Med Ctr 1976; Pathology, Vanderbilt Univ Med Ctr 1981; **Fellow:** Hematopathology, Vanderbilt Univ 1984; **Fac Appt:** Assoc Prof Path, Vanderbilt Univ

Mills, Stacey E MD [Path] - **Spec Exp:** Breast Pathology; Ear, Nose & Throat Pathology; Surgical Pathology; Bone Pathology; **Hospital:** Univ of Virginia Health Sys; **Address:** Univ VA Hlth System, Dept Pathology, PO Box 800214, Charlottesville, VA 22908-0214; **Phone:** 434-982-4406; **Board Cert:** Anatomic Pathology 2009; **Med School:** Univ VA Sch Med 1977; **Resid:** Pathology, Univ Virginia Med Ctr 1980; **Fellow:** Pathology, Univ Virginia Med Ctr 1981; **Fac Appt:** Prof Path, Univ VA Sch Med

Nicosia, Santo MD [Path] - **Spec Exp:** Ovarian Cancer; Cytopathology; **Hospital:** H Lee Moffitt Cancer Ctr & Research Inst; **Address:** 12901 Bruce B Downs Blvd, MDC Box 11, Tampa, FL 33612-4742; **Phone:** 813-974-3133; **Board Cert:** Anatomic Pathology 1978; Cytopathology 1990; **Med School:** Italy 1967; **Resid:** Anatomic Pathology, Michael Reese Hosp 1972; **Fellow:** Hosp Univ Penn 1973; **Fac Appt:** Prof Path, Univ S Fla Coll Med

Sewell, C Whitaker MD [Path] - **Spec Exp:** Breast Pathology; Surgical Pathology; **Hospital:** Emory Univ Hosp; **Address:** Emory Univ Hosp, Dept Pathology, 1364 Clifton Rd NE, rm H185C, Atlanta, GA 30322; **Phone:** 404-712-7003; **Board Cert:** Anatomic & Clinical Pathology 1974; **Med School:** Emory Univ 1969; **Resid:** Pathology, Emory Univ Hosp 1974; **Fac Appt:** Prof Path, Emory Univ

Weiss, Sharon A W MD [Path] - **Spec Exp:** Soft Tissue Pathology; Surgical Pathology; Sarcoma; **Hospital:** Emory Univ Hosp; **Address:** Emory Univ Hosp, Dept Pathology, 1364 Clifton Rd NE, rm H176, Atlanta, GA 30322; **Phone:** 404-712-0708; **Board Cert:** Anatomic Pathology 1974; **Med School:** Johns Hopkins Univ 1971; **Resid:** Pathology, Johns Hopkins Hosp 1975; **Fac Appt:** Prof Path, Emory Univ

Midwest

Allred, D Craig MD [Path] - **Spec Exp:** Breast Cancer; Breast Pathology; Breast Cancer Risk Assessment; **Hospital:** Barnes-Jewish Hosp; **Address:** Washington Univ Sch Med, Path & Immunology, 660 S Euclid Ave, Box 8118, St Louis, MO 63110; **Phone:** 314-362-6313; **Board Cert:** Anatomic Pathology 1984; **Med School:** Univ Utah 1979; **Resid:** Anatomic Pathology, Univ Conn Hlth Ctr 1983; **Fellow:** Immunopathology, Univ Conn Hlth Ctr 1982; **Fac Appt:** Prof Path, Baylor Coll Med

Balla, Andre K MD/PhD [Path] - **Spec Exp:** Prostate Cancer; Gynecologic Pathology; Tumor Banking; **Hospital:** Univ of IL Med Ctr at Chicago; **Address:** Univ Illinois Chicago, Dept Path, 840 S Wood St, 130 CSN Bldg, MC 847, Chicago, IL 60612; **Phone:** 312-996-3879; **Board Cert:** Anatomic & Clinical Pathology 1988; **Med School:** Brazil 1972; **Resid:** Pathology, Hahnemann Univ Hosp 1988; **Fellow:** Clinical Immunology, Scripps Clin Rsch Fdn 1981; **Fac Appt:** Prof Path, Univ IL Coll Med

Behm, Frederick G MD [Path] - **Spec Exp:** Hematopathology; **Hospital:** Univ of IL Med Ctr at Chicago; **Address:** Univ Illinois Chicago, Dept Pathology, 840 S Wood St, 130 CSN Bldg, MC 847, Chicago, IL 60612-7335; **Phone:** 312-996-3150; **Board Cert:** Anatomic & Clinical Pathology 1980; Hematology 1983; **Med School:** Med Coll Wisc 1974; **Resid:** Pathology, Med Coll Va Hosps 1979; **Fac Appt:** Prof Path, Univ IL Coll Med

Bell, Debra A MD [Path] - **Spec Exp:** Gynecologic Pathology; Ovarian Cancer; **Hospital:** Mayo Med Ctr & Clin - Rochester; **Address:** Mayo Clinic-Pathology Dept, 200 First St SW, Rochester, MN 55905; **Phone:** 507-284-1800; **Board Cert:** Anatomic Pathology 1980; Cytopathology 1989; **Med School:** Albany Med Coll 1976; **Resid:** Pathology, NYU Med Ctr 1981; **Fellow:** Cytopathology, Meml Sloan Kettering Cancer Ctr 1982; **Fac Appt:** Assoc Prof Path, Mayo Med Sch

Cho, Kathleen R MD [Path] - **Spec Exp:** Gynecologic Pathology; Ovarian Cancer; Cervical Cancer; **Hospital:** Univ of Michigan Hosp; **Address:** Univ Michigan Med Sch, 109 Zina Pitcher Pl, rm 1506, Ann Arbor, MI 48109-2200; **Phone:** 734-764-1549; **Board Cert:** Anatomic Pathology 1990; **Med School:** Vanderbilt Univ 1984; **Resid:** Pathology, Johns Hopkins Hosp 1988; **Fellow:** Gynecologic Pathology, Johns Hopkins Hosp 1990; **Fac Appt:** Prof Path, Univ Mich Med Sch

Cohen, Michael B MD [Path] - **Spec Exp:** Urologic Cancer; Cytopathology; **Hospital:** Univ Iowa Hosp & Clinics, Iowa City VA Hlth Care Sys; **Address:** Univ Iowa - Dept Pathology, 200 Hawkins Drive, C670GH, Iowa City, IA 52242; **Phone:** 319-384-9609; **Board Cert:** Anatomic Pathology 2008; Cytopathology 1996; **Med School:** Albany Med Coll 1982; **Resid:** Pathology, UCSF Hosps & Clinics 1986; **Fellow:** Cytopathology, UCSF Hosps & Clinics 1987; **Fac Appt:** Prof Path, Univ Iowa Coll Med

Goldblum, John R MD [Path] - **Spec Exp:** Soft Tissue Pathology; Esophageal Cancer; Gastrointestinal Pathology; Sarcoma; **Hospital:** Cleveland Clin (page 70); **Address:** Cleveland Clinic, Anatomic Pathology L25, 9500 Euclid Ave, Cleveland, OH 44195; **Phone:** 216-444-8238; **Board Cert:** Anatomic Pathology 1993; **Med School:** Univ Mich Med Sch 1989; **Resid:** Anatomic Pathology, Univ Michigan Hosps 1993; **Fac Appt:** Prof Path, Cleveland Cl Coll Med/Case West Res

Greenson, Joel K MD [Path] - **Spec Exp:** Liver Cancer; Gastrointestinal Pathology; Liver Pathology; **Hospital:** Univ of Michigan Hosp; **Address:** Univ Michigan Hospitals, Dept Pathology, 1301 Catherine St, Med Sci 1 Bldg - rm 5218, Ann Arbor, MI 48109-5602; **Phone:** 734-936-6770; **Board Cert:** Anatomic & Clinical Pathology 1988; **Med School:** Univ Mich Med Sch 1984; **Resid:** Pathology, Cedars-Sinai Med Ctr 1988; **Fellow:** Gastrointestinal Pathology, Johns Hopkins Hosp 1990; **Fac Appt:** Prof Path, Univ Mich Med Sch

Pathology

Kurtin, Paul J MD [Path] - **Spec Exp:** Lymph Node Pathology; Bone Marrow Pathology; Lymphoma; **Hospital:** Mayo Med Ctr & Clin - Rochester; **Address:** Mayo Clinic - Div Hematopathology, 200 First St SW, Hilton 1160A, Rochester, MN 55905; **Phone:** 507-284-4939; **Board Cert:** Anatomic & Clinical Pathology 1983; Hematology 1988; **Med School:** Med Coll Wisc 1979; **Resid:** Anatomic & Clinical Pathology, Vanderbilt Univ Med Ctr 1983; **Fellow:** Hematopathology, Brigham & Women's Hosp 1984; Surgical Pathology, Brigham & Women's Hosp 1986; **Fac Appt:** Prof Path, Mayo Med Sch

Lucas, David R MD [Path] - **Spec Exp:** Bone Tumors; Soft Tissue Tumors; Surgical Pathology; **Hospital:** Univ of Michigan Hosp; **Address:** 1500 E Medical Ctr Drive, rm 2G332-UH, Ann Arbor, MI 48109; **Phone:** 734-232-0022; **Board Cert:** Anatomic Pathology 1993; **Med School:** Wayne State Univ 1988; **Resid:** Pathology, Wayne State Univ Med Ctr 1991; **Fellow:** Surgical Pathology, Mayo Clinic 1993; **Fac Appt:** Prof Path, Univ Mich Med Sch

Myers, Jeffrey L MD [Path] - **Spec Exp:** Lung Cancer; Lung Pathology; **Hospital:** Univ of Michigan Hosp; **Address:** 1500 E Medical Center Drive, Univ Michigan, 2G332 UH, Ann Arbor, MI 48109-5912; **Phone:** 734-936-1888; **Board Cert:** Anatomic Pathology 1986; **Med School:** Washington Univ, St Louis 1981; **Resid:** Anatomic Pathology, Barnes Jewish Hosp 1984; **Fellow:** Surgical Pathology, Univ Alabama Med Ctr 1985; **Fac Appt:** Prof Path, Univ Mich Med Sch

Rubin, Brian P MD [Path] - **Spec Exp:** Bone & Soft Tissue Pathology; Sarcoma; **Hospital:** Cleveland Clin (page 70); **Address:** Cleveland Clinic, Dept Anatomic Pathology, L25, 9500 Euclid Ave, Cleveland, OH 44195; **Phone:** 216-445-5551; **Board Cert:** Anatomic Pathology 1999; **Med School:** Cornell Univ-Weill Med Coll 1995; **Resid:** Pathology, Brigham & Womens Hosp 2000; **Fac Appt:** Asst Prof Path, Univ Wash

Scheithauer, Bernd W MD [Path] - **Spec Exp:** Brain Tumors; Pituitary Tumors; Neuro-Pathology; **Hospital:** Mayo Med Ctr & Clin - Rochester; **Address:** Mayo Clinic, Dept Pathology, 200 First St SW, Hilton Bldg, Rochester, MN 55905; **Phone:** 507-284-8350; **Board Cert:** Anatomic Pathology 1979; Neuropathology 1979; **Med School:** Loma Linda Univ 1973; **Resid:** Anatomic Pathology, Stanford Univ Med Ctr 1976; Neuropathology, Stanford Univ Med Ctr 1978; **Fellow:** Surgical Pathology, Stanford Univ Med Ctr 1979; **Fac Appt:** Prof Path, Mayo Med Sch

Suster, Saul M MD [Path] - **Spec Exp:** Lung Cancer; Mediastinal Tumors; Surgical Pathology; **Hospital:** Froedtert and Med Ctr of WI; **Address:** Med College of Wisconsin, Dept Pathology, Dynacare Lab Bldg, rm 226, 9200 W Wisconsin Ave, Milwaukee, WI 53226; **Phone:** 414-805-6968; **Board Cert:** Anatomic & Clinical Pathology 1988; **Med School:** Ecuador 1976; **Resid:** Anatomic Pathology, Tel Aviv Univ Med Ctr 1984; Anatomic & Clinical Pathology, Mt Sinai Med Ctr 1988; **Fellow:** Surgical Pathology, Yale-New Haven Hosp 1990; **Fac Appt:** Prof Path, Med Coll Wisc

Ulbright, Thomas M MD [Path] - **Spec Exp:** Testicular Cancer; Gynecologic Pathology; **Hospital:** IU Health Methodist Hosp; **Address:** Clarion Pathology Laboratory, 350 W 11th St, rm 4078, Indianapolis, IN 46202; **Phone:** 317-491-6498; **Board Cert:** Anatomic Pathology 1980; **Med School:** Washington Univ, St Louis 1975; **Resid:** Pathology, Barnes Jewish Hosp 1978; Surgical Pathology, Barnes Jewish Hosp 1979; **Fellow:** Gynecologic Pathology, St Johns Mercy Med Ctr 1980; **Fac Appt:** Prof Path, Indiana Univ

Wollmann, Robert MD [Path] - **Spec Exp:** Neuro-Pathology; Brain Tumors; **Hospital:** Univ of Chicago Med Ctr; **Address:** Univ Chicago Med Ctr, 5841 S Maryland Ave, MC 6101, Chicago, IL 60615-2707; **Phone:** 773-702-6166; **Board Cert:** Anatomic Pathology 1975; Neuropathology 1977; **Med School:** Univ IL Coll Med 1969; **Resid:** Anatomic Pathology, Univ Chicago Med Ctr 1972; **Fellow:** Neuropathology, Max Planck Inst 1972; **Fac Appt:** Prof Path, Univ Chicago-Pritzker Sch Med

Great Plains and Mountains

De Masters, Bette K MD [Path] - **Spec Exp:** Neuro-Pathology; Brain Tumors; **Hospital:** Univ of CO Hosp - Anschutz Inpatient Pav, Chldn's Hosp - Aurora (CO); **Address:** Univ CO Hlth Sci Ctr, Dept Pathology, 12605 East 16th Ave MS F-768, Aurora, CO 80045; **Phone:** 270-848-4421; **Board Cert:** Anatomic & Clinical Pathology 1982; Neuropathology 1985; **Med School:** Univ Wisc 1977; **Resid:** Internal Medicine, Presby Hosp 1979; Pathology, Univ Colo Med Sch 1982; **Fellow:** Neurological Pathology, Univ Colo/Univ Kansas 1984; **Fac Appt:** Prof Path, Univ Colorado

Thor, Ann D MD [Path] - **Spec Exp:** Breast Cancer; Gynecologic Cancer; **Hospital:** Univ of CO Hosp - Anschutz Inpatient Pav; **Address:** Univ CO, Dept Pathology,, Anshutz Med Campus, Box 6511, Aurora, CO 80045-0508; **Phone:** 303-724-3704; **Board Cert:** Anatomic Pathology 1987; Cytopathology 1989; **Med School:** Vanderbilt Univ 1981; **Resid:** Pathology, Vanderbilt Univ 1983; **Fellow:** Immunopathology, Natl Cancer Inst 1986; Gynecologic Pathology, Mass Genl Hosp 1990; **Fac Appt:** Prof Path, Univ Colorado

Weisenburger, Dennis D MD [Path] - **Spec Exp:** Hematopathology; Lymphoma; **Hospital:** Nebraska Med Ctr; **Address:** Dept Pathology and Microbiology, 983135 Nebraska Medical Center, Omaha, NE 68198-3135; **Phone:** 402-559-7688; **Board Cert:** Anatomic & Clinical Pathology 1979; **Med School:** Univ Minn 1974; **Resid:** Anatomic Pathology, Univ Iowa Hosps 1978; **Fellow:** Hematopathology, City of Hope Natl Med Ctr 1980; **Fac Appt:** Prof Path, Univ Nebr Coll Med

Southwest

Bruner, Janet M MD [Path] - **Spec Exp:** Brain Tumors; Neuro-Pathology; **Hospital:** UT MD Anderson Cancer Ctr; **Address:** MD Anderson Cancer Ctr, 1515 Holcombe Blvd, Ste 85, Houston, TX 77030; **Phone:** 713-792-6127; **Board Cert:** Anatomic Pathology 1982; Neuropathology 1984; **Med School:** Med Coll OH 1979; **Resid:** Anatomic & Clinical Pathology, Med Coll Ohio Hosp 1982; **Fellow:** Neurological Pathology, Baylor Coll Med 1984; **Fac Appt:** Prof Path, Univ Tex, Houston

Cagle, Philip MD [Path] - **Spec Exp:** Pulmonary Pathology; Lung Cancer; Mesothelioma; **Hospital:** Methodist Hosp - Houston; **Address:** Methodist Hospital, Dept Pathology, 6565 Fannin St, Ste 227, Houston, TX 77030; **Phone:** 713-441-6478; **Board Cert:** Anatomic & Clinical Pathology 1985; **Med School:** Univ Tenn Coll Med 1981; **Resid:** Pathology, Baylor Coll Med Ctr 1985; **Fellow:** Pulmonary Pathology 1987; **Fac Appt:** Prof Path, Baylor Coll Med

Foucar, M Kathryn MD [Path] - **Spec Exp:** Leukemia; Lymph Node Pathology; Bone Marrow Pathology; **Hospital:** Univ Hosp - New Mexico; **Address:** TriCore Reference Lab, Hematopathology, 1001 Woodward Pl NE, Albuquerque, NM 87102; **Phone:** 505-938-8456; **Board Cert:** Anatomic & Clinical Pathology 1978; **Med School:** Ohio State Univ 1974; **Resid:** Anatomic Pathology, Univ NM Health & Sci Ctr 1976; Anatomic Pathology, Univ Minn Med Ctr 1978; **Fellow:** Surgical Pathology, Univ Minn Med Ctr 1979; **Fac Appt:** Prof Path, Univ New Mexico

Grogan, Thomas M MD [Path] - **Spec Exp:** Immunopathology; Lymphoma; **Hospital:** Univ Med Ctr - Tucson; **Address:** AHSC, Dept Pathology, 1501 N Campbell Ave, rm 5211, Tucson, AZ 85724; **Phone:** 520-626-7477; **Board Cert:** Anatomic Pathology 1976; **Med School:** Geo Wash Univ 1971; **Resid:** Pathology, Letterman Army Med Ctr 1976; **Fellow:** Immunopathology, Stanford Univ Sch Med 1979; **Fac Appt:** Prof Path, Univ Ariz Coll Med

Pathology

Hamilton, Stanley R MD [Path] - **Spec Exp:** Surgical Pathology; Gastrointestinal Pathology; Liver Pathology; **Hospital:** UT MD Anderson Cancer Ctr; **Address:** Univ Texas MD Anderson Cancer Ctr, 1515 Holcombe Blvd, Unit 085, Houston, TX 77030-4009; **Phone:** 713-792-2040; **Board Cert:** Anatomic & Clinical Pathology 1978; **Med School:** Indiana Univ 1973; **Resid:** Pathology, Johns Hopkins Hosp 1978; **Fellow:** St Marks Hosp 1979; **Fac Appt:** Prof Path, Univ Tex, Houston

Kinney, Marsha C MD [Path] - **Spec Exp:** Hematopathology; Lymphoma; Leukemia; **Hospital:** Univ Hlth Syst-San Antonio; **Address:** Univ Texas Hlth & Sci Ctr, Dept Path, 7703 Floyd Curl Drive, MC 7750, San Antonio, TX 78229-3900; **Phone:** 210-567-4072; **Board Cert:** Anatomic & Clinical Pathology 1985; Hematology 1998; **Med School:** Univ Tex SW, Dallas 1981; **Resid:** Pathology, Vanderbilt Univ Med Ctr 1985; **Fellow:** Hematopathology, Vanderbilt Univ Med Ctr 1988; **Fac Appt:** Prof Path, Univ Tex, San Antonio

Leslie, Kevin O MD [Path] - **Spec Exp:** Pulmonary Pathology; Lung Cancer; Surgical Pathology; **Hospital:** Mayo Clinic - Scottsdale; **Address:** Mayo Clinic, Scottsdale, 13400 E Shea Blvd, Dept Pathology, Scottsdale, AZ 85259; **Phone:** 480-301-8021; **Board Cert:** Anatomic & Clinical Pathology 1982; **Med School:** Albert Einstein Coll Med 1976; **Resid:** Anatomic & Clinical Pathology, Univ Colorado Health Sci Ctr 1982; **Fellow:** Surgical Pathology, Stanford Univ Med Ctr 1983; **Fac Appt:** Prof Path, Mayo Med Sch

Moran, Cesar A MD [Path] - **Spec Exp:** Lung Cancer; Mediastinal Tumors; Mesothelioma; **Hospital:** UT MD Anderson Cancer Ctr; **Address:** MD Anderson Cancer Ctr, Dept Pathology, 1515 Holcombe Blvd, rm G1-3738, Houston, TX 77030; **Phone:** 713-792-8134; **Board Cert:** Anatomic Pathology 1992; **Med School:** Guatemala 1981; **Resid:** Anatomic Pathology, Mt Sinai Med Ctr 1988; **Fellow:** Surgical Pathology, Yale-New Haven Med Ctr 1989; **Fac Appt:** Prof Path, Univ Tex, Houston

Prieto, Victor G MD/PhD [Path] - **Spec Exp:** Dermatopathology; Melanoma; Skin Cancer; **Hospital:** UT MD Anderson Cancer Ctr; **Address:** MD Anderson Cancer Ctr, Dept Pathology, 1515 Holcombe Blvd, Box 85, Houston, TX 77030-4000; **Phone:** 713-792-0918; **Board Cert:** Anatomic Pathology 1995; Dermatopathology 1997; **Med School:** Spain 1986; **Resid:** Pathology, New York Hosp-Cornell Med Ctr 1993; **Fellow:** Pathology, Meml Sloan Kettering Cancer Ctr 1995; Dermatopathology, New York Hosp-Cornell Med Ctr 1996; **Fac Appt:** Prof Path, Univ Tex, Houston

Rashid, Asif MD/PhD [Path] - **Spec Exp:** Gastrointestinal Pathology; Liver Pathology; **Hospital:** UT MD Anderson Cancer Ctr; **Address:** MD Anderson Cancer Ctr, Dept Pathology, 1515 Holcombe Blvd, Box 85, Houston, TX 77030; **Phone:** 713-745-1101; **Board Cert:** Anatomic Pathology 1994; **Med School:** Pakistan 1984; **Resid:** Anatomic Pathology, Mass Genl Hosp 1993; **Fellow:** Anatomic Pathology, Mass Genl Hosp 1994; Anatomic Pathology, Johns Hopkins 1996

Sahin, Aysegul MD [Path] - **Spec Exp:** Breast Cancer; **Hospital:** UT MD Anderson Cancer Ctr; **Address:** 1515 Holcombe Blvd, Box 0085, Houston, TX 77030; **Phone:** 713-794-1500; **Board Cert:** Pathology 1987; **Med School:** Turkey 1980; **Resid:** Pathology, Oregon Hlth Sci Univ 1986; **Fellow:** Surgical Pathology, Univ Iowa Hosps & Clins 1987; **Fac Appt:** Prof Path, Univ Tex, Houston

Silva, Elvio G MD [Path] - **Spec Exp:** Gynecologic Pathology; Gynecologic Cancer; **Hospital:** UT MD Anderson Cancer Ctr, Cedars-Sinai Med Ctr; **Address:** MD Anderson Cancer Ctr, Dept Pathology, 1515 Holcombe Blvd, Unit 85, MC G1-3563B, Houston, TX 77030; **Phone:** 713-792-3154; **Board Cert:** Anatomic Pathology 2007; **Med School:** Argentina 1969; **Resid:** Pathology, National Univ Med Ctr 1975; Anatomic Pathology, Univ Toronto 1978; **Fellow:** Surgical Pathology, MD Anderson Cancer Ctr 1979; **Fac Appt:** Prof Path

Wheeler, Thomas M MD [Path] - **Spec Exp:** Thyroid Disorders; Thyroid Cancer; Genitourinary Cancer; **Hospital:** Ben Taub Genl Hosp; **Address:** Baylor Coll Med, Dept Pathology, One Baylor Plaza, rm T203, MS 315, Houston, TX 77030; **Phone:** 713-798-4664; **Board Cert:** Anatomic & Clinical Pathology 1981; Cytopathology 1990; **Med School:** Baylor Coll Med 1977; **Resid:** Pathology, Baylor Affil Hosps 1981; **Fac Appt:** Prof Path, Baylor Coll Med

West Coast and Pacific

Amin, Mahul MD [Path] - **Spec Exp:** Genitourinary Pathology; Bladder Cancer; **Hospital:** Cedars-Sinai Med Ctr; **Address:** Cedars Sinai Med Ctr, 8700 Beverly Blvd, Ste 8728, Los Angeles, CA 90048; **Phone:** 310-423-6631; **Board Cert:** Anatomic & Clinical Pathology 1996; **Med School:** India 1983; **Resid:** Pathology, Henry Ford Hosp 1992; **Fellow:** Surgical Pathology, MD Anderson Cancer Ctr 1993; **Fac Appt:** Prof Path, UCLA-David Geffen Sch Med

Arber, Daniel A MD [Path] - **Spec Exp:** Bone Marrow Pathology; Lymph Node Pathology; Spleen Pathology; **Hospital:** Stanford Univ Hosp & Clinics, Lucile Packard Chldn's Hosp; **Address:** Clinic Laboratories, Stanford Univ Med Ctr, 300 Pasteur Drive, rm H1507, MC 5627, Stanford, CA 94305; **Phone:** 650-725-5604; **Board Cert:** Anatomic & Clinical Pathology 1991; Hematology 1993; **Med School:** Univ Tex, San Antonio 1986; **Resid:** Anatomic & Clinical Pathology, Scott & White Meml Hosp 1991; **Fellow:** Hematopathology, City of Hope Natl Med Ctr 1993; **Fac Appt:** Prof Path, Stanford Univ

Bollen, Andrew W MD [Path] - **Spec Exp:** Neuro-Pathology; Brain Tumors; **Hospital:** UCSF Med Ctr, San Francisco Genl Hosp; **Address:** UCSF School of Medicine, Dept Pathology/Neuropathology, 505 Parnassus Ave, rm M553, Box 0102, San Francisco, CA 94143-0511; **Phone:** 415-476-5236; **Board Cert:** Neuropathology 1992; Anatomic Pathology 1992; Clinical Pathology 1993; **Med School:** UCSD 1985; **Resid:** Anatomic Pathology, UCSF Med Ctr 1991; **Fellow:** Neuropathology, UCSF Med Ctr 1989; **Fac Appt:** Prof Path, UCSF

Chandrasoma, Parakrama T MD [Path] - **Spec Exp:** Gastrointestinal Pathology; Gastrointestinal Cancer; Neuro-Pathology; **Hospital:** LAC & USC Med Ctr; **Address:** LAC-USC Med Ctr, Dept Path, Clinic Tower Fl 7 - rm A7A127, 1100 N State St, Los Angeles, CA 90033; **Phone:** 323-226-4600; **Board Cert:** Anatomic Pathology 1982; **Med School:** Sri Lanka 1971; **Resid:** Anatomic Pathology, Univ Sri Lanka 1978; Anatomic Pathology, LAC-USC Med Ctr 1982; **Fac Appt:** Prof Path, USC Sch Med

Chang, Karen L MD [Path] - **Spec Exp:** Leukemia; **Hospital:** City of Hope Natl Med Ctr (page 69); **Address:** 1500 E Duarte Rd, Duarte, CA 91010-3012; **Phone:** 626-256-4673 x62456; **Board Cert:** Anatomic & Clinical Pathology 1992; **Med School:** Mount Sinai Sch Med 1985; **Resid:** Anatomic Pathology, Stanford Univ Med Ctr 1988; Clinical Pathology, Stanford Univ Med Ctr 1991; **Fellow:** Surgical Pathology, Stanford Univ Med Ctr 1989

Cochran, Alistair J MD [Path] - **Spec Exp:** Melanoma; Dermatopathology; **Hospital:** UCLA Ronald Reagan Med Ctr; **Address:** UCLA Med Ctr, Dept Path & Med, 10833 Le Conte Ave, rm 13-145CHS, MC 173216, Los Angeles, CA 90095-1732; **Phone:** 310-825-2743; **Med School:** Scotland, UK 1959; **Resid:** Dermatopathology, Western Infirmary 1968; Pathology, Western Infirmary 1968; **Fellow:** Immunology, Karolinska Inst 1970; **Fac Appt:** Prof Path, UCLA

Dubeau, Louis MD/PhD [Path] - **Spec Exp:** Ovarian Cancer; Breast Cancer; **Hospital:** USC Norris Cancer Hosp; **Address:** USC Norris Cancer Ctr, Dept Pathology, 1441 Eastlake Ave, rm 6338, Los Angeles, CA 90033-1048; **Phone:** 323-865-0720; **Board Cert:** Anatomic Pathology 1984; **Med School:** McGill Univ 1979; **Resid:** Anatomic Pathology, McGill Univ Med Ctr 1984; **Fac Appt:** Prof Path, USC Sch Med

Pathology

Hammar, Samuel P MD [Path] - **Spec Exp:** Lung Cancer; Pulmonary Pathology; **Hospital:** Harrison Med Ctr; **Address:** Diagnostic Specialties Laboratory, 700 Lebo Blvd, Bremerton, WA 98310; **Phone:** 360-479-7707; **Board Cert:** Anatomic & Clinical Pathology 1975; **Med School:** Univ Wash 1970

Koss, Michael N MD [Path] - **Spec Exp:** Pulmonary Pathology; Lung Cancer; Kidney Pathology; **Hospital:** USC Norris Cancer Hosp, USC Univ Hosp; **Address:** 2222 Ocean View Ave, Ste 212, Los Angeles, CA 90057; **Phone:** 213-381-2260; **Board Cert:** Anatomic Pathology 1979; **Med School:** Stanford Univ 1970; **Resid:** Pathology, Columbia Presby Med Ctr 1974; **Fellow:** Renal Pathology, Columbia Presby Med Ctr 1975; Pulmonary Pathology, Armed Forces Inst Path 1978; **Fac Appt:** Prof Path, USC Sch Med

Le Boit, Philip E MD [Path] - **Spec Exp:** Cutaneous Lymphoma; Skin Cancer; Dermatopathology; **Hospital:** UCSF Med Ctr; **Address:** UCSF - Dermatopathology Section, 1701 Divisadero St, rm 499, San Francisco, CA 94115; **Phone:** 415-353-7546; **Board Cert:** Anatomic Pathology 1983; Dermatopathology 1983; Clinical Pathology 1986; **Med School:** Albany Med Coll 1979; **Resid:** Anatomic Pathology, UCSF Med Ctr 1981; Clinical Pathology, Mt Sinai Hosp 1982; **Fellow:** Dermatopathology, New York Hosp-Cornell Med Ctr 1983; **Fac Appt:** Prof Path, UCSF

Ljung, Britt-Marie E MD [Path] - **Spec Exp:** Breast Cancer; Cytopathology; Fine Needle Aspiration Biopsy; **Hospital:** UCSF - Mt Zion Med Ctr; **Address:** UCSF - Dept Pathology, 1600 Divisadero St, Box 1785, R-200, San Francisco, CA 94143-1785; **Phone:** 415-353-7320; **Board Cert:** Anatomic Pathology 1985; Cytopathology 1989; **Med School:** Sweden 1975; **Resid:** Pathology, Karolinska Hosp 1979; Anatomic Pathology, UCLA Med Ctr 1983; **Fac Appt:** Prof Path, UCSF

Mischel, Paul S MD [Path] - **Spec Exp:** Neuro-Pathology; Brain Tumors; **Hospital:** UCLA Ronald Reagan Med Ctr; **Address:** UCLA Med Ctr, Div Neuropathology, 10833 Le Conte Ave, rm 13-317 CHS, Los Angeles, CA 90095-1732; **Phone:** 310-825-2339; **Board Cert:** Anatomic Pathology 1997; Neuropathology 1997; **Med School:** Cornell Univ-Weill Med Coll 1991; **Resid:** Anatomic & Clinical Pathology, UCLA Med Center 1996; **Fellow:** Neurological Pathology, UCLA 1995; Research, Howard Hughes Med Inst/UCSF 1998; **Fac Appt:** Prof Path, UCLA

Nathwani, Bharat N MD [Path] - **Spec Exp:** Hematopathology; Leukemia; Lymphoma; **Hospital:** Cedars-Sinai Med Ctr; **Address:** Cedars-Sinai Dept Pathology, 8700 Beverly Blvd, South Tower, rm 7706, Los Angeles, CA 90048; **Phone:** 310-248-6659; **Board Cert:** Anatomic Pathology 1977; **Med School:** India 1969; **Resid:** Pathology, JJ Group-Grant Med Ctr 1972; Pathology, Rush-Presby-St Lukes Med Ctr 1974; **Fellow:** Hematopathology, City Hope Natl Med Ctr 1975; **Fac Appt:** Prof Path, USC Sch Med

Perry, Arie MD [Path] - **Spec Exp:** Neuro-Pathology; Brain Tumors; **Hospital:** UCSF Med Ctr; **Address:** UCSF-Dept of Neuropathology, 505 Parnassus Ave, rm M-551, San Francisco, CA 94143; **Phone:** 415-476-5236; **Board Cert:** Anatomic & Clinical Pathology 1995; Neuropathology 1997; **Med School:** Univ Tex SW, Dallas 1990; **Resid:** Pathology, Univ Tex SW 1994; **Fellow:** Surgical Pathology, Mayo Clin 1995; Neurological Pathology, Mayo Clin 1998; **Fac Appt:** Assoc Prof Path, Washington Univ, St Louis

Rutgers, Joanne MD [Path] - **Spec Exp:** Gynecologic Cancer; Gastrointestinal Pathology; **Hospital:** Long Beach Meml Med Ctr; **Address:** 2801 Atlantic Ave, Dept of Pathology, Long Beach, CA 90806; **Phone:** 562-933-0717; **Board Cert:** Clinical Pathology 1992; Anatomic Pathology 1985; Cytopathology 1997; **Med School:** UCSD 1981; **Resid:** Pathology, Montefiore Med Ctr 1983; Pathology, NYU Med Ctr 1985; **Fellow:** Gynecologic Pathology, Mass Genl Hosp 1989; **Fac Appt:** Clin Prof Path, UC Irvine

Sibley, Richard K MD [Path] - **Spec Exp:** Kidney Pathology; Breast Pathology; Liver Pathology; **Hospital:** Stanford Univ Hosp & Clinics; **Address:** Stanford Univ Med Ctr, Surg Path Lab, 300 Pasteur Drive, rm H2110, MC 5324, Stanford, CA 94305; **Phone:** 650-723-7211; **Board Cert:** Anatomic Pathology 1975; **Med School:** Univ Tex SW, Dallas 1971; **Resid:** Anatomic Pathology, Univ Chicago Hosps 1974; **Fellow:** Stanford Univ Med Ctr 1975; **Fac Appt:** Prof Path, Stanford Univ

Triche, Timothy J MD/PhD [Path] - **Spec Exp:** Pediatric Pathology; Pediatric Cancers; Sarcoma; **Hospital:** Chldns Hosp - Los Angeles; **Address:** Chldns Hosp Los Angeles, Dept Patholgy, 4650 Sunset Blvd, MS 133, Los Angeles, CA 90027; **Phone:** 323-361-8898; **Board Cert:** Anatomic Pathology 1975; **Med School:** Tulane Univ 1971; **Resid:** Anatomic Pathology, Barnes Hosp-Wash Univ 1973; Surgical Pathology, Barnes Hosp 1974; **Fellow:** Pathology, Natl Cancer Inst 1975; **Fac Appt:** Prof Path, USC Sch Med

True, Lawrence D MD [Path] - **Spec Exp:** Urologic Pathology; Prostate Cancer; Bladder Cancer; **Hospital:** Univ Wash Med Ctr; **Address:** Univ Wash Med Ctr, Dept Anatomic Path, Campus Box 356100, rm NE110, 1959 NE Pacific St, Seattle, WA 98195-6100; **Phone:** 206-598-6400; **Board Cert:** Anatomic Pathology 1981; **Med School:** Tulane Univ 1971; **Resid:** Pathology, Univ Colo Hlth Sci Ctr 1980; **Fac Appt:** Prof Path, Univ Wash

Warnke, Roger A MD [Path] - **Spec Exp:** Lymphoma; Hematopathology; **Hospital:** Stanford Univ Hosp & Clinics; **Address:** Stanford Hosp, 300 Pasteur, Pathology, rm L235, Stanford, CA 94305-5324; **Phone:** 650-725-5167; **Board Cert:** Anatomic Pathology 1975; **Med School:** Washington Univ, St Louis 1971; **Resid:** Pathology, Stanford Univ Med Ctr 1974; **Fellow:** Surgical Pathology, Stanford Univ Med Ctr 1975; Immunology, Stanford Univ Med Ctr 1976; **Fac Appt:** Prof Path, Stanford Univ

Weiss, Lawrence M MD [Path] - **Spec Exp:** Lymphoma; Hematopathology; Adrenal Pathology; **Hospital:** City of Hope Natl Med Ctr (page 69); **Address:** City of Hope Natl Med Ctr, Div Pathology, 1500 E Duarte Rd, Duarte, CA 91010-0269; **Phone:** 626-256-4673 x62456; **Board Cert:** Anatomic Pathology 1985; **Med School:** Univ MD Sch Med 1981; **Resid:** Pathology, Brigham & Women's Hosp 1983; **Fellow:** Surgical Pathology, Stanford Univ Hosp 1984

Wilczynski, Sharon P MD/PhD [Path] - **Spec Exp:** Gynecologic Cancer; Breast Cancer; Ovarian Cancer; Clinical Trials; **Hospital:** City of Hope Natl Med Ctr (page 69); **Address:** City Hope Natl Med Ctr-Dept of Pathology, 1500 E Duarte Rd, Duarte, CA 91010; **Phone:** 626-256-4673 x62456; **Board Cert:** Anatomic & Clinical Pathology 1985; Cytopathology 1991; **Med School:** Med Coll PA Hahnemann 1981; **Resid:** Pathology, Hosp Univ Penn 1983; Anatomic & Clinical Pathology, Long Beach Meml Hosp 1985; **Fac Appt:** Prof Path, USC-Keck School of Medicine

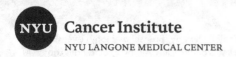

NYU **Cancer Institute**
NYU LANGONE MEDICAL CENTER

NYU Langone Medical Center
550 First Avenue , New York, NY 10016
www.NYULMC.org

NYU Clinical Cancer Center
160 East 34th Street, New York, NY 10016
www.NYUCI.org

**The Stephen D. Hassenfeld Children's Center
for Cancer and Blood Disorders**
160 East 32nd Street, New York, NY 10016
www.NYUMC.org/Hassenfeld

The NYU Cancer Institute is an NCI-designated cancer center and provides personalized patient care that is both compassionate and state of the art. The doctors and researchers work together to develop innovative therapies for patients. The Cancer Institute is world-renowned for excellence in cancer-focused research, personalized care, education and community outreach. Its mission is to discover the origins of human cancer and to use that knowledge to eradicate the personal and societal burden of cancer in our community, the nation and the world. For more information about our expert physicians, call 212-731-5000. *We specialize in the following areas:*

Patient-Focused Setting
The NYU Clinical Cancer Center is the principal outpatient facility of The Cancer Institute and serves as home to our patients and their caregivers. The center and its multidisciplinary team of experts provide access to the latest treatment options and clinical trials along with a variety of programs in cancer risk reduction/prevention, screening, diagnostics, genetic counseling and supportive services. In addition the NYUCI emphasizes the importance of a holistic approach to management services in complementary medicine, psychosocial support, survivorship and palliative care.

Renowned Expertise
The NYU Cancer Institute brings together experts from a variety of disciplines to create collaborative research endeavors and clinical care teams. The Cancer Institute offers a full continuum of personalized care, from prevention through diagnosis, treatment and post-treatment support. The compassion and expertise of our team members helps patients better manage the symptoms of their diseases as well as meet their special needs. Additionally, we have created special emphasis programs in diseases such as breast cancer, melanoma, GI cancer, prostate cancer, hematologic malignancies and lung cancer among others, as well as, translational programs in cancer healthcare disparities, molecularly targeted therapy, and the cell signaling pathways involved in cancer.

A Translational Approach
NYU Langone Medical Center scientists and other researchers excel in uncovering how cancer develops at the molecular level, and how we can harness that knowledge to reduce the risk of cancer and treat the disease. The Medical Center constantly seeks to create new opportunities for collaboration between investigators within our own institution, those located elsewhere in the NYU network of campuses, and researchers at other institutions.

The Stephen D. Hassenfeld Children's Center for Cancer and Blood Disorders
The center is a leading pediatric outpatient facility for the treatment of childhood cancers and blood diseases. Its unique interdisciplinary and family-centered approach combines the most advanced medical treatments with psychosocial and emotional support services for young patients and their families.

Pediatrics

A pediatrician is concerned with the physical, emotional and social health of children from birth to young adulthood. Care encompasses a broad spectrum of health services ranging from preventive health-care to the diagnosis and treatment of acute and chronic diseases.

A pediatrician deals with biological, social and environmental influences on the developing child, and with the impact of disease and dysfunction on development.

Training Required: Three years. Certification in one or more of the following specialties requires additional training

Pediatric Hematology/Oncology: A pediatrician trained in the combination of pediatrics, hematology and oncology to recognize and manage pediatric blood disorders and cancerous diseases.

Pediatric Allergy and Immunology: An allergist-immunologist is trained in evaluation, physical and laboratory diagnosis and management of disorders involving the immune system. Selected examples of such conditions include asthma, anaphylaxis, rhinitis, eczema and adverse reactions to drugs, foods and insect stings as well as immune deficiency diseases (both acquired and congenital), defects in host defense and problems related to autoimmune disease, organ transplantation or malignancies of the immune system. As our understanding of the immune system develops, the scope of this specialty is widening.

Training programs are available at some medical centers to provide individuals with expertise in both allergy/immunology and pediatric pulmonology. Such individuals are candidates for dual certification.

Pediatric Endocrinology: A pediatrician who provides expert care to infants, children and adolescents who have diseases that result from an abnormality in the endocrine glands (glands which secrete hormones) These diseases include diabetes mellitus, growth failure, unusual size for age, early or late pubertal development, birth defects, the genital region and disorders of the thyroid, the adrenal and pituitary glands.

Pediatric Otolaryngology: A subspecialty of Otolaryngology. A pediatric otolaryngologist has special expertise in the management of infants and children with disorders that include congenital and acquired conditions involving the aerodigestive tract, nose and paranasal sinuses, the ear and other areas of the head and neck. The pediatric otolaryngologist has special skills in the diagnosis, treatment and management of childhood disorders of voice, speech, language and hearing.

Pediatric Surgery: A surgeon with expertise in the management of surgical conditions in premature and newborn infants, children and adolescents.

PEDIATRIC HEMATOLOGY-ONCOLOGY

New England

Altman, Arnold MD [PHO] - **Spec Exp:** Leukemia; **Hospital:** CT Chldns Med Ctr; **Address:** CT Childrens Med Ctr, Hematology/Oncology, 282 Washington St, Ste 2J, Hartford, CT 06106; **Phone:** 860-545-9630; **Board Cert:** Pediatrics 1971; Pediatric Hematology-Oncology 1974; **Med School:** Johns Hopkins Univ 1965; **Resid:** Pediatrics, Chldns Hosp Med Ctr 1970; **Fellow:** Pediatric Hematology-Oncology, Chldns Hosp Med Ctr 1972; **Fac Appt:** Prof Ped, Univ Conn

Billett, Amy L MD [PHO] - **Spec Exp:** Hodgkin's Disease; Lymphoma, Non-Hodgkin's; **Hospital:** Children's Hospital - Boston; **Address:** 450 Brookline Ave, Boston, MA 02215; **Phone:** 617-632-5640; **Board Cert:** Pediatric Hematology-Oncology 2009; **Med School:** Harvard Med Sch 1984; **Resid:** Pediatrics, Univ Wash Affil Hosps 1987; **Fellow:** Pediatric Hematology-Oncology, Children's Hosp 1990; **Fac Appt:** Assoc Prof Ped, Harvard Med Sch

Diller, Lisa R MD [PHO] - **Spec Exp:** Neuroblastoma; Cancer Survivors-Late Effects of Therapy; **Hospital:** Children's Hospital - Boston, Dana-Farber Cancer Inst; **Address:** Dana-Farber Cancer Inst, 450 Brookline Ave, MS SW 312, Boston, MA 02115; **Phone:** 617-632-5642; **Board Cert:** Pediatric Hematology-Oncology 2007; **Med School:** UCSD 1985; **Resid:** Pediatrics, Chldns Hosp 1988; **Fellow:** Pediatric Hematology-Oncology, Chldns Hosp-Dana Farber Cancer Inst 1991; **Fac Appt:** Assoc Prof Ped, Harvard Med Sch

Guinan, Eva C MD [PHO] - **Spec Exp:** Bone Marrow Transplant; **Hospital:** Dana-Farber Cancer Inst, Children's Hospital - Boston; **Address:** Dana Faber Cancer Inst, 44 Binney St, Boston, MA 02115; **Phone:** 617-632-4932; **Board Cert:** Pediatrics 1986; Pediatric Hematology-Oncology 1998; **Med School:** Harvard Med Sch 1980; **Resid:** Internal Medicine, Children's Hosp 1982; **Fellow:** Pediatric Hematology-Oncology, Dana Farber Cancer Inst 1985; **Fac Appt:** Assoc Prof Med, Harvard Med Sch

Homans, Alan C MD [PHO] - **Spec Exp:** Leukemia; **Hospital:** Fletcher Allen Health Care-Med Ctr Campus; **Address:** Fletcher Allen Healthcare, 111 Colchester Ave Smith Bldg - Ste 559A, Burlington, VT 05401; **Phone:** 802-847-2850; **Board Cert:** Pediatrics 1985; Pediatric Hematology-Oncology 1987; **Med School:** Ohio State Univ 1979; **Resid:** Pediatrics, Med Ctr Hosp 1981; Pediatrics, Univ Mass Med Ctr 1982; **Fellow:** Pediatric Hematology-Oncology, Rhode Island Hosp 1985; **Fac Appt:** Prof Ped, Univ VT Coll Med

Kieran, Mark W MD/PhD [PHO] - **Spec Exp:** Brain Tumors; Neuro-Oncology; **Hospital:** Dana-Farber Cancer Inst, Children's Hospital - Boston; **Address:** Dana Farber Cancer Inst, 44 Binney St, Shields Warren Ste 331, Boston, MA 02115; **Phone:** 617-632-4386; **Board Cert:** Pediatric Hematology-Oncology 2004; **Med School:** Univ Calgary 1986; **Resid:** Pediatrics, Montreal Chldns Hosp 1992; **Fellow:** Pediatric Hematology-Oncology, Chldns Hosp 1995; **Fac Appt:** Asst Prof Ped, Harvard Med Sch

Sallan, Stephen E MD [PHO] - **Spec Exp:** Pediatric Cancers; Leukemia; **Hospital:** Children's Hospital - Boston, Dana-Farber Cancer Inst; **Address:** Dana Farber Cancer Inst, 450 Brookline Ave, MS Dana 1642, Boston, MA 02215; **Phone:** 617-632-5508; **Board Cert:** Pediatrics 1972; **Med School:** Wayne State Univ 1967; **Resid:** Pediatrics, Chldns Hosp 1969; Pediatrics, Hosp Sick Chldn 1970; **Fellow:** Pediatric Oncology, Chldns Hosp Med Ctr 1975; **Fac Appt:** Prof Ped, Harvard Med Sch

Pediatric Hematology/Oncology

Schwartz, Cindy Lee MD [PHO] - **Spec Exp:** Hodgkin's Disease; Bone Cancer; Cancer Survivors-Late Effects of Therapy; **Hospital:** Rhode Island Hosp; **Address:** RI Hospital, Div Ped Hem/Onc, 593 Eddy St, MPS rm 117, Providence, RI 02903-4923; **Phone:** 401-444-5171; **Board Cert:** Pediatrics 1985; Pediatric Hematology-Oncology 2009; **Med School:** Brown Univ 1979; **Resid:** Pediatrics, Johns Hopkins Hosp 1982; **Fellow:** Pediatric Hematology-Oncology, Johns Hopkins Hosp 1985; **Fac Appt:** Prof Med, Brown Univ

van Hoff, Jack MD [PHO] - **Spec Exp:** Brain Tumors; Clinical Trials; **Hospital:** Dartmouth - Hitchcock Med Ctr; **Address:** DHMC, Dept Pediatric Hem/Onc, One Medical Center Drive, Lebanon, NH 03756; **Phone:** 603-650-5541; **Board Cert:** Pediatrics 1985; Pediatric Hematology-Oncology 1987; **Med School:** UMDNJ-NJ Med Sch, Newark 1981; **Resid:** Pediatrics, Yale New Haven Hosp 1984; **Fellow:** Pediatric Hematology-Oncology, Yale New Haven Hosp 1986

Weinstein, Howard J MD [PHO] - **Spec Exp:** Bone Marrow Transplant; Leukemia; Lymphoma; **Hospital:** Mass Genl Hosp, Dana-Farber Cancer Inst; **Address:** 55 Fruit St, Yawkey 8B-8893, Boston, MA 02114-2622; **Phone:** 617-724-3315; **Board Cert:** Pediatrics 1977; **Med School:** Univ MD Sch Med 1972; **Resid:** Pediatrics, Mass Genl Hosp 1974; **Fellow:** Pediatric Hematology-Oncology, Dana Farber Cancer Inst/Chldns Hosp 1977; **Fac Appt:** Prof Ped, Harvard Med Sch

Mid Atlantic

Adamson, Peter C MD [PHO] - **Spec Exp:** Drug Development; Clinical Trials; Rhabdomyosarcoma; Pediatric Cancers; **Hospital:** Chldns Hosp of Philadelphia; **Address:** Chldns Hosp of Philadelphia, Div Onc, 34th St & Civic Ctr Blvd Abramson Bldg, Philadelphia, PA 19104; **Phone:** 215-590-3025; **Board Cert:** Pediatric Hematology-Oncology 2005; **Med School:** Cornell Univ-Weill Med Coll 1984; **Resid:** Pediatrics, Chldns Hosp 1987; **Fellow:** Pediatric Hematology-Oncology, Natl Cancer Inst 1990; **Fac Appt:** Assoc Prof Pharm, Univ Pennsylvania

Aledo, Alexander MD [PHO] - **Spec Exp:** Leukemia; Lymphoma; Bone Tumors; **Hospital:** NY-Presby Hosp/Weill Cornell (page 78), NY Hosp Queens; **Address:** 525 E 68th St, rm P695, New York, NY 10021-4870; **Phone:** 212-746-3447; **Board Cert:** Pediatric Hematology-Oncology 2004; **Med School:** NYU Sch Med 1984; **Resid:** Pediatrics, NY Hosp 1987; **Fellow:** Pediatric Hematology-Oncology, Meml Sloan Kettering Cancer Ctr 1990; **Fac Appt:** Assoc Clin Prof Ped, Cornell Univ-Weill Med Coll

Angiolillo, Anne L MD [PHO] - **Spec Exp:** Leukemia; Lymphoma; **Hospital:** Chldns Natl Med Ctr; **Address:** Chldns Natl Med Ctr-Hem/Onc, 111 Michigan Ave NW, Washington, DC 20010; **Phone:** 202-884-2800; **Board Cert:** Pediatrics 2001; Pediatric Hematology-Oncology 2004; **Med School:** NY Med Coll 1989; **Resid:** Pediatrics, Chldns Natl Med Ctr 1992; **Fellow:** Pediatric Hematology-Oncology, Chldns Natl Med Ctr 1995

Arceci, Robert J MD/PhD [PHO] - **Spec Exp:** Leukemia; Histiocytoma; Bone Marrow Transplant; **Hospital:** Johns Hopkins Hosp; **Address:** Kimmel Cancer Ctr, Bunting-Blaustein Bldg, 1650 Orleans St, I-207, Baltimore, MD 21231; **Phone:** 410-502-7519; **Board Cert:** Pediatrics 1987; Pediatric Hematology-Oncology 2005; **Med School:** Univ Rochester 1981; **Resid:** Pediatrics, Chldns Hosp 1983; **Fellow:** Pediatric Hematology-Oncology, Chldns Hosp/Dana Farber Cancer Ctr 1986; **Fac Appt:** Prof Ped, Johns Hopkins Univ

Brecher, Martin L MD [PHO] - **Spec Exp:** Brain Tumors; Lymphoma; Hodgkin's Disease; Leukemia; **Hospital:** Roswell Park Cancer Inst, Women's & Chldn's Hosp of Buffalo, The; **Address:** Roswell Park Cancer Inst, Dept Pediatrics, Elm & Carlton Sts, Buffalo, NY 14263; **Phone:** 716-845-2333; **Board Cert:** Pediatrics 1977; Pediatric Hematology-Oncology 1978; **Med School:** SUNY Buffalo 1972; **Resid:** Pediatrics, Buffalo Chldns Hosp 1975; **Fellow:** Hematology & Oncology, Buffalo Chldns Hosp/Roswell Park Cancer Inst 1977; **Fac Appt:** Prof Ped, SUNY Buffalo

Bussel, James MD [PHO] - **Spec Exp:** Bleeding/Coagulation Disorders; Platelet Disorders; **Hospital:** NY-Presby Hosp/Weill Cornell (page 78), Lenox Hill Hosp; **Address:** 525 E 68th St, rm P-695, New York, NY 10065; **Phone:** 212-746-3474; **Board Cert:** Pediatrics 1979; Pediatric Hematology-Oncology 1980; **Med School:** Columbia P&S 1975; **Resid:** Pediatrics, Chldns Hosp 1978; **Fellow:** Pediatric Hematology-Oncology, NY Presby Hosp/Cornell 1981; **Fac Appt:** Prof Ped, Cornell Univ-Weill Med Coll

Cairo, Mitchell S MD [PHO] - **Spec Exp:** Bone Marrow Transplant; Leukemia; Lymphoma; **Hospital:** NYPresby-Morgan Stanley Children's Hosp (page 78); **Address:** Columbia Univ Med Ctr, 3959 Broadway, CHN 10-03, New York, NY 10032; **Phone:** 212-305-8316; **Board Cert:** Pediatrics 1980; Pediatric Hematology-Oncology 1982; **Med School:** UCSF 1976; **Resid:** Pediatrics, UCLA Med Ctr 1979; **Fellow:** Pediatric Hematology-Oncology, Indiana Univ Med Ctr 1981; **Fac Appt:** Prof Ped, Columbia P&S

Carroll, William L MD [PHO] - **Spec Exp:** Leukemia; **Hospital:** NYU Langone Med Ctr (page 79); **Address:** NYU Med Ctr, Div Ped Hem/Onc, 160 E 32nd St, Fl 2, New York, NY 10016; **Phone:** 212-263-8400; **Board Cert:** Pediatrics 1984; Pediatric Hematology-Oncology 1987; **Med School:** UC Irvine 1978; **Resid:** Pediatrics, Chldns Hosp Med Ctr 1981; **Fellow:** Pediatric Hematology-Oncology, Stanford Univ 1987; **Fac Appt:** Prof Ped, NYU Sch Med

Chen, Allen R MD/PhD [PHO] - **Spec Exp:** Bone Marrow Transplant; Hodgkin's Disease; Immunotherapy; Graft vs Host Disease; **Hospital:** Johns Hopkins Hosp; **Address:** Johns Hopkins Hosp, Div Peds Oncology, 1650 Orleans St CRB Bldg Fl 2M - rm 53, Baltimore, MD 21231; **Phone:** 410-955-7385; **Board Cert:** Pediatric Hematology-Oncology 2006; **Med School:** Duke Univ 1986; **Resid:** Pediatrics, Chldns Hosp Med Ctr 1989; **Fellow:** Pediatric Hematology-Oncology, Fred Hutchinson Canc Ctr 1993; Bone Marrow Transplant, Fred Hutchinson Canc Ctr 1994; **Fac Appt:** Assoc Prof Ped, Johns Hopkins Univ

Cheung, Nai-Kong V MD/PhD [PHO] - **Spec Exp:** Neuroblastoma; **Hospital:** Meml Sloan-Kettering Cancer Ctr (page 75); **Address:** 1275 York Ave, Box 170, New York, NY 10065; **Phone:** 212-639-8401; **Board Cert:** Pediatrics 1987; Pediatric Hematology-Oncology 1998; **Med School:** Harvard Med Sch 1978; **Resid:** Pediatrics, Stanford Univ Hosp 1980; **Fellow:** Pediatric Hematology-Oncology, Stanford Univ Hosp 1982; **Fac Appt:** Assoc Prof Ped, Cornell Univ-Weill Med Coll

Civin, Curt I MD [PHO] - **Spec Exp:** Pediatric Cancers; Leukemia; Bone Marrow Transplant; **Hospital:** Univ of MD Med Ctr; **Address:** Univ Maryland Office of Assoc Dean, 655 W Baltimore St, rm 14-023, Baltimore, MD 21201; **Phone:** 410-706-1181; **Board Cert:** Pediatrics 1979; Pediatric Hematology-Oncology 1980; **Med School:** Harvard Med Sch 1974; **Resid:** Pediatrics, Chldns Hosp 1976; **Fellow:** Pediatric Hematology-Oncology, Natl Cancer Inst 1979; **Fac Appt:** Prof Ped, Univ MD Sch Med

Cohen, Kenneth J MD [PHO] - **Spec Exp:** Brain Tumors; Spinal Tumors; **Hospital:** Johns Hopkins Hosp; **Address:** Johns Hopkins Hosp, 600 N Wolfe St, rm CMSC-800, Baltimore, MD 21287; **Phone:** 410-614-5055; **Board Cert:** Pediatrics 1990; Pediatric Hematology-Oncology 2002; **Med School:** SUNY Upstate Med Univ 1987; **Resid:** Pediatrics, Univ Colo Hlth Sci Ctr 1990; **Fellow:** Pediatric Hematology-Oncology, Johns Hopkins Hospital 1994; **Fac Appt:** Assoc Prof Ped, Johns Hopkins Univ

Pediatric Hematology/Oncology

Drachtman, Richard A MD [PHO] - **Spec Exp:** Pediatric Cancers; **Hospital:** Robert Wood Johnson Univ Hosp - New Brunswick, Jersey Shore Univ Med Ctr; **Address:** Cancer Inst of New Jersey, 195 Little Albany St, rm 3507, New Brunswick, NJ 08903; **Phone:** 732-235-5437; **Board Cert:** Pediatric Hematology-Oncology 2007; **Med School:** Ros Franklin Univ/Chicago Med Sch 1984; **Resid:** Pediatrics, N Shore Univ Hosp 1988; **Fellow:** Pediatric Hematology-Oncology, Mount Sinai Hosp 1991; **Fac Appt:** Prof Ped, UMDNJ-RW Johnson Med Sch

Dunkel, Ira J MD [PHO] - **Spec Exp:** Retinoblastoma; Brain & Spinal Cord Tumors; Brain Tumors; Pediatric Cancers; **Hospital:** Meml Sloan-Kettering Cancer Ctr (page 75); **Address:** 1275 York Ave, Box 185, New York, NY 10065; **Phone:** 212-639-2153; **Board Cert:** Pediatric Hematology-Oncology 2007; **Med School:** Duke Univ 1985; **Resid:** Pediatrics, Duke Univ Med Ctr 1988; **Fellow:** Pediatric Hematology-Oncology, Memorial-Sloan Kettering 1992; **Fac Appt:** Assoc Prof Ped, Cornell Univ-Weill Med Coll

Felix, Carolyn A MD [PHO] - **Spec Exp:** Leukemia; Leukemia in Infants; **Hospital:** Chldns Hosp of Philadelphia; **Address:** Colket Translational Research Bldg, 3501 Civic Ctr Blvd, Philadelphia, PA 19104; **Phone:** 215-590-2831; **Board Cert:** Pediatrics 1987; Pediatric Hematology-Oncology 1987; **Med School:** Boston Univ 1981; **Resid:** Pediatrics, Chldns Hosp 1984; **Fellow:** Pediatric Hematology-Oncology, Natl Cancer Inst-Pediatric Br 1987; **Fac Appt:** Assoc Prof Ped, Univ Pennsylvania

Frantz, Christopher N MD [PHO] - **Spec Exp:** Solid Tumors; Neuroblastoma; Leukemia; **Hospital:** Alfred I duPont Hosp for Children, Wilmington Hosp; **Address:** Alfred I duPont Hosp for Chldn, 1600 Rockland Rd, Box 269, Wilmington, DE 19899; **Phone:** 302-651-5500; **Board Cert:** Pediatrics 1977; Pediatric Hematology-Oncology 2005; **Med School:** Albert Einstein Coll Med 1971; **Resid:** Pediatrics, Chldns Hosp 1976; **Fellow:** Pediatric Hematology-Oncology, Chldns Hosp/Dana Farber Cancer Inst 1979

Friedman, Alan D MD [PHO] - **Spec Exp:** Leukemia; **Hospital:** Johns Hopkins Hosp; **Address:** 1650 Orleans St CRB1 Bldg - rm 253, Baltimore, MD 21231; **Phone:** 410-955-8817; **Board Cert:** Pediatrics 1987; Pediatric Hematology-Oncology 2005; **Med School:** Harvard Med Sch 1983; **Resid:** Pediatrics, Childrens Hosp 1986; **Fellow:** Pediatric Hematology-Oncology, Johns Hopkins Hosp 1987; **Fac Appt:** Prof Ped, Johns Hopkins Univ

Garvin, James H MD/PhD [PHO] - **Spec Exp:** Brain Tumors; Pediatric Cancers; Bone Marrow Transplant; **Hospital:** NYPresby-Morgan Stanley Children's Hosp (page 78); **Address:** 161 Fort Washington Ave Fl 7 - rm 708, New York, NY 10032-3729; **Phone:** 212-305-8685; **Board Cert:** Pediatrics 1982; Pediatric Hematology-Oncology 1984; **Med School:** Jefferson Med Coll 1976; **Resid:** Pediatrics, Chldns Hosp 1978; Pediatrics, Middlesex Hosp 1979; **Fellow:** Pediatric Hematology-Oncology, Dana Farber Cancer Inst/Childrens Hosp 1982; **Fac Appt:** Clin Prof Ped, Columbia P&S

Greenberg, Jay N MD [PHO] - **Hospital:** Chldns Natl Med Ctr, Inova Fairfax Hosp; **Address:** Pediatric Hematology/Oncology, 111 Michigan Ave NW Fl 4 W Wing, Washington, DC 20010; **Phone:** 202-476-2140; **Board Cert:** Pediatrics 1981; Pediatric Hematology-Oncology 1982; **Med School:** Univ Pennsylvania 1976; **Resid:** Pediatrics, Univ MI Hosp 1978; Pediatrics, Chldns Hosp 1979; **Fellow:** Pediatric Hematology-Oncology, Chldns Hosp 1982

Grupp, Stephan A MD/PhD [PHO] - **Spec Exp:** Stem Cell Transplant; Neuroblastoma; Bone Marrow Transplant; **Hospital:** Chldns Hosp of Philadelphia; **Address:** Childrens Hosp - Oncology, 34th St & Civic Ctr Blvd Abramson Bldg, Philadelphia, PA 19104; **Phone:** 215-590-2821; **Board Cert:** Pediatric Hematology-Oncology 2009; **Med School:** Univ Cincinnati 1987; **Resid:** Pediatrics, Chldns Hosp 1990; **Fellow:** Pediatric Hematology-Oncology, Dana Farber Cancer Inst/Chldns Hosp 1992; **Fac Appt:** Asst Prof Ped, Univ Pennsylvania

Guarini, Ludovico MD [PHO] - **Spec Exp:** Leukemia; Solid Tumors; **Hospital:** Maimonides Med Ctr (page 74); **Address:** 4802 10th Ave, Dept of Pediatrics, Brooklyn, NY 11219; **Phone:** 718-765-2671; **Board Cert:** Pediatrics 1984; Pediatric Hematology-Oncology 2007; **Med School:** Italy 1974; **Resid:** Pediatrics, Beth Israel Hosp 1981; **Fellow:** Pediatric Hematology-Oncology, Columbia-Presby Med Ctr 1984; **Fac Appt:** Assoc Prof Ped, Mount Sinai Sch Med

Halligan, Gregory E MD [PHO] - **Spec Exp:** Clinical Trials; Solid Tumors; **Hospital:** St. Christopher's Hosp for Chldn; **Address:** St Christophers Hosp for Children, Dept Oncology, 3601 A St, Philadelphia, PA 19134; **Phone:** 215-427-4447; **Board Cert:** Pediatrics 1982; Pediatric Hematology-Oncology 1984; **Med School:** Belgium 1977; **Resid:** Pediatrics, St Christophers Hosp for Chldn 1981; **Fellow:** Pediatric Hematology-Oncology, St Christophers Hosp for Chldn 1984; **Fac Appt:** Assoc Prof Ped, Drexel Univ Coll Med

Halpern, Steven MD [PHO] - **Spec Exp:** Leukemia & Lymphoma; Brain Tumors; Hodgkin's Disease; **Hospital:** Morristown Med Ctr, Overlook Med Ctr; **Address:** 100 Madison Ave, Morristown, NJ 07960; **Phone:** 973-971-6720; **Board Cert:** Pediatrics 1981; Pediatric Hematology-Oncology 1982; **Med School:** Ros Franklin Univ/Chicago Med Sch 1976; **Resid:** Pediatrics, St Christophers Hosp for Children 1979; **Fellow:** Pediatric Hematology-Oncology, Childrens Hosp 1982; **Fac Appt:** Asst Prof Ped, UMDNJ-NJ Med Sch, Newark

Harris, Michael B MD [PHO] - **Spec Exp:** Leukemia & Lymphoma; Bone Tumors; Cancer Survivors-Late Effects of Therapy; **Hospital:** Hackensack Univ Med Ctr (page 73); **Address:** Tomorrows Chldns Inst, JM Sanzari Chldns Hosp, 30 Prospect Ave, Imus 1-TCI, rm PC116, Hackensack, NJ 07601; **Phone:** 201-996-5437; **Board Cert:** Pediatrics 1974; Pediatric Hematology-Oncology 1974; **Med School:** Albert Einstein Coll Med 1969; **Resid:** Pediatrics, Chldns Hosp 1971; **Fellow:** Pediatric Hematology-Oncology, Chldns Hosp 1974; **Fac Appt:** Prof Ped, UMDNJ-NJ Med Sch, Newark

Helman, Lee Jay MD [PHO] - **Spec Exp:** Solid Tumors; **Hospital:** Natl Inst of Hlth - Clin Ctr; **Address:** National Cancer Inst, NIH, 31 Center Drive, rm 3A11, Bethesda, MD 20892; **Phone:** 301-496-4257; **Board Cert:** Internal Medicine 1983; Medical Oncology 1985; **Med School:** Univ MD Sch Med 1980; **Resid:** Internal Medicine, Barnes Hosp 1983; **Fellow:** Oncology, Natl Inst Hlth 1986

Jakacki, Regina I MD [PHO] - **Spec Exp:** Neuro-Oncology; Clinical Trials; Palliative Care; **Hospital:** Chldns Hosp of Pittsburgh - UPMC; **Address:** Children's Hospital Pittsburgh, 45th & Penn Drive, Pittsburgh, PA 15201; **Phone:** 412-692-8864; **Board Cert:** Pediatric Hematology-Oncology 2007; **Med School:** Univ Pennsylvania 1985; **Resid:** Pediatrics, Childrens Hosp 1988; **Fellow:** Pediatric Hematology-Oncology, Childrens Hosp 1991; **Fac Appt:** Assoc Prof Ped, Univ Pittsburgh

Kamen, Barton A MD/PhD [PHO] - **Spec Exp:** Drug Development; Leukemia; **Hospital:** Robert Wood Johnson Univ Hosp - New Brunswick; **Address:** Cancer Inst of New Jersey, 195 Little Albany St, rm 3549, New Brunswick, NJ 08903; **Phone:** 732-235-8864; **Board Cert:** Pediatrics 1981; Pediatric Hematology-Oncology 1987; **Med School:** Case West Res Univ 1976; **Resid:** Pediatrics, Yale-New Haven Hosp 1978; **Fellow:** Pediatric Hematology-Oncology, Yale-New Haven Hosp 1980; **Fac Appt:** Prof Ped, UMDNJ-RW Johnson Med Sch

Korones, David N MD [PHO] - **Spec Exp:** Brain Tumors; Palliative Care; Pediatric Cancers; **Hospital:** Univ of Rochester Strong Meml Hosp; **Address:** Golisano Childrens Hosp at Strong, 601 Elmwood Ave, Box 777, Rochester, NY 14642-8777; **Phone:** 585-275-2981; **Board Cert:** Pediatrics 1987; Pediatric Hematology-Oncology 2006; Hospice & Palliative Medicine 2002; **Med School:** Vanderbilt Univ 1983; **Resid:** Pediatrics, Strong Meml Hosp 1986; **Fellow:** Pediatrics, Yale Univ 1988; Pediatric Hematology-Oncology, Strong Meml Hosp 1991; **Fac Appt:** Prof Ped, Univ Rochester

Pediatric Hematology/Oncology

Kushner, Brian H MD [PHO] - **Spec Exp:** Neuroblastoma; Bone Marrow Transplant; Immunotherapy; **Hospital:** Meml Sloan-Kettering Cancer Ctr (page 75); **Address:** 1275 York Avenue, New York, NY 10065; **Phone:** 800-525-2225; **Board Cert:** Pediatrics 1983; Pediatric Hematology-Oncology 1987; **Med School:** Johns Hopkins Univ 1976; **Resid:** Pediatrics, Columbia-Presby Med Ctr 1978; Pediatrics, NY Hosp 1979; **Fellow:** Pediatric Hematology-Oncology, Boston Chldns Hosp 1980; Pediatric Hematology-Oncology, Meml Sloan Kettering Cancer Ctr 1986; **Fac Appt:** Prof Ped, Cornell Univ-Weill Med Coll

Kuttesch, John F MD [PHO] - **Spec Exp:** Brain Tumors; Brain Tumors-Recurrent; Solid Tumors; **Hospital:** Penn State Chldns Hosp; **Address:** Penn State College of Medicine, Div Ped Hem/Onc & Stem Cell Transplant, 500 University Drive, MC HO85, Hershey, PA 17033-0850; **Phone:** 717-531-6012; **Board Cert:** Pediatrics 2008; Pediatric Hematology-Oncology 2007; **Med School:** Univ Tex, Houston 1985; **Resid:** Pediatrics, Vanderbilt Univ Med Ctr 1988; **Fellow:** Pediatric Hematology-Oncology, St Judes Chldns Hosp 1992; **Fac Appt:** Prof Ped

Lange, Beverly J MD [PHO] - **Spec Exp:** Leukemia; Brain & Spinal Cord Tumors; Cognitive Rehabilitation; **Hospital:** Chldns Hosp of Philadelphia; **Address:** Chldns Hosp Phila, Medical Oncology, 34th St & Civic Ctr Blvd, Wood Center Fl 4, Philadelphia, PA 19104; **Phone:** 215-590-3025; **Board Cert:** Pediatrics 1976; Pediatric Hematology-Oncology 1997; **Med School:** Temple Univ 1971; **Resid:** Pediatrics, Philadelphia Genl Hosp 1973; **Fellow:** Pediatric Oncology, Chldns Hosp; **Fac Appt:** Prof Ped, Univ Pennsylvania

Lipton, Jeffrey M MD/PhD [PHO] - **Spec Exp:** Bone Marrow Failure Disorders; Stem Cell Transplant; Bone Marrow Transplant; **Hospital:** Steven & Alexandra Cohen Chldn's Med Ctr of NY; **Address:** Steven & Alexandra Cohen Chldn's Med Ctr, Division, Hematology/Oncology, 269-01 76th Ave Ave, rm 255, New Hyde Park, NY 11040-1433; **Phone:** 718-470-3460; **Board Cert:** Pediatrics 1981; **Med School:** St Louis Univ 1975; **Resid:** Pediatrics, Boston Chldns Hosp 1977; **Fellow:** Pediatric Hematology-Oncology, Boston Chldns Hosp/Dana Farber Cancer Inst 1979; **Fac Appt:** Prof Ped, Albert Einstein Coll Med

Loeb, David M MD/PhD [PHO] - **Spec Exp:** Bone Marrow Transplantation; Bone Cancer; **Hospital:** Johns Hopkins Hosp; **Address:** 601 N Caroline St, Baltimore, MD 21287; **Phone:** 410-955-8751; **Board Cert:** Pediatrics 2005; Pediatric Hematology-Oncology 2000; **Med School:** Columbia P&S 1994; **Resid:** Pediatrics, John Hopkins Hosp 1997; **Fellow:** Pediatric Oncology, John Hopkins Hosp 1997; **Fac Appt:** Asst Prof Ped, Johns Hopkins Univ

Luchtman-Jones, Lori MD [PHO] - **Spec Exp:** Leukemia; Bleeding/Coagulation Disorders; **Hospital:** Chldns Natl Med Ctr; **Address:** Chldn's Natl Med Ctr, 111 Michigan Ave NW Fl 4 - Ste 4043, Washington, DC 20010; **Phone:** 202-476-2140; **Board Cert:** Pediatric Hematology-Oncology 2004; **Med School:** UCSD 1987; **Resid:** Pediatrics, UCSD School Med 1990; **Fellow:** Pediatric Hematology-Oncology, Washington Univ 1995; **Fac Appt:** Asst Prof Ped, Washington Univ, St Louis

Marcus, Judith R MD [PHO] - **Spec Exp:** Leukemia; Lymphoma; Bleeding/Coagulation Disorders; Solid Tumors-Pediatric; **Hospital:** NYPresby-Morgan Stanley Children's Hosp (page 78), White Plains Hosp Ctr; **Address:** 161 Ft Washington Ave, Ste 7I, New York, NY 10032; **Phone:** 914-684-0220; **Board Cert:** Pediatrics 1997; Pediatric Hematology-Oncology 1997; **Med School:** NYU Sch Med 1971; **Resid:** Pediatrics, Bronx Muni Hosp-Albert Einstein 1974; **Fellow:** Pediatric Hematology-Oncology, Meml Sloan Kettering Cancer Ctr 1979; **Fac Appt:** Clin Prof Ped, Columbia P&S

Maris, John M MD [PHO] - **Spec Exp:** Neuroblastoma; Clinical Trials; **Hospital:** Chldns Hosp of Philadelphia; **Address:** Chldns Hosp Philadelphia - Oncology, 3501 Civic Ctr Blvd CTRB Bldg - rm 3060, Philadelphia, PA 19104-4318; **Phone:** 215-590-5244; **Board Cert:** Pediatric Hematology-Oncology 2004; **Med School:** Univ Pennsylvania 1989; **Resid:** Pediatrics, Chldns Hosp 1992; **Fellow:** Pediatric Hematology-Oncology, Chldns Hosp 1996

Meyers, Paul A MD [PHO] - **Spec Exp:** Pediatric Cancers; Bone Tumors; Sarcoma; **Hospital:** Meml Sloan-Kettering Cancer Ctr (page 75), NY-Presby Hosp/Weill Cornell (page 78); **Address:** 1275 York Ave, New York, NY 10065; **Phone:** 800-525-2225; **Board Cert:** Pediatrics 1978; Pediatric Hematology-Oncology 1978; **Med School:** Mount Sinai Sch Med 1973; **Resid:** Pediatrics, Mt Sinai Hosp 1976; **Fellow:** Pediatric Hematology-Oncology, NY Hosp-Cornell Med Ctr 1979; **Fac Appt:** Prof Ped, Cornell Univ-Weill Med Coll

O'Reilly, Richard MD [PHO] - **Spec Exp:** Bone Marrow Transplant; **Hospital:** Meml Sloan-Kettering Cancer Ctr (page 75), NY-Presby Hosp/Weill Cornell (page 78); **Address:** 1275 York Avenue, New York, NY 10065; **Phone:** 800-525-2225; **Board Cert:** Pediatrics 1974; **Med School:** Univ Rochester 1968; **Resid:** Pediatrics, Chldrns Hosp 1972; **Fellow:** Infectious Disease, Chldrns Hosp 1973; **Fac Appt:** Prof Ped, Cornell Univ-Weill Med Coll

Parker, Robert MD [PHO] - **Spec Exp:** Pediatric Cancers; Bleeding/Coagulation Disorders; Lymphoma; **Hospital:** Stony Brook Univ Med Ctr; **Address:** Stony Brook Univ Hosp, Dept Peds, HSC T-11, Rm 029, Stony Brook, NY 11794-8111; **Phone:** 631-444-7720; **Board Cert:** Pediatrics 1983; Pediatric Hematology-Oncology 1984; **Med School:** Brown Univ 1976; **Resid:** Internal Medicine, Roger Williams Med Ctr 1977; Pediatrics, Rhode Island Hosp 1979; **Fellow:** Pediatric Hematology-Oncology, Natl Cancer Inst 1981; Hematology, Natl Cancer Inst 1984; **Fac Appt:** Prof Ped, SUNY Stony Brook

Reaman, Gregory H MD [PHO] - **Spec Exp:** Leukemia; Lymphoma; Cancer Survivors-Late Effects of Therapy; **Hospital:** Chldns Natl Med Ctr; **Address:** 111 Michigan Ave NW, West Bldg Fl 4 - Ste 600, Washington, DC 20010-2916; **Phone:** 202-476-2800; **Board Cert:** Pediatrics 1978; Pediatric Hematology-Oncology 1978; **Med School:** Loyola Univ-Stritch Sch Med 1973; **Resid:** Hematology, Montreal Chldns Hosp 1975; Pediatrics, Montreal Chldns Hosp 1976; **Fellow:** Pediatric Oncology, Natl Cancer Inst 1979; **Fac Appt:** Prof Ped, Geo Wash Univ

Rheingold, Susan R MD [PHO] - **Spec Exp:** Leukemia; Clinical Trials; **Hospital:** Chldns Hosp of Philadelphia; **Address:** Chldns Hosp Phila - Div Oncology, 3501 Civic Ctr Blvd CTRB Bldg Fl 10, Philadelphia, PA 19104; **Phone:** 215-590-5244; **Board Cert:** Pediatrics 2010; Pediatric Hematology-Oncology 2008; **Med School:** Univ Pennsylvania 1992; **Resid:** Pediatrics, Johns Hopkins Hosp 1995; **Fellow:** Pediatric Hematology-Oncology, Chldns Hosp 1999; **Fac Appt:** Asst Prof Ped, Univ Pennsylvania

Ritchey, A Kim MD [PHO] - **Spec Exp:** Leukemia; Hematologic Malignancies; **Hospital:** Chldns Hosp of Pittsburgh - UPMC; **Address:** Chldns Hosp, Div Hematology/Oncology, One Children's Hosp Drive, 4401 Penn Ave, Faculty Pavilion Fl 8, Pittsburgh, PA 15224; **Phone:** 412-692-5055; **Board Cert:** Pediatrics 1977; Pediatric Hematology-Oncology 2007; **Med School:** Univ Cincinnati 1972; **Resid:** Pediatrics, Johns Hopkins Hosp 1975; **Fellow:** Pediatric Hematology-Oncology, Yale-New Haven Hosp 1980; **Fac Appt:** Prof Ped, Univ Pittsburgh

Rood, Brian R MD [PHO] - **Spec Exp:** Brain Tumors; **Hospital:** Chldns Natl Med Ctr; **Address:** CNMC Div Ped Onc, 111 Michigan Ave NW, Washington, DC 20010; **Phone:** 202-476-2140; **Board Cert:** Pediatrics 2006; Pediatric Hematology-Oncology 2010; **Med School:** Jefferson Med Coll 1995; **Resid:** Pediatrics, Univ VT Hosp 1998; **Fellow:** Pediatric Hematology-Oncology, Chldns Natl Med Ctr 1998; Research, Chldns Natl Med Ctr 2001

Small, Donald MD [PHO] - **Spec Exp:** Leukemia; Lymphoma; **Hospital:** Johns Hopkins Hosp; **Address:** Johns Hopkins Univ, 1650 Orleans St CRB-1 Bldg - rm 251, Baltimore, MD 21231; **Phone:** 410-614-0994; **Board Cert:** Pediatric Hematology-Oncology 2002; **Med School:** Johns Hopkins Univ 1985; **Resid:** Pediatrics, Johns Hopkins Hosp 1987; **Fellow:** Pediatric Hematology-Oncology, Johns Hopkins Hosp 1990; **Fac Appt:** Prof Ped, Johns Hopkins Univ

Pediatric Hematology/Oncology

Steinherz, Peter G MD [PHO] - **Spec Exp:** Leukemia & Lymphoma; Pediatric Cancers; Wilms' Tumor; **Hospital:** Meml Sloan-Kettering Cancer Ctr (page 75), NY-Presby Hosp/Weill Cornell (page 78); **Address:** 1275 York Avenue, New York, NY 10065; **Phone:** 212-639-7951; **Board Cert:** Pediatrics 1973; Pediatric Hematology-Oncology 1978; **Med School:** Albert Einstein Coll Med 1968; **Resid:** Pediatrics, NY Hosp-Cornell 1971; **Fellow:** Pediatric Hematology-Oncology, NY Hosp-Cornell 1975; **Fac Appt:** Prof Ped, Cornell Univ-Weill Med Coll

Weinblatt, Mark E MD [PHO] - **Spec Exp:** Leukemia & Lymphoma; Bleeding/Coagulation Disorders; Solid Tumors; **Hospital:** Winthrop Univ Hosp; **Address:** Winthrop Univ Hosp, 120 Mineola Blvd, Ste 460, Mineola, NY 11501; **Phone:** 516-663-9400; **Board Cert:** Pediatrics 1980; Pediatric Hematology-Oncology 1982; **Med School:** Albert Einstein Coll Med 1976; **Resid:** Pediatrics, Jacobi Med Ctr 1979; **Fellow:** Pediatric Hematology-Oncology, Children's Hosp 1981; **Fac Appt:** Prof Ped, SUNY Stony Brook

Weiner, Michael MD [PHO] - **Spec Exp:** Hodgkin's Disease; Lymphoma; Leukemia; **Hospital:** NY-Presby Hosp/Columbia (page 78); **Address:** 161 Fort Washington Ave, Irving Pavilion-FL 7, New York, NY 10032-3710; **Phone:** 212-305-9770; **Board Cert:** Pediatrics 1980; Pediatric Hematology-Oncology 1980; **Med School:** SUNY Hlth Sci Ctr 1972; **Resid:** Pediatrics, Montefiore Med Ctr 1974; **Fellow:** Pediatric Hematology-Oncology, NYU Med Ctr 1976; Pediatric Hematology-Oncology, Johns Hopkins Hosp 1977; **Fac Appt:** Prof Ped, Columbia P&S

Wexler, Leonard MD [PHO] - **Spec Exp:** Rhabdomyosarcoma; Bone Cancer; Gastrointestinal Stromal Tumors; Sarcoma-Soft Tissue; **Hospital:** Meml Sloan-Kettering Cancer Ctr (page 75); **Address:** 1275 York Avenue, New York, NY 10065; **Phone:** 800-525-2225; **Board Cert:** Pediatrics 2007; Pediatric Hematology-Oncology 2007; **Med School:** Boston Univ 1985; **Resid:** Pediatrics, Montefiore Med Ctr 1988; **Fellow:** Pediatric Hematology-Oncology, National Cancer Inst 1991; **Fac Appt:** Assoc Prof Ped, Columbia P&S

Wiley, Joseph M MD [PHO] - **Hospital:** Sinai Hosp - Baltimore; **Address:** Sinai Hospital, Div Pediattic Hematology/Oncology, 2401 W Belvedrer Ave, Baltimore, MD 21215; **Phone:** 410-601-5864; **Board Cert:** Pediatrics 1986; Pediatric Hematology-Oncology 2005; **Med School:** Univ MD Sch Med 1982; **Resid:** Pediatrics, Johns Hopkins Hosp 1995; **Fellow:** Pediatric Hematology-Oncology, Johns Hopkins Hosp 1998; **Fac Appt:** Assoc Prof Ped, Johns Hopkins Univ

Wolfe, Lawrence C MD [PHO] - **Spec Exp:** Palliative Care; Adrenal Cancer; **Hospital:** Steven & Alexandra Cohen Chldn's Med Ctr of NY; **Address:** Steven & Alexandra Cohen Chldn's Med Ctr, Div Pediatric Hematology/Oncology, 269-01 76th Ave, New Hyde Park, NY 11040; **Phone:** 718-470-3460; **Board Cert:** Pediatrics 1981; Pediatric Hematology-Oncology 1987; Hospice & Palliative Medicine 2011; **Med School:** Harvard Med Sch 1976; **Resid:** Pediatrics, Chldns Hosp 1978; **Fellow:** Pediatric Hematology-Oncology, Chldns Hosp 1991; **Fac Appt:** Prof Ped

York, Teresa A MD [PHO] - **Spec Exp:** Leukemia; **Hospital:** Univ of MD Med Ctr; **Address:** Greenebaum Cancer Center, 22 S Greene St, rm N5E16, Baltimore, MD 21201; **Phone:** 410-328-2808; **Board Cert:** Pediatric Hematology-Oncology 2004; **Med School:** W VA Univ 1997; **Resid:** Pediatrics, W Va Univ Chldns Hosp 2000; **Fellow:** Pediatric Hematology-Oncology, Med Univ SC Hosp 2000; **Fac Appt:** Asst Prof Ped, Univ MD Sch Med

Southeast

Barredo, Julio C MD [PHO] - **Spec Exp:** Leukemia; Bone Marrow Transplant; Cancer Survivors-Late Effects of Therapy; Stem Cell Transplant; **Hospital:** Univ of Miami Hosp & Clins/Sylvester Comp Canc Ctr (page 82); **Address:** Univ Miami Dept Pediatrics (R-131), PO Box 016960, Miami, FL 33101; **Phone:** 305-585-5635; **Board Cert:** Pediatric Hematology-Oncology 2007; **Med School:** Peru 1982; **Resid:** Pediatrics, Kings Co Hosp 1987; **Fellow:** Pediatric Hematology-Oncology, Chldns Hosp/USC 1988; **Fac Appt:** Prof Ped, Univ Miami Sch Med

Bertolone, Salvatore MD [PHO] - **Spec Exp:** Bone Marrow Transplant; **Hospital:** Kosair Chldn's Hosp, Norton Hosp; **Address:** Pediatric Hematology/Oncology, 601 S Floyd St, Ste 403, Louisville, KY 40202; **Phone:** 502-629-7750; **Board Cert:** Pediatrics 1975; Pediatric Hematology-Oncology 1976; **Med School:** Univ Louisville Sch Med 1970; **Resid:** Pediatrics, Univ Louisville 1972; **Fellow:** Pediatric Hematology-Oncology, Univ Colorado 1974; **Fac Appt:** Prof Ped, Univ Louisville Sch Med

Blatt, Julie MD [PHO] - **Spec Exp:** Neuroblastoma; Cancer Survivors-Late Effects of Therapy; **Hospital:** NC Memorial Hosp - UNC; **Address:** UNC, Dept Ped Hematology Oncology, 170 Manning Drive, Campus Box 7236, Chapel Hill, NC 27599-7236; **Phone:** 919-966-1178; **Board Cert:** Pediatrics 1981; Pediatric Hematology-Oncology 1982; **Med School:** Johns Hopkins Univ 1976; **Resid:** Pediatrics, Columbia-Presby Hosp 1978; **Fellow:** Pediatric Oncology, Natl Cancer Inst 1982; **Fac Appt:** Prof Ped, Univ NC Sch Med

Castellino, Sharon M MD [PHO] - **Spec Exp:** Cancer Survivors-Late Effects of Therapy; Leukemia; Lymphoma; **Hospital:** Brenner Chldn's Hosp; **Address:** Wake Forest Univ Baptist Med Ctr, Div Pediatric Hematology/Oncology, Medical Center Blvd, Winston-Salem, NC 27157; **Phone:** 336-716-4324; **Board Cert:** Pediatrics 2003; Pediatric Hematology-Oncology 2006; **Med School:** Duke Univ 1992; **Resid:** Pediatrics, Childrens Hosp 1994; Pediatrics, Duke Univ Med Ctr 1995; **Fellow:** Pediatric Hematology-Oncology, Duke Univ 1997; **Fac Appt:** Asst Prof Ped, Wake Forest Univ

Frangoul, Haydar A MD [PHO] - **Spec Exp:** Stem Cell Transplant; **Hospital:** Vanderbilt Monroe Carrell Jr. Chldn's Hosp; **Address:** 1215 21st Ave S, 397 Preston Rsch Bldg, Nashville, TN 37232-6310; **Phone:** 615-936-1762; **Board Cert:** Pediatric Hematology-Oncology 2008; **Med School:** Amer Univ Beirut 1990; **Resid:** Pediatrics, Duke Univ Med Ctr 1993; **Fellow:** Pediatric Hematology-Oncology, Duke Univ Med Ctr 1994; Pediatric Hematology-Oncology, Seattle Chldns/Fred Hutchinson Cancer Ctr 1996; **Fac Appt:** Assoc Prof Ped, Vanderbilt Univ

Friedman, Debra L MD [PHO] - **Spec Exp:** Cancer Survivors-Late Effects of Therapy; Hodgkin's Disease; Retinoblastoma; **Hospital:** Vanderbilt Monroe Carrell Jr. Chldn's Hosp, Vanderbilt Univ Med Ctr; **Address:** 1215 21st Ave S, 397 Preston Research Bldg, Nashville, TN 37232-6310; **Phone:** 615-936-1762; **Board Cert:** Pediatric Hematology-Oncology 2006; **Med School:** UMDNJ-RW Johnson Med Sch 1991; **Resid:** Pediatrics, Chldns Hosp 1994; **Fellow:** Pediatric Hematology-Oncology, Chldns Hosp 1997; Cancer Epidemiology, Univ Penn; **Fac Appt:** Asst Prof Ped, Vanderbilt Univ

Furman, Wayne L MD [PHO] - **Spec Exp:** Neuroblastoma; Liver Cancer; Drug Development; **Hospital:** St. Jude Children's Research Hosp; **Address:** St Jude Children's Research Hospital, 262 Danny Thomas Pl, Memphis, TN 38105; **Phone:** 901-595-2800; **Board Cert:** Pediatrics 1985; Pediatric Hematology-Oncology 1987; **Med School:** Ohio State Univ 1979; **Resid:** Pediatrics, Children's Hosp 1983; **Fellow:** Pediatric Hematology-Oncology, St Jude Chldn's Rsch Hosp 1985; **Fac Appt:** Prof Ped, Univ Tenn Coll Med

Pediatric Hematology/Oncology

Gajjar, Amar J MD [PHO] - **Spec Exp:** Brain Tumors; Medulloblastoma; Neuro-Oncology; Drug Development; **Hospital:** St. Jude Children's Research Hosp; **Address:** St Judes Children's Hosp, Dept Oncology, 262 Danny Thomas Pl, rm C6024, MS 260, Memphis, TN 38105-2794; **Phone:** 901-595-4599; **Board Cert:** Pediatric Hematology-Oncology 2007; **Med School:** India 1984; **Resid:** Pediatrics, All Chldns Hosp 1989; **Fellow:** Hematology & Oncology, St Jude Chldns Hosp 1990; **Fac Appt:** Prof Ped, Univ Tenn Coll Med

Godder, Kamar MD/PhD [PHO] - **Spec Exp:** Stem Cell Transplant; Leukemia; Palliative Care; **Hospital:** Med Coll of VA Hosp; **Address:** 401-09 N 11th St, Richmond, VA 23298; **Phone:** 804-828-9300; **Board Cert:** Pediatric Hematology-Oncology 2005; **Med School:** Israel 1980; **Resid:** Pediatrics, Hadassah-Mt Scopus 1984; **Fellow:** Pediatric Hematology-Oncology, Meml Sloan Kettering Cancer Ctr 1988; **Fac Appt:** Prof Ped, Va Commonwealth Univ Sch Med

Gold, Stuart H MD [PHO] - **Spec Exp:** Leukemia; Brain Tumors; Cancer Survivors-Late Effects of Therapy; **Hospital:** NC Memorial Hosp - UNC; **Address:** UNC, Dept Ped Hem-Onc, 1185A Physicians Office Bldg, 170 Manning Drive, Campus Box 7236, Chapel Hill, NC 27599-7236; **Phone:** 919-966-1178; **Board Cert:** Pediatrics 1986; Pediatric Hematology-Oncology 1987; **Med School:** Vanderbilt Univ 1981; **Resid:** Pediatrics, Univ Colorado Hlth Sci Ctr 1984; **Fellow:** Pediatric Hematology-Oncology, Univ Colorado Hlth Sci Ctr 1989; **Fac Appt:** Prof Ped, Univ NC Sch Med

Green, Daniel M MD [PHO] - **Spec Exp:** Wilms' Tumor; Fertility in Cancer Survivors; Cancer Survivors-Late Effects of Therapy; **Hospital:** St. Jude Children's Research Hosp; **Address:** Dept Epidemiology & Cancer Control, St Jude Chldn's Rsch Hosp, 262 Danny Thomas Pl, MS 735, Memphis, TN 38105-2794; **Phone:** 901-595-5915; **Board Cert:** Pediatrics 1986; Pediatric Hematology-Oncology 1997; **Med School:** St Louis Univ 1973; **Resid:** Pediatrics, Boston City Hosp 1975; **Fellow:** Pediatric Hematology-Oncology, Chldns Hosp Med Ctr 1978

Gururangan, Sridharan MD [PHO] - **Spec Exp:** Brain Tumors; Spinal Cord Tumors; Neuro-Oncology; **Hospital:** Duke Univ Hosp; **Address:** Robert Tisch Brain Tumor Ctr at Duke, DUMC Box 3624, Durham, NC 27710; **Phone:** 919-684-3506; **Med School:** India 1958; **Resid:** Pediatrics, Le Bonheur Children's Med Ctr 1992; **Fellow:** Pediatric Hematology-Oncology, St Jude Children's Hosp 1993; Pediatric Hematology-Oncology, Meml Sloan Kettering Cancer Ctr 1996

Hudson, Melissa M MD [PHO] - **Spec Exp:** Cancer Survivors-Late Effects of Therapy; Hodgkin's Disease; **Hospital:** St. Jude Children's Research Hosp; **Address:** St Jude Children's Research Hosp, 262 Danny Thomas Pl, MS 735, Memphis, TN 38105; **Phone:** 901-595-3384; **Board Cert:** Pediatrics 1988; Pediatric Hematology-Oncology 2006; **Med School:** Univ Tex SW, Dallas 1983; **Resid:** Pediatrics, Univ Texas Affil Hosps 1986; **Fellow:** Pediatric Hematology-Oncology, MD Anderson Cancer Ctr 1989

Johnston, J Martin MD [PHO] - **Spec Exp:** Leukemia; Lymphoma; **Hospital:** Meml Hlth Univ Med Ctr - Savannah; **Address:** Backus Children's Hosp Outpatient Ctr, 4700 Waters Ave, PO Box 23089, Savannah, GA 31403-3089; **Phone:** 912-350-8194; **Board Cert:** Pediatric Hematology-Oncology 2009; **Med School:** Duke Univ 1984; **Resid:** Pediatrics, Univ Utah Med Ctr 1988; **Fellow:** Pediatric Hematology-Oncology, Barnes Jewish Hosp 1991; **Fac Appt:** Assoc Prof Ped, Mercer Univ Sch Med

Kane, Javier R MD [PHO] - **Spec Exp:** Palliative Care; **Hospital:** St. Jude Children's Research Hosp; **Address:** St Jude Chldns Rsch Hosp, Dept Oncology, 262 Danny Thomas Pl, MS 260, Memphis, TN 38105-2794; **Phone:** 901-595-4152; **Board Cert:** Pediatrics 2007; Pediatric Hematology-Oncology 2004; Hospice & Palliative Medicine 2008; **Med School:** Mexico 1986; **Resid:** Pediatrics, Austin Med Ed Prog 1992; **Fellow:** Pediatric Hematology-Oncology, Univ Tennessee

Keller Jr, Frank G MD [PHO] - **Spec Exp:** Leukemia; Hodgkin's Disease; **Hospital:** Chldns Hlthcare Atlanta @ Egleston; **Address:** Aflac Cancer Ctr at Egleston, 1405 Clifton Rd NE, Tower 1, 4th Fl, Atlanta, GA 30322; **Phone:** 404-785-1200; **Board Cert:** Pediatric Hematology-Oncology 2009; **Med School:** Univ NC Sch Med 1986; **Resid:** Pediatrics, Vanderbilt Univ Med Ctr 1990; **Fellow:** Pediatric Hematology-Oncology, Duke Univ Med Ctr 1993; **Fac Appt:** Assoc Prof Ped, Emory Univ

Kreissman, Susan G MD [PHO] - **Spec Exp:** Neuroblastoma; Clinical Trials; **Hospital:** Duke Univ Hosp; **Address:** Duke Univ Med Ctr, Box 102382, Durham, NC 27710; **Phone:** 919-684-3401; **Board Cert:** Pediatric Hematology-Oncology 2004; **Med School:** Mount Sinai Sch Med 1985; **Resid:** Pediatrics, Chldns Hosp 1988; **Fellow:** Pediatric Hematology-Oncology, Chldns Hosp/Dana Farber Cancer Inst 1991; **Fac Appt:** Assoc Prof Ped, Duke Univ

Kurtzberg, Joanne MD [PHO] - **Spec Exp:** Stem Cell Transplant; Bone Marrow Transplant; **Hospital:** Duke Univ Hosp; **Address:** Duke Univ Med Ctr, 1400 Morreene Rd, Durham, NC 27705; **Phone:** 919-668-1100; **Board Cert:** Pediatrics 1982; Pediatric Hematology-Oncology 1982; **Med School:** NY Med Coll 1976; **Resid:** Pediatrics, Dartmouth Med Ctr 1977; Pediatrics, Upstate Med Ctr 1979; **Fellow:** Pediatric Hematology-Oncology, Upstate Med Ctr 1980; Pediatric Hematology-Oncology, Duke Med Ctr 1983; **Fac Appt:** Prof Ped, Duke Univ

Laver, Joseph H MD [PHO] - **Spec Exp:** Stem Cell Transplant; Lymphoma, Non-Hodgkin's; **Hospital:** St. Jude Children's Research Hosp; **Address:** St Jude's Chldns Rsch Hosp, rm C-7045E, 262 Danny Thomas Pl, Memphis, TN 38105-3678; **Phone:** 901-595-3532; **Board Cert:** Pediatrics 1985; Pediatric Hematology-Oncology 1987; **Med School:** Israel 1979; **Resid:** Pediatrics, Assaf Harofeh Med Ctr 1982; **Fellow:** Pediatric Hematology-Oncology, Meml Slaon Kettering 1985

Leung, Wing-Hang MD/PhD [PHO] - **Spec Exp:** Bone Marrow & Stem Cell Transplant; Cancer Survivors-Late Effects of Therapy; **Hospital:** St. Jude Children's Research Hosp; **Address:** St Judes Chldns Hosp, 262 Danny Thomas Pl, rm C6072, MS 260, Bone Marrow Transplant& Cellular Therapy, Memphis, TN 38105-3678; **Phone:** 901-495-3300; **Board Cert:** Pediatrics 2008; Pediatric Hematology-Oncology 2006; **Med School:** Hong Kong 1988; **Resid:** Internal Medicine, Kings Co Hosp 1994; **Fellow:** Hematology & Oncology, Johns Hopkins Hosp 1997

McLean, Thomas W MD [PHO] - **Hospital:** Wake Forest Univ Baptist Med Ctr; **Address:** Wake Forest Univ Scho Medicine, Dept Ped/Onc, Medical Center Blvd, Winston Salem, NC 27157; **Phone:** 336-716-4085; **Board Cert:** Pediatrics 2009; Pediatric Hematology-Oncology 2006; **Med School:** Med Univ SC 1990; **Resid:** Pediatrics, Chldns Hosp 1993; **Fellow:** Pediatric Hematology-Oncology, Great Ormons St Hosp for Sick Chldn 1994; Pediatric Hematology-Oncology, Dana Farber Chldns Hosp 1997; **Fac Appt:** Assoc Prof Ped, Wake Forest Univ

Moscow, Jeffrey A MD [PHO] - **Spec Exp:** Pediatric Cancers; **Hospital:** Univ of Kentucky Albert B. Chandler Hosp; **Address:** Univ Kentucky - Kentucky Clinic, 740 S Limestone, rm J457, Lexington, KY 40536-0284; **Phone:** 859-323-0239; **Board Cert:** Pediatrics 1988; Pediatric Hematology-Oncology 2007; **Med School:** Dartmouth Med Sch 1982; **Resid:** Pediatrics, Univ Texas SW Med Ctr 1985; **Fellow:** Pediatric Hematology-Oncology, Natl Cancer Inst 1989; **Fac Appt:** Prof Ped, Univ KY Coll Med

Neuberg, Ronnie W MD [PHO] - **Spec Exp:** Pediatric Cancers; Gene Therapy; Clinical Trials; Brain Tumors; **Hospital:** Palmetto Health Richland Mem Hosp, MUSC Chldns Hosp; **Address:** Palmetto Health Richland, 7 Richland Medical Park Drive, Ste 7215, Columbia, SC 29203; **Phone:** 803-434-3533; **Board Cert:** Pediatrics 1982; Pediatric Hematology-Oncology 1982; **Med School:** SUNY Buffalo 1977; **Resid:** Pediatrics, Chldns Hosp 1980; **Fellow:** Pediatric Hematology-Oncology, SUNY Upstate Med Ctr 1982; **Fac Appt:** Assoc Prof Ped, Univ SC Sch Med

Pediatric Hematology/Oncology

Nieder, Michael L MD [PHO] - **Spec Exp:** Bone Marrow Transplant; **Hospital:** All Children's Hosp; **Address:** 601 5th St S, Dept 7865, St Petersburg, FL 33701-4816; **Phone:** 727-767-6856; **Board Cert:** Pediatrics 1986; Pediatric Hematology-Oncology 2009; **Med School:** Univ IL Coll Med 1982; **Resid:** Pediatrics, Chldns Meml Hosp 1985; **Fellow:** Pediatric Hematology-Oncology, Chldns Meml Hosp 1988; **Fac Appt:** Prof Ped, Univ S Fla Coll Med

Olson, Thomas A MD [PHO] - **Spec Exp:** Germ Cell Tumors; Retinoblastoma; Sarcoma; **Hospital:** Chldns Hlthcare Atlanta @ Egleston; **Address:** Childrens at Egleston Aflac Cancer Ctr, 1405 Clifton Rd NE, Tower 1, 4th Fl, Atlanta, GA 30322; **Phone:** 404-785-1200; **Board Cert:** Pediatrics 1982; Pediatric Hematology-Oncology 1984; **Med School:** Loyola Univ-Stritch Sch Med 1978; **Resid:** Pediatrics, Walter Reed AMC 1981; **Fellow:** Pediatric Hematology-Oncology, Walter Reed AMC 1983; **Fac Appt:** Assoc Prof Ped, Emory Univ

Pui, Ching-Hon MD [PHO] - **Spec Exp:** Leukemia; Lymphoma; **Hospital:** St. Jude Children's Research Hosp; **Address:** St Jude Chldns Rsch Hosp, 262 Danny Thomas Pl, Memphis, TN 38105; **Phone:** 901-595-3606; **Board Cert:** Pediatrics 1980; Pediatric Hematology-Oncology 1982; **Med School:** Taiwan 1976; **Resid:** Pediatrics, St Jude Chldns Rsch Hosp 1979; **Fellow:** Hematology & Oncology, St Jude Chldns Rsch Hosp 1981; **Fac Appt:** Prof Ped, Univ Tenn Coll Med

Ribeiro, Raul MD [PHO] - **Spec Exp:** Leukemia & Lymphoma; **Hospital:** St. Jude Children's Research Hosp; **Address:** St Jude's Chldns Rsch Hosp, 262 Danny Thomas Pl, rm S-2012, MS 721, Memphis, TN 38105-3678; **Phone:** 901-595-3694; **Board Cert:** Pediatric Hematology-Oncology 2009; **Med School:** Brazil 1975; **Resid:** Pediatrics, Univ Parana Sch Med 1978; **Fellow:** Hematology & Oncology, St Jude's Chldns Rsch Hosp 1987; **Fac Appt:** Prof Ped, Univ Tenn Coll Med

Rosoff, Philip M MD [PHO] - **Spec Exp:** Cancer Survivors-Late Effects of Therapy; Leukemia; **Hospital:** Duke Univ Hosp; **Address:** Duke Univ Med Ctr, Box 10238, Durham, NC 27710-0001; **Phone:** 919-684-3401; **Board Cert:** Pediatrics 1984; Pediatric Hematology-Oncology 2009; **Med School:** Case West Res Univ 1978; **Resid:** Pediatrics, Chldns Hosp 1980; **Fellow:** Pediatric Hematology-Oncology, Chldns Hosp/Dana Farber Cancer Inst 1984; **Fac Appt:** Assoc Prof Ped, Duke Univ

Russo, Carolyn MD [PHO] - **Spec Exp:** Brain Tumors; Cancer Survivors-Late Effects of Therapy; Palliative Care; **Hospital:** Huntsville Hosp, The; **Address:** 910 Adams St, Ste 310, huntsville, AL 35801; **Phone:** 256-265-5834; **Board Cert:** Pediatric Hematology-Oncology 2005; **Med School:** UCLA 1984; **Resid:** Pediatrics, Harbor-UCLA Med Ctr 1987; **Fellow:** Pediatric Hematology-Oncology, Stanford Med Ctr 1990

Sandler, Eric MD [PHO] - **Spec Exp:** Bone Marrow Transplant; Leukemia; Bone Tumors; **Hospital:** Wolfson Chldns Hosp; **Address:** 807 Childrens Way, Jacksonville, FL 32207; **Phone:** 904-697-3793; **Board Cert:** Pediatrics 2008; Pediatric Hematology-Oncology 2007; **Med School:** Univ VT Coll Med 1985; **Resid:** Pediatrics, UCSF Med Ctr 1988; **Fellow:** Pediatric Hematology-Oncology, Univ Fla Med Sch 1991; **Fac Appt:** Assoc Prof Ped, Mayo Med Sch

Sandlund Jr, John T MD [PHO] - **Spec Exp:** Lymphoma, Non-Hodgkin's; Leukemia & Lymphoma; **Hospital:** St. Jude Children's Research Hosp, Le Bonheur Chldns Med Ctr; **Address:** St Jude Children's Research Hosp, 262 Danny Thomas Pl, MS 260, Memphis, TN 38105; **Phone:** 901-595-2153; **Board Cert:** Pediatrics 1986; Pediatric Hematology-Oncology 1987; **Med School:** Ohio State Univ 1980; **Resid:** Pediatrics, Columbus Chldns Hosp 1983; **Fellow:** Hematology, Natl Cancer Inst 1986; Research, Natl Cancer Inst 1987; **Fac Appt:** Prof Ped, Univ Tenn Coll Med

Santana, Victor M MD [PHO] - **Spec Exp:** Solid Tumors; **Hospital:** St. Jude Children's Research Hosp; **Address:** St Jude Chldn's Rsch Hosp, Dept Oncology, 262 Danny Thomas Pl, rm C6041, MS 274, Memphis, TN 38105-2794; **Phone:** 901-595-2801; **Board Cert:** Pediatrics 1982; Pediatric Hematology-Oncology 1984; **Med School:** Puerto Rico 1978; **Resid:** Pediatrics, Johns Hopkins Hosp 1981; **Fellow:** Pediatric Hematology-Oncology, Johns Hopkins Hosp 1984; **Fac Appt:** Prof Ped, Univ Tenn Coll Med

Shearer, Patricia C MD [PHO] - **Spec Exp:** Cancer Survivors-Late Effects of Therapy; **Hospital:** Shands at Univ of FL; **Address:** Univ Florida/Shands Cancer Ctr, Cancer Survivorship Program, PO Box 103633, Gainesville, FL 32610; **Phone:** 352-273-8021; **Board Cert:** Pediatric Hematology-Oncology 2007; **Med School:** Louisiana State U, New Orleans 1986; **Resid:** Pediatrics, Johns Hopkins Hosp 1989; **Fellow:** Pediatric Hematology-Oncology, St Jude Chldns Rsch Hosp 1992; **Fac Appt:** Assoc Clin Prof Ped, Univ Fla Coll Med

Tebbi, Cameron MD [PHO] - **Spec Exp:** Hodgkin's Disease; Leukemia; Carcinoid Tumors; Histiocytoma; **Hospital:** St. Josephs Chldns Hosp, Tampa Genl Hosp; **Address:** 4019 Carrollwood Village Drive, Tampa, FL 33607; **Phone:** 813-601-4400; **Board Cert:** Pediatrics 1974; Pediatric Hematology-Oncology 1980; **Med School:** Iran 1968; **Resid:** Pediatrics, Cincinnati Chldns Hosp 1972; Pediatric Hematology-Oncology, MD Anderson Cancer Inst 1972; **Fellow:** Pediatric Hematology-Oncology, St Louis Chldns Hosp 1973; Medical Oncology, Ontario Cancer Inst 1974

Wang, Winfred C MD [PHO] - **Spec Exp:** Bone Marrow Failure Disorders; Anemia-Aplastic; **Hospital:** St. Jude Children's Research Hosp, Le Bonheur Chldns Med Ctr; **Address:** St Jude Chldn Rsch Hosp, 262 Danny Thomas Pl, MS 800, Memphis, TN 38105-2729; **Phone:** 901-595-2051; **Board Cert:** Pediatrics 1972; Pediatric Hematology-Oncology 1974; **Med School:** Univ Chicago-Pritzker Sch Med 1967; **Resid:** Pediatrics, Montefiore Med Ctr 1969; Pediatrics, Kauikeolani Chldns Hosp 1970; **Fellow:** Pediatric Hematology-Oncology, UCSF Med Ctr 1975; **Fac Appt:** Prof Ped, Univ Tenn Coll Med

Wechsler, Daniel S MD/PhD [PHO] - **Spec Exp:** Leukemia & Lymphoma; Neuroblastoma; **Hospital:** Duke Univ Hosp; **Address:** Duke Univ Med Ctr-Ped Hem/Onc, Box 102382, Durham, NC 27710; **Phone:** 919-684-3401; **Board Cert:** Pediatric Hematology-Oncology 2009; **Med School:** Canada 1987; **Resid:** Pediatrics, Johns Hopkins Hosp 1990; **Fellow:** Pediatric Hematology-Oncology, Johns Hopkins Hosp 1994; **Fac Appt:** Assoc Prof Ped, Duke Univ

Midwest

Arndt, Carola A MD [PHO] - **Spec Exp:** Sarcoma; Brain Tumors; Stem Cell Transplant; **Hospital:** Mayo Med Ctr & Clin - Rochester; **Address:** Mayo Clinic, Dept Pediatrics, 200 1st St SW, Rochester, MN 55905; **Phone:** 507-284-2652; **Board Cert:** Pediatrics 1982; Pediatric Hematology-Oncology 1987; **Med School:** Boston Univ 1978; **Resid:** Pediatrics, Naval Reg Med Ctr 1981; **Fellow:** Pediatric Hematology-Oncology, Natl Inst Hlth 1984

Beyer, Eric C MD/PhD [PHO] - **Spec Exp:** Pediatric Cancers; Bleeding/Coagulation Disorders; **Hospital:** Univ of Chicago Med Ctr; **Address:** University of Chicago Hospitals, 5841 S Maryland Ave, 900 E 57th St, Chicago, IL 60637; **Phone:** 773-702-6808; **Board Cert:** Pediatrics 1987; **Med School:** UCSD 1982; **Resid:** Pediatrics, Chldns Hosp 1984; **Fellow:** Hematology & Oncology, Dana Farber Cancer Inst 1987; **Fac Appt:** Prof Ped, Univ Chicago-Pritzker Sch Med

Pediatric Hematology/Oncology

Blum, Kristie MD [PHO] - **Spec Exp:** Lymphoma; Lymphoma, Non-Hodgkin's; Lymphomas-Rare; **Hospital:** Ohio St Univ Med Ctr; **Address:** B315 Starling-Loving Hall, 320 W 10th Ave, Columbus, OH 43210; **Phone:** 614-293-8508; **Board Cert:** Internal Medicine 2000; Hematology 2004; Medical Oncology 2004; **Med School:** Univ Miami Sch Med 1997; **Resid:** Internal Medicine, Univ VA Hlth Sci Ctr 2000; **Fellow:** Hematology & Oncology, Vanderbilt Univ Med Ctr 2001; Hematology & Oncology, Wash Univ Affil Hosp 2003; **Fac Appt:** Asst Prof Med, Ohio State Univ

Boxer, Laurence MD [PHO] - **Spec Exp:** Congenital Neutropenia-Severe; Anemias & Red Cell Disorders; Bone Marrow Failure Disorders; Anemia-Aplastic; **Hospital:** Univ of Michigan Hosp; **Address:** Univ Michigan, L-2110 Womens Hosp, 1500 E Medical Ctr Dr, Box 0238, Ann Arbor, MI 48109-0238; **Phone:** 734-764-7126; **Board Cert:** Pediatrics 1971; Pediatric Hematology-Oncology 2010; **Med School:** Stanford Univ 1966; **Resid:** Pediatrics, Yale-New Haven Hosp 1968; Pediatrics, Stanford Univ Hosp 1969; **Fellow:** Hematology & Oncology, Chldns Hosp-Harvard 1974; **Fac Appt:** Prof Ped, Univ Mich Med Sch

Camitta, Bruce M MD [PHO] - **Spec Exp:** Leukemia; Anemia-Aplastic; Bone Marrow Transplant; **Hospital:** Chldns Hosp - Wisconsin; **Address:** MACC Fund Ctr for Cancer/Blood Disorders, 8701 Watertown Plank Rd, Ste 3018, Milwaukee, WI 53226; **Phone:** 414-456-4170; **Board Cert:** Pediatrics 1971; Pediatric Hematology-Oncology 1976; **Med School:** Johns Hopkins Univ 1966; **Resid:** Pediatrics, Chldns Hosp 1968; Pediatrics, Johns Hopkins Hosp 1969; **Fellow:** Pediatric Hematology-Oncology, Chldns Hosp 1973; **Fac Appt:** Prof Ped, Med Coll Wisc

Castle, Valerie P MD [PHO] - **Spec Exp:** Neuroblastoma; Cancer Survivors-Late Effects of Therapy; **Hospital:** Univ of Michigan Hosp; **Address:** Univ Mich Comp Cancer Ctr, 1500 E Medical Center Drive, Level B1-258, Reception B, Ann Arbor, MI 48109-0911; **Phone:** 734-936-9814; **Board Cert:** Pediatric Hematology-Oncology 2006; **Med School:** McMaster Univ 1983; **Resid:** Pediatrics, McMaster Univ Med Ctr 1986; **Fellow:** Pediatric Hematology-Oncology, Univ Mich Hosps 1989; **Fac Appt:** Prof Ped, Univ Mich Med Sch

Cohn, Susan L MD [PHO] - **Spec Exp:** Neuroblastoma; **Hospital:** Univ of Chicago Med Ctr; **Address:** Univ Chicago Medical Ctr, 900 E 57th St, rm 5100, Chicago, IL 60637; **Phone:** 773-702-2571; **Board Cert:** Pediatrics 1985; Pediatric Hematology-Oncology 1987; **Med School:** Univ IL Coll Med 1980; **Resid:** Pediatrics, Michael Reese Hosp 1984; **Fellow:** Hematology & Oncology, Chldns Meml Hosp 1985; **Fac Appt:** Prof Ped, Univ Chicago-Pritzker Sch Med

Corey, Seth J MD [PHO] - **Spec Exp:** Bone Marrow Failure Disorders; Leukemia; Myelodysplastic Syndromes; **Hospital:** Children's Mem Hosp -Chicago; **Address:** Robert Lurie Comp Cancer Ctr, 303 E Superior St, Chicago, IL 60611; **Phone:** 312-503-6694; **Board Cert:** Pediatrics 1986; Pediatric Hematology-Oncology 2004; **Med School:** Tulane Univ 1982; **Resid:** Pediatrics, St Louis Chldns Hosp 1985; **Fellow:** Hematology & Oncology, Tufts Univ 1992; Renal Pathology, Boston Chldns-Dana Farber Ctr 1989; **Fac Appt:** Prof Ped, Northwestern Univ-Feinberg Sch Med

Croop, James M MD/PhD [PHO] - **Spec Exp:** Solid Tumors; Clinical Trials; **Hospital:** Riley Hosp for Children; **Address:** Riley Hosp for Children, Hem/Onc, 702 Barnhill Drive, rm 4340, Indianapolis, IN 46202; **Phone:** 317-944-2143; **Board Cert:** Pediatrics 1985; Pediatric Hematology-Oncology 2005; **Med School:** Univ Pennsylvania 1980; **Resid:** Pediatrics, Childrens Hosp 1983; **Fellow:** Pediatric Hematology-Oncology, Childrens Hosp 1985; **Fac Appt:** Prof Ped, Indiana Univ

Davies, Stella M MD/PhD [PHO] - **Spec Exp:** Leukemia; Bone Marrow Transplant; Stem Cell Transplant; **Hospital:** Cincinnati Chldns Hosp Med Ctr; **Address:** Cincinnati Chldns Hosp Med Ctr, 3333 Burnet Ave, MLC 7015, Cincinnati, OH 45229-3039; **Phone:** 513-636-2469; **Med School:** England, UK 1981; **Resid:** Pediatrics, Univ Newcastle Med Ctr 1985; **Fellow:** Pediatric Hematology-Oncology, Univ Minn Med Ctr 1993; **Fac Appt:** Prof Ped, Univ Cincinnati

Fallon, Robert J MD/PhD [PHO] - **Spec Exp:** Lymphoma; Hodgkin's Disease; Stem Cell Transplant; **Hospital:** Riley Hosp for Children; **Address:** Riley Childrens Hospital, 702 Barnhill Drive, rm 4340, Indianapolis, IN 46202; **Phone:** 317-944-2143; **Board Cert:** Internal Medicine 1983; Medical Oncology 1985; **Med School:** NYU Sch Med 1980; **Resid:** Internal Medicine, Brigham & Womens Hosp 1983; **Fellow:** Hematology & Oncology, Brigham & Womens Hosp/Dana Farber Cancer Inst 1985; **Fac Appt:** Prof Ped, Indiana Univ

Ferrara, James MD [PHO] - **Spec Exp:** Bone Marrow Transplant; Graft vs Host Disease; **Hospital:** Univ of Michigan Hosp; **Address:** Univ Michigan Comprehensive Cancer Ctr, 1500 E Medical Center Drive, Ste 6308, Ann Arbor, MI 48109-5942; **Phone:** 734-615-1340; **Board Cert:** Pediatrics 2005; Pediatric Hematology-Oncology 2006; **Med School:** Georgetown Univ 1980; **Resid:** Pediatrics, Children's Hosp 1982; **Fellow:** Pediatric Hematology-Oncology, Children's Hosp 1985; **Fac Appt:** Prof Ped, Univ Mich Med Sch

Friebert, Sarah E MD [PHO] - **Spec Exp:** Palliative Care; Cancer Survivors-Late Effects of Therapy; **Hospital:** Akron Children's Hosp; **Address:** Children's Hosp Med Ctr of Akron, One Perkins Sq Fl 5, Akron, OH 44308; **Phone:** 330-543-3343; **Board Cert:** Pediatrics 2004; Pediatric Hematology-Oncology 2008; Hospice & Palliative Medicine 2008; **Med School:** Case West Res Univ 1993; **Resid:** Pediatrics, Chldns Hosp 1996; **Fellow:** Pediatric Hematology-Oncology, Rainbow Babies-Chldns Hosp 1999; **Fac Appt:** Asst Prof Ped, NE Ohio Univ

Goldman, Stewart MD [PHO] - **Spec Exp:** Neuro-Oncology; Brain Tumors; Clinical Trials; **Hospital:** Children's Mem Hosp -Chicago; **Address:** Childrens Meml Hosp, Div Hem/Onc, 2300 Childrens Plaza, Box 30, Chicago, IL 60614; **Phone:** 773-880-3004; **Board Cert:** Pediatric Hematology-Oncology 2011; **Med School:** Loyola Univ-Stritch Sch Med 1985; **Resid:** Pediatrics, Univ Chicago Hosps 1988; **Fellow:** Pediatric Hematology-Oncology, Univ Chicago Hosps 1991

Haut, Paul R MD [PHO] - **Spec Exp:** Stem Cell Transplant; Bone Marrow Transplant; Leukemia; **Hospital:** Riley Hosp for Children, IU Health North Hosp; **Address:** Riley Hospital for Children, 702 Barnhill Drive, rm 4340, Indianapolis, IN 46202; **Phone:** 317-944-2143; **Board Cert:** Pediatric Hematology-Oncology 2008; **Med School:** Univ Ark 1990; **Resid:** Pediatrics, Arkansas Children's Hosp 1994; **Fellow:** Pediatric Hematology-Oncology, Children's Meml Hosp 1997; **Fac Appt:** Prof Ped, Indiana Univ

Hayani, Ammar MD [PHO] - **Spec Exp:** Leukemia; Solid Tumors; Lymphoma; **Hospital:** Adv Christ Med Ctr, Adv Good Samaritan Hosp; **Address:** Hope Childrens Hosp, 4440 W 95th St, Oak Lawn, IL 60453-2600; **Phone:** 708-684-4094; **Board Cert:** Pediatric Hematology-Oncology 2005; **Med School:** Syria 1982; **Resid:** Pediatrics, LSU Hosp 1987; **Fellow:** Pediatric Hematology-Oncology, Baylor Affil Hosp 1991

Hayashi, Robert J MD [PHO] - **Spec Exp:** Bone Marrow Transplant; Cancer Survivors-Late Effects of Therapy; Leukemia; **Hospital:** St. Louis Chldns Hosp; **Address:** St Louis Chldns Hosp, Div Ped Hem Onc, One Children's Pl, Ste 9 South, Box 8116, St Louis, MO 63110; **Phone:** 314-454-6018; **Board Cert:** Pediatrics 2007; Pediatric Hematology-Oncology 2007; **Med School:** Washington Univ, St Louis 1986; **Resid:** Pediatrics, St Louis Childrens Hosp 1989; **Fellow:** Pediatric Hematology-Oncology, Johns Hopkins Hosp 1992; **Fac Appt:** Assoc Prof Ped, Washington Univ, St Louis

Hetherington, Maxine MD [PHO] - **Spec Exp:** Brain Tumors; **Hospital:** Chldns Mercy Hosps & Clinics; **Address:** Childrens Mercy Hosptial, 2401 Gillham Rd, Kansas City, MO 64108; **Phone:** 816-234-3265; **Board Cert:** Pediatrics 1983; Pediatric Hematology-Oncology 1987; **Med School:** Univ Tenn Coll Med 1978; **Resid:** Pediatrics, Childrens Med Ctr 1981; **Fellow:** Pediatric Hematology-Oncology, Univ Texas Hlth Sci Ctr 1987; **Fac Appt:** Assoc Prof Ped, Univ MO-Kansas City

Pediatric Hematology/Oncology

Hilden, Joanne M MD [PHO] - **Spec Exp:** Brain Tumors; Leukemia & Lymphoma; Bone Tumors; Soft Tissue Tumors; **Hospital:** St. Vincent Indianapolis Hosp; **Address:** Peyton Manning Chldn's Hosp, at St Vincent, 8402 Harcourt Rd, Ste 603, Indianapolis, IN 46260; **Phone:** 317-338-4673; **Board Cert:** Pediatrics 2006; Pediatric Hematology-Oncology 2009; Hospice & Palliative Medicine 2008; **Med School:** Univ Minn 1988; **Resid:** Pediatrics, Univ Minn Med Ctr 1991; **Fellow:** Pediatric Hematology-Oncology, Univ Minn Med Ctr 1994; **Fac Appt:** Assoc Prof Ped, Indiana Univ

Hord, Jeffrey D MD [PHO] - **Spec Exp:** Hematologic Malignancies; Bone Marrow Failure Disorders; Pediatric Cancers; **Hospital:** Akron Children's Hosp; **Address:** Akron Childrens Hosp, Hematology/Oncology, One Perkins Square, Akron, OH 44308; **Phone:** 330-543-8580; **Board Cert:** Pediatric Hematology-Oncology 2004; **Med School:** Univ KY Coll Med 1989; **Resid:** Pediatrics, Childrens Hosp 1992; **Fellow:** Pediatric Hematology-Oncology, Vanderbilt Univ Med Ctr 1995; **Fac Appt:** Prof Ped, NE Ohio Univ

Hutchinson, Raymond MD [PHO] - **Spec Exp:** Leukemia; Hodgkin's Disease; **Hospital:** Univ of Michigan Hosp; **Address:** Univ Michigan Hosp, 1500 E Med Ctr Drive, rm L2110, Level B1, 258 Reception B, Ann Arbor, MI 48109-5238; **Phone:** 734-936-9814; **Board Cert:** Pediatrics 1979; Pediatric Hematology-Oncology 1980; **Med School:** Harvard Med Sch 1973; **Resid:** Pediatrics, New England Med Ctr 1975; **Fellow:** Pediatric Hematology-Oncology, Childrens Hosp 1978; **Fac Appt:** Prof Ped, Univ Mich Med Sch

Lusher, Jeanne M MD [PHO] - **Hospital:** Chldns Hosp of Michigan; **Address:** Children's Hospital Michigan, Div Hem/Onc, 3901 Beaubien Blvd, Detroit, MI 48201; **Phone:** 313-745-5515; **Board Cert:** Pediatrics 1986; Pediatric Hematology-Oncology 1986; **Med School:** Univ Cincinnati 1960; **Resid:** Pediatrics, Charity Hosp/Tulane Univ 1963; **Fellow:** Hematology & Oncology, Charity Hosp/Tulane Univ 1965; Hematology & Oncology, Saint Louis Children's Hosp 1966; **Fac Appt:** Prof Ped, Wayne State Univ

Manera, Ricarchito B MD [PHO] - **Spec Exp:** Leukemia & Lymphoma; Brain Tumors; **Hospital:** Loyola Univ Med Ctr; **Address:** Loyola University Med Ctr, Div Pediatric Hematology/Oncology, 2160 S First Ave, Maywood, IL 60611; **Phone:** 708-327-9136; **Board Cert:** Pediatrics 2010; Pediatric Hematology-Oncology 2011; **Med School:** Philippines 1984; **Resid:** Pediatrics, Bronx-Lebanon Hosp Ctr 1995; **Fellow:** Pediatric Hematology-Oncology, MD Anderson Cancer Ctr 1994; Pediatric Hematology-Oncology, Columbia-Presby Med Ctr 1996; **Fac Appt:** Assoc Prof Ped, Loyola Univ-Stritch Sch Med

Morgan, Elaine MD [PHO] - **Spec Exp:** Leukemia; Palliative Care; Ethics; Langerhans Cell Histiocytosis (LCH); **Hospital:** Children's Mem Hosp -Chicago; **Address:** Children's Meml Hosp, Div Hem/Onc, 2300 Children's Plaza, Box 30, Chicago, IL 60614; **Phone:** 773-880-4562; **Board Cert:** Pediatrics 1976; Pediatric Hematology-Oncology 2009; Hospice & Palliative Medicine 2008; **Med School:** Univ Pennsylvania 1971; **Resid:** Pediatrics, Chldns Hosp 1974; **Fellow:** Pediatric Hematology-Oncology, Chldns Hosp Med Ctr 1975; Pediatric Hematology-Oncology, Chldns Meml Med Ctr 1976; **Fac Appt:** Prof Ped, Northwestern Univ-Feinberg Sch Med

Neglia, Joseph MD [PHO] - **Spec Exp:** Cancer Survivors-Late Effects of Therapy; **Address:** Univ Minnesota-Div Ped Hem/Oncology, 420 Delaware St SE, MMC 391, PWB 13-118, Minneapolis, MN 55455; **Phone:** 612-624-3113; **Board Cert:** Pediatrics 1986; Pediatric Hematology-Oncology 1987; **Med School:** Loma Linda Univ 1981; **Resid:** Pediatrics, Baylor Coll Med 1984; **Fellow:** Pediatric Hematology-Oncology, Univ Minn Hosp 1987; **Fac Appt:** Prof Ped, Univ Minn

O'Dorisio, M Sue MD/PhD [PHO] - **Spec Exp:** Neuroblastoma; Medulloblastoma; Neuroendocrine Tumors; **Hospital:** Univ Iowa Hosp & Clinics; **Address:** UIHC Dept Pediatrics, Div Hematology/Oncology, 200 Hawkins Drive, 2520 JCP, Iowa City, IA 52242; **Phone:** 319-356-7873; **Board Cert:** Pediatrics 2007; Pediatric Hematology-Oncology 2009; **Med School:** Ohio State Univ 1985; **Resid:** Pediatrics, Chldns Hosp 1988; **Fellow:** Pediatric Hematology-Oncology, Chldns Hosp 1992; **Fac Appt:** Prof Ped, Univ Iowa Coll Med

Olshefski, Randal S MD [PHO] - **Spec Exp:** Brain Tumors; **Hospital:** Nationwide Chldn's Hosp; **Address:** Nationwide Chldn's Hosp: Hemology/Onc, 700 Children's Drive, Columbus, OH 43205; **Phone:** 614-722-3552; **Board Cert:** Pediatric Hematology-Oncology 2004; **Med School:** Univ Pittsburgh 1988; **Resid:** Pediatrics, Nationwide Chldn's Hosp 1991; **Fellow:** Hematology & Oncology, Children's Natl Med Ctr 1995; **Fac Appt:** Clin Prof Ped, Ohio State Univ

Plautz, Gregory E MD [PHO] - **Spec Exp:** Brain Tumors; Leukemia & Lymphoma; Wilms' Tumor; Cancer Survivors-Late Effects of Therapy; **Hospital:** Cleveland Clin (page 70); **Address:** Cleveland Clinic Fdn - Div Ped Hem Onc, 9500 Euclid Ave, Cleveland, OH 44195; **Phone:** 216-445-4044; **Board Cert:** Pediatric Hematology-Oncology 2005; **Med School:** Indiana Univ 1984; **Resid:** Pediatrics, Johns Hopkins Hosp 1987; **Fellow:** Pediatric Hematology-Oncology, Univ Michigan Affil Hosp 1990; **Fac Appt:** Assoc Prof Ped, Case West Res Univ

Puccetti, Diane M MD [PHO] - **Spec Exp:** Brain Tumors; Neuro-Oncology; Cancer Survivors-Late Effects of Therapy; **Hospital:** Univ WI Hosp & Clins; **Address:** Univ Wisconsin Childrens Hosp, 1111 Highland Ave, 4105 WIMR, Madison, WI 53792; **Phone:** 608-263-6420; **Board Cert:** Pediatric Hematology-Oncology 2007; **Med School:** Med Coll OH 1985; **Resid:** Pediatrics, UC-Irvine Med Ctr 1986; Pediatrics, Med Coll Ohio 1988; **Fellow:** Pediatric Hematology-Oncology, Riley Hosp Chldn 1991; **Fac Appt:** Assoc Clin Prof Ped, Univ Wisc

Razzouk, Bassem I MD [PHO] - **Spec Exp:** Leukemia; Clinical Trials; Lymphoma; Langerhans Cell Histiocytosis (LCH); **Hospital:** St. Vincent Indianapolis Hosp; **Address:** Peyton Manning Chldns Hosp, Center for Cancer & Blood Diseases, 2001 W 86th St, Indianapolis, IN 46260; **Phone:** 317-338-4673; **Board Cert:** Pediatrics 2008; Pediatric Hematology-Oncology 2004; **Med School:** Lebanon 1987; **Resid:** Pediatrics, American Univ Med Ctr 1990; Pediatrics, SUNY Hlth Sci Ctr 1992; **Fellow:** Hematology & Oncology, St. Jude Chldns Rsch Hosp 1995

Rubin, Charles M MD [PHO] - **Spec Exp:** Brain Tumors; Retinoblastoma; Bone Marrow Transplant; **Hospital:** Univ Chicago-Comer Chldn's Hosp; **Address:** Univ Chicago Med Ctr, 5841 S Maryland Ave, MC 4060, Chicago, IL 60637; **Phone:** 773-702-6808; **Board Cert:** Pediatrics 1984; Clinical Cytogenetics 1987; Pediatric Hematology-Oncology 1984; **Med School:** Tufts Univ 1979; **Resid:** Pediatrics, Chldn's Hosp 1982; Pediatric Hematology-Oncology, Univ Minnesota Hosp 1985; **Fellow:** Cytogenetics, Univ Chicago-Pritzker School of Med 1987; **Fac Appt:** Assoc Prof Ped, Univ Chicago-Pritzker Sch Med

Salvi, Sharad MD [PHO] - **Spec Exp:** Leukemia & Lymphoma; Solid Tumors; **Hospital:** Adv Christ Med Ctr, Central DuPage Hosp; **Address:** Hope Chldns Hosp, 4440 W 95th St, Oak Lawn, IL 60453; **Phone:** 708-684-4094; **Board Cert:** Pediatrics 1982; Pediatric Hematology-Oncology 1982; **Med School:** India 1974; **Resid:** Pediatrics, Lincoln Meml Hosp 1979; **Fellow:** Pediatric Hematology-Oncology, Chldns Hosp/Roswell Park Meml Cancer Inst 1981

Sencer, Susan F MD [PHO] - **Spec Exp:** Pediatric Cancers; Complementary Medicine; **Hospital:** Chldns Hosp and Clinics - Minneapolis; **Address:** Chldns Specialty Clinic, Hem/Onc Clin, 2525 Chicago Ave S, Ste CSC-175, Minneapolis, MN 55404; **Phone:** 612-813-5940; **Board Cert:** Pediatric Hematology-Oncology 2007; **Med School:** Univ Minn 1984; **Resid:** Pediatrics, Univ Minnesota Affil Hosp 1988; **Fellow:** Pediatric Hematology-Oncology, Univ Minnesota Affil Hosp 1991

Pediatric Hematology/Oncology

Sondel, Paul M MD/PhD [PHO] - **Spec Exp:** Immunotherapy; Stem Cell Transplant; Pediatric Cancers; **Hospital:** Univ WI Hosp & Clins; **Address:** 4159 WIMR, 1111 Highland Ave, Madison, WI 53705; **Phone:** 608-263-6200; **Board Cert:** Pediatrics 1981; **Med School:** Harvard Med Sch 1977; **Resid:** Pediatrics, Univ MN Hosp 1978; Pediatrics, Univ Wisconsin Hosp 1980; **Fellow:** Research, Sidney Farber Cancer Inst/Harvard 1977; **Fac Appt:** Prof Ped, Univ Wisc

Tannous, Raymond MD [PHO] - **Spec Exp:** Wilms' Tumor; Leukemia & Lymphoma; Pain-Cancer; **Hospital:** Univ Iowa Hosp & Clinics; **Address:** Univ Iowa Hosps & Clinics, Dept Peds, 200 Hawkins Drive, rm 2528 JCP, Iowa City, IA 52242; **Phone:** 319-356-2229; **Board Cert:** Pediatrics 1976; Pediatric Hematology-Oncology 1978; **Med School:** France 1972; **Resid:** Pediatrics, St Jude Chldns Rsch Hosp 1976; **Fellow:** Pediatric Hematology-Oncology, St Jude Chldns Rsch Hosp 1977; **Fac Appt:** Assoc Prof Ped, Univ Iowa Coll Med

Vik, Terry A MD [PHO] - **Spec Exp:** Neuroblastoma; Clinical Trials; Cancer Survivors-Late Effects of Therapy; Leukemia; **Hospital:** Riley Hosp for Children; **Address:** Riley Hosp Children, 702 Barnhill Drive, rm 4340, Indianapolis, IN 46202; **Phone:** 317-944-2143; **Board Cert:** Pediatrics 1987; Pediatric Hematology-Oncology 2004; **Med School:** Johns Hopkins Univ 1983; **Resid:** Pediatrics, UCLA Med Ctr 1986; **Fellow:** Pediatric Hematology-Oncology, Chldns Hosp/Dana Farber 1989; **Fac Appt:** Assoc Prof Ped, Indiana Univ

Yaddanapudi, Ravindranath MD [PHO] - **Spec Exp:** Leukemia; **Hospital:** Chldns Hosp of Michigan; **Address:** Children's Hospital Michigan, Div Hem/Onc, 3901 Beaubien Blvd, Detroit, MI 48201; **Phone:** 313-745-5515; **Board Cert:** Pediatrics 1970; Pediatric Hematology-Oncology 1974; **Med School:** India 1964; **Resid:** Pathology, Western Penn Hosp 1967; Pediatrics, Children's Hosp 1969; **Fellow:** Pediatric Hematology-Oncology, Children's Hosp Michigan 1971; **Fac Appt:** Prof Ped, Wayne State Univ

Great Plains and Mountains

Abromowitch, Minnie MD [PHO] - **Hospital:** Children's Hosp - Omaha; **Address:** Children's Hosp & Med Ctr, Dept Pediatric Hem Onc, 8200 Dodge St, Omaha, NE 68114; **Phone:** 402-955-3950; **Board Cert:** Pediatrics 1980; Pediatric Hematology-Oncology 1982; **Med School:** Univ Manitoba 1973; **Resid:** Pediatrics, Hospital for Sick Children 1976; Pediatric Hematology-Oncology, Univ Manitoba 1978; **Fellow:** Pediatric Hematology-Oncology, St Jude Chldns Research Hosp 1980; **Fac Appt:** Assoc Prof Ped, Univ Nebr Coll Med

Bruggers, Carol S MD [PHO] - **Spec Exp:** Brain Tumors; Clinical Trials; **Hospital:** Primary Children's Med Ctr, Univ Utah Hlth Care; **Address:** Primary Children's Medical Ctr, 100 Mario Capecchi Drive, Salt Lake City, UT 84113; **Phone:** 801-662-4700; **Board Cert:** Pediatrics 2008; Pediatric Hematology-Oncology 2008; **Med School:** Mich State Univ 1984; **Resid:** Pediatrics, Univ Colorado Health Sci Ctr 1987; **Fellow:** Pediatric Hematology-Oncology, Duke Univ Med Ctr 1991; **Fac Appt:** Prof Ped, Univ Utah

Coccia, Peter F MD [PHO] - **Spec Exp:** Bone Marrow Transplant; Leukemia & Lymphoma; Solid Tumors; **Hospital:** Nebraska Med Ctr, Children's Hosp - Omaha; **Address:** Univ Nebr Med Ctr, Dept Pediatrics, 982168 Nebraska Med Ctr, Omaha, NE 68198-2168; **Phone:** 402-559-7257; **Board Cert:** Clinical Pathology 1972; Hematology 1975; Pediatrics 1976; Pediatric Hematology-Oncology 1976; **Med School:** SUNY Upstate Med Univ 1968; **Resid:** Pathology, Upstate Med Ctr 1970; Pediatrics, Univ Minn 1973; **Fellow:** Pediatric Hematology-Oncology, Univ Minn 1974; **Fac Appt:** Prof Ped, Univ Nebr Coll Med

Kobrinsky, Nathan L MD [PHO] - **Spec Exp:** Pediatric Cancers; Immunotherapy; **Hospital:** Sanford Med Ctr Fargo; **Address:** Sanford Roger Maris Cancer Ctr, 820 4th St N, Fargo, ND 58122; **Phone:** 701-234-7544; **Board Cert:** Pediatrics 1981; Pediatric Hematology-Oncology 1982; **Med School:** Univ Manitoba 1976; **Resid:** Pediatrics, Chldns Hlth Sci Ctr 1978; **Fellow:** Pediatric Hematology-Oncology, Chldns Hlth Sci Ctr 1979; Pediatric Hematology-Oncology, Univ Minn 1981; **Fac Appt:** Prof Ped, Univ ND Sch Med

Southwest

Albritton, Karen H MD [PHO] - **Spec Exp:** Sarcoma; **Hospital:** Cook Chldns Med Ctr; **Address:** Cook Childrens Med Ctr, Hematology/Oncology Clinic, 901 7th Ave, Ste 220, Fort Worth, TX 76104; **Phone:** 682-885-4007; **Board Cert:** Pediatric Hematology-Oncology 2002; Medical Oncology 2001; **Med School:** Univ Tex, San Antonio 1992; **Resid:** Internal Medicine & Pediatrics, Univ NC Hosps 1996; **Fellow:** Hematology & Oncology, Univ NC Hosps 2000

Berg, Stacey MD [PHO] - **Spec Exp:** Drug Discovery & Development; Brain Tumors; Solid Tumors; **Hospital:** Texas Chldns Hosp; **Address:** Texas Chldns Cancer Ctr, Dept Ped Hem-Onc, 6701 Fannin St, Ste CC 1400, Houston, TX 77030; **Phone:** 832-822-4242; **Board Cert:** Pediatrics 2007; Pediatric Hematology-Oncology 2007; **Med School:** Univ Pittsburgh 1985; **Resid:** Pediatrics, Chldns Hosp 1988; **Fellow:** Pediatric Hematology-Oncology, Natl Inst Hlth 1991; **Fac Appt:** Prof Ped, Baylor Coll Med

Blaney, Susan MD [PHO] - **Spec Exp:** Brain Tumors; Neuro-Oncology; Drug Development; Clinical Trials; **Hospital:** Texas Chldns Hosp; **Address:** 6701 Fannin St, Ste 1410.00, Houston, TX 77030; **Phone:** 832-822-1482; **Board Cert:** Pediatric Hematology-Oncology 2005; **Med School:** Med Coll OH 1984; **Resid:** Pediatrics, Letterman AMC 1987; **Fellow:** Pediatric Oncology, Walter Reed AMC 1990; **Fac Appt:** Prof Ped, Baylor Coll Med

Dreyer, ZoAnn E MD [PHO] - **Spec Exp:** Cancer Survivors-Late Effects of Therapy; Leukemia in Infants; **Hospital:** Texas Chldns Hosp; **Address:** Texas Childrens Hosp, Clinical Care Ctr, 6701 Fannin St Fl 14, MC CC1400, Houston, TX 77030; **Phone:** 832-822-4242; **Board Cert:** Pediatrics 1988; Pediatric Hematology-Oncology 2005; **Med School:** UC Davis 1982; **Resid:** Pediatrics, Baylor Affil Hosps 1985; **Fellow:** Pediatric Hematology-Oncology, Baylor Coll Med 1988; **Fac Appt:** Assoc Prof Ped, Baylor Coll Med

Goldman, Stanton C MD [PHO] - **Spec Exp:** Leukemia; Lymphoma; Stem Cell Transplant; **Hospital:** Med City Dallas Hosp; **Address:** 7777 Forest Ln, Ste D400, Dallas, TX 75230; **Phone:** 972-566-6647; **Board Cert:** Pediatric Hematology-Oncology 2004; Pediatrics 2008; **Med School:** Boston Univ 1990; **Resid:** Pediatrics, Chldns Natl Med Ctr 1996; **Fellow:** Pediatric Hematology-Oncology, Johns Hopkins Hosp

Graham, Michael L MD [PHO] - **Spec Exp:** Bone Marrow Transplant; Leukemia; Stem Cell Transplant; **Hospital:** Banner Desert Med Ctr; **Address:** Cardon Chldns Med Ctr, Div Pediatric Hematology/Oncology, 1432 S Dobson Rd, Ste 107, Mesa, AZ 85202; **Phone:** 480-412-4100; **Board Cert:** Pediatrics 1980; Pediatric Hematology-Oncology 1984; **Med School:** Brown Univ 1975; **Resid:** Pediatrics, Johns Hopkins Hosp 1978; Pediatric Hematology-Oncology, Johns Hopkins Hosp 1980; **Fellow:** Medical Oncology, Yale-New Haven Hosp 1982; **Fac Appt:** Assoc Prof Ped, Univ Ariz Coll Med

Pediatric Hematology/Oncology

Meyer, William H MD [PHO] - **Spec Exp:** Sarcoma; Pediatric Cancers; **Hospital:** Chldns Hosp OU Med Ctr; **Address:** OU Childrens Physicians, 1200 N Phillips Ave, Ste 10000, Oklahoma City, OK 73104; **Phone:** 405-271-4412; **Board Cert:** Pediatrics 1980; Pediatric Hematology-Oncology 1980; **Med School:** Jefferson Med Coll 1974; **Resid:** Pediatrics, Wilmington Med Ctr 1977; **Fellow:** Pediatric Hematology-Oncology, Johns Hopkins Hosp 1980; **Fac Appt:** Prof Ped, Univ Okla Coll Med

Tomlinson, Gail E MD [PHO] - **Spec Exp:** Cancer Survivors-Late Effects of Therapy; Cancer Genetics; Liver Cancer; Kidney Cancer; **Hospital:** Christus Santa Rosa Children's Hosp, Univ Hlth Syst-San Antonio; **Address:** UT HSC at San Antonio, 7703 Floyd Curl Drive, MC 7810, San Antonio, TX 78229; **Phone:** 210-704-3405; **Board Cert:** Pediatrics 2008; Pediatric Hematology-Oncology 2009; **Med School:** Geo Wash Univ 1984; **Resid:** Pediatrics, Chldns Hosp Natl Med Ctr 1987; **Fellow:** Pediatric Hematology-Oncology, MD Anderson Cancer Ctr 1989; Pediatric Hematology-Oncology, Univ Texas SW Med Ctr 1992; **Fac Appt:** Prof Ped, Univ Tex, San Antonio

Williams, James A MD [PHO] - **Spec Exp:** Sarcoma; Leukemia; **Hospital:** Banner Desert Med Ctr, St. Joseph's Hosp & Med Ctr - Phoenix; **Address:** 1919 E Thomas Rd, Phoenix, AZ 85016; **Phone:** 602-546-0920; **Board Cert:** Pediatric Hematology-Oncology 2008; **Med School:** Wayne State Univ 1993; **Resid:** Pediatrics, Wayne St Univ Med Ctr 1996; **Fellow:** Pediatric Hematology-Oncology, Wayne St Univ Med Ctr 1999

Winick, Naomi J MD [PHO] - **Spec Exp:** Leukemia; **Hospital:** Chldns Med Ctr of Dallas; **Address:** Ctr for Cancer & Blood Disorders, 1935 Med District Drive Brides Bldg Fl 3, Dallas, TX 75235-7794; **Phone:** 214-456-2382; **Board Cert:** Pediatrics 1984; Pediatric Hematology-Oncology 1987; **Med School:** Northwestern Univ 1978; **Resid:** Pediatrics, Babies Hosp-Columbia Presbyterian Med Ctr 1981; **Fellow:** Pediatric Hematology-Oncology, Sloan-Kettering Cancer Ctr 1983; **Fac Appt:** Prof Ped, Univ Tex SW, Dallas

West Coast and Pacific

Andrews, Robert G MD [PHO] - **Spec Exp:** Bone Marrow Transplant; Leukemia; Lymphoma; **Hospital:** Seattle Chldns Hosp; **Address:** 1100 Fairview Ave N, D2-373, PO Box 19024, Seattle, WA 98109; **Phone:** 206-667-5000; **Board Cert:** Pediatrics 1984; Pediatric Hematology-Oncology 1984; **Med School:** Univ Minn 1976; **Resid:** Pediatrics, New England Med Ctr 1979; **Fellow:** Pediatric Hematology-Oncology, Children's Hosp Med Ctr 1983; **Fac Appt:** Assoc Prof Ped, Univ Wash

Banerjee, Anuradha MD [PHO] - **Spec Exp:** Brain Tumors; **Hospital:** UCSF Med Ctr; **Address:** UC San Francisco, Div Ped Oncology/Neuro Oncology, 400 Parnassus Ave, rm A808, Box 0372, San Francisco, CA 94107; **Phone:** 415-353-2986; **Board Cert:** Pediatrics 2004; Pediatric Hematology-Oncology 2004; **Med School:** Tulane Univ 1992; **Resid:** Pediatrics, UCSF Med Ctr 1996; **Fellow:** Pediatric Hematology-Oncology, UCSF Med Ctr 1997; **Fac Appt:** Assoc Clin Prof Ped, UCSF

Ducore, Jonathan M MD [PHO] - **Spec Exp:** Brain Tumors; Bone & Soft Tissue Tumors; **Hospital:** UC Davis Med Ctr; **Address:** UC Davis Med Ctr, Dept Pediatrics, Div Pediatric Hematology/Oncology, 2521 Stockton Blvd, Sacramento, CA 95817; **Phone:** 916-734-8336; **Board Cert:** Pediatrics 1978; Pediatric Hematology-Oncology 1978; **Med School:** Duke Univ 1973; **Resid:** Pediatrics, Chldns Med Ctr 1975; **Fellow:** Pediatric Hematology-Oncology, Univ Colorado Med Ctr 1977; Cancer Research, Natl Cancer Inst 1980; **Fac Appt:** Assoc Prof Ped, UC Davis

Finklestein, Jerry Z MD [PHO] - **Spec Exp:** Cancer Survivors-Late Effects of Therapy; Anemias & Red Cell Disorders; **Hospital:** Long Beach Meml Med Ctr, LAC - Harbor - UCLA Med Ctr; **Address:** 2653 Elm Ave, Ste 200, Long Beach, CA 90806-1652; **Phone:** 562-728-5000; **Board Cert:** Pediatrics 1980; Pediatric Hematology-Oncology 1974; **Med School:** McGill Univ 1963; **Resid:** Pediatrics, Montreal Chldns Hosp 1966; **Fellow:** Pediatric Hematology-Oncology, LA Chldns Hosp 1968; **Fac Appt:** Clin Prof Ped, UCLA

Finlay, Jonathan MD [PHO] - **Spec Exp:** Brain Tumors; **Hospital:** Chldns Hosp - Los Angeles, Chldns Hosp - Oakland; **Address:** 4650 Sunset Blvd, MS 54, Los Angeles, CA 90027-6016; **Phone:** 323-361-8147; **Board Cert:** Pediatrics 1984; Pediatric Hematology-Oncology 1987; **Med School:** England, UK 1973; **Resid:** Pediatrics, Univ Birmingham 1975; Pediatrics, Christie Hosp 1976; **Fellow:** Pediatric Allergy & Immunology, Univ Wisconsin Hosp 1978; Pediatric Hematology-Oncology, Univ Wisconsin Hosp 1980; **Fac Appt:** Prof Ped, USC-Keck School of Medicine

Geyer, J Russell MD [PHO] - **Spec Exp:** Pediatric Cancers; Neuro-Oncology; Brain Tumors; **Hospital:** Seattle Chldns Hosp, Univ Wash Med Ctr; **Address:** Seattle Chldns Hosp - Div Hem/Onc, 4800 Sand Point Way NE, MS B-6553, Seattle, WA 98105; **Phone:** 206-987-2106; **Board Cert:** Pediatrics 1983; Pediatric Hematology-Oncology 1987; **Med School:** Wayne State Univ 1977; **Resid:** Pediatrics, Chldns Hosp Michigan 1980; **Fellow:** Pediatric Hematology-Oncology, Univ Michigan Med Ctr 1981; **Fac Appt:** Prof Ped, Univ Wash

Hawkins, Douglas MD [PHO] - **Spec Exp:** Bone Tumors; Ewing's Sarcoma; Leukemia; Rhabdomyosarcoma; **Hospital:** Seattle Chldns Hosp; **Address:** Children's Hosp & Regl Med Ctr, 4800 Sand Point Way NE, MS B6553, Seattle, WA 98105; **Phone:** 206-987-2106; **Board Cert:** Pediatric Hematology-Oncology 2004; **Med School:** Harvard Med Sch 1990; **Resid:** Pediatrics, Univ Washington Med Ctr 1993; **Fellow:** Pediatric Hematology-Oncology, Fred Hutchinson Cancer Research Ctr 1996; **Fac Appt:** Assoc Prof Ped, Univ Wash

Horn, Biljana N MD [PHO] - **Spec Exp:** Bone Marrow Transplant; Brain Tumors; Stem Cell Transplant; Immunotherapy; **Hospital:** UCSF Med Ctr; **Address:** UCSF Med Ctr, Pediatric BMT Prgm, 505 Parnassus Ave, rm M-659, San Francisco, CA 94143; **Phone:** 415-476-2188; **Board Cert:** Pediatrics 2006; Pediatric Hematology-Oncology 2004; **Med School:** Croatia 1983; **Resid:** Pediatrics, Rainbow Babies & Chldns Hosp 1991; **Fellow:** Pediatric Hematology-Oncology, Natl Cancer Inst 1994; Pediatric Neuro-Oncology, UCSF Med Ctr 1998; **Fac Appt:** Assoc Prof Ped, UCSF

Kapoor, Neena MD [PHO] - **Spec Exp:** Bone Marrow Transplant; **Hospital:** Chldns Hosp - Los Angeles; **Address:** Chlds Hosp LA-Rsch Immunology/BMT, 4650 Sunset Blvd, MS 62, Los Angeles, CA 90027; **Phone:** 323-361-2546; **Board Cert:** Pediatrics 1978; **Med School:** India 1972; **Resid:** Pediatrics, Rhode Island Hosp 1976; **Fellow:** Pediatric Hematology-Oncology, Meml Sloan-Kettering Cancer Ctr 1978; **Fac Appt:** Prof Ped, USC Sch Med

Kung, Faith H MD [PHO] - **Spec Exp:** Leukemia & Lymphoma; Bleeding/Coagulation Disorders; Cancer Survivors-Late Effects of Therapy; **Hospital:** Rady Children's Hosp - San Diego; **Address:** UCSD Med Ctr, Div Ped Hem/Oncology, 200 W Arbor Drive, San Diego, CA 92103-8447; **Phone:** 619-543-6844; **Board Cert:** Pediatrics 1967; Pediatric Hematology-Oncology 1974; **Med School:** Univ VA Sch Med 1957; **Resid:** Pediatrics, NC Meml Hosp 1960; **Fellow:** Pediatric Hematology-Oncology, Chldns Hosp/Babies Hosp 1962; **Fac Appt:** Prof Ped, UCSD

Link, Michael P MD [PHO] - **Spec Exp:** Stem Cell Transplant; **Hospital:** Lucile Packard Chldn's Hosp, Stanford Univ Hosp & Clinics; **Address:** 1000 Welch Rd, Ste 300, Palo Alto, CA 94304; **Phone:** 650-723-5535; **Board Cert:** Pediatrics 1979; Pediatric Hematology-Oncology 1980; **Med School:** Stanford Univ 1974; **Resid:** Pediatrics, Chldns Hosp Med Ctr 1976; **Fellow:** Hematology & Oncology, Dana Farber Cancer Inst 1979; **Fac Appt:** Prof Ped, Stanford Univ

Pediatric Hematology/Oncology

Marina, Neyssa MD [PHO] - **Spec Exp:** Sarcoma; Cancer Survivors-Late Effects of Therapy; Germ Cell Tumors; **Hospital:** Lucile Packard Chldn's Hosp; **Address:** Pediatric Hematology & Oncology, 725 Walsh Rd, Palo Alto, CA 94304; **Phone:** 650-497-8953; **Board Cert:** Pediatrics 1987; Pediatric Hematology-Oncology 2005; **Med School:** Puerto Rico 1983; **Resid:** Pediatrics, Univ Pediatric Hosp 1986; **Fellow:** Pediatric Hematology-Oncology, St Jude Children's Hosp 1989; **Fac Appt:** Prof Ped, Stanford Univ

Matthay, Katherine K MD [PHO] - **Spec Exp:** Neuroblastoma; Bone Marrow & Stem Cell Transplant; **Hospital:** UCSF Med Ctr; **Address:** UCSF, Dept Ped Onc, 505 Parnassus Ave, Box 0106, San Francisco, CA 94143; **Phone:** 415-476-0603; **Board Cert:** Pediatrics 1979; Pediatric Hematology-Oncology 1980; **Med School:** Univ Pennsylvania 1973; **Resid:** Pediatrics, Univ Colorado 1976; **Fellow:** Pediatric Hematology-Oncology, UCSF 1979; **Fac Appt:** Prof Ped, UCSF

Nicholson, H Stacy MD [PHO] - **Spec Exp:** Brain Tumors; Cancer Survivors-Late Effects of Therapy; Histiocytoma; **Hospital:** Doernbecher Chldns Hosp/OHSU, OR Hlth & Sci Univ; **Address:** OR Hlth Scis Univ, 707 SW Gaines Rd, CDRCP, Portland, OR 97239; **Phone:** 503-494-4265; **Board Cert:** Pediatrics 2008; Pediatric Hematology-Oncology 2007; **Med School:** Med Coll GA 1985; **Resid:** Pediatrics, Chldns National Med Ctr 1988; **Fellow:** Pediatric Hematology-Oncology, Chldns National Med Ctr 1991; **Fac Appt:** Prof Ped, Oregon Hlth & Sci Univ

Park, Julie MD [PHO] - **Spec Exp:** Pediatric Cancers; Neuroblastoma; Lymphoma, Non-Hodgkin's; **Hospital:** Seattle Chldns Hosp; **Address:** Seattle Chldn's-Hem/Onc Dept, 4800 Sandpoint Way NE, Box B6553, Seattle, WA 98105; **Phone:** 206-987-2106; **Board Cert:** Pediatric Hematology-Oncology 2004; **Med School:** Univ VT Coll Med 1988; **Resid:** Pediatrics, Univ Wash Affil Hosp 1991; **Fellow:** Pediatric Hematology-Oncology, Univ Wash/Fred Hutchinson Cancer Rsch Ctr 1994; Pediatric Hematology-Oncology, Leukemia Soc/Fred Hutchinson Cancer Rsch Ctr 1996; **Fac Appt:** Assoc Prof Ped, Univ Wash

Pendergrass, Thomas W MD [PHO] - **Spec Exp:** Pediatric Cancers; Retinoblastoma; **Hospital:** Seattle Chldns Hosp, Univ Wash Med Ctr; **Address:** Seattle Chldn's Hosp, 4800 Sandpoint Way NE, Box 5371, MS B6553, Seattle, WA 98105; **Phone:** 206-987-2106; **Board Cert:** Pediatrics 1978; **Med School:** Univ Tenn Coll Med 1971; **Resid:** Pediatrics, Children's Memorial Hosp 1973; **Fellow:** Pediatric Hematology-Oncology, Children's Hosp Med Ctr 1977; **Fac Appt:** Prof Ped, Univ Wash

Rosenthal, Joseph MD [PHO] - **Spec Exp:** Bone Marrow Transplant; Clinical Trials; **Hospital:** Chldns Hosp Central CA; **Address:** Valley Children's Hospital, 9300 Valley Children's Pl, Madera, CA 93636; **Phone:** 559-353-5490 x68442; **Board Cert:** Pediatrics 2003; Pediatric Hematology-Oncology 2004; **Med School:** Israel 1984; **Resid:** Pediatrics, Soroka Med Ctr 1988; Pediatrics, Chldn Hosp 1995; **Fellow:** Pediatric Hematology-Oncology, Univ Colorado Affil Hosp 1991; Pediatric Hematology-Oncology, Chldn Hosp 1994; **Fac Appt:** Assoc Prof Ped, USC-Keck School of Medicine

Sakamoto, Kathleen M MD [PHO] - **Spec Exp:** Leukemia; Pediatric Cancers; Bone Marrow Transplant; **Hospital:** Mattel Chldns Hosp at UCLA; **Address:** Mattel Chldns Hosp UCLA, Div Hem-Onc, David Geffen Sch Med, 10833 Le Conte Ave, Los Angeles, CA 90095-1752; **Phone:** 310-825-6708; **Board Cert:** Pediatrics 2007; Pediatric Hematology-Oncology 2007; **Med School:** Univ Cincinnati 1985; **Resid:** Pediatrics, Chldn's Hosp 1988; **Fellow:** Pediatric Hematology-Oncology, Chldn's Hosp 1991; **Fac Appt:** Prof Ped, UCLA

Siegel, Stuart E MD [PHO] - **Spec Exp:** Leukemia & Lymphoma; Infections in Cancer Patients; Psychosocial Support in Childhood Cancer; Solid Tumors; **Hospital:** Chldns Hosp - Los Angeles, Ventura Cnty Med Ctr; **Address:** Chldns Hosp, 4650 Sunset Blvd, MS 54, Los Angeles, CA 90027-6062; **Phone:** 323-361-2205; **Board Cert:** Pediatrics 1973; Pediatric Hematology-Oncology 1976; **Med School:** Boston Univ 1967; **Resid:** Pediatrics, Univ Minnesota Hosps 1969; **Fellow:** Pediatric Hematology-Oncology, Natl Cancer Inst 1972; **Fac Appt:** Prof Ped, USC-Keck School of Medicine

Thomas, Gregory A MD [PHO] - **Spec Exp:** Palliative Care; Anemias & Red Cell Disorders; Bleeding/Coagulation Disorders; **Hospital:** Doernbecher Chldns Hosp/OHSU; **Address:** 707 SW Gaines Rd, MC 1104-CDRCP, Portland, OR 97239; **Phone:** 503-346-0644; **Board Cert:** Pediatrics 1986; Pediatric Hematology-Oncology 2005; **Med School:** Oregon Hlth & Sci Univ 1981; **Resid:** Pediatrics, Univ Utah Med Ctr 1984; **Fellow:** Pediatric Hematology-Oncology, Univ Utah Med Ctr 1987; **Fac Appt:** Assoc Prof Ped, Oregon Hlth & Sci Univ

PEDIATRIC ALLERGY & IMMUNOLOGY

Mid Atlantic

Kamani, Naynesh R MD [PA&I] - **Spec Exp:** Stem Cell Transplant; Immunotherapy; Bone Marrow Transplant; **Hospital:** Chldns Natl Med Ctr; **Address:** Chldns Natl Med Ctr, Div Hematology, 111 Michigan Ave NW, Washington, DC 20010; **Phone:** 202-476-2140; **Board Cert:** Pediatrics 1983; Allergy & Immunology 1983; Diagnostic Lab Immunology 1986; **Med School:** Ethiopia 1975; **Resid:** Pediatrics, Downstate Med Ctr-Kings Co Hosp 1981; **Fellow:** Pediatric Allergy & Immunology, Chldns Hosp 1983; **Fac Appt:** Prof Ped, Geo Wash Univ

West Coast and Pacific

Cowan, Morton J MD [PA&I] - **Spec Exp:** Bone Marrow Transplant; **Hospital:** UCSF Med Ctr; **Address:** UCSF Med Ctr, Peds BMT Program, 505 Parnassus Ave, rm M659, San Francisco, CA 94143-1278; **Phone:** 415-476-2188; **Board Cert:** Pediatrics 1981; Allergy & Immunology 1983; **Med School:** Univ Pennsylvania 1970; **Resid:** Surgery, Duke Univ Med Ctr 1972; Pediatrics, UCSF Med Ctr 1977; **Fellow:** Research, Natl Inst Hlth 1975; Immunology, UCSF Med Ctr 1979; **Fac Appt:** Prof Ped, UCSF

PEDIATRIC CARDIOLOGY

Mid Atlantic

Steinherz, Laurel MD [PCd] - **Spec Exp:** Cardiac Effects of Cancer/Cancer Therapy; **Hospital:** Meml Sloan-Kettering Cancer Ctr (page 75), NY-Presby Hosp/Weill Cornell (page 78); **Address:** 1275 York Avenue, New York, NY 10065; **Phone:** 212-639-8103; **Board Cert:** Pediatrics 1976; Pediatric Cardiology 1978; **Med School:** Albert Einstein Coll Med 1970; **Resid:** Pediatrics, Chldns Hosp 1972; **Fellow:** Pediatric Cardiology, NY Hosp-Cornell Med Ctr 1975; **Fac Appt:** Prof Ped, Cornell Univ-Weill Med Coll

PEDIATRIC ENDOCRINOLOGY

Mid Atlantic

Sklar, Charles A MD [PEn] - Spec Exp: Cancer Survivors-Late Effects of Therapy; Growth Disorders in Childhood Cancer; **Hospital:** Meml Sloan-Kettering Cancer Ctr (page 75); **Address:** 1275 York Avenue, New York, NY 10065; **Phone:** 800-525-2225; **Board Cert:** Pediatrics 1979; Pediatric Endocrinology 1980; **Med School:** USC Sch Med 1974; **Resid:** Pediatrics, Childrens Hosp 1976; **Fellow:** Pediatric Endocrinology, UCSF Med Ctr 1979; **Fac Appt:** Assoc Prof Ped, Cornell Univ-Weill Med Coll

Southeast

Meacham, Lillian R MD [PEn] - **Spec Exp:** Growth Disorders in Childhood Cancer; Cancer Survivors-Late Effects of Therapy; **Hospital:** Chldns Hlthcare Atlanta @ Egleston, Chldns Hlthcare Atlanta @ Scottish Rite; **Address:** Aflac Outpatient Center, 1405 Clifton Rd NE, 4th Fl, Tower 1, Atlanta, GA 30322; **Phone:** 404-785-1200; **Board Cert:** Pediatrics 2006; Pediatric Endocrinology 2006; **Med School:** Emory Univ 1984; **Resid:** Pediatrics, Emory Univ Hosp 1987; **Fellow:** Pediatric Endocrinology, Emory Univ 1990; **Fac Appt:** Prof Ped, Emory Univ

Midwest

Zimmerman, Donald MD [PEn] - **Spec Exp:** Growth Disorders in Childhood Cancer; Thyroid Cancer; Thyroid Disorders; **Hospital:** Children's Mem Hosp -Chicago; **Address:** Children's Memorial Hosp, 2300 Children's Plaza, Div Endocrinology, Box 54, Chicago, IL 60614; **Phone:** 773-327-7740; **Board Cert:** Internal Medicine 1977; Endocrinology 1979; Pediatrics 1983; Pediatric Endocrinology 2001; **Med School:** Univ IL Coll Med 1974; **Resid:** Internal Medicine, Johns Hopkins Hosp 1977; Pediatrics, Mayo Clinic 1981; **Fellow:** Endocrinology, Diabetes & Metabolism, Mayo Clinic 1980; **Fac Appt:** Prof Ped, Northwestern Univ

PEDIATRIC OTOLARYNGOLOGY

New England

McGill, Trevor J MD [PO] - **Spec Exp:** Head & Neck Tumors; **Hospital:** Children's Hospital - Boston; **Address:** Childrens Hosp, Dept Otolaryngology, 300 Longwood Ave, LO-367, Boston, MA 02115; **Phone:** 617-355-6460; **Board Cert:** Otolaryngology 1988; **Med School:** Ireland 1967; **Resid:** Otolaryngology, Royal Natl Throat Nose & Ear Hosp 1974; **Fellow:** Otolaryngology, Mass Eye & Ear Infirm 1976; **Fac Appt:** Prof Oto, Harvard Med Sch

West Coast and Pacific

Crockett, Dennis M MD [PO] - **Spec Exp:** Head & Neck Cancer; **Hospital:** USC Univ Hosp; **Address:** 26726 Crown Valley Pkwy, Ste 200, Mission Viejo, CA 92691; **Phone:** 949-364-4361; **Board Cert:** Otolaryngology 1985; **Med School:** USC Sch Med 1979; **Resid:** Otolaryngology, LAC-USC Med Ctr 1984; **Fellow:** Pediatrics, Boston Chldns Hosp 1985; **Fac Appt:** Assoc Prof Oto, USC Sch Med

Geller, Kenneth Allen MD [PO] - **Spec Exp:** Head & Neck Cancer; **Hospital:** Chldns Hosp - Los Angeles, Huntington Memorial Hosp; **Address:** Chldns Hosp, Div Otolaryngology, 4650 Sunset Blvd, MS 58, Los Angeles, CA 90027; **Phone:** 323-361-2145; **Board Cert:** Otolaryngology 1978; **Med School:** USC Sch Med 1972; **Resid:** Surgery, Wadsworth VA Hosp 1975; Otolaryngology, UCLA Hlth Scis Ctr 1978; **Fellow:** Pediatric Otolaryngology, Chldns Hosp 1979; **Fac Appt:** Assoc Clin Prof Oto, USC Sch Med

PEDIATRIC PULMONOLOGY

West Coast and Pacific

Cooper, Dan M MD [PPul] - **Hospital:** Chldns Hosp Orange Co; **Address:** Chldns Hosp Orange Co, Dept Ped Pulmology, 455 S Main St, Orange, CA 92868; **Phone:** 714-532-7983; **Board Cert:** Pediatrics 1980; Pediatric Pulmonology 2009; **Med School:** UCSF 1974; **Resid:** Internal Medicine, Hadassah Hosp; Pediatrics, Chldns Hosp Med Ctr 1980; **Fellow:** Pediatric Pulmonology, Babies Hosp-Columbia Univ 1994; **Fac Appt:** Prof Ped, UC Irvine

PEDIATRIC SURGERY

New England

Latchaw, Laurie MD [PS] - **Spec Exp:** Pediatric Thoracic Surgery; Cancer Surgery; Neonatal Surgery; **Hospital:** Dartmouth - Hitchcock Med Ctr; **Address:** DHMC, Clinic 6M, One Medical Center Drive, Lebanon, NH 03756; **Phone:** 603-653-9883; **Board Cert:** Surgery 2001; Pediatric Surgery 2003; **Med School:** Rush Med Coll 1976; **Resid:** Surgery, Univ Texas 1981; **Fellow:** Pediatric Surgery, Montreal Chldns Hosp 1983; **Fac Appt:** Assoc Prof S, Dartmouth Med Sch

Shamberger, Robert C MD [PS] - **Spec Exp:** Wilms' Tumor; Neuroblastoma; **Hospital:** Children's Hospital - Boston; **Address:** Children's Hosp-Dept Surgery, 300 Longwood Ave, Fegan - 3, Boston, MA 02115; **Phone:** 617-355-8326; **Board Cert:** Surgery 2002; Pediatric Surgery 2003; Surgical Critical Care 1999; **Med School:** Harvard Med Sch 1975; **Resid:** Surgery, Massachusetts Genl Hosp 1978; Pediatric Surgery, Children's Hosp 1985; **Fellow:** Surgical Oncology, NCI-Surgical Branch 1980; **Fac Appt:** Prof S, Harvard Med Sch

Mid Atlantic

Alexander, Frederick MD [PS] - **Spec Exp:** Solid Tumors; **Hospital:** Hackensack Univ Med Ctr (page 73); **Address:** Joseph M Sanzari Chldns Hosp-HUMC, 30 Prospect Ave, Ste PC311, Hackensack, NJ 07601; **Phone:** 201-996-2921; **Board Cert:** Pediatric Surgery 1999; **Med School:** Columbia P&S 1977; **Resid:** Surgery, Brigham-Womens Hosp 1984; **Fellow:** Pediatric Surgery, Chldns Hosp 1986; **Fac Appt:** Clin Prof S

Colombani, Paul M MD [PS] - **Spec Exp:** Pediatric Thoracic Surgery; Transplant-Kidney; Transplant-Liver; Cancer Surgery; **Hospital:** Johns Hopkins Hosp; **Address:** 600 N Wolfe St, Harvey 319, Baltimore, MD 21287; **Phone:** 410-955-5210; **Board Cert:** Surgery 2003; Pediatric Surgery 2003; **Med School:** Univ KY Coll Med 1976; **Resid:** Surgery, Geo Wash Univ Hosp 1981; **Fellow:** Pediatric Surgery, Johns Hopkins Hosp 1983; **Fac Appt:** Prof S, Johns Hopkins Univ

Pediatric Surgery

Ginsburg, Howard B MD [PS] - **Spec Exp:** Neonatal Surgery; Tumor Surgery; Pediatric Urology; Gastrointestinal Surgery; **Hospital:** NYU Langone Med Ctr (page 79), Bellevue Hosp Ctr; **Address:** 530 First Ave, Ste 10W, New York, NY 10016-6402; **Phone:** 212-263-7391; **Board Cert:** Pediatric Surgery 2001; **Med School:** Univ Cincinnati 1972; **Resid:** Surgery, NYU-Bellvue Hosp 1977; Pediatric Surgery, Columbia-Presby Med Ctr 1979; **Fellow:** Pediatric Surgery, Mass Genl Hosp 1980; **Fac Appt:** Assoc Prof PS, NYU Sch Med

La Quaglia, Michael MD [PS] - **Spec Exp:** Cancer Surgery; Neuroblastoma; Liver Cancer; Colon & Rectal Cancer; **Hospital:** Meml Sloan-Kettering Cancer Ctr (page 75), NY-Presby Hosp/Weill Cornell (page 78); **Address:** 1275 York Ave, Ste H1315, New York, NY 10065; **Phone:** 212-639-7002; **Board Cert:** Surgery 2003; Pediatric Surgery 2007; **Med School:** UMDNJ-NJ Med Sch, Newark 1976; **Resid:** Surgery, Mass Genl Hosp 1983; **Fellow:** Cardiothoracic Surgery, Broadgreen Ctr 1984; Pediatric Surgery, Chldns Hosp 1985; **Fac Appt:** Prof S, Cornell Univ-Weill Med Coll

Spigland, Nitsana A MD [PS] - **Spec Exp:** Congenital Anomalies; Cancer Surgery; Minimally Invasive Surgery; **Hospital:** NY-Presby Hosp/Weill Cornell (page 78); **Address:** NY Hosp-Cornell Med Ctr, 525 E 68th St, Box 209, New York, NY 10021; **Phone:** 212-746-5648; **Board Cert:** Pediatric Surgery 2003; **Med School:** NY Med Coll 1982; **Resid:** Surgery, Lenox Hill Hosp 1987; **Fellow:** Pediatric Surgery, St Justine Chldn's Hosp 1989; **Fac Appt:** Assoc Prof S, Cornell Univ-Weill Med Coll

Stolar, Charles J H MD [PS] - **Spec Exp:** Neonatal Surgery; Pediatric Cancers; **Hospital:** NYPresby-Morgan Stanley Children's Hosp (page 78); **Address:** Morgan Stanley Chldns Hosp NY-Presby, 3959 Broadway, Fl 2 - rm 215 North, New York, NY 10032; **Phone:** 212-342-8586; **Board Cert:** Surgery 2001; Pediatric Surgery 2007; **Med School:** Georgetown Univ 1974; **Resid:** Surgery, Univ Illinois Hosp 1980; **Fellow:** Pediatric Surgery, Chldns Hosp Natl Med Ctr 1982; **Fac Appt:** Prof S, Columbia P&S

Strauch, Eric D MD [PS] - **Spec Exp:** Pediatric Cancers; Neonatal Surgery; **Hospital:** Univ of MD Med Ctr; **Address:** UMMC, Dept Pediatric Surgery, 22 S Greene St, N4E37, Baltimore, MD 21201; **Phone:** 410-328-5730; **Board Cert:** Surgery 2003; Pediatric Surgery 2005; **Med School:** Univ MD Sch Med 1988; **Resid:** Surgery, Univ Maryland Med Ctr; **Fellow:** Pediatric Surgery, jOHNS hOPKINS hOSP 1996; **Fac Appt:** Assoc Prof S, Univ MD Sch Med

Southeast

Davidoff, Andrew M MD [PS] - **Spec Exp:** Neuroblastoma; Cancer Surgery; **Hospital:** St. Jude Children's Research Hosp, Le Bonheur Chldns Med Ctr; **Address:** St Jude Chldns Rsch Hosp, Dept Surg, 262 Danny Thomas Pl, MS 133, Memphis, TN 38105; **Phone:** 901-595-4060; **Board Cert:** Surgery 2005; Pediatric Surgery 2007; **Med School:** Univ Pennsylvania 1987; **Resid:** Surgery, Duke Med Ctr 1994; **Fellow:** Pediatric Surgery, Chldns Hosp 1996; **Fac Appt:** Assoc Prof S, Univ Tenn Coll Med

Morgan III, Walter M MD [PS] - **Spec Exp:** Germ Cell Tumors; Neuroblastoma; Bone Cancer; Laparoscopic Surgery; **Hospital:** Vanderbilt Monroe Carrell Jr. Chldn's Hosp, Vanderbilt Univ Med Ctr; **Address:** Vanderbilt Dept Pediatric Surgery, 2200 Children's Way, 7100 Doctors Office Tower, Nashville, TN 37232-9780; **Phone:** 615-936-1050; **Board Cert:** Pediatric Surgery 2001; **Med School:** Vanderbilt Univ 1982; **Resid:** Surgery, Johns Hopkins Hosp 1988; **Fellow:** Pediatric Surgery, Johns Hopkins Hosp 1990; **Fac Appt:** Asst Prof S, Vanderbilt Univ

Paidas, Charles N MD [PS] - **Spec Exp:** Pediatric Cancers; Laparoscopic Surgery; **Hospital:** Tampa Genl Hosp; **Address:** USF Dept Surgery, 12901 Bruce B Downs Blvd, Box MDC33, Tampa, FL 33612; **Phone:** 813-259-0929; **Board Cert:** Surgery 1999; Pediatric Surgery 2001; Surgical Critical Care 2002; **Med School:** NY Med Coll 1981; **Resid:** Surgery, NY Med Coll Affil Hosps 1987; **Fellow:** Pediatric Surgery, Johns Hopkins Hosp 1991; **Fac Appt:** Prof S, Univ S Fla Coll Med

Rice, Henry MD [PS] - **Spec Exp:** Neonatal Surgery; Cancer Surgery; **Hospital:** Duke Univ Hosp; **Address:** Duke Univ Med Ctr, Dept Ped Surg, DUMC, Box 3815, Durham, NC 27710; **Phone:** 919-681-5077; **Board Cert:** Surgery 2006; Pediatric Surgery 2009; **Med School:** Yale Univ 1988; **Resid:** Surgery, Univ Wash Affil Hosps 1996; **Fellow:** Pediatric Surgery, Chldns Hosp of Buffalo 1998; **Fac Appt:** Assoc Prof S, Duke Univ

Ricketts, Richard R MD [PS] - **Spec Exp:** Neonatal Surgery; Cancer Surgery; Gastrointestinal Surgery; **Hospital:** Chldns Hlthcare Atlanta @ Egleston, Chldns Hlthcare Atlanta @ Scottish Rite; **Address:** Atlanta Pediatric Surgery, 1975 Century Blvd, Ste 6, Atlanta, GA 30345; **Phone:** 404-982-9938; **Board Cert:** Surgery 2004; Pediatric Surgery 2001; **Med School:** Northwestern Univ 1973; **Resid:** Surgery, LAC-USC Med Ctr 1978; **Fellow:** Pediatric Surgery, Chldns Meml Hosp 1980; **Fac Appt:** Prof S, Emory Univ

Shochat, Stephen J MD [PS] - **Spec Exp:** Cancer Surgery; Pediatric Cancers; **Hospital:** St. Jude Children's Research Hosp; **Address:** St Jude Childrens Research Hosp, Dept Surgery, 262 Danny Thomas Pl, Memphis, TN 38105; **Phone:** 901-595-4060; **Board Cert:** Surgery 1969; Thoracic Surgery 1975; Pediatric Surgery 2005; **Med School:** Med Coll VA 1963; **Resid:** Surgery, Barnes Hosp 1968; Pediatric Surgery, Boston Chldns Hosp 1970; **Fellow:** Thoracic Surgery, George Washington Univ Med Ctr 1974; **Fac Appt:** Prof S, Univ Tenn Coll Med

Midwest

Aiken, John J MD [PS] - **Spec Exp:** Tumor Surgery; Solid Tumors; **Hospital:** Chldns Hosp - Wisconsin; **Address:** 999 N 92nd St, Ste C-320, Milwaukee, WI 53226; **Phone:** 414-266-6550; **Board Cert:** Surgery 2004; Pediatric Surgery 2000; **Med School:** Univ Cincinnati 1984; **Resid:** Surgery, Mass Genl Hosp 1991; **Fellow:** Pediatric Surgery, Chldns Hosp 1993; **Fac Appt:** Assoc Prof S, Med Coll Wisc

Ehrlich, Peter F MD [PS] - **Spec Exp:** Pediatric Cancers; Wilms' Tumor; Thyroid Cancer; **Hospital:** Mott Chldns Hosp, Hurley Med Ctr-Mich St Univ; **Address:** Mott Children's Hospital, 1500 E Medical Ctr Drive, rm MOTT F3970, Ann Arbor, MI 48109; **Phone:** 734-764-4151; **Board Cert:** Surgery 2007; Pediatric Surgery 2009; **Med School:** Canada 1989; **Resid:** Surgery, Univ Toronto Med Ctr 1996; **Fellow:** Pediatric Surgery, Children's Natl Med Ctr 1998; **Fac Appt:** Assoc Clin Prof S, Univ Mich Med Sch

Moss, R Lawrence MD [PS] - **Spec Exp:** Congenital Anomalies; Cancer Surgery; Minimally Invasive Surgery; **Hospital:** Nationwide Chldn's Hosp; **Address:** Nationwide Children's Hosp, Dept Surgery, Surgeon-in-Chief, 700 Children's Drive, Columbus, OH 43205; **Phone:** 614-722-3900; **Board Cert:** Surgery 1999; Pediatric Surgery 2003; Surgical Critical Care 2000; **Med School:** UCSD 1986; **Resid:** Surgery, Virginia Mason Med Ctr 1991; Surgical Critical Care, Chldns Meml Hosp 1992; **Fellow:** Pediatric Surgery, Chldns Meml Hosp 1994; **Fac Appt:** Prof S, Yale Univ

Rescorla, Frederick J MD [PS] - **Spec Exp:** Cancer Surgery; Head & Neck Cancer; Gastrointestinal Surgery; Laparoscopic Surgery; **Hospital:** Riley Hosp for Children; **Address:** Riley Hospital for Children, 702 Barnhill Drive, rm 2500, Indianapolis, IN 46202; **Phone:** 317-274-4681; **Board Cert:** Surgery 2004; Surgical Critical Care 2009; Pediatric Surgery 2007; **Med School:** Univ Wisc 1981; **Resid:** Surgery, Indiana Univ Med Ctr 1986; Pediatric Surgery, Indiana Univ Med Ctr 1988; **Fac Appt:** Prof S, Indiana Univ

Pediatric Surgery

Warner, Brad MD [PS] - **Spec Exp:** Gastrointestinal Surgery; Neonatal Surgery; Pediatric Cancers; **Hospital:** St. Louis Chldns Hosp; **Address:** 1 Children's Pl, Ste 5S40, St Louis, MO 63110; **Phone:** 314-454-6022; **Board Cert:** Surgery 2009; Pediatric Surgery 2001; **Med School:** Univ MO-Kansas City 1982; **Resid:** Surgery, Univ Cincinnati Med Ctr 1989; **Fellow:** Pediatric Surgery, Chldns Hosp Med Ctr 1991; **Fac Appt:** Prof S, Univ Cincinnati

Great Plains and Mountains

Meyers, Rebecka L MD [PS] - **Spec Exp:** Transplant-Liver; Tumor Surgery; Biliary Surgery; Pancreatic Surgery; **Hospital:** Primary Children's Med Ctr, Univ Utah Hlth Care; **Address:** Primary Chlds Med Ctr, Dept Ped Surg, 100 N Mario Capecchi Drive, Ste 2600, Salt Lake City, UT 84113-1103; **Phone:** 801-662-2950; **Board Cert:** Surgery 2003; Pediatric Surgery 2005; **Med School:** Oregon Hlth & Sci Univ 1985; **Resid:** Surgery, UCSF Med Ctr 1990; **Fellow:** Research, Cardio Rsch Inst-UCSF 1992; Pediatric Surgery, St Christophers Hosp for Chldn 1994; **Fac Appt:** Assoc Prof S, Univ Utah

Southwest

Jackson, Richard J MD [PS] - **Spec Exp:** Pediatric Cancers; Neonatal Surgery; Robotic Surgery; **Hospital:** Arkansas Chldns Hosp; **Address:** Arkansas Children's Hospital, 1 Children's Way, Slot 837, Little Rock, AR 72202-3591; **Phone:** 501-364-1446; **Board Cert:** Surgery 2008; Pediatric Surgery 2001; Surgical Critical Care 1998; **Med School:** W VA Univ 1983; **Resid:** Surgery, W Va Univ Hosps 1988; Pediatric Surgery, Chldns Hosp 1989; **Fellow:** Surgical Critical Care, Chldns Hosp-Univ Pittsburgh 1990; Pediatric Surgery, Chldns Hosp-Univ Pittsburgh 1992

Nuchtern, Jed MD [PS] - **Spec Exp:** Pediatric Thoracic Surgery; Cancer Surgery; Laparoscopic Surgery; **Hospital:** Texas Chldns Hosp, Ben Taub Genl Hosp; **Address:** Texas Children's Hosp, 6621 Fannin St, MC CC650, Houston, TX 77030; **Phone:** 832-822-3135; **Board Cert:** Surgery 2003; Surgical Critical Care 2002; Pediatric Surgery 2007; **Med School:** Harvard Med Sch 1985; **Resid:** Surgery, Univ Washington 1992; Pediatric Surgery, Baylor Coll Med 1995; **Fellow:** Cellular Molecular Biology, Natl Inst Hlth 1990; **Fac Appt:** Prof S, Baylor Coll Med

Skinner, Michael A MD [PS] - **Spec Exp:** Endocrine Cancers; Thyroid Cancer; **Hospital:** UT Southwestern Med Ctr at Dallas; **Address:** UT Southwestern Med Ctr at Dallas, 1935 Med District Drive, Ste B3250, Dallas, TX 75235; **Phone:** 214-456-6040; **Board Cert:** Surgery 2000; Pediatric Surgery 2003; **Med School:** Rush Med Coll 1984; **Resid:** Surgery, Duke Univ Med Ctr 1991; **Fellow:** Pediatric Surgery, Indiana Univ 1993; **Fac Appt:** Assoc Prof S, Univ Tex SW, Dallas

West Coast and Pacific

Farmer, Diana MD [PS] - **Spec Exp:** Pediatric Cancers; **Hospital:** UCSF Med Ctr; **Address:** 513 Parnassus Ave, Ste HNW1601, Box 0570, San Francisco, CA 94143-0570; **Phone:** 415-476-2538; **Board Cert:** Surgery 2001; Pediatric Surgery 2005; **Med School:** Univ Wash 1983; **Resid:** Surgery, UCSF Med Ctr 1993; **Fellow:** Pediatric Surgery, Childrens Hosp 1995; **Fac Appt:** Assoc Prof S, UCSF

Healey, Patrick J MD [PS] - **Spec Exp:** Transplant Surgery-Pediatric; Transplant-Kidney; Transplant-Liver; Tumor Surgery; **Hospital:** Seattle Chldns Hosp; **Address:** 4800 Sand Point Way, Dept Surgery, Box 359300, MS W7800, Seattle, WA 98105; **Phone:** 206-987-1800; **Board Cert:** Surgery 2002; Pediatric Surgery 2009; **Med School:** Boston Univ 1987; **Resid:** Surgery, Hartford Hosp 1992; **Fellow:** Transplant Surgery, Univ WA Med Ctr 1995; Pediatric Surgery, Chldns Hosp 1997; **Fac Appt:** Asst Prof S, Univ Wash

Sawin, Robert S MD [PS] - **Spec Exp:** Pediatric Cancers; Pediatric Thoracic Surgery; Transplant-Liver; **Hospital:** Seattle Chldns Hosp; **Address:** Seattle Chldn's Hosp, 4800 Sand Point Way NE, MS W7729, Seattle, WA 98145-5005; **Phone:** 206-987-2039; **Board Cert:** Surgical Critical Care 2001; Pediatric Surgery 2009; **Med School:** Univ Pittsburgh 1982; **Resid:** Surgery, Brigham Women's Hosp 1987; **Fellow:** Pediatric Surgery, Chldns Hosp 1989; **Fac Appt:** Prof S, Univ Wash

PEDIATRICS

Mid Atlantic

Oeffinger, Kevin MD [Ped] - **Spec Exp:** Cancer Survivors-Late Effects of Therapy; **Hospital:** Meml Sloan-Kettering Cancer Ctr (page 75); **Address:** 300 E 66th St, New York, NY 10065; **Phone:** 800-525-2225; **Board Cert:** Family Medicine 2006; **Med School:** Univ Tex, San Antonio 1984; **Resid:** Family Medicine, Baylor Coll Med 1985; **Fellow:** Family Medicine, Fam Practice Faculty Dev Ctr 1999; Natl Cancer Inst 2000

Southwest

Kleinerman, Eugenie S MD [Ped] - **Spec Exp:** Ewing's Sarcoma; Cancer Survivors-Late Effects of Therapy; **Hospital:** UT MD Anderson Cancer Ctr; **Address:** MD Anderson Cancer Ctr, Dept Pediatrics, 1515 Holcombe Blvd, Unit 87, Houston, TX 77030; **Phone:** 713-792-8110; **Board Cert:** Pediatrics 1980; **Med School:** Duke Univ 1975; **Resid:** Pediatrics, Chldns Hosp-Natl Med Ctr 1978; **Fellow:** Immunology, Natl Cancer Inst 1981; **Fac Appt:** Prof Ped, Univ Tex, Houston

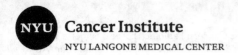

Cancer Institute
NYU LANGONE MEDICAL CENTER

NYU Langone Medical Center
550 First Avenue , New York, NY 10016
www.NYULMC.org

NYU Clinical Cancer Center
160 East 34th Street, New York, NY 10016
www.NYUCI.org

The Stephen D. Hassenfeld Children's Center
for Cancer and Blood Disorders
160 East 32nd Street, New York, NY 10016
www.NYUMC.org/Hassenfeld

The NYU Cancer Institute is an NCI-designated cancer center and provides personalized patient care that is both compassionate and state of the art. The doctors and researchers work together to develop innovative therapies for patients. The Cancer Institute is world-renowned for excellence in cancer-focused research, personalized care, education and community outreach. Its mission is to discover the origins of human cancer and to use that knowledge to eradicate the personal and societal burden of cancer in our community, the nation and the world. For more information about our expert physicians, call 212-731-5000. *We specialize in the following areas:*

Patient-Focused Setting
The NYU Clinical Cancer Center is the principal outpatient facility of The Cancer Institute and serves as home to our patients and their caregivers. The center and its multidisciplinary team of experts provide access to the latest treatment options and clinical trials along with a variety of programs in cancer risk reduction/prevention, screening, diagnostics, genetic counseling and supportive services. In addition the NYUCI emphasizes the importance of a holistic approach to management services in complementary medicine, psychosocial support, survivorship and palliative care.

Renowned Expertise
The NYU Cancer Institute brings together experts from a variety of disciplines to create collaborative research endeavors and clinical care teams. The Cancer Institute offers a full continuum of personalized care, from prevention through diagnosis, treatment and post-treatment support. The compassion and expertise of our team members helps patients better manage the symptoms of their diseases as well as meet their special needs. Additionally, we have created special emphasis programs in diseases such as breast cancer, melanoma, GI cancer, prostate cancer, hematologic malignancies and lung cancer among others, as well as, translational programs in cancer healthcare disparities, molecularly targeted therapy, and the cell signaling pathways involved in cancer.

A Translational Approach
NYU Langone Medical Center scientists and other researchers excel in uncovering how cancer develops at the molecular level, and how we can harness that knowledge to reduce the risk of cancer and treat the disease. The Medical Center constantly seeks to create new opportunities for collaboration between investigators within our own institution, those located elsewhere in the NYU network of campuses, and researchers at other institutions.

The Stephen D. Hassenfeld Children's Center for Cancer and Blood Disorders
The center is a leading pediatric outpatient facility for the treatment of childhood cancers and blood diseases. Its unique interdisciplinary and family-centered approach combines the most advanced medical treatments with psychosocial and emotional support services for young patients and their families.

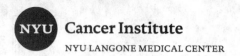

Cancer Institute
NYU LANGONE MEDICAL CENTER

NYU Langone Medical Center
550 First Avenue , New York, NY 10016
www.NYULMC.org

NYU Clinical Cancer Center
160 East 34th Street, New York, NY 10016
www.NYUCI.org

**The Stephen D. Hassenfeld Children's Center
for Cancer and Blood Disorders**
160 East 32nd Street, New York, NY 10016
www.NYUMC.org/Hassenfeld

The NYU Cancer Institute is an NCI-designated cancer center and provides personalized patient care that is both compassionate and state of the art. The doctors and researchers work together to develop innovative therapies for patients. The Cancer Institute is world-renowned for excellence in cancer-focused research, personalized care, education and community outreach. Its mission is to discover the origins of human cancer and to use that knowledge to eradicate the personal and societal burden of cancer in our community, the nation and the world. For more information about our expert physicians, call 212-731-5000. *We specialize in the following areas:*

Patient-Focused Setting
The NYU Clinical Cancer Center is the principal outpatient facility of The Cancer Institute and serves as home to our patients and their caregivers. The center and its multidisciplinary team of experts provide access to the latest treatment options and clinical trials along with a variety of programs in cancer risk reduction/prevention, screening, diagnostics, genetic counseling and supportive services. In addition the NYUCI emphasizes the importance of a holistic approach to management services in complementary medicine, psychosocial support, survivorship and palliative care.

Renowned Expertise
The NYU Cancer Institute brings together experts from a variety of disciplines to create collaborative research endeavors and clinical care teams. The Cancer Institute offers a full continuum of personalized care, from prevention through diagnosis, treatment and post-treatment support. The compassion and expertise of our team members helps patients better manage the symptoms of their diseases as well as meet their special needs. Additionally, we have created special emphasis programs in diseases such as breast cancer, melanoma, GI cancer, prostate cancer, hematologic malignancies and lung cancer among others, as well as, translational programs in cancer healthcare disparities, molecularly targeted therapy, and the cell signaling pathways involved in cancer.

A Translational Approach
NYU Langone Medical Center scientists and other researchers excel in uncovering how cancer develops at the molecular level, and how we can harness that knowledge to reduce the risk of cancer and treat the disease. The Medical Center constantly seeks to create new opportunities for collaboration between investigators within our own institution, those located elsewhere in the NYU network of campuses, and researchers at other institutions.

The Stephen D. Hassenfeld Children's Center for Cancer and Blood Disorders
The center is a leading pediatric outpatient facility for the treatment of childhood cancers and blood diseases. Its unique interdisciplinary and family-centered approach combines the most advanced medical treatments with psychosocial and emotional support services for young patients and their families.

The Best in American Medicine
www.CastleConnolly.com

Plastic Surgery

A plastic surgeon deals with the repair, reconstruction or replacement of physical defects of form or function involving the skin, musculoskeletal system, craniomaxillofacial structures, hand, extremities, breast and trunk and external genitalia. He/she uses aesthetic surgical principles not only to improve undesirable qualities of normal structures (commonly called "cosmetic surgery") but in all reconstructive procedures as well.

A plastic surgeon possesses special knowledge and skill in the design and surgery of grafts, flaps, free tissue transfer and replantation. Competence in the management of complex wounds, the use of implantable materials, and in tumor surgery is required.

Training Required: Five to seven years

Plastic Surgery within the Head and Neck: A plastic surgeon with additional training in plastic and reconstructive procedures within the head, face, neck and associated structures, including cutaneous head and neck oncology and reconstruction, management of maxillofacial trauma, soft tissue repair and neural surgery.

The field is diverse and involved a wide range of patients, from the newborn to the aged. While both cosmetic and reconstructive surgery are practiced, there are many additional procedures which interface with them.

Surgery of the Hand:
(See Hand Surgery under Orthopaedic Surgery)

PLASTIC SURGERY

New England

Collins, Dale MD [PlS] - **Spec Exp:** Breast Cancer; Breast Reconstruction; **Hospital:** Dartmouth - Hitchcock Med Ctr; **Address:** Div Plastic Surgery, 1 Medical Center Drive, Lebanon, NH 03756; **Phone:** 603-653-3500; **Board Cert:** Plastic Surgery 2007; **Med School:** Emory Univ 1989; **Resid:** Plastic Surgery, Washington Univ Med Ctr 1994; **Fellow:** Microsurgery, Washington Univ Med Ctr 1995; **Fac Appt:** Prof S, Dartmouth Med Sch

Stadelmann, Wayne K MD [PlS] - **Spec Exp:** Melanoma-Head & Neck; Breast Reconstruction; **Hospital:** Concord Hospital, New London Hosp; **Address:** 246 Pleasant St, Ste 210, MS 03301, Concord, NH 03301; **Phone:** 603-224-5200; **Board Cert:** Plastic Surgery 2009; **Med School:** Univ Chicago-Pritzker Sch Med 1990; **Resid:** Surgery, Univ Chicago Hosps 1994; Plastic Surgery, Univ S Florida/H Lee Moffit Cancer Ctr 1997

Stahl, Richard S MD [PlS] - **Spec Exp:** Abdominal Wall Reconstruction; Chest Wall Reconstruction; Breast Reconstruction; **Hospital:** Yale-New Haven Hosp, Hosp of St Raphael; **Address:** 5 Durham Rd, Guilford, CT 06437; **Phone:** 203-458-4440; **Board Cert:** Surgery 2001; Plastic Surgery 1984; **Med School:** Vanderbilt Univ 1976; **Resid:** Surgery, Yale New Haven Hosp 1981; **Fellow:** Plastic Surgery, Emory Univ Med Ctr 1983; **Fac Appt:** Clin Prof S, Yale Univ

Mid Atlantic

Cordeiro, Peter G MD [PlS] - **Spec Exp:** Reconstructive Surgery; Breast Reconstruction; Facial Plastic & Reconstructive Surgery; **Hospital:** Meml Sloan-Kettering Cancer Ctr (page 75), Lenox Hill Hosp (Manh Eye, Ear & Throat Hosp); **Address:** 1275 York Avenue, New York, NY 10065; **Phone:** 800-525-2225; **Board Cert:** Surgery 2008; Plastic Surgery 1994; **Med School:** Harvard Med Sch 1983; **Resid:** Surgery, New Eng Deaconess Hosp-Harvard 1989; Plastic Surgery, NYU Med Ctr 1991; **Fellow:** Microsurgery, Meml Sloan-Kettering Cancer Ctr. 1992; Craniofacial Surgery, Univ Miami 1992; **Fac Appt:** Prof S, Cornell Univ-Weill Med Coll

Disa, Joseph MD [PlS] - **Spec Exp:** Cancer Reconstruction; Breast Reconstruction; Head & Neck Reconstruction; Microsurgery; **Hospital:** Meml Sloan-Kettering Cancer Ctr (page 75); **Address:** 1275 York Ave, New York, NY 10065; **Phone:** 212-639-5022; **Board Cert:** Surgery 2005; Plastic Surgery 2009; **Med School:** Univ Mass Sch Med 1988; **Resid:** Surgery, Univ Md Med Ctr 1994; Plastic Surgery, Johns Hopkins Univ 1996; **Fellow:** Reconstructive Microsurgery, Meml Sloan-Kettering Cancer Ctr.; **Fac Appt:** Prof PlS, Cornell Univ-Weill Med Coll

Hoffman, Lloyd A MD [PlS] - **Spec Exp:** Breast Reconstruction; **Hospital:** NY-Presby Hosp/Columbia (page 78), Lenox Hill Hosp; **Address:** 12A E 68th St, New York, NY 10021; **Phone:** 212-861-1640; **Board Cert:** Plastic Surgery 1989; **Med School:** Northwestern Univ 1978; **Resid:** Surgery, New York Hosp 1983; Plastic Surgery, NYU Med Ctr 1986; **Fellow:** Hand Surgery, NYU Med Ctr 1987; **Fac Appt:** Assoc Prof PlS, Cornell Univ-Weill Med Coll

Levine, Joshua L MD [PlS] - **Spec Exp:** Breast Reconstruction; Microsurgery; **Hospital:** New York Eye & Ear Infirm (page 77), Montefiore Med Ctr - Div. Weiler; **Address:** 1776 Broadway at 57th St, Ste 1200, New York, NY 10019; **Phone:** 212-245-8140; **Board Cert:** Plastic Surgery 2005; **Med School:** Med Coll GA 1994; **Resid:** Plastic Surgery, Montefiore Med Ctr 2000; Plastic Surgery, Montefiore Med Ctr 2001; **Fellow:** Cosmetic Plastic Surgery, NY Eye & Ear Infirm 2003; Reconstructive Microsurgery, Louisiana State Univ 2004

Loree, Thom R MD [PlS] - **Spec Exp:** Head & Neck Cancer; Thyroid Cancer; Reconstructive Surgery; **Hospital:** Roswell Park Cancer Inst, Sisters of Charity Hosp, Buffalo; **Address:** Roswell Park Cancer Inst, Dept Head & Neck Surgery, Elm & Carlton Sts, Buffalo, NY 14263; **Phone:** 716-845-3158; **Board Cert:** Surgery 1997; Plastic Surgery 2004; **Med School:** Geo Wash Univ 1982; **Resid:** Surgery, St Lukes-Roosevelt Hosp 1987; Plastic Surgery, St Lukes-Roosevelt Hosp 1989; **Fellow:** Head & Neck Surgical Oncology, Meml Sloan-Kettering Cancer Ctr 1990; **Fac Appt:** Assoc Prof S, SUNY Buffalo

Manson, Paul MD [PlS] - **Spec Exp:** Skin Cancer; Reconstructive Surgery; **Hospital:** Johns Hopkins Hosp, Univ of MD Med Ctr; **Address:** 601 N Caroline St, McElderry-8152F, Baltimore, MD 21287; **Phone:** 410-955-9470; **Board Cert:** Plastic Surgery 1979; **Med School:** Northwestern Univ 1968; **Resid:** Surgery, New Eng Deaconess Hosp 1971; Plastic Surgery, Johns Hopkins Hosp 1978; **Fellow:** Surgery, Lahey Clinic 1974; **Fac Appt:** Prof PlS, Johns Hopkins Univ

Mehrara, Babak J MD [PlS] - **Spec Exp:** Breast Reconstruction; Cancer Reconstruction; Microsurgery; Reconstructive Surgery-Face; **Hospital:** Meml Sloan-Kettering Cancer Ctr (page 75); **Address:** 1275 York Ave, New York, NY 10065; **Phone:** 212-639-8639; **Board Cert:** Plastic Surgery 2003; **Med School:** Columbia P&S 1993; **Resid:** Surgery, NYU Med Ctr 1996; Plastic Surgery, NYU Med Ctr 2001; **Fellow:** Microsurgery, UCLA Med Ctr 2002; **Fac Appt:** Assoc Prof S, Cornell Univ-Weill Med Coll

Serletti, Joseph M MD [PlS] - **Spec Exp:** Breast Reconstruction; Reconstructive Surgery; **Hospital:** Hosp Univ Penn - UPHS (page 80); **Address:** Hosp Univ Penn, Dept Plastic Surgery, 10 Penn Tower, 3400 Spruce St, Philadelphia, PA 19104; **Phone:** 215-662-3743; **Board Cert:** Plastic Surgery 2003; **Med School:** Univ Rochester 1982; **Resid:** Surgery, Strong Meml Hosp 1986; Plastic Surgery, Strong Meml Hosp 1988; **Fellow:** Reconstructive Surgery, Johns Hopkins Hosp 1990; **Fac Appt:** Prof PlS, Univ Pennsylvania

Slezak, Sheri MD [PlS] - **Spec Exp:** Breast Reconstruction; **Hospital:** Univ of MD Med Ctr; **Address:** Univ Maryland, Dept Plastic Surgery, 22 S Greene St, rm S8D18, Baltimore, MD 21201; **Phone:** 410-328-2360; **Board Cert:** Plastic Surgery 1991; **Med School:** Harvard Med Sch 1980; **Resid:** Surgery, Columbia-Presby Med Ctr 1985; Plastic Surgery, Johns Hopkins Hosp 1989; **Fac Appt:** Assoc Prof PlS, Univ MD Sch Med

Sultan, Mark R MD [PlS] - **Spec Exp:** Breast Reconstruction; **Hospital:** St. Luke's - Roosevelt Hosp Ctr - Roosevelt Div (page 71); **Address:** 1100 Park Ave, New York, NY 10128; **Phone:** 212-360-0700; **Board Cert:** Plastic Surgery 1992; **Med School:** Columbia P&S 1982; **Resid:** Surgery, Columbia-Presby Hosp 1987; Plastic Surgery, Columbia-Presby Hosp 1990; **Fellow:** Head and Neck Surgery, Emory Univ Hosp 1989; **Fac Appt:** Assoc Prof S, Columbia P&S

Ting, Jess MD [PlS] - **Spec Exp:** Breast Reconstruction; **Hospital:** Mount Sinai Med Ctr (page 76), Mount Sinai Hosp of Queens (page 76); **Address:** 5 E 98th St, Fl 14, Ste B, Box 1259, New York, NY 10029; **Phone:** 212-241-4410; **Board Cert:** Plastic Surgery 2002; Hand Surgery 2003; **Med School:** Columbia P&S 1995; **Resid:** Surgery, Columbia Presby Med Ctr 1998; Plastic Surgery, Univ Pittsburgh Med Ctr 2000; **Fellow:** Hand Surgery, Hosp Special Surgery 2001; **Fac Appt:** Asst Prof S, Mount Sinai Sch Med

Topham, Neal MD [PlS] - **Spec Exp:** Breast Reconstruction; Head & Neck Reconstruction; Reconstructive Surgery; Microsurgery; **Hospital:** Fox Chase Cancer Ctr (page 72); **Address:** Fox Chase Cancer Center, Dept Surgical Oncology, 333 Cottman Ave, C308, Philadelphia, PA 19111; **Phone:** 215-728-2662; **Board Cert:** Plastic Surgery 2005; **Med School:** Case West Res Univ 1994; **Resid:** Surgery, Akron Med Ctr 1998; Plastic Surgery, Case Western Reserve Univ 2000; **Fellow:** Microvascular Surgery, MD Anderson Cancer Ctr 2003; **Fac Appt:** Assoc Prof S, Univ Pennsylvania

Plastic Surgery

Tufaro, Anthony P MD/DDS [PlS] - **Spec Exp:** Head & Neck Cancer; Skin Cancer-Head & Neck; Merkel Cell Carcinoma; Craniofacial Surgery/Reconstruction; **Hospital:** Johns Hopkins Hosp; **Address:** Johns Hopkins Plastic Surgery, 601 N Caroline St Fl 8, Baltimore, MD 21287; **Phone:** 410-955-9846; **Board Cert:** Plastic Surgery 2000; **Med School:** Hahnemann Univ 1993; **Resid:** Surgery, Johns Hopkins Hosp 1995; **Fellow:** Plastic Surgery, Johns Hopkins Hosp 1997; Head and Neck Surgery, Meml Sloan Kettering Cancer Ctr 1999; **Fac Appt:** Assoc Prof S, Johns Hopkins Univ

Southeast

Allen, Robert J MD [PlS] - **Spec Exp:** Breast Reconstruction; Microsurgery; **Hospital:** Roper Hosp; **Address:** 125 Doughty St, Ste 590, Charleston, SC 29403; **Phone:** 888-890-3437; **Board Cert:** Plastic Surgery 1985; **Med School:** Med Univ SC 1976; **Resid:** Surgery, LSU Med Ctr 1982; Plastic Surgery, LSU Med Ctr 1981; **Fellow:** Microsurgery, NYU Med Ctr 1983; **Fac Appt:** Assoc Clin Prof PlS, Louisiana State U, New Orleans

Fix, R Jobe MD [PlS] - **Spec Exp:** Breast Reconstruction; Microsurgery; **Hospital:** Univ of Ala Hosp at Birmingham, Children's Hospital - Birmingham; **Address:** Univ of Alabama Hosp, Div Plastic Surg, 1530 3rd Ave S, Ste FOT-1102, Birmingham, AL 35294; **Phone:** 205-801-8500; **Board Cert:** Surgery 2009; Plastic Surgery 1991; Hand Surgery 2001; **Med School:** Univ Nebr Coll Med 1982; **Resid:** Surgery, Valley Med Ctr 1987; Plastic Surgery, Univ Ala Hosp 1989; **Fac Appt:** Prof PlS, Univ Alabama

Georgiade, Gregory S MD [PlS] - **Spec Exp:** Breast Reconstruction; **Hospital:** Duke Univ Hosp; **Address:** Duke Univ Med Ctr, Box 3960, Durham, NC 27710; **Phone:** 919-684-3039; **Board Cert:** Surgery 2001; Plastic Surgery 1981; **Med School:** Duke Univ 1973; **Resid:** Surgery, Duke Univ Med Ctr 1978; Plastic Surgery, Duke Univ Med Ctr 1980; **Fac Appt:** Prof S, Duke Univ

Maxwell, G Patrick MD [PlS] - **Spec Exp:** Breast Reconstruction; **Hospital:** Baptist Hosp - Nashville, Centennial Med Ctr; **Address:** 2020 21st Ave S, Nashville, TN 37212; **Phone:** 615-932-7700; **Board Cert:** Plastic Surgery 1981; **Med School:** Vanderbilt Univ 1972; **Resid:** Surgery, Johns Hopkins Hosp 1976; Plastic Surgery, Johns Hopkins Hosp 1979; **Fellow:** Microsurgery, Davies Med Ctr 1975; **Fac Appt:** Asst Clin Prof PlS, Vanderbilt Univ

McCraw, John MD [PlS] - **Spec Exp:** Breast Reconstruction; **Hospital:** Univ Mississippi Med Ctr; **Address:** Univ Mississippi Med Ctr, Div Plastic Surg, 2500 N State St, Jackson, MS 39216; **Phone:** 601-815-1343; **Board Cert:** Surgery 1972; Plastic Surgery 1974; **Med School:** Univ MO-Columbia Sch Med 1966; **Resid:** Orthopaedic Surgery, Duke U Med Ctr 1969; Surgery, Univ Florida Med Ctr 1971; **Fellow:** Plastic Surgery, Univ Florida Med Ctr 1973; **Fac Appt:** Prof PlS, Univ Miss

Smith Jr, David J MD [PlS] - **Spec Exp:** Breast Reconstruction; Reconstructive Surgery; **Hospital:** Tampa Genl Hosp; **Address:** USF Dept Plastic Surgery, 2 Tampa General Circle Fl 7, Tampa, FL 33606; **Phone:** 813-259-0842; **Board Cert:** Plastic Surgery 1981; **Med School:** Indiana Univ 1973; **Resid:** Surgery, Grady Hosp 1988; Plastic Surgery, Indiana Univ Med Ctr 1980; **Fellow:** Hand Surgery, Univ Louisville 1979; **Fac Appt:** Prof S, Univ S Fla Coll Med

Smith, Paul D MD [PlS] - **Spec Exp:** Reconstructive Surgery-Face; Breast Reconstruction; **Hospital:** H Lee Moffitt Cancer Ctr & Research Inst; **Address:** 2 Tampa Genl Cir Fl 7, Tampa, FL 33606-3589; **Phone:** 813-259-0964; **Board Cert:** Plastic Surgery 2002; **Med School:** Univ IL Coll Med 1994; **Resid:** Surgery, Univ IL Med Ctr 1999; **Fellow:** Plastic Surgery, Univ Texas SW Med Ctr 2001; **Fac Appt:** Prof PlS, Univ S Fla Coll Med

Midwest

Brandt, Keith E MD [PlS] - **Spec Exp:** Breast Reconstruction; Cancer Reconstruction; **Hospital:** Barnes-Jewish Hosp, Barnes-Jewish West County Hosp; **Address:** 4921 Parkview Pl, Ste 6G, St Louis, MO 63110-1010; **Phone:** 314-362-7388; **Board Cert:** Surgery 1999; Plastic Surgery 2003; Hand Surgery 2005; **Med School:** Univ Tex, Houston 1983; **Resid:** Surgery, Univ Nebraska Med Ctr 1989; Plastic Surgery, Univ Tennessee 1991; **Fellow:** Hand Surgery, Wash Univ 1992; Microsurgery, Wash Univ 1993; **Fac Appt:** Prof S, Washington Univ, St Louis

Coleman III, John J MD [PlS] - **Spec Exp:** Cancer Reconstruction; Breast Reconstruction; Head & Neck Surgery; Facial Plastic & Reconstructive Surgery; **Hospital:** IU Health Methodist Hosp, Riley Hosp for Children; **Address:** 545 Barnhill Dr, Emerson Hall, Ste 232, Indianapolis, IN 46202-5120; **Phone:** 317-274-8106; **Board Cert:** Surgery 1998; Plastic Surgery 1981; **Med School:** Harvard Med Sch 1973; **Resid:** Surgery, Emory Univ Affil Hosp 1978; Plastic Surgery, Emory Univ Affil Hosp 1979; **Fellow:** Surgical Oncology, Univ Maryland Med Ctr 1981; **Fac Appt:** Prof S, Indiana Univ

Hammond, Dennis C MD [PlS] - **Spec Exp:** Breast Reconstruction; **Hospital:** Spectrum Hlth Blodgett Campus; **Address:** 4070 Lake Drive SE, Ste 202, Grand Rapids, MI 49546; **Phone:** 616-464-4420; **Board Cert:** Plastic Surgery 1994; **Med School:** Univ Mich Med Sch 1985; **Resid:** Surgery, Blodgett Meml Med Ctr 1988; Plastic/Reconstructive Surgery, Grand Rapids Area Med Educ Ctr 1990; **Fellow:** Plastic Surgery, Baptist Hosp 1991; Hand & Microvascular Surgery, Med Coll Wisconsin 1992; **Fac Appt:** Prof PlS, Univ Mich Med Sch

Miller, Michael J MD [PlS] - **Spec Exp:** Cancer Reconstruction; Breast Reconstruction; Head & Neck Reconstruction; **Hospital:** Ohio St Univ Med Ctr; **Address:** OSU Div of Plastic Surgery, 915 Olentangy River Rd, Ste 2100, Columbus, OH 43212; **Phone:** 614-293-8566; **Board Cert:** Plastic Surgery 1993; **Med School:** Univ Mass Sch Med 1983; **Resid:** Surgery, Berkshire Med Ctr 1987; **Fellow:** Plastic Surgery, Ohio State Univ Med Ctr 1989; **Fac Appt:** Prof S, Ohio State Univ

Walton Jr, Robert L MD [PlS] - **Spec Exp:** Nasal Reconstruction; Breast Reconstruction; **Hospital:** Resurrection Hlth Care St Joseph Hosp, Children's Mem Hosp -Chicago; **Address:** 60 E Delaware Place, Ste 1430, Chicago, IL 60611-1495; **Phone:** 312-337-7795; **Board Cert:** Plastic Surgery 1980; **Med School:** Univ Kansas 1972; **Resid:** Surgery, Johns Hopkins Hosp 1974; Plastic Surgery, Yale-New Haven Hosp 1978; **Fellow:** Hand Surgery, Hartford Hosp 1978; **Fac Appt:** Prof PlS, Northwestern Univ-Feinberg Sch Med

Wilkins, Edwin G MD [PlS] - **Spec Exp:** Breast Reconstruction; Microsurgery; **Hospital:** Univ of Michigan Hosp; **Address:** Univ Mich, Div Plastic Surg, 1500 E Med Ctr Drive, rm 2130 Taubman Ctr, Ann Arbor, MI 48109-5340; **Phone:** 734-998-6022; **Board Cert:** Plastic Surgery 1991; **Med School:** Wake Forest Univ 1981; **Resid:** Surgery, Charlotte Meml Hosp 1986; Plastic Surgery, Vanderbilt Univ Med Ctr 1988; **Fellow:** Reconstructive Microsurgery, Univ Louisville Sch Med 1989; **Fac Appt:** Assoc Prof PlS, Univ Mich Med Sch

Yetman, Randall MD [PlS] - **Spec Exp:** Breast Reconstruction; Melanoma; Microsurgery; **Hospital:** Cleveland Clin (page 70); **Address:** 9500 Euclid Ave, Desk A60, Cleveland, OH 44195; **Phone:** 216-444-6908; **Board Cert:** Plastic Surgery 1984; **Med School:** Univ Miami Sch Med 1975; **Resid:** Surgery, Montefiore Med Ctr 1979; Plastic Surgery, NY Cornell Med Ctr 1981; **Fellow:** Plastic Surgery, Cleveland Clin Fdn 1982

Plastic Surgery

Great Plains and Mountains

Rockwell, William MD [PlS] - **Spec Exp:** Microsurgery; Sarcoma; Breast Reconstruction; **Hospital:** Univ Utah Hlth Care; **Address:** 30 N 1900 E, rm 3B400, Salt Lake City, UT 84132; **Phone:** 801-585-3253; **Board Cert:** Plastic Surgery 1994; Hand Surgery 2006; **Med School:** Washington Univ, St Louis 1984; **Resid:** Surgery, Univ Washington/Barnes Hosp 1987; Plastic Surgery, Univ Rochester Affil Hosp 1991; **Fellow:** Hand Surgery, Univ Rochester Affil Hosp 1992; **Fac Appt:** Assoc Prof PlS, Univ Utah

Southwest

Butler, Charles E MD [PlS] - **Spec Exp:** Breast Reconstruction; **Hospital:** UT MD Anderson Cancer Ctr; **Address:** Univ Texas- M.D. Anderson Cancer Ctr, 1515 Holcombe Blvd, Ste 1488, P.O. Box 301402, Houston, TX 77030; **Phone:** 713-794-1247; **Board Cert:** Plastic Surgery 2010; Surgery 2008; **Med School:** Univ Pennsylvania 1990; **Resid:** Surgery, Mass Genl Hosp 1993; Plastic Surgery, Brigham & Women's Hosp 1995; **Fellow:** Research, Brigham & Women's Hosp 1998; **Fac Appt:** Prof PlS, Case West Res Univ

Menick, Frederick J MD [PlS] - **Spec Exp:** Reconstructive Surgery-Face; Nasal Reconstruction; Cancer Reconstruction; **Hospital:** St. Joseph's Hosp - Tucson; **Address:** 1102 N Eldorado Pl, Tucson, AZ 85715; **Phone:** 520-881-4525; **Board Cert:** Plastic Surgery 1983; **Med School:** Yale Univ 1970; **Resid:** Surgery, Stanford Med Ctr 1974; Surgery, Univ Ariz Med Ctr 1979; **Fellow:** Plastic Surgery, UC Irvine 1981; Plastic Surgery, Univ Miami 1982; **Fac Appt:** Assoc Clin Prof S, Univ Ariz Coll Med

Robb, Geoffrey L MD [PlS] - **Spec Exp:** Breast Reconstruction; Head & Neck Cancer Reconstruction; Facial Plastic & Reconstructive Surgery; **Hospital:** UT MD Anderson Cancer Ctr, St. Luke's Episcopal Hosp-Houston; **Address:** 1515 Holcombe Blvd, Unit 1488, Houston, TX 77030; **Phone:** 713-794-1247; **Board Cert:** Otolaryngology 1979; Plastic Surgery 1986; **Med School:** Univ Miami Sch Med 1974; **Resid:** Otolaryngology, Naval Reg Med Ctr 1979; Plastic Surgery, Univ Pittsburgh 1985; **Fellow:** Microvascular Surgery, Univ Pittsburgh 1986; **Fac Appt:** Prof PlS, Univ Tex, Houston

Schusterman, Mark A MD [PlS] - **Spec Exp:** Breast Reconstruction; Cancer Reconstruction; **Hospital:** Methodist Hosp - Houston, St. Luke's Episcopal Hosp-Houston; **Address:** 1200 Binz St, Ste 1200, Houston, TX 77004; **Phone:** 713-794-0368; **Board Cert:** Plastic Surgery 1989; **Med School:** Univ Louisville Sch Med 1980; **Resid:** Surgery, Univ Hosp 1985; Plastic Surgery, Univ Pittsburgh Med Ctr 1987; **Fellow:** Microsurgery, Univ Pittsburgh 1988; **Fac Appt:** Clin Prof PlS, Baylor Coll Med

Yuen, James C MD [PlS] - **Spec Exp:** Breast Reconstruction; Head & Neck Cancer Reconstruction; Chest Wall Reconstruction; Limb Sparing Surgery; **Hospital:** UAMS Med Ctr; **Address:** 4301 W Markham, Ste 720, Little Rock, AR 72205; **Phone:** 501-686-8711; **Board Cert:** Surgery 2001; Plastic Surgery 2004; **Med School:** Med Coll VA 1985; **Resid:** Surgery, West Va Med Ctr 1990; Plastic/Reconstructive Surgery, Duke Univ Med Ctr 1993; **Fellow:** Hand & Microvascular Surgery, Kleinert Inst of Hand & Microsurgery 1991; **Fac Appt:** Assoc Prof S, Univ Ark

West Coast and Pacific

Andersen, James S MD [PlS] - **Spec Exp:** Breast Reconstruction; Head & Neck Reconstruction; Microsurgery; **Hospital:** City of Hope Natl Med Ctr (page 69), Huntington Memorial Hosp; **Address:** City Hope Natl Cancer Ctr, Div Plastic Surgery, 1500 E Duarte Rd, Duarte, CA 91010; **Phone:** 626-471-7100; **Board Cert:** Plastic Surgery 1994; **Med School:** Jefferson Med Coll 1983; **Resid:** Surgery, Hosp Univ Penn 1989; Plastic Surgery, Hosp Univ Penn 1991; **Fellow:** Microsurgery, USC Med Ctr 1992; **Fac Appt:** Assoc Clin Prof S, USC Sch Med

Hansen, Juliana MD [PlS] - **Spec Exp:** Breast Reconstruction; Cancer Reconstruction; **Hospital:** OR Hlth & Sci Univ; **Address:** 3303 SW Bond Ave, MC CH5P, Portland, OR 97239; **Phone:** 503-494-6687; **Board Cert:** Plastic Surgery 2008; **Med School:** Univ Wash 1988; **Resid:** Surgery, UCSF Med Ctr 1994; Plastic Surgery, UCSF Med Ctr 1996

Isik, Ferda Frank MD [PlS] - **Spec Exp:** Breast Reconstruction; **Hospital:** Swedish Med Ctr-First Hill-Seattle; **Address:** The Polyclinic, 1145 Broadway, Seattle, WA 98122; **Phone:** 206-860-4566; **Board Cert:** Surgery 2001; Plastic Surgery 2007; **Med School:** Mount Sinai Sch Med 1985; **Resid:** Surgery, Boston Univ Hosps 1990; Plastic Surgery, Univ Wash Affil Hosp 1995; **Fellow:** Research, NIH / Univ Washington 1992

Jewell, Mark L MD [PlS] - **Spec Exp:** Breast Reconstruction; **Hospital:** Sacred Heart Med Ctr; **Address:** 10 Coburg Rd, Ste 300, Eugene, OR 97401; **Phone:** 541-683-3234; **Board Cert:** Plastic Surgery 1981; **Med School:** Univ Kansas 1973; **Resid:** Surgery, LAC-Harbor Med Ctr 1976; Plastic Surgery, Erlanger Hosp 1979; **Fellow:** Burn Surgery, LAC-USC Med Ctr 1977; **Fac Appt:** Asst Clin Prof PlS, Oregon Hlth & Sci Univ

Miller, Timothy A MD [PlS] - **Spec Exp:** Eyelid Cancer & Reconstruction; Skin Cancer; Nasal Reconstruction; **Hospital:** UCLA Ronald Reagan Med Ctr; **Address:** 200 UCLA Medical Plaza, Ste 465, Los Angeles, CA 90095-8344; **Phone:** 310-825-5644; **Board Cert:** Surgery 1971; Plastic Surgery 1973; **Med School:** UCLA 1963; **Resid:** Surgery, Johns Hopkins Hosp 1967; Thoracic Surgery, UCLA Med Ctr 1969; **Fellow:** Plastic Surgery, Univ Pittsburgh 1971; **Fac Appt:** Prof S, UCLA

Sherman, Randolph MD [PlS] - **Spec Exp:** Breast Reconstruction; **Hospital:** Cedars-Sinai Med Ctr; **Address:** 8635 W 3rd St, Ste 650-W, Los Angeles, CA 90048; **Phone:** 310-423-2129; **Board Cert:** Surgery 2004; Plastic Surgery 1986; Hand Surgery 2000; **Med School:** Univ MO-Columbia Sch Med 1977; **Resid:** Surgery, UCSF Hosps 1981; Surgery, State Univ of New York 1983; **Fellow:** Plastic Surgery, USC Med Ctr 1985; **Fac Appt:** Prof S, USC Sch Med

The Best in American Medicine
www.CastleConnolly.com

Psychiatry

A psychiatrist specializes in the prevention, diagnosis and treatment of mental, addictive and emotional disorders such as schizophrenia and other psychotic disorders, mood disorders, anxiety disorders, substance-related disorders, sexual and gender identity disorders and adjustment disorders. The psychiatrist is able to understand the biologic, psychologic and social components of illness, and therefore is uniquely prepared to treat the whole person. A psychiatrist is qualified to order diagnostic laboratory tests and to prescribe medications, evaluate and treat psychologic and interpersonal problems and to intervene with families who are coping with stress, crises and other problems in living.

Training Required: Four years

Certification in one of the following subspecialties requires additional training and examination.

Addiction Psychiatry: A psychiatrist who focuses on the evaluation and treatment of individuals with alcohol, drug, or other substancerelated disorders and of individuals with the dual diagnosis of substance-related and other psychiatric disorders.

Child & Adolescent Psychiatry: A psychiatrist with additional training in the diagnosis and treatment of developmental, behavioral, emotional and mental disorders of childhood and adolescence

Geriatric Psychiatry: A psychiatrist with expertise in the prevention, evaluation, diagnosis and treatment of mental and emotional disorders in the elderly. The geriatric psychiatrist seeks to improve the psychiatric care of the elderly both in health and in disease.

PSYCHIATRY

New England

Block, Susan D MD [Psyc] - **Spec Exp:** Psychiatry in Cancer; Palliative Care; **Hospital:** Dana-Farber Cancer Inst, Brigham & Women's Hosp; **Address:** Dana Farber Cancer Inst, 450 Brookline Ave, Shields Warren, Boston, MA 02115; **Phone:** 617-632-5788; **Board Cert:** Internal Medicine 1981; Psychiatry 1984; Hospice & Palliative Medicine 2003; **Med School:** Case West Res Univ 1977; **Resid:** Internal Medicine, Beth Israel Hosp 1980; Psychiatry, Beth Israel Hosp 1982; **Fac Appt:** Prof Psyc, Harvard Med Sch

Greenberg, Donna B MD [Psyc] - **Spec Exp:** Psychiatry in Cancer; **Hospital:** Mass Genl Hosp; **Address:** Mass General Hosp, 55 Fruit St, Yawkey 9A- Psych, Fatigue Dept, Boston, MA 02114-2696; **Phone:** 617-724-4800; **Board Cert:** Internal Medicine 1978; Psychiatry 1990; **Med School:** Univ Rochester 1975; **Resid:** Internal Medicine, Boston City Hosp 1978; Psychiatry, Mass Genl Hosp 1989; **Fellow:** Psychiatry, Mass Genl Hosp 1979; **Fac Appt:** Assoc Prof Psyc, Harvard Med Sch

Rauch, Paula K MD [Psyc] - **Spec Exp:** Psychiatry in Childhood Cancer; Children/Families with Severe Illness; Parent Guidance in Parental Cancer; Psychiatry in Physical Illness; **Hospital:** Mass Genl Hosp; **Address:** Mass General Hosp, Dept Child Psychiatry, 55 Fruit St, Yawkey 6A, Boston, MA 02114; **Phone:** 617-724-5600; **Board Cert:** Psychiatry 1990; Child & Adolescent Psychiatry 1991; **Med School:** Univ Cincinnati 1981; **Resid:** Psychiatry, Mass Genl Hosp 1984; **Fac Appt:** Asst Prof Psyc, Harvard Med Sch

Mid Atlantic

Basch, Samuel MD [Psyc] - **Spec Exp:** Psychiatry in Physical Illness; Psychiatry in Cancer; **Hospital:** Mount Sinai Med Ctr (page 76); **Address:** 10 E 85th St, Ste 1B, New York, NY 10028-0412; **Phone:** 212-427-0344; **Board Cert:** Psychiatry 1970; **Med School:** Hahnemann Univ 1961; **Resid:** Psychiatry, Mount Sinai Hosp 1965; **Fellow:** Psychoanalysis, Columbia Presby Hosp 1976; **Fac Appt:** Clin Prof Psyc, Mount Sinai Sch Med

Breitbart, William MD [Psyc] - **Spec Exp:** Psychiatry in Cancer; AIDS Related Cancers; Pain-Cancer; Palliative Care; **Hospital:** Meml Sloan-Kettering Cancer Ctr (page 75); **Address:** 1275 York Avenue, New York, NY 10065; **Phone:** 646-888-0100; **Board Cert:** Internal Medicine 1982; Psychiatry 1986; Psychosomatic Medicine 2005; **Med School:** Albert Einstein Coll Med 1978; **Resid:** Internal Medicine, Bronx Muni Hosp Ctr 1982; Psychiatry, Bronx Muni Hosp Ctr 1984; **Fellow:** Psychiatric Oncology, Meml Sloan Kettering Cancer Ctr 1986; **Fac Appt:** Prof Psyc, Cornell Univ-Weill Med Coll

Klagsbrun, Samuel C MD [Psyc] - **Spec Exp:** Psychiatry in Cancer; Psychiatry in Terminal Illness; **Hospital:** Four Winds Hosp; **Address:** Four Winds Hospital, 800 Cross River Rd, Katonah, NY 10536; **Phone:** 914-763-8151 x2222; **Board Cert:** Psychiatry 1977; **Med School:** Ros Franklin Univ/Chicago Med Sch 1962; **Resid:** Psychiatry, Yale-New Haven Hosp 1966; **Fac Appt:** Clin Prof Psyc, Albert Einstein Coll Med

Kunkel, Elisabeth J MD [Psyc] - **Spec Exp:** Psychiatry in Cancer; Psychiatry in Physical Illness; **Hospital:** Thomas Jefferson Univ Hosp (page 81), Methodist Hosp; **Address:** Thomas Jefferson Univ, 1020 Samson St, Thompson Bldg, Ste 1652, Philadelphia, PA 19107; **Phone:** 215-955-9545; **Board Cert:** Psychiatry 1989; Psychosomatic Medicine 2005; **Med School:** McGill Univ 1983; **Resid:** Psychiatry, NYU Med Ctr 1987; **Fellow:** Liaison Psychiatry, Meml Sloan Kettering Cancer Ctr 1989; Consultation Psychiatry, Meml Sloan Kettering Cancer Ctr 1989; **Fac Appt:** Prof Psyc, Jefferson Med Coll

Roth, Andrew J MD [Psyc] - **Spec Exp:** Psychiatry of Prostate Cancer; **Hospital:** Meml Sloan-Kettering Cancer Ctr (page 75); **Address:** 641 Lexington Ave Fl 7, New York, NY 10022; **Phone:** 646-888-0024; **Board Cert:** Psychiatry 1993; Geriatric Psychiatry 2007; Psychosomatic Medicine 2005; **Med School:** NY Med Coll 1988; **Resid:** Psychiatry, Mt Sinai Med Ctr 1992; **Fellow:** Liaison Psychiatry, Meml Sloan-Kettering Canc Ctr 1994; **Fac Appt:** Clin Prof Psyc, Cornell Univ-Weill Med Coll

Midwest

Riba, Michelle B MD [Psyc] - **Spec Exp:** Psychiatry in Cancer; **Hospital:** Univ of Michigan Hosp; **Address:** Comprehensive Depression Ctr, 4250 Plymouth Rd, 1533 Rachel Upjohn Bldg, MC 5763, Ann Arbor, MI 48109-0295; **Phone:** 734-764-6879; **Board Cert:** Psychiatry 1991; Psychosomatic Medicine 2005; **Med School:** Univ Conn 1985; **Resid:** Psychiatry, Univ Connecticut 1988; **Fac Appt:** Clin Prof Psyc, Univ Mich Med Sch

Great Plains and Mountains

Greiner, Carl B MD [Psyc] - **Spec Exp:** Psychiatry in Cancer; Psychiatry in Physical Illness; Palliative Care; Ethics; **Hospital:** Nebraska Med Ctr; **Address:** UNMC, dept Psychiatry, 985575 Nebraska Medical Ctr, Omaha, NE 68198-5575; **Phone:** 402-552-6002; **Board Cert:** Psychiatry 1984; Forensic Psychiatry 2008; **Med School:** Univ Cincinnati 1978; **Resid:** Psychiatry, Univ Cincinnati Med Ctr 1982; **Fac Appt:** Prof Psyc, Univ Nebr Coll Med

Southwest

Baile, Walter F MD [Psyc] - **Spec Exp:** Psychiatry in Cancer; **Hospital:** UT MD Anderson Cancer Ctr; **Address:** PO Box 301402, Unit 1426, Texas, TX 77230; **Phone:** 713-563-1484; **Board Cert:** Psychiatry 1980; **Med School:** Italy 1973; **Resid:** Psychiatry, Johns Hopkins Hosp 1976; **Fellow:** Behavioral Medicine, Natl Inst Aging 1978; **Fac Appt:** Prof Psyc, Univ Tex, Houston

Valentine, Alan D MD [Psyc] - **Spec Exp:** Psychiatry in Cancer; Palliative Care; **Hospital:** UT MD Anderson Cancer Ctr; **Address:** MD Anderson Cancer Center, Dept Psychiatry Unit 1454, PO Box 301402, Houston, TX 77230-1402; **Phone:** 713-745-3344; **Board Cert:** Psychiatry 1992; Geriatric Psychiatry 2006; Psychosomatic Medicine 2005; **Med School:** Univ Tex, Houston 1986; **Resid:** Psychiatry, Univ Texas Affil Hosps; **Fac Appt:** Assoc Prof Psyc, Univ Tex, Houston

Psychiatry

West Coast and Pacific

Fann, Jesse R MD [Psyc] - **Spec Exp:** Psychiatry in Physical Illness; Psychiatry in Cancer; **Hospital:** Univ Wash Med Ctr, Harborview Med Ctr; **Address:** 1959 NE Pacific St, Box 356560, Seattle, WA 98195-6560; **Phone:** 206-685-4280; **Board Cert:** Psychiatry 2005; **Med School:** Northwestern Univ 1989; **Resid:** Psychiatry, Univ Washington Med Ctr 1993; **Fellow:** Liaison Psychiatry, Univ Washington Med Ctr 1995; Epidemiology, Univ Washington Med Ctr 1996; **Fac Appt:** Assoc Prof Psyc, Univ Wash

Kerrihard, Thomas N MD [Psyc] - **Spec Exp:** Psychiatry in Physical Illness; Psychiatry in Cancer; **Hospital:** Cedars-Sinai Med Ctr; **Address:** Cedars Sinai Medical Ctr, Dept Psychiatry, 8700 Beverly Blvd, Ste AC1004, Los Angeles, CA 90048; **Phone:** 310-423-8030; **Board Cert:** Psychiatry 2009; Pain Medicine 2005; Hospice & Palliative Medicine 2008; **Med School:** Harvard Med Sch 1994; **Resid:** Psychiatry, Mass Genl Hosp 1998; **Fellow:** Liaison Psychiatry, Meml Sloan Kettering Cancer Ctr 1999

Spiegel, David MD [Psyc] - **Spec Exp:** Psychiatry in Cancer; **Hospital:** Stanford Univ Hosp & Clinics; **Address:** Stanford Univ School of Medicine, Dept Psychiatry & Behavioral Sciences, 401 Quarry Rd PBS Bldg - rm 2325, Stanford, CA 94305-5718; **Phone:** 650-723-6421; **Board Cert:** Psychiatry 1976; **Med School:** Harvard Med Sch 1971; **Resid:** Psychiatry, Harvard Univ/Mass Mental Hlth Ctr 1974; Psychiatry, Cambridge Hosp-Harvard Med Sch 1974; **Fellow:** Community Psychiatry, Harvard Univ Med School 1974; **Fac Appt:** Prof Psyc, Stanford Univ

Strouse, Thomas B MD [Psyc] - **Spec Exp:** Psychiatry in Cancer; Pain-Cancer; Psychiatry in Physical Illness; Palliative Care; **Hospital:** UCLA Ronald Reagan Med Ctr, Cedars-Sinai Med Ctr; **Address:** UCLA Resnick Neuropsychiatric Hosp, 757 Westwood Plaza, Ste 4230B, Los Angeles, CA 90095; **Phone:** 310-267-9159; **Board Cert:** Psychiatry 1993; Pain Medicine 2000; Hospice & Palliative Medicine 2008; Psychosomatic Medicine 2009; **Med School:** Case West Res Univ 1987; **Resid:** Psychiatry, UCLA Med Ctr 1991; **Fac Appt:** Clin Prof Psyc, UCLA

Pulmonary Disease

a subspecialty of Internal Medicine

An internist who treats diseases of the lungs and airways. The pulmonologist diagnoses and treats cancer, pneumonia, pleurisy, asthma, occupational diseases, bronchitis, sleep disorders, emphysema and other complex disorders of the lungs.

Training Required: Three years in internal medicine plus additional training and examination for certification in pulmonary disease.

PULMONARY DISEASE

Mid Atlantic

King, Earl D MD [Pul] - **Spec Exp:** Lung Cancer; **Hospital:** Fox Chase Cancer Ctr (page 72); **Address:** Fox Chase Cancer Center, 333 Cottman Ave, Philadelphia, PA 19111; **Phone:** 215-728-5703; **Board Cert:** Internal Medicine 1989; Pulmonary Disease 2002; Critical Care Medicine 2003; Sleep Medicine 1995; **Med School:** Penn State Coll Med 1986; **Resid:** Internal Medicine, Temple Univ Med Ctr 1989; **Fellow:** Pulmonary Critical Care Medicine, Johns Hopkins Hosp 1993; Sleep Medicine, Johns Hopkins Hosp 1993

Libby, Daniel M MD [Pul] - **Spec Exp:** Lung Cancer; **Hospital:** NY-Presby Hosp/Weill Cornell (page 78); **Address:** 635 Madison Ave, Ste 1101, New York, NY 10022; **Phone:** 212-628-6611; **Board Cert:** Internal Medicine 1977; Pulmonary Disease 1980; **Med School:** Baylor Coll Med 1974; **Resid:** Internal Medicine, NY Hosp 1977; **Fellow:** Pulmonary Disease, NY Hosp 1979; **Fac Appt:** Clin Prof Med, Cornell Univ-Weill Med Coll

Nelson, Judith E MD [Pul] - **Spec Exp:** Palliative Care; **Hospital:** Mount Sinai Med Ctr (page 76); **Address:** Mt Sinai Medical Ctr, One Gustave Levy Pl, Box 1232, New York, NY 10029; **Phone:** 212-241-2587; **Board Cert:** Internal Medicine 1989; Pulmonary Disease 2002; Critical Care Medicine 2003; Hospice & Palliative Medicine 2005; **Med School:** NYU Sch Med 1986; **Resid:** Internal Medicine, Mt Sinai Med Ctr 1989; **Fellow:** Pulmonary Critical Care Medicine, Mt Sinai Med Ctr 1992; **Fac Appt:** Assoc Prof Med, Mount Sinai Sch Med

Steinberg, Harry MD [Pul] - **Spec Exp:** Lung Cancer; **Hospital:** Long Island Jewish Med Ctr, N Shore Univ Hosp; **Address:** LI Jewish Med Ctr, Dept Med, 270-05 76th Ave, New Hyde Park, NY 11040-1433; **Phone:** 516-465-5400; **Med School:** Temple Univ 1966; **Resid:** Internal Medicine, LI Jewish Med Ctr 1969; Pulmonary Critical Care Medicine, LI Jewish Med Ctr 1970; **Fellow:** Pulmonary Disease, Hosp Univ Penn 1974; **Fac Appt:** Clin Prof Med, Albert Einstein Coll Med

Teirstein, Alvin S MD [Pul] - **Spec Exp:** Lung Cancer; **Hospital:** Mount Sinai Med Ctr (page 76), James J. Peters VA Med Ctr-Bronx; **Address:** Mount Sinai Med Ctr, 1 Gustave Levy Pl, Box 1232, New York, NY 10029; **Phone:** 212-241-5656; **Board Cert:** Internal Medicine 1961; Pulmonary Disease 1969; **Med School:** SUNY Downstate 1953; **Resid:** Internal Medicine, Mt Sinai Med Ctr 1957; **Fellow:** Pulmonary Disease, Mt Sinai Med Ctr 1954; Pulmonary Disease, VA Med Ctr 1956; **Fac Appt:** Prof Med, Mount Sinai Sch Med

Unger, Michael MD [Pul] - **Spec Exp:** Lung Cancer; Cancer Prevention; **Hospital:** Fox Chase Cancer Ctr (page 72); **Address:** Fox Chase Cancer Center, 333 Cottman Ave, Philadelphia, PA 19111; **Phone:** 215-728-6900; **Board Cert:** Internal Medicine 1977; Pulmonary Disease 1978; **Med School:** France 1971; **Resid:** Internal Medicine, Mt Sinai Hosp 1974; **Fellow:** Pulmonary Disease, NY Hosp-Cornell 1976; **Fac Appt:** Clin Prof Med, Thomas Jefferson Univ

Southeast

Alberts, W Michael MD [Pul] - **Spec Exp:** Lung Cancer; **Hospital:** H Lee Moffitt Cancer Ctr & Research Inst; **Address:** H Lee Moffitt Cancer Ctr, Thoracic Onc, 12902 Magnolia Drive, MCC VP Suite, Tampa, FL 33612; **Phone:** 813-979-3067; **Board Cert:** Internal Medicine 1980; Pulmonary Disease 1982; **Med School:** Univ IL Coll Med 1977; **Resid:** Internal Medicine, Ohio State Univ Hosp 1980; **Fellow:** Pulmonary Critical Care Medicine, UCSD Med Ctr 1983; **Fac Appt:** Prof Med, Univ S Fla Coll Med

Garver Jr, Robert MD [Pul] - **Spec Exp:** Lung Cancer; **Hospital:** Mobile Infirmary Med Ctr; **Address:** 109 Med Park Drive, Ste C, Andalusia, AL 36420; **Phone:** 888-681-5864; **Board Cert:** Internal Medicine 1984; Pulmonary Disease 1986; **Med School:** Johns Hopkins Univ 1981; **Resid:** Internal Medicine, Johns Hopkins Hosp 1984; **Fellow:** Pulmonary Disease, NHLBI 1985; **Fac Appt:** Prof Med, Univ Alabama

Goldman, Allan L MD [Pul] - **Spec Exp:** Lung Cancer; **Hospital:** Tampa Genl Hosp, James A Haley VA Hosp; **Address:** USF Coll Med, Dept Internal Medicine, 12901 Bruce B Downs Blvd, Box MDC19, Tampa, FL 33612-4742; **Phone:** 813-974-2271; **Board Cert:** Internal Medicine 1972; Pulmonary Disease 1972; **Med School:** Univ Minn 1968; **Resid:** Internal Medicine, Brooke Army Hosp 1970; **Fellow:** Pulmonary Disease, Walter Reed Army Hosp 1972; **Fac Appt:** Prof Med, Univ S Fla Coll Med

Midwest

Silver, Michael R MD [Pul] - **Spec Exp:** Lung Cancer; **Hospital:** Rush Univ Med Ctr, Rush Oak Park Hosp; **Address:** Rush Univ Med Ctr, Professional Office Bldg 3, 1725 W Harrison St, Ste 054, Chicago, IL 60612; **Phone:** 312-942-6744; **Board Cert:** Internal Medicine 1984; Pulmonary Disease 1988; Critical Care Medicine 2009; **Med School:** Albany Med Coll 1981; **Resid:** Internal Medicine, Rush-Presby-St Lukes Med Ctr 1985; **Fellow:** Pulmonary Critical Care Medicine, Rush-Presby-St Lukes Med Ctr 1987; **Fac Appt:** Assoc Prof Med, Rush Med Coll

Great Plains and Mountains

Kern, Jeffrey A MD [Pul] - **Spec Exp:** Lung Cancer; **Hospital:** Natl Jewish Med & Rsch Ctr; **Address:** National Jewish Health, 1400 Jackson St, Denver, CO 80206; **Phone:** 877-225-5654; **Board Cert:** Internal Medicine 1982; Pulmonary Disease 1986; **Med School:** Univ Wisc 1979; **Resid:** Internal Medicine, Parkland Meml Hosp 1982; **Fellow:** Pulmonary Critical Care Medicine, Hosp Univ of Penn 1984

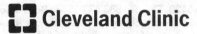 **Cleveland Clinic**

Every life deserves world class care.

Coordinated Focus on Lung Cancer

At Cleveland Clinic Taussig Cancer Institute, more than 250 top cancer specialists, researchers, nurses and technicians are dedicated to delivering the most effective medical treatments and offering access to the latest clinical trials for more than 13,000 new cancer patients every year. Our doctors are nationally and internationally known for their contributions to cancer breakthroughs and their ability to deliver superior outcomes for our patients. In recognition of these and other achievements, *U.S.News & World Report* has ranked Cleveland Clinic as one of the top cancer centers in the nation.

Chest Cancer Center

The Chest Cancer Center at Cleveland Clinic, which includes specialists from the Respiratory Institute, Taussig Cancer Institute and Heart and Vascular Institute, uses a multidisciplinary approach to cancer care. Patients with lung cancer, mesothelioma and rare tumors of the chest wall and mediastinum (mid-chest cavity), can benefit from this comprehensive, coordinated care.

Treatment Advances

Cleveland Clinic doctors identified and validated exhaled breath biomarkers for the development of a breath test that may help to identify and diagnose someone with early stage lung cancer.

Doctors and researchers also developed a blood bio-repository to study tests that are capable of assisting with the screening, diagnosis and management of patients with lung nodules and lung cancer.

Lung cancer patients also benefit from video-assisted thoracoscopy designed to assist patients who develop dangerous fluid levels in the pleural space.

Stereotactic radiation is being advanced for the treatment of patients who are not candidates for surgery, sometimes only requiring a single radiation treatment.

Cleveland Clinic
Taussig Cancer Institute
9500 Euclid Avenue
Cleveland, OH 44195

clevelandclinic.org/lungTCD

**Appointments | Information:
Call the Cancer Answer Line at
866.223.8100.**

Cancer Treatment Guides
Cleveland Clinic has developed comprehensive treatment guides for many cancers. To download our free treatment guides, visit clevelandclinic.org/cancertreatmentguides.

Comprehensive Online Medical Second Opinion
Cleveland Clinic experts can review your medical records and render an opinion that includes treatment options and recommendations. Call 216.444.3223 or 800.223.2273 ext. 43223; email eclevelandclinic@ccf.org.

Special Assistance for Out-of-State Patients
Cleveland Clinic Global Patient Services offers a complimentary Medical Concierge service for patients who travel from outside of Ohio. Call 800.223.2273, ext. 55580, or email medicalconcierge@ccf.org.

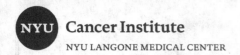
Cancer Institute

NYU LANGONE MEDICAL CENTER

NYU Langone Medical Center
550 First Avenue , New York, NY 10016
www.NYULMC.org

NYU Clinical Cancer Center
160 East 34th Street, New York, NY 10016
www.NYUCI.org

**The Stephen D. Hassenfeld Children's Center
for Cancer and Blood Disorders**
160 East 32nd Street, New York, NY 10016
www.NYUMC.org/Hassenfeld

The NYU Cancer Institute is an NCI-designated cancer center and provides personalized patient care that is both compassionate and state of the art. The doctors and researchers work together to develop innovative therapies for patients. The Cancer Institute is world-renowned for excellence in cancer-focused research, personalized care, education and community outreach. Its mission is to discover the origins of human cancer and to use that knowledge to eradicate the personal and societal burden of cancer in our community, the nation and the world. For more information about our expert physicians, call 212-731-5000. *We specialize in the following areas:*

Patient-Focused Setting
The NYU Clinical Cancer Center is the principal outpatient facility of The Cancer Institute and serves as home to our patients and their caregivers. The center and its multidisciplinary team of experts provide access to the latest treatment options and clinical trials along with a variety of programs in cancer risk reduction/prevention, screening, diagnostics, genetic counseling and supportive services. In addition the NYUCI emphasizes the importance of a holistic approach to management services in complementary medicine, psychosocial support, survivorship and palliative care.

Renowned Expertise
The NYU Cancer Institute brings together experts from a variety of disciplines to create collaborative research endeavors and clinical care teams. The Cancer Institute offers a full continuum of personalized care, from prevention through diagnosis, treatment and post-treatment support. The compassion and expertise of our team members helps patients better manage the symptoms of their diseases as well as meet their special needs. Additionally, we have created special emphasis programs in diseases such as breast cancer, melanoma, GI cancer, prostate cancer, hematologic malignancies and lung cancer among others, as well as, translational programs in cancer healthcare disparities, molecularly targeted therapy, and the cell signaling pathways involved in cancer.

A Translational Approach
NYU Langone Medical Center scientists and other researchers excel in uncovering how cancer develops at the molecular level, and how we can harness that knowledge to reduce the risk of cancer and treat the disease. The Medical Center constantly seeks to create new opportunities for collaboration between investigators within our own institution, those located elsewhere in the NYU network of campuses, and researchers at other institutions.

The Stephen D. Hassenfeld Children's Center for Cancer and Blood Disorders
The center is a leading pediatric outpatient facility for the treatment of childhood cancers and blood diseases. Its unique interdisciplinary and family-centered approach combines the most advanced medical treatments with psychosocial and emotional support services for young patients and their families.

The Best in American Medicine
www.CastleConnolly.com

Radiology

A radiologist is a physician who utilizes imaging methodologies to diagnose and manage patients and provide therapeutic options. They specialize in Diagnostic Radiology or Radiation Oncology.

Radiation Oncology: A subspecialist in radiation oncology deals with the therapeutic applications of radiant energy and its modifiers and the study and management of disease, especially malignant tumors.

Diagnostic Radiology: A radiologist who utilizes X-ray, radionuclides, ultrasound and electromagnetic radiation to diagnose and treat disease.

Training Required: Four years. Subspecialties which include Interventional Radiology and Neuroradiology, require additional training and examination.

Interventional Radiology: A radiologist who diagnoses and treats diseases by various radiologic imaging modalities. These include fluoroscopy, digital radiography, computed tomography, sonography and magnetic resonance imaging.

Neuroradiology: A radiologist who diagnoses and treats diseases utilizing imaging procedures as they relate to the brain, spine and spinal cord, head, neck and organs of special sense in adults and children.

Additional certification in subspecialties such as Pediatric Radiology and Interventional Radiology require additional training and examination.

Nuclear Medicine: A nuclear medicine specialist employs the properties of radioactive atoms and molecules in the diagnosis and treatment of disease, and in research. Radiation detection and imaging instrument systems are used to detect disease as it changes the function and metabolism of normal cells, tissues and organs. A wide variety of diseases can be found in this way, usually before the structure of the organ involved by the disease can be seen to be abnormal by any other techniques. Early detection of coronary artery disease (including acute heart attack); early cancer detection and evaluation of the effect of tumor treatment; diagnosis of infection and inflammation anywhere in the body; and early detection of blood clot in the lungs, are all possible with these techniques. Unique forms or radioactive molecules can attack and kill cancer cells (e.g., lymphoma, thyroid cancer) or can relieve the severe pain of cancer that has spread to bone.

The nuclear medicine specialist has special knowledge in the biologic effects of radiation exposure, the fundamentals of the physical sciences and the principles and operation of radiation detection and imaging instrumentation systems.

Training Required: Three years

RADIATION ONCOLOGY

New England

Choi, Noah C MD [RadRO] - **Spec Exp:** Lung Cancer; Esophageal Cancer; Mesothelioma; **Hospital:** Mass Genl Hosp; **Address:** Mass Genl Hosp, Dept Rad Oncology, 100 Blossom St, Cox 3, Boston, MA 02114; **Phone:** 617-726-6050; **Board Cert:** Therapeutic Radiology 1970; **Med School:** South Korea 1963; **Resid:** Radiation Oncology, Princess Margaret Hosp 1970; **Fac Appt:** Prof RadRO, Harvard Med Sch

D'Amico, Anthony V MD/PhD [RadRO] - **Spec Exp:** Prostate Cancer; Brachytherapy; Urologic Cancer; **Hospital:** Dana-Farber Cancer Inst, Brigham & Women's Hosp; **Address:** Brigham & Women's Hosp, Radiation Oncology, L2, 75 Francis St, Boston, MA 02115; **Phone:** 617-632-6328; **Board Cert:** Radiation Oncology 2010; **Med School:** Univ Pennsylvania 1990; **Resid:** Radiation Oncology, Hosp Univ Penn 1994; **Fac Appt:** Prof RadRO, Harvard Med Sch

DeLaney, Thomas F MD [RadRO] - **Spec Exp:** Sarcoma; Proton Beam Therapy; **Hospital:** Mass Genl Hosp; **Address:** Francis H. Burr Proton Therapy Ctr, MGH Radiation Oncology, 30 Fruit St, Boston, MA 02114; **Phone:** 617-726-6876; **Board Cert:** Therapeutic Radiology 1986; Radiation Oncology 1999; **Med School:** Harvard Med Sch 1982; **Resid:** Therapeutic Radiology, Mass Genl Hosp 1986; **Fac Appt:** Assoc Prof RadRO, Harvard Med Sch

Harris, Jay R MD [RadRO] - **Spec Exp:** Breast Cancer; **Hospital:** Brigham & Women's Hosp, Dana-Farber Cancer Inst; **Address:** Dana Farber Cancer Inst, 44 Binney St, Dana 1622, Boston, MA 02115; **Phone:** 617-632-2291; **Board Cert:** Therapeutic Radiology 1976; **Med School:** Stanford Univ 1970; **Resid:** Radiation Therapy, Joint Ctr Rad Ther 1976; **Fellow:** Radiation Therapy, Harvard Med Sch 1977; **Fac Appt:** Prof RadRO, Harvard Med Sch

Hartford, Alan C MD/PhD [RadRO] - **Spec Exp:** Prostate Cancer; Brain & Spinal Tumors; **Hospital:** Dartmouth - Hitchcock Med Ctr; **Address:** Darthmouth-Hitchcock Med Ctr, 1 Med Ctr Drive, Lebanon, NH 03756; **Phone:** 603-650-6602; **Board Cert:** Radiation Oncology 2010; **Med School:** Harvard Med Sch 1992; **Resid:** Radiation Oncology, Mass Genl Hosp 1998; **Fellow:** Radiation Oncology, Mass Genl Hosp 1999; **Fac Appt:** Assoc Prof RadRO, Dartmouth Med Sch

Heimann, Ruth MD [RadRO] - **Spec Exp:** Breast Cancer; Gastrointestinal Cancer; Lung Cancer; **Hospital:** Fletcher Allen Health Care- Med Ctr Campus; **Address:** Fletcher Allen Radiation Medicine, 111 Colchester Ave, Burlington, VT 05401; **Phone:** 802-847-3506; **Board Cert:** Radiation Oncology 1995; **Med School:** UMDNJ-NJ Med Sch, Newark 1989; **Resid:** Radiation Oncology, Meml Sloan-Kettering Cancer Ctr 1993; **Fac Appt:** Prof Med, Univ VT Coll Med

Kachnic, Lisa A MD [RadRO] - **Spec Exp:** Breast Cancer; Gastrointestinal Cancer; Thoracic Cancers; **Hospital:** Boston Med Ctr; **Address:** Boston Medical Ctr, Dept Rad/Onc, 830 Harrison Ave, lower level, Boston, MA 02118; **Phone:** 617-638-7070; **Board Cert:** Radiation Oncology 2006; **Med School:** Tufts Univ 1991; **Resid:** Radiation Oncology, Mass Genl Hosp 1996; **Fac Appt:** Assoc Prof RadRO, Boston Univ

Kaplan, Irving D MD [RadRO] - **Spec Exp:** Prostate Cancer; Brachytherapy; **Hospital:** Beth Israel Deaconess Med Ctr - Boston; **Address:** Beth Israel Deaconess Med Ctr, Dept Radiation Oncology, 330 Brookline Ave, Boston, MA 02215; **Phone:** 617-667-2345; **Board Cert:** Radiation Oncology 1989; **Med School:** Stanford Univ 1985; **Resid:** Radiation Oncology, Stanford Univ Med Ctr 1989; **Fac Appt:** Asst Prof RadRO, Harvard Med Sch

Radiation Oncology

Mauch, Peter M MD [RadRO] - **Spec Exp:** Lymphoma; Hodgkin's Disease; **Hospital:** Dana-Farber Cancer Inst; **Address:** Brigham & Womens Hosp, 75 Francis St, Radiation Oncology ASB1/L2, Boston, MA 02115; **Phone:** 617-732-6310; **Board Cert:** Therapeutic Radiology 1978; **Med School:** St Louis Univ 1974; **Resid:** Radiation Therapy, Harvard Joint Ctr 1978; **Fac Appt:** Prof RadRO, Harvard Med Sch

Peschel, Richard E MD [RadRO] - **Spec Exp:** Prostate Cancer; Testicular Cancer; **Hospital:** Yale-New Haven Hosp, Yale Med Group; **Address:** Yale-New Haven Hosp, Dept Therapeutic Radiology, 15 York St, rm HRT 142, New Haven, CT 06510; **Phone:** 203-785-2957; **Board Cert:** Therapeutic Radiology 1982; **Med School:** Yale Univ 1977; **Resid:** Radiation Oncology, Yale-New Haven Hosp 1981; **Fac Appt:** Prof RadRO, Yale Univ

Recht, Abram MD [RadRO] - **Spec Exp:** Breast Cancer; Gastrointestinal Cancer; Gynecologic Cancer; **Hospital:** Beth Israel Deaconess Med Ctr - Boston; **Address:** 330 Brookline Ave Finard Bldg - rm B25, Beth Israel Deaconess Med Ctr, Boston, MA 02215; **Phone:** 617-667-2345; **Board Cert:** Therapeutic Radiology 1984; **Med School:** Johns Hopkins Univ 1980; **Resid:** Radiation Oncology, Joint Ctr Radiation Therapy 1984; **Fac Appt:** Prof RadRO, Harvard Med Sch

Roberts, Kenneth MD [RadRO] - **Spec Exp:** Pediatric Cancers; Lymphoma; Hodgkin's Disease; **Hospital:** Yale-New Haven Hosp, Yale Med Group; **Address:** Yale Univ Sch Med, Dept Radiation Therapy, 15 York St, New Haven, CT 06520-8040; **Phone:** 203-785-2957; **Board Cert:** Internal Medicine 1987; Medical Oncology 1989; Radiation Oncology 1995; **Med School:** Duke Univ 1984; **Resid:** Internal Medicine, Ohio State Univ Hosps 1987; Radiation Oncology, Duke Univ Med Ctr 1992; **Fellow:** Hematology & Oncology, Duke Univ Med Ctr 1989; **Fac Appt:** Assoc Prof Rad, Yale Univ

Russell, Anthony Henryk MD [RadRO] - **Spec Exp:** Gynecologic Cancer; Intensity Modulated Radiotherapy (IMRT); Proton Beam Therapy; **Hospital:** Mass Genl Hosp; **Address:** Clark Ctr for Radiology, 100 Blossom St, COX 3, Boston, MA 02114; **Phone:** 617-726-5184; **Board Cert:** Therapeutic Radiology 1978; **Med School:** Harvard Med Sch 1974; **Resid:** Radiation Oncology, Mass Genl Hosp 1978

Taghian, Alphonse G MD/PhD [RadRO] - **Spec Exp:** Breast Cancer; **Hospital:** Mass Genl Hosp; **Address:** MGH Dept Radiation Oncology, 100 Blossom St, COX 3, Boston, MA 02114; **Phone:** 617-726-6050; **Board Cert:** Radiation Oncology 2006; **Med School:** Egypt 1980; **Resid:** Radiation Oncology, Vautrin Cancer Ctr 1987; Radiation Oncology, Inst Gustave Roussy 1989; **Fellow:** Radiation Oncology, Mass Genl Hosp 1993; **Fac Appt:** Assoc Prof RadRO, Harvard Med Sch

Tarbell, Nancy MD [RadRO] - **Spec Exp:** Brain Tumors-Pediatric; Proton Beam Therapy; **Hospital:** Mass Genl Hosp; **Address:** Massachusetts Genl Hosp, Proton Ctr, 55 Fruit St, Boston, MA 02114; **Phone:** 617-724-1836; **Board Cert:** Therapeutic Radiology 1983; **Med School:** SUNY Upstate Med Univ 1979; **Resid:** Radiation Therapy, Harvard Med School 1983; **Fac Appt:** Prof RadRO, Harvard Med Sch

Wazer, David E MD [RadRO] - **Spec Exp:** Breast Cancer; Melanoma; **Hospital:** Rhode Island Hosp, Tufts Med Ctr; **Address:** 593 Eddy St, Providence, RI 02903; **Phone:** 401-444-8311; **Board Cert:** Radiation Oncology 1988; **Med School:** NYU Sch Med 1982; **Resid:** Radiation Oncology, Tufts New Eng Med Ctr 1988; **Fellow:** Neurological Chemistry, NYU Med Ctr 1984; **Fac Appt:** Prof RadRO, Tufts Univ

Wilson, Lynn D MD [RadRO] - **Spec Exp:** Lymphoma, Cutaneous T Cell (CTCL); Lymphoma, Cutaneous B Cell (CBCL); Lung Cancer; Head & Neck Cancer; **Hospital:** Yale-New Haven Hosp, Yale Med Group; **Address:** Yale Univ Sch Med, Dept Therapeutic Rad, PO Box 208040, New Haven, CT 06520-8040; **Phone:** 203-688-4344; **Board Cert:** Radiation Oncology 2004; **Med School:** Geo Wash Univ 1990; **Resid:** Therapeutic Radiology, Yale-New Haven Hosp 1994; **Fac Appt:** Prof RadRO, Yale Univ

Zietman, Anthony L MD [RadRO] - **Spec Exp:** Prostate Cancer; Urologic Cancer; Proton Beam Therapy; **Hospital:** Mass Genl Hosp; **Address:** Mass General Hosp, Yawkey Ste 7E, 55 Fruit St, Boston, MA 02114; **Phone:** 617-724-1158; **Board Cert:** Radiation Oncology 1994; **Med School:** England, UK 1983; **Resid:** Internal Medicine, St Stephens & Westminster Hosp 1986; Radiation Oncology, Mass Genl Hosp 1989; **Fellow:** Radiation Oncology, Middlesex Hosp 1991; Radiation Oncology, Mass Genl Hosp; **Fac Appt:** Prof RadRO, Harvard Med Sch

Mid Atlantic

Berg, Christine D MD [RadRO] - **Spec Exp:** Breast Cancer-Early Detection; Breast Cancer-High Risk Women; **Hospital:** Natl Inst of Hlth - Clin Ctr; **Address:** 6130 Executive Blvd, Bethesda, MD 20892; **Phone:** 301-496-8544; **Board Cert:** Internal Medicine 1980; Medical Oncology 1983; Therapeutic Radiology 1986; Radiation Oncology 1999; **Med School:** Northwestern Univ 1977; **Resid:** Internal Medicine, Northwestern Meml Hosp 1981; Radiation Oncology, Georgetown Univ Hosp 1986; **Fellow:** Medical Oncology, Natl Cancer Inst-NIH 1984

Bogart, Jeffrey A MD [RadRO] - **Spec Exp:** Lung Cancer; Thoracic Cancers; Prostate Cancer; Clinical Trials; **Hospital:** SUNY Upstate Med Univ Shos; **Address:** SUNY Upstate Medical Ctr, Dept Radiation Oncology, 750 E Adams St, Syracuse, NY 13210; **Phone:** 315-464-5276; **Board Cert:** Radiation Oncology 1994; **Med School:** SUNY Upstate Med Univ 1989; **Resid:** Radiation Oncology, SUNY Hlth Sci Ctr 1993; **Fac Appt:** Prof RadRO, SUNY Upstate Med Univ

Constine, Louis Sanders MD [RadRO] - **Spec Exp:** Pediatric Cancers; Lymphoma; Cancer Survivors-Late Effects of Therapy; Sarcoma; **Hospital:** Univ of Rochester Strong Meml Hosp; **Address:** 601 Elmwood Ave, Box 647, Rochester, NY 14642; **Phone:** 585-275-5622; **Board Cert:** Pediatrics 1978; Therapeutic Radiology 1981; Pediatric Hematology-Oncology 1978; **Med School:** Johns Hopkins Univ 1973; **Resid:** Pediatrics, Moffitt Hosp-UCSF Med Ctr 1975; Pediatrics, Stanford Hosp Med Ctr 1976; **Fellow:** Therapeutic Radiology, Stanford Hosp Med Ctr 1981; Pediatric Hematology-Oncology, Univ Wash/Chldns Ortho Hosp 1978; **Fac Appt:** Prof RadRO, Univ Rochester

Cooper, Jay MD [RadRO] - **Spec Exp:** Head & Neck Cancer; Skin Cancer; Chemo-Radiation Combined Therapy; **Hospital:** Maimonides Med Ctr (page 74); **Address:** 6300 8th Ave, Brooklyn, NY 11220; **Phone:** 718-765-2700; **Board Cert:** Therapeutic Radiology 1977; **Med School:** NYU Sch Med 1973; **Resid:** Radiation Oncology, NYU Med Ctr 1977; **Fac Appt:** Prof RadRO, Albert Einstein Coll Med

DeWeese, Theodore L MD [RadRO] - **Spec Exp:** Urologic Cancer; Prostate Cancer; Testicular Cancer; **Hospital:** Johns Hopkins Hosp; **Address:** Johns Hopkins Hosp, Weinberg Bldg, 401 N Broadway, rm 1363, Baltimore, MD 21231; **Phone:** 410-955-8964; **Board Cert:** Radiation Oncology 2005; **Med School:** Univ Colorado 1990; **Resid:** Radiation Oncology, Johns Hopkins Hosp 1994; **Fellow:** Urologic Oncology, Johns Hopkins Hosp 1995; **Fac Appt:** Prof RadRO, Johns Hopkins Univ

Radiation Oncology

Dicker, Adam P MD/PhD [RadRO] - **Spec Exp:** Prostate Cancer; **Hospital:** Thomas Jefferson Univ Hosp (page 81); **Address:** Bodine Cancer Treatment Ctr, 111 South 11th St, Philadelphia, PA 19107-5097; **Phone:** 215-955-6527; **Board Cert:** Radiation Oncology 2000; **Med School:** Cornell Univ-Weill Med Coll 1992; **Resid:** Surgery, Lenox Hill Hosp 1994; Radiation Oncology, Meml Sloan Kettering Cancer Ctr 1997; **Fac Appt:** Prof RadRO, Thomas Jefferson Univ

Dritschilo, Anatoly MD [RadRO] - **Spec Exp:** Prostate Cancer; **Hospital:** Georgetown Univ Hosp; **Address:** Georgetown Univ Hosp, Dept Radiation Medicine, LL-Bles, 3800 Reservoir Rd NW, Washington, DC 20007; **Phone:** 202-687-2144; **Board Cert:** Therapeutic Radiology 1977; **Med School:** UMDNJ-NJ Med Sch, Newark 1973; **Resid:** Radiation Therapy, Harvard Joint Rad Ther Ctr 1977; **Fac Appt:** Prof Med, Georgetown Univ

Ennis, Ronald D MD [RadRO] - **Spec Exp:** Prostate Cancer; Brachytherapy; Breast Cancer; **Hospital:** St. Luke's - Roosevelt Hosp Ctr - Roosevelt Div (page 71), Beth Israel Med Ctr - Petrie Division (page 71); **Address:** 1000 10th Ave, Lower Level, New York, NY 10019; **Phone:** 212-523-7165; **Board Cert:** Radiation Oncology 2005; **Med School:** Yale Univ 1990; **Resid:** Therapeutic Radiology, Yale-New Haven Hosp 1994

Flickinger, John C MD [RadRO] - **Spec Exp:** Neuro-Oncology; Brain & Spinal Tumors; **Hospital:** UPMC Presby, Pittsburgh; **Address:** UPMC Cancer Ctr, Radiation Oncology, 5230 Centre Ave, Pittsburgh, PA 15213; **Phone:** 412-647-3600; **Board Cert:** Therapeutic Radiology 1985; **Med School:** Univ Chicago-Pritzker Sch Med 1981; **Resid:** Radiation Therapy, Mass Genl Hosp 1985; **Fac Appt:** Prof RadRO, Univ Pittsburgh

Formenti, Silvia C MD [RadRO] - **Spec Exp:** Breast Cancer; Chemo-Radiation Combined Therapy; **Hospital:** NYU Langone Med Ctr (page 79); **Address:** NYU Med Ctr, Dept Radiation Oncology, 160 E 34th St, New York, NY 10016; **Phone:** 212-263-2601; **Board Cert:** Radiation Oncology 1991; **Med School:** Italy 1980; **Resid:** Internal Medicine, San Carlo Borromeo Hosp 1983; Medical Oncology, Univ of Pavia Med Ctr 1985; **Fellow:** Radiation Oncology, USC Med Ctr 1990; **Fac Appt:** Prof RadRO, NYU Sch Med

Freedman, Gary M MD [RadRO] - **Spec Exp:** Breast Cancer; **Hospital:** Hosp Univ Penn - UPHS (page 80); **Address:** Hosp U Penn, Dept Radiation Oncology, 3400 Spruce St, Philadelphia, PA 19104; **Phone:** 215-615-6767; **Board Cert:** Radiation Oncology 2000; **Med School:** Temple Univ 1993; **Resid:** Radiation Oncology, Fox Chase Cancer Ctr 1997

Gejerman, Glen MD [RadRO] - **Spec Exp:** Prostate Cancer; Intensity Modulated Radiotherapy (IMRT); Breast Cancer; Brachytherapy; **Hospital:** Hackensack Univ Med Ctr (page 73); **Address:** Hackensack Univ Med Ctr, Radiation Onc, 30 Prospect Ave, Hackensack, NJ 07601; **Phone:** 201-996-2464; **Board Cert:** Radiation Oncology 2006; **Med School:** UMDNJ-NJ Med Sch, Newark 1990; **Resid:** Radiation Oncology, Montefiore Med Ctr 1995; **Fac Appt:** Asst Clin Prof RadRO, Albert Einstein Coll Med

Goodman, Robert L MD [RadRO] - **Spec Exp:** Breast Cancer; Lymphoma; Prostate Cancer; Brain Tumors; **Hospital:** Saint Barnabas Med Ctr; **Address:** St Barnabas Med Ctr, Dept Rad Oncology, 94 Old Short Hills Rd, Livingston, NJ 07039; **Phone:** 973-322-5133; **Board Cert:** Internal Medicine 1971; Therapeutic Radiology 1974; Medical Oncology 1975; **Med School:** Columbia P&S 1966; **Resid:** Internal Medicine, Beth Israel Hosp 1970; Radiation Therapy, Harvard Joint Ctr Rad Therapy 1974; **Fellow:** Hematology, NY-Presby Hosp 1969

Greenberger, Joel S MD [RadRO] - **Spec Exp:** Lung Cancer; Esophageal Cancer; **Hospital:** UPMC Presby, Pittsburgh; **Address:** UPMC Cancer Ctr, Cancer Pavilion, 5230 Centre Ave, Pittsburgh, PA 15232; **Phone:** 412-647-3600; **Board Cert:** Therapeutic Radiology 1977; **Med School:** Harvard Med Sch 1971; **Resid:** Radiation Therapy, Mass General Hosp 1977; **Fac Appt:** Prof RadRO, Univ Pittsburgh

Haffty, Bruce MD [RadRO] - **Spec Exp:** Breast Cancer; Head & Neck Cancer; Lung Cancer; **Hospital:** Robert Wood Johnson Univ Hosp - New Brunswick, Robert Wood Johnson Univ Hosp Hamilton; **Address:** The Cancer Institute of New Jersey, 195 Little Albany St, rm 2038, New Brunswick, NJ 08903; **Phone:** 732-253-3939; **Board Cert:** Radiation Oncology 1988; **Med School:** Yale Univ 1984; **Resid:** Radiation Oncology, Yale-New Haven Hosp 1988; **Fac Appt:** Prof RadRO

Hahn, Stephen M MD [RadRO] - **Spec Exp:** Lung Cancer; Prostate Cancer; Sarcoma; Photodynamic Therapy; **Hospital:** Hosp Univ Penn - UPHS (page 80), Penn Presby Med Ctr - UPHS (page 80); **Address:** Hosp of the Univ of Penn, 3400 Spruce St Donner Bldg Fl 2, Philadelphia, PA 19104; **Phone:** 215-662-7296; **Board Cert:** Internal Medicine 1987; Medical Oncology 2001; Radiation Oncology 2004; **Med School:** Temple Univ 1984; **Resid:** Internal Medicine, UCSF Med Ctr 1988; Medical Oncology, Natl Inst Hlth 1991; **Fellow:** Radiation Oncology, Natl Inst Hlth 1994; **Fac Appt:** Prof RadRO, Univ Pennsylvania

Harrison, Louis B MD [RadRO] - **Spec Exp:** Brachytherapy; Head & Neck Cancer; Radiation Therapy-Intraoperative; **Hospital:** Beth Israel Med Ctr - Petrie Division (page 71), St. Luke's - Roosevelt Hosp Ctr - Roosevelt Div (page 71); **Address:** Beth Israel Med Ctr, Dept Rad Onc, 10 Union Square East, Ste 4G, New York, NY 10003-3314; **Phone:** 212-844-8087; **Board Cert:** Therapeutic Radiology 1986; **Med School:** SUNY Downstate 1982; **Resid:** Therapeutic Radiology, Yale-New Haven Hosp 1986; **Fac Appt:** Prof RadRO, Albert Einstein Coll Med

Horwitz, Eric MD [RadRO] - **Spec Exp:** Prostate Cancer; Intensity Modulated Radiotherapy (IMRT); Brachytherapy; **Hospital:** Fox Chase Cancer Ctr (page 72); **Address:** Fox Chase Cancer Ctr, Dept Radiation Oncology, 333 Cottman Ave, Philadelphia, PA 19111; **Phone:** 215-728-2995; **Board Cert:** Radiation Oncology 2010; **Med School:** Albany Med Coll 1992; **Resid:** Radiation Oncology, William Beaumont Hosp 1997

Isaacson, Steven R MD [RadRO] - **Spec Exp:** Brain Tumors; Neuro-Oncology; Stereotactic Radiosurgery; Gliomas; **Hospital:** NY-Presby Hosp/Columbia (page 78); **Address:** NY Presbyterian-Columbia Med Ctr, Dept Radiation Oncology, 622 W 168th St BHN Bldg - rm B-11, New York, NY 10032-3720; **Phone:** 212-305-2611; **Board Cert:** Radiation Oncology 1988; Otolaryngology 1978; **Med School:** Jefferson Med Coll 1973; **Resid:** Otolaryngology, Hosp Univ Penn 1978; Radiation Oncology, SUNY Hlth Sci Ctr 1988; **Fac Appt:** Clin Prof RadRO, Columbia P&S

Kleinberg, Lawrence MD [RadRO] - **Spec Exp:** Brain & Spinal Cord Tumors; Brain Tumors-Metastatic; Stereotactic Radiosurgery; Esophageal Cancer; **Hospital:** Johns Hopkins Hosp; **Address:** Johns Hopkins Oncology Ctr Weinberg Bldg, 401 N Broadway, Ste 1440, Baltimore, MD 21231; **Phone:** 410-614-2597; **Board Cert:** Radiation Oncology 1994; **Med School:** Yale Univ 1989; **Resid:** Radiation Oncology, Meml Sloan-Kettering Canc Ctr 1993; **Fac Appt:** Assoc Prof RadRO, Johns Hopkins Univ

Kuettel, Michael MD/PhD [RadRO] - **Spec Exp:** Prostate Cancer; **Hospital:** Roswell Park Cancer Inst; **Address:** Roswell Park Cancer Inst, Radiation Med, Elm and Carlton St, Buffalo, NY 14263; **Phone:** 716-845-1562; **Board Cert:** Radiation Oncology 1992; **Med School:** Northwestern Univ-Feinberg Sch Med 1985; **Resid:** Internal Medicine, Northwestern Hosp 1986; Radiation Oncology, Johns Hopkins Hosp 1990; **Fac Appt:** Prof RadRO, SUNY Buffalo

Lepanto, Philip B MD [RadRO] - **Hospital:** St. Mary's Med Ctr - Huntington, Cabell Huntington Hosp; **Address:** St Mary's Med Ctr, Dept Radiation Oncology, 2900 First Ave, Huntington, WV 25702; **Phone:** 304-526-1143; **Board Cert:** Therapeutic Radiology 1975; **Med School:** Univ Louisville Sch Med 1970; **Resid:** Diagnostic Radiology, Graduate Hosp 1972; Radiation Therapy, Hosp Univ Penn 1975; **Fac Appt:** Clin Prof Rad, Marshall Univ

McCormick, Beryl MD [RadRO] - **Spec Exp:** Breast Cancer; Eye Tumors/Cancer; **Hospital:** Meml Sloan-Kettering Cancer Ctr (page 75), NY-Presby Hosp/Weill Cornell (page 78); **Address:** 1275 York Avenue, New York, NY 10065; **Phone:** 800-525-2225; **Board Cert:** Therapeutic Radiology 1977; **Med School:** UMDNJ-NJ Med Sch, Newark 1973; **Resid:** Therapeutic Radiology, Meml Sloan Kettering Cancer Ctr 1977; **Fac Appt:** Prof RadRO, Cornell Univ-Weill Med Coll

Nicolaou, Nicos MD [RadRO] - **Spec Exp:** Lymphoma; Hodgkin's Disease; Urologic Cancer; Breast Cancer; **Address:** Phila Cancer Treatment, 1 Presidential Blvd, Ste 100, Bala Cynwyd, PA 19004; **Phone:** 610-632-4100; **Board Cert:** Radiation Oncology 2010; **Med School:** South Africa 1984; **Resid:** Radiation Oncology, Univ British Columbia Cancer Ctr 1994; **Fellow:** Radiation Oncology, Fox Chase Cancer Ctr 1995; **Fac Appt:** Assoc Prof RadRO, Univ Pennsylvania

Nori, Dattatreyudu MD [RadRO] - **Spec Exp:** Prostate Cancer; Brachytherapy; Lung Cancer; Breast Cancer; **Hospital:** NY-Presby Hosp/Weill Cornell (page 78), NY Hosp Queens; **Address:** 525 E 68th St, Box 575, New York, NY 10065; **Phone:** 212-746-3679; **Board Cert:** Therapeutic Radiology 1979; **Med School:** India 1970; **Resid:** Radiation Oncology, Meml Sloan Kettering Cancer Ctr 1975; **Fellow:** Radiation Oncology, Meml Sloan Kettering Cancer Ctr 1978; **Fac Appt:** Prof RadRO, Cornell Univ-Weill Med Coll

Porrazzo, Michael S MD [RadRO] - **Spec Exp:** Prostate Cancer; Central Nervous System Cancer; Breast Cancer; Stereotactic Radiosurgery; **Hospital:** Washington Hosp Ctr; **Address:** Wash Hosp Ctr-Dept. Radiation Onc, 110 Irving St NW, Rm CG-107, Washington, DC 20010; **Phone:** 202-877-3925; **Board Cert:** Radiation Oncology 1990; **Med School:** Meharry Med Coll 1985; **Resid:** Radiation Oncology, SUNY Hlth Sci Ctr 1989

Randolph-Jackson, Pamela D MD [RadRO] - **Spec Exp:** Breast Cancer; Lung Cancer; Gastrointestinal Cancer; **Hospital:** Washington Hosp Ctr; **Address:** 110 Irving St NW, CG 116, Washington, DC 20010; **Phone:** 202-877-3925; **Board Cert:** Radiation Oncology 2004; **Med School:** E Tenn State Univ 1988; **Resid:** Radiology, Howard Univ Hosp 1992; **Fellow:** Radiation Oncology, Jefferson Med Coll 1993

Regine, William F MD [RadRO] - **Spec Exp:** Stereotactic Radiosurgery; Brain & Spinal Tumors; Gastrointestinal Cancer; **Hospital:** Univ of MD Med Ctr; **Address:** Univ MD Med System-Greenbaum Cancer Ctr, 22 S Green St Guldelsky Bldg, Baltimore, MD 21201; **Phone:** 410-328-6080; **Board Cert:** Radiation Oncology 1992; **Med School:** SUNY Upstate Med Univ 1987; **Resid:** Radiation Oncology, Thomas Jefferson Univ Hosp 1991; **Fellow:** Radiation Oncology, Thomas Jefferson Univ Hosp 1992; **Fac Appt:** Prof RadRO, Univ MD Sch Med

Rotman, Marvin MD [RadRO] - **Spec Exp:** Bladder Cancer; Gynecologic Cancer; Eye Tumors/Cancer; Prostate Cancer; **Hospital:** SUNY Downstate Med Ctr, Univ Hosp of Bklyn at Long Island Coll Hosp (page 71); **Address:** 450 Clarkson Ave, Box 1211, Brooklyn, NY 11203-2056; **Phone:** 718-270-2181; **Board Cert:** Diagnostic Radiology 1966; Radiation Oncology 1999; **Med School:** Jefferson Med Coll 1958; **Resid:** Internal Medicine, Albert Einstein Med Ctr 1960; Radiation Oncology, Montefiore Hosp Med Ctr 1965; **Fac Appt:** Prof RadRO, SUNY Downstate

Schiff, Peter B MD/PhD [RadRO] - **Spec Exp:** Prostate Cancer; Gynecologic Cancer; Breast Cancer; **Hospital:** NYU Langone Med Ctr (page 79); **Address:** NYU Clinical Cancer Ctr, 160 E 34th St Fl 1, New York, NY 10016; **Phone:** 212-731-5003; **Board Cert:** Radiation Oncology 1990; **Med School:** Albert Einstein Coll Med 1984; **Resid:** Radiation Oncology, Meml Sloan Kettering Cancer Ctr 1988; **Fac Appt:** Prof RadRO, NYU Sch Med

Solin, Lawrence J MD [RadRO] - **Spec Exp:** Breast Cancer; **Hospital:** Albert Einstein Med Ctr; **Address:** Albert Einstein Medical Center, Dept Radiation Oncology, 5501 Old York Rd, Philadelphia, PA 19141; **Phone:** 215-456-6280; **Board Cert:** Therapeutic Radiology 1984; **Med School:** Brown Univ 1978; **Resid:** Surgery, Thos Jefferson Univ Hosp 1981; Radiation Oncology, Thos Jefferson Univ Hosp 1982; **Fellow:** Radiation Oncology, Hosp Univ Penn 1984; **Fac Appt:** Prof Emeritus RadRO, Univ Pennsylvania

Stock, Richard MD [RadRO] - **Spec Exp:** Prostate Cancer; **Hospital:** Mount Sinai Med Ctr (page 76); **Address:** Dept Radiation Oncology, 1184 5th Ave, Box 1236, New York, NY 10029; **Phone:** 212-241-7502; **Board Cert:** Radiation Oncology 1993; **Med School:** Mount Sinai Sch Med 1988; **Resid:** Radiation Oncology, Meml Sloan Kettering Cancer Ctr 1992; **Fac Appt:** Prof RadRO, Mount Sinai Sch Med

Streeter Jr, Oscar E MD [RadRO] - **Spec Exp:** Lung Cancer; Head & Neck Cancer; **Hospital:** Howard Univ Hosp; **Address:** Howard Univ Hosp, Dept Radiation Onc, 2041 Georgia Ave NW, Washington, DC 20060; **Phone:** 202-865-6100; **Board Cert:** Radiation Oncology 1989; **Med School:** Howard Univ 1982; **Resid:** Radiation Oncology, Howard Univ 1986; Radiation Oncology, USC Sch Med 1994; **Fac Appt:** Assoc Prof RadRO, USC Sch Med

Suntharalingam, Mohan MD [RadRO] - **Spec Exp:** Head & Neck Cancer; Lung Cancer; Esophageal Cancer; **Hospital:** Univ of MD Med Ctr; **Address:** 22 S Greene St, Baltimore, MD 21201; **Phone:** 410-328-2331; **Board Cert:** Radiation Oncology 2005; **Med School:** Thomas Jefferson Univ 1990; **Resid:** Radiation Oncology, Univ Maryland Med Ctr 1993; **Fellow:** Radiation Oncology, Univ Maryland Med Ctr 1994; **Fac Appt:** Prof RadRO, Univ MD Sch Med

Weiss, Marisa C MD [RadRO] - **Spec Exp:** Breast Cancer; **Hospital:** Lankenau Hosp; **Address:** Lankenau Hospital, Dept Rad Oncology, 100 E Lancaster Ave, Wynnewood, PA 19096; **Phone:** 484-476-2433; **Board Cert:** Radiation Oncology 1988; **Med School:** Univ Pennsylvania 1984; **Resid:** Radiation Oncology, Hosp Univ Penn 1988; **Fellow:** Radiological Biology, Hosp Univ Penn 1990

Werner-Wasik, Maria MD [RadRO] - **Spec Exp:** Brain Tumors; Lung Cancer; Melanoma; Breast Cancer; **Hospital:** Thomas Jefferson Univ Hosp (page 81); **Address:** Thomas Jefferson Univ Hosp, Dept Radiation Oncology, 111 S 11 St, Philadelphia, PA 19107; **Phone:** 215-955-6702; **Board Cert:** Radiation Oncology 1994; **Med School:** Poland 1979; **Resid:** Internal Medicine, Framingham Union Hosp 1990; Radiation Oncology, Tufts/New England Med Ctr 1993; **Fellow:** Radiation Oncology, Hosp Univ Penn 1994; **Fac Appt:** Assoc Prof RadRO, Thomas Jefferson Univ

Wharam Jr, Moody D MD [RadRO] - **Spec Exp:** Pediatric Cancers; Brain Tumors; Sarcoma-Soft Tissue; **Hospital:** Johns Hopkins Hosp; **Address:** Kimmel Cancer Ctr, Dept Rad Oncology, 401 N Broadway St, Ste 1440, Baltimore, MD 21231-2410; **Phone:** 410-955-8964; **Board Cert:** Therapeutic Radiology 1974; **Med School:** Univ VA Sch Med 1969; **Resid:** Radiation Oncology, UCSF Med Ctr 1973; **Fac Appt:** Prof RadRO, Johns Hopkins Univ

Yahalom, Joachim MD [RadRO] - **Spec Exp:** Lymphoma; Hodgkin's Disease; Multiple Myeloma; **Hospital:** Meml Sloan-Kettering Cancer Ctr (page 75); **Address:** 1275 York Ave, SM03, Dept Radiation Onc, New York, NY 10065; **Phone:** 212-639-5999; **Board Cert:** Radiation Oncology 1988; **Med School:** Israel 1976; **Resid:** Internal Medicine, Hadassah Hosp 1979; Radiation Oncology, Hadassah Hosp 1984; **Fellow:** Radiation Oncology, Meml Sloan Kettering Canc Ctr 1986; **Fac Appt:** Prof RadRO, Cornell Univ-Weill Med Coll

Radiation Oncology

Zelefsky, Michael J MD [RadRO] - **Spec Exp:** Prostate Cancer; Brachytherapy; Head & Neck Cancer; **Hospital:** Meml Sloan-Kettering Cancer Ctr (page 75); **Address:** 1275 York Avenue, New York, NY 10065; **Phone:** 800-525-2225; **Board Cert:** Radiation Oncology 1991; **Med School:** Albert Einstein Coll Med 1986; **Resid:** Radiation Oncology, Meml Sloan Kettering Cancer Ctr 1990; **Fac Appt:** Prof RadRO, Cornell Univ-Weill Med Coll

Southeast

Anscher, Mitchell S MD [RadRO] - **Spec Exp:** Prostate Cancer; Brachytherapy; Penile Cancer; Testicular Cancer; **Hospital:** Med Coll of VA Hosp, Hunter Holmes McGuire VA Med Ctr - Richmond; **Address:** 401 College St, Box 980058, Department of Radiation Oncology, Richmond, VA 23298-0058; **Phone:** 804-828-7238; **Board Cert:** Internal Medicine 1984; Radiation Oncology 1987; **Med School:** Med Coll VA 1981; **Resid:** Internal Medicine, St Marys Hosp 1984; Radiation Oncology, Duke Univ Med Ctr 1987; **Fac Appt:** Prof RadRO, Va Commonwealth Univ Sch Med

Beitler, Jonathan J MD [RadRO] - **Spec Exp:** Head & Neck Cancer; Breast Cancer; Lung Cancer; Brachytherapy; **Hospital:** Emory Univ Hosp; **Address:** Winship Cancer Institute, Dept Radiation Oncology, 1365C Clifton Rd NE, Atlanta, GA 30322; **Phone:** 404-778-3473; **Board Cert:** Radiation Oncology 2000; **Med School:** Med Coll PA Hahnemann 1982; **Resid:** Surgery, Downstate Med Ctr 1985; Radiation Oncology, Meml Sloan Kettering Cancer Ctr 1988; **Fac Appt:** Prof RadRO, Emory Univ

Blackstock, A William MD [RadRO] - **Spec Exp:** Lung Cancer; Gastrointestinal Cancer; Clinical Trials; **Hospital:** Wake Forest Univ Baptist Med Ctr; **Address:** Wake Forest, Comprehensive Cancer Ctr, Dept Radiation Oncology, Medical Center Blvd, Winston-Salem, NC 27157; **Phone:** 336-713-3600; **Board Cert:** Radiation Oncology 2006; **Med School:** E Carolina Univ 1989; **Resid:** Radiation Oncology, Univ NC Hosps 1994; **Fac Appt:** Prof RadRO, Wake Forest Univ

Bonner, James Alan MD [RadRO] - **Spec Exp:** Head & Neck Cancer; Lung Cancer; **Hospital:** Univ of Ala Hosp at Birmingham; **Address:** UAB- Birmingham, Dept Rad Onc, 1700 6th Ave S, rm 2262, Birmingham, AL 35294; **Phone:** 205-934-2761; **Board Cert:** Radiation Oncology 1990; **Med School:** Wayne State Univ 1985; **Resid:** Radiation Oncology, Univ Michigan Med Ctr 1989; **Fac Appt:** Prof RadRO, Univ Alabama

Brizel, David M MD [RadRO] - **Spec Exp:** Head & Neck Cancer; Sarcoma; **Hospital:** Duke Univ Hosp; **Address:** Duke Univ Med Ctr, Dept Rad Onc, Box 3085, Durham, NC 27710-0001; **Phone:** 919-668-5637; **Board Cert:** Radiation Oncology 1987; **Med School:** Northwestern Univ 1983; **Resid:** Radiation Oncology, Harvard Joint Ctr Radiation Ther 1987; **Fac Appt:** Prof RadRO, Duke Univ

Chakravarthy, Anuradha M MD [RadRO] - **Spec Exp:** Breast Cancer; Gastrointestinal Cancer; **Hospital:** Vanderbilt Univ Med Ctr; **Address:** Vanderbilt Radiation Oncology, 22nd St at Pierce Ave, B-1003 TVC Bldg, Nashville, TN 37232; **Phone:** 615-322-2555; **Board Cert:** Radiation Oncology 1994; Internal Medicine 1986; Medical Oncology 1989; **Med School:** Geo Wash Univ 1983; **Resid:** Internal Medicine, Mayo Clinic 1986; Medical Oncology, Univ MD Cancer Ctr 1990; **Fellow:** Radiation Oncology, Johns Hopkins Hosp 1993; **Fac Appt:** Assoc Prof RadRO, Vanderbilt Univ

Cmelak, Anthony J MD [RadRO] - **Spec Exp:** Brain Cancer; Stereotactic Radiosurgery; **Hospital:** Vanderbilt Univ Med Ctr; **Address:** Vanderbilt Dept of Radiation Oncology, B-1003 TVC, 22nd Pierce Ave, Nashville, TN 37232-5671; **Phone:** 615-322-2555; **Board Cert:** Radiation Oncology 2008; **Med School:** Northwestern Univ 1992; **Resid:** Radiation Oncology, Stanford Univ Med Ctr 1996; **Fac Appt:** Assoc Prof RadRO, Vanderbilt Univ

Crocker, Ian R MD [RadRO] - **Spec Exp:** Brain Tumors; Eye Tumors/Cancer; Melanoma-Choroidal (eye); **Hospital:** Emory Univ Hosp, Emory Univ Hosp Midtown; **Address:** The Emory Clinic, Dept Radiation Onc, 1365C Clifton Rd NE, CT-104, Atlanta, GA 30322; **Phone:** 404-778-3473; **Board Cert:** Therapeutic Radiology 1983; Internal Medicine 1980; **Med School:** Univ Saskatchewan 1976; **Resid:** Internal Medicine, Univ Hosp-Univ West Ontario 1980; **Fellow:** Radiation Oncology, Princess Margaret Hosp-Univ Toronto 1983; **Fac Appt:** Prof RadRO, Emory Univ

Fiveash, John MD [RadRO] - **Spec Exp:** Brain Tumors; Pediatric Cancers; **Hospital:** Univ of Ala Hosp at Birmingham; **Address:** Hazelrig-Salter Radiation-Oncology Ctr, 1700 6th Ave, Birmingham, AL 35249; **Phone:** 205-934-9999; **Board Cert:** Radiation Oncology 2009; **Med School:** Med Coll GA 1993; **Resid:** Radiation Oncology, GA Hlth Sci Univ 1997

Halle, Jan MD [RadRO] - **Spec Exp:** Breast Cancer; Lung Cancer; **Hospital:** NC Memorial Hosp - UNC, Rex HlthCare; **Address:** Univ North Carolina Sch Med, Dept Rad Onc, 101 Manning Drive, CB 7512, Chapel Hill, NC 27514; **Phone:** 919-445-5218; **Board Cert:** Therapeutic Radiology 1982; **Med School:** Tufts Univ 1975; **Resid:** Radiation Oncology, North Carolina Meml Hosp 1981; **Fac Appt:** Assoc Prof RadRO, Univ NC Sch Med

Henderson, Randal H MD [RadRO] - **Spec Exp:** Gynecologic Cancer; Prostate Cancer; Brachytherapy; Proton Beam Therapy; **Hospital:** Shands at Univ of FL; **Address:** Univ Florida Proton Therapy Inst, 2015 N Jefferson St, Jacksonville, FL 32206; **Phone:** 904-588-1800; **Board Cert:** Therapeutic Radiology 1984; **Med School:** Texas Tech Univ 1979; **Resid:** Radiation Oncology, Univ Florida/Shands Hosp 1983; **Fac Appt:** Prof RadRO, Univ Fla Coll Med

Jose, Baby Oliapuram MD [RadRO] - **Spec Exp:** Head & Neck Cancer; Lung Cancer; Gynecologic Cancer; Prostate Cancer; **Hospital:** Univ of Louisville Hosp, Floyd Meml Hosp & Hlth Svcs; **Address:** James G Brown Cancer Center, 529 S Jackson St Fl 4, Louisville, KY 40202; **Phone:** 502-562-4759; **Board Cert:** Therapeutic Radiology 1978; **Med School:** India 1971; **Resid:** Surgery, CMC Hosp 1974; Radiation Oncology, CMC Hosp 1976; **Fellow:** Radiation Oncology, Brown Univ-RI Hosp 1979; **Fac Appt:** Prof RadRO, Univ Louisville Sch Med

Kudrimoti, Mahesh R MD [RadRO] - **Spec Exp:** Lung Cancer; Head & Neck Cancer; Brachytherapy; **Hospital:** Univ of Kentucky Albert B. Chandler Hosp; **Address:** UKMC, Dept Radiation Oncology, 800 Rose St, C-113, Lexington, KY 40536; **Phone:** 859-323-6486; **Board Cert:** Radiation Oncology 2003; **Med School:** India 1992; **Resid:** Radiation Oncology, Univ KY Chandler Med Ctr 2001; **Fac Appt:** Assoc Prof RadRO, Univ KY Coll Med

Kun, Larry E MD [RadRO] - **Spec Exp:** Brain Tumors; Pediatric Cancers; **Hospital:** St. Jude Children's Research Hosp, Le Bonheur Chldns Med Ctr; **Address:** St Jude Chldns Research Hosp, 262 Danny Thomas Pl, MS 220, Memphis, TN 38105; **Phone:** 901-595-3565; **Board Cert:** Therapeutic Radiology 1973; **Med School:** Jefferson Med Coll 1968; **Resid:** Therapeutic Radiology, Penrose Cancer Hosp 1972; **Fellow:** Radiation Oncology, Natl Cancer Inst 1974; Radiation Oncology, Rotterdam Radiotherapy Inst 1975; **Fac Appt:** Prof, Univ Tenn Coll Med

Landry, Jerome C MD [RadRO] - **Spec Exp:** Gastrointestinal Cancer; Sarcoma-Soft Tissue; **Hospital:** Emory Univ Hosp, Grady Hlth Sys; **Address:** Emory Dept Radiation Oncology, 1365C Clifton Rd NE, Atlanta, GA 30322; **Phone:** 404-778-3473; **Board Cert:** Radiation Oncology 1988; **Med School:** Harvard Med Sch 1983; **Resid:** Radiation Oncology, Mass Genl Hosp 1987; **Fac Appt:** Prof RadRO, Emory Univ

Larner, James M MD [RadRO] - **Spec Exp:** Neuro-Oncology; Brain Tumors; **Hospital:** Univ of Virginia Health Sys; **Address:** Univ Virginia Medical Ctr, Dept Radiation Oncology, 1240 Lee St, PO Box 800383, Charlottesville, VA 22908; **Phone:** 434-924-5191; **Board Cert:** Internal Medicine 1983; Medical Oncology 1987; Hematology 1988; Radiation Oncology 1989; **Med School:** Univ VA Sch Med 1980; **Resid:** Internal Medicine, Thos Jefferson Univ Hosp 1983; Radiation Oncology, Montefiore-Einstein Med Ctr 1989; **Fellow:** Hematology & Oncology, Thos Jefferson Univ Hosp 1986; **Fac Appt:** Assoc Prof Med, Univ VA Sch Med

Lee, W Robert MD [RadRO] - **Spec Exp:** Prostate Cancer; Brachytherapy; Intensity Modulated Radiotherapy (IMRT); **Hospital:** Duke Univ Hosp; **Address:** Duke Univ Med Ctr, Div Radiation Oncology, Box 3085, Durham, NC 27710; **Phone:** 919-668-5640; **Board Cert:** Radiation Oncology 1994; **Med School:** Univ VA Sch Med 1989; **Resid:** Radiation Oncology, Univ Florida 1993; **Fac Appt:** Prof RadRO, Duke Univ

Lewin, Alan A MD [RadRO] - **Spec Exp:** Breast Cancer; Lung Cancer; Brain & Spinal Cord Tumors; **Hospital:** Baptist Hosp of Miami; **Address:** Baptist Hosp Miami, Dept Radiation Oncology, 8900 N Kendall Drive, Miami, FL 33176-2118; **Phone:** 786-596-6566; **Board Cert:** Therapeutic Radiology 1982; Internal Medicine 1976; Hematology 1978; Medical Oncology 1981; **Med School:** Geo Wash Univ 1973; **Resid:** Internal Medicine, Mt Sinai Hosp 1976; **Fellow:** Hematology & Oncology, Beth Israel Med Ctr 1978; Radiation Oncology, Joint Ctr Radiation Therapy 1980; **Fac Appt:** Clin Prof RadRO, Univ Miami Sch Med

Malcolm, Arnold MD [RadRO] - **Spec Exp:** Prostate Cancer; Gynecologic Cancer; Brachytherapy; **Hospital:** Vanderbilt Univ Med Ctr; **Address:** Vanderbilt Radiation Oncology, 22nd St At Pierce Ave, B-1003 TVC Bldg, Nashville, TN 37232; **Phone:** 615-322-2555; **Board Cert:** Radiation Oncology 1977; **Med School:** Meharry Med Coll 1973; **Resid:** Radiation Oncology, Joint Ctr Radiation Therapy 1977; **Fac Appt:** Assoc Prof RadRO, Vanderbilt Univ

Marcus Jr, Robert B MD [RadRO] - **Spec Exp:** Prostate Cancer; Sarcoma; Bone Cancer; Brain & Spinal Cord Tumors; **Hospital:** Shands Jacksonville; **Address:** Univ Florida Proton Therapy Inst, 2015 N Jefferson St, Jacksonville, FL 32206; **Phone:** 904-588-1800; **Board Cert:** Therapeutic Radiology 1980; **Med School:** Univ Fla Coll Med 1975; **Resid:** Radiation Oncology, Shands Hosp 1979; **Fac Appt:** Prof RadRO, Univ Fla Coll Med

Markoe, Arnold M MD [RadRO] - **Spec Exp:** Eye Tumors/Cancer; Orbital Tumors/Cancer; Central Nervous System Cancer; Lymphoma; **Hospital:** Univ of Miami Hosp & Clins/Sylvester Comp Canc Ctr (page 82), Jackson Meml Hosp (page 82); **Address:** Univ of Miami Sylvester Comp Cancer Ctr, 1475 NW 12th Ave Ave NW, MC D-31, Miami, FL 33136; **Phone:** 305-243-4319; **Board Cert:** Therapeutic Radiology 1983; **Med School:** Hahnemann Univ 1977; **Resid:** Radiation Oncology, Hahnemann Hosp 1981; **Fac Appt:** Prof RadRO, Univ Miami Sch Med

Marks, Lawrence MD [RadRO] - **Spec Exp:** Breast Cancer; Lung Cancer; **Hospital:** NC Memorial Hosp - UNC; **Address:** UNC Cancer Hosp, Dept Rad Onc, 101 Manning Drive, rm CB 295, Level B, Campus Box 7512, Chapel Hill, NC 27514; **Phone:** 919-966-0400; **Board Cert:** Radiation Oncology 1989; **Med School:** Univ Rochester 1985; **Resid:** Radiation Oncology, Mass Genl Hosp 1989; **Fac Appt:** Prof RadRO, Univ NC Sch Med

McGarry, Ronald C MD/PhD [RadRO] - **Spec Exp:** Lung Cancer; Lymphoma; Clinical Trials; Stereotactic Radiosurgery; **Hospital:** Univ of Kentucky Albert B. Chandler Hosp; **Address:** Chandler Medical Ctr, Radiation Medicine, 800 Rose St, rm C114C, Lexington, KY 40536; **Phone:** 859-323-6486; **Board Cert:** Radiation Oncology 1999; **Med School:** Canada 1992; **Resid:** Radiation Oncology, Univ W Ontario Regl Cancer Ctr 1997; **Fac Appt:** Prof RadRO, Univ KY Coll Med

Mendenhall, Nancy P MD [RadRO] - **Spec Exp:** Breast Cancer; Lymphoma; Hodgkin's Disease; Prostate Cancer; **Hospital:** Shands at Univ of FL; **Address:** Univ Florida, Proton Therapy Inst, 2015 N Jefferson St, Jacksonville, FL 32206; **Phone:** 904-588-1800; **Board Cert:** Therapeutic Radiology 1985; **Med School:** Univ Fla Coll Med 1980; **Resid:** Diagnostic Radiology, Shands-Univ of Florida 1984; **Fac Appt:** Prof RadRO, Univ Fla Coll Med

Mendenhall, William M MD [RadRO] - **Spec Exp:** Head & Neck Cancer; Stereotactic Radiosurgery; Gastrointestinal Cancer; Gynecologic Cancer; **Hospital:** Shands at Univ of FL; **Address:** Univ Florida, Dept Radiation Oncology, Box 100385, Gainesville, FL 32610-0385; **Phone:** 352-265-0287; **Board Cert:** Therapeutic Radiology 1983; **Med School:** Univ S Fla Coll Med 1978; **Resid:** Radiation Oncology, Univ Fla Affil Hosp 1983; **Fac Appt:** Prof RadRO, Univ Fla Coll Med

Merchant, Thomas E DO [RadRO] - **Spec Exp:** Brain Tumors-Pediatric; **Hospital:** St. Jude Children's Research Hosp; **Address:** St Jude Chldns Rsch Hosp, 262 Danny Thomas Pl, MS 220, Memphis, TN 38105; **Phone:** 901-595-3565; **Board Cert:** Radiation Oncology 2004; **Med School:** Chicago Coll Osteo Med 1989; **Resid:** Radiation Oncology, Meml Sloan Kettering Cancer Ctr 1994

Meredith, Ruby F MD [RadRO] - **Spec Exp:** Multiple Myeloma; Breast Cancer; Radionuclide Therapy; Bone Tumors-Metastatic; **Hospital:** Univ of Ala Hosp at Birmingham; **Address:** Univ Alabama Hosps-Radiation Oncology, 619 19th St S, 1700 6th Ave S, Birmingham, AL 35249; **Phone:** 205-934-2763; **Board Cert:** Radiation Oncology 1987; **Med School:** Ohio State Univ 1983; **Resid:** Radiation Oncology, Med College Va Hosps 1987; **Fac Appt:** Prof RadRO, Univ Alabama

Morris, Monica M MD [RadRO] - **Spec Exp:** Breast Cancer; Lung Cancer; **Hospital:** Univ of Virginia Health Sys; **Address:** Univ VA Hlth Sciences-Radiation Onc, PO Box 800383, Charlottesville, VA 22908; **Phone:** 434-924-5192; **Board Cert:** Radiation Oncology 2008; **Med School:** Baylor Coll Med 1993; **Resid:** Radiation Oncology, Mass Genl Hosp 1998; **Fac Appt:** Assoc Prof RadRO, Univ VA Sch Med

Pollack, Alan MD/PhD [RadRO] - **Spec Exp:** Prostate Cancer; Genitourinary Cancer; Sarcoma; **Hospital:** Univ of Miami Hosp & Clins/Sylvester Comp Canc Ctr (page 82); **Address:** 1475 NW 12th Ave, Ste 1501, Miami, FL 33136; **Phone:** 305-243-4916; **Board Cert:** Radiation Oncology 1993; **Med School:** Univ Miami Sch Med 1987; **Resid:** Radiation Oncology, MD Anderson Cancer Ctr 1992; **Fac Appt:** Prof RadRO, Univ Miami Sch Med

Prosnitz, Leonard MD [RadRO] - **Spec Exp:** Lymphoma; Breast Cancer; Hyperthermia Treatment of Cancer; Sarcoma; **Hospital:** Duke Univ Hosp; **Address:** Duke Univ Med Ctr, Dept Rad Onc, Box 3085, Durham, NC 27710; **Phone:** 919-668-5637; **Board Cert:** Therapeutic Radiology 1970; **Med School:** SUNY Downstate 1961; **Resid:** Internal Medicine, Dartmouth Affil Hosps 1963; Radiation Oncology, Yale-New Haven Hosp 1969; **Fellow:** Hematology & Oncology, Yale-New Haven Hosp 1967; **Fac Appt:** Prof RadRO, Duke Univ

Randall, Marcus E MD [RadRO] - **Spec Exp:** Gynecologic Cancer; Stereotactic Radiosurgery; **Hospital:** Univ of Kentucky Albert B. Chandler Hosp; **Address:** Univ Kentucky Medical Ctr, 800 Rose St, rm C11-14D, Office of Radiation Medicine, Lexington, KY 40536-0001; **Phone:** 859-323-6487; **Board Cert:** Therapeutic Radiology 1986; **Med School:** Univ NC Sch Med 1982; **Resid:** Radiation Oncology, Univ Va Med Ctr 1986; **Fellow:** Radiation Oncology, Univ Va Med Ctr 1986; **Fac Appt:** Prof RadRO, Univ KY Coll Med

Radiation Oncology

Rich, Tyvin A MD [RadRO] - **Spec Exp:** Colon & Rectal Cancer; Chemo-Radiation Combined Therapy; Gastrointestinal Cancer; Gallbladder & Biliary Cancer; **Hospital:** Univ of Virginia Health Sys; **Address:** Univ Va Hlth Sys, Dept Rad Onc, 1240 Lee St, PO Box 800383, Charlottesville, VA 22908-0383; **Phone:** 434-924-5191; **Board Cert:** Radiation Oncology 1978; **Med School:** Univ VA Sch Med 1973; **Resid:** Radiation Oncology, Mass Genl Hosp 1978; **Fellow:** Radiation Oncology, Mt Vernon Hosp/Gray Lab 1978; **Fac Appt:** Prof RadRO, Univ VA Sch Med

Rosenman, Julian MD/PhD [RadRO] - **Spec Exp:** Lung Cancer; Breast Cancer; Prostate Cancer; **Hospital:** NC Memorial Hosp - UNC; **Address:** UNC Cancer Hosp, Dept Rad Onc, 101 Manning Drive, rm CB 295, Level B, Campus Box 7512, Chapel Hill, NC 27514; **Phone:** 919-966-0400; **Board Cert:** Therapeutic Radiology 1981; **Med School:** Univ Tex SW, Dallas 1977; **Resid:** Therapeutic Radiology, Mass Genl Hosp 1981; **Fac Appt:** Prof RadRO, Univ NC Sch Med

Sailer, Scott MD [RadRO] - **Spec Exp:** Breast Cancer; Genitourinary Cancer; Head & Neck Cancer; **Hospital:** WakeMed Cary, WakeMed-Raleigh Campus; **Address:** 300 Ashville Ave, Ste 110, Cary, NC 27518; **Phone:** 919-854-4588; **Board Cert:** Radiation Oncology 1988; **Med School:** Harvard Med Sch 1984; **Resid:** Radiation Therapy, Mass Genl Hosp 1988

Shaw, Edward G MD [RadRO] - **Spec Exp:** Stereotactic Radiosurgery; Brain Tumors; **Hospital:** Wake Forest Univ Baptist Med Ctr; **Address:** Wake Forest Baptist Health, Research Base Fl 4, Piedmont Plaza Two, Winston-Salem, NC 27104; **Phone:** 336-713-6506; **Board Cert:** Radiation Oncology 1987; **Med School:** Rush Med Coll 1983; **Resid:** Radiation Oncology, Mayo Grad Sch Med 1987; **Fac Appt:** Prof RadRO, Wake Forest Univ

Song, Shiyu MD/PhD [RadRO] - **Spec Exp:** Head & Neck Cancer; **Hospital:** VCU Med Ctr; **Address:** 401 College St, Box 980058, Richmond, VA 23298-0037; **Phone:** 804-828-7232; **Board Cert:** Radiation Oncology 2006; **Med School:** China 1983; **Resid:** Radiation Oncology, Univ Wisc Hosp & Clins; **Fellow:** Radiation Oncology, Johns Hopkins Hosp; **Fac Appt:** Asst Prof RadRO, Va Commonwealth Univ Sch Med

St Clair, William H MD/PhD [RadRO] - **Hospital:** Univ of Kentucky Albert B. Chandler Hosp; **Address:** 800 Rose St, Lexington, KY 40536; **Phone:** 859-323-6486; **Board Cert:** Radiation Oncology 2000; **Med School:** Univ KY Coll Med 1995; **Resid:** Radiation Oncology, Mass Genl Hosp 2000; **Fellow:** Radiation Oncology, Mass Genl Hosp 2000

Tepper, Joel E MD [RadRO] - **Spec Exp:** Gastrointestinal Cancer; Sarcoma; Rectal Cancer; **Hospital:** NC Memorial Hosp - UNC; **Address:** UNC Cancer Hosp, Dept Rad Onc, 101 Manning Drive, rm CB 295, Level B, Campus Box 7512, Chapel Hill, NC 27514; **Phone:** 919-966-0400; **Board Cert:** Therapeutic Radiology 1976; **Med School:** Washington Univ, St Louis 1972; **Resid:** Therapeutic Radiology, Mass Genl Hosp 1976; **Fellow:** Therapeutic Radiology, Mass Genl Hosp 1977; **Fac Appt:** Prof RadRO, Univ NC Sch Med

Toonkel, Leonard M MD [RadRO] - **Spec Exp:** Prostate Cancer; Breast Cancer; Brachytherapy; **Hospital:** Mount Sinai Med Ctr - Miami; **Address:** Dept Radiation Oncology, 4300 Alton Rd, Miami Beach, FL 33140; **Phone:** 305-535-3400; **Board Cert:** Therapeutic Radiology 1979; **Med School:** Univ Miami Sch Med 1975; **Resid:** Radiation Therapy, Jackson Meml Hosp 1977; Diagnostic Radiology, MD Anderson Hosp 1978; **Fellow:** Radiation Oncology, MD Anderson Hosp 1979; **Fac Appt:** Assoc Clin Prof Rad, Univ Miami Sch Med

Vijayakumar, Srinivasan MD [RadRO] - **Spec Exp:** Brachytherapy; Prostate Cancer; **Hospital:** Univ Mississippi Med Ctr; **Address:** 350 Woodrow Wilson Drive, Jackson, MS 39213; **Phone:** 601-984-2550; **Board Cert:** Therapeutic Radiology 1986; **Med School:** India 1978; **Resid:** Radiation Oncology, Madras Univ Med Ctr 1981; Radiation Oncology, Michael Reese Hosp 1984; **Fellow:** Brachytherapy, Univ Chicago Hosps 1985; **Fac Appt:** Prof RadRO, Univ Miss

Willett, Christopher MD [RadRO] - **Spec Exp:** Gastrointestinal Cancer; Clinical Trials; **Hospital:** Duke Univ Hosp; **Address:** Duke Univ Med Ctr, PO Box 3085, Durham, NC 27710; **Phone:** 919-668-5640; **Board Cert:** Therapeutic Radiology 1985; **Med School:** Tufts Univ 1981; **Resid:** Radiation Oncology, Mass Genl Hosp 1986; **Fac Appt:** Prof RadRO, Duke Univ

Wolfson, Aaron H MD [RadRO] - **Spec Exp:** Gynecologic Cancer; Sarcoma; Gastrointestinal Cancer; **Hospital:** Univ of Miami Hosp & Clins/Sylvester Comp Canc Ctr (page 82); **Address:** UMHC Sylvester Comp Cancer Ctr, 1475 NW 12th Ave, Box D31, Miami, FL 33136; **Phone:** 305-243-4210; **Board Cert:** Radiation Oncology 1999; **Med School:** Univ Fla Coll Med 1982; **Resid:** Radiation Oncology, Med Coll of Virginia 1989; **Fac Appt:** Prof RadRO, Univ Miami Sch Med

Woo, Shiao Y MD [RadRO] - **Spec Exp:** Brain Tumors-Adult & Pediatric; Proton Beam Therapy; Stereotactic Radiosurgery; Pediatric Cancers; **Hospital:** Univ of Louisville Hosp; **Address:** Univ Louisville-Radiation Onc, 5295 S Jackson St, Louisville, KY 40202; **Phone:** 502-562-4759; **Board Cert:** Radiation Oncology 1988; Pediatrics 1980; **Med School:** Malaysia 1972; **Resid:** Pediatrics, Georgetown Univ Hosp 1978; **Fellow:** Pediatric Hematology-Oncology, Georgetown Univ Hosp 1980; Radiation Oncology, Georgetown Univ Hosp 1988; **Fac Appt:** Prof RadRO, Univ Louisville Sch Med

Midwest

Abrams, Ross A MD [RadRO] - **Spec Exp:** Gastrointestinal Cancer; Lymphoma; **Hospital:** Rush Univ Med Ctr; **Address:** Women's Center for Radiation Therapy, 500 S Paulina, Ground Floor Atrium, Chicago, IL 60612; **Phone:** 312-942-5751; **Board Cert:** Internal Medicine 1976; Medical Oncology 1979; Hematology 1982; Radiation Oncology 1987; **Med School:** Univ Pennsylvania 1973; **Resid:** Internal Medicine, Pennsylvania Hosp 1975; Hematology & Oncology, Hosp Univ Penn 1976; **Fellow:** Hematology & Oncology, Natl Cancer Inst 1978; Radiation Oncology, Med Coll Wisconsin 1987; **Fac Appt:** Prof RadRO, Rush Med Coll

Awan, Azhar M MD [RadRO] - **Spec Exp:** Brain Tumors; Prostate Cancer; Breast Cancer; **Hospital:** Sherman Hosp; **Address:** Sherman Hosp Cancer Care Ctr, 1425 N Randall Rd, Elgin, IL 60123; **Phone:** 224-783-8746; **Board Cert:** Therapeutic Radiology 1985; **Med School:** Loyola Univ-Stritch Sch Med 1981; **Resid:** Therapeutic Radiology, Rush Med Ctr 1985; **Fac Appt:** Assoc Prof RadRO, Univ Chicago-Pritzker Sch Med

Ben-Josef, Edgar MD [RadRO] - **Spec Exp:** Bone Cancer; Gastrointestinal Cancer; Pancreatic Cancer; Intensity Modulated Radiotherapy (IMRT); **Hospital:** Univ of Michigan Hosp; **Address:** Univ of Mich Hosp, 1500 E Medical Ctr Drive, rm UH B2C490, Ann Arbor, MI 48109-0010; **Phone:** 734-936-8207; **Board Cert:** Radiation Oncology 1994; **Med School:** Israel 1986; **Resid:** Radiation Oncology, Wayne State Univ Hosp 1994; **Fellow:** Cancer Biology, Wayne State Univ Hosp 1995; **Fac Appt:** Assoc Prof RadRO, Univ Mich Med Sch

Bradley, Jeffrey D MD [RadRO] - **Spec Exp:** Lung Cancer; Esophageal Cancer; Thoracic Cancers; Clinical Trials; **Hospital:** Barnes-Jewish Hosp; **Address:** Ctr for Advanced Medicine, Rad Oncology, 4921 Parkview Pl Fl LL, St Louis, MO 63110; **Phone:** 314-747-7236; **Board Cert:** Radiation Oncology 2008; **Med School:** Univ Ark 1993; **Resid:** Radiation Oncology, Univ Chicago 1998; **Fac Appt:** Assoc Prof RadRO, Washington Univ, St Louis

Buatti, John M MD [RadRO] - **Spec Exp:** Central Nervous System Cancer; **Hospital:** Univ Iowa Hosp & Clinics; **Address:** 200 Hawkins Drive, rm 01626 PFP, Iowa City, IA 52242; **Phone:** 319-356-2699; **Board Cert:** Radiation Oncology 1994; **Med School:** Georgetown Univ 1986; **Resid:** Internal Medicine, Georgetown Univ 1989; **Fellow:** Radiation Oncology, Univ Arizona 1993; **Fac Appt:** Prof RadRO, Univ Iowa Coll Med

Radiation Oncology

Charboneau, J William MD [RadRO] - **Spec Exp:** Radiofrequency Tumor Ablation; Liver Cancer; Thyroid Cancer; **Hospital:** Mayo Med Ctr & Clin - Rochester; **Address:** Mayo Clinic Dept of Radiology, 200 First St SW, Rochester, MN 55905-0002; **Phone:** 507-284-2097; **Board Cert:** Diagnostic Radiology 1980; **Med School:** Univ Wisc 1976; **Resid:** Diagnostic Radiology, Mayo Clin 1980; **Fac Appt:** Prof, Mayo Med Sch

Ciezki, Jay P MD [RadRO] - **Spec Exp:** Brachytherapy; Prostate Cancer; Genitourinary Cancer; **Hospital:** Cleveland Clin (page 70); **Address:** Cleveland Clinic Fdn, 9500 Euclid Ave, MC T28, Cleveland, OH 44195; **Phone:** 216-445-9465; **Board Cert:** Radiation Oncology 2005; **Med School:** Med Coll Wisc 1991; **Resid:** Radiation Oncology, Cleveland Clinic 1995; **Fellow:** Brachytherapy, Cleveland Clinic 1996

Eisbruch, Avraham MD [RadRO] - **Spec Exp:** Head & Neck Cancer; **Hospital:** Univ of Michigan Hosp; **Address:** Univ MI Hlth Sys, 1500 E Med Ctr Drive, Fl B2 - rm C490, Ann Arbor, MI 48109; **Phone:** 734-936-4319; **Board Cert:** Radiation Oncology 1992; **Med School:** Israel 1979; **Resid:** Radiology, Washington Univ 1992; **Fellow:** Medical Oncology, Univ TX MD Anderson Cancer Ctr 1996; **Fac Appt:** Assoc Clin Prof RadRO, Univ Mich Med Sch

Emami, Bahman MD [RadRO] - **Spec Exp:** Head & Neck Cancer; Lung Cancer; **Hospital:** Loyola Univ Med Ctr, Edward Hines, Jr. VA Hosp; **Address:** Loyola Univ Med Ctr, Dept Rad Onc, 2160 S First Ave Bldg 150 - rm 0300, Maywood, IL 60153-3328; **Phone:** 708-216-2729; **Board Cert:** Therapeutic Radiology 1976; **Med School:** Iran 1968; **Resid:** Radiation Therapy, St Vincents Hosp 1973; Radiation Therapy, New England Med Ctr 1977; **Fac Appt:** Prof RadRO, Loyola Univ-Stritch Sch Med

Forman, Jeffrey D MD [RadRO] - **Spec Exp:** Neutron Therapy for Advanced Cancer; Genitourinary Cancer; Prostate Cancer; **Address:** 70 Fulton St, Pontiac, MI 48341; **Phone:** 248-338-0300; **Board Cert:** Radiation Oncology 1986; **Med School:** NYU Sch Med 1982; **Resid:** Radiation Oncology, Johns Hopkins Hosp 1986; **Fellow:** Therapeutic Radiology, Johns Hopkins Hosp 1987; **Fac Appt:** Prof RadRO, Wayne State Univ

Grigsby, Perry W MD [RadRO] - **Spec Exp:** Gynecologic Cancer; Thyroid Cancer; **Hospital:** Barnes-Jewish Hosp, St. Louis Chldns Hosp; **Address:** Ctr for Advanced Medicine, Rad Oncology, 4921 Parkview Pl Fl LL, St Louis, MO 63110; **Phone:** 314-747-7236; **Board Cert:** Radiation Oncology 1987; **Med School:** Univ KY Coll Med 1982; **Resid:** Radiation Oncology, Barnes Jewish Hosp 1985; **Fac Appt:** Prof RadRO, Washington Univ, St Louis

Halpern, Howard J MD/PhD [RadRO] - **Spec Exp:** Breast Cancer; Esophageal Cancer; Gynecologic Cancer; **Hospital:** Univ of Chicago Med Ctr, Univ of IL Med Ctr at Chicago; **Address:** Univ Chicago Dept Radiation Oncology, 5758 S Maryland Ave, MC 9006, Chicago, IL 60637; **Phone:** 773-702-6870; **Board Cert:** Therapeutic Radiology 1984; **Med School:** Univ Miami Sch Med 1980; **Resid:** Therapeutic Radiology, Harvard Jnt Ctr Rad Ther 1984; **Fellow:** Therapeutic Radiology, Harvard Jnt Ctr Rad Ther 1985; **Fac Appt:** Prof RadRO, Univ Chicago-Pritzker Sch Med

Haraf, Daniel J MD [RadRO] - **Spec Exp:** Head & Neck Cancer; Lung Cancer; Prostate Cancer; **Hospital:** Univ of Chicago Med Ctr; **Address:** Univ Chicago Medical Center, 5841 S Maryland Ave, Chicago, IL 60637; **Phone:** 773-702-6870; **Board Cert:** Internal Medicine 1985; Radiation Oncology 1990; **Med School:** Ros Franklin Univ/Chicago Med Sch 1982; **Resid:** Internal Medicine, Michael Reese Hosp 1985; **Fellow:** Radiation Oncology, Michael Reese Hosp 1988; **Fac Appt:** Prof RadRO, Univ Chicago-Pritzker Sch Med

Harari, Paul M MD [RadRO] - **Spec Exp:** Head & Neck Cancer; **Hospital:** Univ WI Hosp & Clins; **Address:** Dept of Human Oncology, 600 Highland Ave, Ste K4/336, Madison, WI 53792; **Phone:** 608-263-5009; **Board Cert:** Radiation Oncology 1990; **Med School:** Univ VA Sch Med 1984; **Resid:** Radiation Oncology, Univ Arizona Med Ctr 1990; **Fac Appt:** Prof RadRO, Univ Wisc

America's Top Doctors® for Cancer 7th Edition

Hayman, James A MD [RadRO] - **Spec Exp:** Breast Cancer; Stomach Cancer; Lung Cancer; Brain Tumors; **Hospital:** Univ of Michigan Hosp; **Address:** Univ Michigan Hosp, 1500 E Medical Ctr Drive, rm UH B2C490, Ann Arbor, MI 48109-0010; **Phone:** 734-647-9956; **Board Cert:** Radiation Oncology 2004; **Med School:** Univ Chicago-Pritzker Sch Med 1991; **Resid:** Radiation Therapy, Joint Ctr for Radiation Therapy 1996; **Fac Appt:** Assoc Prof RadRO, Univ Mich Med Sch

Johnstone, Peter A S MD [RadRO] - **Spec Exp:** Prostate Cancer; Proton Beam Therapy; Head & Neck Cancer; **Hospital:** IU Health University Hosp; **Address:** IU Dept Radiation Oncology, 535 Barnhill Drive, RT 041, Indianapolis, IN 46202; **Phone:** 317-944-2524; **Board Cert:** Radiation Oncology 2010; **Med School:** Uniformed Srvs Univ, Bethesda 1989; **Resid:** Radiation Oncology, Natl Cancer Inst 1993; **Fac Appt:** Prof RadRO, Indiana Univ

Kim, Jae Ho MD [RadRO] - **Spec Exp:** Brain Tumors; Spinal Cord Tumors; Breast Cancer; Lymphoma; **Hospital:** Henry Ford Hosp; **Address:** Radiation Oncology, 2799 W Grand Blvd, Detroit, MI 48202; **Phone:** 313-916-1029; **Board Cert:** Therapeutic Radiology 1973; **Med School:** Korea 1959; **Resid:** Therapeutic Radiology, Meml-Sloan-Kettering 1972; **Fellow:** Medical Biophysics, Meml-Sloan-Kettering 1968; **Fac Appt:** Prof RadRO, Wayne State Univ

Konski, Andre MD [RadRO] - **Spec Exp:** Esophageal Cancer; Rectal Cancer; Pancreatic Cancer; Gastrointestinal Cancer; **Hospital:** Barbara Ann Karmanos Cancer Inst; **Address:** Dept Radiation Oncology, 4100 John R, Detroit, MI 48201; **Phone:** 313-745-2560; **Board Cert:** Radiation Oncology 2000; **Med School:** NY Med Coll 1984; **Resid:** Radiation Oncology, Stong Meml/Genesee Hosp 1988; **Fac Appt:** Prof RadRO, Wayne State Univ

Lawrence, Theodore S MD/PhD [RadRO] - **Spec Exp:** Gastrointestinal Cancer; Liver Cancer; Pancreatic Cancer; **Hospital:** Univ of Michigan Hosp; **Address:** Univ of Mich Hosp, Dept Rad Onc, 1500 E Med Ctr Dr, SPC5010, Box 5010, UH-B2-C502, Ann Arbor, MI 48109-5010; **Phone:** 734-936-4300; **Board Cert:** Internal Medicine 1983; Medical Oncology 1985; Radiation Oncology 1987; **Med School:** Cornell Univ-Weill Med Coll 1980; **Resid:** Internal Medicine, Stanford Univ Hosp 1983; Radiation Oncology, Natl Cancer Inst 1987; **Fellow:** Medical Oncology, Natl Cancer Inst 1986; **Fac Appt:** Prof RadRO, Univ Mich Med Sch

Lee, Chung K MD [RadRO] - **Spec Exp:** Head & Neck Cancer; Breast Cancer; Lymphoma; Gastrointestinal Cancer; **Address:** Univ Minn, Dept Radiation Oncology, 420 Delaware St SE, MMC 400, Minneapolis, MN 55455; **Phone:** 612-273-6700; **Board Cert:** Therapeutic Radiology 1976; **Med School:** Korea 1965; **Resid:** Radiation Oncology, Yonsei Univ Hosp 1971; Therapeutic Radiology, Univ of Minn Hosp 1976; **Fellow:** Yonsei Univ Hosp; **Fac Appt:** Prof RadRO, Univ Minn

Machtay, Mitchell MD [RadRO] - **Spec Exp:** Head & Neck Cancer; Skin Cancer; Skull Base Tumors; **Hospital:** Univ Hosps Case Med Ctr; **Address:** UH Case Med Ctr, Dept Rad Oncology, 11100 Euclid Ave, Lerner Tower B-181, Cleveland, OH 44106; **Phone:** 216-844-2530; **Board Cert:** Radiation Oncology 1994; **Med School:** NYU Sch Med 1989; **Resid:** Radiation Oncology, Hosp Univ Penn 1993; **Fac Appt:** Assoc Prof RadRO, Jefferson Med Coll

Macklis, Roger M MD [RadRO] - **Spec Exp:** Radioimmunotherapy of Cancer; Breast Cancer; Lymphoma; **Hospital:** Cleveland Clin (page 70); **Address:** Cleveland Cin Fdn, Dept Rad Onc, 9500 Euclid Ave, Desk T28, Cleveland, OH 44195; **Phone:** 216-444-5576; **Board Cert:** Radiation Oncology 1989; **Med School:** Harvard Med Sch 1983; **Resid:** Radiation Oncology, Joint Ctr Radiotherapy Inst 1987; **Fellow:** Research, Dana Farber Cancer Inst 1987; **Fac Appt:** Prof RadRO, Case West Res Univ

Radiation Oncology

Mansur, David B MD [RadRO] - **Spec Exp:** Pediatric Cancers; Breast Cancer; Genitourinary Cancer; **Hospital:** St. Louis Chldns Hosp, Barnes-Jewish Hosp; **Address:** Washington University School of Medicine, Dept Radiation Oncology, 4921 Parkview Pl, St Louis, MO 63110; **Phone:** 314-362-4633; **Board Cert:** Radiation Oncology 2009; **Med School:** Univ Kansas 1992; **Resid:** Radiation Oncology, Unic Chicago Hosps 1997; **Fac Appt:** Assoc Prof RadRO, Washington Univ, St Louis

Martenson Jr, James A MD [RadRO] - **Spec Exp:** Mucositis; Esophageal Cancer; **Hospital:** Mayo Med Ctr & Clin - Rochester; **Address:** Mayo Clinic, Dept Rad/Onc, 200 First St SW, Rochester, MN 55905; **Phone:** 507-284-4561; **Board Cert:** Therapeutic Radiology 1985; **Med School:** Univ Wash 1981; **Resid:** Radiation Oncology, Mayo Clinic 1985; **Fac Appt:** Assoc Prof, Mayo Med Sch

Michalski, Jeff M MD [RadRO] - **Spec Exp:** Prostate Cancer; Sarcoma; Pediatric Cancers; **Hospital:** Barnes-Jewish Hosp, St. Louis Chldns Hosp; **Address:** Ctr for Advanced Medicine, Rad Oncology, 4921 Parkview Pl Fl LL, St Louis, MO 63110; **Phone:** 314-747-7236; **Board Cert:** Radiation Oncology 1991; **Med School:** Med Coll Wisc 1986; **Resid:** Radiation Oncology, Columbia Presby Med Ctr 1988; Radiation Oncology, Mallinckrodt Inst of Radiology 1990; **Fellow:** Radiation Oncology, Mallinckrodt Inst of Radiology 1991; **Fac Appt:** Prof RadRO, Washington Univ, St Louis

Minsky, Bruce MD [RadRO] - **Spec Exp:** Gastrointestinal Cancer; Esophageal Cancer; Colon & Rectal Cancer; Pancreatic Cancer; **Hospital:** Univ of Chicago Med Ctr; **Address:** Univ Chicago Hosp, 5841 S Maryland Ave, Chicago, IL 60637; **Phone:** 773-834-1180; **Board Cert:** Radiation Oncology 1987; **Med School:** Univ Mass Sch Med 1982; **Resid:** Radiation Oncology, Harvard Jt Ctr Rad Ther 1986; **Fac Appt:** Prof RadRO, Univ Chicago-Pritzker Sch Med

Mittal, Bharat B MD [RadRO] - **Spec Exp:** Head & Neck Cancer; Lymphoma; Skin Cancer; **Hospital:** Northwestern Meml Hosp; **Address:** 251 E Huron St, Galter LC-178, Chicago, IL 60611; **Phone:** 312-926-2520; **Board Cert:** Therapeutic Radiology 1981; **Med School:** India 1975; **Resid:** Internal Medicine, Christian Med Coll 1976; Radiation Oncology, Northwestern Meml Hosp 1980; **Fellow:** Radiation Oncology, Mallinckrodt Inst 1981; **Fac Appt:** Prof RadRO, Northwestern Univ

Movsas, Benjamin MD [RadRO] - **Spec Exp:** Lung Cancer; Brain Tumors; Prostate Cancer; Stereotactic Radiosurgery; **Hospital:** Henry Ford Hosp; **Address:** Henry Ford Health Sys, Dept Rad Oncology, 2799 W Grand Blvd, Detroit, MI 48202-2608; **Phone:** 313-916-1029; **Board Cert:** Radiation Oncology 2010; **Med School:** Washington Univ, St Louis 1990; **Resid:** Radiation Oncology, National Cancer Inst 1995

Myerson, Robert J MD [RadRO] - **Spec Exp:** Gastrointestinal Cancer; Breast Cancer; Hyperthermia Treatment of Cancer; **Hospital:** Barnes-Jewish Hosp; **Address:** Ctr for Advanced Med, Rad Oncology, 4921 Parkview Pl Fl LL, St Louis, MO 63110; **Phone:** 314-747-7236; **Board Cert:** Therapeutic Radiology 1985; **Med School:** Univ Miami Sch Med 1980; **Resid:** Radiation Therapy, Hosp Univ Penn 1984; **Fac Appt:** Prof RadRO, Washington Univ, St Louis

Pierce, Lori J MD [RadRO] - **Spec Exp:** Breast Cancer; **Hospital:** Univ of Michigan Hosp; **Address:** Univ Hosp, Dept Radiation Oncology, 1500 E Med Ctr, rm B2C440, Box 5010, Ann Arbor, MI 48109-5099; **Phone:** 734-936-4300; **Board Cert:** Radiation Oncology 1989; **Med School:** Duke Univ 1985; **Resid:** Radiation Oncology, Hosp Univ Penn 1989; **Fac Appt:** Prof RadRO, Univ Mich Med Sch

Schomberg, Paula J MD [RadRO] - **Spec Exp:** Brain Tumors; Pediatric Cancers; **Hospital:** Mayo Med Ctr & Clin - Rochester; **Address:** Mayo Clinic - Charlton Bldg, Desk R, 200 1st St SW, Rochester, MN 55905; **Phone:** 507-284-4561; **Board Cert:** Therapeutic Radiology 1984; **Med School:** Med Coll Wisc 1979; **Resid:** Radiation Therapy, Mayo Clinic 1983; **Fac Appt:** Prof RadRO, Mayo Med Sch

Small Jr, William MD [RadRO] - **Spec Exp:** Gynecologic Cancer; Gastrointestinal Cancer; Breast Cancer; Pancreatic Cancer; **Hospital:** Northwestern Meml Hosp; **Address:** Northwestern Meml Hosp, Rad Oncology, 251 E Huron St Galter Bldg - Ste L178, Chicago, IL 60611; **Phone:** 312-472-3650; **Board Cert:** Radiation Oncology 2004; **Med School:** Northwestern Univ 1990; **Resid:** Radiation Oncology, Northwestern Univ 1994; **Fac Appt:** Prof RadRO, Northwestern Univ

Suh, John H MD [RadRO] - **Spec Exp:** Brain Tumors-Adult & Pediatric; Stereotactic Radiosurgery; Stereotactic Body Radiation Therapy; **Hospital:** Cleveland Clin (page 70); **Address:** Cleveland Clinic, Dept Rad/Onc, 9500 Euclid Ave, Desk T28, Cleveland, OH 44195-0001; **Phone:** 216-444-5574; **Board Cert:** Radiation Oncology 2000; **Med School:** Univ Miami Sch Med 1990; **Resid:** Radiation Oncology, Cleveland Clinic 1994; **Fellow:** Radiation Oncology, Cleveland Clinic 1995

Taylor, Marie E MD [RadRO] - **Spec Exp:** Breast Cancer; **Hospital:** Barnes-Jewish Hosp, Barnes-Jewish West County Hosp; **Address:** Center for Advanced Med, Rad Oncology, 4921 Parkview Pl Fl LL, St Louis, MO 63110; **Phone:** 314-747-7236; **Board Cert:** Radiation Oncology 1987; **Med School:** Univ Wash 1982; **Resid:** Radiation Oncology, Univ Wash Med Ctr 1986

Vicini, Frank A MD [RadRO] - **Spec Exp:** Breast Cancer; Prostate Cancer; Brachytherapy; **Hospital:** Beaumont Hosp-Royal Oak; **Address:** William Beaumont Hospital, 3601 W 13 Mile Rd, Royal Oak, MI 48073; **Phone:** 248-551-1219; **Board Cert:** Radiation Oncology 1999; **Med School:** Wayne State Univ 1985; **Resid:** Radiation Oncology, William Beaumont Hosp 1989; **Fellow:** Radiation Oncology, Harvard Med Sch/Joint Ctr for Rad Ther 1990; **Fac Appt:** Clin Prof RadRO, Oakland Univ-William Beaumont Med Sch

Videtic, Gregory M MD [RadRO] - **Spec Exp:** Lung Cancer; Mesothelioma; Esophageal Cancer; Thymoma; **Hospital:** Cleveland Clin (page 70); **Address:** Cleveland Clinic, Radiation Oncology, 9500 Euclid Ave, Cleveland, OH 44195; **Phone:** 216-444-9797; **Board Cert:** Radiation Oncology 2008; **Med School:** McGill Univ 1986; **Resid:** Radiation Oncology, Dalhousie Univ 1988; Radiation Oncology, London Regl Cancer Ctr 1997; **Fellow:** Radiation Oncology, Wayne State Univ 1998; **Fac Appt:** Assoc Prof Rad, Cleveland Cl Coll Med/Case West Res

Weichselbaum, Ralph R MD [RadRO] - **Spec Exp:** Gene Targeted Radiotherapy; Pancreatic Cancer; Rectal Cancer; **Hospital:** Univ of Chicago Med Ctr; **Address:** Univ Chicago Medical Center, 5841 S Maryland Ave, MC 9006, Chicago, IL 60637; **Phone:** 773-702-6870; **Board Cert:** Therapeutic Radiology 1975; **Med School:** Univ IL Coll Med 1971; **Resid:** Therapeutic Radiology, Harvard Jt Ctr Rad Therapy 1975; **Fellow:** Harvard Univ 1976; **Fac Appt:** Prof RadRO, Univ Chicago-Pritzker Sch Med

Wilson, J Frank MD [RadRO] - **Spec Exp:** Breast Cancer; Skin Cancer; **Hospital:** Froedtert and Med Ctr of WI; **Address:** Dept Radiation Oncology, 9200 W Wisconsin Ave, Milwaukee, WI 53226; **Phone:** 414-805-4400; **Board Cert:** Therapeutic Radiology 1971; **Med School:** Univ MO-Columbia Sch Med 1965; **Resid:** Radiation Therapy, Penrose Cancer Hosp 1969; **Fellow:** Radiation Therapy, Natl Cancer Inst/NIH 1971; **Fac Appt:** Prof RadRO, Med Coll Wisc

Great Plains and Mountains

Gaffney, David K MD/PhD [RadRO] - **Spec Exp:** Breast Cancer; Gynecologic Cancer; **Hospital:** Univ Utah Hlth Care; **Address:** Huntsman Cancer Hosp, Dept Rad Oncology, 1950 Circle of Hope, rm 1440, Salt Lake City, UT 84112-5560; **Phone:** 801-581-2396; **Board Cert:** Radiation Oncology 2007; **Med School:** Med Coll Wisc 1992; **Resid:** Radiation Oncology, Univ Utah Hosps 1996; **Fac Appt:** Assoc Prof, Univ Utah

Radiation Oncology

Rabinovitch, Rachel A MD [RadRO] - **Spec Exp:** Breast Cancer; Lymphoma; **Hospital:** Univ of CO Hosp - Anschutz Inpatient Pav; **Address:** Anschutz Cancer Pavilion, Dept Rad Oncology, 1665 Aurora Court, Ste 1032, MS F-706, Aurora, CO 80045; **Phone:** 720-848-0156; **Board Cert:** Radiation Oncology 1994; **Med School:** Albert Einstein Coll Med 1989; **Resid:** Radiation Oncology, Meml Sloan Kettering Cancer Ctr 1993; **Fac Appt:** Assoc Prof RadRO, Univ Colorado

Shrieve, Dennis C MD [RadRO] - **Spec Exp:** Brain Tumors-Adult & Pediatric; Genitourinary Cancer; Gastrointestinal Cancer; **Hospital:** Univ Utah Hlth Care, Primary Children's Med Ctr; **Address:** Huntsman Cancer Inst, Dept Rad Oncology, 1950 Circle of Hope, rm 1440, Salt Lake City, UT 84112; **Phone:** 801-581-2396; **Board Cert:** Radiation Oncology 1993; **Med School:** Univ Miami Sch Med 1989; **Resid:** Radiation Oncology, UCSF Med Ctr; **Fac Appt:** Prof RadRO, Univ Utah

Smalley, Stephen R MD [RadRO] - **Spec Exp:** Colon Cancer; Gastrointestinal Cancer; **Hospital:** Olathe Med Ctr; **Address:** Olathe Medical Center, 20375 W 151st St, Doctors Bldg - Ste 180, Olathe, KS 66061-4575; **Phone:** 913-768-7200; **Board Cert:** Internal Medicine 1982; Radiation Oncology 1987; Medical Oncology 1985; **Med School:** Univ MO-Kansas City 1979; **Resid:** Internal Medicine, Mayo Clinic 1982; Radiation Oncology, Mayo Clinic 1986; **Fellow:** Medical Oncology, Mayo Clinic 1984; **Fac Appt:** Prof RadRO, Univ Kansas

Southwest

Ang, Kie-Kian MD/PhD [RadRO] - **Spec Exp:** Head & Neck Cancer; **Hospital:** UT MD Anderson Cancer Ctr; **Address:** UT MD Anderson Cancer Ctr, 1515 Holcombe Blvd, Unit 97, Houston, TX 77030; **Phone:** 713-563-8400; **Board Cert:** Radiation Oncology 1987; **Med School:** Belgium 1975; **Resid:** Radiation Oncology, Univ Hosp Louvian 1980; **Fac Appt:** Prof, Univ Tex, Houston

Buchholz, Thomas A MD [RadRO] - **Spec Exp:** Breast Cancer; **Hospital:** UT MD Anderson Cancer Ctr; **Address:** Univ Texas MD Anderson Cancer Ctr, 1515 Holcombe Blvd, Unit 97, Houston, TX 77030; **Phone:** 713-794-4892; **Board Cert:** Radiation Oncology 1993; **Med School:** Tufts Univ 1988; **Resid:** Radiation Oncology, Univ Washington Med Ctr 1993; **Fellow:** Research, Univ Washington Med Ctr 1994; **Fac Appt:** Prof RadRO, Univ Tex, Houston

Choy, Hak MD [RadRO] - **Spec Exp:** Lung Cancer; **Hospital:** UT Southwestern Med Ctr at Dallas; **Address:** UT SW Med Ctr - Dallas, Dept Rad-Onc, 5801 Forest Park Rd, Dallas, TX 75390-9183; **Phone:** 214-645-7600; **Board Cert:** Radiation Oncology 1993; **Med School:** Univ Tex Med Br, Galveston 1987; **Resid:** Radiation Oncology, Ohio State Univ Hosp 1989; Radiation Oncology, Univ Texas Hlth Sci Ctr 1991; **Fac Appt:** Prof RadRO, Univ Tex SW, Dallas

Cox, James D MD [RadRO] - **Spec Exp:** Lung Cancer; Esophageal Cancer; Thymoma; Thoracic Cancers; **Hospital:** UT MD Anderson Cancer Ctr; **Address:** Univ Tex MD Anderson Cancer Ctr, 1515 Holcombe Blvd, Unit 97, Houston, TX 77030; **Phone:** 713-563-2316; **Board Cert:** Therapeutic Radiology 1971; **Med School:** Univ Rochester 1965; **Resid:** Diagnostic Radiology, Penrose Cancer Hosp 1969; **Fellow:** Therapeutic Radiology, Inst Gustave-Roussy 1970; **Fac Appt:** Prof RadRO, Univ Tex, Houston

Eifel, Patricia J MD [RadRO] - **Spec Exp:** Cervical Cancer; Uterine Cancer; Vulvar Disease/Cancer; Vaginal Cancer; **Hospital:** UT MD Anderson Cancer Ctr; **Address:** MD Anderson Cancer Ctr, Dept Rad Onc, 1515 Holcombe Blvd, Unit 1202, Houston, TX 77030-4009; **Phone:** 713-563-6900; **Board Cert:** Therapeutic Radiology 1983; **Med School:** Stanford Univ 1977; **Resid:** Radiation Oncology, Stanford Univ Med Ctr 1981; **Fellow:** Therapeutic Radiology, Stanford Univ Med Ctr 1982

Grado, Gordon L MD [RadRO] - **Spec Exp:** Prostate Cancer; Brachytherapy; **Hospital:** Scottsdale Hlthcare - Shea; **Address:** 2926 N Civic Center Plaza, Scottsdale, AZ 85251; **Phone:** 480-614-6300; **Board Cert:** Therapeutic Radiology 1981; Radiation Oncology 1999; **Med School:** Southern IL Univ 1977; **Resid:** Therapeutic Radiology, Mayo Clinic 1981; **Fac Appt:** Assoc Prof RadRO, Univ Minn

Halyard, Michele MD [RadRO] - **Spec Exp:** Breast Cancer; Head & Neck Cancer; **Hospital:** Mayo Clinic - Scottsdale; **Address:** Mayo Clinic, Dept Radiation Oncology, 13400 E Shea Blvd, Scottsdale, AZ 85259-5404; **Phone:** 480-301-8120; **Board Cert:** Radiation Oncology 1989; **Med School:** Howard Univ 1984; **Resid:** Radiation Therapy, Howard Univ Hosp 1987; **Fellow:** Radiation Oncology, Mayo Clinic 1989

Herman, Terence S MD [RadRO] - **Spec Exp:** Breast Cancer; Sarcoma; Brain Tumors; **Hospital:** OU Med Ctr; **Address:** Oklahoma Univ Health Sci Ctr, 825 NE 10th St, Ste 1430, Oklahoma City, OK 73104-5417; **Phone:** 405-271-5641; **Board Cert:** Internal Medicine 1975; Medical Oncology 1977; Therapeutic Radiology 1985; **Med School:** Univ Conn 1972; **Resid:** Internal Medicine, Univ Arizona Med Ctr 1975; Radiation Oncology, Stanford Univ Med Ctr 1985; **Fellow:** Medical Oncology, Univ Arizona 1977; **Fac Appt:** Prof RadRO, Univ Okla Coll Med

Jhingran, Anuja MD [RadRO] - **Spec Exp:** Gynecologic Cancer; Brachytherapy; **Hospital:** UT MD Anderson Cancer Ctr; **Address:** MD Anderson Cancer Ctr, 1515 Holcombe Blvd, Box 1202, Houston, TX 77030; **Phone:** 713-563-6900; **Board Cert:** Radiation Oncology 1993; **Med School:** Texas Tech Univ 1988; **Resid:** Radiation Oncology, Baylor College Med 1993; **Fac Appt:** Assoc Prof RadRO, Univ Tex, Houston

Komaki, Ritsuko U MD [RadRO] - **Spec Exp:** Lung Cancer; Thymoma; Esophageal Cancer; **Hospital:** UT MD Anderson Cancer Ctr; **Address:** UT-MD Anderson Cancer Ctr, Dept Rad Onc, 1515 Holcombe Blvd, Unit 97, Houston, TX 77030; **Phone:** 713-563-2300; **Board Cert:** Therapeutic Radiology 1977; Radiation Oncology 2001; **Med School:** Japan 1969; **Resid:** Radiation Oncology, Med Coll Wisc 1978; **Fac Appt:** Prof RadRO, Univ Tex, Houston

Kuske, Robert R MD [RadRO] - **Spec Exp:** Breast Cancer; **Hospital:** Scottsdale Hlthcare - Shea; **Address:** 9055 E Del Camino Drive, Ste 200, Scottsdale, AZ 85258; **Phone:** 480-922-4600; **Board Cert:** Therapeutic Radiology 1985; **Med School:** Univ Cincinnati 1980; **Resid:** Radiation Oncology, Univ Cincinnati Med Ctr 1984

Lee, Andrew K MD [RadRO] - **Spec Exp:** Prostate Cancer; Proton Beam Therapy; Genitourinary Cancer; **Hospital:** UT MD Anderson Cancer Ctr; **Address:** MD Anderson Cancer Ctr, 1515 Holcombe Blvd, Unit 1150, Houston, TX 77030; **Phone:** 713-563-2348; **Board Cert:** Radiation Oncology 2001; **Med School:** Univ Minn 1996; **Resid:** Radiation Oncology, Joint Ctr for Radiation Therapy/Harvard 2001; **Fac Appt:** Assoc Prof RadRO, Univ Tex, Houston

Medbery, Clinton A MD [RadRO] - **Spec Exp:** Breast Cancer; Prostate Cancer; Brachytherapy; Stereotactic Radiosurgery; **Hospital:** St. Anthony Hosp -Oklahoma City; **Address:** Southwest Radiation Oncology, 1011 N Dewey Ave, Ste 101, Oklahoma City, OK 73101; **Phone:** 405-272-7311; **Board Cert:** Internal Medicine 1980; Medical Oncology 1983; Radiation Oncology 1987; **Med School:** Med Univ SC 1976; **Resid:** Internal Medicine, Naval Hosp 1980; Radiation Oncology, Natl Cancer Inst 1987; **Fellow:** Medical Oncology, Naval Hosp 1982

Morrison, William H MD [RadRO] - **Spec Exp:** Head & Neck Cancer; **Hospital:** UT MD Anderson Cancer Ctr; **Address:** 1515 Holcombe Blvd, Unit 97, Houston, TX 77030-4000; **Phone:** 713-794-1974; **Board Cert:** Internal Medicine 1981; Therapeutic Radiology 1985; **Med School:** Johns Hopkins Univ 1978; **Resid:** Internal Medicine, Rush Presby/St Lukes Med Ctr 1981; **Fellow:** Therapeutic Radiology, Stanford Univ Hosp 1985; **Fac Appt:** Prof RadRO, Univ Tex, Houston

Radiation Oncology

Schild, Steven E MD [RadRO] - **Spec Exp:** Lung Cancer; Prostate Cancer; Clinical Trials; **Hospital:** Mayo Clinic - Scottsdale; **Address:** Mayo Clinic, Dept Radiation Oncology, 13400 E Shea Blvd, Scottsdale, AZ 85259; **Phone:** 480-342-1262; **Board Cert:** Radiation Oncology 1989; **Med School:** Creighton Univ 1985; **Resid:** Radiation Oncology, Mayo Clin 1989; **Fac Appt:** Prof RadRO, Mayo Med Sch

Senzer, Neil N MD [RadRO] - **Spec Exp:** Clinical Trials; Gene Therapy; **Hospital:** Med City Dallas Hosp, Baylor Univ Medical Ctr; **Address:** Mary Crowley Cancer Research Ctr, 7777 Forest Ln C Bldg - Ste 707, Dallas, TX 75230; **Phone:** 972-566-3000; **Board Cert:** Pediatrics 1976; Pediatric Hematology-Oncology 1978; Therapeutic Radiology 1985; **Med School:** SUNY Buffalo 1971; **Resid:** Pediatrics, Johns Hopkins Hosp 1974; Radiation Oncology, St Barnabas Med Ctr 1985; **Fellow:** Pediatric Hematology-Oncology, St Jude Chldns Rsch Hosp 1978

Shina, Donald C MD [RadRO] - **Spec Exp:** Breast Cancer; **Hospital:** Christus St Vincent Reg Med Ctr-Santa Fe; **Address:** Santa Fe Cancer Ctr at St Vincent Hosp, 455 Saint Michael's Drive, Santa Fe, NM 87505; **Phone:** 505-820-5233; **Board Cert:** Internal Medicine 1977; Medical Oncology 1979; Therapeutic Radiology 1981; **Med School:** Case West Res Univ 1974; **Resid:** Internal Medicine, Univ Hosps 1977; **Fellow:** Radiation Oncology, Univ Hosps 1980; Medical Oncology, Univ Hosps 1980

Stea, Baldassarre MD/PhD [RadRO] - **Spec Exp:** Brain Tumors; Stereotactic Radiosurgery; Pediatric Cancers; Lymphoma; **Hospital:** Univ Med Ctr - Tucson, St. Joseph's Hosp - Tucson; **Address:** Univ Hlth Scis Ctr, Dept Rad Onc, 1501 N Campbell Ave, Tucson, AZ 85724-0001; **Phone:** 520-626-6724; **Board Cert:** Radiation Oncology 1987; **Med School:** Geo Wash Univ 1983; **Resid:** Radiation Oncology, Natl Cancer Inst 1987; **Fac Appt:** Prof RadRO, Univ Ariz Coll Med

West Coast and Pacific

Donaldson, Sarah S MD [RadRO] - **Spec Exp:** Pediatric Cancers; Hodgkin's Disease; Sarcoma; Breast Cancer; **Hospital:** Stanford Univ Hosp & Clinics; **Address:** 875 Blake Wilbur Drive, CC Bldg Fl G - rm 226, MC 5847, Stanford, CA 94305-5847; **Phone:** 650-723-6195; **Board Cert:** Therapeutic Radiology 1974; **Med School:** Harvard Med Sch 1968; **Resid:** Radiation Oncology, Stanford Univ Med Ctr 1972; **Fellow:** Pediatric Hematology-Oncology, Inst Gustave-Roussy 1973; Pediatric Hematology-Oncology, MD Anderson Cancer Ctr 1971; **Fac Appt:** Prof RadRO, Stanford Univ

Fowble, Barbara MD [RadRO] - **Spec Exp:** Breast Cancer; **Hospital:** UCSF Med Ctr; **Address:** 1600 Divisadero St, Ste H1031, San Francisco, CA 94115; **Phone:** 415-353-9819; **Board Cert:** Therapeutic Radiology 1976; **Med School:** Jefferson Med Coll 1972; **Resid:** Therapeutic Radiology, Bellevue Hosp Ctr-NYU 1975; Therapeutic Radiology, Hahnemann 1976; **Fellow:** Radiation Therapy, Jefferson Hosp 1977; **Fac Appt:** Prof RadRO, UCSF

Halberg, Francine MD [RadRO] - **Spec Exp:** Breast Cancer; **Hospital:** Marin Genl Hosp, UCSF Med Ctr; **Address:** Marin Cancer Inst-Dept of Rad.Oncology, 1350 S Eliseo Drive, Ste 100, Greenbrae, CA 94904; **Phone:** 415-925-7326; **Board Cert:** Internal Medicine 1981; Therapeutic Radiology 1984; **Med School:** Cornell Univ-Weill Med Coll 1978; **Resid:** Internal Medicine, USPHS Hosp 1981; **Fellow:** Radiation Oncology, Stanford Univ Med Ctr 1984; **Fac Appt:** Assoc Prof RadRO, UCSF

Hancock, Steven MD [RadRO] - **Spec Exp:** Prostate Cancer; Breast Cancer; Cancer Survivors-Late Effects of Therapy; **Hospital:** Stanford Univ Hosp & Clinics; **Address:** Stanford Cancer Center-Dept Rad Onc, 875 Blake Wilbur Drive, MC 5847, Stanford, CA 94305; **Phone:** 650-723-6440; **Board Cert:** Internal Medicine 1980; Therapeutic Radiology 1982; **Med School:** Stanford Univ 1976; **Resid:** Radiation Therapy, Stanford Univ Med Ctr 1981; Internal Medicine, Stanford Univ Med Ctr 1979; **Fac Appt:** Prof RadRO, Stanford Univ

Hoppe, Richard T MD [RadRO] - **Spec Exp:** Lymphoma; Hodgkin's Disease; Cutaneous Lymphoma; **Hospital:** Stanford Univ Hosp & Clinics; **Address:** 875 Blake Wilbur Drive, rm CC-G224, Stanford, CA 94305-5847; **Phone:** 650-723-5510; **Board Cert:** Therapeutic Radiology 1976; **Med School:** Cornell Univ-Weill Med Coll 1971; **Resid:** Radiation Therapy, Stanford Univ Med Ctr 1976; **Fac Appt:** Prof, Stanford Univ

Koh, Wui-Jin MD [RadRO] - **Spec Exp:** Gynecologic Cancer; Brachytherapy; Clinical Trials; **Hospital:** Univ Wash Med Ctr; **Address:** Seattle Cancer Care Alliance, 825 Eastlake Ave E, Box 19023, MS G1-101, Seattle, WA 98109; **Phone:** 206-288-7318; **Board Cert:** Radiation Oncology 1988; **Med School:** Loma Linda Univ 1984; **Resid:** Radiation Oncology, Univ Washington Med Ctr 1988; **Fellow:** Tumor Imaging, Univ Washington Med Ctr 1988; **Fac Appt:** Prof RadRO, Univ Wash

Laramore, George E MD/PhD [RadRO] - **Spec Exp:** Neutron Therapy for Advanced Cancer; Salivary Gland Tumors; Head & Neck Cancer; Skin Cancer; **Hospital:** Univ Wash Med Ctr, Harborview Med Ctr; **Address:** Univ Washington Med Ctr, Dept Rad Onc Box 356043, Seattle, WA 98195; **Phone:** 206-598-4121; **Board Cert:** Therapeutic Radiology 1980; Radiation Oncology 2000; **Med School:** Univ Miami Sch Med 1976; **Resid:** Radiation Oncology, Univ Washington Med Ctr 1980; **Fac Appt:** Prof RadRO, Univ Wash

Larson, David A MD/PhD [RadRO] - **Spec Exp:** Neuro-Oncology; Brain Tumors; Stereotactic Radiosurgery; **Hospital:** UCSF Med Ctr; **Address:** UCSF Med Ctr, Dept Rad Onc, 505 Parnassus Ave, rm L-08, San Francisco, CA 94143-0226; **Phone:** 415-353-8900; **Board Cert:** Therapeutic Radiology 1986; **Med School:** Univ Miami Sch Med 1981; **Resid:** Radiation Therapy, Joint Ctr RadTherapy 1985; **Fac Appt:** Prof RadRO, UCSF

Le, Quynh-Thu Xuan MD [RadRO] - **Spec Exp:** Head & Neck Cancer; Lung Cancer; Thoracic Cancers; Clinical Trials; **Hospital:** Stanford Univ Hosp & Clinics; **Address:** Stanford Univ, Dept Rad Oncology, 875 Blake Wilbur Drive, MC 5847, Ground Flr, Stanford, CA 94305; **Phone:** 650-498-5032; **Board Cert:** Radiation Oncology 2008; **Med School:** UCSF 1993; **Resid:** Radiation Oncology, UCSF Med Ctr 1997; **Fac Appt:** Prof RadRO, Stanford Univ

Mundt, Arno J MD [RadRO] - **Spec Exp:** Gynecologic Cancer; Intensity Modulated Radiotherapy (IMRT); **Hospital:** UCSD Med Ctr-Hillcrest; **Address:** Moores UCSD Cancer Ctr, Radiation Oncology Dept, 3855 Health Sciences Drive, MC 0843, La Jolla, CA 92093-0843; **Phone:** 858-822-6046; **Board Cert:** Radiation Oncology 1994; **Med School:** Univ Mich Med Sch 1987; **Resid:** Physical Medicine & Rehabilitation, George Washington Univ Hosp 1990; Radiation Oncology, Univ Chicago Hosps 1993; **Fellow:** Physical Medicine & Rehabilitation, Univ Chicago Hosps 1994; **Fac Appt:** Assoc Prof RadRO, Univ Chicago-Pritzker Sch Med

Park, Catherine C MD [RadRO] - **Spec Exp:** Breast Cancer; Lymphoma; **Hospital:** UCSF Med Ctr; **Address:** UCSF Radiation Oncology, 1600 Divisadero St, Ste H1031, San Francisco, CA 94115; **Phone:** 415-353-7175; **Board Cert:** Radiation Oncology 2000; **Med School:** UCLA 1995; **Resid:** Radiation Oncology, Mass Genl Hosp 2000; **Fac Appt:** Assoc Prof RadRO, UCSF

Pezner, Richard D MD [RadRO] - **Spec Exp:** Sarcoma-Soft Tissue; Breast Cancer; Stereotactic Radiosurgery; **Hospital:** City of Hope Natl Med Ctr (page 69); **Address:** City of Hope Med Ctr-Div Radiation Onc, 1500 E Duarte Rd, Duarte, CA 91010-3000; **Phone:** 626-301-8247; **Board Cert:** Therapeutic Radiology 1979; **Med School:** Northwestern Univ 1975; **Resid:** Radiation Oncology, Oregon Health Sci Ctr 1979; **Fac Appt:** Clin Prof RadRO, UC Irvine

Quivey, Jeanne M MD [RadRO] - **Spec Exp:** Head & Neck Cancer; Breast Cancer; Eye Tumors/Cancer; Intensity Modulated Radiotherapy (IMRT); **Hospital:** UCSF Med Ctr; **Address:** UCSF Med Ctr @ Mt Zion, Radiation Onc Dept, 1600 Divisadero St, Ste H1031, Box 1708, San Francisco, CA 94115-3010; **Phone:** 415-353-7175; **Board Cert:** Therapeutic Radiology 1974; **Med School:** UCSF 1970; **Resid:** Radiation Therapy, UCSF Med Ctr 1974; **Fac Appt:** Prof RadRO, UCSF

Radiation Oncology

Roach III, Mack MD [RadRO] - **Spec Exp:** Prostate Cancer; Genitourinary Cancer; Lung Cancer; **Hospital:** UCSF - Mt Zion Med Ctr, UCSF Med Ctr; **Address:** UCSF Radiation Oncology, 1600 Divisadero St, Ste H1031, San Francisco, CA 94143-1708; **Phone:** 415-353-7181; **Board Cert:** Internal Medicine 1984; Medical Oncology 1985; Radiation Oncology 1987; **Med School:** Stanford Univ 1979; **Resid:** Internal Medicine, ML King Genl Hosp 1981; Radiation Oncology, Stanford Univ Med Ctr 1987; **Fellow:** Medical Oncology, UCSF Med Ctr 1983; **Fac Appt:** Prof RadRO, UCSF

Rose, Christopher M MD [RadRO] - **Spec Exp:** Prostate Cancer; Breast Cancer; Intensity Modulated Radiotherapy (IMRT); **Hospital:** Providence St Joseph Med Ctr, Providence Tarzana Med Ctr; **Address:** Valley Radiotherapy Assocs, The Ctr for Radiation Therapy, 9229 Wilshire Blvd, Beverly Hills, CA 90210; **Phone:** 310-205-5777; **Board Cert:** Radiation Oncology 1999; **Med School:** Harvard Med Sch 1974; **Resid:** Internal Medicine, Beth Israel Deaconess 1976; Radiation Oncology, Joint Ctr Rad Therapy 1979; **Fellow:** Cancer Research, British Inst Cancer Rsch 1979; **Fac Appt:** Clin Prof RadRO, USC Sch Med

Rossi, Carl John MD [RadRO] - **Spec Exp:** Prostate Cancer; Proton Beam Therapy; **Hospital:** Loma Linda Univ Med Ctr; **Address:** Loma Linda Univ Med Ctr, 11234 Anderson St, rm B124, Loma Linda, CA 92354; **Phone:** 909-558-4280; **Board Cert:** Radiation Oncology 1994; **Med School:** Loyola Univ-Stritch Sch Med 1988; **Resid:** Radiation Oncology, Loma Linda Univ Med Ctr 1992; **Fac Appt:** Asst Prof RadRO, Loma Linda Univ

Russell, Kenneth J MD [RadRO] - **Spec Exp:** Genitourinary Cancer; Prostate Cancer; Lymphoma; **Hospital:** Univ Wash Med Ctr; **Address:** Seattle Cancer Care Alliance, 825 Eastlake Ave E, Box 19023, MS G1-101, Seattle, WA 98109; **Phone:** 206-288-7318; **Board Cert:** Therapeutic Radiology 1984; **Med School:** Harvard Med Sch 1979; **Resid:** Radiation Therapy, Stanford Univ Med Ctr 1983; **Fellow:** Radiological Biology, Stanford Univ Med Ctr 1985; **Fac Appt:** Prof Rad, Univ Wash

Sandler, Howard M MD [RadRO] - **Spec Exp:** Prostate Cancer; Genitourinary Cancer; Brain Tumors; **Hospital:** Cedars-Sinai Med Ctr; **Address:** S Oschin Comprehensive Cancer Inst, Cedars-Sinai Med Ctr, 8700 Beverly Blvd, Los Angeles, CA 90048; **Phone:** 310-423-4234; **Board Cert:** Radiation Oncology 1989; **Med School:** Univ Conn 1985; **Resid:** Radiation Oncology, Hosp Univ Penn 1989

Seung, Steven K MD/PhD [RadRO] - **Spec Exp:** Stereotactic Radiosurgery; Brain Tumors; Esophageal Cancer; Lung Cancer; **Hospital:** Providence Portland Med Ctr; **Address:** 4805 NE Glisan St, Garden Level, Portland, OR 97213; **Phone:** 503-215-6029; **Board Cert:** Radiation Oncology 2010; **Med School:** Univ Chicago-Pritzker Sch Med 1994; **Resid:** Radiation Oncology, UCSF Med Ctr 1998

Thomas Jr, Charles R MD [RadRO] - **Spec Exp:** Gastrointestinal Cancer; Esophageal Cancer; Colon & Rectal Cancer; **Hospital:** OR Hlth & Sci Univ; **Address:** 3181 SW Sam Jackson Park Rd, MC KPV4, Portland, OR 97239; **Phone:** 503-494-8756; **Board Cert:** Internal Medicine 2010; Radiation Oncology 1999; **Med School:** Univ IL Coll Med 1985; **Resid:** Internal Medicine, Baylor Coll Med 1988; Radiation Oncology, Univ Wash Med Ctr 1997; **Fellow:** Medical Oncology, Rush Univ Med Ctr 1999; **Fac Appt:** Prof RadRO, Oregon Hlth & Sci Univ

Tripuraneni, Prabhakar MD [RadRO] - **Spec Exp:** Prostate Cancer; Head & Neck Cancer; Lymphoma; **Hospital:** Scripps Green Hosp, Scripps Meml Hosp - La Jolla; **Address:** Scripps Clinic, Div Radiation Oncology, 10666 N Torrey Pines Rd, MSB 1, La Jolla, CA 92037; **Phone:** 858-554-2000; **Board Cert:** Therapeutic Radiology 1983; **Med School:** India 1976; **Resid:** Radiation Oncology, Univ Alberta 1981; Radiation Oncology, UCSF Med Ctr 1983; **Fac Appt:** Clin Prof RadRO, UCSD

Wara, William M MD [RadRO] - **Spec Exp:** Brain & Spinal Tumors; Sarcoma; Pediatric Cancers; **Hospital:** Kaiser Permanente S San Francisco Med Ctr; **Address:** Cancer Treatment Ctr, 220 Oyster Pt Blvd, South San Francisco, CA 94080; **Phone:** 650-827-6500; **Board Cert:** Therapeutic Radiology 1974; **Med School:** UC Irvine 1969; **Resid:** Therapeutic Radiology, UCSF Medical Ctr 1973; **Fac Appt:** Prof RadRO, UCSF

Wong, Jeffrey Y C MD [RadRO] - **Spec Exp:** Radioimmunotherapy of Cancer; Prostate Cancer; Intensity Modulated Radiotherapy (IMRT); Multiple Myeloma; **Hospital:** City of Hope Natl Med Ctr (page 69); **Address:** City of Hope Med Ctr-Dept Radiation Onc, 1500 E Duarte Rd, Duarte, CA 91768-3012; **Phone:** 626-359-8111 x62969; **Board Cert:** Therapeutic Radiology 1985; **Med School:** Johns Hopkins Univ 1981; **Resid:** Radiation Oncology, UCSF Med Ctr 1985; **Fac Appt:** Prof RadRO, UC Irvine

DIAGNOSTIC RADIOLOGY

New England

Kopans, Daniel B MD [DR] - **Spec Exp:** Breast Imaging; Breast Cancer; **Hospital:** Mass Genl Hosp; **Address:** Mass Genl Hosp, Avon Comprehensive Breast Ctr, 15 Parkman St, WAC 240, Boston, MA 02114; **Phone:** 617-726-3093; **Board Cert:** Diagnostic Radiology 1977; **Med School:** Harvard Med Sch 1973; **Resid:** Diagnostic Radiology, Mass Genl Hosp 1977; **Fac Appt:** Prof Rad, Harvard Med Sch

McCarthy, Shirley M MD/PhD [DR] - **Spec Exp:** Gynecologic Cancer; **Hospital:** Yale-New Haven Hosp, Yale Med Group; **Address:** Yale-New Haven Hosp, 333 Cedar St, Ste TE2, PO Box 208042, New Haven, CT 06520-3206; **Phone:** 203-785-2384; **Board Cert:** Diagnostic Radiology 1983; **Med School:** Yale Univ 1979; **Resid:** Diagnostic Radiology, Yale-New Haven Hosp 1983; **Fellow:** Cross Sectional Imaging, UCSF Med Ctr 1984; **Fac Appt:** Prof Rad, Yale Univ

Weinreb, Jeffrey C MD [DR] - **Spec Exp:** Breast Cancer; Abdominal Imaging; CT Body Scan; **Hospital:** Yale-New Haven Hosp, Yale Med Group; **Address:** Yale Univ Sch Medicine, Dept Radiology, 333 Cedar St, rm MRC147, Box 208042, New Haven, CT 06520-8042; **Phone:** 203-785-5913; **Board Cert:** Diagnostic Radiology 1983; **Med School:** Mount Sinai Sch Med 1978; **Resid:** Diagnostic Radiology, LI Jewish Med Ctr 1982; **Fellow:** Ultrasound/CT, Hosp Univ Penn 1983; **Fac Appt:** Prof Rad, Yale Univ

Mid Atlantic

Austin, John H M MD [DR] - **Spec Exp:** Lung Cancer; Thoracic Radiology; **Hospital:** NY-Presby Hosp/Columbia (page 78); **Address:** Columbia Presby Hosp, Dept Radiology, 622 W 168th St, HP 3-305, New York, NY 10032-3784; **Phone:** 212-305-2986; **Board Cert:** Diagnostic Radiology 1970; **Med School:** Yale Univ 1965; **Resid:** Diagnostic Radiology, UCSF Med Ctr 1968; **Fellow:** Diagnostic Radiology, UCSF Med Ctr 1970; **Fac Appt:** Prof Emeritus Rad, Columbia P&S

Brem, Rachel F MD [DR] - **Spec Exp:** Breast Imaging; Breast Cancer; **Hospital:** G Washington Univ Hosp; **Address:** Mammography Clinic, 2150 Pennsylvania Ave NW, DC Level, Washington, DC 20037; **Phone:** 202-741-3031; **Board Cert:** Diagnostic Radiology 1990; **Med School:** Columbia P&S 1984; **Resid:** Diagnostic Radiology, Johns Hopkins Hosp 1989; **Fellow:** Mammography, Johns Hopkins Hosp 1990; **Fac Appt:** Prof Rad, Geo Wash Univ

Diagnostic Radiology

Conant, Emily F MD [DR] - **Spec Exp:** Breast Cancer; Breast Imaging; **Hospital:** Hosp Univ Penn - UPHS (page 80); **Address:** Dept Radiology (Breast Imaging), 3400 Spruce St, 1 Silverstein, Philadelphia, PA 19104; **Phone:** 215-662-4032; **Board Cert:** Diagnostic Radiology 1989; **Med School:** Univ Pennsylvania 1984; **Resid:** Diagnostic Radiology, Hosp Univ Penn 1986; **Fellow:** Breast Imaging, Hosp Univ Penn 1989; **Fac Appt:** Prof Rad, Univ Pennsylvania

Dershaw, D David MD [DR] - **Spec Exp:** Breast Imaging; Breast Cancer; Mammography; **Hospital:** Meml Sloan-Kettering Cancer Ctr (page 75); **Address:** 300 E 66th St, New York, NY 10065; **Phone:** 800-525-2225; **Board Cert:** Diagnostic Radiology 1978; **Med School:** Jefferson Med Coll 1974; **Resid:** Diagnostic Radiology, New York Hosp 1978; **Fellow:** Ultrasound, Thos Jefferson Univ Hosp 1979; **Fac Appt:** Prof Rad, Cornell Univ-Weill Med Coll

Edelstein, Barbara A MD [DR] - **Spec Exp:** Breast Cancer; **Address:** 1045 Park Ave, New York, NY 10028; **Phone:** 212-860-7700; **Board Cert:** Diagnostic Radiology 1983; **Med School:** NY Med Coll 1977; **Resid:** Diagnostic Radiology, Montefiore Hosp 1982

Evers, Kathryn A MD [DR] - **Spec Exp:** Breast Cancer; Mammography; **Hospital:** Fox Chase Cancer Ctr (page 72); **Address:** Fox Chase Cancer Ctr, Diagnostic Imaging, 333 Cottman Ave, Philadelphia, PA 19111; **Phone:** 215-728-2646; **Board Cert:** Diagnostic Radiology 1980; **Med School:** NYU Sch Med 1975; **Resid:** Diagnostic Radiology, Hosp Univ Penn 1980; **Fellow:** Diagnostic Radiology, Hosp Univ Penn 1981; **Fac Appt:** Asst Clin Prof Rad, Temple Univ

Fishman, Elliot MD [DR] - **Spec Exp:** CT Body Scan; Abdominal Imaging; Cancer Imaging; **Hospital:** Johns Hopkins Hosp; **Address:** Johns Hopkins Hosp, Dept Radiology, 601 N Caroline St, JHOC 3254, Baltimore, MD 21287-0006; **Phone:** 410-955-5173; **Board Cert:** Diagnostic Radiology 1981; **Med School:** Univ MD Sch Med 1977; **Resid:** Diagnostic Radiology, Sinai Hosp 1980; **Fellow:** Computerized Tomography, Johns Hopkins Hosp 1981; **Fac Appt:** Prof Rad, Johns Hopkins Univ

Henschke, Claudia L MD/PhD [DR] - **Spec Exp:** Lung Cancer; Thoracic Radiology; **Hospital:** Mount Sinai Med Ctr (page 76); **Address:** Mt Sinai Med Ctr, Radiology Dept, 1 Gustave Levy Pl, Box 1234, New York, NY 10029; **Phone:** 212-241-2420; **Board Cert:** Diagnostic Radiology 1981; **Med School:** Howard Univ 1977; **Resid:** Diagnostic Radiology, Brigham & Womens Hosp 1983; **Fac Appt:** Prof Rad, Cornell Univ-Weill Med Coll

Hricak, Hedvig MD/PhD [DR] - **Spec Exp:** Prostate Cancer-MR Spectroscopy (MRSI); Breast Imaging; Breast Cancer; **Hospital:** Meml Sloan-Kettering Cancer Ctr (page 75); **Address:** 1275 York Ave, Ste C278, New York, NY 10065; **Phone:** 800-525-2225; **Board Cert:** Diagnostic Radiology 1978; **Med School:** Yugoslavia 1970; **Resid:** Diagnostic Radiology, St Joseph Mercy Hosp 1977; **Fellow:** Ultrasound/CT, Henry Ford Hosp 1978; **Fac Appt:** Prof Rad, Cornell Univ-Weill Med Coll

Levy, Angela D MD [DR] - **Spec Exp:** Abdominal Imaging; **Hospital:** Georgetown Univ Hosp, Armed Forces Inst of Path; **Address:** Georgetown University Hospital, 3800 Reservoir Rd NW, Ground Floor, Washington, DC 20007; **Phone:** 202-444-3380; **Board Cert:** Diagnostic Radiology 1993; **Med School:** Uniformed Srvs Univ, Bethesda 1988; **Resid:** Diagnostic Radiology, Walter Reed Army Hosp 1992; **Fac Appt:** Assoc Prof Rad, Uniformed Srvs Univ, Bethesda

Mitnick, Julie MD [DR] - **Spec Exp:** Mammography; Breast Cancer; **Address:** 650 1st Ave, New York, NY 10016; **Phone:** 212-686-4440; **Board Cert:** Diagnostic Radiology 1977; **Med School:** NYU Sch Med 1973; **Resid:** Diagnostic Radiology, NYU Med Ctr 1977; **Fellow:** Pediatric Radiology, NYU Med Ctr 1978; **Fac Appt:** Assoc Clin Prof Rad, NYU Sch Med

Panicek, David M MD [DR] - **Spec Exp:** Bone Cancer; Soft Tissue Tumors; Musculoskeletal Tumor Imaging; **Hospital:** Meml Sloan-Kettering Cancer Ctr (page 75); **Address:** Department of Radiology, 1275 York Ave, New York, NY 10065; **Phone:** 800-525-2225; **Board Cert:** Diagnostic Radiology 1984; **Med School:** Cornell Univ-Weill Med Coll 1980; **Resid:** Diagnostic Radiology, NY Hosp-Cornell Med Ctr 1984; **Fac Appt:** Prof Rad, Cornell Univ-Weill Med Coll

Parsons, Rosaleen B MD [DR] - **Spec Exp:** CT Body Scan; Genitourinary Cancer; Genitourinary Radiology; **Hospital:** Fox Chase Cancer Ctr (page 72); **Address:** Fox Chase Cancer Ctr, Dept of Diagnostic Imaging, 333 Cottman Ave, Philadelphia, PA 19111; **Phone:** 215-728-3024; **Board Cert:** Diagnostic Radiology 1991; **Med School:** Med Coll PA Hahnemann 1986; **Resid:** Diagnostic Radiology, Med Coll Penn Affil Hosp 1991; **Fac Appt:** Assoc Clin Prof Rad, Temple Univ

Rao, Vijay M MD [DR] - **Spec Exp:** Head & Neck Tumors Imaging; **Hospital:** Thomas Jefferson Univ Hosp (page 81); **Address:** 132 S 10th St, 1087 Main Bldg, Philadelphia, PA 19107-4824; **Phone:** 215-955-4804; **Board Cert:** Diagnostic Radiology 1978; **Med School:** India 1973; **Resid:** Diagnostic Radiology, Thomas Jefferson Univ Hosp 1978; **Fac Appt:** Prof Rad, Thomas Jefferson Univ

Roth, Susan G MD [DR] - **Spec Exp:** Breast Imaging; Breast Cancer; **Hospital:** Hosp Univ Penn - UPHS (page 80); **Address:** Hosp Univ Penn, Dept Radiology, 3400 Spruce St, Philadelphia, PA 19104; **Phone:** 215-614-0124; **Board Cert:** Diagnostic Radiology 1989; **Med School:** Univ Pennsylvania 1986; **Resid:** Diagnostic Radiology, Johns Hopkins Hosp 1989; **Fac Appt:** Prof Rad, Univ Pennsylvania

Yankelevitz, David MD [DR] - **Spec Exp:** Lung Cancer; Thoracic Radiology; **Hospital:** Mount Sinai Med Ctr (page 76); **Address:** Mt Sinai Med Ctr, Radiology Dept, 1 Gustave Levy Pl, Box 1234, New York, NY 10029; **Phone:** 212-241-2420; **Board Cert:** Diagnostic Radiology 1987; Nuclear Medicine 1987; **Med School:** SUNY Hlth Sci Ctr 1981; **Resid:** Diagnostic Radiology, Long Island Coll Hosp 1984; Nuclear Medicine, NY-Cornell Med Ctr 1987; **Fellow:** Diagnostic Radiology, NY-Cornell Med Ctr 1987; **Fac Appt:** Prof Rad, Cornell Univ-Weill Med Coll

Southeast

Abbitt, Patricia L MD [DR] - **Spec Exp:** Breast Imaging; Breast Cancer; **Hospital:** Shands at Univ of FL; **Address:** Shands Healthcare, Dept Radiology, 1600 SW Archer Rd, PO Box 100374, Gainesville, FL 32610; **Phone:** 352-265-0291; **Board Cert:** Diagnostic Radiology 1986; **Med School:** Tufts Univ 1981; **Resid:** Diagnostic Radiology, Univ VA Med Ctr 1986; **Fellow:** Breast Imaging, Univ VA Med Ctr 1987; **Fac Appt:** Prof Rad, Univ Fla Coll Med

Cardenosa, Gilda MD [DR] - **Spec Exp:** Breast Imaging; **Hospital:** Med Coll of VA Hosp; **Address:** VCU Med Ctr at Stony Point, Dept Radiology, 9000 Stony Point Pkwy, Richmond, VA 23235; **Phone:** 804-560-8906 x7862; **Board Cert:** Diagnostic Radiology 1989; **Med School:** Columbia P&S 1984; **Resid:** Diagnostic Radiology, Mass Genl Hosp 1989; **Fac Appt:** Prof Rad, Med Coll VA

Chiles, Caroline MD [DR] - **Spec Exp:** Thoracic Radiology; Lung Cancer; **Hospital:** Wake Forest Univ Baptist Med Ctr; **Address:** Medical Center Blvd, Winston-Salem, NC 27157; **Phone:** 336-716-4316; **Board Cert:** Diagnostic Radiology 1984; **Med School:** Duke Univ 1979; **Resid:** Diagnostic Radiology, Stanford Univ Hosp 1984; **Fellow:** Thoracic Radiology, Duke Univ Med Ctr 1985; **Fac Appt:** Assoc Prof Rad, Bowman Gray

Diagnostic Radiology

Elster, Allen D MD [DR] - **Spec Exp:** MRI; Neurologic Imaging; Brain Tumors; Spinal Tumors; **Hospital:** Wake Forest Univ Baptist Med Ctr; **Address:** Wake Forest Univ Baptist Med Ctr, 1 Medical Center Blvd, Dept Radiology, Winston Salem, NC 27157-1088; **Phone:** 336-716-7095; **Board Cert:** Diagnostic Radiology 1987; Neuroradiology 2005; **Med School:** Baylor Coll Med 1980; **Resid:** Surgery, Mass Genl Hosp 1983; Diagnostic Radiology, Univ Texas 1986; **Fellow:** Neuroradiology, Bowman Gray Sch Med 1987; **Fac Appt:** Prof Rad, Wake Forest Univ

Freimanis, Rita I MD [DR] - **Spec Exp:** Breast Cancer; Breast Imaging; **Hospital:** Wake Forest Univ Baptist Med Ctr; **Address:** Wake Forest Univ Bapt Med Ctr, One Medical Center Blvd, Winston-Salem, NC 27157; **Phone:** 336-713-4019; **Board Cert:** Diagnostic Radiology 1990; **Med School:** Bowman Gray 1985; **Resid:** Diagnostic Radiology, NC Bapt Hosp 1990; **Fac Appt:** Assoc Prof Rad, Wake Forest Univ

Patz, Edward F MD [DR] - **Spec Exp:** Thoracic Radiology; PET Imaging; Lung Cancer; **Hospital:** Duke Univ Hosp; **Address:** Duke Univ Med Ctr, Dept Radiology, Box 3808, Durham, NC 27710; **Phone:** 919-684-7999; **Board Cert:** Diagnostic Radiology 1990; **Med School:** Univ MD Sch Med 1985; **Resid:** Diagnostic Radiology, Brigham & Womens Hosp 1990; **Fellow:** Thoracic Radiology, Brigham & Womens Hosp 1990; **Fac Appt:** Prof, Duke Univ

Zagoria, Ronald J MD [DR] - **Spec Exp:** Abdominal Imaging; Genitourinary Radiology; MRI; **Hospital:** Wake Forest Univ Baptist Med Ctr; **Address:** Wake Forest Univ Bapt Med Ctr, Medical Center Blvd, MRI Bldg Fl 3, Winston-Salem, NC 27157; **Phone:** 336-716-2471; **Board Cert:** Diagnostic Radiology 1987; Vascular & Interventional Radiology 2004; **Med School:** Univ MD Sch Med 1983; **Resid:** Radiology, Bowman Gray Med Ctr 1987; **Fellow:** Abdominal Imaging, Bowman Gray Med Ctr 1987; **Fac Appt:** Prof Rad, Wake Forest Univ

Midwest

Helvie, Mark A MD [DR] - **Spec Exp:** Breast Imaging; Breast Cancer; Mammography; **Hospital:** Univ of Michigan Hosp; **Address:** Univ Of Michigan Hospital, Taubman Center, rm 2910N, 1500 E Medical Center Drive, Ann Arbor, MI 48109-0326; **Phone:** 734-936-4367; **Board Cert:** Internal Medicine 1983; Diagnostic Radiology 1986; **Med School:** Univ NC Sch Med 1980; **Resid:** Internal Medicine, Univ Michigan Hosps 1983; Diagnostic Radiology, Univ Michigan Hosps 1986; **Fellow:** Breast Imaging, Univ Michigan Hosps 1987; **Fac Appt:** Prof, Univ Mich Med Sch

Jackson, Valerie P MD [DR] - **Spec Exp:** Breast Imaging; **Hospital:** IU Health Methodist Hosp, Wishard Hlth Srvs; **Address:** Indiana Univ Hosp, Dept Radiology, 550 N University Blvd, rm 0663, Indianapolis, IN 46202; **Phone:** 317-944-1866; **Board Cert:** Diagnostic Radiology 1982; **Med School:** Indiana Univ 1978; **Resid:** Diagnostic Radiology, Indiana Univ Med Ctr 1982; **Fac Appt:** Prof Rad, Indiana Univ

Monsees, Barbara MD [DR] - **Spec Exp:** Mammography; Breast Cancer; **Hospital:** Barnes-Jewish Hosp; **Address:** 510 S Kingshighway Blvd, Campus Box 8131, St Louis, MO 63110; **Phone:** 314-454-7500; **Board Cert:** Diagnostic Radiology 1980; **Med School:** Washington Univ, St Louis 1975; **Resid:** Pediatrics, St Louis Chldns Hosp 1977; Diagnostic Radiology, Mallinckrodt Inst Radiology 1980; **Fac Appt:** Prof, Washington Univ, St Louis

Sagel, Stuart S MD [DR] - **Spec Exp:** Lung Cancer; Occupational Lung Disease; **Hospital:** Barnes-Jewish Hosp, Barnes-Jewish West County Hosp; **Address:** Mallinckrodt Inst Rad-Barnes Hosp, 510 S Kingshighway Blvd, Box 8131, St Louis, MO 63110-1016; **Phone:** 314-362-2927; **Board Cert:** Diagnostic Radiology 1970; **Med School:** Temple Univ 1965; **Resid:** Diagnostic Radiology, Yale New Haven Hosp 1968; Diagnostic Radiology, UCSF Med Ctr 1970; **Fac Appt:** Prof Rad, Washington Univ, St Louis

Swensen, Stephen J MD [DR] - **Spec Exp:** Lung Cancer; **Hospital:** Mayo Med Ctr & Clin - Rochester; **Address:** Mayo Clinic - Diagnostic Radiology, 200 1st St SW, Rochester, MN 55905; **Phone:** 507-284-8550; **Board Cert:** Diagnostic Radiology 1986; **Med School:** Univ Wisc 1981; **Resid:** Diagnostic Radiology, Mayo Clinic 1986; **Fellow:** Pulmonary Radiology, Brigham & Womens Hosp 1987; **Fac Appt:** Prof Rad, Mayo Med Sch

Southwest

Erasmus, Jeremy J MD [DR] - **Spec Exp:** Lung Cancer; CT Body Scan; PET Imaging; **Hospital:** UT MD Anderson Cancer Ctr; **Address:** MD Anderson Cancer Ctr, Dept of Rad, 1515 Holcombe Blvd, Unit 1478, Houston, TX 77030; **Phone:** 713-792-5878; **Board Cert:** Diagnostic Radiology 1993; **Med School:** South Africa 1982; **Resid:** Diagnostic Radiology, Queens Univ 1993; **Fac Appt:** Prof Rad, Univ Tex, Houston

Huynh, Phan Tuong MD [DR] - **Spec Exp:** Mammography; Breast Cancer; **Hospital:** St. Luke's Episcopal Hosp-Houston; **Address:** 6624 Fannin St, St Luke's Tower, Womens Ctr Fl 10, Houston, TX 77030; **Phone:** 832-355-8130; **Board Cert:** Diagnostic Radiology 1994; **Med School:** Univ VA Sch Med 1989; **Resid:** Diagnostic Radiology, Univ Virginia Med Ctr 1994; **Fellow:** Mammography, Univ Virginia 1995; **Fac Appt:** Assoc Clin Prof Rad, Baylor Coll Med

Otto, Pamela MD [DR] - **Spec Exp:** Breast Imaging; Breast Cancer; **Hospital:** Univ Hlth Syst-San Antonio, Audie L Murphy Meml Vets Hosp - San Antonio; **Address:** 7703 Floyd Curl Drive, MC 7800, San Antonio, TX 78229; **Phone:** 210-567-3448; **Board Cert:** Diagnostic Radiology 1993; **Med School:** Univ MO-Columbia Sch Med 1988; **Resid:** Diagnostic Radiology, Univ Texas Hlth Sci Ctr 1993; **Fellow:** Breast Imaging, Univ Texas Hlth Sci Ctr 1993; **Fac Appt:** Assoc Prof Rad, Univ Tex, San Antonio

Ulissey, Michael J MD [DR] - **Spec Exp:** Breast Imaging; Breast Cancer; Mammography; **Hospital:** UT Southwestern Med Ctr at Dallas; **Address:** Univ SW Med Ctr, 5701 Maple Drive, Ste 300, Dallas, TX 75235; **Phone:** 214-266-3300; **Board Cert:** Diagnostic Radiology 1998; **Med School:** Texas A&M Univ 1991; **Resid:** Diagnostic Radiology, Univ Oklahoma Hlth Ctr 1998; **Fellow:** Radiology, Univ TX SW Clin Breast Radiology 1999; Magnetic Resonance Imaging, UT Southwestern Med Ctr 2004; **Fac Appt:** Assoc Prof Rad, Univ Tex SW, Dallas

West Coast and Pacific

Bahn, Duke K MD [DR] - **Spec Exp:** Prostate Cancer-Cryosurgery; Immunotherapy; **Hospital:** Comm Meml Hosp - Ventura; **Address:** Prostate Inst of America, 168 N Brent St, Ste 402, Ventura, CA 93003; **Phone:** 805-585-3082; **Board Cert:** Diagnostic Radiology 1978; **Med School:** Korea 1970; **Resid:** Diagnostic Radiology, Wayne State Univ Med Ctr 1978; **Fac Appt:** Clin Prof Rad

Bassett, Lawrence W MD [DR] - **Spec Exp:** Breast Imaging; **Hospital:** UCLA Ronald Reagan Med Ctr; **Address:** 200 UCLA Med Plaza, rm 165-47, Los Angeles, CA 90095; **Phone:** 310-206-9608; **Board Cert:** Diagnostic Radiology 1975; **Med School:** UC Irvine 1968; **Resid:** Diagnostic Radiology, UCLA Med Ctr 1972; **Fac Appt:** Prof, UCLA

Coakley, Fergus V MD [DR] - **Spec Exp:** Abdominal Imaging; Anal Cancer; Liver Cancer; Esophageal Cancer; **Hospital:** UCSF Med Ctr; **Address:** UCSF Medical Ctr, 505 Parnassus Ave Fl 3 - rm M372, San Francisco, CA 94143; **Phone:** 415-353-1821; **Board Cert:** Diagnostic Radiology 2001; **Med School:** Ireland 1988; **Resid:** Internal Medicine, Mater & St. Vincents Hosp 1991; Radiology, Leicester Univ Hosp 1996; **Fellow:** Body Imaging, Meml Sloan-Kettering Cancer Ctr 1997; **Fac Appt:** Prof Rad, UCSF

Diagnostic Radiology

Feig, Stephen Albert MD [DR] - **Spec Exp:** Breast Imaging; Breast Cancer; **Hospital:** UC Irvine Med Ctr; **Address:** UCI Medical Ctr, 101 City Drive South Route 140, Orange, CA 92868-3298; **Phone:** 714-456-6905; **Board Cert:** Diagnostic Radiology 1972; **Med School:** NYU Sch Med 1967; **Resid:** Radiology, Bronx Muni Hosp-Einstein 1971; **Fac Appt:** Prof Rad, UC Irvine

Lehman, Constance D MD/PhD [DR] - **Spec Exp:** Breast Imaging; Breast Cancer; MRI-Breast; Mammography; **Hospital:** Univ Wash Med Ctr, Swedish Med Ctr-First Hill-Seattle; **Address:** Seattle Cancer Care Alliance, 825 Eastlake Ave E, MS G2600, Seattle, WA 98109-1023; **Phone:** 206-288-2046; **Board Cert:** Diagnostic Radiology 1995; **Med School:** Yale Univ 1990; **Resid:** Diagnostic Radiology, Univ Washington Med Ctr 1995; **Fellow:** Breast Imaging, Univ Washington Med Ctr 1996; **Fac Appt:** Prof Rad, Univ Wash

Parikh, Jay Rajendra MD [DR] - **Spec Exp:** Breast Imaging; Breast Cancer; Mammography; **Hospital:** Swedish Med Ctr-First Hill-Seattle; **Address:** 1221 Madison St, Ste 520, Seattle, WA 98104; **Phone:** 206-215-3939; **Board Cert:** Diagnostic Radiology 1996; **Med School:** Univ Ottawa 1990; **Resid:** Diagnostic Radiology, Queens Univ Faculty Hlth Scics 1996; **Fac Appt:** Assoc Clin Prof Rad, Univ Wash

NEURORADIOLOGY

New England

Sze, Gordon K MD [NRad] - **Spec Exp:** Brain Tumors; Spinal Cord Tumors; Head & Neck Cancer; MRI; **Hospital:** Yale-New Haven Hosp, Yale Med Group; **Address:** Yale-New Haven Hospital, Yale Diagnostic Radiology, 20 York St, New Haven, CT 06510; **Phone:** 203-785-3667; **Board Cert:** Diagnostic Radiology 1985; Neuroradiology 2008; **Med School:** Harvard Med Sch 1981; **Resid:** Diagnostic Radiology, UCSF Med Ctr 1985; **Fellow:** Neuroradiology, UCSF Med Ctr 1986; **Fac Appt:** Prof Rad, Yale Univ

Mid Atlantic

Faro, Scott H MD [NRad] - **Spec Exp:** Brain Mapping; Brain Tumors; MRI-Functional; **Hospital:** Temple Univ Hosp; **Address:** 3401 N Broad St, Philadelphia, PA 19140; **Phone:** 215-707-5003; **Board Cert:** Diagnostic Radiology 1993; Neuroradiology 2006; **Med School:** UMDNJ-Rutgers Med Sch 1986; **Resid:** Diagnostic Radiology, Med Ctr Delaware 1991; **Fellow:** Neuroradiology, Jefferson Med Ctr 1992; Neuroradiology, Hosp U Penn 1993; **Fac Appt:** Prof Rad, Temple Univ

Loevner, Laurie A MD [NRad] - **Spec Exp:** Head & Neck Cancer; Thyroid Cancer; Brain Tumor Imaging; Spinal Tumor Imaging; **Hospital:** Hosp Univ Penn - UPHS (page 80), Pennsylvania Hosp (page 80); **Address:** 3400 Spruce St Dulles Bldg Fl 2nd, Philadelphia, PA 19104; **Phone:** 215-662-3020; **Board Cert:** Diagnostic Radiology 1993; Neuroradiology 2006; **Med School:** Univ Pennsylvania 1988; **Resid:** Diagnostic Radiology, Univ Michigan Hosps 1993; **Fellow:** Neuroradiology, Hosp Univ Penn 1995; **Fac Appt:** Prof Rad, Univ Pennsylvania

Vezina, L Gilbert MD [NRad] - **Spec Exp:** Brain Tumors; **Hospital:** Chldns Natl Med Ctr; **Address:** Chldns Natl Med Ctr, Dept Radiology, 111 Michigan Ave NW, Washington, DC 20010-2970; **Phone:** 202-476-3651; **Board Cert:** Diagnostic Radiology 1987; Neuroradiology 2008; **Med School:** McGill Univ 1983; **Resid:** Diagnostic Radiology, Mass Genl Hosp 1987; **Fellow:** Neurological Radiology, Mass Genl Hosp 1989; Pediatric Neuroradiology, Chldns Natl Med Ctr 1991; **Fac Appt:** Prof, Geo Wash Univ

Southeast

Johnson, Annette MD [NRad] - **Spec Exp:** Brain Tumors; MRI; **Hospital:** Wake Forest Univ Baptist Med Ctr; **Address:** Medical Center Blvd, Wake Forest Baptist Hlth, Dept Radiology, Winston-Salem, NC 27157; **Phone:** 336-716-2872; **Board Cert:** Diagnostic Radiology 1996; Neuroradiology 2008; **Med School:** Med Coll VA 1992; **Resid:** Diagnostic Radiology, Geisinger Med Ctr 1996; **Fellow:** Diagnostic Radiology, Mallinckrodt Inst Radiology/Washingtno Univ 1998; **Fac Appt:** Assoc Prof Rad, Wake Forest Univ

Maldjian, Joseph MD [NRad] - **Spec Exp:** Brain Tumors; **Hospital:** Wake Forest Univ Baptist Med Ctr; **Address:** Wake Forest Univ Med Ctr, Dept Radiology, Medical Center Blvd MRI Bldg Fl 3, Winston-Salem, NC 27157; **Phone:** 336-716-7849; **Board Cert:** Diagnostic Radiology 1993; Neuroradiology 2005; **Med School:** UMDNJ-NJ Med Sch, Newark 1988; **Resid:** Diagnostic Radiology, Mount Sinai Med Ctr 1993; **Fellow:** Neuroradiology, Hosp U Penn 1995

Murtagh, F Reed MD [NRad] - **Spec Exp:** Neuro-Oncology; Brain Tumor Imaging; Spinal Tumor Imaging; **Hospital:** H Lee Moffitt Cancer Ctr & Research Inst; **Address:** Univ Diagnostic Institute-USF, 3301 Alumni Drive, Tampa, FL 33612; **Phone:** 813-975-0725; **Board Cert:** Diagnostic Radiology 1978; Neuroradiology 2004; **Med School:** Temple Univ 1971; **Resid:** Diagnostic Radiology, Jackson Meml Hosp 1978; **Fellow:** Neurological Radiology, Univ Miami 1979; **Fac Appt:** Prof Rad, Univ S Fla Coll Med

Provenzale, James M MD [NRad] - **Spec Exp:** Brain Tumor Imaging; **Hospital:** Duke Univ Hosp, Durham VA Med Ctr; **Address:** Duke University Medical Ctr, Dept Radiology, Box 3808, Durham, NC 27710; **Phone:** 919-684-7218; **Board Cert:** Neurology 1988; Diagnostic Radiology 1991; Neuroradiology 2001; **Med School:** Albany Med Coll 1983; **Resid:** Neurology, NC Memorial Hosp 1987; Diagnostic Radiology, Mass Genl Hosp 1991; **Fellow:** Neuroradiology, Mass Genl Hosp 1992; **Fac Appt:** Prof Rad, Duke Univ

Midwest

Koeller, Kelly K MD [NRad] - **Spec Exp:** Brain Tumor Imaging; Head & Neck Tumors Imaging; Spinal Tumor Imaging; **Hospital:** Mayo Med Ctr & Clin - Rochester; **Address:** Mayo Clinic, 200 First St SW, Charlton Bldg, rm 2-290, Rochester, MN 55905; **Phone:** 507-266-3412; **Board Cert:** Diagnostic Radiology 1990; Neuroradiology 2004; **Med School:** Univ Tenn Coll Med 1982; **Resid:** Diagnostic Radiology, Naval Hosp 1990; **Fellow:** Neuroradiology, UCSF Med Ctr 1992

Mukherji, Suresh K MD [NRad] - **Spec Exp:** Head & Neck Radiology; Head & Neck Tumors Imaging; **Hospital:** Univ of Michigan Hosp; **Address:** Univ of Michigan-Dept Radiology, 1500 E Medical Ctr Drive, UH-B2A209B, Ann Arbor, MI 48109-0030; **Phone:** 734-936-8865; **Board Cert:** Diagnostic Radiology 1992; Neuroradiology 2006; **Med School:** Georgetown Univ 1987; **Resid:** Diagnostic Radiology, Brigham & Women's Hosp 1992; **Fellow:** Neuroradiology, Univ Florida 1994; **Fac Appt:** Prof Rad, Univ Mich Med Sch

West Coast and Pacific

Cha, Soonmee MD [NRad] - **Spec Exp:** Brain Tumors; **Hospital:** UCSF Med Ctr; **Address:** 350 Parnassus Ave, Ste 307, Neuroradiology Section, San Francisco, CA 94117; **Phone:** 415-353-8913; **Board Cert:** Diagnostic Radiology 1996; Neuroradiology 2008; **Med School:** Georgetown Univ 1991; **Resid:** Diagnostic Radiology, North Shore Univ Hosp 1996; **Fellow:** Neuroradiology, NYU Med Ctr 1998; **Fac Appt:** Assoc Prof Rad, UCSF

Neuroradiology

Dillon, William P MD [NRad] - **Spec Exp:** Brain Tumors; **Hospital:** UCSF Med Ctr; **Address:** 505 Parnassus Ave, rm L 371, San Francisco, CA 94143-0628; **Phone:** 415-353-1668; **Board Cert:** Diagnostic Radiology 1982; Neuroradiology 2006; **Med School:** Loyola Univ-Stritch Sch Med 1978; **Resid:** Diagnostic Radiology, Univ Utah Hosp 1982; **Fellow:** Neuroradiology, UCSF Med Ctr 1983; **Fac Appt:** Prof, UCSF

Hesselink, John R MD [NRad] - **Spec Exp:** MRI & CT of Brain & Spine; Brain Tumor Imaging; **Hospital:** UCSD Med Ctr-Hillcrest; **Address:** UCSD Med Ctr, Div Neuroradiology, 200 W Arbor Drive, MC 8749, San Diego, CA 92013; **Phone:** 619-543-3856; **Board Cert:** Diagnostic Radiology 1975; Neuroradiology 2005; **Med School:** Univ Wisc 1971; **Resid:** Diagnostic Radiology, Univ Wisconsin-Madison 1975; **Fellow:** Neuroradiology, Mass Genl Hosp- Harvard Univ 1979; **Fac Appt:** Prof Rad, UCSD

VASCULAR & INTERVENTIONAL RADIOLOGY

New England

Hallisey, Michael J MD [VIR] - **Spec Exp:** Liver Cancer/Chemoembolization; **Hospital:** Hartford Hosp; **Address:** 399 Farmington Ave, Farmington, CT 06032; **Phone:** 860-676-0110; **Board Cert:** Diagnostic Radiology 1991; Vascular & Interventional Radiology 2008; **Med School:** Univ Conn 1986; **Resid:** Diagnostic Radiology, Hospital of St Raphael 1991

Mid Atlantic

Brown, Karen T MD [VIR] - **Spec Exp:** Liver Cancer; Radiofrequency Tumor Ablation; **Hospital:** Meml Sloan-Kettering Cancer Ctr (page 75); **Address:** 1275 York Avenue, New York, NY 10065; **Phone:** 800-525-2225; **Board Cert:** Diagnostic Radiology 1984; Vascular & Interventional Radiology 2004; **Med School:** Boston Univ 1979; **Resid:** Diagnostic Radiology, Mass Genl Hosp 1984; **Fellow:** Vascular & Interventional Radiology, Mass Genl Hosp 1985; **Fac Appt:** Prof Rad, Cornell Univ-Weill Med Coll

Cohen, Gary S MD [VIR] - **Spec Exp:** Cancer Chemoembolization; Liver Cancer/Chemoembolization; **Hospital:** Temple Univ Hosp, Jeanes Hosp; **Address:** 3401 N Broad St, MS 19140, Parkinson Bldg Fl 1 - Ste C, Philadelphia, PA 19140; **Phone:** 215-707-7002; **Board Cert:** Diagnostic Radiology 1992; Vascular & Interventional Radiology 2006; **Med School:** Mount Sinai Sch Med 1988; **Resid:** Diagnostic Radiology, Temple Univ Hosp 1992; **Fellow:** Vascular & Interventional Radiology, Temple Univ Hosp 1993; **Fac Appt:** Prof Rad, Temple Univ

Geschwind, Jean-Francois H MD [VIR] - **Spec Exp:** Liver Cancer/Chemoembolization; Cancer Chemoembolization; Cancer Radiotherapy; **Hospital:** Johns Hopkins Hosp; **Address:** Interventional Radiology, 600 N Wolfe St Blalock Bldg - rm 545, Baltimore, MD 21287; **Phone:** 410-614-2227; **Board Cert:** Diagnostic Radiology 1998; **Med School:** Boston Univ 1991; **Resid:** Diagnostic Radiology, UCSF Med Ctr 1996; **Fellow:** Interventional Radiology, Johns Hopkins Hosp 1998; **Fac Appt:** Assoc Prof, Johns Hopkins Univ

Haskal, Ziv MD [VIR] - **Spec Exp:** Liver Cancer/Chemoembolization; **Hospital:** Univ of MD Med Ctr; **Address:** 22 S Greene St, rm G2K14, Baltimore, MD 21201; **Phone:** 410-328-7467; **Board Cert:** Diagnostic Radiology 1991; Vascular & Interventional Radiology 2010; **Med School:** Boston Univ 1986; **Resid:** Diagnostic Radiology, UCSF Med Ctr 1991; **Fellow:** Vascular & Interventional Radiology, UCSF Med Ctr 1992; **Fac Appt:** Prof Rad, Univ MD Sch Med

Soulen, Michael C MD [VIR] - **Spec Exp:** Liver Cancer/Chemoembolization; Kidney Cancer; Radiofrequency Tumor Ablation; **Hospital:** Hosp Univ Penn - UPHS (page 80); **Address:** Hosp Univ Penn, Interventional Radiology, 3400 Spruce St Dulles Bldg Fl Ground, Philadelphia, PA 19104; **Phone:** 215-615-4135; **Board Cert:** Diagnostic Radiology 1989; Vascular & Interventional Radiology 2006; **Med School:** Univ Pennsylvania 1984; **Resid:** Diagnostic Radiology, Johns Hopkins Med Inst 1989; **Fellow:** Vascular & Interventional Radiology, Thomas Jefferson Univ Hosp 1991; **Fac Appt:** Prof Rad, Univ Pennsylvania

Weintraub, Joshua L MD [VIR] - **Spec Exp:** Gastrointestinal Cancer; Chemoembolization & Tumor Ablation; **Hospital:** Mount Sinai Med Ctr (page 76); **Address:** Mount Sinai Medical Ctr, Dept Radiology, One Gustave L Levy Pl, Box 1234, New York, NY 10029; **Phone:** 212-241-7409; **Board Cert:** Diagnostic Radiology 1996; Vascular & Interventional Radiology 1998; **Med School:** Wayne State Univ 1991; **Resid:** Diagnostic Radiology, Beth Israel Hosp 1996; **Fellow:** Vascular & Interventional Radiology, Hosp Univ Penn 1997; **Fac Appt:** Assoc Prof Rad, Mount Sinai Sch Med

Wood, Bradford J MD [VIR] - **Spec Exp:** Radiofrequency Tumor Ablation; Liver Cancer; Kidney Cancer; Gene Therapy Delivery Systems; **Hospital:** Natl Inst of Hlth - Clin Ctr; **Address:** National Inst Health, 9000 Rockville Pike, msc 1182, Bldg 10, rm 1C364, Bethesda, MD 20892; **Phone:** 301-594-4511; **Board Cert:** Diagnostic Radiology 1996; Vascular & Interventional Radiology 2000; **Med School:** Univ VA Sch Med 1991; **Resid:** Diagnostic Radiology, Georgetown Univ Med Ctr 1996; **Fellow:** Abdominal/Interventional Radiology, Mass General Hosp 1997

Southeast

Mauro, Matthew A MD [VIR] - **Spec Exp:** Cancer Chemoembolization; Cancer Radiotherapy; Gastrointestinal Cancer; **Hospital:** NC Memorial Hosp - UNC; **Address:** University NC Hosps, Dept Radiology, CB 7510, 2006 Old Clinic Bldg, Chapel Hill, NC 27514-7590; **Phone:** 919-966-4238; **Board Cert:** Diagnostic Radiology 1981; Vascular & Interventional Radiology 2003; **Med School:** Cornell Univ-Weill Med Coll 1977; **Resid:** Diagnostic Radiology, Univ NC Hosps 1980; **Fellow:** Interventional Radiology, Univ NC Hosp 1981; Abdominal/Interventional Radiology, Mallinckrodt Inst 1982; **Fac Appt:** Prof Rad, Univ NC Sch Med

Midwest

Rilling, William S MD [VIR] - **Spec Exp:** Liver Cancer/Chemoembolization; **Hospital:** Froedtert and Med Ctr of WI; **Address:** Froedtert Hosp, Dept Radiology, 9200 W Wisconsin Ave, Milwaukee, WI 53226; **Phone:** 414-805-3028; **Board Cert:** Diagnostic Radiology 1995; Vascular & Interventional Radiology 2007; **Med School:** Univ Wisc 1990; **Resid:** Diagnostic Radiology, Univ Wisc Affil Hosps 1995; **Fellow:** Vascular & Interventional Radiology, Northwestern Meml Hosp 1996; **Fac Appt:** Assoc Prof Rad, Univ Wisc

Salem, Riad MD [VIR] - **Spec Exp:** Cancer Radiotherapy; Cancer Chemoembolization; Liver Cancer/Chemoembolization; **Hospital:** Northwestern Meml Hosp; **Address:** Northwestern Univ Dept Radiology, 676 N St Clair St, Ste 800, Chicago, IL 60611; **Phone:** 312-695-5753; **Board Cert:** Diagnostic Radiology 1997; Vascular & Interventional Radiology 2010; **Med School:** McGill Univ 1993; **Resid:** Diagnostic Radiology, Geo Washington Univ Hosp 1997; **Fellow:** Interventional Radiology, Chldns Hosp 1998; Interventional Radiology, Hosp Univ Penn 1998; **Fac Appt:** Assoc Prof Rad, Northwestern Univ

Vascular & Interventional Radiology

West Coast and Pacific

Goodwin, Scott C MD [VIR] - **Spec Exp:** Liver Cancer/Chemoembolization; **Hospital:** UC Irvine Med Ctr; **Address:** 333 City Blvd W, Ste 1405, MC 5005, Orange, CA 92868; **Phone:** 714-456-7517; **Board Cert:** Diagnostic Radiology 1989; Vascular & Interventional Radiology 2007; **Med School:** Harvard Med Sch 1984; **Resid:** Diagnostic Radiology, UCLA Medical Ctr 1988; **Fellow:** Vascular & Interventional Radiology, UCLA Medical Ctr 1989; **Fac Appt:** Prof Rad, UCLA

McGahan, John P MD [VIR] - **Spec Exp:** Radiofrequency Tumor Ablation; Liver Cancer; Kidney Cancer; **Hospital:** UC Davis Med Ctr; **Address:** UC Davis Medical Ctr, Dept Radiology, 4860 Y St ACC3100, Sacramento, CA 95817; **Phone:** 916-734-3606; **Board Cert:** Diagnostic Radiology 1979; **Med School:** Oregon Hlth & Sci Univ 1974; **Resid:** Surgery, UC Davis Med Ctr 1976; Diagnostic Radiology, UC Davis Med Ctr 1979; **Fac Appt:** Prof Rad, UC Davis

NUCLEAR MEDICINE

Mid Atlantic

Agress Jr, Harry MD [NuM] - **Spec Exp:** PET Imaging; Cancer Detection & Staging; Nuclear Oncology; **Hospital:** Hackensack Univ Med Ctr (page 73); **Address:** Hackensack Univ Med Ctr, 30 Prospect Ave, Hackensack, NJ 07601; **Phone:** 201-996-2196; **Board Cert:** Nuclear Medicine 1976; Diagnostic Radiology 1978; **Med School:** Tufts Univ 1972; **Resid:** Radiology, Columbia-Presby Med Ctr 1978; **Fellow:** Nuclear Medicine, Natl Inst Hlth 1975; **Fac Appt:** Clin Prof Rad, Columbia P&S

Alavi, Abass MD [NuM] - **Spec Exp:** Brain Tumors; Neurologic Imaging; PET Imaging-Brain; **Hospital:** Hosp Univ Penn - UPHS (page 80), Chldns Hosp of Philadelphia; **Address:** Hosp Univ Penn, Div Nuclear Med, 3400 Spruce St, Donner Bldg rm 110, Philadelphia, PA 19104; **Phone:** 215-662-3069; **Board Cert:** Internal Medicine 1972; Nuclear Medicine 1973; **Med School:** Iran 1964; **Resid:** Internal Medicine, Albert Einstein Med Ctr/Phila VA Hosp 1969; Hematology, Hosp Univ Penn 1970; **Fellow:** Nuclear Medicine, Hosp Univ Penn 1973; **Fac Appt:** Prof Rad, Univ Pennsylvania

Carrasquillo, Jorge A MD [NuM] - **Spec Exp:** Radioimmunotherapy of Cancer; PET Imaging; **Hospital:** Meml Sloan-Kettering Cancer Ctr (page 75); **Address:** 1275 York Avenue, Nuclear Medicine Svc, Box 77, New York, NY 10065; **Phone:** 212-639-2459; **Board Cert:** Internal Medicine 1977; Nuclear Medicine 1982; **Med School:** Univ Puerto Rico 1974; **Resid:** Internal Medicine, Univ Dist Hosp 1977; Nuclear Medicine, Univ Wash Hosp 1982

Goldsmith, Stanley J MD [NuM] - **Spec Exp:** Thyroid Cancer; PET Imaging; Neuroendocrine Tumors; **Hospital:** NY-Presby Hosp/Weill Cornell (page 78); **Address:** 525 E 68th St Starr Bldg - rm 2-21, New York, NY 10021-9800; **Phone:** 212-746-4588; **Board Cert:** Internal Medicine 1969; Nuclear Medicine 1972; Endocrinology 1972; **Med School:** SUNY Downstate 1962; **Resid:** Internal Medicine, Kings Co Hosp 1967; **Fellow:** Endocrinology, Diabetes & Metabolism, Mt Sinai Hosp 1968; Nuclear Medicine, Bronx VA Hosp 1969; **Fac Appt:** Prof Rad, Cornell Univ-Weill Med Coll

Lamonica, Dominick M MD [NuM] - **Spec Exp:** Thyroid Cancer; Lymphoma, Non-Hodgkin's; **Hospital:** Roswell Park Cancer Inst; **Address:** Roswell Park Cancer Inst, Elm & Carlton St, Dept of Nuclear Medicine, Buffalo, NY 14263; **Phone:** 716-845-3282; **Board Cert:** Internal Medicine 2005; Nuclear Medicine 2006; **Med School:** Mount Sinai Sch Med 1987; **Resid:** Internal Medicine, Univ Hosp-SUNY Stony Brook 1991; Diagnostic Radiology, Nassau City Med Ctr 1992; **Fellow:** Nuclear Medicine, DVAMC North Port-SUNY Stony Brook 1994; Nuclear Medicine, SUNY Buffalo-RPCI 1995; **Fac Appt:** Asst Prof, SUNY Buffalo

Larson, Steven M MD [NuM] - **Spec Exp:** Thyroid Cancer; PET Imaging; **Hospital:** Meml Sloan-Kettering Cancer Ctr (page 75); **Address:** 1275 York Ave, New York, NY 10065; **Phone:** 800-525-2225; **Board Cert:** Nuclear Medicine 1972; Internal Medicine 1973; **Med School:** Univ Wash 1965; **Resid:** Internal Medicine, Virginia Mason Hosp 1970; Nuclear Medicine, Natl Inst Hlth 1972; **Fac Appt:** Prof NuM, Cornell Univ-Weill Med Coll

Strauss, H William MD [NuM] - **Spec Exp:** Cardiac Imaging in Cancer Therapy; Thyroid Cancer; **Hospital:** Meml Sloan-Kettering Cancer Ctr (page 75); **Address:** 1275 York Avenue, New York, NY 10065; **Phone:** 212-639-7238; **Board Cert:** Nuclear Medicine 1988; **Med School:** SUNY Downstate 1965; **Resid:** Internal Medicine, Downstate Med Ctr 1967; Internal Medicine, Bellevue Hosp 1968; **Fellow:** Nuclear Medicine, Johns Hopkins Hosp 1970; **Fac Appt:** Prof NuM, Cornell Univ-Weill Med Coll

Wahl, Richard L MD [NuM] - **Spec Exp:** Radioimmunotherapy of Cancer; PET Imaging; PET Imaging-Breast; **Hospital:** Johns Hopkins Hosp; **Address:** Johns Hopkins Hosp, Radiology Dept, Nuclear Medicine Fl 3, 601 N Caroline St, JHOC-3223, Baltimore, MD 21287; **Phone:** 410-955-5465; **Board Cert:** Diagnostic Radiology 1982; Nuclear Medicine 1983; **Med School:** Washington Univ, St Louis 1978; **Resid:** Diagnostic Radiology, Mallinckrodt Inst 1982; **Fellow:** Nuclear Radiology, Mallinckrodt Inst 1983; **Fac Appt:** Prof Rad, Johns Hopkins Univ

Southeast

Alazraki, Naomi P MD [NuM] - **Spec Exp:** Nuclear Oncology; **Hospital:** Atlanta VA Med Ctr, Emory Univ Hosp; **Address:** VA Medical Ctr - Atlanta, 1670 Clairmont Rd, MC 115, Decatur, GA 30033; **Phone:** 404-321-6111; **Board Cert:** Nuclear Medicine 1972; Diagnostic Radiology 1972; **Med School:** Albert Einstein Coll Med 1966; **Resid:** Diagnostic Radiology, Univ Hospital 1971; **Fac Appt:** Prof Rad, Emory Univ

Coleman, R Edward MD [NuM] - **Spec Exp:** PET Imaging; Tumor Imaging; **Hospital:** Duke Univ Hosp; **Address:** Duke Univ Med Ctr, Erwin Rd, Box 3949, Durham, NC 27710-0001; **Phone:** 919-684-7244; **Board Cert:** Internal Medicine 1973; Nuclear Medicine 1974; **Med School:** Washington Univ, St Louis 1968; **Resid:** Internal Medicine, Royal Victoria Hosp 1970; **Fellow:** Nuclear Medicine, Mallinckrodt Inst Radiology 1974; **Fac Appt:** Prof Rad, Duke Univ

Midwest

Dillehay, Gary L MD [NuM] - **Spec Exp:** Lymphoma; PET Imaging; Thyroid Cancer; **Hospital:** Northwestern Meml Hosp; **Address:** Northwestern Meml Hosp, Dept Nuclear Medicine, 675 N St Clair St, Galter 8-110, Chicago, IL 60611; **Phone:** 312-926-5119; **Board Cert:** Nuclear Medicine 1985; Nuclear Radiology 1987; **Med School:** Mayo Med Sch 1979; **Resid:** Diagnostic Radiology, Northwestern Meml Hosp 1983; Nuclear Medicine, Northwestern Meml Hosp 1984; **Fac Appt:** Prof Rad, Northwestern Univ-Feinberg Sch Med

Neumann, Donald R MD [NuM] - **Spec Exp:** Nuclear Oncology; Parathyroid Disease; **Hospital:** Cleveland Clin (page 70); **Address:** 9500 Euclid Ave, MS Jb3, Cleveland, OH 44195; **Phone:** 216-444-2193; **Board Cert:** Diagnostic Radiology 1987; Nuclear Radiology 1990; **Med School:** Wright State Univ 1980; **Resid:** Diagnostic Radiology, Mount Sinai Med Ctr 1987; **Fellow:** Magnetic Resonance Imaging, Mount Sinai Med Ctr 1988

Nuclear Medicine

Siegel, Barry A MD [NuM] - **Spec Exp:** Cancer Detection & Staging; PET Imaging; **Hospital:** Barnes-Jewish Hosp, St. Louis Chldns Hosp; **Address:** 510 S Kingshighway Blvd, St Louis, MO 63110-1016; **Phone:** 314-362-2809; **Board Cert:** Nuclear Medicine 1973; Diagnostic Radiology 1977; Nuclear Radiology 1981; **Med School:** Washington Univ, St Louis 1969; **Resid:** Diagnostic Radiology, Mallinckrodt Inst Radiology 1973; **Fellow:** Nuclear Medicine, Mallinckrodt Inst Radiology 1973; **Fac Appt:** Prof Rad, Washington Univ, St Louis

Wiseman, Gregory MD [NuM] - **Spec Exp:** Lymphoma, Non-Hodgkin's; Multiple Myeloma; Radioimmunotherapy of Cancer; **Hospital:** Mayo Med Ctr & Clin - Rochester; **Address:** Mayo Clinic, Dept Nuc Med, 200 First St SW, Charlton Bldg, Rochester, MN 55905; **Phone:** 507-284-9599; **Board Cert:** Internal Medicine 1986; Hematology 1988; Nuclear Medicine 2002; **Med School:** Univ Utah 1983; **Resid:** Internal Medicine, Mayo Clinic 1986; Nuclear Medicine, Univ Washington Med Ctr 1992; **Fellow:** Hematology, Mayo Clinic 1989; Medical Oncology, Univ Washington 1991; **Fac Appt:** Asst Prof, Mayo Med Sch

Southwest

Podoloff, Donald A MD [NuM] - **Spec Exp:** Prostate Cancer; Breast Cancer; **Hospital:** UT MD Anderson Cancer Ctr; **Address:** UT MD Anderson Cancer Ctr, 1515 Holcombe Blvd, Box 57, Houston, TX 77030; **Phone:** 713-745-1160; **Board Cert:** Diagnostic Radiology 1973; Nuclear Medicine 1975; Nuclear Radiology 1975; **Med School:** SUNY Downstate 1964; **Resid:** Internal Medicine, Beth Israel Med Ctr 1968; Diagnostic Radiology, Wilford Hall USAF Med Ctr 1973; **Fac Appt:** Prof Rad, Univ Tex, Houston

West Coast and Pacific

Scheff, Alice M MD [NuM] - **Spec Exp:** PET Imaging; Thyroid Disorders; **Hospital:** Santa Clara Vly Med Ctr; **Address:** 751 S Bascom Ave, Nuclear Med, San Jose, CA 95128; **Phone:** 408-885-6970; **Board Cert:** Nuclear Medicine 1982; Nuclear Radiology 1983; **Med School:** Penn State Coll Med 1978; **Resid:** Diagnostic Radiology, Penn State-Hershey Med Ctr 1982; Nuclear Medicine, Penn State-Hershey Med Ctr 1982; **Fellow:** Magnetic Resonance Imaging, Long Beach Meml Med Ctr 1993

Waxman, Alan D MD [NuM] - **Spec Exp:** PET Imaging-Brain; Thyroid Cancer; Cancer Detection & Staging; **Hospital:** Cedars-Sinai Med Ctr, USC Univ Hosp; **Address:** Cedars-Sinai Med Ctr, Taper Imaging, 8700 Beverly Blvd, rm 1258, Los Angeles, CA 90048-1804; **Phone:** 310-423-4216; **Board Cert:** Nuclear Medicine 1972; **Med School:** USC Sch Med 1963; **Resid:** Nuclear Medicine, Wadsworth VA Hosp 1965; **Fellow:** Internal Medicine, Natl Inst Hlth 1967; **Fac Appt:** Clin Prof, USC Sch Med

City of Hope™

canswer.

Radiation Oncology Experts

Technological advances are making a difference for cancer patients. TomoTherapy provides City of Hope oncologists with the unprecedented ability to incorporate 3-D imaging and radiation treatment in one machine, to target tumors with the utmost precision. This means more effective tumor eradication and less radiation to healthy organs, resulting in significantly reduced side effects.

To learn more, call 800-826-HOPE
www.cityofhope.org/radonc
1500 East Duarte Road, Duarte, California 91010

City of Hope is recognized as one of only 40 National Cancer Institute-designated Comprehensive Cancer Centers and is ranked by *U.S.News & World Report* as one of "America's Best Hospitals" in cancer and urology.

City of Hope's *Helford Clinical Research Hospital* integrates lifesaving research and superior clinical care. Multidisciplinary teams of medical professionals work together to deliver promising new therapies to patients quickly, safely and effectively. They care for the whole patient, including their emotional, psychological, spiritual and nutritional needs.

A recognized leader in compassionate patient care, innovative science and translational research, City of Hope collaborates with other top institutions around the globe, rapidly developing laboratory breakthroughs into revolutionary new treatments.

City of Hope welcomes patient referrals from physicians throughout the world. Please contact specialists directly or call **800-826-HOPE**.

City of Hope has answers to cancer.

FOX CHASE
CANCER CENTER

333 Cottman Avenue
Philadelphia, PA 19111-2497
Phone: 1-888-FOX CHASE • Fax: 215-728-2702
www.foxchase.org

RADIATION ONCOLOGY

Fox Chase Cancer Center has one of the country's largest, most experienced programs in radiation oncology. Recognized as international leaders in developing the most advanced treatment technologies, our radiation oncologists are experts in treating patients with prostate, breast, lung and gastrointestinal cancers. Other major treatment interests include central nervous system cancers, head and neck cancers, and sarcomas.

We treat patients with radiation therapy alone, in combination with surgery and/or chemotherapy and through Fox Chase and national clinical trials offering the newest treatments. We also conduct research in medical physics and radiation biology to enhance the effectiveness of therapy.

Radiation treatment highlights:

- Fox Chase physicians are among the nation's most experienced in treating patients with intensity-modulated radiation therapy (IMRT) and are developing the image-guided radiation therapies of the future.
- Advances in brachytherapy, such as real-time intraoperative planning, mean our patients receive the most precise prostate implants, either permanent low-dose-rate or temporary high-dose-rate.
- Stereotactic radiosurgery and stereotactic radiotherapy permit sub-millimeter precision for brain, lung, and head and neck cancers.

Fox Chase uses sophisticated imaging tools during treatment planning and daily treatment sessions to target cancer precisely and spare any healthy surrounding tissue undue exposure to radiation. We were the first in the Philadelphia region to offer many advanced planning tools—such as the Calypso 4-D Localization System, High Intensity Focused Ultrasound (HIFU), and the Trilogy Stereotactic System—to provide the most targeted treatment.

Because of our outstanding reputation as a leader in cancer therapy, we frequently work with the world's foremost makers of medical equipment to test prototypes and develop the best applications—long before they are available elsewhere.

World-Class Radiation Therapy

In addition to providing world-class radiation therapy at Fox Chase Cancer Center, we serve patients at Fox Chase Cancer Center Buckingham—our radiation oncology facility in Bucks County, Pa. An experienced Fox Chase team of clinicians offers patients here the latest radiation treatments.

The facility features advanced technologies that decrease treatment time, improve precision and reduce possible side effects.

CyberKnife Robotic Radiosurgery System
- Painless, non-surgical option for inoperable or complex tumors
- Image-guided approach offers sub-millimeter accuracy

Trilogy Linear Accelerator with Rapid Arc
- Power and precision for more comfortable treatments and shorter treatment times

LightSpeed RT 16 slice 4D CT Simulator
- One of the most important tools for radiation treatment planning allowing assessment of tumor motion

For more about Fox Chase physicians and services, visit our website, www.foxchase.org, or call 1-888-FOX CHASE.

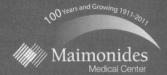

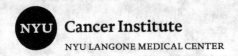

Cancer Institute

NYU LANGONE MEDICAL CENTER

NYU Langone Medical Center
550 First Avenue , New York, NY 10016
www.NYULMC.org

NYU Clinical Cancer Center
160 East 34th Street, New York, NY 10016
www.NYUCI.org

**The Stephen D. Hassenfeld Children's Center
for Cancer and Blood Disorders**
160 East 32nd Street, New York, NY 10016
www.NYUMC.org/Hassenfeld

The NYU Cancer Institute is an NCI-designated cancer center and provides personalized patient care that is both compassionate and state of the art. The doctors and researchers work together to develop innovative therapies for patients. The Cancer Institute is world-renowned for excellence in cancer-focused research, personalized care, education and community outreach. Its mission is to discover the origins of human cancer and to use that knowledge to eradicate the personal and societal burden of cancer in our community, the nation and the world. For more information about our expert physicians, call 212-731-5000. *We specialize in the following areas:*

Patient-Focused Setting
The NYU Clinical Cancer Center is the principal outpatient facility of The Cancer Institute and serves as home to our patients and their caregivers. The center and its multidisciplinary team of experts provide access to the latest treatment options and clinical trials along with a variety of programs in cancer risk reduction/prevention, screening, diagnostics, genetic counseling and supportive services. In addition the NYUCI emphasizes the importance of a holistic approach to management services in complementary medicine, psychosocial support, survivorship and palliative care.

Renowned Expertise
The NYU Cancer Institute brings together experts from a variety of disciplines to create collaborative research endeavors and clinical care teams. The Cancer Institute offers a full continuum of personalized care, from prevention through diagnosis, treatment and post-treatment support. The compassion and expertise of our team members helps patients better manage the symptoms of their diseases as well as meet their special needs. Additionally, we have created special emphasis programs in diseases such as breast cancer, melanoma, GI cancer, prostate cancer, hematologic malignancies and lung cancer among others, as well as, translational programs in cancer healthcare disparities, molecularly targeted therapy, and the cell signaling pathways involved in cancer.

A Translational Approach
NYU Langone Medical Center scientists and other researchers excel in uncovering how cancer develops at the molecular level, and how we can harness that knowledge to reduce the risk of cancer and treat the disease. The Medical Center constantly seeks to create new opportunities for collaboration between investigators within our own institution, those located elsewhere in the NYU network of campuses, and researchers at other institutions.

The Stephen D. Hassenfeld Children's Center for Cancer and Blood Disorders
The center is a leading pediatric outpatient facility for the treatment of childhood cancers and blood diseases. Its unique interdisciplinary and family-centered approach combines the most advanced medical treatments with psychosocial and emotional support services for young patients and their families.

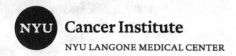

Cancer Institute
NYU LANGONE MEDICAL CENTER

NYU Langone Medical Center
550 First Avenue , New York, NY 10016
www.NYULMC.org

NYU Clinical Cancer Center
160 East 34th Street, New York, NY 10016
www.NYUCI.org

**The Stephen D. Hassenfeld Children's Center
for Cancer and Blood Disorders**
160 East 32nd Street, New York, NY 10016
www.NYUMC.org/Hassenfeld

The NYU Cancer Institute is an NCI-designated cancer center and provides personalized patient care that is both compassionate and state of the art. The doctors and researchers work together to develop innovative therapies for patients. The Cancer Institute is world-renowned for excellence in cancer-focused research, personalized care, education and community outreach. Its mission is to discover the origins of human cancer and to use that knowledge to eradicate the personal and societal burden of cancer in our community, the nation and the world. For more information about our expert physicians, call 212-731-5000. *We specialize in the following areas:*

Patient-Focused Setting
The NYU Clinical Cancer Center is the principal outpatient facility of The Cancer Institute and serves as home to our patients and their caregivers. The center and its multidisciplinary team of experts provide access to the latest treatment options and clinical trials along with a variety of programs in cancer risk reduction/prevention, screening, diagnostics, genetic counseling and supportive services. In addition the NYUCI emphasizes the importance of a holistic approach to management services in complementary medicine, psychosocial support, survivorship and palliative care.

Renowned Expertise
The NYU Cancer Institute brings together experts from a variety of disciplines to create collaborative research endeavors and clinical care teams. The Cancer Institute offers a full continuum of personalized care, from prevention through diagnosis, treatment and post-treatment support. The compassion and expertise of our team members helps patients better manage the symptoms of their diseases as well as meet their special needs. Additionally, we have created special emphasis programs in diseases such as breast cancer, melanoma, GI cancer, prostate cancer, hematologic malignancies and lung cancer among others, as well as, translational programs in cancer healthcare disparities, molecularly targeted therapy, and the cell signaling pathways involved in cancer.

A Translational Approach
NYU Langone Medical Center scientists and other researchers excel in uncovering how cancer develops at the molecular level, and how we can harness that knowledge to reduce the risk of cancer and treat the disease. The Medical Center constantly seeks to create new opportunities for collaboration between investigators within our own institution, those located elsewhere in the NYU network of campuses, and researchers at other institutions.

The Stephen D. Hassenfeld Children's Center for Cancer and Blood Disorders
The center is a leading pediatric outpatient facility for the treatment of childhood cancers and blood diseases. Its unique interdisciplinary and family-centered approach combines the most advanced medical treatments with psychosocial and emotional support services for young patients and their families.

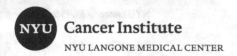

NYU Cancer Institute
NYU LANGONE MEDICAL CENTER

NYU Langone Medical Center
550 First Avenue , New York, NY 10016
www.NYULMC.org

NYU Clinical Cancer Center
160 East 34th Street, New York, NY 10016
www.NYUCI.org

**The Stephen D. Hassenfeld Children's Center
for Cancer and Blood Disorders**
160 East 32nd Street, New York, NY 10016
www.NYUMC.org/Hassenfeld

The NYU Cancer Institute is an NCI-designated cancer center and provides personalized patient care that is both compassionate and state of the art. The doctors and researchers work together to develop innovative therapies for patients. The Cancer Institute is world-renowned for excellence in cancer-focused research, personalized care, education and community outreach. Its mission is to discover the origins of human cancer and to use that knowledge to eradicate the personal and societal burden of cancer in our community, the nation and the world. For more information about our expert physicians, call 212-731-5000. *We specialize in the following areas:*

Patient-Focused Setting
The NYU Clinical Cancer Center is the principal outpatient facility of The Cancer Institute and serves as home to our patients and their caregivers. The center and its multidisciplinary team of experts provide access to the latest treatment options and clinical trials along with a variety of programs in cancer risk reduction/prevention, screening, diagnostics, genetic counseling and supportive services. In addition the NYUCI emphasizes the importance of a holistic approach to management services in complementary medicine, psychosocial support, survivorship and palliative care.

Renowned Expertise
The NYU Cancer Institute brings together experts from a variety of disciplines to create collaborative research endeavors and clinical care teams. The Cancer Institute offers a full continuum of personalized care, from prevention through diagnosis, treatment and post-treatment support. The compassion and expertise of our team members helps patients better manage the symptoms of their diseases as well as meet their special needs. Additionally, we have created special emphasis programs in diseases such as breast cancer, melanoma, GI cancer, prostate cancer, hematologic malignancies and lung cancer among others, as well as, translational programs in cancer healthcare disparities, molecularly targeted therapy, and the cell signaling pathways involved in cancer.

A Translational Approach
NYU Langone Medical Center scientists and other researchers excel in uncovering how cancer develops at the molecular level, and how we can harness that knowledge to reduce the risk of cancer and treat the disease. The Medical Center constantly seeks to create new opportunities for collaboration between investigators within our own institution, those located elsewhere in the NYU network of campuses, and researchers at other institutions.

The Stephen D. Hassenfeld Children's Center for Cancer and Blood Disorders
The center is a leading pediatric outpatient facility for the treatment of childhood cancers and blood diseases. Its unique interdisciplinary and family-centered approach combines the most advanced medical treatments with psychosocial and emotional support services for young patients and their families.

PENN RADIATION ONCOLOGY

Advancing Cancer Care

At Penn Medicine, the Department of Radiation Oncology is a national leader in clinical care, research, and education and is one of the largest and most respected clinical services in the Philadelphia region.

Excellence and Expertise

At Penn, patient care is backed by a nationally recognized research and teaching program. The department conducts basic research to better understand tumor response to radiation and to increase that response, enabling the development of new treatment approaches.

The department offers a wide range of services, including many that combine radiation therapy with chemotherapy and/or surgery. Penn provides complete evaluation, treatment and follow-up care for patients whose cancer can be effectively treated with radiation and also sees patients with benign (noncancerous) diseases that can be treated with radiation. Understanding the emotional implications of cancer, support services are available for patients and their loved ones.

Imaging procedures for treatment planning include X-ray filming and fluoroscopy, and CT linkage with computerized dosimetry. Treatment options include Intensity-Modulated Radiation Therapy (IMRT), Image-Guided Radiation Therapy (IGRT), Conformal Radiation Therapy, CyberKnife® and Gamma Knife®. Symptom management and access to innovative treatments, such as photodynamic therapy, further differentiates Penn Radiation Oncology from other radiation oncology centers.

Leaders in Research

Penn radiation oncologists are experts in cancer treatment and research, and have contributed many important advances in the field.

Penn Radiation Oncology also conducts a wide range of clinical trials involving the innovative use of radiation therapy in combination with other therapies in order to find better ways to treat patients with different types of cancer. In addition, Penn Radiation Oncology's advanced treatment options offer the possibility of retreatment when other radiation therapy treatments have failed.

Penn Radiation Oncology Network

The Penn Radiation Oncology Network offers convenient locations throughout Southeastern Pennsylvania and New Jersey. At each facility, full-time, board-certified Penn radiation oncologists provide outstanding clinical and patient-focused care. Patients can be evaluated for proton therapy, CyberKnife and Gamma Knife at all network sites.

The Roberts Proton Therapy Center

The Roberts Proton Therapy Center is the world's largest proton therapy center and the first to be associated with an academic medical center. It offers the unique ability to fully integrate conventional radiation treatment with proton radiation for certain types of cancer. In addition, the Center is connected to the Ruth and Raymond Perelman Center for Advanced Medicine, home of Penn's Abramson Cancer Center.

Because of its proximity to the Abramson Cancer Center, all cancer diagnostic and treatment services are available in one location.
This allows patients to easily navigate from one department to the next, ensuring exceptional and timely care.

The Stereotactic Center at Pennsylvania Hospital

The Stereotactic Center offers both CyberKnife and Gamma Knife. These non-invasive radiosurgery therapy treatment options provide extremely accurate high dose radiation for many types of tumors. CyberKnife treats tumors throughout the body including spine, lung, liver, pancreas and prostate. Gamma Knife provides powerful treatment for brain and head and neck tumors.

For more information or to schedule an appointment with Penn's Department of Radiation Oncology, call 800.789.PENN or visit PennMedicine.org.

Hospital of the University of Pennsylvania | Penn Presbyterian Medical Center | Pennsylvania Hospital

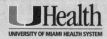
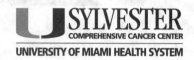

Surgery

A surgeon manages a broad spectrum of surgical conditions affecting almost any area of the body. The surgeon establishes the diagnosis and provides the preoperative, operative and postoperative care to surgical patients and is usually responsible for the comprehensive management of the trauma victim and the critically ill surgical patient.

The surgeon uses a variety of diagnostic techniques, including endoscopy, for observing internal structures and may use specialized instruments during operative procedures. A general surgeon is expected to be familiar with the salient features of other surgical specialties in order to recognize problems in those areas and to know when to refer a patient to another specialist.

Training Required: Five years

SURGERY

New England

Ashley, Stanley W MD [S] - **Spec Exp:** Gastrointestinal Cancer & Surgery; **Hospital:** Brigham & Women's Hosp, Dana-Farber Cancer Inst; **Address:** Brigham & Womens Hosp, Dept Surgery, 75 Francis St, Boston, MA 02115; **Phone:** 617-732-6730; **Board Cert:** Surgery 2004; Surgical Critical Care 1999; **Med School:** Cornell Univ-Weill Med Coll 1981; **Resid:** Surgery, Barnes Jewish Med Ctr 1989; **Fac Appt:** Prof S, Harvard Med Sch

Ballantyne, Garth H MD [S] - **Spec Exp:** Laparoscopic Surgery; Colon Cancer; **Hospital:** Lawrence & Meml Hosp; **Address:** 4 Shaw's Cove, Ste 201, New London, CT 06320; **Phone:** 860-444-7675; **Board Cert:** Surgery 2006; Colon & Rectal Surgery 1985; **Med School:** Columbia P&S 1977; **Resid:** Surgery, UCLA Med Ctr 1980; Surgery, Northwestern Meml Hosp 1982; **Fellow:** Colon & Rectal Surgery, Mayo Clinic 1984

Becker, James M MD [S] - **Spec Exp:** Gastrointestinal Cancer; Gastrointestinal Surgery; **Hospital:** Boston Med Ctr; **Address:** 88 E Newton St, rm C500, Boston, MA 02118-2393; **Phone:** 617-638-8600; **Board Cert:** Surgery 1999; **Med School:** Case West Res Univ 1975; **Resid:** Surgery, Univ Utah Med Ctr 1980; **Fellow:** Research, Mayo Clinic 1982; **Fac Appt:** Prof S, Boston Univ

Callery, Mark P MD [S] - **Spec Exp:** Pancreatic Cancer; Liver Cancer; Laparoscopic Surgery; **Hospital:** Beth Israel Deaconess Med Ctr - Boston; **Address:** Beth Israel Deaconess Med Ctr, Dept Surgery, 330 Brookline Ave, Ste 928, Boston, MA 02215; **Phone:** 617-667-3798; **Board Cert:** Surgery 2004; **Med School:** Albany Med Coll 1985; **Resid:** Surgery, Albany Med Coll Hosp 1987; Surgery, Barnes Jewish Med Ctr 1992; **Fellow:** Research, Wash Univ Sch Med 1990; **Fac Appt:** Assoc Prof S, Harvard Med Sch

Cioffi, William G MD [S] - **Spec Exp:** Cancer Surgery; **Hospital:** Rhode Island Hosp; **Address:** Rhode Island Hosp, Dept Surg, 2 Dudley St, Ste 470, Providence, RI 02905; **Phone:** 401-553-8348; **Board Cert:** Surgery 2007; Surgical Critical Care 2008; **Med School:** Univ VT Coll Med 1981; **Resid:** Surgery, Med Ctr Hosp 1986; **Fac Appt:** Prof S, Brown Univ

Cusack Jr, James C MD [S] - **Spec Exp:** Gastrointestinal Cancer; Liver & Biliary Cancer; Melanoma; **Hospital:** Mass Genl Hosp; **Address:** Mass Genl Hosp, Div Surgical Oncology, 55 Fruit St Yawkey Bldg Fl 7, Boston, MA 02114-2621; **Phone:** 617-724-4093; **Board Cert:** Surgery 2001; **Med School:** Emory Univ 1986; **Resid:** Surgery, Tufts-New England Med Ctr 1991; **Fellow:** Surgical Oncology, Brigham & Women's Hosp 1992; Surgical Oncology, MD Anderson Cancer Ctr 1992; **Fac Appt:** Assoc Prof S, Harvard Med Sch

Eisenberg, Burton L MD [S] - **Spec Exp:** Breast Cancer; Melanoma; Sarcoma; **Hospital:** Dartmouth - Hitchcock Med Ctr; **Address:** DHMC, Dept General Surgery, One Medical Center Drive, Lebanon, NH 03756; **Phone:** 603-650-9479; **Board Cert:** Surgery 1999; **Med School:** Univ Tenn Coll Med 1974; **Resid:** Surgery, Wilford Hall USAF Med Ctr 1979; **Fellow:** Surgical Oncology, Meml Sloan-Kettering Cancer Ctr 1981; **Fac Appt:** Prof S, Dartmouth Med Sch

Gawande, Atul A MD [S] - **Spec Exp:** Endocrine Surgery; Cancer Surgery; Gastrointestinal Surgery; **Hospital:** Brigham & Women's Hosp, Dana-Farber Cancer Inst; **Address:** Brigham & Womens Hosp, Div Gnl Surgery, ASB2-3rd Fl, 75 Francis St, Boston, MA 02115; **Phone:** 617-732-6830; **Board Cert:** Surgery 2004; **Med School:** Harvard Med Sch 1995; **Resid:** Surgery, Brigham & Womens Hosp 2003; **Fac Appt:** Assoc Prof S, Harvard Med Sch

Goodman, Martin D MD [S] - **Spec Exp:** Gastrointestinal Cancer; Peritoneal Carcinomatosis; **Hospital:** Tufts Med Ctr; **Address:** Tufts Med Ctr, Surgical Oncology, 800 Washington St, Box 9248, Boston, MA 02111; **Phone:** 617-636-9248; **Board Cert:** Surgery 2001; **Med School:** UMDNJ-RW Johnson Med Sch 1994; **Resid:** Surgery, Cooper Hosp 2000; **Fellow:** Surgical Oncology, UPMC 2002

Hodin, Richard A MD [S] - **Spec Exp:** Thyroid Cancer; Parathyroid Cancer; Adrenal Tumors; Endocrine Surgery; **Hospital:** Mass Genl Hosp; **Address:** Mass Genl Hosp, Dept Surgery, Wang Bldg-#460, 15 Parkman Street, Boston, MA 02114; **Phone:** 617-724-2570; **Board Cert:** Surgery 2001; **Med School:** Tulane Univ 1984; **Resid:** Surgery, Beth Israel Med Ctr 1990; **Fellow:** Endocrine Surgery, Brigham & Women's Hosp 1989; **Fac Appt:** Prof S, Harvard Med Sch

Hughes, Kevin S MD [S] - **Spec Exp:** Breast Cancer; Ovarian Cancer; Breast Cancer-High Risk Women; Hereditary Cancer; **Hospital:** Mass Genl Hosp, Newton - Wellesley Hosp; **Address:** Mass Genl Hosp, Dept Surgery, 55 Fruit St, Yawkey Center Fl 7 - Ste B, Boston, MA 02114; **Phone:** 617-724-0048; **Board Cert:** Surgery 2006; **Med School:** Dartmouth Med Sch 1979; **Resid:** Surgery, Mercy Hosp 1984; **Fellow:** Surgical Oncology, National Cancer Inst 1986; **Fac Appt:** Assoc Prof S, Harvard Med Sch

Iglehart, J Dirk MD [S] - **Spec Exp:** Breast Cancer; **Hospital:** Brigham & Women's Hosp, Dana-Farber Cancer Inst; **Address:** Dana-Farber Cancer Inst, 450 Brookline Ave, Smith 1058, Boston, MA 02215; **Phone:** 617-632-5178 x1; **Board Cert:** Surgery 2005; **Med School:** Harvard Med Sch 1975; **Resid:** Surgery, Duke Univ Med Ctr 1981; Thoracic Surgery, Duke Univ Med Ctr 1984; **Fac Appt:** Prof S, Harvard Med Sch

Jenkins, Roger L MD [S] - **Spec Exp:** Transplant-Liver; Liver & Biliary Cancer; Pancreatic Cancer; **Hospital:** Lahey Clin, Children's Hospital - Boston; **Address:** 41 Mall Rd, Fl 4, Ste West, Burlington, MA 01805; **Phone:** 781-744-2500; **Board Cert:** Surgery 2005; **Med School:** Univ VT Coll Med 1977; **Resid:** Surgery, New Eng Deaconess Hosp 1982; **Fellow:** Cardiac Surgery, New Eng Deaconess Hosp 1983; Transplant Surgery, Univ Pittsburgh Hosp 1983; **Fac Appt:** Prof S, Tufts Univ

Kavanah, Maureen MD [S] - **Spec Exp:** Breast Cancer; Gynecologic Cancer; Melanoma; **Hospital:** Boston Med Ctr; **Address:** Boston Medical Ctr, 820 Harrison Ave, rm 5009, Bldg FGH, Boston, MA 02118; **Phone:** 617-638-8473; **Board Cert:** Surgery 2009; **Med School:** Tufts Univ 1975; **Resid:** Surgery, St Elizabeths Hosp 1979; **Fellow:** Surgical Oncology, Boston Univ Med Ctr 1981; **Fac Appt:** Assoc Prof S, Boston Univ

Krag, David N MD [S] - **Spec Exp:** Sentinel Node Surgery; Breast Cancer; Cancer Surgery; Melanoma; **Hospital:** Fletcher Allen Health Care- Med Ctr Campus; **Address:** Univ Vermont Coll Med, Dept Surgery, 89 Beaumont Ave, Given Bldg - E309C, Burlington, VT 05405; **Phone:** 802-656-5830; **Board Cert:** Surgery 2006; **Med School:** Loyola Univ-Stritch Sch Med 1980; **Resid:** Surgery, UC Davis Med Ctr 1983; **Fellow:** Surgical Oncology, UCLA Med Ctr 1984; **Fac Appt:** Assoc Prof S, Univ VT Coll Med

Lannin, Donald R MD [S] - **Spec Exp:** Breast Cancer; Breast Surgery; **Hospital:** Yale-New Haven Hosp, Yale Med Group; **Address:** Yale-New Haven Breast Ctr, 20 York St, New Haven, CT 06510; **Phone:** 203-785-2328; **Board Cert:** Surgery 2002; **Med School:** Univ Minn 1974; **Resid:** Surgery, Univ Minnesota Med Ctr 1982; **Fac Appt:** Prof S, Yale Univ

Lillemoe, Keith D MD [S] - **Spec Exp:** Pancreatic Cancer; Colon Cancer; Pancreatic & Biliary Surgery; Gastrointestinal Cancer; **Hospital:** Mass Genl Hosp; **Address:** Mass General Hosp, Dept Surgery, 55 Fruit St, White 506, Boston, MA 02114; **Phone:** 617-643-1010; **Board Cert:** Surgery 2007; **Med School:** Johns Hopkins Univ 1978; **Resid:** Surgery, Johns Hopkins Hosp 1985; **Fac Appt:** Prof S, Harvard Med Sch

McAneny, David B MD [S] - **Spec Exp:** Gastrointestinal Cancer & Surgery; Endocrine Tumors; Pancreatic Cancer; Biliary Surgery; **Hospital:** Boston Med Ctr; **Address:** Boston Med Ctr, FGH Bldg - Ste 5008, 820 Harrison Ave, Boston, MA 02118; **Phone:** 617-638-8446; **Board Cert:** Surgery 2008; **Med School:** Georgetown Univ 1983; **Resid:** Surgery, Boston Med Ctr 1988; **Fellow:** Gastrointestinal Surgery, Lahey Clinic 1989; **Fac Appt:** Assoc Prof S, Boston Univ

McFadden, David W MD [S] - **Spec Exp:** Pancreatic Cancer; **Hospital:** Fletcher Allen Health Care- Med Ctr Campus; **Address:** Fletcher Allen Hlthcare, Fletcher House 301, 111 Colchester Ave, Burlington, VT 05401; **Phone:** 802-847-5354; **Board Cert:** Surgery 2007; Surgical Critical Care 2003; **Med School:** Univ VA Sch Med 1980; **Resid:** Surgery, Johns Hopkins Hosp 1986; **Fellow:** Surgery, Johns Hopkins Hosp 1988; **Fac Appt:** Prof S, Univ VT Coll Med

Moore Jr, Francis D MD [S] - **Spec Exp:** Endocrine Surgery; Thyroid Cancer; **Hospital:** Brigham & Women's Hosp; **Address:** Brigham & Womens Hosp, 75 Francis St, ASB11-3rd Fl, Boston, MA 02115; **Phone:** 617-732-6830; **Board Cert:** Surgery 2004; **Med School:** Harvard Med Sch 1976; **Resid:** Surgery, Brigham & Womens Hosp 1984; **Fellow:** Immunology, Harvard Med Sch 1981; **Fac Appt:** Prof S, Harvard Med Sch

Ponn, Teresa MD [S] - **Spec Exp:** Breast Cancer; **Hospital:** Elliot Hosp; **Address:** Elliot Breast Health Center, 275 Mammoth Rd, Manchester, NH 03109; **Phone:** 603-668-3067; **Board Cert:** Surgery 2000; **Med School:** Univ Fla Coll Med 1976; **Resid:** Surgery, Stanford Univ Med Ctr 1982

Salem, Ronald R MD [S] - **Spec Exp:** Cancer Surgery; Liver & Biliary Surgery; Gastrointestinal Cancer; Liver Cancer; **Hospital:** Yale-New Haven Hosp, Yale Med Group; **Address:** Dept Surgery, 333 Cedar St, TMP 203, New Haven, CT 06520-8062; **Phone:** 203-785-3577; **Board Cert:** Surgery 2000; **Med School:** Zimbabwe 1978; **Resid:** Surgery, Hammersmith Hosp 1985; Surgery, New England Deaconess Hosp 1989; **Fac Appt:** Prof S, Yale Univ

Smith, Barbara L MD/PhD [S] - **Spec Exp:** Breast Cancer; Breast Cancer-High Risk Women; **Hospital:** Mass Genl Hosp; **Address:** MGH Cancer Center, Yawkey 9A, 55 Fruit St, Boston, MA 02114; **Phone:** 617-724-4800; **Board Cert:** Surgery 2009; **Med School:** Harvard Med Sch 1983; **Resid:** Surgery, Brigham & Women's Hosp 1989; **Fac Appt:** Asst Prof S, Harvard Med Sch

Sosa, Julie A MD [S] - **Spec Exp:** Thyroid Cancer; Parathyroid Cancer; Endocrine Cancers; **Hospital:** Yale-New Haven Hosp; **Address:** Yale Univ Sch Med, Dept Surgery, 333 Cedar St, Box 208062, New Haven, CT 06520; **Phone:** 203-785-2314; **Board Cert:** Surgery 2004; **Med School:** Johns Hopkins Univ 1994; **Resid:** Surgery, Johns Hopkins Hosp 2001; **Fellow:** Surgical Oncology, Johns Hoplins Hosp 2002; **Fac Appt:** Assoc Prof S, Yale Univ

Sutton, John E MD [S] - **Spec Exp:** Esophageal Cancer; Liver & Biliary Surgery; Pancreatic Cancer; **Hospital:** Dartmouth - Hitchcock Med Ctr; **Address:** One Medical Center Drive, Lebanon, NH 03756; **Phone:** 603-650-8022; **Board Cert:** Surgery 2001; Surgical Critical Care 2007; **Med School:** Georgetown Univ 1974; **Resid:** Surgery, Dartmouth-Hitchcock Med Ctr 1981; **Fellow:** Surgical Critical Care, Dartmouth-Hitchcock Med Ctr 1983; **Fac Appt:** Prof S, Dartmouth Med Sch

Tanabe, Kenneth K MD [S] - **Spec Exp:** Liver Cancer; Colon & Rectal Cancer; Melanoma; **Hospital:** Mass Genl Hosp, Newton - Wellesley Hosp; **Address:** Mass General Hosp, Div Surgical Oncology, 55 Fruit St, Yawkey 7B, Boston, MA 02114; **Phone:** 617-724-3868; **Board Cert:** Surgery 2000; **Med School:** UCSD 1985; **Resid:** Surgery, New York Hosp-Cornell 1990; **Fellow:** Surgical Oncology, MD Anderson Cancer Ctr 1993; **Fac Appt:** Assoc Prof S, Harvard Med Sch

Thayer, Sarah P MD/PhD [S] - **Spec Exp:** Pancreatic Cancer; Gastrointestinal Cancer & Surgery; Hepatobiliary Surgery; Breast Cancer & Surgery; **Hospital:** Mass Genl Hosp; **Address:** Mass Genl Hosp, 15 Parkman St, WAC 460, Boston, MA 02114; **Phone:** 617-726-0624; **Board Cert:** Surgery 2001; **Med School:** Univ VA Sch Med 1991; **Resid:** Surgery, Mass Genl Hosp 1994; Surgery, Mass Genl Hosp 2001; **Fellow:** Research, Meml Sloan Kettering Cancer Ctr 1998; **Fac Appt:** Assoc Prof Surg & Onc, Harvard Med Sch

Udelsman, Robert MD [S] - **Spec Exp:** Parathyroid Cancer; Adrenal Tumors; Thyroid Cancer; **Hospital:** Yale-New Haven Hosp, Yale Med Group; **Address:** Yale School Medicine, Dept Surgery, PO Box 208062, New Haven, CT 06520-8062; **Phone:** 203-785-2697; **Board Cert:** Surgery 2009; **Med School:** Geo Wash Univ 1981; **Resid:** Surgery, Natl Inst Hlth 1986; Surgery, Johns Hopkins Hosp 1989; **Fellow:** Gastrointestinal Surgery, Johns Hopkins Hosp 1990; Surgical Oncology, Natl Cancer Inst 1985; **Fac Appt:** Prof S, Yale Univ

Ward, Barbara MD [S] - **Spec Exp:** Breast Cancer; Breast Surgery; **Hospital:** Greenwich Hosp; **Address:** 77 Lafayette Pl, Ste 302, Greenwich, CT 06830-5426; **Phone:** 203-863-4250; **Board Cert:** Surgery 2002; **Med School:** Temple Univ 1983; **Resid:** Surgery, Yale-New Haven Hosp 1990; **Fellow:** Surgical Oncology, Natl Cancer Inst 1987; **Fac Appt:** Assoc Clin Prof S, Yale Univ

Zinner, Michael MD [S] - **Spec Exp:** Colon & Rectal Cancer & Surgery; Pancreatic Cancer; Stomach Cancer; Gastrointestinal Stromal Tumors; **Hospital:** Brigham & Women's Hosp, Dana-Farber Cancer Inst; **Address:** Brigham & Women's Hosp, Dept Surg, 75 Francis St, Twr 1, Ste 220, Boston, MA 02115; **Phone:** 617-732-8181; **Board Cert:** Surgery 2000; **Med School:** Univ Fla Coll Med 1971; **Resid:** Surgery, Johns Hopkins Hosp 1974; Surgery, Johns Hopkins Hosp 1980; **Fac Appt:** Prof S, Harvard Med Sch

Mid Atlantic

Alexander Jr, H Richard MD [S] - **Spec Exp:** Gastrointestinal Cancer & Surgery; Liver Cancer-Metastatic; Pancreatic Cancer; **Hospital:** Univ of MD Med Ctr; **Address:** UMMC, Dept Surgery, 22 S Greene St, rm S4B05, Baltimore, MD 21201; **Phone:** 410-328-2999; **Board Cert:** Surgery 2004; **Med School:** Georgetown Univ 1979; **Resid:** Surgery, Bethesda Naval Hosp 1985; **Fellow:** Surgical Oncology, Meml Sloan Kettering Cancer Ctr 1989; **Fac Appt:** Prof S, Univ MD Sch Med

Alfonso, Antonio E MD [S] - **Spec Exp:** Breast Cancer; Head & Neck Surgery; Thyroid Cancer; **Hospital:** Univ Hosp of Bklyn at Long Island Coll Hosp (page 71), SUNY Downstate Med Ctr; **Address:** Long Island Coll Hosp, 339 Hicks St, Brooklyn, NY 11201; **Phone:** 718-875-3244; **Board Cert:** Surgery 1973; **Med School:** Philippines 1968; **Resid:** Surgery, Temple Univ Hosp 1972; **Fellow:** Surgical Oncology, Meml Sloan Kettering Cancer Ctr 1974; **Fac Appt:** Prof S, SUNY Downstate

August, David MD [S] - **Spec Exp:** Pancreatic Cancer; Esophageal Cancer; Stomach Cancer; Sarcoma-Soft Tissue; **Hospital:** Robert Wood Johnson Univ Hosp - New Brunswick; **Address:** Cancer Institute of NJ, 195 Little Albany St, New Brunswick, NJ 08903; **Phone:** 732-235-7701; **Board Cert:** Surgery 2005; **Med School:** Yale Univ 1980; **Resid:** Surgery, Yale-New Haven Hosp 1986; **Fellow:** Surgical Oncology, Natl Cancer Inst 1984; **Fac Appt:** Prof S, UMDNJ-RW Johnson Med Sch

Axelrod, Deborah MD [S] - **Spec Exp:** Breast Cancer; **Hospital:** NYU Langone Med Ctr (page 79); **Address:** NYU Clinical Cancer Ctr, 160 E 34th St, New York, NY 10016; **Phone:** 212-731-5366; **Board Cert:** Surgery 2008; **Med School:** Israel 1982; **Resid:** Surgery, Beth Israel Med Ctr 1988; **Fellow:** Surgical Oncology, Meml Sloan Kettering Cancer Ctr 1986; **Fac Appt:** Assoc Prof S, NYU Sch Med

Surgery

Bartlett, David L MD [S] - **Spec Exp:** Peritoneal Carcinomatosis; Pancreatic Cancer; Liver Cancer; Appendix Cancer; **Hospital:** UPMC Shadyside; **Address:** UPMC Cancer Pavilion, 5150 Centre Ave Fl 4 - rm 415, Pittsburgh, PA 15232; **Phone:** 412-692-2852; **Board Cert:** Surgery 2004; **Med School:** Univ Tex, Houston 1987; **Resid:** Surgery, Hosp Univ Penn 1993; **Fellow:** Surgical Oncology, Meml Sloan-Kettering Cancer Ctr 1995; **Fac Appt:** Assoc Prof S, Univ Pittsburgh

Boraas, Marcia MD [S] - **Spec Exp:** Breast Cancer; **Hospital:** Fox Chase Cancer Ctr (page 72); **Address:** Fox Chase Cancer Ctr, Dept Surgery, 333 Cotman Ave, rm P2131, Philadelphia, PA 19111; **Phone:** 215-728-2982; **Board Cert:** Surgery 2005; **Med School:** Univ Pennsylvania 1977; **Resid:** Surgery, Hosp U Penn 1983

Borgen, Patrick I MD [S] - **Spec Exp:** Breast Cancer; Breast Cancer & Surgery; **Hospital:** Maimonides Med Ctr (page 74); **Address:** Maimonides Breast Ctr, 6300 8th Ave, Brooklyn, NY 11220; **Phone:** 718-765-2570; **Board Cert:** Surgery 2002; **Med School:** Louisiana State U, New Orleans 1984; **Resid:** Surgery, Ochsner Fdn Hosp 1989; **Fellow:** Surgical Oncology, Meml Sloan Kettering Canc Ctr 1990; **Fac Appt:** Prof S, Cornell Univ-Weill Med Coll

Brennan, Murray F MD [S] - **Spec Exp:** Sarcoma; Pancreatic Cancer; Stomach Cancer; Endocrine Cancers; **Hospital:** Meml Sloan-Kettering Cancer Ctr (page 75); **Address:** 1275 York Ave, New York, NY 10065; **Phone:** 212-639-6586; **Board Cert:** Surgery 1975; **Med School:** New Zealand 1964; **Resid:** Surgery, Univ Otago Hosp 1969; **Fellow:** Surgery, Harvard Med Sch 1972; Surgery, Peter Bent Brigham Hosp 1975; **Fac Appt:** Prof S, Cornell Univ-Weill Med Coll

Brooks, Ari D MD [S] - **Spec Exp:** Breast Cancer; **Hospital:** Hahnemann Univ Hosp; **Address:** Drexel Surgical Assocs, 219 N Broad St Fl 8, Philadelphia, PA 19107; **Phone:** 215-762-2295; **Board Cert:** Surgery 2000; **Med School:** Hahnemann Univ 1992; **Resid:** Surgery, NYU Med Ctr 1999; **Fellow:** Surgical Oncology, Meml Sloan-Kettering Cancer Ctr 2001; **Fac Appt:** Assoc Prof S, Drexel Univ Coll Med

Cameron, John L MD [S] - **Spec Exp:** Pancreatic Cancer; Pancreatic Surgery; Biliary Cancer; Liver Cancer; **Hospital:** Johns Hopkins Hosp; **Address:** 600 N Wolfe St Blalock Bldg - Ste 679, Baltimore, MD 21287; **Phone:** 410-955-5166; **Board Cert:** Surgery 1970; Thoracic Surgery 1971; **Med School:** Johns Hopkins Univ 1962; **Resid:** Surgery, Johns Hopkins Hosp 1970; **Fellow:** Thoracic Surgery, Johns Hopkins Hosp 1971; **Fac Appt:** Prof S, Johns Hopkins Univ

Cance, William G MD [S] - **Spec Exp:** Pancreatic Cancer; Endocrine Cancers; Colon & Rectal Cancer; **Hospital:** Roswell Park Cancer Inst; **Address:** Department of Surgical Oncology, Elm and Carlton Streets, Buffalo, NY 14263; **Phone:** 716-845-8204; **Board Cert:** Surgery 2009; **Med School:** Duke Univ 1982; **Resid:** Surgery, Barnes Jewish Hosp 1988; **Fellow:** Surgical Oncology, Meml Sloan Kettering Canc Ctr 1990; **Fac Appt:** Prof S, SUNY Buffalo

Carty, Sally E MD [S] - **Spec Exp:** Endocrine Surgery; Endocrine Tumors; Parathyroid Surgery; **Hospital:** UPMC Presby, Pittsburgh, UPMC Shadyside; **Address:** 3471 Fifth Ave, Ste 101, Pittsburgh, PA 15213; **Phone:** 412-647-0467; **Board Cert:** Surgery 1999; **Med School:** Penn State Coll Med 1984; **Resid:** Surgery, Penn State Hershey Med Ctr 1989; **Fellow:** Surgical Oncology, Natl Cancer Inst 1991; **Fac Appt:** Prof S, Univ Pittsburgh

Chabot, John A MD [S] - **Spec Exp:** Liver & Biliary Surgery; Pancreatic Cancer; Pancreatic Surgery; Thyroid & Parathyroid Surgery; **Hospital:** NY-Presby Hosp/Columbia (page 78); **Address:** NY Presby-Columbia Medical Ctr, 161 Ft Washington Ave Fl 8 - Ste 819, New York, NY 10032; **Phone:** 212-305-9468; **Board Cert:** Surgery 2000; **Med School:** Dartmouth Med Sch 1983; **Resid:** Surgery, Columbia-Presby Med Ctr 1990; **Fac Appt:** Prof S, Columbia P&S

Cherqui, Daniel MD [S] - **Spec Exp:** Transplant-Liver; Hepatobiliary Surgery; Liver Cancer; Minimally Invasive Surgery; **Hospital:** NY-Presby Hosp/Weill Cornell (page 78); **Address:** 525 E 68th St, Box 287, New York, NY 10065; **Phone:** 212-746-2127; **Med School:** France 1980; **Resid:** Surgery, Hospitaux de Paris 1986; **Fellow:** Hepatobiliary Surgery, Paul Brousse Hosp 1987; Transplant Surgery, Univ Chicago Med Ctr; **Fac Appt:** Prof S, Cornell Univ-Weill Med Coll

Choti, Michael A MD [S] - **Spec Exp:** Pancreatic Cancer; Liver Cancer-Metastatic; Carcinoid Tumors; **Hospital:** Johns Hopkins Hosp; **Address:** Johns Hopkins Hosp, 600 N Wolfe St Blalock Bldg - rm 665, Baltimore, MD 21287; **Phone:** 410-955-7113; **Board Cert:** Surgery 2002; **Med School:** Yale Univ 1983; **Resid:** Surgery, Hosp Univ Penn 1990; **Fellow:** Surgical Oncology, Meml Sloan-Kettering Canc Ctr 1992; **Fac Appt:** Prof S, Johns Hopkins Univ

Coit, Daniel G MD [S] - **Spec Exp:** Melanoma; Pancreatic Cancer; Stomach Cancer; **Hospital:** Meml Sloan-Kettering Cancer Ctr (page 75); **Address:** 1275 York Avenue, New York, NY 10065; **Phone:** 800-525-2225; **Board Cert:** Surgery 2004; **Med School:** Univ Cincinnati 1976; **Resid:** Internal Medicine, New Eng Deaconess Hosp 1978; Surgery, New Eng Deaconess Hosp 1983; **Fellow:** Surgical Oncology, Meml Sloan Kettering Canc Ctr 1985; **Fac Appt:** Prof S, Cornell Univ-Weill Med Coll

Curcillo, Paul G MD [S] - **Spec Exp:** Minimally Invasive Surgery; Gastrointestinal Cancer & Surgery; Natural Orifice Surgery (NOTES); **Hospital:** Fox Chase Cancer Ctr (page 72); **Address:** Fox Chase Cancer Ctr, Dept Surgery, 333 Cottman Ave, Philadelphia, PA 19111; **Phone:** 215-728-5363; **Board Cert:** Surgery 2007; **Med School:** Univ Pennsylvania 1989; **Resid:** Surgery, Thomas Jefferson Univ Hosp 1995; **Fac Appt:** Assoc Prof S, Drexel Univ Coll Med

Drebin, Jeffrey A MD/PhD [S] - **Spec Exp:** Pancreatic Cancer; Liver Cancer; Biliary Cancer; Gastrointestinal Cancer; **Hospital:** Hosp Univ Penn - UPHS (page 80); **Address:** Hosp Univ Penn, Dept Surgery, 3400 Spruce St, 4 Silverstein Pavilion, Philadelphia, PA 19104; **Phone:** 215-662-2165; **Board Cert:** Surgery 2004; **Med School:** Harvard Med Sch 1987; **Resid:** Surgery, Johns Hopkins Hosp 1994; **Fellow:** Medical Oncology, Johns Hopkins Hosp 1991; Surgical Oncology, Johns Hopkins Hosp 1995; **Fac Appt:** Prof S, Univ Pennsylvania

Duncan, Mark D MD [S] - **Spec Exp:** Gastrointestinal Cancer & Surgery; Minimally Invasive Surgery; **Hospital:** Johns Hopkins Bayview Med Ctr; **Address:** Johns Hopkins Bayview Med Ctr, 4940 Eastern Ave, Baltimore, MD 21224; **Phone:** 410-550-1226; **Board Cert:** Surgery 1997; **Med School:** Mayo Med Sch 1987; **Resid:** Surgery, Georgetown Univ Hosp 1994; **Fellow:** Surgery, VA Medical Ctr 1991

Edge, Stephen B MD [S] - **Spec Exp:** Breast Cancer; Cancer Surgery; **Hospital:** Roswell Park Cancer Inst; **Address:** Roswell Park Cancer Inst, Dept Surg Onc, Elm & Carlton Streets, Buffalo, NY 14263; **Phone:** 716-845-2918; **Board Cert:** Surgery 2006; **Med School:** Case West Res Univ 1979; **Resid:** Surgery, Univ Hosp 1986; **Fellow:** Surgical Oncology, Natl Cancer Inst 1984; **Fac Appt:** Prof S, SUNY Buffalo

Edington, Howard D MD [S] - **Spec Exp:** Melanoma; Breast Reconstruction; Reconstructive Surgery; **Hospital:** Magee-Womens Hosp - UPMC; **Address:** Magee-Women's Hospital, Dept Surgery, 300 Halket St, rm 2502, Pittsburgh, PA 15213; **Phone:** 412-641-1342; **Board Cert:** Surgery 2008; Plastic Surgery 1993; **Med School:** Temple Univ 1983; **Resid:** Surgery, Univ Pittsburgh Med Ctr 1989; Plastic Surgery, Univ Pittsburgh Med Ctr 1990; **Fellow:** Hand Surgery, Univ Pittsburgh Med Ctr 1991; Surgical Oncology, National Cancer Inst 1993; **Fac Appt:** Assoc Prof S, Univ Pittsburgh

Surgery

Emond, Jean C MD [S] - **Spec Exp:** Transplant-Liver; Liver Cancer; Liver & Biliary Cancer; Hepatobiliary Surgery; **Hospital:** NY-Presby Hosp/Columbia (page 78), Holy Name Med Ctr; **Address:** 622 W 168th St, PH - Fl 14, New York, NY 10032; **Phone:** 212-305-9691; **Board Cert:** Surgery 2006; **Med School:** Univ Chicago-Pritzker Sch Med 1979; **Resid:** Surgery, Cook Cty Hosp 1984; **Fellow:** Surgery, Hopital P Brousse/Univ de Paris Sud 1985; Transplant Surgery, Univ Chicago Hosps 1987; **Fac Appt:** Prof S, Columbia P&S

Estabrook, Alison MD [S] - **Spec Exp:** Breast Cancer; Breast Cancer-High Risk Women; **Hospital:** St. Luke's - Roosevelt Hosp Ctr - Roosevelt Div (page 71); **Address:** 425 W 59th St, Ste 7A, New York, NY 10019-1104; **Phone:** 212-523-7500; **Board Cert:** Surgery 2004; **Med School:** NYU Sch Med 1978; **Resid:** Surgery, Columbia Presby Med Ctr 1984; **Fellow:** Surgical Oncology, Columbia Presby Med Ctr 1982; **Fac Appt:** Prof S, Columbia P&S

Fahey III, Thomas J MD [S] - **Spec Exp:** Endocrine Surgery; Pancreatic Cancer; Minimally Invasive Surgery; **Hospital:** NY-Presby Hosp/Weill Cornell (page 78); **Address:** NY Presby Cornell Med Ctr, Dept Surgery, 525 E 68 St, rm F2024, Box 249, New York, NY 10065; **Phone:** 212-746-5130; **Board Cert:** Surgery 2002; **Med School:** Cornell Univ-Weill Med Coll 1986; **Resid:** Surgery, New York Hosp 1992; **Fellow:** Endocrine Surgery, Royal North Shore Hosp 1993; **Fac Appt:** Prof S, Cornell Univ-Weill Med Coll

Fong, Yuman MD [S] - **Spec Exp:** Pancreatic Cancer; Liver & Biliary Cancer; Stomach Cancer; **Hospital:** Meml Sloan-Kettering Cancer Ctr (page 75), NY-Presby Hosp/Weill Cornell (page 78); **Address:** 1275 York Ave, rm C887, New York, NY 10065; **Phone:** 800-525-2225; **Board Cert:** Surgery 2002; **Med School:** Cornell Univ-Weill Med Coll 1984; **Resid:** Surgery, NY Hosp-Cornell Med Ctr 1992; **Fellow:** Surgical Oncology, Meml Sloan-Kettering Cancer Ctr 1994; **Fac Appt:** Prof S, Cornell Univ-Weill Med Coll

Fraker, Douglas L MD [S] - **Spec Exp:** Melanoma; Endocrine Tumors; Liver Cancer; Sarcoma; **Hospital:** Hosp Univ Penn - UPHS (page 80); **Address:** Hosp Univ Penn, Dept Surgery, 3400 Spruce St, 4 Silverstein Pavilion, Philadelphia, PA 19104; **Phone:** 215-662-7866; **Board Cert:** Surgery 2002; **Med School:** Harvard Med Sch 1983; **Resid:** Surgery, UCSF Med Ctr 1986; Surgery, UCSF Med Ctr 1991; **Fellow:** Surgical Oncology, National Cancer Inst 1989; **Fac Appt:** Prof S, Univ Pennsylvania

Frazier, Thomas G MD [S] - **Spec Exp:** Breast Cancer; **Hospital:** Bryn Mawr Hosp; **Address:** 101 S Bryn Mawr Ave, Ste 201, Bryn Mawr, PA 19010; **Phone:** 610-520-0700; **Board Cert:** Surgery 2004; **Med School:** Univ Pennsylvania 1968; **Resid:** Surgery, Hosp Univ Penn 1975; **Fellow:** Surgical Oncology, MD Anderson Cancer Ctr 1976; **Fac Appt:** Clin Prof S, Drexel Univ Coll Med

Geller, David A MD [S] - **Spec Exp:** Liver Cancer; Laparoscopic Surgery; Liver & Biliary Cancer; **Hospital:** UPMC Presby, Pittsburgh, UPMC Passavant-McCandless; **Address:** UPMC Liver Cancer Center, 3459 5th Ave, Pittsburgh, PA 15213-2582; **Phone:** 412-692-2001; **Board Cert:** Surgery 2005; **Med School:** Northwestern Univ-Feinberg Sch Med 1988; **Resid:** Surgery, UPMC-Presbyterian 1993; **Fellow:** Hepatobiliary Surgery, UPMC-Presbyterian 1998; Transplant Surgery, UPMC-Presbyterian 1998; **Fac Appt:** Prof S, Univ Pittsburgh

Gibbs, John F MD [S] - **Spec Exp:** Liver Cancer; Biliary Cancer; Pancreatic Cancer; Neuroendocrine Tumors; **Hospital:** Roswell Park Cancer Inst; **Address:** Roswell Park Cancer Inst, Dept Surgical Oncology, Elm & Carlton Streets, Buffalo, NY 14263-0001; **Phone:** 716-845-5807; **Board Cert:** Surgery 2009; **Med School:** UCSD 1985; **Resid:** Surgery, Rush Presby-St Lukes Med Ctr 1990; **Fellow:** Transplant Surgery, Baylor Univ Med Ctr 1992; Surgical Oncology, Roswell Park Cancer Inst 1996; **Fac Appt:** Assoc Prof S, SUNY Buffalo

Hanna, Nader N MD [S] - **Spec Exp:** Pancreatic Cancer; Adrenal Tumors; Peritoneal Carcinomatosis; Sarcoma-Soft Tissue; **Hospital:** Univ of MD Med Ctr; **Address:** 22 S Greene St, Ste S4B-07, Baltimore, MD 21201; **Phone:** 410-328-7320; **Board Cert:** Surgery 2005; **Med School:** Egypt 1985; **Resid:** Surgery, St. Elizabeth's Med Ctr-Tuft's Univ 1994; **Fellow:** Surgical Oncology, Univ Chicago 1997; Research, Univ Chicago; **Fac Appt:** Assoc Prof S, Univ MD Sch Med

Hiotis, Spiros P MD/PhD [S] - **Spec Exp:** Liver Cancer; Gallbladder & Biliary Cancer; Pancreatic Cancer; Stomach Cancer; **Hospital:** Mount Sinai Med Ctr (page 76); **Address:** Surgical Oncology Assocs, 5 E 98th St Fl 12, Box 1259, New York, NY 100 129; **Phone:** 212-241-2891; **Board Cert:** Surgery 2000; **Med School:** Univ MD Sch Med 1992; **Resid:** Surgery, USF Med Ctr 1998; **Fellow:** Surgical Oncology, Meml Sloan Kettering Cancer Ctr 2000; **Fac Appt:** Asst Prof S, Mount Sinai Sch Med

Hoffman, John P MD [S] - **Spec Exp:** Pancreatic Cancer; Gastrointestinal Cancer; Hepatobiliary Surgery; Liver Cancer; **Hospital:** Fox Chase Cancer Ctr (page 72); **Address:** Fox Chase Cancer Ctr, 333 Cottman Ave, Philadelphia, PA 19111-2497; **Phone:** 215-728-3518; **Board Cert:** Surgery 1998; **Med School:** Case West Res Univ 1970; **Resid:** Surgery, Virginia Mason Hosp 1977; **Fellow:** Surgical Oncology, Meml Sloan Kettering Cancer Ctr 1980; **Fac Appt:** Prof S, Temple Univ

Jarnagin, William MD [S] - **Spec Exp:** Hepatobiliary Surgery; Liver Cancer; Pancreatic Cancer; Gallbladder & Biliary Cancer; **Hospital:** Meml Sloan-Kettering Cancer Ctr (page 75); **Address:** 1275 York Ave, New York, NY 10065; **Phone:** 212-639-7601; **Board Cert:** Surgery 2006; **Med School:** Rush Med Coll 1988; **Resid:** Surgery, Univ Calif San Francisco 1996; **Fellow:** Hepatopancreatobiliary Surgery, Meml Sloan-Kettering Cancer Ctr 1997; **Fac Appt:** Prof S, Cornell Univ

Johnson, Ronald R MD [S] - **Spec Exp:** Breast Cancer; **Hospital:** Magee-Womens Hosp - UPMC; **Address:** Magee-Womens Hosp - UPMC, 300 Halket St, Ste 2601, Pittsburgh, PA 15213; **Phone:** 412-641-1225; **Board Cert:** Surgery 1999; **Med School:** Univ Pittsburgh 1983; **Resid:** Surgery, Univ Pittsburgh Med Ctr 1989; **Fac Appt:** Asst Prof S, Univ Pittsburgh

Julian, Thomas B MD [S] - **Spec Exp:** Breast Cancer & Surgery; Clinical Trials; **Hospital:** Allegheny General Hosp; **Address:** Allegheny Cancer Ctr, 320 E North Ave, Cancer Center Fl 5, Pittsburgh, PA 15212; **Phone:** 412-359-8229; **Board Cert:** Surgery 2001; **Med School:** Univ Pittsburgh 1976; **Resid:** Surgery, Univ Pittsburgh Med Ctr 1982; **Fac Appt:** Assoc Prof S, Drexel Univ Coll Med

Karpeh Jr, Martin S MD [S] - **Spec Exp:** Gastrointestinal Cancer; Esophageal Cancer; Pancreatic Cancer; Liver Cancer; **Hospital:** Beth Israel Med Ctr - Petrie Division (page 71); **Address:** Beth Israel Med Ctr, Philips Ambulatory Ctr, 10 Union Square E, Ste 4D, New York, NY 10003; **Phone:** 212-420-4041; **Board Cert:** Surgery 1998; **Med School:** Penn State Coll Med 1983; **Resid:** Surgery, Hosp Univ Penn 1989; **Fellow:** Surgical Oncology, Meml Sloan Kettering Cancer Ctr 1991; **Fac Appt:** Prof S, Mount Sinai Sch Med

Leach, Steven D MD [S] - **Spec Exp:** Pancreatic Cancer; **Hospital:** Johns Hopkins Hosp; **Address:** Johns Hopkins Med Outpatient Ctr, 601 N Caroline St, Baltimore, MD 21287; **Phone:** 410-933-1233; **Board Cert:** Surgery 2004; **Med School:** Emory Univ 1986; **Resid:** Surgery, Yale-New Haven Hosp 1993; **Fellow:** Surgical Oncology, MD Anderson Cancer Ctr 1995; **Fac Appt:** Prof S, Johns Hopkins Univ

Lee, Kenneth K W MD [S] - **Spec Exp:** Pancreatic Cancer; Gastrointestinal Cancer & Surgery; **Hospital:** UPMC Presby, Pittsburgh, UPMC Shadyside; **Address:** UPMC Presbyterian, 200 Lothrop St, Ste 497, Scaife Hall, Pittsburgh, PA 15261; **Phone:** 412-647-0457; **Board Cert:** Surgery 2008; **Med School:** Univ Chicago-Pritzker Sch Med 1981; **Resid:** Surgery, Univ Chicago Hosps 1988; **Fac Appt:** Assoc Prof S, Univ Pittsburgh

Surgery

Libutti, Steven K MD [S] - **Spec Exp:** Liver Cancer; Neuroendocrine Tumors; Gastrointestinal Cancer; **Hospital:** Montefiore Med Ctr - Div. Weiler, Montefiore Med Ctr - Div. Moses; **Address:** 3400 Bainbridge Ave Fl 4th, Bronx, NY 10467; **Phone:** 718-920-4231; **Board Cert:** Surgery 2004; **Med School:** Columbia P&S 1990; **Resid:** Surgery, Columbia Presby Med Ctr 1995; **Fellow:** Surgical Oncology, Natl Cancer Inst 1996; **Fac Appt:** Prof S, Albert Einstein Coll Med

Lieberman, Michael D MD [S] - **Spec Exp:** Gastrointestinal Cancer; Colon & Rectal Cancer & Surgery; Hepatobiliary Surgery; Pancreatic Cancer; **Hospital:** NY-Presby Hosp/Weill Cornell (page 78); **Address:** 1315 York Ave, Box 216, New York, NY 10021; **Phone:** 212-746-5434; **Board Cert:** Surgery 2003; **Med School:** UMDNJ-NJ Med Sch, Newark 1985; **Resid:** Surgery, Hosp Univ Penn 1992; **Fellow:** Surgical Oncology, Hosp Univ Penn 1990; Surgical Oncology, Meml Sloan-Kettering Cancer Ctr 1994; **Fac Appt:** Assoc Prof S, Cornell Univ-Weill Med Coll

Marsh Jr, James W MD [S] - **Spec Exp:** Transplant-Liver; Liver Cancer; Pancreatic Cancer; **Hospital:** UPMC Presby, Pittsburgh, Monongahela Valley Hosp; **Address:** UPMC, Starzl Transplantation Inst, 3459 Fifth Ave 7 South, Pittsburgh, PA 15213-2582; **Phone:** 412-647-5800; **Board Cert:** Surgery 2003; **Med School:** Univ Ark 1979; **Resid:** Surgery, St Paul Hosp 1984; **Fellow:** Transplant Surgery, Mayo Clinic 1985; Transplant Surgery, Univ Pittsburgh Hosps 1986; **Fac Appt:** Prof S, Univ Pittsburgh

Michelassi, Fabrizio MD [S] - **Spec Exp:** Gastrointestinal Cancer; Colon Cancer; **Hospital:** NY-Presby Hosp/Weill Cornell (page 78); **Address:** Weill Cornell Med College, Surg Dept, 525 E 68th St, rm F-739, New York, NY 10021; **Phone:** 212-746-6006; **Board Cert:** Surgery 2002; **Med School:** Italy 1975; **Resid:** Surgery, NYU Med Ctr 1981; **Fellow:** Research, Mass Genl Hosp 1983; **Fac Appt:** Prof S, Cornell Univ-Weill Med Coll

Morrow, Monica MD [S] - **Spec Exp:** Breast Cancer; **Hospital:** Meml Sloan-Kettering Cancer Ctr (page 75); **Address:** 300 E 66th St, New York, NY 10065; **Phone:** 646-888-5350; **Board Cert:** Surgery 2001; **Med School:** Jefferson Med Coll 1976; **Resid:** Surgery, Med Ctr Hosp Vermont 1981; **Fellow:** Surgical Oncology, Meml Sloan Kettering Cancer Ctr 1983; **Fac Appt:** Prof S, Cornell Univ-Weill Med Coll

Nava-Villarreal, Hector MD [S] - **Spec Exp:** Esophageal Cancer; Stomach Cancer; Barrett's Esophagus; **Hospital:** Roswell Park Cancer Inst; **Address:** Roswell Park Cancer Inst, Elm & Carlton Sts, Buffalo, NY 14263; **Phone:** 716-845-5915; **Board Cert:** Surgery 2001; **Med School:** Mexico 1967; **Resid:** Surgery, Buffalo Genl Hosp 1974; **Fellow:** Surgical Oncology, Roswell Park Cancer Inst 1976; **Fac Appt:** Assoc Prof S, SUNY Buffalo

Newman, Elliot MD [S] - **Spec Exp:** Gastrointestinal Cancer; Pancreatic Cancer; Liver Cancer; Colon & Rectal Cancer; **Hospital:** NYU Langone Med Ctr (page 79); **Address:** NYU Medical Ctr, 530 1st Ave, Ste 6C, New York, NY 10016-6402; **Phone:** 212-263-7302; **Board Cert:** Surgery 2004; **Med School:** NYU Sch Med 1986; **Resid:** Surgery, NYU Med Ctr 1989; Surgery, NYU Med Ctr 1993; **Fellow:** Research, Meml Sloan Kettering Cancer Ctr 1991; Surgical Oncology, Meml Sloan Kettering Cancer Ctr 1995; **Fac Appt:** Assoc Prof S, NYU Sch Med

Nowak, Eugene J MD [S] - **Spec Exp:** Breast Cancer; Gastrointestinal Surgery; Sentinel Node Surgery; **Hospital:** NY-Presby Hosp/Weill Cornell (page 78); **Address:** 325 E 79th St, Ground Fl, New York, NY 10075-0954; **Phone:** 212-517-6693; **Board Cert:** Surgery 2002; **Med School:** UMDNJ-NJ Med Sch, Newark 1975; **Resid:** Surgery, New York Hosp 1980; **Fac Appt:** Asst Clin Prof S, Cornell Univ-Weill Med Coll

O'Hea, Brian J MD [S] - **Spec Exp:** Breast Cancer; Sentinel Node Surgery; **Hospital:** Stony Brook Univ Med Ctr; **Address:** SUNY Stony Brook, Dept Surgery, 3 Edmund D Pelligrino Rd, Stony Brook, NY 11794-8191; **Phone:** 631-444-1795; **Board Cert:** Surgery 2002; **Med School:** Georgetown Univ 1986; **Resid:** Surgery, St Vincent's Hosp 1991; **Fellow:** Breast Disease, Meml Sloan-Kettering Cancer Ctr 1996; **Fac Appt:** Asst Prof S, SUNY Stony Brook

Olthoff, Kim M MD [S] - **Spec Exp:** Transplant-Liver-Adult & Pediatric; Liver & Biliary Surgery; Liver Cancer; **Hospital:** Hosp Univ Penn - UPHS (page 80), Chldns Hosp of Philadelphia; **Address:** Hosp Univ Penn - Dept Surgery, 3400 Spruce St Dulles Bldg Fl 2, Philadelphia, PA 19104; **Phone:** 215-662-6136; **Board Cert:** Surgery 2003; **Med School:** Univ Chicago-Pritzker Sch Med 1986; **Resid:** Surgery, UCLA Med Ctr 1990; **Fellow:** Transplant Surgery, UCLA Med Ctr; **Fac Appt:** Prof S, Univ Pennsylvania

Osborne, Michael P MD [S] - **Spec Exp:** Breast Cancer & Surgery; Breast Reconstruction; **Hospital:** Beth Israel Med Ctr - Petrie Division (page 71); **Address:** Beth Israel Comprehensive Cancer Center, 10 Union Square Ave E, Ste 4E, MS 10003, New York, NY 10011; **Phone:** 212-367-0133; **Med School:** England, UK 1970; **Resid:** Surgery, Charing Cross Hosp 1977; Surgery, Royal Marsden Hosp 1980; **Fellow:** Surgical Oncology, Meml Sloan-Kettering Canc Ctr 1981; **Fac Appt:** Prof S, Cornell Univ-Weill Med Coll

Paty, Philip B MD [S] - **Spec Exp:** Colon & Rectal Cancer; Pelvic Tumors; Appendix Cancer; **Hospital:** Meml Sloan-Kettering Cancer Ctr (page 75); **Address:** 1275 York Avenue, New York, NY 10065; **Phone:** 800-525-2225; **Board Cert:** Surgery 2001; **Med School:** Stanford Univ 1983; **Resid:** Surgery, UCSF Med Ctr 1990; **Fellow:** Surgical Oncology, Meml Sloan Kettering Cancer Ctr 1992; **Fac Appt:** Prof S, Cornell Univ-Weill Med Coll

Pawlik, Timothy M MD [S] - **Spec Exp:** Liver Cancer; Pancreatic Cancer; Gastrointestinal Cancer; Gallbladder & Biliary Cancer; **Hospital:** Johns Hopkins Hosp; **Address:** Johns Hopkins Hospital, 600 N Wolfe St, Harvey Bldg - rm 611, Baltimore, MD 21287; **Phone:** 410-502-2387; **Board Cert:** Surgery 2004; **Med School:** Tufts Univ 1995; **Resid:** Surgery, Univ Michigan Hosp 2002; **Fellow:** Research, Mass Genl Hosp 2004; Surgical Oncology, UT MD Anderson Cancert Ctr 2006; **Fac Appt:** Assoc Prof S, Johns Hopkins Univ

Philosophe, Benjamin MD [S] - **Spec Exp:** Transplant-Liver; Transplant-Pancreas; Hepatobiliary Surgery; Liver Cancer; **Hospital:** Univ of MD Med Ctr; **Address:** UMMC Transplant Ctr, 29 S Greene St, rm 200, Baltimore, MD 21201; **Phone:** 410-328-1145; **Board Cert:** Surgery 2001; **Med School:** Boston Univ 1990; **Resid:** Surgery, Barnes Jewish Hosp 1995; **Fellow:** Hepatopancreatobiliary Surgery, Toronto Hosp 1996; Transplant Surgery, Toronto Hosp 1997; **Fac Appt:** Assoc Prof S, Univ MD Sch Med

Reich, David J MD [S] - **Spec Exp:** Transplant-Liver; Hepatobiliary Surgery; Liver Cancer; **Hospital:** Hahnemann Univ Hosp; **Address:** 216 N Broad St Fl 5, Philadelphia, PA 19102; **Phone:** 215-762-8153; **Board Cert:** Surgery 2003; **Med School:** McGill Univ 1989; **Resid:** Surgery, Beth Israel Med Ctr 1994; **Fellow:** Hepatobiliary Surgery, Mt Sinai Med Ctr 1996

Ridge, John Andrew MD/PhD [S] - **Spec Exp:** Head & Neck Cancer & Surgery; Thyroid Cancer & Surgery; Laryngeal Cancer; **Hospital:** Fox Chase Cancer Ctr (page 72); **Address:** 333 Cottman Ave, Philadelphia, PA 19111; **Phone:** 215-728-3517; **Board Cert:** Surgery 2007; **Med School:** Stanford Univ 1982; **Resid:** Surgery, Univ Colorado Med Ctr 1987; **Fellow:** Surgical Oncology, Meml Sloan-Kettering Cancer Ctr 1989; **Fac Appt:** Prof S, Temple Univ

Rosenberg, Steven A MD [S] - **Spec Exp:** Melanoma; Kidney Cancer; **Hospital:** Natl Inst of Hlth - Clin Ctr; **Address:** National Cancer Inst, 9000 Rockville Pike CRC Bldg, rm 3W-3940, Bethesda, MD 20892; **Phone:** 301-496-4164; **Board Cert:** Surgery 1975; **Med School:** Johns Hopkins Univ 1964; **Resid:** Surgery, Peter Bent Brigham Hosp 1974

Surgery

Roses, Daniel F MD [S] - **Spec Exp:** Breast Cancer; Melanoma; Thyroid & Parathyroid Surgery; **Hospital:** NYU Langone Med Ctr (page 79); **Address:** 530 First Ave, Ste 6B, New York, NY 10016-6402; **Phone:** 212-263-7329; **Board Cert:** Surgery 1975; **Med School:** NYU Sch Med 1969; **Resid:** Surgery, NYU-Bellevue Hosp 1974; **Fellow:** Surgical Oncology, NYU-Bellevue Hosp 1978; **Fac Appt:** Prof Surg & Onc, NYU Sch Med

Sataloff, Dahlia M MD [S] - **Spec Exp:** Breast Cancer; **Hospital:** Pennsylvania Hosp (page 80); **Address:** 700 Spruce St, Ste B03, Philadelphia, PA 19106; **Phone:** 215-829-8461; **Board Cert:** Surgery 2005; **Med School:** Univ Mich Med Sch 1978; **Resid:** Surgery, St Joseph Mercy Hosp 1980; Surgery, Pennsylvania Hosp 1985; **Fac Appt:** Clin Prof S, Univ Pennsylvania

Saunders Jr, John R MD [S] - **Spec Exp:** Head & Neck Cancer; Thyroid Cancer; **Hospital:** Greater Baltimore Med Ctr; **Address:** Johns Hopkins Head & Neck Ctr at GBMC, 6569 N Charles St, Ste 401, Physicians Pavilion West, Baltimore, MD 21204; **Phone:** 443-849-8940; **Board Cert:** Surgery 2008; **Med School:** Georgetown Univ 1971; **Resid:** Surgery, Walter Reed Army Hosp 1976; **Fellow:** Head and Neck Surgery, Walter Reed Army Hosp 1980; **Fac Appt:** Assoc Prof S, Johns Hopkins Univ

Schnabel, Freya MD [S] - **Spec Exp:** Breast Cancer; Breast Cancer-High Risk Women; **Hospital:** NYU Langone Med Ctr (page 79); **Address:** 160 E 34th St Fl 3, New York, NY 10016; **Phone:** 212-731-5367; **Board Cert:** Surgery 2008; **Med School:** NYU Sch Med 1982; **Resid:** Surgery, NYU Med Ctr 1987; **Fellow:** Research, SUNY Hlth Sci Ctr 1988; **Fac Appt:** Prof S, NYU Sch Med

Schraut, Wolfgang H MD [S] - **Spec Exp:** Gastrointestinal Surgery; Colon & Rectal Cancer & Surgery; Laparoscopic Surgery; **Hospital:** UPMC Presby, Pittsburgh, Magee-Womens Hosp - UPMC; **Address:** Univ Pittsburgh Med Ctr, Dept Surgery, 200 Lothrop St, Ste 497, Scaife Hall, Pittsburgh, PA 15261; **Phone:** 412-647-0457; **Board Cert:** Surgery 2009; **Med School:** Germany 1970; **Resid:** Surgery, Univ Chicago Hosps 1978; **Fac Appt:** Prof S, Univ Pittsburgh

Schulick, Richard D MD [S] - **Spec Exp:** Liver Cancer; Biliary Cancer; Pancreatic Cancer; Adrenal Tumors; **Hospital:** Johns Hopkins Hosp; **Address:** Johns Hopkins Hosp-Dept Surgery, 600 N Wolfe St, Blalock 685, Baltimore, MD 21287; **Phone:** 410-614-9879; **Board Cert:** Surgery 2007; **Med School:** Johns Hopkins Univ 1989; **Resid:** Surgery, Johns Hopkins Hosp 1994; **Fellow:** Clinical Pharmacology, NIH 1995; Thyroid Oncology, Maml Sloan Kettering Cancer Ctr 1996; **Fac Appt:** Prof Surg & Onc, Johns Hopkins Univ

Shah, Jatin P MD/PhD [S] - **Spec Exp:** Head & Neck Cancer & Surgery; Thyroid Cancer; Skull Base Tumors; Salivary Gland Tumors & Surgery; **Hospital:** Meml Sloan-Kettering Cancer Ctr (page 75); **Address:** 1275 York Ave, New York, NY 10065; **Phone:** 212-639-7604; **Board Cert:** Surgery 1975; **Med School:** India 1964; **Resid:** Surgery, SSG Hosp 1967; Surgery, NY Eye & Ear Infirm 1974; **Fellow:** Head & Neck Surgical Oncology, Meml Sloan-Kettering Hosp 1972; **Fac Appt:** Prof S, Cornell Univ-Weill Med Coll

Shapiro, Richard L MD [S] - **Spec Exp:** Breast Cancer; Melanoma; Thyroid & Parathyroid Surgery; Cancer Surgery; **Hospital:** NYU Langone Med Ctr (page 79); **Address:** NYU Medical Clinical Cancer Center, 160 E 34th St Fl 4, New York, NY 10016; **Phone:** 212-731-5347; **Board Cert:** Surgery 2004; **Med School:** NYU Sch Med 1988; **Resid:** Surgery, NYU Langone Med Ctr 1993; **Fellow:** Surgical Oncology, NYU Langone Med Ctr 1995; **Fac Appt:** Assoc Prof S, NYU Sch Med

Sigurdson, Elin R MD [S] - **Spec Exp:** Breast Cancer; Colon & Rectal Cancer; Melanoma; Gastrointestinal Cancer; **Hospital:** Fox Chase Cancer Ctr (page 72); **Address:** 333 Cottman Ave, Philadelphia, PA 19111-2412; **Phone:** 215-728-3519; **Board Cert:** Surgery 2006; **Med School:** Univ Toronto 1980; **Resid:** Surgery, Univ Toronto Med Ctr 1984; **Fellow:** Surgical Oncology, Meml Sloan-Kettering Cancer Ctr 1987; **Fac Appt:** Assoc Prof S

Simmons, Rache M MD [S] - **Spec Exp:** Breast Cancer & Surgery; Minimally Invasive Surgery; **Hospital:** NY-Presby Hosp/Weill Cornell (page 78); **Address:** Weill Cornell Breast Ctr, 425 E 61st St Fl 10, New York, NY 10065; **Phone:** 212-821-0853; **Board Cert:** Surgery 2005; **Med School:** Duke Univ 1988; **Resid:** Surgery, Univ NC Hosp 1993; **Fellow:** Surgical Oncology, NY Hosp-Cornell Hosp 1994; **Fac Appt:** Assoc Prof S, Cornell Univ-Weill Med Coll

Skinner, Kristin A MD [S] - **Spec Exp:** Breast Cancer; **Hospital:** Univ of Rochester Strong Meml Hosp; **Address:** Univ Rochester Med Ctr, 601 Elmwood Ave, Box SURG, Rochester, NY 14642; **Phone:** 585-276-3332; **Board Cert:** Surgery 2005; **Med School:** Johns Hopkins Univ 1988; **Resid:** Surgery, UCLA Med Ctr 1995; **Fellow:** Surgical Oncology, UCLA Med Ctr 1994; **Fac Appt:** Assoc Prof S, Univ Rochester

Sugarbaker, Paul H MD [S] - **Spec Exp:** Appendix Cancer; Peritoneal Carcinomatosis; Cystadenocarcinoma; Ovarian Cancer; **Hospital:** Washington Hosp Ctr; **Address:** Washington Hosp Ctr, 106 Irving St NW, Ste 3900N, Washington, DC 20010; **Phone:** 202-877-3908; **Board Cert:** Surgery 1973; **Med School:** Cornell Univ-Weill Med Coll 1967; **Resid:** Surgery, Peter Bent Brigham Hosp 1973; **Fellow:** Surgical Oncology, Mass Genl Hosp 1976; **Fac Appt:** Prof S, Univ Wash

Sundaram, Magesh MD [S] - **Spec Exp:** Gastrointestinal Cancer & Surgery; Pancreatic Cancer; Stomach Cancer; Liver & Biliary Cancer; **Hospital:** Ruby Memorial - WVU Hosp; **Address:** WV Univ Hosp-Dept Surgery, PO Box 9238, Morgantown, WV 26506; **Phone:** 304-293-7095; **Board Cert:** Surgery 2006; **Med School:** Univ MD Sch Med 1990; **Resid:** Surgery, Delaware Med Ctr 1995; **Fellow:** Surgical Oncology, Jackson Meml Hosp 1997; **Fac Appt:** Assoc Prof Surg & Onc, W VA Univ

Swistel, Alexander J MD [S] - **Spec Exp:** Breast Cancer; Sentinel Node Surgery; Nipple Sparing Mastectomy; Cancer Reconstruction; **Hospital:** NY-Presby Hosp/Weill Cornell (page 78), St. Luke's - Roosevelt Hosp Ctr - Roosevelt Div (page 71); **Address:** 425 E 61st St, Fl 10, New York, NY 10065; **Phone:** 212-821-0602; **Board Cert:** Surgery 2005; **Med School:** Brown Univ 1975; **Resid:** Surgery, St Luke's Roosevelt Hosp Ctr 1981; **Fellow:** Surgical Oncology, Meml Sloan Kettering Canc Ctr 1983; **Fac Appt:** Assoc Clin Prof S, Cornell Univ-Weill Med Coll

Tafra, Lorraine MD [S] - **Spec Exp:** Breast Cancer; **Hospital:** Anne Arundel Med Ctr; **Address:** 2000 Medical Parkway, Ste 200, Annapolis, MD 21401; **Phone:** 443-481-5300; **Board Cert:** Surgery 2005; **Med School:** Case West Res Univ 1986; **Resid:** Surgery, Rhode Island Hosp 1988; Surgery, Hosp Univ Penn 1992; **Fellow:** Surgical Oncology, John Wayne Cancer Inst 1994

Tartter, Paul MD [S] - **Spec Exp:** Breast Cancer; Breast Cancer in Elderly; Sentinel Node Surgery; **Hospital:** St. Luke's - Roosevelt Hosp Ctr - Roosevelt Div (page 71), Mount Sinai Med Ctr (page 76); **Address:** 425 W 59th St, Ste 7A, New York, NY 10019-1104; **Phone:** 212-523-7500; **Board Cert:** Surgery 2003; **Med School:** Brown Univ 1977; **Resid:** Surgery, Mt Sinai Hosp 1982; **Fac Appt:** Assoc Prof S, Columbia P&S

Tchou, Julia Chok-Moua MD/PhD [S] - **Spec Exp:** Breast Cancer; Breast Cancer Risk Assessment; **Hospital:** Hosp Univ Penn - UPHS (page 80); **Address:** Abramson Cancer Ctr, Rena Rowan Breast Ctr Fl 3 West, 3400 Civic Ctr Blvd, Philadelphia, PA 19104; **Phone:** 215-615-7575; **Board Cert:** Surgery 2002; **Med School:** SUNY Stony Brook 1995; **Resid:** Surgery, Johns Hopkins Hosp 2001; **Fellow:** Gastrointestinal Surgery, Johns Hopkins Hosp 2002; Breast Surgery, Northwestern Meml Hosp 2003; **Fac Appt:** Asst Prof S, Univ Pennsylvania

Teperman, Lewis W MD [S] - **Spec Exp:** Transplant-Liver; Transplant-Kidney; Liver Cancer; **Hospital:** NYU Langone Med Ctr (page 79); **Address:** 403 E 34th St Fl 3, Transplant Assocs, New York, NY 10016; **Phone:** 212-263-8134; **Board Cert:** Surgery 2007; **Med School:** Mount Sinai Sch Med 1981; **Resid:** Surgery, Columbia Presby Med Ctr 1984; Surgery, LI Jewish Med Ctr 1986; **Fellow:** Transplant Surgery, Univ Pittsburgh 1988; **Fac Appt:** Assoc Prof S, NYU Sch Med

Surgery

Tsangaris, Theodore N MD [S] - **Spec Exp:** Breast Cancer; **Hospital:** Johns Hopkins Hosp; **Address:** Johns Hopkins Hospital, 600 N Wolfe St, Carnegie 686, Baltimore, MD 21287; **Phone:** 410-955-2615; **Board Cert:** Surgery 2005; **Med School:** Geo Wash Univ 1983; **Resid:** Surgery, Geo Washington Univ Med Ctr 1989; **Fellow:** Surgical Oncology, Baylor Univ Med Ctr 1990; **Fac Appt:** Assoc Prof S, Johns Hopkins Univ

Van Zee, Kimberly J MD [S] - **Spec Exp:** Breast Cancer; **Hospital:** Meml Sloan-Kettering Cancer Ctr (page 75); **Address:** Meml Sloan Kettering Cancer Ctr, Evelyn H Lauder Breast Center, 300 E 66th St, New York, NY 10065; **Phone:** 800-525-2225; **Board Cert:** Surgery 2003; **Med School:** Harvard Med Sch 1987; **Resid:** Surgery, New York Hosp-Cornell 1990; Surgery, New York Hosp-Cornell 1994; **Fellow:** Research, New York Hosp-Cornell 1993; **Fac Appt:** Prof S, Cornell Univ-Weill Med Coll

Willey, Shawna C MD [S] - **Spec Exp:** Breast Cancer; Clinical Trials; **Hospital:** Georgetown Univ Hosp; **Address:** 3800 Reservoir Rd NW, PHC Bldg Fl 4, Washington, DC 20007; **Phone:** 202-444-0241; **Board Cert:** Surgery 2009; **Med School:** Univ Iowa Coll Med 1982; **Resid:** Surgery, George Washington Univ Med Ctr 1988; **Fac Appt:** Asst Prof S, Georgetown Univ

Yang, James C MD [S] - **Spec Exp:** Kidney Cancer; Kidney Cancer Clinical Trials; Clinical Trials; Immunotherapy; **Hospital:** Natl Inst of Hlth - Clin Ctr; **Address:** National Cancer Inst, 9000 Rockville Pike CRC Bldg - rm 3-5952, Bethesda, MD 20892; **Phone:** 301-496-1574; **Board Cert:** Surgery 2005; **Med School:** UCSD 1978; **Resid:** Surgery, UCSD Med Ctr 1984; **Fellow:** Surgical Oncology, Natl Cancer Inst 1986

Yeo, Charles J MD [S] - **Spec Exp:** Pancreatic Cancer; Biliary Cancer; Gastrointestinal Surgery; Pancreatic Endocrine Tumors; **Hospital:** Thomas Jefferson Univ Hosp (page 81); **Address:** 1015 Walnut St, Ste 620, Philadelphia, PA 19107; **Phone:** 215-955-9402; **Board Cert:** Surgery 2005; **Med School:** Johns Hopkins Univ 1979; **Resid:** Surgery, Johns Hopkins Hosp 1985; **Fellow:** Research, SUNY Downstate 1982; **Fac Appt:** Prof S, Thomas Jefferson Univ

Southeast

Adams, Reid B MD [S] - **Spec Exp:** Hepatobiliary Surgery; Liver Cancer; Pancreatic & Biliary Surgery; **Hospital:** Univ of Virginia Health Sys; **Address:** UVA Health System, Dept Surgery, PO Box 800709, Charlottesville, VA 22908; **Phone:** 434-924-2839; **Board Cert:** Surgery 2003; **Med School:** Univ VA Sch Med 1987; **Resid:** Surgery, Univ Va Hlth Sci Ctr 1994; **Fellow:** Hepatopancreatobiliary Surgery, Univ Toronto Med Ctr 1995; **Fac Appt:** Assoc Prof S, Univ VA Sch Med

Bear, Harry D MD/PhD [S] - **Spec Exp:** Breast Cancer; Melanoma; Gastrointestinal Cancer; **Hospital:** Med Coll of VA Hosp; **Address:** Med Coll Virginia - VCU, PO Box 980011, Richmond, VA 23298; **Phone:** 804-828-9325; **Board Cert:** Surgery 2003; **Med School:** Med Coll VA 1975; **Resid:** Surgery, Brigham & Women's Hosp 1983; **Fellow:** Surgical Oncology, Med Coll Virgina 1984; **Fac Appt:** Prof Surg & Onc, Med Coll VA

Beauchamp, Robert D MD [S] - **Spec Exp:** Esophageal Cancer; Colon & Rectal Cancer; Gastrointestinal Cancer; Breast Cancer; **Hospital:** Vanderbilt Univ Med Ctr, TN Valley Healthcare Sys-Nashville; **Address:** Vanderbilt Dept Surgery, Medical Center North D-4316, 1161 21st Ave S, Nashville, TN 37232-2730; **Phone:** 615-322-2363; **Board Cert:** Surgery 2007; **Med School:** Univ Tex Med Br, Galveston 1982; **Resid:** Surgery, Univ Tex Med Br 1987; **Fellow:** Cellular Molecular Biology, Vanderbilt Univ 1989; **Fac Appt:** Prof S, Vanderbilt Univ

Behrns, Kevin E MD [S] - **Spec Exp:** Pancreatic Cancer; Gastrointestinal Cancer & Surgery; **Hospital:** Shands at Univ of FL; **Address:** Shands Healthcare at Univ Florida, PO Box 100109, Gainesville, FL 32610-0109; **Phone:** 352-265-0604; **Board Cert:** Surgery 2005; **Med School:** Mayo Med Sch 1988; **Resid:** Surgery, Mayo Clinic 1995; **Fac Appt:** Prof S, Univ Fla Coll Med

Bland, Kirby MD [S] - **Spec Exp:** Breast Cancer; Colon Cancer; Thyroid & Parathyroid Cancer & Surgery; **Hospital:** Univ of Ala Hosp at Birmingham; **Address:** UAB, Dept Surgery, 1530 3rd Ave S, BDB 502, Birmingham, AL 35294-0002; **Phone:** 205-975-2193; **Board Cert:** Surgery 2000; **Med School:** Univ Alabama 1968; **Resid:** Surgery, Univ Fla Hosp 1970; Surgery, Univ Fla Hosp 1976; **Fellow:** Surgical Oncology, MD Anderson Cancer Ctr 1977; **Fac Appt:** Prof S, Univ Alabama

Calvo, Benjamin MD [S] - **Spec Exp:** Colon Cancer; Endocrine Cancers; Breast Cancer; **Hospital:** NC Memorial Hosp - UNC; **Address:** UNC, Dept of Surgery, 170 Manning Drive, 1150 POB, CB #7213, Chapel Hill, NC 27599; **Phone:** 919-966-5221; **Board Cert:** Surgery 1999; **Med School:** Univ MD Sch Med 1981; **Resid:** Surgery, George Washington Univ Hosp 1988; Surgery, Natl Inst Hlth 1991; **Fellow:** Surgery, Meml Sloan Kettering Cancer Ctr 1993; **Fac Appt:** Assoc Prof S, Univ NC Sch Med

Chari, Ravi S MD [S] - **Spec Exp:** Liver Cancer; Biliary Cancer; Transplant-Liver; **Hospital:** Centennial Med Ctr; **Address:** Centennial Med Ctr, 2300 Patterson St, Nashville, TN 37203; **Phone:** 615-342-1050; **Board Cert:** Surgery 2005; **Med School:** Canada 1989; **Resid:** Surgery, Duke Univ Med Ctr 1996; **Fellow:** Transplant Surgery, Univ Toronto-Toronto Hosp 1998; **Fac Appt:** Prof S, Vanderbilt Univ

Cole, David J MD [S] - **Spec Exp:** Breast Brachytherapy; Gastrointestinal Cancer; Vaccine Therapy; Gene Therapy; **Hospital:** MUSC Med Ctr; **Address:** 96 Jonathan Lucas St, MSC 613 /CSB 420, Charleston, SC 29425; **Phone:** 843-792-4638; **Board Cert:** Surgery 2000; **Med School:** Cornell Univ-Weill Med Coll 1986; **Resid:** Surgery, Emory Univ Affil Hosp 1991; **Fellow:** Surgical Oncology, Natl Cancer Institute 1994; **Fac Appt:** Prof S, Med Univ SC

Daneker, George W MD/PhD [S] - **Spec Exp:** Gastrointestinal Surgery; Cancer Surgery; Melanoma; Laparoscopic Surgery; **Hospital:** St. Joseph's Hosp - Atlanta, Northside Hosp; **Address:** 5673 Peachtree Dunwoody Rd, Ste 300, Atlanta, GA 30342; **Phone:** 404-252-6118; **Board Cert:** Surgery 2002; **Med School:** Univ MD Sch Med 1983; **Resid:** Surgery, Univ Cincinnati Med Ctr 1990; **Fellow:** Cancer Research, New Engl Deaconess Med Ctr 1988; Surgical Oncology, UT MD Anderson Cancer Ctr 1992

Eason, James D MD [S] - **Spec Exp:** Transplant-Kidney; Transplant-Pancreas & Liver; Liver Cancer; **Hospital:** Methodist Univ Hosp - Memphis; **Address:** Transplant Inst, 1265 Union Ave, rm S1011, Memphis, TN 38104; **Phone:** 901-516-7469; **Board Cert:** Surgery 2002; **Med School:** Univ Tenn Coll Med 1987; **Resid:** Surgery, Wilford Hall USAF Med Ctr 1992; **Fellow:** Transplant Surgery, Mass Genl Hosp 1994; **Fac Appt:** Prof S, Univ Tenn Coll Med

Flynn, Michael B MD [S] - **Spec Exp:** Head & Neck Cancer; Head & Neck Surgery; Thyroid & Parathyroid Surgery; **Hospital:** Univ of Louisville Hosp, Norton Hosp; **Address:** 401 E Chestnut St, Ste 710, Louisville, KY 40202; **Phone:** 502-583-8303; **Board Cert:** Surgery 1972; **Med School:** Ireland 1962; **Resid:** Surgery, Univ Maryland Hosp 1969; **Fellow:** Surgical Oncology, MD Anderson Hosp 1970; Head and Neck Surgery, MD Anderson Hosp 1971; **Fac Appt:** Prof S, Univ Louisville Sch Med

Gabram, Sheryl G A MD [S] - **Spec Exp:** Breast Cancer; Breast Cancer-High Risk Women; **Hospital:** Emory Univ Hosp, Grady Hlth Sys; **Address:** Winship Cancer Institute, 1365 Clifton Rd NE C Bldg Fl 2, Atlanta, GA 30322; **Phone:** 404-778-1230; **Board Cert:** Surgery 2006; **Med School:** Georgetown Univ 1982; **Resid:** Surgery, Washington Hosp Ctr 1987; **Fellow:** Trauma, Hartford Hosp 1988; **Fac Appt:** Prof S, Emory Univ

Greene, Frederick L MD [S] - **Spec Exp:** Gastrointestinal Surgery; Gastrointestinal Cancer; **Hospital:** Carolinas Med Ctr; **Address:** Carolinas Medical Ctr, 1025 Morehead Medical Drive, Ste 300, Charlotte, NC 28204; **Phone:** 704-355-1813; **Board Cert:** Surgery 2009; **Med School:** Univ VA Sch Med 1970; **Resid:** Surgery, Yale-New Haven Hosp 1976; **Fellow:** Surgical Oncology, Yale-New Haven Hosp 1973; **Fac Appt:** Prof S, Univ NC Sch Med

Hanks, John B MD [S] - **Spec Exp:** Endocrine Cancers; Breast Cancer; Thyroid Cancer & Surgery; **Hospital:** Univ of Virginia Health Sys; **Address:** Univ VA Hlth Sys, Dept Surgery, PO Box 800709, Charlottesville, VA 22908-0709; **Phone:** 434-924-0376; **Board Cert:** Surgery 2001; **Med School:** Univ Rochester 1973; **Resid:** Surgery, Duke Univ Med Ctr 1982; **Fac Appt:** Prof S, Univ VA Sch Med

Herrmann, Virginia M MD [S] - **Spec Exp:** Breast Cancer; Nutrition & Cancer Prevention/Control; **Hospital:** Hilton Head Reg Med Ctr, MUSC Med Ctr; **Address:** Hilton Head Reg Med Ctr, 25 Hospital Center Blvd, Ste 300, Hilton Head Isl, SC 29926; **Phone:** 843-682-7377; **Board Cert:** Surgery 2009; **Med School:** St Louis Univ 1974; **Resid:** Surgery, St Louis Univ Hosps 1979; **Fellow:** Surgery, Brigham & Women's Hosp 1980; **Fac Appt:** Prof S, Med Univ SC

Heslin, Martin J MD [S] - **Spec Exp:** Gastrointestinal Cancer; Pancreatic Cancer; Biliary Cancer; Sarcoma-Soft Tissue; **Hospital:** Univ of Ala Hosp at Birmingham; **Address:** Univ Alabama, 1922 7th Ave S, Ste 321, Birmingham, AL 35294-0016; **Phone:** 205-934-3064; **Board Cert:** Surgery 2006; **Med School:** SUNY Upstate Med Univ 1987; **Resid:** Surgery, NYU Med Ctr 1994; Surgery, Meml Sloan-Kettering Canc Ctr 1991; **Fellow:** Surgical Oncology, Meml Sloan-Kettering Cancer Ctr 1996; **Fac Appt:** Prof S, Univ Alabama

Kelley, Mark C MD [S] - **Spec Exp:** Breast Cancer; Melanoma; **Hospital:** Vanderbilt Univ Med Ctr, TN Valley Healthcare Sys-Nashville; **Address:** Vanderbilt Div Surgical Oncology, 2220 Pierce Ave, 597 Preston Rsch Bldg, Nashville, TN 37232-6860; **Phone:** 615-322-2391; **Board Cert:** Surgery 2005; **Med School:** Univ Fla Coll Med 1989; **Resid:** Surgery, Shands Hosp 1995; **Fellow:** Surgical Oncology, John Wayne Cancer Inst 1997; **Fac Appt:** Assoc Prof S, Vanderbilt Univ

Krontiras, Helen MD [S] - **Spec Exp:** Breast Cancer; **Hospital:** Univ of Ala Hosp at Birmingham; **Address:** The Kirklin Clinic, 2000 6th Ave S, Birmingham, AL 35233; **Phone:** 205-801-8266; **Board Cert:** Surgery 2010; **Med School:** Univ Alabama 1991; **Resid:** Surgery, Univ AL Hosp 2000; **Fellow:** Surgical Oncology, Northwestern Univ Med Ctr 2001; **Fac Appt:** Assoc Prof S, Univ Alabama

Levi, Joe U MD [S] - **Spec Exp:** Pancreatic Cancer; Liver Cancer; Biliary Surgery; **Hospital:** Jackson Meml Hosp (page 82), Univ of Miami Hosp & Clins/Sylvester Comp Canc Ctr (page 82); **Address:** 1120 NW 14th St, M875, Clinical Research Bldg, Miami, FL 33136; **Phone:** 305-243-4211; **Board Cert:** Surgery 1975; **Med School:** Univ Fla Coll Med 1967; **Resid:** Surgery, Johns Hopkins Hosp 1969; Surgery, Jackson Meml Hosp 1974; **Fac Appt:** Prof S, Univ Miami Sch Med

Levine, Edward A MD [S] - **Spec Exp:** Breast Cancer; Esophageal Cancer; Peritoneal Carcinomatosis; Sarcoma; **Hospital:** Wake Forest Univ Baptist Med Ctr; **Address:** Wake Forest Univ Baptist Med Ctr, Dept Surgery, Med Ctr Blvd Fl 5, Winston-Salem, NC 27157; **Phone:** 336-716-4276; **Board Cert:** Surgery 1999; **Med School:** Ros Franklin Univ/Chicago Med Sch 1985; **Resid:** Surgery, Michael Reese Hosp 1990; **Fellow:** Surgical Oncology, Univ Illinois 1992; **Fac Appt:** Prof S, Wake Forest Univ

Lind, David S MD [S] - **Spec Exp:** Breast Cancer; Melanoma; Sarcoma; **Hospital:** Med Coll of GA Hosp and Clin (MCG Health Inc); **Address:** MCG Health, Div Surgical Oncology, 1120 15th St, Augusta, GA 30912; **Phone:** 706-721-6744; **Board Cert:** Surgery 2000; **Med School:** Eastern VA Med Sch 1984; **Resid:** Surgery, Univ Texas Affil Hosp 1989; **Fellow:** Medical Oncology, Med Coll Virginia 1992; **Fac Appt:** Prof S, Med Coll GA

Livingstone, Alan S MD [S] - **Spec Exp:** Liver & Biliary Cancer; Stomach Cancer; Esophageal Cancer; Pancreatic Cancer; **Hospital:** Jackson Meml Hosp (page 82), Univ of Miami Hosp & Clins/Sylvester Comp Canc Ctr (page 82); **Address:** 1150 NW 14th St Fl 4, Miami, FL 33136; **Phone:** 305-243-4902; **Board Cert:** Surgery 2007; **Med School:** McGill Univ 1971; **Resid:** Surgery, Montreal Genl Hosp 1976; Surgery, Jackson Meml Hosp 1975; **Fac Appt:** Prof S, Univ Miami Sch Med

Lyerly, H Kim MD [S] - **Spec Exp:** Breast Cancer; Immunotherapy; **Hospital:** Duke Univ Hosp, Durham Regional Hosp; **Address:** Duke Comprehensive Cancer Center, DUMC Box 2714, Durham, NC 27710; **Phone:** 919-684-5613; **Board Cert:** Surgery 2001; **Med School:** UCLA 1983; **Resid:** Surgery, Duke Univ Med Ctr 1990; **Fac Appt:** Prof S, Duke Univ

McGrath, Patrick C MD [S] - **Spec Exp:** Breast Cancer; Cancer Surgery; **Hospital:** Univ of Kentucky Albert B. Chandler Hosp; **Address:** Univ Kentucky Hospital, Dept General Surgery, 800 Rose St, rm C224, Lexington, KY 40536-0293; **Phone:** 859-323-6346 x240; **Board Cert:** Surgery 2008; **Med School:** Univ IL Coll Med 1980; **Resid:** Surgery, Med Coll Virginia Hosp 1986; **Fellow:** Surgical Oncology, Med Coll Virginia Hosp 1988; **Fac Appt:** Prof S, Univ KY Coll Med

McMasters, Kelly M MD [S] - **Spec Exp:** Melanoma; Breast Cancer; Liver Cancer; **Hospital:** Univ of Louisville Hosp; **Address:** 401 S Chestnut St, Ste 710, Louisville, KY 40202; **Phone:** 502-583-8303; **Board Cert:** Surgery 2005; **Med School:** UMDNJ-RW Johnson Med Sch 1989; **Resid:** Surgery, Univ Louisville Sch Med 1994; **Fellow:** Surgical Oncology, Texas-MD Anderson Cancer Ctr 1995; **Fac Appt:** Prof S, Univ Louisville Sch Med

Neifeld, James P MD [S] - **Spec Exp:** Melanoma; Head & Neck Cancer; Gastrointestinal Cancer; Cancers-Rare & Unusual; **Hospital:** Med Coll of VA Hosp; **Address:** Medical College Virginia Hosp, PO Box 980645, Richmond, VA 23298-0645; **Phone:** 804-828-9324; **Board Cert:** Surgery 2008; **Med School:** Med Coll VA 1972; **Resid:** Surgery, Med Coll Va Hosps 1978; **Fac Appt:** Prof S, Va Commonwealth Univ Sch Med

Olson, John A MD [S] - **Spec Exp:** Endocrine Cancers; Breast Cancer; Melanoma; Clinical Trials; **Hospital:** Duke Univ Hosp; **Address:** Duke Univ Med Ctr, Box 2945, Durham, NC 27710; **Phone:** 919-684-6849; **Board Cert:** Surgery 2009; **Med School:** Univ Fla Coll Med 1992; **Resid:** Surgery, Barnes Hospital/Wash Univ 1998; **Fellow:** Endocrine Surgery, Royal Infirmary 1997; Surgical Oncology, Meml Sloan-Kettering Cancer Ctr 2000; **Fac Appt:** Assoc Prof S, Duke Univ

Pappas, Theodore N MD [S] - **Spec Exp:** Pancreatic Surgery; Laparoscopic Surgery; **Hospital:** Duke Univ Hosp; **Address:** Duke Univ Med Ctr, Dept Surgery, DUMC Box 3479, Durham, NC 27710; **Phone:** 919-681-3442; **Board Cert:** Surgery 1997; **Med School:** Ohio State Univ 1981; **Resid:** Surgery, Brigham & Womens Hosp 1988; **Fellow:** Research, Wadworth VA Med Ctr 1985; **Fac Appt:** Prof S, Duke Univ

Pinson, C Wright MD [S] - **Spec Exp:** Transplant-Liver; Liver & Biliary Cancer; Pancreatic Cancer; **Hospital:** Vanderbilt Univ Med Ctr; **Address:** Vanderbilt Univ Med Ctr, TVC 3810A, 1301 Med Center Drive, Nashville, TN 37232-5545; **Phone:** 615-343-9324; **Board Cert:** Surgery 2007; Surgical Critical Care 2007; **Med School:** Vanderbilt Univ 1980; **Resid:** Surgery, Oregon Health Sci Ctr 1986; **Fellow:** Gastrointestinal Surgery, Lahey Clinic 1987; Transplant Surgery, Deaconess Hosp 1988; **Fac Appt:** Prof S, Vanderbilt Univ

Roh, Mark S MD [S] - **Spec Exp:** Liver Cancer; Cancer Surgery; **Hospital:** MD Anderson Cancer Ctr-Orlando; **Address:** 1400 S Orange Ave, MP 760, Orlando, FL 32806; **Phone:** 321-841-5134; **Board Cert:** Surgery 2006; **Med School:** Ohio State Univ 1979; **Resid:** Surgery, Univ Pittsburgh Med Ctr 1982; Surgery, Univ Pittsburgh Med Ctr 1986; **Fellow:** Surgical Oncology, Meml Sloan-Kettering Cancer Ctr 1984; Surgical Oncology, Meml Sloan-Kettering Cancer Ctr 1987; **Fac Appt:** Prof S, Drexel Univ Coll Med

Rosemurgy, Alexander S MD [S] - **Spec Exp:** Pancreatic Cancer; Gastrointestinal Surgery; Minimally Invasive Surgery; **Hospital:** Tampa Genl Hosp; **Address:** Digestive Disorders Ctr, Tampa General Hospital, 2 Columbia Drive, rm F145, Tampa, FL 33601; **Phone:** 813-844-7393; **Board Cert:** Surgery 2005; **Med School:** Univ Mich Med Sch 1979; **Resid:** Surgery, Univ Chicago Hosps 1984; **Fac Appt:** Prof S, Univ S Fla Coll Med

Salo, Jonathan C MD [S] - **Spec Exp:** Gastrointestinal Cancer; Esophageal Cancer; **Hospital:** Carolinas Med Ctr; **Address:** Blumenthal Cancer Center, PO Box 32861, Charlotte, NC 28203; **Phone:** 704-355-2884; **Board Cert:** Surgery 2005; **Med School:** UCSF 1981; **Resid:** Surgery, UCSF Med Ctr 1993; **Fellow:** Surgical Oncology, Natl Cancer Inst 1991; Surgical Oncology, Meml Sloan-Kettering Cancer Ctr 1998; **Fac Appt:** Asst Prof S, Univ NC Sch Med

Shen, Perry MD [S] - **Spec Exp:** Liver & Biliary Cancer; Pancreatic Cancer; Gastrointestinal Cancer; Melanoma; **Hospital:** Wake Forest Univ Baptist Med Ctr; **Address:** Wake Forest Univ Baptist Med Ctr, Dept Surgery, Medical Center Blvd Fl 5, Winston-Salem, NC 27157; **Phone:** 336-716-0545; **Board Cert:** Surgery 2008; **Med School:** USC Sch Med 1992; **Resid:** Surgery, LAC-USC Med Ctr 1998; **Fellow:** Surgical Oncology, John Wayne Cancer Inst 2000; **Fac Appt:** Assoc Prof S, Wake Forest Univ

Slingluff Jr, Craig L MD [S] - **Spec Exp:** Melanoma; Immunotherapy; **Hospital:** Univ of Virginia Health Sys; **Address:** UVA Health System, Dept Surgery, PO Box 800709, Charlottesville, VA 22908; **Phone:** 434-924-1730; **Board Cert:** Surgery 2002; **Med School:** Univ VA Sch Med 1984; **Resid:** Surgery, Duke Univ Med Ctr 1991; **Fellow:** Surgical Research, Duke Univ Med Ctr 1992; **Fac Appt:** Prof S, Univ VA Sch Med

Solorzano, Carmen C MD [S] - **Spec Exp:** Endocrine Cancers; Minimally Invasive Surgery; Thyroid & Parathyroid Cancer & Surgery; Adrenal Cancer; **Hospital:** Vanderbilt Univ Med Ctr; **Address:** 2220 Pierce Ave PRB Bldg Fl 5 - Ste 97, Ave, Nashville, TN 37232; **Phone:** 615-322-2391; **Board Cert:** Surgery 2009; **Med School:** Univ Fla Coll Med 1993; **Resid:** Surgery, Univ Florida Affil Hosp 1999; **Fellow:** Surgical Oncology, UT MD Anderson Cancer Ctr 2002; **Fac Appt:** Assoc Prof S, Vanderbilt Univ

Sondak, Vernon K MD [S] - **Spec Exp:** Cancer Surgery; Melanoma; Sarcoma; **Hospital:** H Lee Moffitt Cancer Ctr & Research Inst; **Address:** H Lee Moffitt Cancer Ctr, Cutaneous Program, 12902 Magnolia Drive, Tampa, FL 33612; **Phone:** 813-745-1968; **Board Cert:** Surgery 2008; **Med School:** Boston Univ 1980; **Resid:** Surgery, UCLA Med Ctr 1987; **Fellow:** Surgical Oncology, UCLA Med Ctr 1984; **Fac Appt:** Prof S, Univ S Fla Coll Med

Staley, Charles A MD [S] - **Spec Exp:** Gastrointestinal Cancer & Rare Tumors; Pancreatic Cancer; Liver & Biliary Cancer; **Hospital:** Emory Univ Hosp; **Address:** Emory - Winship Cancer Inst, 1365 Clifton Rd NE, C Bldg Fl 2, Atlanta, GA 30322; **Phone:** 404-778-3307; **Board Cert:** Surgery 2001; **Med School:** Dartmouth Med Sch 1987; **Resid:** Surgery, Univ Pittsburgh Med Ctr 1992; **Fellow:** Surgical Oncology, MD Anderson Cancer Ctr 1995; **Fac Appt:** Prof S, Emory Univ

Tyler, Douglas S MD [S] - **Spec Exp:** Pancreatic Cancer; Colon & Rectal Cancer; Rectal Cancer/Sphincter Preservation; Melanoma; **Hospital:** Duke Univ Hosp, Durham VA Med Ctr; **Address:** Duke University Med Ctr, Box 3118, Durham, NC 27710; **Phone:** 919-684-6858; **Board Cert:** Surgery 2010; **Med School:** Dartmouth Med Sch 1985; **Resid:** Surgery, Duke Univ Med Ctr 1992; **Fellow:** Surgical Oncology, MD Anderson Cancer Ctr 1994; **Fac Appt:** Prof S, Duke Univ

Urist, Marshall M MD [S] - **Spec Exp:** Cancer Surgery; Breast Cancer; Melanoma; **Hospital:** Univ of Ala Hosp at Birmingham; **Address:** Univ Alabama Sch Med, Dept Surgery, 1922 7th Ave S, Kracke Bldg, Ste 321, Birmingham, AL 35294; **Phone:** 205-934-3065; **Board Cert:** Surgery 2000; **Med School:** Univ Chicago-Pritzker Sch Med 1971; **Resid:** Surgery, Johns Hopkins Hosp 1978; **Fellow:** Surgical Oncology, UCLA Med Ctr 1976; **Fac Appt:** Prof S, Univ Alabama

White Jr, Richard L MD [S] - **Spec Exp:** Breast Cancer; Melanoma; Sarcoma; Immunotherapy; **Hospital:** Carolinas Med Ctr; **Address:** Carolinas Medical Center, 1000 Blythe Blvd, Box 32861, Charlotte, NC 28203; **Phone:** 704-355-2884; **Board Cert:** Surgery 2002; **Med School:** Columbia P&S 1986; **Resid:** Surgery, Georgetown Univ Hosp 1992; **Fellow:** Surgical Oncology, NIH-Natl Cancer Inst 1995; **Fac Appt:** Clin Prof S, Univ NC Sch Med

Whitworth, Pat W MD [S] - **Spec Exp:** Breast Cancer; **Hospital:** Baptist Hosp - Nashville, Centennial Med Ctr; **Address:** 300 20th Ave N, Ste 401, Nashville, TN 37203; **Phone:** 615-620-5535; **Board Cert:** Surgery 2009; **Med School:** Univ Tenn Coll Med 1983; **Resid:** Surgery, Univ Louisville Med Ctr 1988; **Fellow:** Surgical Oncology, MD Anderson Cancer Ctr 1991; **Fac Appt:** Assoc Clin Prof S, Vanderbilt Univ

Wood, William C MD [S] - **Spec Exp:** Breast Cancer; **Hospital:** Emory Univ Hosp; **Address:** Winship Cancer Institute, 1365C Clifton Rd NE, Ste B206, Atlanta, GA 30322; **Phone:** 404-778-3301; **Board Cert:** Surgery 1974; **Med School:** Harvard Med Sch 1966; **Resid:** Surgery, Mass Genl Hosp 1968; Surgery, Mass Genl Hosp 1974; **Fellow:** Surgical Oncology, Natl Cancer Inst 1970; **Fac Appt:** Prof S, Emory Univ

Yeatman, Timothy J MD [S] - **Spec Exp:** Liver Cancer; **Hospital:** H Lee Moffitt Cancer Ctr & Research Inst; **Address:** H Lee Moffitt Cancer Ctr, 12902 Magnolia Drive, Tampa, FL 33612-9497; **Phone:** 813-979-7292; **Board Cert:** Surgery 2000; **Med School:** Emory Univ 1984; **Resid:** Surgery, Univ Florida 1990; **Fellow:** Surgical Oncology, MD Anderson Cancer Ctr 1992; **Fac Appt:** Prof S, Univ S Fla Coll Med

Midwest

Abouljoud, Marwan S MD [S] - **Spec Exp:** Transplant-Liver; Liver Cancer; **Hospital:** Henry Ford Hosp; **Address:** Henry Ford Hospital, 2799 W Grand Blvd, CFP2, Detroit, MI 48202; **Phone:** 313-916-2941; **Board Cert:** Surgery 2002; **Med School:** Lebanon 1985; **Resid:** Surgery, Univ of Mich igan Med Ctr 1988; Surgery, Henry Ford Hosp 1992; **Fellow:** Transplant Surgery, Univ Alabama 1994; Transplant Surgery, Baylor Univ Med Ctr 1996; **Fac Appt:** Prof S, Wayne State Univ

Angelos, Peter MD/PhD [S] - **Spec Exp:** Thyroid & Parathyroid Cancer & Surgery; Adrenal Tumors; Ethics; **Hospital:** Univ of Chicago Med Ctr; **Address:** 5841 S Maryland Ave, MS 4052, Chicago, IL 60637; **Phone:** 773-702-4429; **Board Cert:** Surgery 2004; **Med School:** Boston Univ 1989; **Resid:** Surgery, Northwestern Univ 1995; **Fellow:** Medical Ethics, Univ of Chicago Hosps 1992; Endocrine Surgery, Univ of Michigan Med Sch 1996; **Fac Appt:** Prof S, Univ Chicago-Pritzker Sch Med

Surgery

Aranha, Gerard V MD [S] - **Spec Exp:** Pancreatic & Biliary Surgery; Stomach Cancer; Esophageal Cancer; **Hospital:** Loyola Univ Med Ctr, Edward Hines, Jr. VA Hosp; **Address:** 2160 S first Ave, Bldg 110, rm 3236, Maywood, IL 60153-3328; **Phone:** 708-327-2391; **Board Cert:** Surgery 2006; **Med School:** India 1969; **Resid:** Surgery, Loyola Univ Med Ctr 1975; **Fellow:** Surgical Oncology, Univ Minn Hosp 1977; **Fac Appt:** Prof S, Loyola Univ-Stritch Sch Med

Averbook, Bruce J MD [S] - **Spec Exp:** Melanoma; Cancer Surgery; Clinical Trials; **Hospital:** MetroHealth Med Ctr; **Address:** Metrohealth Medical Ctr, Surgical Oncology, 2500 Metrohealth Drive, rm C2110, Cleveland, OH 44109; **Phone:** 216-778-4795; **Board Cert:** Surgery 2000; **Med School:** Geo Wash Univ 1983; **Resid:** Surgery, UC Irvine Med Ctr 1990; **Fellow:** Surgical Oncology, NCI, NIH Surg Br 1993; **Fac Appt:** Assoc Prof S, Case West Res Univ

Brems, John J MD [S] - **Spec Exp:** Pancreatic Cancer; Liver Cancer; Transplant-Liver; Colon Cancer; **Hospital:** Sherman Hosp; **Address:** 745 Fletcher Drive, Ste 302, Elgin, IL 60123; **Phone:** 847-695-6600; **Board Cert:** Surgery 2004; Surgical Critical Care 2000; **Med School:** St Louis Univ 1981; **Resid:** Surgery, St Louis Univ 1986; **Fellow:** Transplant Surgery, UCLA Med Ctr 1987; **Fac Appt:** Prof S, Loyola Univ-Stritch Sch Med

Brown, Charles K MD [S] - **Spec Exp:** Melanoma; Sarcoma; **Hospital:** CTCA at Midwestern Reg Med Ctr; **Address:** Cancer Treatments Ctrs America, 2520 Elishe Ave, Zion, IL 60099; **Phone:** 800-955-2822; **Board Cert:** Surgery 2000; **Med School:** Univ Fla Coll Med 1992; **Resid:** Surgery, Univ Arizona Med Ctr 1998; **Fellow:** Surgical Oncology, UPMC Med Ctr 1999; Surgical Oncology, Univ Chicago Med Ctr 2000

Brunt, L Michael MD [S] - **Spec Exp:** Minimally Invasive Surgery; Adrenal Tumors; **Hospital:** Barnes-Jewish Hosp; **Address:** Washington Univ Sch Med, Dept Surgery, 660 S Euclid Ave, Box 8109, St Louis, MO 63110; **Phone:** 314-454-7194 x2; **Board Cert:** Surgery 2006; **Med School:** Johns Hopkins Univ 1980; **Resid:** Surgery, Barnes Jewish Hosp 1987; **Fellow:** Surgery, Barnes Jewish Hosp 1984; **Fac Appt:** Prof S, Washington Univ, St Louis

Chang, Alfred E MD [S] - **Spec Exp:** Cancer Surgery; Breast Cancer; Gastrointestinal Cancer; Melanoma; **Hospital:** Univ of Michigan Hosp; **Address:** 1500 E Medical Center Drive, 3302 Cancer Geriatric Ctr SPC 5932, Ann Arbor, MI 48109-5932; **Phone:** 734-936-4392; **Board Cert:** Surgery 2001; **Med School:** Harvard Med Sch 1974; **Resid:** Surgery, Duke Univ Med Ctr 1976; Surgery, Hosp Univ Penn 1982; **Fellow:** Surgical Oncology, Natl Cancer Inst 1979; **Fac Appt:** Prof S, Univ Mich Med Sch

Chapman, William C MD [S] - **Spec Exp:** Transplant-Liver-Adult & Pediatric; Liver Cancer; Liver & Biliary Surgery; **Hospital:** Barnes-Jewish Hosp, St. Louis Chldns Hosp; **Address:** Washington Univ Sch Med, 660 S Euclid Ave, Box 8109, St Louis, MO 63110; **Phone:** 314-362-7792; **Board Cert:** Surgery 2001; Surgical Critical Care 2001; **Med School:** Med Univ SC 1984; **Resid:** Surgery, Vanderbilt Univ Med Ctr 1991; **Fellow:** Hepatobiliary Surgery, Kings College Hosp 1992; **Fac Appt:** Prof S, Washington Univ, St Louis

Crowe Jr, Joseph P MD [S] - **Spec Exp:** Breast Cancer; Tumor Surgery; **Hospital:** Cleveland Clin (page 70); **Address:** Cleveland Clinic Fdn, Dept Surg, 9500 Euclid Ave, Desk A10, Cleveland, OH 44195; **Phone:** 216-444-3024; **Board Cert:** Surgery 2004; **Med School:** Case West Res Univ 1978; **Resid:** Surgery, Univ Hosp-Case West Reserve 1983; **Fellow:** Surgical Oncology, Meml Sloan Kettering Cancer Ctr 1985

Donohue, John H MD [S] - **Spec Exp:** Gastrointestinal Cancer; Breast Cancer; Stomach Cancer; **Hospital:** Mayo Med Ctr & Clin - Rochester; **Address:** Mayo Clinic, Dept General Surgery, 200 First St SW, Rochester, MN 55905; **Phone:** 507-284-0362; **Board Cert:** Surgery 2005; **Med School:** Harvard Med Sch 1978; **Resid:** Surgery, UCSF Med Ctr 1981; Surgery, UCSF Med Ctr 1985; **Fellow:** Surgery, Natl Inst Hlth 1983; Surgical Oncology, Meml Sloan-Kettering Canc Ctr 1987; **Fac Appt:** Prof S, Mayo Med Sch

Eberlein, Timothy J MD [S] - **Spec Exp:** Breast Cancer; Melanoma; Immunotherapy; **Hospital:** Barnes-Jewish Hosp, St. Louis Chldns Hosp; **Address:** Wash Univ School Med, Dept Surgery, 660 S Euclid Ave, Box 8109, St Louis, MO 63110-1093; **Phone:** 314-362-8020; **Board Cert:** Surgery 2006; **Med School:** Univ Pittsburgh 1977; **Resid:** Surgery, Peter Bent Brigham Hosp 1979; Surgery, Brigham-Womens Hosp 1985; **Fellow:** Immunology, Natl Inst Hlth 1982; **Fac Appt:** Prof S, Washington Univ, St Louis

Edwards, Michael J MD [S] - **Spec Exp:** Breast Cancer; Melanoma; **Hospital:** Univ Hosp - Cincinnati; **Address:** 234 Goodman St, ML 0772, Cincinnati, OH 45219; **Phone:** 513-584-8900; **Board Cert:** Surgery 2005; **Med School:** Emory Univ 1981; **Resid:** Surgery, Univ Louisville Hosp 1986; **Fellow:** Surgical Oncology, MD Anderson Cancer Ctr 1987; **Fac Appt:** Prof S, Univ Ark

Ellison, E Christopher MD [S] - **Spec Exp:** Biliary Cancer; Pancreatic Cancer; **Hospital:** Ohio St Univ Med Ctr; **Address:** 1654 Upham Drive, Ste 327 Means Hall, Columbus, OH 43210-1236; **Phone:** 614-293-4499; **Board Cert:** Surgery 2001; **Med School:** Univ Wisc 1976; **Resid:** Surgery, Ohio State Univ 1981; **Fac Appt:** Prof S, Ohio State Univ

Evans, Douglas B MD [S] - **Spec Exp:** Pancreatic Cancer; Thyroid Cancer; Endocrine Cancers; **Hospital:** Froedtert and Med Ctr of WI; **Address:** Medical Coll Wisconsin, Dept Surgery, 9200 W Wisconsin Ave, Ste 3510, Milwaukee, WI 53226-6533; **Phone:** 414-805-5706; **Board Cert:** Surgery 2008; **Med School:** Boston Univ 1983; **Resid:** Surgery, Dartmouth-Hitchcock Med Ctr 1988; **Fellow:** Surgical Oncology, MD Anderson Cancer Ctr 1990; **Fac Appt:** Prof S, Med Coll Wisc

Farrar, William B MD [S] - **Spec Exp:** Breast Cancer; Thyroid Cancer; **Hospital:** Arthur G James Cancer Hosp & Research Inst, Ohio St Univ Med Ctr; **Address:** 410 W 10th Ave, N924 Doan Hall, Columbus, OH 43210-1240; **Phone:** 614-293-8890; **Board Cert:** Surgery 2000; **Med School:** Univ VA Sch Med 1975; **Resid:** Surgery, Ohio State Univ Hosps 1980; **Fellow:** Surgical Oncology, Meml Sloan-Kettering Cancer Ctr 1982; **Fac Appt:** Prof S, Ohio State Univ

Fung, John J MD/PhD [S] - **Spec Exp:** Transplant-Liver; Transplant-Kidney; Liver & Biliary Cancer; **Hospital:** Cleveland Clin (page 70), Euclid Hosp; **Address:** Cleveland Clinic, Dept Surgery, 9500 Euclid Ave, Desk A80, Cleveland, OH 44195-0001; **Phone:** 216-444-3776; **Board Cert:** Surgery 2008; **Med School:** Univ Chicago-Pritzker Sch Med 1982; **Resid:** Surgery, Strong Memorial Hosp 1988; **Fellow:** Transplant Surgery, Univ Pittsburgh 1986; **Fac Appt:** Prof S, Cleveland Cl Coll Med/Case West Res

Goulet Jr, Robert J MD [S] - **Spec Exp:** Breast Cancer; Breast Surgery; **Hospital:** Commun Hosp E - Indianapolis; **Address:** Community Hospital Breast Care, 1400 N Ritter Ave, Ste 485, Indianapolis, IN 46219; **Phone:** 317-355-2727; **Board Cert:** Surgery 2006; **Med School:** SUNY Downstate 1979; **Resid:** Surgery, SUNY-Downstate Med Ctr 1986; **Fellow:** Surgical Research, SUNY-Downstate Med Ctr 1983; **Fac Appt:** Prof S, Indiana Univ

Grant, Clive S S MD [S] - **Spec Exp:** Thyroid & Parathyroid Cancer & Surgery; Adrenal Tumors; Breast Cancer; **Hospital:** Mayo Med Ctr & Clin - Rochester; **Address:** Mayo Clinic, Dept Surgery, 200 First St SW, Rochester, MN 55905-0001; **Phone:** 507-284-2644; **Board Cert:** Surgery 2001; **Med School:** Univ Colorado 1975; **Resid:** Surgery, Mayo Clinic 1980; **Fac Appt:** Prof S, Mayo Med Sch

Hansen, Nora M MD [S] - **Spec Exp:** Sentinel Node Surgery; Breast Cancer-High Risk Women; Breast Cancer Risk Assessment; **Hospital:** Northwestern Meml Hosp; **Address:** Lynn Sage Breast Surgery Ctr, 250 E Superior St Fl 4 - Ste 420, Chicago, IL 60611; **Phone:** 312-695-1156; **Board Cert:** Surgery 2006; **Med School:** NY Med Coll 1988; **Resid:** Surgery, Univ Chicago Hosps 1995; **Fellow:** Surgical Oncology, Univ Chicago Hosps 1996; **Fac Appt:** Assoc Prof S, Northwestern Univ

Hinshaw, Daniel B MD [S] - **Spec Exp:** Palliative Care; **Hospital:** VA Ann Arbor Healthcare Sys, Univ of Michigan Hosp; **Address:** VA Medical Ctr, 2215 Fuller Rd, rm 530, MS 112, Ann Arbor, MI 48105; **Phone:** 734-769-7100 x5939; **Board Cert:** Surgery 2003; Hospice & Palliative Medicine 2008; **Med School:** Loma Linda Univ 1978; **Resid:** Surgery, Loma Linda U Med Ctr 1983; **Fellow:** Immunology, Scripps Clinic Rsch Fdn 1985; Cleveland Clin 2001; **Fac Appt:** Clin Prof S, Univ Mich Med Sch

Howe, James R. MD [S] - **Spec Exp:** Endocrine Surgery; Gastrointestinal Cancer; Colon & Rectal Cancer; **Hospital:** Univ Iowa Hosp & Clinics; **Address:** 200 Hawkins Drive JCP Bldg - rm 4645, Iowa City, IA 52242-1086; **Phone:** 319-356-1727; **Board Cert:** Surgery 2006; **Med School:** Univ VT Coll Med 1987; **Resid:** Surgery, Barnes Hosp-Wash Univ 1994; **Fellow:** Research, Wash Univ-NCI 1991; Surgical Oncology, Meml Sloan Kettering Cancer Ctr 1996; **Fac Appt:** Prof S, Univ Iowa Coll Med

Johnson Miller, Denise L MD [S] - **Spec Exp:** Breast Cancer; Breast Cancer-High Risk Women; Melanoma; **Hospital:** Franciscan St. Francis Hlth-Indianapolis; **Address:** St Francis Breast Specialists, 5255 E Stop 11 Rd, Ste 250, Indianapolis, IN 46237; **Phone:** 317-781-7391; **Board Cert:** Surgery 2001; **Med School:** Washington Univ, St Louis 1978; **Resid:** Surgery, Univ Illinois Med Ctr 1986; Immunology, Univ Texas SW Med Ctr 1982; **Fellow:** Surgical Oncology, City of Hope Med Ctr 1989

Kaufman, Howard L MD [S] - **Spec Exp:** Cancer Surgery; Vaccine Therapy; Melanoma; Immunotherapy; **Hospital:** Rush Univ Med Ctr; **Address:** 1725 W Harrison St, Ste 845, Chicago, IL 60612-3244; **Phone:** 312-942-0600; **Board Cert:** Surgery 2007; **Med School:** Loyola Univ-Stritch Sch Med 1986; **Resid:** Surgery, Boston Univ Hosp 1995; **Fellow:** Surgical Oncology, Natl Cancer Inst 1996; **Fac Appt:** Prof S, Loyola Univ-Stritch Sch Med

Kendrick, Michael L MD [S] - **Spec Exp:** Pancreatic Cancer; Liver Cancer; Hepatobiliary Surgery; Laparoscopic Surgery; **Hospital:** Mayo Med Ctr & Clin - Rochester; **Address:** Mayo Clinic Atten: Dept of Surgery, 200 First St SW, Rochester, MN 55905; **Phone:** 507-284-2511; **Board Cert:** Surgery 2004; **Med School:** Geo Wash Univ 1997; **Resid:** Surgery, Mayo Clinic 2003; **Fellow:** Hepatopancreatobiliary Surgery, Mayo Clinic 2004; Laparoscopic Surgery, Mt Sinai Med Ctr 2005; **Fac Appt:** Assoc Prof S, Mayo Med Sch

Kim, Julian A MD [S] - **Spec Exp:** Melanoma; Breast Cancer; Gastrointestinal Cancer; Immunotherapy; **Hospital:** Univ Hosps Case Med Ctr; **Address:** 11100 Euclid Ave, LKS 5047, Cleveland, OH 44106-1716; **Phone:** 216-844-8247; **Board Cert:** Surgery 2002; **Med School:** Med Univ Ohio at Toledo 1986; **Resid:** Surgery, Univ Maryland Hosps 1991; **Fellow:** Surgical Oncology, Arthur James Cancer Hosp & Rsch Inst 1993; Immunotherapy, Ohio State Univ Comp Cancer Ctr 1994; **Fac Appt:** Assoc Prof S, Case West Res Univ

Leeming, Rosemary A MD [S] - **Spec Exp:** Breast Cancer & Surgery; Clinical Trials; **Hospital:** Univ Hosps Case Med Ctr; **Address:** 3909 Orange Pl, Ste 4400, Orange Village, OH 44122; **Phone:** 216-591-1909; **Board Cert:** Surgery 2009; **Med School:** Hahnemann Univ 1983; **Resid:** Surgery, Mt Sinai Med Ctr 1989; **Fellow:** Breast Disease, Univ Pitts-Shadyside Hosp 1989; **Fac Appt:** Asst Prof S, Case West Res Univ

Mahvi, David M MD [S] - **Spec Exp:** Gastrointestinal Cancer & Surgery; Liver Cancer; Pancreatic Cancer; **Hospital:** Northwestern Meml Hosp; **Address:** NMH/ Arkes Family Pavilion, Ste 650, 676 N St Clair, Chicago, IL 60611; **Phone:** 312-695-1419; **Board Cert:** Surgery 2007; **Med School:** Med Univ SC 1981; **Resid:** Surgery, Duke Univ Med Ctr 1989; **Fac Appt:** Prof S, Northwestern Univ

Mamounas, Eleftherios P MD [S] - **Spec Exp:** Breast Cancer; **Hospital:** Aultman Hosp; **Address:** Aultman Cancer Ctr, 2600 6th St SW, Canton, OH 44710; **Phone:** 330-363-6281; **Board Cert:** Surgery 2009; **Med School:** Greece 1983; **Resid:** Surgery, McKeesport Hosp 1989; **Fellow:** Clinical Oncology, Univ Pittsburgh 1991; Surgical Oncology, Roswell Park Cancer Inst 1992; **Fac Appt:** Prof S, NE Ohio Univ

Melvin, W Scott MD [S] - **Spec Exp:** Liver & Biliary Surgery; Pancreatic Cancer; Laparoscopic Surgery; **Hospital:** Ohio St Univ Med Ctr; **Address:** 410 W 10th Ave, rm N729, North Doan Hall, Columbus, OH 43210; **Phone:** 614-293-4499; **Board Cert:** Surgery 2002; **Med School:** Med Coll OH 1987; **Resid:** Surgery, Univ Maryland 1992; **Fellow:** Gastrointestinal Surgery, Grant Med Ctr 1993; **Fac Appt:** Prof S, Ohio State Univ

Millis, J Michael MD [S] - **Spec Exp:** Transplant-Liver-Adult & Pediatric; Liver Cancer; Transplant-Pancreas; **Hospital:** Univ of Chicago Med Ctr; **Address:** 5841 S Maryland Ave, MS 5027, Chicago, IL 60637; **Phone:** 773-702-6319; **Board Cert:** Surgery 2001; Surgical Critical Care 2001; **Med School:** Univ Tenn Coll Med 1985; **Resid:** Surgery, UCLA Med Ctr 1992; **Fellow:** Transplant Surgery, UCLA Med Ctr 1994; **Fac Appt:** Prof S, Univ Chicago-Pritzker Sch Med

Moley, Jeffrey F MD [S] - **Spec Exp:** Thyroid Cancer & Surgery; Endocrine Cancers; Melanoma; **Hospital:** Barnes-Jewish Hosp; **Address:** Washington Univ School Med, Dept Surgery, 660 S Euclid Ave, Box 8109, St Louis, MO 63110; **Phone:** 314-362-2280; **Board Cert:** Surgery 2005; **Med School:** Columbia P&S 1980; **Resid:** Surgery, Yale-New Haven Hosp 1985; **Fellow:** Surgical Oncology, National Cancer Inst 1987; **Fac Appt:** Prof S, Washington Univ, St Louis

Nagorney, David M MD [S] - **Spec Exp:** Pancreatic Cancer; Hepatobiliary Surgery; Gastrointestinal Cancer; **Hospital:** Mayo Med Ctr & Clin - Rochester; **Address:** Mayo Clin, Dept Surgery, 200 1st St SW, Mayo E12, Rochester, MN 55905; **Phone:** 507-284-0362; **Board Cert:** Surgery 2001; **Med School:** Univ Kansas 1975; **Resid:** Surgery, Mayo Clin 1982; **Fellow:** Hepatobiliary Surgery, Hammersmith Hosp 1985; **Fac Appt:** Prof S, Mayo Med Sch

Nathanson, S David MD [S] - **Spec Exp:** Breast Cancer; Breast Cancer Risk Assessment; Melanoma; Sarcoma; **Hospital:** Henry Ford Hosp, Henry Ford- W Bloomfield Hosp; **Address:** 2799 W Grand Blvd, Detroit, MI 48202; **Phone:** 313-916-2917; **Board Cert:** Surgery 2002; **Med School:** South Africa 1966; **Resid:** Surgery, Univ Witwaterstrand 1974; Surgical Oncology, UCLA Med Ctr 1980; **Fellow:** Surgery, UC Davis 1982; **Fac Appt:** Prof S, Case West Res Univ

Newman, Lisa A MD [S] - **Spec Exp:** Breast Cancer; **Hospital:** Univ of Michigan Hosp; **Address:** Univ Michigan Cancer Center, 1500 E Medical Center Drive, rm 3308-CGC, Ann Arbor, MI 48109-5932; **Phone:** 734-936-8771; **Board Cert:** Surgery 2001; **Med School:** SUNY Downstate 1985; **Resid:** Surgery, Downstate Med Ctr 1990; **Fac Appt:** Assoc Prof S, Univ Mich Med Sch

Onders, Raymond P MD [S] - **Spec Exp:** Laparoscopic Surgery; Gastrointestinal Cancer; **Hospital:** Univ Hosps Case Med Ctr; **Address:** 11100 Euclid Ave, MS LKS 5047, Cleveland, OH 44106-5047; **Phone:** 216-844-5797; **Board Cert:** Surgery 2001; **Med School:** NE Ohio Univ 1988; **Resid:** Surgery, Case Western Reserve Univ 1993; **Fac Appt:** Assoc Prof S, NE Ohio Univ

Posner, Mitchell C MD [S] - **Spec Exp:** Pancreatic Cancer; Gastrointestinal Cancer; Esophageal Cancer; **Hospital:** Univ of Chicago Med Ctr; **Address:** Univ Chicago Medical Center, 5841 S Maryland Ave, Ste G209, MC 5094, Chicago, IL 60637-1447; **Phone:** 773-834-4007; **Board Cert:** Surgery 2006; **Med School:** SUNY Buffalo 1981; **Resid:** Surgery, Univ Colorado Med Ctr 1986; **Fellow:** Surgical Oncology, Meml Sloan Kettering Cancer Ctr 1988; **Fac Appt:** Prof S, Univ Chicago-Pritzker Sch Med

Saha, Sukamal MD [S] - **Spec Exp:** Sentinel Node Surgery; Colon Cancer; Head & Neck Cancer & Surgery; **Hospital:** McLaren Reg Med Ctr, Genesys Reg Med Ctr - St Joseph Campus; **Address:** 3500 Calkins Rd, Ste A, Flint, MI 48532; **Phone:** 810-230-9600 x500; **Board Cert:** Surgery 2000; **Med School:** India 1977; **Resid:** Surgery, Hahnemann Univ Hosp 1985; Surgery, Easton Hosp 1987; **Fellow:** Surgical Oncology, Tulane Univ Med Ctr 1989; Head and Neck Surgery, Roswell Park Meml Hosp 1990; **Fac Appt:** Asst Prof S, Mich State Univ

Sarr, Michael G MD [S] - **Spec Exp:** Pancreatic Cancer; Gastrointestinal Cancer; **Hospital:** Mayo Med Ctr & Clin - Rochester; **Address:** Mayo Clinic, 200 First St SW, Dept Surg, Desk West 12A, Rochester, MN 55905; **Phone:** 507-284-0362; **Board Cert:** Surgery 2001; **Med School:** Johns Hopkins Univ 1976; **Resid:** Surgery, Johns Hopkins Hosp 1982; **Fellow:** Surgery, Mayo Clinic 1984; Surgery, Johns Hopkins Hosp 1985; **Fac Appt:** Prof S, Mayo Med Sch

Schwartzentruber, Douglas J MD [S] - **Spec Exp:** Cancer Surgery; Melanoma; Kidney Cancer; **Hospital:** Indiana Univ Hlth Goshen Hosp; **Address:** Cancer Ctr at Goshen Health System, 200 High Park Ave, Goshen, IN 46526; **Phone:** 574-535-2888; **Board Cert:** Surgery 2008; **Med School:** Indiana Univ 1982; **Resid:** Surgery, Indiana Univ Med Ctr 1987; **Fellow:** Surgical Oncology, Natl Cancer Inst 1990; **Fac Appt:** Assoc Clin Prof S, Indiana Univ

Scott-Conner, Carol E H MD/PhD [S] - **Spec Exp:** Breast Cancer; Cancer Surgery; Laparoscopic Surgery; **Hospital:** Univ Iowa Hosp & Clinics, Iowa City VA Hlth Care Sys; **Address:** Univ Iowa, Dept Surg, 200 Hawkins Drive, 4622 JCP, Iowa City, IA 52242-1086; **Phone:** 319-356-0330; **Board Cert:** Surgery 2000; Surgical Critical Care 1998; **Med School:** NYU Sch Med 1976; **Resid:** Surgery, NYU Med Ctr 1981; **Fac Appt:** Prof S, Univ Iowa Coll Med

Shenk, Robert R MD [S] - **Spec Exp:** Breast Cancer; Melanoma; Pancreatic Cancer; Stomach Cancer; **Hospital:** Univ Hosps Case Med Ctr; **Address:** Univ Hosp Case Med Ctr, 11100 Euclid Ave, Dept General Surgery, Cleveland, OH 44106; **Phone:** 216-844-3026; **Board Cert:** Surgery 2004; **Med School:** Case West Res Univ 1978; **Resid:** Surgery, Univ Hosp 1985; Immunology, Natl Cancer Inst 1982; **Fellow:** Surgical Oncology, Anderson Hosp 1987; **Fac Appt:** Assoc Prof S, Case West Res Univ

Sielaff, Timothy D MD/PhD [S] - **Spec Exp:** Liver Cancer; Pancreatic Cancer; Gallbladder & Biliary Cancer; **Hospital:** Abbott - Northwestern Hosp; **Address:** Virginia Piper Cancer Inst, Liver and Pancreas Clinic, 800 E 28th St, Minneapolis, MN 55407; **Phone:** 612-863-7553; **Board Cert:** Surgery 2008; **Med School:** Med Coll VA 1989; **Resid:** Surgery, Univ Minn Hosps 1997; **Fellow:** Transplant Surgery, Univ Toronto Affil Hosp 1998; **Fac Appt:** Assoc Prof S, Univ Minn

Simeone, Diane M MD [S] - **Spec Exp:** Pancreatic Cancer; Cancer Surgery; **Hospital:** Univ of Michigan Hosp; **Address:** Univ Michigan Hlth Sys, 1500 E Med Ctr Drive, 2210B Taubman Center SPC 5343, Ann Arbor, MI 48109-5343; **Phone:** 734-615-1600; **Board Cert:** Surgery 2005; **Med School:** Duke Univ 1988; **Resid:** Surgery, Univ Mich Med Ctr 1995; **Fac Appt:** Prof S, Univ Mich Med Sch

Siperstein, Allan E MD [S] - **Spec Exp:** Laparoscopic Surgery; Endocrine Tumors; Thyroid & Parathyroid Cancer & Surgery; **Hospital:** Cleveland Clin (page 70); **Address:** Cleveland Clinic, Dept Endocrine Surg, 9500 Euclid Ave, MC F20, Cleveland, OH 44195; **Phone:** 216-444-5664; **Board Cert:** Surgery 2007; **Med School:** Univ Tex SW, Dallas 1983; **Resid:** Surgery, UCSF Med Ctr 1990; **Fellow:** Research, UCSF Med Ctr 1988

Stahl, Donna L MD [S] - **Spec Exp:** Breast Cancer; Breast Surgery; **Hospital:** Jewish Hosp - Kenwood - Cincinnati; **Address:** 4750 E Galbraith Rd, Ste 112, Cincinnati, OH 45236; **Phone:** 513-686-3109; **Board Cert:** Surgery 2000; **Med School:** Univ Iowa Coll Med 1971; **Resid:** Surgery, Univ Cincinnati Hosps 1978

Staren, Edgar MD/PhD [S] - **Spec Exp:** Breast Cancer; Endocrine Cancers; Liver Cancer; **Hospital:** CTCA at Midwestern Reg Med Ctr; **Address:** Cancer Treatment Ctrs America, 2610 Sheridan Rd, Zion, IL 60099; **Phone:** 847-731-5805; **Board Cert:** Surgery 2006; **Med School:** Loyola Univ-Stritch Sch Med 1982; **Resid:** Surgery, Rush-Presby-St Lukes Med Ctr 1987; **Fellow:** Surgical Oncology, Rush-Presby-St Lukes Med Ctr 1988

Talamonti, Mark S MD [S] - **Spec Exp:** Pancreatic Cancer; Liver Cancer; Gastrointestinal Cancer & Surgery; Melanoma; **Hospital:** Evanston/North Shore Univ Hlth Sys, Highland Park/North Shore Univ Hlth Syst; **Address:** North Shore Univ Health System, 2560 Ridge Ave, Evanston, IL 60201; **Phone:** 847-570-1700; **Board Cert:** Surgery 2009; **Med School:** Northwestern Univ 1983; **Resid:** Surgery, Northwestern Meml Hosp 1989; **Fellow:** Surgical Oncology, MD Anderson Cancer Ctr 1991; **Fac Appt:** Clin Prof S, Univ Chicago-Pritzker Sch Med

Tuttle, Todd M MD [S] - **Spec Exp:** Breast Cancer; Minimally Invasive Surgery; Cancer Surgery; **Address:** Univ Minn, Dept Surgery, 420 Delaware St SE, MMC 195, Minneapolis, MN 55455; **Phone:** 612-625-2991; **Board Cert:** Surgery 2004; **Med School:** Johns Hopkins Univ 1988; **Resid:** Surgery, Med Coll Virginia Hosps 1994; **Fellow:** Surgical Oncology, MD Anderson Cancer Ctr 1996; **Fac Appt:** Assoc Prof S

Vickers, Selwyn M MD [S] - **Spec Exp:** Pancreatic Cancer; Liver Cancer; Gastrointestinal Surgery; **Address:** University of Minnesota, 420 Delaware St SE, Phillips Wangensteen Bldg, MMC 195, Minneapolis, MN 55455; **Phone:** 612-626-1999; **Board Cert:** Surgery 2003; **Med School:** Johns Hopkins Univ 1986; **Resid:** Surgery, Johns Hopkins Hosp 1992; **Fellow:** NIH-Dept Aging 1987; **Fac Appt:** Prof S, Johns Hopkins Univ

Walker, Alonzo P MD [S] - **Spec Exp:** Breast Cancer; **Hospital:** Froedtert and Med Ctr of WI; **Address:** Dept Surgery, 9200 W Wisconsin Ave, Milwaukee, WI 53226-3522; **Phone:** 414-805-5737; **Board Cert:** Surgery 2004; **Med School:** Univ Fla Coll Med 1976; **Resid:** Surgery, Univ Maryland Hosps 1983; **Fac Appt:** Prof S, Med Coll Wisc

Walsh, R Matthew MD [S] - **Spec Exp:** Pancreatic Cancer; Gastrointestinal Surgery; Hepatobiliary Surgery; **Hospital:** Cleveland Clin (page 70); **Address:** Cleveland Clin, Dept Surgery, 9500 Euclid Ave, Desk A100, Cleveland, OH 44195; **Phone:** 216-445-7576; **Board Cert:** Surgery 1999; **Med School:** Med Coll Wisc 1985; **Resid:** Surgery, Loyola Univ Hosp 1990; **Fellow:** Endoscopy, Mass General Hosp 1991; Hepatopancreatobiliary Surgery, Cleveland Clinic; **Fac Appt:** Assoc Prof S, Cleveland Cl Coll Med/Case West Res

Weber, Sharon M MD [S] - **Spec Exp:** Liver Cancer; Pancreatic & Biliary Surgery; Colon & Rectal Cancer; Sarcoma; **Hospital:** Univ WI Hosp & Clins, Wm S Middleton Mem Vet Hosp-Madison; **Address:** 600 Highland Ave, Madison, WI 53792; **Phone:** 608-265-0500; **Board Cert:** Surgery 2009; **Med School:** Med Coll Wisc 1993; **Resid:** Surgery, Univ Wisc Med Ctr 1999; **Fellow:** Tumor Immunology, Univ Wisc Med Ctr 1997; Hepatobiliary Surgery, Meml Sloan Kettering Cancer Ctr 2001; **Fac Appt:** Assoc Prof S, Univ Wisc

Surgery

Weigel, Ronald J MD/PhD [S] - **Spec Exp:** Breast Cancer; Endocrine Surgery; **Hospital:** Univ Iowa Hosp & Clinics; **Address:** Univ Iowa Carver Coll Med-Dept Surgery, 200 Hawkins Drive, 1516 JCP, Iowa City, IA 52242; **Phone:** 319-356-4200; **Board Cert:** Surgery 2001; **Med School:** Yale Univ 1986; **Resid:** Surgery, Duke Univ Med Ctr 1992; **Fellow:** Immunology, Duke Univ Med Ctr; **Fac Appt:** Prof S, Univ Iowa Coll Med

Witt, Thomas R MD [S] - **Spec Exp:** Breast Cancer; **Hospital:** Rush Univ Med Ctr; **Address:** Surgical Oncology Group, 1725 W Harrison St, Ste 409, Chicago, IL 60612-3828; **Phone:** 312-942-2302; **Board Cert:** Surgery 2000; **Med School:** Northwestern Univ 1975; **Resid:** Surgery, Rush Presby-St Lukes Med Ctr 1980; **Fellow:** Surgical Oncology, Meml Sloan Kettering Cancer Ctr 1982; **Fac Appt:** Assoc Prof S, Rush Med Coll

Great Plains and Mountains

Edney, James A MD [S] - **Spec Exp:** Breast Cancer; Thyroid & Parathyroid Cancer & Surgery; Cancer Surgery; Melanoma; **Hospital:** Nebraska Med Ctr; **Address:** Univ Nebraska Med Ctr, Dept Surgery, 984030 Nebraska Medical Ctr, Omaha, NE 68198-4030; **Phone:** 402-559-7272; **Board Cert:** Surgery 2000; **Med School:** Univ Nebr Coll Med 1975; **Resid:** Surgery, Univ Nebraska Med Ctr 1980; **Fellow:** Surgical Oncology, Univ Colorado Med Ctr 1981; **Fac Appt:** Prof S, Univ Nebr Coll Med

Finlayson, Christina A MD [S] - **Spec Exp:** Breast Cancer; **Hospital:** Univ of CO Hosp - Anschutz Inpatient Pav; **Address:** 12631 E 17th Ave, P.O. Box 6511, Auora, CO 80045; **Phone:** 303-724-2728; **Board Cert:** Surgery 2004; **Med School:** Univ Utah 1989; **Resid:** Surgery, Univ Colorado Hlth Sci Ctr 1994; **Fellow:** Surgical Oncology, Fox Chase Cancer Ctr 1996; **Fac Appt:** Prof S, Univ Colorado

Mulvihill, Sean J MD [S] - **Spec Exp:** Gastrointestinal Surgery; Liver & Biliary Cancer; Pancreatic Cancer; **Hospital:** Univ Utah Hlth Care; **Address:** Univ Utah, Dept Surgery, 30 N 1900 E, rm 3B110, Salt Lake City, UT 84132; **Phone:** 801-581-7304; **Board Cert:** Surgery 2008; **Med School:** USC Sch Med 1981; **Resid:** Surgery, UCLA Med Ctr 1987; **Fac Appt:** Prof S, Univ Utah

Nelson, Edward W MD [S] - **Spec Exp:** Breast Cancer; **Hospital:** Univ Utah Hlth Care; **Address:** Univ Utah Med Ctr, Div Genl Surgery, 30 N 1900 E, rm 3B322, Salt Lake City, UT 84132; **Phone:** 801-581-7738; **Board Cert:** Surgery 2008; **Med School:** Univ Utah 1974; **Resid:** Surgery, Univ Utah Med Ctr 1979; **Fac Appt:** Prof S, Univ Utah

Pearlman, Nathan W MD [S] - **Spec Exp:** Gastrointestinal Cancer; Melanoma; Head & Neck Cancer; **Hospital:** Univ of CO Hosp - Anschutz Inpatient Pav; **Address:** 12631 E 17th Ave, MS C-313, Aurora, CO 80045; **Phone:** 303-724-2728; **Board Cert:** Surgery 1974; **Med School:** Univ IL Coll Med 1966; **Resid:** Surgery, Univ Colorado Med Ctr 1973; **Fellow:** Surgical Oncology, Sloan-Kettering Cancer Ctr 1975; **Fac Appt:** Prof S, Univ Colorado

Sasson, Aaron R MD [S] - **Spec Exp:** Gastrointestinal Cancer; Pancreatic Cancer; Liver Cancer; Neuroendocrine Tumors; **Hospital:** Nebraska Med Ctr; **Address:** 984030 Univ Nebraska Med Ctr, Omaha, NE 68198-4030; **Phone:** 402-559-8941; **Board Cert:** Surgery 2000; **Med School:** UMDNJ-NJ Med Sch, Newark 1993; **Resid:** Surgery, UCSD Med Ctr 1999; **Fellow:** Surgical Oncology, Fox Chase Cancer Ctr 2001; **Fac Appt:** Assoc Prof S, Univ Nebr Coll Med

Sauter, Edward R MD/PhD [S] - **Spec Exp:** Breast Cancer; Breast Cancer Risk Assessment; Clinical Trials; **Hospital:** Fargo VA Med Ctr, Sanford Med Ctr Fargo; **Address:** Univ North Dakota Dept Surgery, 501 N Columbia Rd, MS 9037, Grand Forks, ND 58202; **Phone:** 701-777-4862; **Board Cert:** Surgery 2000; **Med School:** Louisiana State U, New Orleans 1986; **Resid:** Surgery, Ochsner Fdn Hosp 1991; **Fellow:** Surgical Oncology, Fox Chase Cancer Ctr 1993; **Fac Appt:** Prof S, Univ ND Sch Med

Southwest

Ames, Frederick C MD [S] - **Spec Exp:** Breast Cancer; **Hospital:** UT MD Anderson Cancer Ctr; **Address:** MD Anderson Cancer Ctr, Dept Surgery, 1515 Holcombe Blvd, Unit 444, Houston, TX 77030-4009; **Phone:** 713-792-6929; **Board Cert:** Surgery 1975; **Med School:** Univ Tex Med Br, Galveston 1969; **Resid:** Surgery, Univ Texas Med Branch 1971; Surgery, St Joseph Hosp 1974; **Fellow:** Surgical Oncology, MD Anderson Cancer Ctr 1975; **Fac Appt:** Prof S, Univ Tex, Houston

Babiera, Gildy V MD [S] - **Spec Exp:** Breast Cancer; **Hospital:** UT MD Anderson Cancer Ctr; **Address:** MD Anderson Cancer Ctr, Dept Surgical Oncology, Unit 444, PO Box 301402, Houston, TX 77230-1402; **Phone:** 713-792-2121; **Board Cert:** Surgery 2007; **Med School:** NY Med Coll 1991; **Resid:** Surgery, NYU Med Ctr 1995; Surgery, NYU Med Ctr 1997; **Fellow:** Surgical Oncology, MD Anderson Cancer Ctr 1996; **Fac Appt:** Assoc Prof Surg & Onc, Univ Tex, Houston

Beitsch, Peter D MD [S] - **Spec Exp:** Breast Cancer; **Hospital:** Med City Dallas Hosp; **Address:** 7777 Forrest Ln C Bldg - Ste 760, Dallas, TX 75230; **Phone:** 972-566-8039; **Board Cert:** Surgery 2002; **Med School:** Univ Tex SW, Dallas 1986; **Resid:** Surgery, Univ TX SW Med Ctr 1993; **Fellow:** Surgical Oncology, MD Anderson Cancer Ctr 1990; Surgical Oncology, John Wayne Cancer Inst 1994

Bolton, John S MD [S] - **Spec Exp:** Cancer Surgery; Esophageal Cancer; Pancreatic Cancer; Liver Cancer; **Hospital:** Ochsner Med Ctr-New Orleans; **Address:** Ochsner Clin, Dept Surg, 1514 Jefferson Hwy, New Orleans, LA 70121; **Phone:** 504-842-4072; **Board Cert:** Surgery 2002; **Med School:** Louisiana State U, New Orleans 1976; **Resid:** Surgery, Charity Hosp 1981; **Fellow:** Hepatopancreatobiliary Surgery, Lahey Clinic 1980; Surgical Oncology, Meml Sloan Kettering Cancer Ctr 1982; **Fac Appt:** Asst Clin Prof S, Louisiana State U, New Orleans

Brunicardi, F Charles MD [S] - **Spec Exp:** Pancreatic Cancer; **Hospital:** St. Luke's Episcopal Hosp-Houston; **Address:** 6620 Main St, Ste 1475, Houston, TX 77030; **Phone:** 713-798-8070; **Board Cert:** Surgery 2009; **Med School:** UMDNJ-Rutgers Med Sch 1980; **Resid:** Surgery, SUNY Brooklyn Hlth Sci Ctr 1989; **Fellow:** Pancreatic Physiology, SUNY Brooklyn Hlth Sci Ctr 1986; **Fac Appt:** Prof S, Baylor Coll Med

Curley, Steven A MD [S] - **Spec Exp:** Colon & Rectal Cancer; Liver Cancer; Hepatobiliary Surgery; **Hospital:** UT MD Anderson Cancer Ctr; **Address:** MD Anderson Cancer Ctr, Dept Surg Oncology, 1515 Holcome Blvd, Unit 1484, Houston, TX 77230-1402; **Phone:** 713-792-2022; **Board Cert:** Surgery 2008; **Med School:** Univ Tex, Houston 1982; **Resid:** Surgery, Univ New Mexico Hosps 1988; **Fellow:** Surgical Oncology, MD Anderson Cancer Ctr 1990; **Fac Appt:** Prof S, Univ Tex, Houston

Dooley, William C MD [S] - **Spec Exp:** Breast Cancer; Tumors-Rare & Multiple; Sarcoma; Melanoma; **Hospital:** OU Med Ctr; **Address:** 825 NE 10th St, Ste 4500, Oklahoma City, OK 73104; **Phone:** 405-271-7867; **Board Cert:** Surgery 2011; **Med School:** Vanderbilt Univ 1982; **Resid:** Surgery, Johns Hopkins Hosp 1987; Surgical Oncology, Oxford Univ 1986; **Fellow:** Surgical Oncology, Johns Hopkins 1988; **Fac Appt:** Prof S, Univ Okla Coll Med

Ellis, Lee M MD [S] - **Spec Exp:** Colon & Rectal Cancer; Metastatic Cancer; Peritoneal Carcinomatosis; **Hospital:** UT MD Anderson Cancer Ctr; **Address:** MD Anderson Cancer Ctr, Dept Surgery & Cancer Biology, 1515 Holcombe Blvd, Box 173, Houston, TX 77030; **Phone:** 713-792-6926; **Board Cert:** Surgery 2009; **Med School:** Univ VA Sch Med 1983; **Resid:** Surgery, Univ Fla-Shands Hosp 1990; **Fellow:** Surgical Oncology, MD Anderson Cancer Ctr 1992; **Fac Appt:** Prof S, Univ Tex, Houston

Euhus, David M MD [S] - **Spec Exp:** Breast Cancer; **Hospital:** UT Southwestern Med Ctr at Dallas; **Address:** Univ Texas SW Med Ctr - Div Surg Oncology, 5323 Harry Hines Blvd, MC 9155, Dallas, TX 75390; **Phone:** 214-648-6467; **Board Cert:** Surgery 2001; **Med School:** St Louis Univ 1984; **Resid:** Surgery, UCLA Med Ctr 1991; **Fellow:** Surgical Oncology, UCLA Med Ctr 1988; Breast Disease, Queens Med Ctr 1990; **Fac Appt:** Prof S, Univ Tex SW, Dallas

Feig, Barry W MD [S] - **Spec Exp:** Gastrointestinal Cancer; Sarcoma; Breast Cancer; **Hospital:** UT MD Anderson Cancer Ctr; **Address:** UT MD Anderson Cancer Ctr, Dept Surg Onc, 1400 Pressler St, Unit 1484, Houston, TX 77030; **Phone:** 713-792-2022; **Board Cert:** Surgery 2008; **Med School:** SUNY Upstate Med Univ 1984; **Resid:** Surgery, Northwestern Univ Med Ctr 1990; **Fellow:** Trauma, Univ Minnesota Affil Hosp 1991; Surgical Oncology, UT MD Anderson Cancer Ctr 1994; **Fac Appt:** Prof S, Univ Tex, Houston

Fisher, William E MD [S] - **Spec Exp:** Pancreatic Cancer; **Hospital:** St. Luke's Episcopal Hosp-Houston; **Address:** 6620 Main St, Ste 1475, Houston, TX 77030; **Phone:** 713-798-8070; **Board Cert:** Surgery 2006; **Med School:** Univ Cincinnati 1990; **Resid:** Surgery, Ohio State U Hosps 1996; **Fellow:** Cancer Research, Ohio State U Hosps 1998; **Fac Appt:** Asst Prof S, Baylor Coll Med

Grant, Michael D MD [S] - **Spec Exp:** Breast Cancer; Breast Surgery; **Hospital:** Baylor Univ Medical Ctr; **Address:** 3900 Junius St, Ste 220, Baylor Med Pavillion, Dallas, TX 75246; **Phone:** 214-826-7300; **Board Cert:** Surgery 2001; **Med School:** Univ Tex, Houston 1987; **Resid:** Surgery, Baylor Univ Med Ctr 1992; **Fellow:** Breast Cancer, Baylor Univ Med Ctr 1993

Gray, Richard J MD [S] - **Spec Exp:** Breast Cancer; Melanoma; **Hospital:** Mayo Clinic - Phoenix, Mayo Clinic - Scottsdale; **Address:** Mayo Clinic, 5777 E Mayo Blvd, Phoenix, AZ 85054; **Phone:** 480-342-2849; **Board Cert:** Surgery 2001; **Med School:** Mich State Univ 1995; **Resid:** Surgery, Mayo Clinic 2000; **Fellow:** Surgical Oncology, H Lee Moffitt Cancer Ctr 2001; **Fac Appt:** Assoc Prof S, Mayo Med Sch

Hunt, Kelly K MD [S] - **Spec Exp:** Breast Cancer; Sarcoma-Soft Tissue; Gene Therapy; **Hospital:** UT MD Anderson Cancer Ctr; **Address:** MD Anderson Cancer Ctr, 1400 Pressler St, Unit 1484, Houston, TX 77030-4000; **Phone:** 713-792-7216; **Board Cert:** Surgery 2001; **Med School:** Univ Tenn Coll Med 1986; **Resid:** Surgery, UCLA Med Ctr 1993; **Fellow:** Surgical Oncology, MD Anderson Cancer Ctr 1996; **Fac Appt:** Prof Surg & Onc, Univ Tex, Houston

Jackson, Gilchrist MD [S] - **Spec Exp:** Thyroid & Parathyroid Surgery; Head & Neck Cancer & Surgery; Endocrine Tumors; Gastrointestinal Cancer & Surgery; **Hospital:** St. Luke's Episcopal Hosp-Houston, Woman's Hosp TX; **Address:** 2727 W Holcombe Blvd Fl 3-A, Houston, TX 77025; **Phone:** 713-442-1132; **Board Cert:** Surgery 2008; **Med School:** Univ Louisville Sch Med 1974; **Resid:** Surgery, Parkland Hosp 1979; **Fellow:** Surgical Oncology, MD Anderson Hosp 1980; **Fac Appt:** Assoc Clin Prof S, Baylor Coll Med

Klimberg, Vicki S MD [S] - **Spec Exp:** Breast Cancer; Radiofrequency Tumor Ablation; Sentinel Node Surgery; **Hospital:** UAMS Med Ctr; **Address:** Univ Arkansas Medical Sciences, 4301 W Markham, MS 725, Little Rock, AR 72205-7199; **Phone:** 501-686-5669; **Board Cert:** Surgery 1999; **Med School:** Univ Fla Coll Med 1984; **Resid:** Surgery, Univ Fla Med Ctr 1989; **Fellow:** Clinical Oncology, Univ Fla 1990; Breast Disease, Univ Arkansas for Med Scis 1991; **Fac Appt:** Prof S, Univ Ark

Krouse, Robert S MD [S] - **Spec Exp:** Cancer Surgery; Gastrointestinal Cancer; Palliative Care; **Hospital:** Southern AZ VA Health Care Sys - Tucson; **Address:** Southern AZ VA Hosp Care System, Surg Care Line, 2-112, 3601 S 6th Ave, Tucson, AZ 85723; **Phone:** 520-792-1450 x6145; **Board Cert:** Surgery 2007; **Med School:** Hahnemann Univ 1991; **Resid:** Surgery, Univ Hawaii Integrated Surg Prog 1993; Immunotherapy, Natl Cancer Inst 1994; **Fellow:** Surgery, W Virginia Univ Sch Med 1997; Surgical Oncology, City of Hope Natl Med Ctr 2000; **Fac Appt:** Asst Prof S, Univ Ariz Coll Med

Kuhn, Joseph A MD [S] - **Spec Exp:** Liver Cancer; Peritoneal Carcinomatosis; Melanoma; Thyroid Cancer; **Hospital:** Baylor Univ Medical Ctr; **Address:** 7777 Forest Lane St, Ste C-410, Dallas, TX 75230; **Phone:** 214-823-5000; **Board Cert:** Surgery 2009; Surgical Critical Care 2003; **Med School:** Univ Tex Med Br, Galveston 1984; **Resid:** Surgery, Baylor Univ Med Ctr 1989; **Fellow:** Surgical Oncology, City Hosp Natl Med Ctr 1992

Lee, Jeffrey E MD [S] - **Spec Exp:** Melanoma; Pancreatic Cancer; Endocrine Tumors; **Hospital:** UT MD Anderson Cancer Ctr; **Address:** UT MD Anderson Cancer Ctr, 1400 Holcombe Blvd, Unit 444 Fl 12, Houston, TX 77030-4009; **Phone:** 713-792-7218; **Board Cert:** Surgery 1999; **Med School:** Stanford Univ 1984; **Resid:** Surgery, Stanford Univ Hosp 1987; Surgery, Stanford Univ Hosp 1991; **Fellow:** Immunology, Stanford Univ Sch Med 1989; Surgical Oncology, Univ Tex-MD Anderson Cancer Ctr 1993; **Fac Appt:** Prof S, Univ Tex, Houston

Leitch, A Marilyn MD [S] - **Spec Exp:** Breast Cancer & Surgery; Melanoma; Sarcoma; **Hospital:** UT Southwestern Med Ctr at Dallas; **Address:** UT Southwestern Med Ctr - Dept Surgery, 5323 Harry Hines Blvd, Dallas, TX 75390-9155; **Phone:** 214-648-3039; **Board Cert:** Surgery 2003; **Med School:** Univ Tex SW, Dallas 1978; **Resid:** Surgery, UCLA Med Ctr 1984; **Fellow:** Surgical Oncology, MD Anderson Cancer Ctr 1985; **Fac Appt:** Prof S, Univ Tex SW, Dallas

Li, Benjamin D L MD [S] - **Spec Exp:** Gastrointestinal Cancer; Sarcoma; Breast Cancer; **Hospital:** Louisiana State Univ Hosp, Willis-Knighton Med Ctr; **Address:** LSU Hlth Scis Ctr, Dept Surgery, 1501 Kings Hwy, Shreveport, LA 71130; **Phone:** 318-675-6100; **Board Cert:** Surgery 2002; **Med School:** Yale Univ 1986; **Resid:** Surgery, Northwestern Univ-McGraw Med Ctr 1992; **Fellow:** Surgical Oncology, Roswell Park Cancer Inst 1995; **Fac Appt:** Prof S, Louisiana State U, New Orleans

Mansfield, Paul F MD [S] - **Spec Exp:** Appendix Cancer; Stomach Cancer; Colon Cancer; Melanoma; **Hospital:** UT MD Anderson Cancer Ctr; **Address:** UT MD Anderson Cancer Ctr, 1400 Pressler St, Ste FCT18.5000, Unit 1485, Houston, TX 77030; **Phone:** 713-794-5499; **Board Cert:** Surgery 2006; **Med School:** Jefferson Med Coll 1983; **Resid:** Surgery, Pennsylvania Hosp 1988; **Fellow:** Surgical Oncology, MD Anderson Cancer Ctr 1991; **Fac Appt:** Prof Surg & Onc, Univ Tex, Houston

McCabe, Daniel P MD [S] - **Spec Exp:** Cancer Surgery; **Hospital:** Tucson Med Ctr; **Address:** Southwestern Surgical Assoc, 1951 N Wilmot Rd Bldg 2, Tucson, AZ 85712; **Phone:** 520-795-5845; **Board Cert:** Surgery 2002; **Med School:** Creighton Univ 1979; **Resid:** Surgery, St Joseph Hosp 1982; Surgery, Baystate Med Ctr 1984; **Fellow:** Surgical Oncology, James Cancer Ctr/Ohio State 1986; **Fac Appt:** Asst Clin Prof S, Univ Ariz Coll Med

Meric-Bernstam, Funda MD [S] - **Spec Exp:** Breast Cancer & Surgery; Clinical Trials; **Hospital:** UT MD Anderson Cancer Ctr; **Address:** UT MD Anderson Cancer Center, 1400 Pressler St, Unit 1484, Houston, TX 77030; **Phone:** 713-563-6104; **Board Cert:** Surgery 2007; **Med School:** Yale Univ 1991; **Resid:** Surgery, Univ Mich Med Ctr 1998; **Fellow:** Surgical Oncology, UT MD Anderson Cancer Ctr 2001; **Fac Appt:** Prof Surg & Onc, Univ Tex, Houston

Surgery

Pisters, Peter MD [S] - **Spec Exp:** Pancreatic Cancer; Sarcoma-Soft Tissue; Gastrointestinal Cancer; **Hospital:** UT MD Anderson Cancer Ctr; **Address:** MD Anderson Cancer Ctr, 1515 Holcombe Blvd, Unit 1484, Houston, TX 77230-1402; **Phone:** 713-792-2022; **Board Cert:** Surgery 2001; **Med School:** Univ Western Ontario 1985; **Resid:** Surgery, NYU/Bellevue Hosp 1992; **Fellow:** Surgical Research, Meml Sloan-Kettering Cancer Ctr 1989; Surgical Oncology, Meml Sloan-Kettering Cancer Ctr 1994; **Fac Appt:** Prof S, Univ Tex, Houston

Pockaj, Barbara A MD [S] - **Spec Exp:** Melanoma; Breast Cancer; Stomach Cancer; Clinical Trials; **Hospital:** Mayo Clinic - Scottsdale; **Address:** Mayo Clinic, Dept Surgery, 5777 E Mayo Blvd, Phoenix, AZ 85054; **Phone:** 480-342-2849; **Board Cert:** Surgery 2005; **Med School:** Vanderbilt Univ 1987; **Resid:** Surgery, Case Western Res Univ Affil Hosps 1995; **Fellow:** Surgical Oncology, Natl Inst Hlth 1992; **Fac Appt:** Assoc Prof S, Mayo Med Sch

Pollock, Raphael E MD/PhD [S] - **Spec Exp:** Sarcoma; **Hospital:** UT MD Anderson Cancer Ctr; **Address:** MD Anderson Cancer Ctr, Dept Surg Oncology, 1515 Holcombe Blvd, Unit 1447, Houston, TX 77030; **Phone:** 713-792-6928; **Board Cert:** Surgery 2003; **Med School:** St Louis Univ 1977; **Resid:** Surgery, Univ Chicago 1979; Surgery, Rush Presby-St Lukes Hosp 1982; **Fellow:** Surgical Oncology, MD Anderson Cancer Ctr 1984; **Fac Appt:** Prof S, Univ Tex, Houston

Postier, Russell G MD [S] - **Spec Exp:** Cancer Surgery; Pancreatic Cancer; Biliary Surgery; Gastrointestinal Surgery; **Hospital:** OU Med Ctr; **Address:** OU Physicians, Dept Surgery, 825 NE 10th St, Ste 4500, Oklahoma City, OK 73104; **Phone:** 405-271-1400; **Board Cert:** Surgery 2000; **Med School:** Univ Okla Coll Med 1975; **Resid:** Surgery, Johns Hopkins Hosp 1981; **Fac Appt:** Prof S, Univ Okla Coll Med

Ross, Merrick I MD [S] - **Spec Exp:** Sentinel Node Surgery; Breast Cancer; Melanoma; **Hospital:** UT MD Anderson Cancer Ctr; **Address:** UT MD Anderson Cancer Ctr, Dept Surg Onc, 1515 Holcombe Blvd, Unit 1484, Houston, TX 77030; **Phone:** 713-792-2022; **Board Cert:** Surgery 2007; **Med School:** Univ IL Coll Med 1980; **Resid:** Surgery, Univ Illinois Hosp & Clin 1982; Surgery, Univ Illinois Hosp & Clin 1987; **Fellow:** Research, Scripps Clin & Rsch 1984; Surgical Oncology, Univ TX-MD Anderson Cancer Ctr 1989; **Fac Appt:** Prof S, Univ Tex, Houston

Skibber, John M MD [S] - **Spec Exp:** Rectal Cancer/Sphincter Preservation; Colon & Rectal Cancer-Familial Polyposis; **Hospital:** UT MD Anderson Cancer Ctr; **Address:** 1400 Pressler St, PO Box 301402, Unit 1484, Houston, TX 77230-1402; **Phone:** 713-792-5165; **Board Cert:** Surgery 2009; **Med School:** Jefferson Med Coll 1981; **Resid:** Surgery, NYU Med Ctr 1989; **Fellow:** Surgical Oncology, UT MD Anderson Cancer Ctr 1991; **Fac Appt:** Prof S, Univ Tex, Houston

Stolier, Alan J MD [S] - **Spec Exp:** Breast Cancer; **Hospital:** Ochsner Baptist Med Ctr; **Address:** 2525 Severn Ave, Metairie, LA 70002; **Phone:** 504-832-4200; **Board Cert:** Surgery 2006; **Med School:** Louisiana State U, New Orleans 1970; **Resid:** Surgery, Charity Hosp 1974; **Fellow:** Surgical Oncology, MD Anderson Hosp 1976; **Fac Appt:** Clin Prof S, Tulane Univ

Vauthey, Jean Nicholas MD [S] - **Spec Exp:** Hepatobiliary Surgery; Liver Cancer; Gallbladder & Biliary Cancer; **Hospital:** UT MD Anderson Cancer Ctr; **Address:** UT MD Anderson Cancer Ctr -Surg Oncology, 1515 Holcombe Blvd, Unit 1484, Houston, TX 77030; **Phone:** 713-792-2022; **Board Cert:** Surgery 2000; **Med School:** Switzerland 1979; **Resid:** Surgery, Ochsner Med Fdn 1989; **Fellow:** Hepatobiliary Surgery, Med Fac Univ Bern 1991; Surgical Oncology, Meml Sloan-Kettering Cancer Ctr 1993; **Fac Appt:** Prof S, Univ Tex, Houston

Woltering, Eugene MD [S] - **Spec Exp:** Carcinoid Tumors; **Hospital:** Ochsner Med Ctr-New Orleans; **Address:** 200 W Esplanade, Ste 200, Kenner, LA 70062; **Phone:** 504-464-8500; **Board Cert:** Surgery 2002; **Med School:** Ohio State Univ 1975; **Resid:** Surgery, Vanderbilt Med Ctr 1982; Surgical Oncology, Natl Inst Hlth 1979; **Fellow:** Surgical Oncology, Ohio State Univ 1984; **Fac Appt:** Prof S, Louisiana State U, New Orleans

Wood, R Patrick MD [S] - **Spec Exp:** Liver Cancer; **Hospital:** St. Luke's Episcopal Hosp-Houston; **Address:** 6624 Fannin St, Ste 1200, Houston, TX 77030; **Phone:** 713-795-8994; **Board Cert:** Surgery 2004; **Med School:** Univ Rochester 1979; **Resid:** Surgery, NYU/Bellevue Hosp Ctr 1984; **Fellow:** Transplant Surgery, Univ Pittsburgh 1985; **Fac Appt:** Clin Prof S, Univ Tex, Houston

Zannis, Victor J MD [S] - **Spec Exp:** Breast Cancer; **Hospital:** Phoenix Baptist Hosp & Med Ctr, J C Lincoln Hosp - North Mountain; **Address:** 2525 W Greenway Rd, Ste 130, Phoenix, AZ 85023; **Phone:** 602-942-8000; **Board Cert:** Surgery 2000; **Med School:** UCLA 1976; **Resid:** Surgery, Maricopa Med Ctr 1982

West Coast and Pacific

Anderson, Benjamin O MD [S] - **Spec Exp:** Breast Cancer & Surgery; **Hospital:** Univ Wash Med Ctr; **Address:** Univ Washington Dept Surgery, 1959 NE Pacific St, Box 356410, Seattle, WA 98195-6410; **Phone:** 206-288-6806; **Board Cert:** Surgery 2002; **Med School:** Albert Einstein Coll Med 1985; **Resid:** Surgery, Univ Colorado Affil Hosp 1992; **Fellow:** Surgical Oncology, Meml Sloan Kettering Cancer Ctr 1994; **Fac Appt:** Prof S, Univ Wash

Bilchik, Anton J MD/PhD [S] - **Spec Exp:** Gastrointestinal Cancer; Laparoscopic Surgery; **Hospital:** St. John's Hlth Ctr, Santa Monica, Cedars-Sinai Med Ctr; **Address:** 2336 Santa Monica Blvd, Ste 206, Santa Monica, CA 90404; **Phone:** 310-696-0716; **Board Cert:** Surgery 2004; **Med School:** South Africa 1985; **Resid:** Surgery, UCLA Med Ctr 1996; **Fellow:** John Wayne Cancer Inst. 1998; **Fac Appt:** Asst Clin Prof S, UCLA

Bouvet, Michael MD [S] - **Spec Exp:** Endocrine Surgery; Pancreatic Cancer; Biliary Cancer; **Hospital:** UCSD Med Ctr-Hillcrest; **Address:** UCSD Moores Cancer Ctr, 3855 Health Science Drive, La Jolla, CA 92093-0987; **Phone:** 858-822-6191; **Board Cert:** Surgery 2004; **Med School:** Univ Wash 1989; **Resid:** Surgery, UCSD Med Ctr 1995; **Fellow:** Surgical Oncology, MD Anderson Cancer Ctr 1998; **Fac Appt:** Assoc Prof S, UCSD

Busuttil, Ronald W MD/PhD [S] - **Spec Exp:** Transplant-Liver; Liver Cancer; **Hospital:** UCLA Ronald Reagan Med Ctr; **Address:** 757 WestWood Plaza, Ste 8236, Los Angeles, CA 90095-7430; **Phone:** 310-825-5318; **Board Cert:** Surgery 2007; **Med School:** Tulane Univ 1971; **Resid:** Surgery, UCLA Med Ctr 1976; **Fellow:** Surgery, UCLA Med Ctr 1975; **Fac Appt:** Prof S, UCLA

Butler, John A MD [S] - **Spec Exp:** Breast Cancer; Thyroid Cancer; Adrenal Tumors; Small Bowel Cancer; **Hospital:** UC Irvine Med Ctr; **Address:** UC-Irvine Medical Ctr-Zot 5376, 101 City Drive S, Rte 81 Bldg 56 - Ste 256, Orange, CA 92868-3298; **Phone:** 714-456-8030; **Board Cert:** Surgery 2003; **Med School:** Loyola Univ-Stritch Sch Med 1976; **Resid:** Surgery, LAC-USC Med Ctr 1982; Surgery, Harbor-UCLA Med Ctr 1982; **Fellow:** Surgical Oncology, Meml Sloan-Kettering Cancer Ctr 1984; **Fac Appt:** Prof S, UC Irvine

Byrd, David MD [S] - **Spec Exp:** Cancer Surgery; Tumor Surgery; Melanoma; Breast Cancer & Surgery; **Hospital:** Univ Wash Med Ctr; **Address:** Univ Washington Med Ctr, Dept Surgical Specialites Center, 1959 NE Pacific St, Box 356165, Seattle, WA 98195; **Phone:** 206-598-4477; **Board Cert:** Surgery 2008; **Med School:** Tulane Univ 1982; **Resid:** Surgery, Univ Wash Med Ctr 1987; **Fellow:** Surgical Oncology, Univ Tex-MD Anderson Cancer Ctr 1992; **Fac Appt:** Assoc Prof S, Univ Wash

Chang, Helena MD [S] - **Spec Exp:** Breast Cancer; Cancer Surgery; **Hospital:** UCLA Ronald Reagan Med Ctr; **Address:** 200 UCLA Medical Plaza Drive, Ste B265-1, Revlon Breast Clinic, Los Angeles, CA 90095-7028; **Phone:** 310-825-2144; **Board Cert:** Surgery 1997; **Med School:** Temple Univ 1981; **Resid:** Surgery, Episcopal Hosp 1986; **Fellow:** Cellular Molecular Biology, Temple Univ 1977; Surgical Oncology, Meml Sloan-Kettering Cancer Ctr 1988; **Fac Appt:** Prof S, UCLA

Clark, Orlo H MD [S] - **Spec Exp:** Thyroid Cancer & Surgery; Neuroendocrine Tumors; Parathyroid Cancer; **Hospital:** UCSF - Mt Zion Med Ctr, UCSF Med Ctr; **Address:** UCSF Mt Zion Med Ctr, 1600 Divisadero St, C-347, Box 1674, San Francisco, CA 94115-1926; **Phone:** 415-353-7687; **Board Cert:** Surgery 1974; **Med School:** Cornell Univ-Weill Med Coll 1967; **Resid:** Surgery, UCSF Med Ctr 1970; Surgery, UCSF Med Ctr 1973; **Fellow:** Surgery, Royal Med Sch London 1971; **Fac Appt:** Prof S, UCSF

Colquhoun, Steven D MD [S] - **Spec Exp:** Liver Cancer; Transplant-Liver; Pancreatic Cancer; Hepatobiliary Surgery; **Hospital:** Cedars-Sinai Med Ctr; **Address:** Cedars-Sinai Med Center, 8635 W 3rd St, Ste 590-W, Los Angeles, CA 90048; **Phone:** 310-423-2641; **Board Cert:** Surgery 2003; Surgical Critical Care 2008; **Med School:** Loyola Univ-Stritch Sch Med 1984; **Resid:** Surgery, UCLA Med Ctr 1990; **Fellow:** Surgical Oncology, UCLA Med Ctr 1993; Transplant Surgery, UCLA Med Ctr 1994; **Fac Appt:** Assoc Clin Prof S, UCLA

Duh, Quan-Yang MD [S] - **Spec Exp:** Endocrine Surgery; Thyroid & Parathyroid Cancer & Surgery; Adrenal Tumors; Minimally Invasive Surgery; **Hospital:** UCSF Med Ctr, VA Med Ctr - San Francisco; **Address:** UCSF Medical Ctr, 1600 Divisadero St, Box 1926, San Francisco, CA 94115; **Phone:** 415-353-7687; **Board Cert:** Surgery 2007; **Med School:** UCSF 1981; **Resid:** Surgery, UCSF Med Ctr 1988; **Fellow:** Endocrine Surgery, UCSF Med Ctr 1987; **Fac Appt:** Prof S, UCSF

Eilber, Frederick R MD [S] - **Spec Exp:** Tumor Surgery; Sarcoma; **Hospital:** UCLA Ronald Reagan Med Ctr; **Address:** 10833 Le Conte Ave CHS Bldg - rm 54-140, Los Angeles, CA 90095; **Phone:** 310-825-7086; **Board Cert:** Surgery 1973; **Med School:** Univ Mich Med Sch 1965; **Resid:** Surgery, Univ Maryland Hosp 1972; **Fellow:** Surgery, Univ Tex-MD Anderson Hosp 1973; **Fac Appt:** Prof S, UCLA

Ellenhorn, Joshua DI MD [S] - **Spec Exp:** Gastrointestinal Cancer; Pancreatic Surgery; Cancer Surgery; **Hospital:** City of Hope Natl Med Ctr (page 69), Huntington Memorial Hosp; **Address:** 1500 E Duarte Rd, Duarte, CA 91010; **Phone:** 626-471-7100; **Board Cert:** Surgery 2000; **Med School:** Boston Univ 1984; **Resid:** Surgery, Univ Cincinnati Hosp 1991; **Fellow:** Surgical Oncology, Meml Sloan-Kettering Cancer Ctr 1993; **Fac Appt:** Prof S

Esserman, Laura J MD [S] - **Spec Exp:** Breast Cancer; **Hospital:** UCSF - Mt Zion Med Ctr, UCSF Med Ctr; **Address:** UCSF-Helen Diller Family Comp Cancer Ctr, 1600 Divisadero St Fl 2, Box 1710, San Francisco, CA 94115; **Phone:** 415-353-7070; **Board Cert:** Surgery 2001; **Med School:** Stanford Univ 1983; **Resid:** Surgery, Stanford Univ Med Ctr 1991; **Fellow:** Oncology, Stanford Univ Med Ctr 1988; **Fac Appt:** Assoc Prof S, UCSF

Essner, Richard MD [S] - **Spec Exp:** Sentinel Node Surgery; Melanoma; Gastrointestinal Surgery; **Hospital:** St. John's Hlth Ctr, Santa Monica; **Address:** 2336 Santa Monica Blvd, Ste 206, Santa Monica, CA 90404-2302; **Phone:** 310-696-0716; **Board Cert:** Surgery 2002; **Med School:** Emory Univ 1985; **Resid:** Surgery, Univ NC Hosps 1992; **Fac Appt:** Asst Clin Prof S, USC Sch Med

Giuliano, Armando E MD [S] - **Spec Exp:** Breast Cancer; Sentinel Node Surgery; Thyroid & Parathyroid Surgery; **Hospital:** Cedars-Sinai Med Ctr; **Address:** Saul & Joyce Brandman Breast Ctr, 310 N San Vincente Blvd, Los Angeles, CA 90048; **Phone:** 310-423-9331 x0; **Board Cert:** Surgery 2009; **Med School:** Univ Chicago-Pritzker Sch Med 1973; **Resid:** Surgery, UCSF Med Ctr 1980; **Fellow:** Surgical Oncology, UCLA Med Ctr 1978; **Fac Appt:** Prof S, UCLA

Goodnight, James E MD [S] - **Spec Exp:** Melanoma; Breast Cancer; Bone & Soft Tissue Tumors; **Hospital:** UC Davis Med Ctr; **Address:** 4501 X St, Sacramento, CA 95817; **Phone:** 916-734-5959; **Board Cert:** Surgery 2007; **Med School:** Baylor Coll Med 1968; **Resid:** Surgery, Univ Utah Hosp 1976; **Fellow:** Surgical Oncology, UCLA Med Ctr 1978; **Fac Appt:** Prof S, UC Davis

Goodson III, William H MD [S] - **Spec Exp:** Breast Cancer; **Hospital:** CA Pacific Med Ctr-Pacific Campus, UCSF - Mt Zion Med Ctr; **Address:** 2100 Webster St, Ste 401, San Francisco, CA 94115-2378; **Phone:** 415-923-3925; **Board Cert:** Surgery 2006; **Med School:** Harvard Med Sch 1971; **Resid:** Surgery, Univ Hosps 1976; Surgery, Childrens Hosp 1977

Hemming, Alan W MD [S] - **Spec Exp:** Liver Cancer; Transplant-Liver; Hepatobiliary Surgery; Pancreatic Cancer; **Hospital:** UCSD Med Ctr-Hillcrest, Rady Children's Hosp - San Diego; **Address:** UCSD Ctr-Hepatobiliary Dis & Transplant, 200 W Arbor Drive, Ste 2 - rm 280, MS 8401, San Diego, CA 92103-8401; **Phone:** 619-543-5870; **Board Cert:** Surgery 2004; **Med School:** Univ British Columbia Fac Med 1987; **Resid:** Surgery, Univ British Columbia Med Ctr 1994; **Fellow:** Transplant Surgery, Univ Toronto/Hosp for Sick Children 1995; Hepatobiliary Surgery, Univ Toronto 1996; **Fac Appt:** Prof S, UCSD

Karlan, Scott R MD [S] - **Spec Exp:** Breast Cancer & Surgery; **Hospital:** Cedars-Sinai Med Ctr; **Address:** 310 N San Vicente Blvd Fl 3, Los Angeles, CA 90048; **Phone:** 310-423-9331; **Board Cert:** Surgery 2005; **Med School:** Harvard Med Sch 1982; **Resid:** Surgery, Yale-New Haven Hosp 1987; **Fac Appt:** Clin Prof S, UCLA

Kaufman, Cary S MD [S] - **Spec Exp:** Breast Cancer & Surgery; **Hospital:** St. Joseph Hosp - Bellingham; **Address:** 2940 Squalicum Pkwy, Ste 101, Bellingham, WA 98225; **Phone:** 360-671-9877; **Board Cert:** Surgery 2000; **Med School:** UCLA 1973; **Resid:** Surgery, Univ Wash Med Ctr 1975; Surgery, Harbor-UCLA Med Ctr 1979; **Fac Appt:** Asst Clin Prof S, Univ Wash

Kirgan, Daniel MD [S] - **Spec Exp:** Cancer Surgery; Breast Cancer & Surgery; **Hospital:** Univ Med Ctr - Las Vegas; **Address:** 1707 W Charleston Blvd, Ste 160, Las Vegas, NV 89102; **Phone:** 702-671-5150; **Board Cert:** Surgery 2004; **Med School:** Geo Wash Univ 1986; **Resid:** Surgery, Univ Med Ctr 1992; **Fellow:** Surgical Oncology, John Wayne Cancer Inst 1994; **Fac Appt:** Assoc Prof S, Univ Nevada

Klein, Andrew S MD [S] - **Spec Exp:** Transplant-Liver; Liver Cancer; **Hospital:** Cedars-Sinai Med Ctr; **Address:** Liver & Transplant Ctr at Cedars-Sinai, 8635 W Third St, Ste 590W, Los Angeles, CA 90048; **Phone:** 310-423-2641; **Board Cert:** Surgery 2007; **Med School:** Johns Hopkins Univ 1979; **Resid:** Surgery, Johns Hopkins Hosp 1982; Surgery, Johns Hopkins Hosp 1986; **Fellow:** Transplant Surgery, UCLA-CHS 1988; **Fac Appt:** Clin Prof S, UCLA

Knudson, Mary Margaret MD [S] - **Spec Exp:** Breast Cancer; **Hospital:** UCSF Med Ctr, San Francisco Genl Hosp; **Address:** 1001 Potrero Ave, Ste 3A, San Francisco, CA 94110; **Phone:** 415-206-4623; **Board Cert:** Surgery 2002; Surgical Critical Care 2008; **Med School:** Univ Mich Med Sch 1976; **Resid:** Surgery, Beth Israel Hosp 1979; Surgery, Univ Mich Med Ctr 1982; **Fellow:** Pediatric Surgery, Stanford Univ Hosps 1983; **Fac Appt:** Assoc Prof S, UCSF

Lowy, Andrew M MD [S] - **Spec Exp:** Pancreatic Cancer; Gastrointestinal Cancer; Peritoneal Carcinomatosis; Clinical Trials; **Hospital:** UCSD Med Ctr-Hillcrest; **Address:** Moores UCSD Cancer Ctr, 3855 Health Sciences Drive, La Jolla, CA 92093-0987; **Phone:** 858-822-2124; **Board Cert:** Surgery 2003; **Med School:** Cornell Univ-Weill Med Coll 1988; **Resid:** Surgery, NY-Cornell Med Ctr 1996; **Fellow:** Surgical Oncology, MD Anderson Cancer Ctr 1996; **Fac Appt:** Prof S, UCSD

Moossa, AR MD [S] - **Spec Exp:** Pancreatic Cancer; Gastrointestinal Cancer; Hepatobiliary Surgery; **Hospital:** UCSD Med Ctr-Hillcrest; **Address:** 9300 Campus Point Drive, La Jolla, CA 92037; **Phone:** 858-657-6113; **Med School:** England, UK 1965; **Resid:** Surgery, Liverpool Univ Hosps 1970; **Fellow:** Surgical Oncology, Johns Hopkins Hosp 1972; **Fac Appt:** Prof S, UCSD

Surgery

Nakakura, Eric MD/PhD [S] - **Spec Exp:** Pancreatic Cancer; Liver Cancer; Gastrointestinal Cancer; Sarcoma; **Hospital:** UCSF Med Ctr; **Address:** 1600 Divisadero St Fl 4, Box 1705, San Francisco, CA 94115; **Phone:** 415-353-9888; **Board Cert:** Surgery 2004; **Med School:** Stanford Univ 1995; **Resid:** Surgery, Johns Hopkins Hosp 2000; **Fellow:** Surgical Oncology, Johns Hopkins Hosp 2004; **Fac Appt:** Asst Prof S, UCSF

Nissen, Nicholas N MD [S] - **Spec Exp:** Liver Cancer; Transplant-Liver; Pancreatic Cancer; Minimally Invasive Surgery; **Hospital:** Cedars-Sinai Med Ctr; **Address:** Cedars-Sinai Medical Center, 8635 W 3rd St, Ste 590-W, Los Angeles, CA 90048; **Phone:** 310-423-2641; **Board Cert:** Surgery 1999; Surgical Critical Care 1999; **Med School:** Univ Minn 1991; **Resid:** Surgery, Loyola Univ Med Ctr 1998; **Fellow:** Surgical Critical Care, Univ Pittsburgh Med Ctr 1999; Hepatobiliary Surgery, UCLA Med Ctr 2001

Norton, Jeffrey A MD [S] - **Spec Exp:** Pancreatic Cancer; Gastrointestinal Cancer & Surgery; Endocrine Surgery; **Hospital:** Stanford Univ Hosp & Clinics; **Address:** 875 Blake Wilbur Drive, Clin F, Stanford, CA 94305; **Phone:** 650-723-5461; **Board Cert:** Surgery 2001; **Med School:** SUNY Upstate Med Univ 1973; **Resid:** Surgery, Duke Univ Med Ctr 1982; **Fellow:** Research, Natl Cancer Inst 1989; **Fac Appt:** Prof S, Stanford Univ

Paz, Isaac Benjamin MD [S] - **Spec Exp:** Breast Cancer; Esophageal Cancer; **Hospital:** City of Hope Natl Med Ctr (page 69); **Address:** 1500 E Duarte Rd, Duarte, CA 91010; **Phone:** 626-256-4673 x67100; **Board Cert:** Surgery 2000; **Med School:** Chile 1981; **Resid:** Surgery, Univ Catolica de Chile 1985; Surgery, Univ Arizona 1990; **Fellow:** Surgical Oncology, City of Hope Med Ctr 1993

Pellegrini, Carlos MD [S] - **Spec Exp:** Esophageal Cancer; Esophageal Surgery; Gastrointestinal Cancer & Surgery; Minimally Invasive Surgery; **Hospital:** Univ Wash Med Ctr; **Address:** Univ Washington Medical Ctr, Dept Surgery, 1959 NE Pacific St, Box 356165, Seattle, WA 98195; **Phone:** 206-598-4547; **Board Cert:** Surgery 1998; **Med School:** Argentina 1971; **Resid:** Surgery, Granadero Hosp 1975; Surgery, Univ Chicago Hosps 1979; **Fac Appt:** Prof S, Univ Wash

Peterson, Laura D MD [S] - **Spec Exp:** Breast Cancer; Breast Surgery; **Hospital:** Kapiolani Med Ctr for Women & Chldn, Straub Clinic & Hosp; **Address:** Kapi'olani Womens Ctr, 1907 S Beretania St, Ste 501, Honolulu, HI 96826; **Phone:** 808-949-3444; **Board Cert:** Surgery 2004; **Med School:** UCSD 1998; **Resid:** Surgery, Univ Hawaii Affil Hosp 2004; **Fellow:** Minimally Invasive Surgery, Kaiser Permanente 2005; Surgical Oncology, Kaiser Permanente 2005

Reber, Howard A MD [S] - **Spec Exp:** Pancreatic Cancer; Gastrointestinal Cancer; **Hospital:** UCLA Ronald Reagan Med Ctr; **Address:** UCLA General Surgery, 10833 Le Cone Ave CHS Bldg - rm 72-215, Los Angeles, CA 90095; **Phone:** 310-794-7788; **Board Cert:** Surgery 1971; **Med School:** Univ Pennsylvania 1964; **Resid:** Surgery, Hosp Univ Penn 1970; **Fac Appt:** Prof S, UCLA

Sener, Stephen F MD [S] - **Spec Exp:** Breast Cancer; Lymphedema; Thyroid Cancer; Melanoma; **Hospital:** USC Univ Hosp; **Address:** USC Norris Comprehensive Cancer Ctr, 1441 Eastlake Ave, Ste 7415, Los Angeles, CA 90033; **Phone:** 323-865-3535; **Board Cert:** Surgery 2001; **Med School:** Northwestern Univ 1977; **Resid:** Surgery, Northwestern Univ 1982; **Fellow:** Surgery, Meml Sloan Kettering Cancer Ctr 1984; **Fac Appt:** Prof S, USC-Keck School of Medicine

Silverstein, Melvin J MD [S] - **Spec Exp:** Breast Cancer; **Hospital:** Hoag Meml Hosp Presby; **Address:** 1 Hoag Drive, Breast Care Ctr, Newport Beach, CA 92658; **Phone:** 949-764-8281; **Board Cert:** Surgery 1971; **Med School:** Albany Med Coll 1965; **Resid:** Surgery, Boston City Hosp-Tufts Univ 1970; **Fellow:** Surgical Oncology, UCLA Med Ctr 1975

Sinanan, Mika N MD [S] - **Spec Exp:** Gastrointestinal Surgery; Gastrointestinal Cancer; Liver & Biliary Cancer; Laparoscopic Surgery; **Hospital:** Univ Wash Med Ctr; **Address:** Univ Washington, Dept Surgery, 1959 NE Pacific St, Box 356165, Seattle, WA 98195-6410; **Phone:** 206-598-4477; **Board Cert:** Surgery 2008; **Med School:** Johns Hopkins Univ 1980; **Resid:** Surgery, Univ Washington Hosp 1988; **Fellow:** Gastrointestinal Surgery, Univ Brit Columbia Med Ctr 1986; **Fac Appt:** Prof S, Univ Wash

Trisal, Vijay MD [S] - **Spec Exp:** Skin Cancer; **Hospital:** City of Hope Natl Med Ctr (page 69); **Address:** City of Hope Med Ctr, Dept Surgery, 1500 E Duarte Rd, Duarte, CA 91010; **Phone:** 626-256-4673 x67100; **Board Cert:** Surgery 2003; **Med School:** India 1993; **Resid:** Surgery, Providence Hosp & Med Ctrs 2002; **Fellow:** Surgical Oncology, City of Hope Natl Med Ctr 2004

Vetto, John MD [S] - **Spec Exp:** Cancer Surgery; **Hospital:** OR Hlth & Sci Univ; **Address:** 3181 SW Sam Jackson Park Rd, MC L619, Portland, OR 97239; **Phone:** 503-494-5501; **Board Cert:** Surgery 2009; **Med School:** Oregon Hlth & Sci Univ 1982; **Resid:** Surgery, Brigham & Women's Hosp 1984; Surgery, UCLA Med Ctr 1989; **Fellow:** Surgical Oncology, Natl Cancer Inst 1986; Surgical Oncology, Meml Sloan Kettering Cancer Ctr 1991; **Fac Appt:** Assoc Prof S, Oregon Hlth & Sci Univ

Wagman, Lawrence D MD [S] - **Spec Exp:** Liver Cancer; Gastrointestinal Cancer; Breast Cancer; Carcinoid Tumors; **Hospital:** St. Joseph's Hosp - Orange, City of Hope Natl Med Ctr (page 69); **Address:** 1010 W La Veta Ave, Fl 4, Ste 470, Orange, CA 92868; **Phone:** 714-835-8300; **Board Cert:** Surgery 2004; **Med School:** Columbia P&S 1978; **Resid:** Surgery, Med Coll Virginia Hosp 1985; **Fellow:** Surgical Oncology, NIH/NCI 1982; **Fac Appt:** Assoc Clin Prof S, UCSD

Wallace, Anne Marie MD [S] - **Spec Exp:** Breast Cancer; Breast Reconstruction; Melanoma; **Hospital:** UCSD Med Ctr-Hillcrest; **Address:** UCSD Moores Cancer Ctr, 3855 Health Sciences Drive #0987, La Jolla, CA 92093; **Phone:** 858-822-6193; **Board Cert:** Surgery 2001; Plastic Surgery 2005; **Med School:** Creighton Univ 1987; **Resid:** Surgery, Washington Hosp Ctr 1992; Plastic Surgery, UCSD Med Ctr 1994; **Fellow:** Surgical Breast Oncology, MD Anderson Cancer Ctr 1995; **Fac Appt:** Clin Prof S, UCSD

Wapnir, Irene L MD [S] - **Spec Exp:** Breast Surgery; Breast Cancer; **Hospital:** Stanford Univ Hosp & Clinics; **Address:** Stanford Univ Medical Ctr, 300 Pasteur Drive, rm H3625, Palo Alto, CA 94305; **Phone:** 650-736-1353; **Board Cert:** Surgery 2008; **Med School:** Mexico 1980; **Resid:** Surgery, Lincoln Hosp 1985; **Fellow:** Breast Disease, RW Johnson Univ Med Ctr 1986; **Fac Appt:** Assoc Prof S, Stanford Univ

Yeung, Raymond S W MD [S] - **Spec Exp:** Liver & Biliary Cancer; Liver Cancer; Melanoma; Breast Cancer; **Hospital:** Univ Wash Med Ctr; **Address:** Univ of Washington, Dept Surgery, 1959 NE Pacific St, Box 356165, Seattle, WA 98195; **Phone:** 206-598-4477; **Board Cert:** Surgery 2009; **Med School:** Univ Toronto 1982; **Resid:** Surgery, University of Toronto 1987; **Fellow:** Surgical Oncology, Fox Chase Cancer Ctr 1992; **Fac Appt:** Prof S, Univ Wash

canswer.

Non-profit cancer research and treatment center ~ 183 beds ~ Accredited by The Joint Commission

Surgical Oncology Experts

As a recognized leader in the field of laparoscopic and robotic-assisted surgery, City of Hope uses the most advanced *da Vinci S*® robotic system. Guided by skilled surgeons, *da Vinci* goes beyond the reach of humans and performs with greater precision, removing tumors without disturbing the healthy tissue around them. The result is less blood loss, minimal discomfort and faster recovery times. Robotic-assisted surgery is used for many cancers, including colon, kidney, liver, lung and prostate cancer. And City of Hope is one of only two hospitals in the U.S. using this method to treat head and neck cancers.

To learn more, call 800-826-HOPE
www.cityofhope.org/davinci

1500 East Duarte Road, Duarte, California 91010

City of Hope is recognized as one of only 40 National Cancer Institute-designated Comprehensive Cancer Centers and is ranked by *U.S.News & World Report* as one of "America's Best Hospitals" in cancer and urology.

City of Hope's *Helford Clinical Research Hospital* integrates lifesaving research and superior clinical care. Multidisciplinary teams of medical professionals work together to deliver promising new therapies to patients quickly, safely and effectively. They care for the whole patient, including their emotional, psychological, spiritual and nutritional needs.

A recognized leader in compassionate patient care, innovative science and translational research, City of Hope collaborates with other top institutions around the globe, rapidly developing laboratory breakthroughs into revolutionary new treatments.

City of Hope welcomes patient referrals from physicians throughout the world. Please contact specialists directly or call **800-826-HOPE**.

City of Hope has answers to cancer.

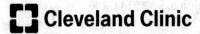
Cleveland Clinic
Every life deserves world class care.

Recognized Leader in Breast Cancer

At Cleveland Clinic Taussig Cancer Institute, more than 250 top cancer specialists, researchers, nurses and technicians are dedicated to delivering the most effective medical treatments and offering access to the latest clinical trials for more than 13,000 new cancer patients every year. Our doctors are nationally and internationally known for their contributions to cancer breakthroughs and their ability to deliver superior outcomes for our patients. In recognition of these and other achievements, *U.S.News & World Report* has ranked Cleveland Clinic as one of the top cancer centers in the nation.

Breast Center Services

Patients have access to the latest breast imaging capabilities, including digital mammography, expert interpretation by dedicated breast imaging physicians and special care for high-risk patients. Breast Center specialists use breast magnetic resonance imaging to complement existing screening, diagnostic and surgical strategies.

Treatment and Reconstruction

The Breast Center offers patients the latest treatments, including techniques and reconstructive surgery performed alone or together with therapeutic cancer surgery, including a nipple-sparing procedure and innovative flap reconstruction using the patient's own tissue to create a more natural-looking breast. Chemotherapy, hormonal therapy and novel targeted therapies may be used to prevent recurrence or as primary treatment for breast cancer. Patients undergoing radiation therapy are fitted with a unique device developed at Cleveland Clinic that shields the opposite breast from scatter radiation.

Cleveland Clinic
Taussig Cancer Institute
9500 Euclid Avenue
Cleveland, OH 44195

clevelandclinic.org/breastTCD

**Appointments | Information:
Call the Cancer Answer Line at
866.223.8100.**

Cancer Treatment Guides
Cleveland Clinic has developed comprehensive treatment guides for many cancers. To download our free treatment guides, visit clevelandclinic.org/cancertreatmentguides.

**Comprehensive Online
Medical Second Opinion**
Cleveland Clinic experts can review your medical records and render an opinion that includes treatment options and recommendations. Call 216.444.3223 or 800.223.2273 ext. 43223; email eclevelandclinic@ccf.org.

**Special Assistance for
Out-of-State Patients**
Cleveland Clinic Global Patient Services offers a complimentary Medical Concierge service for patients who travel from outside of Ohio. Call 800.223.2273, ext. 55580, or email medicalconcierge@ccf.org.

FOX CHASE
CANCER CENTER

333 Cottman Avenue
Philadelphia, PA 19111-2497
Phone: 1-888-FOX CHASE • Fax: 215-728-2702
www.foxchase.org

SURGICAL ONCOLOGY

Studies show that experienced surgeons provide better surgical outcomes. At Fox Chase, our surgeons are fellowship-trained, meaning they have up to four years of additional training in the highly complex techniques of cancer surgery. They have extensive experience, focused entirely on cancer care and treat nearly all types of cancers with minimally invasive techniques. In addition, our plastic and reconstructive surgeons specialize in restoring form and function with excellent results for patients needing reconstructive surgery after cancer treatment.

Breast Cancer: We offer the most advanced diagnostic techniques, including digital mammography, stereotactic breast biopsy and sentinel lymph-node surgery. Treatment options include breast-preserving surgery with radiation therapy as well as skin-sparing mastectomy with cosmetic reconstructive surgery.

Gastrointestinal Cancers: Our gastrointestinal surgeons have extensive expertise with colorectal, pancreatic, stomach, liver and other bowel cancers and are the most experienced laparoscopic and robotic experts in the region. We also offer the most advanced endoscopic and minimally invasive techniques to avoid major surgery. In addition, Fox Chase offers personalized care for patients with Barrett's esophagus—a condition that increases the risk of gastrointestinal cancer—to prevent the need for surgery and the development of cancer.

Genitourinary Cancers: Our urologic surgical oncologists have extensive expertise in the treatment of prostate, bladder, kidney, ureteral, adrenal, testicular and penile cancers. Our urologists emphasize organ preservation, quality of life and minimally invasive/robotic approaches to cancer surgery.

Gynecologic Cancers: Our gynecologic surgeons offer the most advanced laparoscopic and robotic techniques as well as complex open surgery for women with cancers of the uterus, ovary and cervix.

Head and Neck Cancers: Fox Chase provides patients with one-stop consultations with surgical, radiation and medical oncologists. Expertise includes otolaryngology, transoral laser surgery, plastic and microvascular reconstruction as well as robotic surgery.

Lung and Esophageal Cancers: Our thoracic surgeons offer a variety of minimally invasive techniques for patients with lung and esophageal cancers, including video-assisted thoracic surgery (VATS) and laparoscopic esophageal surgery. Fox Chase is one of only a few centers in the country offering these options.

Minimally Invasive Surgery

At Fox Chase, we offer the broadest range of minimally invasive treatment options for your cancer. Minimally invasive procedures allow the surgeon to reach the tumor through tiny incisions and with pinpoint accuracy. This benefits patients because it means less scarring, reduced pain, less bleeding, fewer complications, and a faster recovery.

Fox Chase is one of only a few institutions worldwide using robot-assisted surgery to treat nearly all types of cancers, including prostate, gynecologic, kidney, bladder, colon, lung, and head and neck cancers. In addition, Fox Chase's highly skilled surgeons have extensive experience performing laparoscopic surgery for cancers of the liver, pancreas, bile ducts, and gallbladder; video-assisted thoracic surgery (VATS) for lung and other thoracic cancers; and transoral laser surgery for cancers of the head and neck.

For more about Fox Chase physicians and services, visit our website, www.foxchase.org, or call 1-888-FOX CHASE.

THE TISCH CANCER INSTITUTE
AT THE MOUNT SINAI MEDICAL CENTER

One Gustave L. Levy Place
Fifth Avenue and 100th Street
New York, NY 10029-6574
Physician Referral: 1-800-MD-SINAI (637-4624)
www.tischcancerinstitute.org

THE TISCH CANCER INSTITUTE is embedded within a renowned medical center that has world-class research facilities, one of the nation's top-ranked hospitals, and an outstanding medical school. Patients have access to the best possible cancer care across a variety of disciplines, including medical, surgical, and radiation treatments; palliative care; behavioral medicine; physical therapy; psychosocial services—and cutting-edge cancer research. For fully integrated, multidisciplinary care, our patients are also treated by the best specialists in every field at Mount Sinai and can receive seamless referrals.

Services and Programs – The Tisch Cancer Institute employs a multidisciplinary treatment approach, providing access to clinical breakthroughs, innovative techniques, leading-edge technologies, and a wide range of diagnostic, therapeutic, and support services for all types of cancer. The Institute treats: breast cancer; hematological malignancies (including multiple myeloma, myelodysplastic syndrome, and myeloproliferative disorders); genitourinary cancers (including prostate, bladder, and kidney); head and neck cancers; thoracic cancer (including lung and esophagus); gynecologic cancers; brain tumors; and other diagnoses. In addition to surgical treatment, the Institute provides radiation and medical oncology therapies, as well as bone marrow transplantation. The Dubin Breast Center, consisting of 15,000 square feet, is a newly constructed facility that opened in April 2011 and significantly expands the treatment space for breast cancer patients.

THE RUTTENBERG TREATMENT CENTER
The Derald H. Ruttenberg Treatment Center houses the ambulatory cancer program of The Tisch Cancer Institute and is operated by the Mount Sinai Hospital.

THE DUBIN BREAST CARE CENTER
The Dubin Breast Care Center offers the latest, most innovative approaches available for breast health and the treatment of breast cancer.

The Tisch Cancer Institute encourages collaboration with colleagues across the Medical Center, drawing upon the knowledge of a vast network of specialists who are outstanding in their fields. These experts consist of award-winning physicians and surgeons specializing in cardiac care, neurology, urology, pediatrics, digestive diseases, obstetrics and gynecology, and other therapeutic areas. Oncologists, surgeons, radiation oncologists, and specialists from across the medical spectrum work together to provide the highest quality care to all cancer patients. Furthermore, Mount Sinai's nursing staff is an important part of the Medical Center's focus on delivering exceptional patient care, and it has received the prestigious Magnet Award for nursing excellence. Mount Sinai is also renowned for its palliative care program, which provides the highest level of care, focusing on the relief of pain, symptoms, and stress in cancer patients in both an inpatient and outpatient setting.

A Heritage of Breakthroughs – Teams of physicians and scientists at The Tisch Cancer Institute at Mount Sinai work together to rapidly translate laboratory research into new patient treatments. Among the advances pioneered at Mount Sinai are the first successful treatment of tumors of the bladder by transurethral electrocoagulation, the first demonstration of how asbestos can cause cancerous changes in the DNA of cells, and the first development of an ultrasound-guided technique to insert radioactive seeds into the prostate to treat prostate cancer.

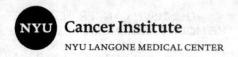

NYU Cancer Institute
NYU LANGONE MEDICAL CENTER

NYU Langone Medical Center
550 First Avenue , New York, NY 10016
www.NYULMC.org

NYU Clinical Cancer Center
160 East 34th Street, New York, NY 10016
www.NYUCI.org

**The Stephen D. Hassenfeld Children's Center
for Cancer and Blood Disorders**
160 East 32nd Street, New York, NY 10016
www.NYUMC.org/Hassenfeld

The NYU Cancer Institute is an NCI-designated cancer center and provides personalized patient care that is both compassionate and state of the art. The doctors and researchers work together to develop innovative therapies for patients. The Cancer Institute is world-renowned for excellence in cancer-focused research, personalized care, education and community outreach. Its mission is to discover the origins of human cancer and to use that knowledge to eradicate the personal and societal burden of cancer in our community, the nation and the world. For more information about our expert physicians, call 212-731-5000. *We specialize in the following areas:*

Patient-Focused Setting
The NYU Clinical Cancer Center is the principal outpatient facility of The Cancer Institute and serves as home to our patients and their caregivers. The center and its multidisciplinary team of experts provide access to the latest treatment options and clinical trials along with a variety of programs in cancer risk reduction/prevention, screening, diagnostics, genetic counseling and supportive services. In addition the NYUCI emphasizes the importance of a holistic approach to management services in complementary medicine, psychosocial support, survivorship and palliative care.

Renowned Expertise
The NYU Cancer Institute brings together experts from a variety of disciplines to create collaborative research endeavors and clinical care teams. The Cancer Institute offers a full continuum of personalized care, from prevention through diagnosis, treatment and post-treatment support. The compassion and expertise of our team members helps patients better manage the symptoms of their diseases as well as meet their special needs. Additionally, we have created special emphasis programs in diseases such as breast cancer, melanoma, GI cancer, prostate cancer, hematologic malignancies and lung cancer among others, as well as, translational programs in cancer healthcare disparities, molecularly targeted therapy, and the cell signaling pathways involved in cancer.

A Translational Approach
NYU Langone Medical Center scientists and other researchers excel in uncovering how cancer develops at the molecular level, and how we can harness that knowledge to reduce the risk of cancer and treat the disease. The Medical Center constantly seeks to create new opportunities for collaboration between investigators within our own institution, those located elsewhere in the NYU network of campuses, and researchers at other institutions.

The Stephen D. Hassenfeld Children's Center for Cancer and Blood Disorders
The center is a leading pediatric outpatient facility for the treatment of childhood cancers and blood diseases. Its unique interdisciplinary and family-centered approach combines the most advanced medical treatments with psychosocial and emotional support services for young patients and their families.

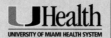
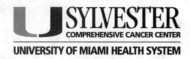

UNIVERSITY OF MIAMI HEALTH SYSTEM

DRIVEN TO BEAT CANCER

Sylvester Comprehensive Cancer Center serves as the cancer research diagnosis and treatment hub of UHealth – University of Miami Health System. Over the past decade and a half, Sylvester has grown with unstoppable momentum and singular focus – to develop and implement cancer breakthroughs and save lives.

Gaining the attention and respect of physicians and scientists from around the world, Sylvester has emerged as a magnet for today's leading cancer experts, attracting among the most innovative cancer professionals across a full spectrum of disciplines. Drawn to its entrepreneurial spirit, its unique international flair, and its awe-inspiring knowledge base, the team at Sylvester represents the future of university-based cancer care and research. It represents the real-world possibility to find the cure.

MORE CANCER SPECIALISTS. MORE SPECIALIZED CARE.

Patients who receive care from specialized hospitals often have better outcomes. At Sylvester we recognize the value of specialization, so we maintain a singular focus on cancer…only cancer. With more cancer experts than any other South Florida facility – more than 250 physicians and scientists, all faculty of the Miller School of Medicine – we have earned a reputation for delivering the most advanced treatment options available. This recognition has contributed to intense demand for care at Sylvester and more than a quarter million patient visits annually.

PHASE I CLINICAL TRIALS PROGRAM

Sylvester created South Florida's only academic phase I testing center dedicated to drug development for cancer patients. This novel program provides the necessary foundation to speed promising therapies from the laboratory to patients in need of care.

Phase I trials are the first studies in humans and, as a result, an important step to transition novel treatments from the bench to the bedside. The Phase I Clinical Trials Program assists physicians and scientists to establish important collaborative relationships that often translate into more treatment choices for patients.

Sylvester has assembled 15 multidisciplinary teams with focused expertise in specific types of cancers, including:

- Bone & Soft Tissue Cancers
- Breast Cancer
- Colorectal Cancer
- Eye Cancer
- Gynecologic Cancer
- Head & Neck Cancer
- Leukemia, Lymphoma & Myeloma
- Lung Cancer
- Melanoma & Related Skin Cancers
- Neurological Cancer
- Pancreatic, Liver & Related Cancers
- Pediatric Cancer
- Prostate, Bladder & Kidney Cancers
- Stomach & Esophageal Cancers
- Thyroid & Other Endocrine Cancers

As a leader in cancer research and treatment, Sylvester Comprehensive Cancer Center, with outpatient locations in Deerfield Beach and Kendall, is part of UHealth – University of Miami Health System, which includes more than 1,200 physicians, 30 outpatient locations, University of Miami Hospital, and the nation's top-ranked eye hospital, Bascom Palmer Eye Institute.

1475 N.W. 12th Avenue
Miami, Florida 33136
800-545-2292
www.sylvester.org

The Best in American Medicine
www.CastleConnolly.com

Thoracic Surgery

A thoracic surgeon provides the operative, perioperative care and critical care of patients with pathologic conditions within the chest. Included is the surgical care of coronary artery disease, cancers of the lung, esophagus and chest wall, abnormalities of the trachea, abnormalities of the great vessels and heart valves, congenital anomalies, tumors of the mediastinum and diseases of the diaphragm. The management of the airway and injuries of the chest is within the scope of the specialty.

Thoracic surgeons have the knowledge, experience and technical skills to accurately diagnose, operate upon safely and effectively manage patients with thoracic diseases of the chest. This requires substantial knowledge of cardiorespiratory physiology and oncology, as well as capability in the use of heart assist devices, management of abnormal heart rhythms and drainage of the chest cavity, respiratory support systems, endoscopy and invasive and noninvasive diagnostic techniques.

Training Required: Six to eight years

THORACIC SURGERY

New England

Brinckerhoff, Laurence H MD [TS] - **Spec Exp:** Lung Cancer; Esophageal Cancer; Minimally Invasive Thoracic Surgery; **Hospital:** Tufts Med Ctr; **Address:** Tufts Dept Thoracic Surgery, 750 Washington St, Box 5589, Boston, MA 02111; **Phone:** 617-636-5589; **Board Cert:** Surgery 2002; Thoracic Surgery 2006; **Med School:** Dartmouth Med Sch 1994; **Resid:** Surgery, Univ Virginia Med Ctr 2001; **Fellow:** Cardiothoracic Surgery, Univ Colorado Hlth Sci Ctr 2004

Bueno, Raphael MD [TS] - **Spec Exp:** Lung Cancer; Minimally Invasive Thoracic Surgery; Minimally Invasive Esophageal Surgery; Endoscopic Surgery; **Hospital:** Brigham & Women's Hosp, Dana-Farber Cancer Inst; **Address:** Brigham and Women's Hospital, Division of Thoracic Surgery Clin, 75 Francis St, Boston, MA 02115; **Phone:** 617-732-6824; **Board Cert:** Thoracic Surgery 2006; Surgery 2002; Surgical Critical Care 2003; **Med School:** Harvard Med Sch 1985; **Resid:** Surgery, Brigham & Women's Hosp 1992; **Fellow:** Surgical Critical Care, Brigham & Women's Hosp 1993; Thoracic Surgery, Mass Genl Hosp 1995; **Fac Appt:** Assoc Prof S, Harvard Med Sch

Fernando, Hiran C MD [TS] - **Spec Exp:** Esophageal Cancer; Lung Cancer; Minimally Invasive Thoracic Surgery; **Hospital:** Boston Med Ctr; **Address:** Boston Med Ctr Thoracic Surgery, 88 E Newton St, Robinson B402, Boston, MA 02118; **Phone:** 617-638-5600; **Board Cert:** Surgery 2005; Thoracic Surgery 2009; **Med School:** England, UK 1986; **Resid:** Surgery, Harbor/UCLA Med Ctr 1993; Thoracic Surgery, UC Davis Med Ctr 1998; **Fellow:** Minimally Invasive Surgery, Univ Pittsburgh 2001; **Fac Appt:** Assoc Prof TS, Boston Univ

Gaissert, Henning A MD [TS] - **Spec Exp:** Esophageal Cancer; Tracheal Surgery; Lung Cancer; Thymoma; **Hospital:** Mass Genl Hosp, Newton - Wellesley Hosp; **Address:** Mass Genl Hosp, 55 Fruit St, BLK 1570, Boston, MA 02114; **Phone:** 617-726-5341; **Board Cert:** Surgery 2011; Thoracic Surgery 2004; **Med School:** Germany 1984; **Resid:** Surgery, Mass Genl Hosp 1989; Surgery, Barnes Jewish Hosp 1991; **Fellow:** Research, Harvard Med Sch 1993; Cardiothoracic Surgery, Barnes Jewish Hosp 1996; **Fac Appt:** Assoc Prof S, Harvard Med Sch

Mathisen, Douglas MD [TS] - **Spec Exp:** Tracheal Surgery; Lung Cancer; Esophageal Cancer; **Hospital:** Mass Genl Hosp, Newton - Wellesley Hosp; **Address:** Mass Genl Hosp, Thoracic Surgery, 55 Fruit St, Blake 1570, Boston, MA 02114; **Phone:** 617-726-6826; **Board Cert:** Thoracic Surgery 2002; **Med School:** Univ IL Coll Med 1974; **Resid:** Surgery, Mass Genl Hosp 1981; Thoracic Surgery, Mass Genl Hosp 1982; **Fellow:** Surgical Oncology, Natl Cancer Inst 1979; **Fac Appt:** Prof S, Harvard Med Sch

Nugent, William C MD [TS] - **Spec Exp:** Thoracic Cancers; **Hospital:** Dartmouth - Hitchcock Med Ctr; **Address:** Dartmouth-Hitchcock Med Ctr, Dept Cardiothoracic Surgery, 1 Medical Center Drive, Lebanon, NH 03756; **Phone:** 603-650-8572; **Board Cert:** Thoracic Surgery 2002; **Med School:** Albany Med Coll 1975; **Resid:** Surgery, Beth Israel Hosp 1980; Thoracic Surgery, Univ Michigan Med Ctr 1983; **Fellow:** Cardiothoracic Surgery, Mass Genl Hosp 1981; **Fac Appt:** Prof S, Dartmouth Med Sch

Sugarbaker, David J MD [TS] - **Spec Exp:** Mesothelioma; Transplant-Lung; Esophageal Cancer; **Hospital:** Brigham & Women's Hosp, Dana-Farber Cancer Inst; **Address:** Brigham & Women's Hosp, 75 Francis St, Division of Thoracic Surgery, Boston, MA 02115-6110; **Phone:** 617-732-6824; **Board Cert:** Thoracic Surgery 1999; **Med School:** Cornell Univ-Weill Med Coll 1979; **Resid:** Surgery, Brigham & Women's Hosp 1982; Surgery, Brigham & Women's Hosp 1986; **Fellow:** Thoracic Surgery, Toronto Genl Hosp 1988; **Fac Appt:** Prof S, Harvard Med Sch

Swanson, Scott J MD [TS] - **Spec Exp:** Lung Cancer; Video Assisted Thoracic Surgery (VATS); Esophageal Cancer; **Hospital:** Brigham & Women's Hosp, Dana-Farber Cancer Inst; **Address:** Div Thoracic Surgery, Brigham & Women's Hosp, 75 Francis St, Boston, MA 02115; **Phone:** 617-525-7532; **Board Cert:** Surgery 2003; Thoracic Surgery 2006; **Med School:** Harvard Med Sch 1985; **Resid:** Surgery, Brigham & Womens Hosp 1990; **Fellow:** Cardiothoracic Surgery, Brigham & Womens Hosp 1994

Wain, John MD [TS] - **Spec Exp:** Lung Cancer; Esophageal Cancer; **Hospital:** Mass Genl Hosp; **Address:** Mass Genl Hosp, Deiv Thoracic Surg, 55 Fruit St, Blake 1570, Boston, MA 02114; **Phone:** 617-726-5200; **Board Cert:** Thoracic Surgery 2000; **Med School:** Jefferson Med Coll 1980; **Resid:** Surgery, Mass Genl Hosp 1985; **Fellow:** Cardiothoracic Surgery, Mass Genl Hosp 1988; **Fac Appt:** Asst Prof TS, Harvard Med Sch

Wright, Cameron D MD [TS] - **Spec Exp:** Lung Cancer; Esophageal Cancer; Tracheal Surgery; **Hospital:** Mass Genl Hosp; **Address:** Mass Genl Hosp, Div Thoracic Surg, 55 Fruit St, Blake 1570, Boston, MA 02114; **Phone:** 617-726-5801; **Board Cert:** Surgery 2006; Thoracic Surgery 2007; **Med School:** Univ Mich Med Sch 1980; **Resid:** Surgery, Mass Genl Hosp 1986; Thoracic Surgery, Mass Genl Hosp 1988; **Fac Appt:** Assoc Prof S, Harvard Med Sch

Mid Atlantic

Altorki, Nasser MD [TS] - **Spec Exp:** Esophageal Cancer; Lung Cancer; Thoracic Cancers; Vaccine Therapy; **Hospital:** NY-Presby Hosp/Weill Cornell (page 78); **Address:** 525 E 68th St, M-404, New York, NY 10065; **Phone:** 212-746-5156; **Board Cert:** Surgery 2006; Thoracic Surgery 2007; **Med School:** Egypt 1978; **Resid:** Surgery, Univ Chicago Hosps 1985; **Fellow:** Cardiothoracic Surgery, Univ Chicago Hosps 1987; **Fac Appt:** Prof S, Cornell Univ-Weill Med Coll

Bains, Manjit MD [TS] - **Spec Exp:** Esophageal Cancer; Lung Cancer; **Hospital:** Meml Sloan-Kettering Cancer Ctr (page 75); **Address:** 1275 York Ave, rm C681, New York, NY 10065; **Phone:** 212-639-7450; **Board Cert:** Surgery 1971; Thoracic Surgery 1972; **Med School:** India 1963; **Resid:** Surgery, Rochester Genl Hosp 1970; **Fellow:** Thoracic Surgery, Sloan Kettering Cancer Ctr 1972; **Fac Appt:** Clin Prof S, Cornell Univ-Weill Med Coll

Battafarano, Richard J MD [TS] - **Spec Exp:** Lung Cancer; Barrett's Esophagus; Esophageal Surgery; Mesothelioma; **Hospital:** Univ of MD Med Ctr; **Address:** Univ MD Med Ctr, Greenebaum Cancer Ctr-Dept Thoracic Surgery, 29 S Greene St, Ste 504, Baltimore, MD 21201; **Phone:** 410-328-6366; **Board Cert:** Surgery 2008; Thoracic Surgery 2000; **Med School:** Hahnemann Univ 1988; **Resid:** Surgery, Univ Minn Hosp & Clin 1997; **Fellow:** Thoracic Surgery, Meml Sloan Kettering Cancer Ctr 1999; **Fac Appt:** Assoc Prof S, Univ MD Sch Med

Demmy, Todd L MD [TS] - **Spec Exp:** Lung Cancer; Thoracic Cancers; Esophageal Cancer; Minimally Invasive Thoracic Surgery; **Hospital:** Roswell Park Cancer Inst, Buffalo General Hosp; **Address:** Roswell Park Cancer Inst, Dept Thoracic Surgery, Elm & Carlton Sts, Buffalo, NY 14263; **Phone:** 716-845-5873; **Board Cert:** Surgery 2008; Thoracic Surgery 2000; Surgical Critical Care 2001; **Med School:** Jefferson Med Coll 1983; **Resid:** Surgery, Baylor Univ Medical Ctr 1988; Thoracic Surgery, Allegheny Genl Hosp 1991; **Fac Appt:** Assoc Prof S, SUNY Buffalo

Downey, Robert MD [TS] - **Spec Exp:** Lung Cancer; Thoracic Cancers; **Hospital:** Meml Sloan-Kettering Cancer Ctr (page 75); **Address:** 1275 York Avenue, New York, NY 10065; **Phone:** 800-525-2225; **Board Cert:** Surgery 2002; Thoracic Surgery 2005; Thoracic Surgery 2005; **Med School:** Columbia P&S 1985; **Resid:** Surgery, Columbia-Presby Med Ctr 1991; **Fellow:** Thoracic Surgery, Mayo Clinic 1992; Thoracic Surgery, Columbia-Presby Med Ctr 1994

Thoracic Surgery

Flores, Raja M MD [TS] - **Spec Exp:** Mesothelioma; Lung Cancer; Video Assisted Thoracic Surgery (VATS); Esophageal Cancer; **Hospital:** Mount Sinai Med Ctr (page 76); **Address:** Chief, Div Thoracic Surgery, Mount Sinai Med Ctr, 1190 Fifth Ave, New York, NY 10029; **Phone:** 212-241-9466; **Board Cert:** Surgery 1999; Thoracic Surgery 2001; **Med School:** Albert Einstein Coll Med 1992; **Resid:** Surgery, Columbia Presby Med Ctr 1997; **Fellow:** Thoracic Surgery, Brigham & Womens Hosp/Dana Faber Cancer Inst 2000; **Fac Appt:** Assoc Prof TS, Cornell Univ-Weill Med Coll

Friedberg, Joseph MD [TS] - **Spec Exp:** Mesothelioma; Lung Cancer; Thoracic Cancers; Photodynamic Therapy; **Hospital:** Penn Presby Med Ctr - UPHS (page 80), Hosp Univ Penn - UPHS (page 80); **Address:** Penn-Presbyterian Medical Ctr, 51 N 39th St, rm W250, Philadelphia, PA 19104; **Phone:** 215-662-9195; **Board Cert:** Surgery 2006; Thoracic Surgery 2006; **Med School:** Harvard Med Sch 1986; **Resid:** Surgery, Mass General Hosp 1994; **Fellow:** Cardiothoracic Surgery, Brigham & Womens Hosp 1996; **Fac Appt:** Assoc Prof TS, Univ Pennsylvania

Gharagozloo, Farid MD [TS] - **Spec Exp:** Video Assisted Thoracic Surgery (VATS); Lung Cancer; **Hospital:** G Washington Univ Hosp, Harbor Hosp; **Address:** 2175 K St NW, Ste 300, Washington, DC 20037; **Phone:** 202-775-8600; **Board Cert:** Thoracic Surgery 2001; **Med School:** Johns Hopkins Univ 1983; **Resid:** Surgery, Mayo Clinic 1989; Research, Harvard Med Sch 1986; **Fellow:** Cardiothoracic Surgery, Mayo Clinic 1992; **Fac Appt:** Prof S, Geo Wash Univ

Heitmiller, Richard F MD [TS] - **Spec Exp:** Esophageal Surgery; Esophageal Cancer; Lung Cancer; **Hospital:** Union Meml Hosp-Baltimore; **Address:** 3333 N Calvert St, Ste 610, Baltimore, MD 21218; **Phone:** 410-554-2063; **Board Cert:** Therapeutic Radiology 2008; **Med School:** Johns Hopkins Univ 1979; **Resid:** Surgery, Mass Genl Hosp 1985; **Fellow:** Thoracic Surgery, Mass Genl Hosp 1987; **Fac Appt:** Assoc Prof Surg & Onc, Johns Hopkins Univ

Kaiser, Larry R MD [TS] - **Spec Exp:** Lung Cancer; Esophageal Cancer; Mediastinal Tumors; **Hospital:** Temple Univ Hosp; **Address:** 3500 N Broad St, MERB Bldg - Fl 11, PO Box 20036, Philadelphia, PA 19140; **Phone:** 215-707-8773; **Board Cert:** Surgery 2005; Thoracic Surgery 2006; **Med School:** Tulane Univ 1977; **Resid:** Surgery, UCLA Med Ctr 1983; Cardiothoracic Surgery, Univ Toronto Hosps 1985; **Fellow:** Surgical Oncology, UCLA Med Ctr 1981; **Fac Appt:** Prof TS, Temple Univ

Keenan, Robert J MD [TS] - **Spec Exp:** Lung Cancer; Esophageal Cancer; Mediastinal Tumors; **Hospital:** Allegheny General Hosp, West Penn Hosp-Forbes Campus; **Address:** Allegheny General Hospital, 320 E North Ave, Pittsburgh, PA 15212; **Phone:** 412-359-6137; **Board Cert:** Surgery 2010; **Med School:** Canada 1984; **Resid:** Surgery, Univ Toronto Med Ctr 1989; **Fellow:** Thoracic Surgery, Univ Pittsburgh Med Ctr 1990; Thoracic Surgery, Univ Toronto Med Ctr 1992; **Fac Appt:** Prof TS, Drexel Univ Coll Med

Keller, Steven M MD [TS] - **Spec Exp:** Lung Cancer; Esophageal Cancer; Mediastinal Tumors; **Hospital:** Montefiore Med Ctr - Div. Moses, Montefiore Med Ctr - Div. Weiler; **Address:** 1575 Blondell St, Ste 125, Bronx, NY 10461; **Phone:** 718-405-8378; **Board Cert:** Thoracic Surgery 2007; **Med School:** Albany Med Coll 1977; **Resid:** Surgery, Mount Sinai Hosp 1985; Thoracic Surgery, Mem Sloan Kettering Cancer Ctr 1987; **Fellow:** Surgical Oncology, NIH/National Cancer Inst 1983; **Fac Appt:** Prof TS, Albert Einstein Coll Med

Kiev, Jonathan MD [TS] - **Spec Exp:** Chest Wall Tumors; Esophageal Cancer; Lung Cancer; **Hospital:** Anne Arundel Med Ctr; **Address:** Annapolis Thoracic Surgery, 2002 Medical Pkwy, Ste 660, Annapolis, MD 21401; **Phone:** 877-503-2609; **Board Cert:** Surgery 2005; Thoracic Surgery 2002; **Med School:** Tulane Univ 1989; **Resid:** Surgery, Hahnemann Univ Hosp 1996; Cardiothoracic Surgery, Loma Linda Univ 2000; **Fellow:** Thoracic Surgery, Univ Pittsburgh 2001; Thoracic Surgery, Mayo Clinic 2001

Krasna, Mark MD [TS] - **Spec Exp:** Esophageal Cancer; Lung Cancer; **Hospital:** St. Joseph Med Ctr, Univ of MD Med Ctr; **Address:** 7501 Osler Drive, Odea Bldg, Ste 104, Towson, MD 21204; **Phone:** 410-427-2220; **Board Cert:** Thoracic Surgery 2000; **Med School:** Israel 1982; **Resid:** Surgery, UMDNJ-Rutgers Med Sch 1988; **Fellow:** Cardiothoracic Surgery, New England Deaconess-Harvard 1990; **Fac Appt:** Prof S, Univ MD Sch Med

Krellenstein, Daniel J MD [TS] - **Spec Exp:** Lung Cancer; Minimally Invasive Thoracic Surgery; **Hospital:** Mount Sinai Med Ctr (page 76), Lenox Hill Hosp; **Address:** 16 E 98th St, Ste 1F, New York, NY 10029-6545; **Phone:** 212-423-9311; **Board Cert:** Surgery 1974; Thoracic Surgery 2006; **Med School:** SUNY Buffalo 1964; **Resid:** Surgery, SUNY Downstate Med Ctr 1972; **Fac Appt:** Assoc Clin Prof TS, Mount Sinai Sch Med

Kucharczuk, John C MD [TS] - **Spec Exp:** Lung Cancer; Esophageal Cancer; Mesothelioma; Mediastinal Tumors; **Hospital:** Hosp Univ Penn - UPHS (page 80); **Address:** Penn Surgery, 3400 Spruce St, 6 White Bldg, Philadelphia, PA 19104; **Phone:** 215-662-4988; **Board Cert:** Surgery 2008; Thoracic Surgery 2002; **Med School:** Univ Pennsylvania 1992; **Resid:** Surgery, Hosp Univ Penn 1999; **Fellow:** Cardiothoracic Surgery, Hosp Univ Penn 2001; **Fac Appt:** Asst Prof S, Univ Pennsylvania

Landreneau, Rodney MD [TS] - **Spec Exp:** Lung Cancer; Esophageal Cancer; **Hospital:** UPMC Passavant-McCandless, UPMC St Margaret; **Address:** 5200 Centre Ave, Ste 715, Pittsburgh, PA 15232; **Phone:** 412-623-2025; **Board Cert:** Thoracic Surgery 1994; **Med School:** Louisiana State U, New Orleans 1965; **Resid:** Surgery, Parkland Meml Hosp 1983; **Fellow:** Cardiothoracic Surgery, Univ Mich Med Ctr 1985; **Fac Appt:** Prof S, Univ Pittsburgh

Marshall, Margaret Blair MD [TS] - **Spec Exp:** Lung Cancer; Esophageal Cancer; Thymoma; Chest Wall Tumors; **Hospital:** Georgetown Univ Hosp, Sibley Mem Hosp; **Address:** Georgetown Univ Hosp, 3800 Reservoir Rd NW, 4PHC, Washington, DC 20007; **Phone:** 202-444-5045; **Board Cert:** Surgery 2009; Thoracic Surgery 2002; **Med School:** Georgetown Univ 1991; **Resid:** Surgery, Georgetown Univ Med Ctr 1995; Cardiothoracic Surgery, Hosp Univ Penn 2001; **Fellow:** Research, Chldn's Hosp 1998; **Fac Appt:** Assoc Prof S, Georgetown Univ

Pass, Harvey MD [TS] - **Spec Exp:** Lung Cancer; Mesothelioma; Clinical Trials; **Hospital:** NYU Langone Med Ctr (page 79); **Address:** NYU Cancer Ctr, 160 E 34th St Fl 8, New York, NY 10016; **Phone:** 212-731-5414; **Board Cert:** Thoracic Surgery 2001; **Med School:** Duke Univ 1973; **Resid:** Surgery, Duke Univ Med Ctr 1975; Surgery, Univ Miss Med Ctr 1980; **Fellow:** Cardiothoracic Surgery, MUSC Med Ctr 1982; **Fac Appt:** Prof S, NYU Sch Med

Pierson III, Richard N MD [TS] - **Spec Exp:** Transplant-Lung; Lung Cancer; **Hospital:** Univ of MD Med Ctr; **Address:** Univ Md Med Ctr, Dept Cardiothoracic Surg, 22 S Greene St, rm N4W94, Baltimore, MD 21201; **Phone:** 410-328-5842; **Board Cert:** Surgery 2000; Thoracic Surgery 2002; **Med School:** Columbia P&S 1983; **Resid:** Surgery, Univ Mich Med Ctr 1990; **Fellow:** Cardiothoracic Surgery, Mass Genl Hosp 1992; **Fac Appt:** Assoc Prof TS, Univ MD Sch Med

Scott, Walter J MD [TS] - **Spec Exp:** Lung Cancer; Esophageal Cancer; Mediastinal Tumors; Video Assisted Thoracic Surgery (VATS); **Hospital:** Fox Chase Cancer Ctr (page 72); **Address:** Fox Chase Cancer Ctr, 333 Cottman Ave, rm C308, Philadelphia, PA 19111; **Phone:** 215-214-1427; **Board Cert:** Thoracic Surgery 1998; **Med School:** Univ Chicago-Pritzker Sch Med 1981; **Resid:** Surgery, Univ Chicago Med Ctr 1987; **Fellow:** Cardiothoracic Surgery, Univ Chicago Med Ctr 1989

Soberman, Mark S MD [TS] - **Spec Exp:** Thoracic Cancers; Lung Cancer; Esophageal Cancer; Esophageal Surgery; **Hospital:** Washington Hosp Ctr; **Address:** 110 Irving St NW, rm 1218, Unit 1F, Washington, DC 20010; **Phone:** 202-877-8115; **Board Cert:** Thoracic Surgery 2003; **Med School:** Emory Univ 1983; **Resid:** Surgery, Emory Univ 1986; **Fellow:** Cardiothoracic Surgery, George Washington Univ 1992; Thoracic Surgery, Cleveland Clinic Fdn 1993

Thoracic Surgery

Sonett, Joshua R MD [TS] - **Spec Exp:** Minimally Invasive Thoracic Surgery; Transplant-Lung; Thoracic Cancers; **Hospital:** NY-Presby Hosp/Columbia (page 78); **Address:** 161 Fort Washington Ave, Ste 301, New York, NY 10032; **Phone:** 212-305-8086; **Board Cert:** Surgery 2004; Thoracic Surgery 2007; **Med School:** E Carolina Univ 1988; **Resid:** Surgery, Univ Mass Med Ctr 1993; **Fellow:** Cardiothoracic Surgery, Univ Pittsburgh Med Ctr 1994; Thoracic Surgery, Meml Sloan Kettering Cancer Ctr; **Fac Appt:** Assoc Prof S, Columbia P&S

Watson, Thomas J MD [TS] - **Spec Exp:** Esophageal Cancer; Lung Cancer; **Hospital:** Univ of Rochester Strong Meml Hosp, Highland Hosp of Rochester; **Address:** 601 Elmwood Ave, Box SURG, Rochester, NY 14642; **Phone:** 585-275-1509; **Board Cert:** Thoracic Surgery 2007; Surgery 2003; **Med School:** Univ SC Sch Med 1988; **Resid:** Surgery, LAC-USC Med Ctr 1993; Cardiothoracic Surgery, LAC-USC Med Ctr 1996; **Fellow:** Esophageal Surgery, LAC-USC Med Ctr 1994; **Fac Appt:** Assoc Prof S, Univ Rochester

Weksler, Benny MD [TS] - **Spec Exp:** Thoracic Cancers; Cancer Surgery; Esophageal Cancer; Minimally Invasive Thoracic Surgery; **Hospital:** UPMC Presby, Pittsburgh; **Address:** UPMC-Presbyterian Med Ctr, 200 Lothrop St, PUCH 800, Pittsburgh, PA 15213; **Phone:** 412-648-6271; **Board Cert:** Surgery 2007; Thoracic Surgery 2007; **Med School:** Brazil 1987; **Resid:** Surgery, NY Med Coll/ Lincoln Med Ctr 1991; Surgery, NY Med Coll/Lincoln Med Ctr 1995; **Fellow:** Cardiothoracic Surgery, Meml Sloan Kettering Cancer Ctr 1997; Minimally Invasive Surgery, Univ Pittsburgh Med Ctr 2008; **Fac Appt:** Assoc Prof S, Thomas Jefferson Univ

Yang, Stephen C MD [TS] - **Spec Exp:** Mesothelioma; Lung Cancer; Esophageal Cancer; Robotic Surgery; **Hospital:** Johns Hopkins Hosp, Johns Hopkins Bayview Med Ctr; **Address:** Johns Hopkins Hosp, 600 N Wolfe St Blalock Bldg - rm 240, Baltimore, MD 21287; **Phone:** 410-933-1233; **Board Cert:** Surgery 2003; Thoracic Surgery 2005; **Med School:** Med Coll VA 1984; **Resid:** Surgery, Univ Tex Hlth Sci Ctr 1990; **Fellow:** Thoracic Surgery, MD Anderson Cancer Ctr 1992; Cardiothoracic Surgery, Med Coll Virginia 1994; **Fac Appt:** Assoc Prof TS, Johns Hopkins Univ

Southeast

Cerfolio, Robert J MD [TS] - **Spec Exp:** Lung Cancer; Tracheal Surgery; Chest Wall Tumors; Esophageal Cancer; **Hospital:** Univ of Ala Hosp at Birmingham; **Address:** 703 19th St S, Ste 739, Zigler Rsch Bldg, Birmingham, AL 35294-0007; **Phone:** 205-934-5937; **Board Cert:** Surgery 2003; Thoracic Surgery 2006; **Med School:** Univ Rochester 1988; **Resid:** Surgery, Cornell-NY Hosp 1990; Surgery, Mayo Clinic 1993; **Fellow:** Cardiothoracic Surgery, Mayo Clinic 1996; **Fac Appt:** Prof TS, Univ Alabama

D'Amico, Thomas MD [TS] - **Spec Exp:** Lung Cancer; Esophageal Cancer; **Hospital:** Duke Univ Hosp; **Address:** Duke Univ Med Ctr, Dept Thoracic Surg, Box 3496, Durham, NC 27710; **Phone:** 919-684-4891; **Board Cert:** Surgery 2004; Thoracic Surgery 2006; **Med School:** Columbia P&S 1987; **Resid:** Surgery, Duke Univ Med Ctr 1989; Cardiothoracic Surgery, Duke Univ Med Ctr 1996; **Fellow:** Thoracic Oncology, Meml Sloan Kettering Cancer Ctr; **Fac Appt:** Assoc Prof S, Duke Univ

Feins, Richard H MD [TS] - **Spec Exp:** Thoracic Cancers; Lung Cancer; Robotic Surgery; Esophageal Surgery; **Hospital:** NC Memorial Hosp - UNC; **Address:** UNC Dept Surgery, Div Cardiothoracic Surgery, 3040 Burnett-Womack Bldg, CB#7065, Chapel Hill, NC 27599-7065; **Phone:** 919-966-3383; **Board Cert:** Thoracic Surgery 2003; **Med School:** Univ VT Coll Med 1973; **Resid:** Surgery, Strong Meml Hosp 1980; Cardiothoracic Surgery, Univ Rochester Affil Hosp 1982; **Fac Appt:** Prof S, Univ NC Sch Med

Harpole Jr, David H MD [TS] - **Spec Exp:** Lung Cancer; Mesothelioma; Esophageal Cancer; **Hospital:** Duke Univ Hosp; **Address:** 3627 DUMC, Durham, NC 27705; **Phone:** 919-668-8413; **Board Cert:** Surgery 2002; Thoracic Surgery 2003; **Med School:** Univ VA Sch Med 1984; **Resid:** Surgery, Duke Univ Med Ctr 1991; **Fellow:** Thoracic Surgery, Duke Univ Med Ctr 1993; **Fac Appt:** Prof S, Duke Univ

Jones, David R MD [TS] - **Spec Exp:** Lung Cancer; Esophageal Cancer; Minimally Invasive Thoracic Surgery; **Hospital:** Univ of Virginia Health Sys; **Address:** Univ Virginnia Hlth Sys, Dept Surgery, PO Box 800679, Charlottesville, VA 22908; **Phone:** 434-243-6443; **Board Cert:** Surgery 2005; Thoracic Surgery 2007; **Med School:** W VA Univ 1989; **Resid:** Surgery, West Va Univ 1995; **Fellow:** Thoracic Surgery, Univ North Carolina 1998; **Fac Appt:** Assoc Prof S, Univ VA Sch Med

Kiernan, Paul D MD [TS] - **Spec Exp:** Lung Cancer; Esophageal Cancer; Mediastinal Tumors; **Hospital:** Inova Fairfax Hosp, Inova Alexandria Hosp; **Address:** 2921 Telestar Court Fl 2, Falls Church, VA 22042; **Phone:** 703-280-5858; **Board Cert:** Thoracic Surgery 2002; **Med School:** Georgetown Univ 1974; **Resid:** Surgery, Mayo Clinic 1979; Cardiothoracic Surgery, Mayo Clinic 1981; **Fellow:** Vascular Surgery, Mayo Clinic 1982; **Fac Appt:** Assoc Clin Prof S, Georgetown Univ

Lau, Christine L MD [TS] - **Spec Exp:** Lung Cancer; Transplant-Lung; Esophageal Cancer; **Hospital:** Univ of Virginia Health Sys; **Address:** Univ VA Hlth System, Div Thoracic & Cardiovascular Surg, P.O. Box 800679, Charlottesville, VA 22908; **Phone:** 434-924-8016; **Board Cert:** Surgery 2003; Thoracic Surgery 2007; **Med School:** Dartmouth Med Sch 1995; **Resid:** Surgery, Duke Affil Hosp; **Fellow:** Cardiothoracic Surgery, Washington Univ Affil Hosps 2005; **Fac Appt:** Assoc Prof S, Univ VA Sch Med

Miller, Daniel L MD [TS] - **Spec Exp:** Esophageal Cancer; Lung Cancer; Mesothelioma; **Hospital:** Emory Univ Hosp, Emory Univ Hosp Midtown; **Address:** The Emory Clinic, 1365A Clifton Rd NE, Ste 2219, Atlanta, GA 30322; **Phone:** 404-778-3755; **Board Cert:** Thoracic Surgery 2005; Surgery 2001; **Med School:** Univ KY Coll Med 1985; **Resid:** Surgery, Georgetown Univ Hosp 1991; **Fellow:** Cardiothoracic Surgery, Mayo Clinic 1994; **Fac Appt:** Prof S, Emory Univ

Mullett, Timothy W MD [TS] - **Spec Exp:** Lung Cancer; Esophageal Surgery; **Hospital:** Univ of Kentucky Albert B. Chandler Hosp; **Address:** Charles T. Wethington Bld, 900 S Limestone St, rm 326, Lexington, KY 40536; **Phone:** 859-323-6494; **Board Cert:** Thoracic Surgery 2007; Surgery 2005; **Med School:** Univ Fla Coll Med 1987; **Resid:** Surgery, Shands/Univ of FL 1993; **Fellow:** Pediatric Surgery, Shands/Univ of FL 1994; Cardiothoracic Surgery, Shands/Univ of FL 1995; **Fac Appt:** Assoc Prof S, Univ KY Coll Med

Nesbitt, Jonathan C MD [TS] - **Spec Exp:** Lung Cancer; Esophageal Cancer; Minimally Invasive Thoracic Surgery; Thoracic Cancers; **Hospital:** Vanderbilt Univ Med Ctr, Saint Thomas Hosp - Nashville; **Address:** Vanderbilt-Ingram Cancer Center, 1301 Medical Center Drive, Ste 1710, Nashville, TN 37232; **Phone:** 615-322-0064; **Board Cert:** Thoracic Surgery 2009; **Med School:** Georgetown Univ 1981; **Resid:** Surgery, Vanderbilt Univ Med Ctr 1987; Cardiothoracic Surgery, Albany Med Ctr 1989; **Fac Appt:** Assoc Prof TS, Vanderbilt Univ

Ninan, Mathews MD [TS] - **Spec Exp:** Lung Cancer; Transplant-Lung; Esophageal Cancer; **Hospital:** Centennial Med Ctr; **Address:** 2410 Patterson St, Ste 212, Nashville, TN 37203; **Phone:** 615-342-7345; **Med School:** India 1988; **Resid:** Surgery, Univ London Affil Hosp 1994; **Fellow:** Cardiothoracic Surgery, Univ Pittsburgh Affil Hosp 1998; **Fac Appt:** Assoc Prof TS, Vanderbilt Univ

Thoracic Surgery

Putnam Jr, Joe B MD [TS] - **Spec Exp:** Lung Cancer; Esophageal Cancer; Sarcoma-Soft Tissue; **Hospital:** Vanderbilt Univ Med Ctr, TN Valley Healthcare Sys-Nashville; **Address:** Vanderbilt Univ Med Ctr - Thoracic Surgery, 609 Oxford House, 1313 21st Ave S, Nashville, TN 37232-4682; **Phone:** 615-343-9202; **Board Cert:** Thoracic Surgery 2007; **Med School:** Univ NC Sch Med 1979; **Resid:** Surgery, Univ Rochester 1986; Thoracic Surgery, Univ Mich Med Ctr 1988; **Fellow:** Surgical Oncology, NCI/NIH-Surg Branch 1984; **Fac Appt:** Prof TS, Vanderbilt Univ

Reed, Carolyn E MD [TS] - **Spec Exp:** Esophageal Cancer; Lung Cancer; **Hospital:** MUSC Med Ctr; **Address:** 25 Coourteney Drive, Ste 7018, MSC 295, Charleston, SC 29425; **Phone:** 843-876-4845; **Board Cert:** Thoracic Surgery 2004; **Med School:** Univ Rochester 1977; **Resid:** Surgery, NY Hosp 1982; Thoracic Surgery, NY Hosp 1985; **Fellow:** Surgical Oncology, Meml Sloan Kettering Cancer Ctr 1983; **Fac Appt:** Prof S, Med Univ SC

Robinson, Lary A MD [TS] - **Spec Exp:** Lung Cancer; Mesothelioma; **Hospital:** H Lee Moffitt Cancer Ctr & Research Inst, Tampa Genl Hosp; **Address:** H Lee Moffitt Cancer Ctr, Div Thoracic Oncology, 12902 Magnolia Drive, Tampa, FL 33612-9497; **Phone:** 813-745-7282; **Board Cert:** Thoracic Surgery 2003; Surgery 2002; Surgical Critical Care 2000; **Med School:** Washington Univ, St Louis 1972; **Resid:** Surgery, Duke Univ Med Ctr 1974; Thoracic Surgery, Duke Univ Med Ctr 1981; **Fellow:** Cardiothoracic Surgery, St Thomas Hosp 1982; Cardiothoracic Surgery, Duke Univ Med Ctr 1983; **Fac Appt:** Prof S, Univ S Fla Coll Med

Zwischenberger, Joseph B MD [TS] - **Spec Exp:** Thoracic Cancers; Lung Cancer; Esophageal Cancer; **Hospital:** Univ of Kentucky Albert B. Chandler Hosp; **Address:** MN264 A B Chandler Med Ctr, 800 Rose St, Lexington, KY 40536; **Phone:** 859-257-1000; **Board Cert:** Surgery 2002; Thoracic Surgery 2005; Surgical Critical Care 1996; **Med School:** Univ KY Coll Med 1977; **Resid:** Surgery, Univ Michigan Hosp 1984; Cardiothoracic Surgery, Univ Michigan Hosp 1985; **Fellow:** Cardiac Surgery, Natl Inst Hlth 1981; **Fac Appt:** Prof S, Univ KY Coll Med

Midwest

Deschamps, Claude MD [TS] - **Spec Exp:** Esophageal Cancer; Lung Cancer; **Hospital:** St. Mary's Hosp - Rochester MN (Mayo); **Address:** Mayo Clinic, Div Thoracic Surgery, 200 First St SW, Rochester, MN 55905; **Phone:** 507-284-8462; **Board Cert:** Surgery 2004; **Med School:** Univ Montreal 1979; **Resid:** Surgery, Univ Montreal Hosps 1984; Thoracic Surgery, Univ Montreal Hosps 1985; **Fellow:** Thoracic Surgery, Mayo Clinic 1987; **Fac Appt:** Prof S, Mayo Med Sch

Ferguson, Mark K MD [TS] - **Spec Exp:** Lung Cancer; Esophageal Cancer; Barrett's Esophagus; Minimally Invasive Surgery; **Hospital:** Univ of Chicago Med Ctr; **Address:** Univ Chicago Medical Ctr, 5841 S Maryland Ave, MC 5035, Chicago, IL 60637; **Phone:** 773-702-3551; **Board Cert:** Thoracic Surgery 2003; **Med School:** Univ Chicago-Pritzker Sch Med 1977; **Resid:** Surgery, Univ Chicago Hosps 1982; **Fellow:** Cardiothoracic Surgery, Univ Chicago Hosps 1984; **Fac Appt:** Prof S, Univ Chicago-Pritzker Sch Med

Howington, John A MD [TS] - **Spec Exp:** Lung Cancer; Esophageal Cancer; Thymoma; Minimally Invasive Thoracic Surgery; **Hospital:** Evanston/North Shore Univ Hlth Sys, Highland Park/North Shore Univ Hlth Syst; **Address:** Evanston NorthShore Health System, 2650 Ridge Ave, Walgreen Bldg - Ste 3507, Evanston, IL 60201; **Phone:** 847-570-2868; **Board Cert:** Thoracic Surgery 2006; Surgery 2004; **Med School:** Univ Tenn Coll Med 1989; **Resid:** Surgery, Truman Med Ctr 1994; **Fellow:** Cardiothoracic Surgery, Vanderbilt Univ Med Ctr 1997; **Fac Appt:** Assoc Prof S, Northwestern Univ

Iannettoni, Mark D MD [TS] - **Spec Exp:** Transplant-Lung; Lung Cancer; Esophageal Surgery; **Hospital:** Univ Iowa Hosp & Clinics; **Address:** Univ Iowa Hosp & Clinics, 200 Hawkins Drive, rm SE514GH, Iowa City, IA 52242; **Phone:** 319-356-1133; **Board Cert:** Surgery 2002; Thoracic Surgery 2002; **Med School:** SUNY Upstate Med Univ 1985; **Resid:** Surgery, SUNY Upstate Med Ctr 1991; Thoracic Surgery, Univ Mich Med Ctr 1993; **Fellow:** Thoracic Surgery, Univ Mich Med Sch 1994

Love, Robert B MD [TS] - **Spec Exp:** Transplant-Heart & Lung; Lung Cancer; Esophageal Cancer; Heart Valve Surgery; **Hospital:** Loyola Univ Med Ctr; **Address:** Loyola Univ Med Ctr, 2160 S First Ave Bldg 110 - rm 6243, Maywood, IL 60153; **Phone:** 708-327-2488; **Board Cert:** Surgery 2007; Thoracic Surgery 2000; Surgical Critical Care 2001; **Med School:** Rush Med Coll 1982; **Resid:** Surgery, Univ of Wisconsin Hosp 1988; Thoracic Surgery, Gloucestershire Royal Hosp 1989; **Fellow:** Cardiothoracic Surgery, Univ of Wisconsin Hosp 1991; **Fac Appt:** Prof TS, Loyola Univ-Stritch Sch Med

Maddaus, Michael A MD [TS] - **Spec Exp:** Esophageal Cancer; Lung Cancer; Minimally Invasive Thoracic Surgery; **Hospital:** Abbott - Northwestern Hosp; **Address:** Univ Minn Med Ctr, Div Thoracic Surgery, 420 Delaware St SE, MMC 207, Minneapolis, MN 55455; **Phone:** 612-624-9461; **Board Cert:** Surgery 2000; Thoracic Surgery 2003; **Med School:** Univ Minn 1982; **Resid:** Surgery, Univ Minn Affil Hosp 1990; Thoracic Surgery, Univ Toronto Affil Hosp 1991; **Fellow:** Cardiac Surgery, St Michael's Hosp/Hosp Sick Chldn 1992; Thoracic Oncology, Meml Sloan Kettering Cancer Ctr 1992; **Fac Appt:** Prof S, Univ Minn

Mason, David P MD [TS] - **Spec Exp:** Minimally Invasive Thoracic Surgery; Lung Cancer; Mesothelioma; Transplant-Lung; **Hospital:** Cleveland Clin (page 70); **Address:** Cleveland Clinic, 9500 Euclid Ave, MC J41, Cleveland, OH 44195; **Phone:** 216-444-4053; **Board Cert:** Surgery 2002; Thoracic Surgery 2004; **Med School:** Columbia P&S 1994; **Resid:** Surgery, Brigham & Womens Hosp 2001; **Fellow:** Vascular Surgery, Univ Washington 1999; Thoracic Surgery, Brigham & Womens Hosp 2003

Meyers, Bryan MD [TS] - **Spec Exp:** Lung Cancer; Esophageal Cancer; Transplant-Lung; **Hospital:** Barnes-Jewish Hosp, Barnes-Jewish West County Hosp; **Address:** 4921 Parkview Pl, Ste 8B, St Louis, MO 63110; **Phone:** 314-362-8598; **Board Cert:** Thoracic Surgery 2007; **Med School:** Univ Chicago-Pritzker Sch Med 1986; **Resid:** Surgery, Mass Genl Hosp 1996; **Fellow:** Cardiothoracic Surgery, Barnes Hosp-Wash Univ 1998; **Fac Appt:** Assoc Prof S, Washington Univ, St Louis

Naunheim, Keith S MD [TS] - **Spec Exp:** Lung Cancer; Esophageal Cancer; Chest Wall Tumors; Video Assisted Thoracic Surgery (VATS); **Hospital:** St. Louis Univ Hosp, SSM St Mary's Hlth Ctr - St Louis; **Address:** 3655 Vista Ave Fl 1, St Louis, MO 63110; **Phone:** 314-577-8360; **Board Cert:** Thoracic Surgery 2004; **Med School:** Univ Chicago-Pritzker Sch Med 1978; **Resid:** Surgery, Univ Chicago Hosp 1983; **Fellow:** Cardiothoracic Surgery, Univ Chicago Hosp 1985; **Fac Appt:** Prof TS, St Louis Univ

Orringer, Mark B MD [TS] - **Spec Exp:** Esophageal Cancer; Lung Cancer; Mediastinal Tumors; Lung Cancer; **Hospital:** Univ of Michigan Hosp; **Address:** Univ Mich, Taubman Ctr, 1500 E Medical Center Drive, 2120 TC, SPC 5344, Ann Arbor, MI 48109; **Phone:** 734-936-4975; **Board Cert:** Surgery 1973; Thoracic Surgery 1974; **Med School:** Univ Pittsburgh 1967; **Resid:** Thoracic Surgery, Johns Hopkins Hosp 1973; **Fac Appt:** Prof S, Univ Mich Med Sch

Patterson, G Alexander MD [TS] - **Spec Exp:** Lung Cancer; Esophageal Cancer; Transplant-Lung; **Hospital:** Barnes-Jewish Hosp; **Address:** 660 S Euclid Ave, Box 8234, St Louis, MO 63110; **Phone:** 314-362-6025; **Board Cert:** Surgery 1978; Thoracic Surgery 1981; Vascular Surgery 1982; **Med School:** Canada 1974; **Resid:** Surgery, Queens Univ Med Ctr 1978; Vascular Surgery, Univ Toronto Med Ctr 1979; **Fellow:** Research, Toronto Genl Hosp 1981; Surgical Critical Care, Johns Hopkins Hosp 1982; **Fac Appt:** Prof S, Washington Univ, St Louis

Thoracic Surgery

Rice, Thomas W MD [TS] - **Spec Exp:** Esophageal Surgery; Minimally Invasive Thoracic Surgery; Lung Cancer; **Hospital:** Cleveland Clin (page 70); **Address:** Cleveland Clinic, 9500 Euclid Ave, Desk J4-1, Cleveland, OH 44195; **Phone:** 216-444-1921; **Board Cert:** Surgery 2004; Thoracic Surgery 2005; **Med School:** Univ Toronto 1978; **Resid:** Surgery, Univ Toronto Med Ctr 1983; Thoracic Surgery, Univ Toronto Med Ctr 1986; **Fellow:** Pulmonary Disease, UCSF Med Ctr 1984; **Fac Appt:** Prof S, Cleveland Cl Coll Med/Case West Res

Weigel, Tracey MD [TS] - **Spec Exp:** Esophageal Cancer; Lung Cancer; Mesothelioma; Thymoma; **Hospital:** Univ WI Hosp & Clins; **Address:** Univ Wisconsin Hosp - Thoracic Surg, 600 Highland Ave, H4/316 CSS, Madison, WI 53792-7375; **Phone:** 608-265-0499; **Board Cert:** Surgery 2003; Thoracic Surgery 2006; **Med School:** Univ Rochester 1986; **Resid:** Surgery, Rhode Island Hosp 1993; **Fellow:** Surgical Oncology, Meml Sloan Kettering Cancer Ctr 1995; Cardiothoracic Surgery, Univ Wisconsin 1996; **Fac Appt:** Assoc Prof S, Univ Wisc

Great Plains and Mountains

Bull, David A MD [TS] - **Spec Exp:** Esophageal Cancer; **Hospital:** Univ Utah Hlth Care; **Address:** Univ Utah, Dept Cardiothoracic Surgery, 30 N 1900 East, Ste 3C127, Salt Lake City, UT 84132; **Phone:** 801-581-5311; **Board Cert:** Surgery 2008; Surgical Critical Care 1999; Vascular Surgery 2003; Thoracic Surgery 2004; **Med School:** UCSF 1985; **Resid:** Surgery, UCSF Medical Ctr 1987; Surgery, Univ Arizona Hosps 1990; **Fellow:** Vascular Surgery, Univ Arizona Hosps 1992; Cardiothoracic Surgery, Univ Arizona Hosps 1994; **Fac Appt:** Assoc Prof TS, Univ Utah

Karwande, Shreekanth V MD [TS] - **Spec Exp:** Thoracic Cancers; Lung Cancer; **Hospital:** St. Mark's Hosp - Salt Lake City; **Address:** MountainStar Cardiovascular Surgery, 1160 E 3900 St S, Ste 3500, Salt Lake City, UT 84124; **Phone:** 801-743-4750; **Board Cert:** Thoracic Surgery 2003; **Med School:** India 1973; **Resid:** Surgery, Erie Co Med Ctr 1981; Cardiothoracic Surgery, NY Hosp 1985; **Fellow:** Cardiothoracic Surgery, Meml Sloan Kettering Cancer Ctr

Southwest

Johnson, Scott B MD [TS] - **Spec Exp:** Thoracic Cancers; **Hospital:** Univ Hlth Syst-San Antonio; **Address:** UT Hlth-San Antonio, Cardiac Surgery, 7703 Floyd Curl Drive, MSC7841, San Antonio, TX 78229; **Phone:** 210-567-5615; **Board Cert:** Surgery 2000; Surgical Critical Care 2001; Thoracic Surgery 2004; **Med School:** Univ New Mexico 1987; **Resid:** Surgery, LAC-USC Hosp 1992; Surgery, UTHSC V Hosp 1995; **Fellow:** Cardiothoracic Surgery, LAC-USC Hosp 1993

Kernstine, Kemp H MD/PhD [TS] - **Spec Exp:** Lung Cancer; Esophageal Cancer; Tracheal Surgery; Esophageal Surgery; **Hospital:** UT Southwestern Med Ctr at Dallas; **Address:** U Texas SW Med Ctr, Cardiothoracic Surgery, 5323 Harry Hines Blvd Fl 9, Ste HA09.134, Dallas, TX 75390-8879; **Phone:** 214-645-7748; **Board Cert:** Thoracic Surgery 2004; Surgery 2001; **Med School:** Duke Univ 1982; **Resid:** Surgery, Univ Minn Med Ctr 1988; **Fellow:** Cardiothoracic Surgery, Brigham & Women's Hosp 1994; **Fac Appt:** Prof TS, Univ Tex SW, Dallas

Lanza, Louis MD [TS] - **Spec Exp:** Lung Cancer; **Hospital:** Mayo Clinic - Scottsdale; **Address:** Mayo Clinic Hosp, 5779 E Mayo Blvd MCSB Bldg Fl 1, Phoenix, AZ 85054; **Phone:** 480-342-2270; **Board Cert:** Thoracic Surgery 2002; **Med School:** Loyola Univ-Stritch Sch Med 1981; **Resid:** Surgery, Univ Michigan Med Ctr 1988; Cardiovascular Surgery, Texas Heart Inst 1991; **Fellow:** Surgical Oncology, Natl Cancer Inst 1986; Thoracic Oncology, MD Anderson Cancer Ctr 1989

Reardon, Michael J MD [TS] - **Spec Exp:** Cardiac Tumors/Cancer; **Hospital:** Methodist Hosp - Houston, UT MD Anderson Cancer Ctr; **Address:** 6550 Fannin St, Ste 1401, Houston, TX 77030; **Phone:** 713-441-5200; **Board Cert:** Thoracic Surgery 2006; **Med School:** Baylor Coll Med 1978; **Resid:** Surgery, Baylor Affil Hosps 1983; Thoracic Surgery, Texas Heart Inst 1985; **Fac Appt:** Prof TS, Cornell Univ-Weill Med Coll

Rice, David C MD [TS] - **Spec Exp:** Mesothelioma; Thoracic Cancers; Minimally Invasive Surgery; **Hospital:** UT MD Anderson Cancer Ctr; **Address:** MD Anderson Cancer Ctr, 1515 Holcombe Blvd, Box 1489, Houston, TX 77030; **Phone:** 713-794-1477; **Board Cert:** Surgery 2002; Thoracic Surgery 2004; **Med School:** Ireland 1991; **Resid:** Surgery, Mayo Clinic 1998; Cardiothoracic Surgery, Baylor Affil Hosps 2001; **Fellow:** Thoracic Surgery, Mayo Clinic 1999

Roth, Jack MD [TS] - **Spec Exp:** Esophageal Cancer; Lung Cancer; Gene Therapy; **Hospital:** UT MD Anderson Cancer Ctr; **Address:** Dept Thoracic & Cardiovasc Surg, 1515 Holcombe Blvd, Unit 1489, Houston, TX 77030-4000; **Phone:** 713-792-7664; **Board Cert:** Thoracic Surgery 2002; **Med School:** Johns Hopkins Univ 1971; **Resid:** Surgery, Johns Hopkins Hosp 1973; Thoracic Surgery, UCLA Ctr Hlth Sci 1979; **Fellow:** Surgical Oncology, UCLA Div Surg Onc 1975; **Fac Appt:** Prof TS, Univ Tex, Houston

Smythe, W Roy MD [TS] - **Spec Exp:** Lung Cancer; Mesothelioma; **Hospital:** Scott & White Mem Hosp; **Address:** 2401 S 31st St, Temple, TX 76508; **Phone:** 254-724-2334; **Board Cert:** Thoracic Surgery 2000; **Med School:** Texas A&M Univ 1989; **Resid:** Surgery, Hosp Univ Penn 1996; **Fellow:** Cardiothoracic Surgery, Hosp Univ Penn 1998; Surgical Oncology, Am Cancer Soc 1996; **Fac Appt:** Asst Prof S, Univ Tex, Houston

Swisher, Stephen G MD [TS] - **Spec Exp:** Esophageal Cancer; Lung Cancer; Mesothelioma; Thoracic Cancers; **Hospital:** UT MD Anderson Cancer Ctr; **Address:** Dept of Thoracic & Cardiovasc Surg, 1515 Holcombe Blvd, Unit 1489, Houston, TX 77030; **Phone:** 713-792-8659; **Board Cert:** Surgery 2002; Thoracic Surgery 2006; **Med School:** UCSD 1986; **Resid:** Surgery, UCLA Med Ctr 1993; **Fellow:** Surgical Oncology, UCLA Med Ctr 1990; Cardiothoracic Surgery, MD Anderson Canc Ctr 1996; **Fac Appt:** Prof TS, Univ Tex, Houston

Walsh, Garrett MD [TS] - **Spec Exp:** Esophageal Cancer; **Hospital:** UT MD Anderson Cancer Ctr; **Address:** 1515 Holcombe Blvd, Unit 1489, Houston, TX 77030; **Phone:** 713-792-6849; **Board Cert:** Surgery 2009; Thoracic Surgery 2009; **Med School:** Queens Univ 1983; **Resid:** Surgery, Royal Victoria Hosp-McGill 1988; Cardiovascular Surgery, McGill Univ 1990

West Coast and Pacific

Cameron, Robert Brian MD [TS] - **Spec Exp:** Lung Cancer; Mesothelioma; **Hospital:** UCLA Ronald Reagan Med Ctr; **Address:** UCLA Medical Ctr-Dept of Thoracic Surg, 10833 Le Conte Ave, rm 64-128CHS, Los Angeles, CA 90095; **Phone:** 310-470-8980; **Board Cert:** Surgery 2002; Thoracic Surgery 2005; **Med School:** UCLA 1984; **Resid:** Surgery, UCLA Hosp & Clinic 1992; **Fellow:** Surgical Oncology, National Inst Health 1989; Cardiothoracic Surgery, NY Hosp/Cornell 1994

De Meester, Tom R MD [TS] - **Spec Exp:** Stomach Cancer; Esophageal Cancer; Lung Cancer; Tracheal Surgery; **Hospital:** USC Univ Hosp; **Address:** 1510 San Pablo St, Ste 514, Los Angeles, CA 90033; **Phone:** 323-442-5925; **Board Cert:** Surgery 1971; Thoracic Surgery 1971; **Med School:** Univ Mich Med Sch 1963; **Resid:** Surgery, Johns Hopkins Hosp 1966; **Fellow:** Thoracic Surgery, Johns Hopkins Hosp 1968; **Fac Appt:** Prof S, USC Sch Med

Thoracic Surgery

Grannis Jr, Frederic W MD [TS] - **Spec Exp:** Lung Cancer; Thoracic Cancers; Palliative Care; Mediastinal Tumors; **Hospital:** City of Hope Natl Med Ctr (page 69), Methodist Hosp - Southern California; **Address:** Thor Surg-City of Hope Natl Med Ctr, 1500 E Duarte Rd, Duarte, CA 91010; **Phone:** 626-359-8111 x62669; **Board Cert:** Surgery 1975; Thoracic Surgery 2000; **Med School:** NY Med Coll 1969; **Resid:** Surgery, Mayo Clinic 1974; Thoracic Surgery, Mayo Clinic 1977; **Fac Appt:** Assoc Prof TS, UCSD

Handy Jr, John R MD [TS] - **Spec Exp:** Lung Cancer; Esophageal Cancer; Mesothelioma; Chest Wall Tumors; **Hospital:** Providence Portland Med Ctr; **Address:** Oregon Clinic-Cardiothoracic Surgery, 1111 NE 99th Ave, Ste 201, Portland, OR 97220; **Phone:** 503-963-3030; **Board Cert:** Surgery 1999; Thoracic Surgery 2001; **Med School:** Duke Univ 1983; **Resid:** Surgery, Brown Univ Hosp 1990; **Fellow:** Cardiothoracic Surgery, MUSC Med Ctr 1993

Jablons, David M MD [TS] - **Spec Exp:** Lung Cancer; Mesothelioma; Esophageal Surgery; **Hospital:** UCSF - Mt Zion Med Ctr; **Address:** UCSF Thoracic Surgery, 1600 Divisadero St Fl 4, San Francisco, CA 94115; **Phone:** 415-885-3882; **Board Cert:** Thoracic Surgery 2002; **Med School:** Albany Med Coll 1984; **Resid:** Surgery, New Eng Med Ctr-Tufts Univ 1986; Surgery, New Eng Med Ctr-Tufts Univ 1991; **Fellow:** Surgical Oncology, Natl Cancer Inst-NIH 1989; Cardiothoracic Surgery, New York Hosp-Cornell 1993; **Fac Appt:** Prof S, UCSF

Shrager, Joseph B MD [TS] - **Spec Exp:** Lung Cancer; Thymoma; Chest Wall Tumors; Esophageal Cancer; **Hospital:** Stanford Univ Hosp & Clinics, VA Hlth Care Sys - Palo Alto; **Address:** Stanford Univ Medical Ctr, Falk Bldg, 300 Pasteur, Fl 2, rm CV207, Stanford, CA 94305-5407; **Phone:** 650-721-2086; **Board Cert:** Thoracic Surgery 2008; Surgery 2009; **Med School:** Harvard Med Sch 1988; **Resid:** Surgery, Hosp Univ Penn 1995; Thoracic Surgery, Mass Genl Hosp 1997; **Fac Appt:** Prof TS, Stanford Univ

Vallieres, Eric MD [TS] - **Spec Exp:** Lung Cancer; Mesothelioma; Mediastinal Tumors; Thoracic Cancers; **Hospital:** Swedish Med Ctr-First Hill-Seattle; **Address:** 1101 Madison St, Ste 850, Seattle, WA 98104; **Phone:** 206-215-6800; **Board Cert:** Surgery 1988; Thoracic Surgery 1990; **Med School:** Canada 1982; **Resid:** Surgery, Univ Toronto Affil Hosp 1988; Thoracic Surgery, Univ Toronto Affil Hosp 1989; **Fellow:** Cardiovascular Surgery, Univ Montreal 1990

Whyte, Richard MD [TS] - **Spec Exp:** Lung Cancer; Esophageal Cancer; Chest Wall Tumors; **Hospital:** Stanford Univ Hosp & Clinics; **Address:** Stanford Univ Sch Med, Div Thor Surg, 300 Pasteur Dr, Bldg CVRB - rm 205, Stanford, CA 94305-5407; **Phone:** 650-723-6649; **Board Cert:** Surgery 2001; Thoracic Surgery 2003; **Med School:** Univ Pittsburgh 1983; **Resid:** Surgery, Mass Genl Hosp 1990; Thoracic Surgery, Univ Michigan Hosp 1992; **Fac Appt:** Prof TS, Stanford Univ

Wood, Douglas E MD [TS] - **Spec Exp:** Lung Cancer; Esophageal Cancer; Tracheal Surgery; Mesothelioma; **Hospital:** Univ Wash Med Ctr, Northwest Hosp - Seattle; **Address:** Univ Washington, Div Cardiothoracic Surg, 1959 NE Pacific St, rm AA-115, MS 356310, AA Bldg, rm 115, Box 356310, Seattle, WA 98195-6310; **Phone:** 206-685-3228; **Board Cert:** Surgery 2009; Thoracic Surgery 2001; **Med School:** Harvard Med Sch 1983; **Resid:** Surgery, Mass Genl Hosp 1989; Thoracic Surgery, Mass Genl Hosp 1991; **Fellow:** Surgical Critical Care, Mass Genl Hosp 1991; **Fac Appt:** Prof TS, Univ Wash

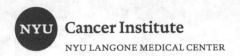

NYU Cancer Institute

NYU LANGONE MEDICAL CENTER

NYU Langone Medical Center
550 First Avenue , New York, NY 10016
www.NYULMC.org

NYU Clinical Cancer Center
160 East 34th Street, New York, NY 10016
www.NYUCI.org

**The Stephen D. Hassenfeld Children's Center
for Cancer and Blood Disorders**
160 East 32nd Street, New York, NY 10016
www.NYUMC.org/Hassenfeld

The NYU Cancer Institute is an NCI-designated cancer center and provides personalized patient care that is both compassionate and state of the art. The doctors and researchers work together to develop innovative therapies for patients. The Cancer Institute is world-renowned for excellence in cancer-focused research, personalized care, education and community outreach. Its mission is to discover the origins of human cancer and to use that knowledge to eradicate the personal and societal burden of cancer in our community, the nation and the world. For more information about our expert physicians, call 212-731-5000. *We specialize in the following areas:*

Patient-Focused Setting
The NYU Clinical Cancer Center is the principal outpatient facility of The Cancer Institute and serves as home to our patients and their caregivers. The center and its multidisciplinary team of experts provide access to the latest treatment options and clinical trials along with a variety of programs in cancer risk reduction/prevention, screening, diagnostics, genetic counseling and supportive services. In addition the NYUCI emphasizes the importance of a holistic approach to management services in complementary medicine, psychosocial support, survivorship and palliative care.

Renowned Expertise
The NYU Cancer Institute brings together experts from a variety of disciplines to create collaborative research endeavors and clinical care teams. The Cancer Institute offers a full continuum of personalized care, from prevention through diagnosis, treatment and post-treatment support. The compassion and expertise of our team members helps patients better manage the symptoms of their diseases as well as meet their special needs. Additionally, we have created special emphasis programs in diseases such as breast cancer, melanoma, GI cancer, prostate cancer, hematologic malignancies and lung cancer among others, as well as, translational programs in cancer healthcare disparities, molecularly targeted therapy, and the cell signaling pathways involved in cancer.

A Translational Approach
NYU Langone Medical Center scientists and other researchers excel in uncovering how cancer develops at the molecular level, and how we can harness that knowledge to reduce the risk of cancer and treat the disease. The Medical Center constantly seeks to create new opportunities for collaboration between investigators within our own institution, those located elsewhere in the NYU network of campuses, and researchers at other institutions.

The Stephen D. Hassenfeld Children's Center for Cancer and Blood Disorders
The center is a leading pediatric outpatient facility for the treatment of childhood cancers and blood diseases. Its unique interdisciplinary and family-centered approach combines the most advanced medical treatments with psychosocial and emotional support services for young patients and their families.

The Best in American Medicine
www.CastleConnolly.com

Urology

A urologist manages benign and malignant medical and surgical disorders of the genitourinary system and the adrenal gland. This specialist has comprehensive knowledge of, and skills in, endoscopic, percutaneous and open surgery of congenital and acquired conditions of the urinary and reproductive systems and their contiguous structures.

Training Required: Five years

UROLOGY

New England

Albertsen, Peter C MD [U] - **Spec Exp:** Prostate Cancer; **Hospital:** Univ of Conn Hlth Ctr, John Dempsey Hosp; **Address:** 263 Farmington Ave, Dowling South Fl 2 - Ste 220, Farmington, CT 06030; **Phone:** 860-679-4100; **Board Cert:** Urology 2004; **Med School:** Columbia P&S 1978; **Resid:** Surgery, New England Deaconess Hosp 1980; Urology, Johns Hopkins Hospital 1984; **Fellow:** Preventive Medicine, Univ WI Affil Hosp 1990; **Fac Appt:** Prof U, Univ Conn

Colberg, John W MD [U] - **Spec Exp:** Prostate Cancer; Bladder Cancer; Kidney Cancer; Testicular Cancer; **Hospital:** Yale-New Haven Hosp, Yale Med Group; **Address:** Yale Urology Group, 800 Howard Ave Fl 3, New Haven, CT 06519; **Phone:** 203-785-2815; **Board Cert:** Urology 2001; **Med School:** Washington Univ, St Louis 1985; **Resid:** Surgery, Yale-New Haven Hosp 1987; Urology, Yale-New Haven Hosp 1990; **Fac Appt:** Assoc Prof U, Yale Univ

Heney, Niall M MD [U] - **Spec Exp:** Urologic Cancer; Prostate Cancer; **Hospital:** Mass Genl Hosp; **Address:** Mass Genl Hosp, Dept Urology, 55 Fruit St, GRB 1102, Boston, MA 02114; **Phone:** 617-726-3011; **Board Cert:** Urology 1977; **Med School:** Ireland 1965; **Resid:** Urology, Regional Hosp 1972; Urology, Mass Genl Hosp 1976; **Fac Appt:** Prof U, Harvard Med Sch

Janeiro Jr, John J MD [U] - **Spec Exp:** Urologic Cancer; **Hospital:** Southern NH Med Ctr, St. Joseph Hosp & Trauma Ctr; **Address:** Urology Center Southern New Hampshire, 17 Riverside St, Ste 201, Nashua, NH 03062; **Phone:** 603-883-1550; **Board Cert:** Urology 2008; **Med School:** Univ Mass Sch Med 1982; **Resid:** Urology, Lahey Clinic 1987; **Fellow:** Pediatric Urology, Childrens Hosp 1989

Libertino, John A MD [U] - **Spec Exp:** Kidney Cancer; Prostate Cancer; Adrenal Tumors; **Hospital:** Lahey Clin; **Address:** Lahey Clinic, Dept Urology, 41 Mall Rd, Burlington, MA 01805-0001; **Phone:** 781-744-2511; **Board Cert:** Urology 1973; **Med School:** Georgetown Univ 1965; **Resid:** Surgery, Strong Meml Hosp 1967; Urology, Yale-New Haven Hosp 1970; **Fellow:** Urology, Yale-New Haven Hosp 1969; **Fac Appt:** Prof S, Harvard Med Sch

Loughlin, Kevin R MD [U] - **Spec Exp:** Prostate Cancer; Bladder Cancer; Penile Cancer; **Hospital:** Brigham & Women's Hosp, Dana-Farber Cancer Inst; **Address:** Brigham & Women's Hosp, Div Urology, 45 Francis St, ASB2-3, Boston, MA 02115; **Phone:** 617-732-6325; **Board Cert:** Urology 2004; **Med School:** NY Med Coll 1975; **Resid:** Pediatrics, New York Hosp 1978; Surgery, Bellevue Hosp Ctr 1979; **Fellow:** Urology, Brigham & Women's Hosp 1983; Urologic Oncology, Meml Sloan Kettering Cancer Ctr 1983; **Fac Appt:** Prof S, Harvard Med Sch

McDougal, W Scott MD [U] - **Spec Exp:** Penile Cancer; Prostate Cancer; Bladder Cancer; Urologic Cancer; **Hospital:** Mass Genl Hosp; **Address:** Mass Genl Hosp, 55 Fruit St GRB Bldg - rm 1102, Boston, MA 02114; **Phone:** 617-726-3010; **Board Cert:** Surgery 1975; Urology 1992; **Med School:** Cornell Univ-Weill Med Coll 1968; **Resid:** Surgery, Univ Hosps Cleveland 1975; Urology, Univ Hosps Cleveland 1975; **Fellow:** Physiology, Yale Med Sch 1972; **Fac Appt:** Prof U, Harvard Med Sch

McGovern, Francis J MD [U] - **Spec Exp:** Prostate Cancer; Urologic Cancer; **Hospital:** Mass Genl Hosp; **Address:** One Hawthorne Pl, Ste 109, Boston, MA 02114; **Phone:** 617-726-3560; **Board Cert:** Urology 2009; **Med School:** Case West Res Univ 1983; **Resid:** Urology, Mass Genl Hosp 1989

Olumi, Aria F MD [U] - **Spec Exp:** Prostate Cancer; Testicular Cancer; Kidney Cancer; Bladder Cancer; **Hospital:** Mass Genl Hosp; **Address:** Mass General Urology Associates, 55 Fruit St, Yawkey Bldg, Ste 7E, Boston, MA 02114; **Phone:** 617-643-0237; **Board Cert:** Urology 2002; **Med School:** Univ SC Sch Med 1992; **Resid:** Surgery, Brigham & Women's Hosp 1994; Urology, Brigham & Women's Hosp 2000; **Fellow:** Research, UCSF Affil Hosp 1998; **Fac Appt:** Assoc Prof S, Harvard Med Sch

Richie, Jerome P MD [U] - **Spec Exp:** Prostate Cancer; Testicular Cancer; Kidney Cancer; **Hospital:** Brigham & Women's Hosp, Dana-Farber Cancer Inst; **Address:** Brigham & Womens Hosp, 45 Francis St, Ste ASB2, Boston, MA 02115; **Phone:** 617-732-6227; **Board Cert:** Urology 1977; **Med School:** Univ Tex Med Br, Galveston 1969; **Resid:** Surgery, UCLA Med Ctr 1971; Urology, UCLA Med Ctr 1975; **Fac Appt:** Prof S, Harvard Med Sch

Sanda, Martin G MD [U] - **Spec Exp:** Prostate Cancer; Bladder Cancer; Kidney Cancer; Urologic Cancer; **Hospital:** Beth Israel Deaconess Med Ctr - Boston; **Address:** Beth Israel Deaconess Medical Ctr, 330 Brookline Ave, Rabb 440, Boston, MA 02115; **Phone:** 617-735-2100; **Board Cert:** Urology 2007; **Med School:** Columbia P&S 1987; **Resid:** Surgery, Med Coll Virginia 1989; Urology, Johns Hopkins Hosp 1994; **Fellow:** Surgical Oncology, Natl Cancer Inst 1991; **Fac Appt:** Assoc Prof U, Harvard Med Sch

Singh, Dinesh MD [U] - **Spec Exp:** Laparoscopic Surgery; Robotic Surgery; Kidney Cancer; Prostate Cancer; **Hospital:** Yale Med Group; **Address:** Yale Urologic Group, Yale Physicians Bldg, 800 Howard Ave Fl 3, New Haven, CT 06519; **Phone:** 203-785-2815; **Board Cert:** Urology 2006; **Med School:** Columbia P&S 1997; **Resid:** Surgery, Brigham & Women's Hosp 1999; Urology, Harvard Med Sch Affil Hosp 2003; **Fellow:** Research, Dana Farber Cancer Inst 2001; Laparoscopic Surgery, Cleveland Clin 2004; **Fac Appt:** Asst Prof U, Yale Univ

Weiss, Robert M MD [U] - **Spec Exp:** Pediatric Urology; Testicular Cancer; Penile Cancer; Bladder Cancer; **Hospital:** Yale-New Haven Hosp, Yale Med Group; **Address:** Yale Univ Sch Med, Dept Urology, 800 Howard Ave, Box 208041, New Haven, CT 06520-8041; **Phone:** 203-785-2815; **Board Cert:** Urology 1970; **Med School:** SUNY Downstate 1960; **Resid:** Surgery, Beth Israel Hosp 1962; Urology, Columbia Presby Hosp 1967; **Fellow:** Pharmacology, Columbia Presby Hosp 1965; **Fac Appt:** Prof U, Yale Univ

Mid Atlantic

Albala, David M MD [U] - **Spec Exp:** Prostate Cancer/Robotic Surgery; Laparoscopic Surgery; **Hospital:** Crouse Hosp, St. Joseph's Hosp Hlth Ctr; **Address:** Associated Medical Professionals, 1226 E Water St, Syracuse, NY 13210; **Phone:** 315-478-4185; **Board Cert:** Urology 2002; **Med School:** Mich State Univ 1983; **Resid:** Surgery, Dartmouth-Hitchcock Med Ctr 1985; Urology, Dartmouth-Hitchcock Med Ctr 1990; **Fellow:** Endourology, Wash Univ Med Ctr 1991

Alexander, Richard B MD [U] - **Spec Exp:** Prostate Cancer; **Hospital:** Univ of MD Med Ctr; **Address:** 419 W Redwood St, Ste 320, Baltimore, MD 21201; **Phone:** 410-328-5109; **Board Cert:** Urology 1999; **Med School:** Johns Hopkins Univ 1981; **Resid:** Surgery, Vanderbilt Univ Affl Hosps 1983; Urology, Johns Hopkins Hosp 1988; **Fellow:** Cancer Immunology, Natl Cancer Inst 1989; **Fac Appt:** Prof U, Univ MD Sch Med

Bagley, Demetrius H MD [U] - **Spec Exp:** Kidney Cancer; Ureter & Renal Pelvis Cancer; Minimally Invasive Urologic Surgery; **Hospital:** Thomas Jefferson Univ Hosp (page 81); **Address:** 833 Chestnut St, Fl 7, Ste 703, Philadelphia, PA 19107; **Phone:** 215-955-1000; **Board Cert:** Urology 1981; **Med School:** Johns Hopkins Univ 1970; **Resid:** Surgery, Yale-New Haven Hosp 1972; Urology, Yale-New Haven Hosp 1979; **Fellow:** Surgery, NCI-USPHS 1975; **Fac Appt:** Prof U, Thomas Jefferson Univ

Urology

Benson, Mitchell C MD [U] - **Spec Exp:** Prostate Cancer/Robotic Surgery; Bladder Cancer; Kidney Cancer; Continent Urinary Diversions; **Hospital:** NY-Presby Hosp/Columbia (page 78); **Address:** NY Presby Hosp-Columbia, Dept Urology, 161 Ft Washington Ave Fl 11 - rm 1102, New York, NY 10032-3713; **Phone:** 212-305-5201; **Board Cert:** Urology 1984; **Med School:** Columbia P&S 1977; **Resid:** Surgery, Mount Sinai Med Ctr 1979; Urology, Columbia-Presby Hosp 1982; **Fellow:** Oncology, Johns Hopkins Hosp 1984; **Fac Appt:** Prof U, Columbia P&S

Burnett II, Arthur L MD [U] - **Spec Exp:** Prostate Cancer; Erectile Dysfunction; **Hospital:** Johns Hopkins Hosp; **Address:** 600 N Wolfe St, Marburg Bldg, Ste 407, Baltimore, MD 21287; **Phone:** 410-955-6100; **Board Cert:** Urology 2007; **Med School:** Johns Hopkins Univ 1988; **Resid:** Surgery, Johns Hopkins Hosp 1990; Urology, Johns Hopkins Hosp 1994; **Fac Appt:** Prof U, Johns Hopkins Univ

Carter, H Ballentine MD [U] - **Spec Exp:** Prostate Cancer; **Hospital:** Johns Hopkins Hosp; **Address:** Brady Urological Inst, Johns Hopkins Hosp, 600 N Wolfe St Marburg Bldg - rm 143, Baltimore, MD 21287; **Phone:** 410-955-6100; **Board Cert:** Urology 1999; **Med School:** Med Univ SC 1981; **Resid:** Surgery, New York Hosp 1983; Urology, New York Hosp 1987; **Fellow:** Research, Johns Hopkins Hosp 1989; **Fac Appt:** Prof U, Johns Hopkins Univ

Chen, David Y T MD [U] - **Spec Exp:** Kidney Cancer; Prostate Cancer; Robotic Surgery; Bladder Cancer; **Hospital:** Fox Chase Cancer Ctr (page 72); **Address:** Fox Chase Cancer Ctr, 8 Huntingdon Pike Fl 3 Urology, Rockledge, PA 19046; **Phone:** 215-728-1111; **Board Cert:** Urology 2006; **Med School:** Cornell Univ 1997; **Resid:** Urology, NY Presby/Cornell Hosp; **Fellow:** NIH/Howard Hughes Med Inst; Urologic Oncology, NY Presby/Cornell Hosp

Cohen, Jeffrey K MD [U] - **Spec Exp:** Urologic Cancer; Prostate Cancer; **Hospital:** Allegheny General Hosp; **Address:** Triangle Urological Group, 1307 Federal St, Ste 300, Pittsburgh, PA 15212-1757; **Phone:** 412-281-1757; **Board Cert:** Urology 2005; **Med School:** SUNY Upstate Med Univ 1979; **Resid:** Surgery, Case Western Reserve Univ Hosp 1981; Urology, Case Western Reserve Univ Hosp 1984; **Fellow:** Urologic Oncology, MD Anderson Cancer Ctr 1985; **Fac Appt:** Assoc Prof U, Drexel Univ Coll Med

Droller, Michael J MD [U] - **Spec Exp:** Urologic Cancer; Bladder Cancer; Prostate Cancer; Kidney Cancer; **Hospital:** Mount Sinai Med Ctr (page 76); **Address:** 5 E 98th St Fl 6, Box 1272, New York, NY 10029-6501; **Phone:** 212-241-3868; **Board Cert:** Urology 2001; **Med School:** Harvard Med Sch 1968; **Resid:** Surgery, Peter Bent Brigham Hosp 1970; Urology, Stanford Univ Med Ctr 1976; **Fellow:** Immunology, Univ Stockholm 1977; **Fac Appt:** Prof U, Mount Sinai Sch Med

Gomella, Leonard G MD [U] - **Spec Exp:** Prostate Cancer; Minimally Invasive Urologic Surgery; Urologic Cancer; **Hospital:** Thomas Jefferson Univ Hosp (page 81); **Address:** Thomas Jefferson Univ, 833 Chestnut St Fl 7 - Ste 703, Philadelphia, PA 19107-5001; **Phone:** 215-955-1000; **Board Cert:** Urology 2008; **Med School:** Univ KY Coll Med 1980; **Resid:** Surgery, Univ Kentucky Med Ctr 1982; Urology, Univ Kentucky Med Ctr 1986; **Fellow:** Urologic Oncology, Natl Cancer Inst 1988; **Fac Appt:** Prof U, Jefferson Med Coll

Grasso, Michael MD [U] - **Spec Exp:** Urologic Cancer; Laparoscopic Surgery; Testicular Cancer; Ureter & Renal Pelvis Cancer; **Hospital:** Lenox Hill Hosp, Westchester Med Ctr; **Address:** 100 E 77 th St, East Bldg - Fl 4th, Dept Urology - Cronin 205, New York, NY 10075; **Phone:** 212-434-6300; **Board Cert:** Urology 2004; **Med School:** Jefferson Med Coll 1986; **Resid:** Surgery, Jefferson Univ Hosp 1988; Urology, Jefferson Univ Hosp 1992; **Fac Appt:** Prof U, NY Med Coll

486

Greenberg, Richard E MD [U] - **Spec Exp:** Prostate Cancer; Bladder Cancer; Kidney Cancer; Prostate Cancer/Robotic Surgery; **Hospital:** Fox Chase Cancer Ctr (page 72), Abington Mem Hosp; **Address:** Fox Chase Cancer Ctr, Div Urol-Dept Surg, 333 Cottman Ave, Ste H3 - rm H3-116, Philadelphia, PA 19111; **Phone:** 215-728-5341; **Board Cert:** Urology 2004; **Med School:** Cornell Univ-Weill Med Coll 1976; **Resid:** Surgery, New York Hosp 1979; Urology, New York Hosp 1983; **Fac Appt:** Prof U, Temple Univ

Hall, Simon J MD [U] - **Spec Exp:** Urologic Cancer; Minimally Invasive Urologic Surgery; Continent Urinary Diversions; Prostate Cancer; **Hospital:** Mount Sinai Med Ctr (page 76); **Address:** Mount Sinai Medical Ctr, 5 98th St, Box 1272, New York, NY 10029; **Phone:** 212-241-4812; **Board Cert:** Urology 2009; **Med School:** Columbia P&S 1988; **Resid:** Surgery, Mt Sinai Med Ctr 1990; Urology, Boston Univ 1994; **Fellow:** Urology, Baylor Coll Med 1996; **Fac Appt:** Assoc Prof U, Mount Sinai Sch Med

Herr, Harry W MD [U] - **Spec Exp:** Bladder Cancer; Prostate Cancer; Testicular Cancer; **Hospital:** Meml Sloan-Kettering Cancer Ctr (page 75), NY-Presby Hosp/Weill Cornell (page 78); **Address:** 1275 York Avenue, New York, NY 10065; **Phone:** 800-525-2225; **Board Cert:** Urology 1976; **Med School:** UCSF 1969; **Resid:** Urology, UC Irvine Med Ctr 1974; **Fellow:** Urology, Meml Sloan Kettering Cancer Ctr 1976; **Fac Appt:** Assoc Prof S, Cornell Univ-Weill Med Coll

Hrebinko Jr, Ronald L MD [U] - **Spec Exp:** Urologic Cancer; Kidney Cancer; Bladder Cancer; Testicular Cancer; **Hospital:** UPMC Presby, Pittsburgh; **Address:** Univ Pittsburgh Dept of Urology, Shadyside Med Bldg, Ste 209, 5200 Centre Ave, Pittsburgh, PA 15232; **Phone:** 412-605-3022; **Board Cert:** Urology 2004; **Med School:** Univ Pittsburgh 1986; **Resid:** Urology, Univ Pittsburgh Med Ctr 1992; **Fellow:** Urologic Oncology, Roswell Park Cancer Ctr 1993; **Fac Appt:** Assoc Prof U, Univ Pittsburgh

Huben, Robert P MD [U] - **Spec Exp:** Bladder Cancer; Prostate Cancer; Kidney Cancer; Urologic Cancer; **Hospital:** Roswell Park Cancer Inst; **Address:** Roswell Park Cancer Inst, Dept Urology, Elm & Carlton Sts, Buffalo, NY 14263-0001; **Phone:** 716-845-3389; **Board Cert:** Urology 1983; **Med School:** Cornell Univ-Weill Med Coll 1976; **Resid:** Urology, East Virginia Med Ctr 1981; **Fellow:** Urologic Oncology, Roswell Park Meml Inst 1982; **Fac Appt:** Assoc Prof U, SUNY Buffalo

Jackman, Stephen V MD [U] - **Spec Exp:** Prostate Cancer/Robotic Surgery; Laparoscopic Surgery; **Hospital:** UPMC Shadyside, UPMC Presby, Pittsburgh; **Address:** 3471 Fifth Ave, Ste 700, Univ Pittsburgh Med Ctr, Dept Urology, Pittsburgh, PA 15213; **Phone:** 412-692-4095; **Board Cert:** Urology 2002; **Med School:** Yale Univ 1994; **Resid:** Urology, Johns Hopkins Hosp 2000; **Fac Appt:** Assoc Prof U, Univ Pittsburgh

Kaplan, Steven A MD [U] - **Spec Exp:** Incontinence after Prostate Cancer; **Hospital:** NY-Presby Hosp/Weill Cornell (page 78); **Address:** NY Presbyterian-Weill Cornell Med Ctr, 525 E 68th St, rm F9West, New York, NY 10021-4870; **Phone:** 212-746-4811; **Board Cert:** Urology 2001; **Med School:** Mount Sinai Sch Med 1982; **Resid:** Surgery, Mount Sinai Hosp 1984; Urology, Columbia Presby Med Ctr 1988; **Fellow:** Urology, Columbia Presby Med Ctr 1990; **Fac Appt:** Prof U, Cornell Univ-Weill Med Coll

Katz, Aaron E MD [U] - **Spec Exp:** Prostate Cancer-Cryosurgery; Kidney Cancer-Cryosurgery; Complementary Medicine; Nutrition & Cancer Prevention; **Hospital:** NY-Presby Hosp/Columbia (page 78); **Address:** NY Presby Med Ctr, Herbert Irving Pav, 161 Ft Washington Ave Fl 11, New York, NY 10032; **Phone:** 212-305-6408; **Board Cert:** Urology 2006; **Med School:** NY Med Coll 1986; **Resid:** Urology, Maimonides Med Ctr 1992; **Fellow:** Urologic Oncology, Columbia Presby Med Ctr 1993; **Fac Appt:** Assoc Clin Prof U, Columbia P&S

Urology

Kavoussi, Louis R MD [U] - **Spec Exp:** Laparoscopic Surgery; Urologic Cancer; Prostate Cancer; Kidney Cancer; **Hospital:** Long Island Jewish Med Ctr, N Shore Univ Hosp; **Address:** 450 Lakeville Rd, Ste M-41, New Hyde Park, NY 11040; **Phone:** 516-734-8558; **Board Cert:** Urology 2009; **Med School:** SUNY Buffalo 1983; **Resid:** Surgery, Barnes Jewish Hosp 1985; Urology, Barnes Jewish Hosp 1989; **Fac Appt:** Prof U, NYU Sch Med

Kirschenbaum, Alexander M MD [U] - **Spec Exp:** Prostate Cancer; Bladder Cancer; Kidney Cancer; **Hospital:** Mount Sinai Med Ctr (page 76); **Address:** 58A E 79th St, New York, NY 10021; **Phone:** 646-422-0926; **Board Cert:** Urology 2006; **Med School:** Mount Sinai Sch Med 1980; **Resid:** Surgery, Mt Sinai Hosp 1982; Urology, Mt Sinai Hosp 1985; **Fellow:** Urologic Oncology, Mt Sinai Hosp 1987; **Fac Appt:** Assoc Prof U, Mount Sinai Sch Med

Lanteri, Vincent J MD [U] - **Spec Exp:** Prostate Cancer/Robotic Surgery; Urologic Cancer; Minimally Invasive Urologic Surgery; **Hospital:** Hackensack Univ Med Ctr (page 73), Monmouth Med Ctr; **Address:** 255 W Spring Valley Ave, Ste 101, Maywood, NJ 07607; **Phone:** 201-487-8866; **Board Cert:** Urology 1982; **Med School:** Mexico 1974; **Resid:** Surgery, UMDNJ Med Ctr 1977; Urology, UMDNJ Med Ctr 1980; **Fellow:** Urologic Oncology, Roswell Park Cancer Inst 1981

Lepor, Herbert MD [U] - **Spec Exp:** Prostate Cancer; **Hospital:** NYU Langone Med Ctr (page 79); **Address:** 150 E 32nd St Fl 2, New York, NY 10016; **Phone:** 646-825-6327; **Board Cert:** Urology 2006; **Med School:** Johns Hopkins Univ 1975; **Resid:** Urology, Johns Hopkins Hosp 1986; **Fac Appt:** Prof U, NYU Sch Med

Lowe, Franklin MD [U] - **Spec Exp:** Complementary Medicine; Prostate Cancer; **Hospital:** St. Luke's - Roosevelt Hosp Ctr - Roosevelt Div (page 71), NY-Presby Hosp/Columbia (page 78); **Address:** 425 W 59th St, Ste 3A, New York, NY 10019-1104; **Phone:** 212-523-7790; **Board Cert:** Urology 2006; **Med School:** Columbia P&S 1979; **Resid:** Surgery, Johns Hopkins Hosp 1981; Urology, Johns Hopkins Hosp 1984; **Fac Appt:** Clin Prof U, Columbia P&S

Malkowicz, S Bruce MD [U] - **Spec Exp:** Prostate Cancer; Bladder Cancer; Kidney Cancer; Gene Therapy; **Hospital:** Hosp Univ Penn - UPHS (page 80); **Address:** 3400 Civic Blvd Perelman Bldg Fl 3W, Philadelphia, PA 19104; **Phone:** 215-662-2891 x7330; **Board Cert:** Urology 2009; **Med School:** Univ Pennsylvania 1981; **Resid:** Surgery, Hosp Univ Penn 1983; Urology, Hosp Univ Penn 1987; **Fellow:** Urologic Oncology, USC Med Ctr 1998; Urologic Oncology, Hosp Univ Penn/Wistar Inst 1990; **Fac Appt:** Prof U, Univ Pennsylvania

Mohler, James L MD [U] - **Spec Exp:** Prostate Cancer; **Hospital:** Roswell Park Cancer Inst; **Address:** Department of Urology, Elm & Carlton Streets, Buffalo, NY 14263; **Phone:** 716-845-3159; **Board Cert:** Urology 2007; **Med School:** Med Coll GA 1980; **Resid:** Surgery, Univ Kentucky Med Ctr 1982; Urology, Univ Kentucky Med Ctr 1985; **Fellow:** Urologic Oncology, Johns Hopkins Hosp 1987; **Fac Appt:** Prof U, SUNY Buffalo

Mostwin, Jacek L MD/PhD [U] - **Spec Exp:** Prostate Cancer; **Hospital:** Johns Hopkins Hosp; **Address:** Johns Hopkins Hosp, 600 N Wolfe St Park 207 Bldg, Baltimore, MD 21287; **Phone:** 410-955-6100; **Board Cert:** Urology 2007; **Med School:** Univ MD Sch Med 1975; **Resid:** Surgery, Univ Michigan Med Ctr 1978; Urology, Johns Hopkins Hosp 1983; **Fac Appt:** Prof U, Johns Hopkins Univ

Naslund, Michael MD [U] - **Spec Exp:** Prostate Cancer; **Hospital:** Univ of MD Med Ctr; **Address:** Maryland Prostate Ctr, 419 W Redwood St, Ste 320, Baltimore, MD 21201; **Phone:** 410-328-0800; **Board Cert:** Urology 2008; **Med School:** Johns Hopkins Univ 1981; **Resid:** Surgery, Johns Hopkins Hosp 1983; Urology, Johns Hopkins Hosp 1987; **Fac Appt:** Prof U, Univ MD Sch Med

Nelson, Joel B MD [U] - **Spec Exp:** Prostate Cancer; **Hospital:** UPMC Shadyside; **Address:** UPMC Shadyside Med Ctr, 5200 Centre Ave, Ste 209, Pittsburgh, PA 15232-1312; **Phone:** 412-605-3013; **Board Cert:** Urology 2008; **Med School:** Northwestern Univ 1988; **Resid:** Surgery, Northwestern MemL Hosp 1990; Urology, Northwestern Meml Hosp 1994; **Fellow:** Urology, Johns Hopkins Hosp; **Fac Appt:** Prof U, Univ Pittsburgh

Partin, Alan W MD/PhD [U] - **Spec Exp:** Prostate Cancer; **Hospital:** Johns Hopkins Hosp; **Address:** Johns Hopkins Hosp, 600 N Wolfe St Marburg Bldg - rm 134, Baltimore, MD 21287-2101; **Phone:** 410-955-6100; **Board Cert:** Urology 2007; **Med School:** Johns Hopkins Univ 1989; **Resid:** Surgery, Johns Hopkins Hosp 1991; Urology, Johns Hopkins Hosp 1996; **Fac Appt:** Prof U, Johns Hopkins Univ

Samadi, David B MD [U] - **Spec Exp:** Prostate Cancer/Robotic Surgery; Kidney Cancer; Bladder Cancer; Urologic Cancer; **Hospital:** Mount Sinai Med Ctr (page 76); **Address:** 625 Madison Ave Fl 2, New York, NY 10022; **Phone:** 212-241-8779; **Board Cert:** Urology 2004; **Med School:** SUNY Stony Brook 1994; **Resid:** Surgery, Montefiore Med Ctr 1996; Urology, Montefiore Med Ctr 2000; **Fellow:** Urologic Oncology, Meml Sloan Kettering Cancer Ctr 2001; Laparoscopic Surgery, Henri Mondor Hosp 2003; **Fac Appt:** Asst Prof U, Mount Sinai Sch Med

Sawczuk, Ihor S MD [U] - **Spec Exp:** Bladder Cancer; Kidney Cancer; Prostate Cancer/Robotic Surgery; Kidney-Sparing Cancer Surgery; **Hospital:** Hackensack Univ Med Ctr (page 73), NY-Presby Hosp/Columbia (page 78); **Address:** Hackensack Univ Med Ctr, 360 Essex St, Ste 403, Hackensack, NJ 07601; **Phone:** 201-336-8090; **Board Cert:** Urology 2005; **Med School:** Med Coll PA Hahnemann 1979; **Resid:** Surgery, St Vincents Hosp 1981; Urology, Columbia-Presby Med Ctr 1984; **Fellow:** Urologic Oncology, Columbia-Presby Med Ctr 1986; **Fac Appt:** Prof U, Columbia P&S

Scardino, Peter T MD [U] - **Spec Exp:** Prostate Cancer; Bladder Cancer; Urologic Cancer; Urinary Reconstruction; **Hospital:** Meml Sloan-Kettering Cancer Ctr (page 75); **Address:** 1275 York Avenue, New York, NY 10065; **Phone:** 646-422-4329; **Board Cert:** Urology 1981; **Med School:** Duke Univ 1971; **Resid:** Surgery, Mass Genl Hosp 1973; Urology, UCLA Med Ctr 1979; **Fellow:** Urology, Natl Cancer Inst 1976; **Fac Appt:** Prof U, Cornell Univ-Weill Med Coll

Scherr, Douglas S MD [U] - **Spec Exp:** Prostate Cancer/Robotic Surgery; Bladder Cancer; Robotic Surgery; Testicular Cancer; **Hospital:** NY-Presby Hosp/Weill Cornell (page 78); **Address:** NY Cornell Medical Ctr, Dept Urology, 525 E 68th St Starr 900, New York, NY 10021; **Phone:** 212-746-5788; **Board Cert:** Urology 2003; **Med School:** Geo Wash Univ 1994; **Resid:** Urology, NY Hosp-Cornell Med Ctr 1999; **Fellow:** Urologic Oncology, Meml Sloan-Kettering Canc Ctr 2002; **Fac Appt:** Assoc Prof U, Cornell Univ-Weill Med Coll

Schlegel, Peter N MD [U] - **Spec Exp:** Prostate Cancer; **Hospital:** NY-Presby Hosp/Weill Cornell (page 78), Hosp For Special Surgery; **Address:** 525 E 68th St, Starr Bldg - Fl 9th - Ste 900, New York, NY 10021-4870; **Phone:** 212-746-5491; **Board Cert:** Urology 2001; **Med School:** Univ Mass Sch Med 1983; **Resid:** Surgery, Johns Hopkins Hosp 1985; Urology, Johns Hopkins Hosp 1989; **Fellow:** Medical Oncology, Johns Hopkins Hosp 1987; Male Reproduction, NY Hosp-Cornell Med Ctr 1991; **Fac Appt:** Prof U, Cornell Univ-Weill Med Coll

Schoenberg, Mark P MD [U] - **Spec Exp:** Bladder Cancer; Urinary Reconstruction; **Hospital:** Johns Hopkins Hosp; **Address:** Johns Hopkins Hosp, 150 Marburg Bldg, 600 N Wolfe St, Baltimore, MD 21287; **Phone:** 410-955-6100; **Board Cert:** Urology 2005; **Med School:** Univ Tex, Houston 1986; **Resid:** Surgery, Hosp U Penn 1988; Urologic Surgery, Hosp U Penn 1992; **Fellow:** Urologic Oncology, Brady Inst/Johns Hopkins 1994; **Fac Appt:** Prof U, Johns Hopkins Univ

Urology

Sheinfeld, Joel MD [U] - **Spec Exp:** Testicular Cancer; Bladder Cancer; Fertility Preservation in Cancer; **Hospital:** Meml Sloan-Kettering Cancer Ctr (page 75); **Address:** 353 E 68th St, New York, NY 10065; **Phone:** 646-422-4311; **Board Cert:** Urology 2009; **Med School:** Univ Fla Coll Med 1981; **Resid:** Urology, Strong Meml Hosp 1986; **Fellow:** Urologic Oncology, Meml Sloan Kettering Cancer Ctr 1989; **Fac Appt:** Assoc Prof U, Cornell Univ-Weill Med Coll

Siegelbaum, Marc MD [U] - **Spec Exp:** Prostate Cancer/Robotic Surgery; Laparoscopic Surgery; Kidney Cancer; Pediatric Urology; **Hospital:** St. Joseph Med Ctr; **Address:** Chesapeake Urology Assocs, 7505 Osler Drive, Ste 506, Towson, MD 21204; **Phone:** 410-296-0167; **Board Cert:** Urology 2009; **Med School:** Univ MD Sch Med 1982; **Resid:** Surgery, Sinai Hosp 1989; Urology, Temple Univ Hlth Sci Ctr 1991

Taneja, Samir S MD [U] - **Spec Exp:** Prostate Cancer; Kidney Cancer; Bladder Cancer; **Hospital:** NYU Langone Med Ctr (page 79); **Address:** NYU Urology Associates, 150 E 32nd St Fl 2, New York, NY 10016-6024; **Phone:** 646-825-6321; **Board Cert:** Urology 2009; **Med School:** Northwestern Univ 1990; **Resid:** Urology, UCLA Med Ctr 1996; **Fellow:** Urologic Oncology, NYU Med Ctr 1998; **Fac Appt:** Assoc Prof U, NYU Sch Med

Tewari, Ashutosh MD [U] - **Spec Exp:** Prostate Cancer/Robotic Surgery; **Hospital:** NY-Presby Hosp/Weill Cornell (page 78); **Address:** Weill Cornell Brady Urologic Health Ct, 525 E 68th St, Starr 900, New York, NY 10021; **Phone:** 212-746-5638; **Board Cert:** Urology 2006; **Med School:** India 1984; **Resid:** Surgery, GSVM Medical College 1990; Urology, Henry Ford Hosp 2003; **Fellow:** Transplant Surgery, Liverpool Univ Med Ctr 1993; Urologic Oncology, Shands Healthcare 1995; **Fac Appt:** Assoc Prof U, Cornell Univ-Weill Med Coll

Trabulsi, Edouard J MD [U] - **Spec Exp:** Minimally Invasive Urologic Surgery; Urologic Cancer; Prostate Cancer; **Hospital:** Thomas Jefferson Univ Hosp (page 81); **Address:** 833 Chesnut St, Ste 703, Philadelphia, PA 19107; **Phone:** 215-955-1000; **Board Cert:** Urology 2005; **Med School:** SUNY Buffalo 1995; **Resid:** Surgery, Thomas Jefferson Univ Hosp 1997; Urology, Thomas Jefferson Univ Hosp 2001; **Fellow:** Urologic Oncology, Meml Sloan Kettering Cancer Ctr 2003; **Fac Appt:** Assoc Prof U, Thomas Jefferson Univ

Uzzo, Robert MD [U] - **Spec Exp:** Bladder Cancer; Prostate Cancer; Robotic Surgery; Minimally Invasive Urologic Surgery; **Hospital:** Fox Chase Cancer Ctr (page 72); **Address:** Fox Chase Cancer Ctr, 333 Cottman Ave, Philadelphia, PA 19111; **Phone:** 215-728-3501; **Board Cert:** Urology 2009; **Med School:** Cornell Univ-Weill Med Coll 1991; **Resid:** Surgery, New York Hosp-Cornell Med Ctr 1993; Urology, New York Hosp-Cornell Med Ctr 1997; **Fellow:** Urologic Oncology, Cleveland Clinic 1999; Renal Transplant, Cleveland Clinic 2000; **Fac Appt:** Assoc Prof S, Temple Univ

Van Arsdalen, Keith N MD [U] - **Spec Exp:** Urologic Cancer; **Hospital:** Hosp Univ Penn - UPHS (page 80), Chldns Hosp of Philadelphia; **Address:** Hosp Univ Penn, Div Urology, 3400 Civic Ctr Blvd, Perelman Center Fl 3W, Philadelphia, PA 19104-4283; **Phone:** 215-662-2891; **Board Cert:** Urology 1984; **Med School:** Med Coll VA 1977; **Resid:** Surgery, Univ Maryland Hosp 1979; Urology, Med Coll Virginia 1982; **Fellow:** Urodynamics, Hosp Univ Penn 1983; **Fac Appt:** Prof U, Univ Pennsylvania

Verghese, Mohan MD [U] - **Spec Exp:** Urologic Cancer; **Hospital:** Washington Hosp Ctr; **Address:** 110 Irving St NW, Ste 3B19, Washington, DC 20010; **Phone:** 202-877-3968; **Board Cert:** Urology 2005; **Med School:** India 1976; **Resid:** Surgery, Bay State Med Ctr 1980; Urology, Washington Hosp Ctr 1984; **Fellow:** Urologic Oncology, Roswell Park Meml Inst 1992

Walsh, Patrick MD [U] - **Spec Exp:** Prostate Cancer; **Hospital:** Johns Hopkins Hosp; **Address:** Brady Urological Inst, 600 N Wolfe St, Park 224, Baltimore, MD 21287-2101; **Phone:** 410-955-6100; **Board Cert:** Urology 1975; **Med School:** Case West Res Univ 1964; **Resid:** Surgery, Peter Bent Brigham Hosp/Childrens Hosp 1967; Urology, UCLA Med Ctr 1971; **Fellow:** Endocrinology, Harbor Genl Hosp 1970; **Fac Appt:** Prof U, Johns Hopkins Univ

Wein, Alan J MD [U] - **Spec Exp:** Prostate Cancer; Testicular Cancer; Bladder Cancer; Kidney Cancer; **Hospital:** Hosp Univ Penn - UPHS (page 80), Pennsylvania Hosp (page 80); **Address:** Univ Penn Hlth Sys, Div Uro, Penn Med, 34th & Civic Ctr Blvd, Perelman Ctr, West Pavilion, Fl 3, Philadelphia, PA 19104-4283; **Phone:** 215-662-2891; **Board Cert:** Urology 1995; **Med School:** Univ Pennsylvania 1966; **Resid:** Surgery, Hosp Univ Penn 1968; Urology, Hosp Univ Penn 1972; **Fellow:** Urology, Hosp Univ Penn 1969; **Fac Appt:** Prof U, Univ Pennsylvania

Weiss, Robert E MD [U] - **Spec Exp:** Bladder Cancer; Kidney Cancer; Testicular Cancer; Robotic Surgery; **Hospital:** Robert Wood Johnson Univ Hosp - New Brunswick, Univ Med Ctr - Princeton; **Address:** 1 Robert Wood Johnson Pl Ste MB588, New Brunswick, NJ 08901-1928; **Phone:** 732-235-9843; **Board Cert:** Urology 2004; **Med School:** NYU Sch Med 1985; **Resid:** Surgery, Mount Sinai Med Ctr 1987; Urology, Mount Sinai Med Ctr 1991; **Fellow:** Urologic Oncology, Meml Sloan Kettering Cancer Ctr 1994; **Fac Appt:** Assoc Prof U, UMDNJ-RW Johnson Med Sch

Yu, George W MD [U] - **Spec Exp:** Nutrition & Disease Prevention/Control; Nutrition & Cancer Prevention/Control; **Hospital:** G Washington Univ Hosp, Anne Arundel Med Ctr; **Address:** 122 Defense Hwy, Ste 224, Annapolis, MD 21401; **Phone:** 410-897-0540; **Board Cert:** Urology 1981; **Med School:** Tufts Univ 1973; **Resid:** Surgery, Brigham & Women's Hosp 1976; Urology, Johns Hopkins Hosp 1981; **Fac Appt:** Prof U, Geo Wash Univ

Southeast

Balaji, K C MD [U] - **Spec Exp:** Prostate Cacner; Urologic Cancer; Robotic Surgery; Minimally Invasive Surgery; **Hospital:** Wake Forest Univ Baptist Med Ctr; **Address:** Wake Forest Univ School of Medicine, Urology Clinic, 140 Charlois Blvd, Winston-Salem, NC 27103; **Phone:** 336-716-4131; **Board Cert:** Urology 2009; **Med School:** India 1986; **Resid:** Surgery, Lebanon Hosp Ctr 1993; Urology, Univ Massachusetts Med Ctr 1997; **Fellow:** Urologic Oncology, Meml Sloan Kettering 1999; **Fac Appt:** Prof U, Wake Forest Univ

Beall, Michael E MD [U] - **Spec Exp:** Prostate Cancer; Testicular Cancer; **Hospital:** Inova Fairfax Hosp, Reston Hosp Ctr; **Address:** 8503 Arlington Blvd, Ste 310, Fairfax, VA 22031; **Phone:** 703-208-4200; **Board Cert:** Urology 1979; **Med School:** Geo Wash Univ 1972; **Resid:** Urology, Geo Wash Univ Hosp 1977; **Fac Appt:** Assoc Clin Prof U, Geo Wash Univ

Busby, J Erik MD [U] - **Spec Exp:** Prostate Cancer; Robotic Surgery; **Hospital:** Univ of Ala Hosp at Birmingham; **Address:** 1530 3rd Ave S, SOT 1105, Birmingham, AL 35294; **Phone:** 205-996-8765; **Board Cert:** Urology 2009; **Med School:** Med Univ SC 1998; **Resid:** Urology, UC Davis Hlth Ctr 2004; **Fellow:** Urologic Oncology, UT MD Anderson Cancer Ctr 2007; **Fac Appt:** Asst Prof S, Univ Alabama

Chang, Sam S MD [U] - **Spec Exp:** Urologic Cancer; Prostate Cancer; Bladder Cancer; Kidney Cancer; **Hospital:** Vanderbilt Univ Med Ctr; **Address:** A1302 Vanderbilt University Med Ctr N, Nashville, TN 37232-2765; **Phone:** 615-322-2101; **Board Cert:** Urology 2010; **Med School:** Vanderbilt Univ 1992; **Resid:** Urology, Vanderbilt Univ Med Ctr 1998; **Fellow:** Urologic Oncology, Meml Sloan Kettering Cancer Ctr 1999; **Fac Appt:** Prof U, Vanderbilt Univ

Cookson, Michael S MD [U] - **Spec Exp:** Urologic Cancer; Bladder Cancer; Prostate Cancer; Testicular Cancer; **Hospital:** Vanderbilt Univ Med Ctr, Saint Thomas Hosp - Nashville; **Address:** Vanderbilt Univ Med Ctr, Urol Surg A1302 MCN, Nashville, TN 37232-2765; **Phone:** 615-322-2101; **Board Cert:** Urology 2006; **Med School:** Univ Okla Coll Med 1988; **Resid:** Urology, UTSA Med Ctr 1994; **Fellow:** Urologic Oncology, Meml Sloan-Kettering Cancer Ctr 1996; **Fac Appt:** Prof U, Vanderbilt Univ

El-Galley, Rizk MD [U] - **Spec Exp:** Urologic Cancer; Laparoscopic Surgery; Bladder Cancer; **Hospital:** Univ of Ala Hosp at Birmingham; **Address:** UAB Hosp FOT-1105, 1530 3rd Ave S, Birmingham, AL 35294-3411; **Phone:** 205-996-8765; **Board Cert:** Urology 2003; **Med School:** Egypt 1983; **Resid:** Urology, Emory Univ Hosp 1999; **Fac Appt:** Asst Prof U, Univ Alabama

Fraser Jr, Lionel B MD [U] - **Spec Exp:** Prostate Cancer; Incontinence after Prostate Cancer; Erectile Dysfunction; **Hospital:** Baptist Med Ctr-Jackson; **Address:** Metropolitan Urology, St Dominics West Med Tower, 971 Lakeland Drive, Ste 360, Jackson, MS 39216; **Phone:** 601-982-0982; **Board Cert:** Urology 2005; **Med School:** Univ Mich Med Sch 1977; **Resid:** Surgery, New England Deaconness Hosp 1979; **Fellow:** Urology, Brigham & Womens Hosp 1983

Greene, Graham MD [U] - **Spec Exp:** Urologic Cancer; **Hospital:** Lakeland Regl Med Ctr; **Address:** Lakeland Regl Cancer Ctr, 3525 Lakeland Hills Blvd, Lakeland, FL 33805; **Phone:** 863-603-6565; **Board Cert:** Urology 2007; **Med School:** Dalhousie Univ 1989; **Resid:** Urology, Victoria Genl Hosp 1994; **Fellow:** Urologic Oncology, M.D. Anderson Cancer Ctr 1997; **Fac Appt:** Assoc Prof

Hemal, Ashok K MD [U] - **Spec Exp:** Urologic Cancer; Robotic Surgery; Reconstructive Urologic Surgery; Laparoscopic Surgery; **Hospital:** Wake Forest Univ Baptist Med Ctr; **Address:** Department of Urology, Medical Center Blvd, Winston-Salem, NC 27157; **Phone:** 336-716-5702; **Med School:** India 1981; **Resid:** Surgery, G R Med College 1985; Urology, Post Grad Inst Med Ed & Rsch 1988; **Fellow:** Robotic Surgery, Henry Ford Hosp; **Fac Appt:** Prof U, Wake Forest Univ

Keane, Thomas E MD [U] - **Spec Exp:** Urologic Cancer; Genitourinary Cancer; Prostate Cancer; Clinical Trials; **Hospital:** MUSC Med Ctr; **Address:** MUSC-Urology Dept, 96 Jonathan Lucas St, Ste CSB644, Charleston, SC 29425; **Phone:** 843-792-1666; **Board Cert:** Urology 2003; **Med School:** Ireland 1981; **Resid:** Urology, St Vincents Hosp 1986; Urology, N Tees Gen Hosp 1988; **Fellow:** Urology, Duke Univ Med Ctr 1993; **Fac Appt:** Prof U, Univ SC Sch Med

Kim, Edward D MD [U] - **Spec Exp:** Prostate Cancer; Bladder Cancer; **Hospital:** Univ of Tennesee Med Ctr; **Address:** University Urology, 1928 Alcoa Hwy, Med Office B Bldg - Ste 222, Knoxville, TN 37920; **Phone:** 865-305-9254; **Board Cert:** Urology 2007; **Med School:** Northwestern Univ 1989; **Resid:** Urology, Northwestern Meml Hosp 1995; **Fellow:** Baylor Coll Med 1996; **Fac Appt:** Assoc Prof U, Univ Tenn Coll Med

Lockhart, Jorge L MD [U] - **Spec Exp:** Bladder Cancer; Urinary Reconstruction; Pelvic Reconstruction; **Hospital:** Tampa Genl Hosp, H Lee Moffitt Cancer Ctr & Research Inst; **Address:** USF Dept Urology, 2 Tampa General Circle Fl 7, Tampa, FL 33606; **Phone:** 813-250-2213; **Board Cert:** Urology 1980; **Med School:** Uruguay 1973; **Resid:** Urology, Duke Univ Med Ctr 1977; **Fellow:** Urodynamics, Duke Univ Med Ctr 1978; **Fac Appt:** Prof S, Univ S Fla Coll Med

Marshall, Fray F MD [U] - **Spec Exp:** Prostate Cancer; **Hospital:** Emory Univ Hosp; **Address:** Emory Urology, 1365 Clifton Rd NE B Bldg - Ste 1400, Atlanta, GA 30322; **Phone:** 404-778-4898; **Board Cert:** Urology 1977; **Med School:** Univ VA Sch Med 1969; **Resid:** Surgery, Univ Mich Hosps 1972; Urology, Mass Genl Hosp 1975; **Fac Appt:** Prof U, Emory Univ

McConnell, John D MD [U] - **Spec Exp:** Prostate Cancer; **Hospital:** Wake Forest Univ Baptist Med Ctr; **Address:** Wake Forest Univ Baptist Med Ctr, Medical Center Blvd, Winston-Salem, NC 27157; **Phone:** 336-716-3408; **Board Cert:** Urology 2004; **Med School:** Loyola Univ-Stritch Sch Med 1978; **Resid:** Surgery, Parkland Hosp 1980; Urology, Parkland Hosp 1984; **Fac Appt:** Prof U, Wake Forest Univ

Miller, Scott D MD [U] - **Spec Exp:** Robotic Surgery; Prostate Cancer/Robotic Surgery; Minimally Invasive Urologic Surgery; Reconstructive Surgery; **Hospital:** Northside Hosp, St. Joseph's Hosp - Atlanta; **Address:** Georgia Urology, 5670 Peachtree Dunwoody Rd, Ste 1250, Atlanta, GA 30342; **Phone:** 404-256-1844; **Board Cert:** Urology 2005; **Med School:** Med Coll GA 1990; **Resid:** Urology, Univ Kentucky Med Ctr 1995

Moul, Judd W MD [U] - **Spec Exp:** Prostate Cancer; Testicular Cancer; Minimally Invasive Urologic Surgery; Clinical Trials; **Hospital:** Duke Univ Hosp, Durham VA Med Ctr; **Address:** Duke Univ Med Ctr, Duke South Bldg - rm 1573, Box 3707, Durham, NC 27710; **Phone:** 919-668-8108; **Board Cert:** Urology 2008; **Med School:** Jefferson Med Coll 1982; **Resid:** Urology, Walter Reed Army Med Ctr 1987; **Fellow:** Urologic Oncology, Duke Univ Med Ctr 1989; **Fac Appt:** Prof S, Duke Univ

Patel, Vipul R MD [U] - **Spec Exp:** Prostate Cancer/Robotic Surgery; Kidney Cancer; **Hospital:** Florida Hosp Celebration Hlth; **Address:** 410 Celebration Pl, Ste 200, Celebration, FL 34747; **Phone:** 407-303-4673; **Board Cert:** Urology 2004; **Med School:** Baylor Coll Med 1995; **Resid:** Urology, Univ Miami; **Fellow:** Urologic Laparoscopic Surg-Endourology, Univ Miami

Penson, David F MD [U] - **Spec Exp:** Urologic Cancer; Bladder Cancer; Erectile Dysfunction; **Hospital:** TN Valley Healthcare Sys-Nashville; **Address:** 2525 W End Ave, Ste 600, Nashville, TN 37203-1738; **Phone:** 615-343-1529; **Board Cert:** Urology 2009; **Med School:** Boston Univ 1991; **Resid:** Urology, UCLA Med Ctr 1997; **Fellow:** Urologic Oncology, Yale-New Haven Hosp 1999; **Fac Appt:** Assoc Prof U, USC-Keck School of Medicine

Pow-Sang, Julio M MD [U] - **Spec Exp:** Prostate Cancer; **Hospital:** H Lee Moffitt Cancer Ctr & Research Inst; **Address:** H Lee Moffitt Cancer Ctr, GU Clinic, 12902 Magnolia Drive, Tampa, FL 33612-9416; **Phone:** 813-972-8418; **Board Cert:** Urology 1999; **Med School:** Mexico 1978; **Resid:** Surgery, Univ Miami Sch Med 1983; Urology, Univ Miami Sch Med 1986; **Fellow:** Urologic Oncology, Univ Fla Coll Med 1987; **Fac Appt:** Prof S, Univ S Fla Coll Med

Pruthi, Raj S MD [U] - **Spec Exp:** Urologic Cancer; Robotic Surgery; **Hospital:** NC Memorial Hosp - UNC; **Address:** UNC Dept Surgery, Urologic Surgery, 2113 POB, rm CB 7235, 170 Manning Drive, Chapel Hill, NC 27514; **Phone:** 919-966-2571; **Board Cert:** Urology 2002; **Med School:** Duke Univ 1992; **Resid:** Surgery, Stanford Univ Hosp 1993; Urology, Stanford Univ Hosp 1998; **Fac Appt:** Assoc Prof U, Univ NC Sch Med

Robertson, Cary N MD [U] - **Spec Exp:** Prostate Cancer; Kidney Cancer; Testicular Cancer; **Hospital:** Duke Univ Hosp; **Address:** Duke Univ Med Ctr, rm 1108, Box 3833, Green Zone Duke South, Durham, NC 27710; **Phone:** 919-684-2446; **Board Cert:** Urology 2006; **Med School:** Tulane Univ 1977; **Resid:** Urology, Duke Univ Med Ctr 1985; **Fellow:** Urologic Oncology, Natl Inst Hlth 1987; **Fac Appt:** Assoc Prof U, Duke Univ

Rowland, Randall MD [U] - **Spec Exp:** Urologic Cancer; **Hospital:** Univ of Kentucky Albert B. Chandler Hosp; **Address:** Univ Kentucky Med Ctr, Div Urology, 800 Rose St, rm MS283, Lexington, KY 40536-0001; **Phone:** 859-323-6677; **Board Cert:** Urology 1980; **Med School:** Northwestern Univ 1972; **Resid:** Urology, Northwestern Meml Hosp 1978; **Fellow:** Urology, Northwestern Meml Hosp 1977; **Fac Appt:** Prof U, Univ KY Coll Med

Urology

Sanders, William Holt MD [U] - **Spec Exp:** Prostate Cancer; Kidney Cancer; **Hospital:** Northside Hosp; **Address:** 980 Johnson Ferry Rd NE, Ste 490, Atlanta, GA 30342-1767; **Phone:** 404-257-0133; **Board Cert:** Urology 2006; **Med School:** Emory Univ 1988; **Resid:** Surgery, Emory Affil Hosp 1990; Urology, Yale-New Haven Hosp 1993; **Fellow:** Urologic Oncology, Emory Univ Hosp 1994

Smith, Joseph A MD [U] - **Spec Exp:** Prostate Cancer/Robotic Surgery; Bladder Cancer; Kidney Cancer; **Hospital:** Vanderbilt Univ Med Ctr; **Address:** Vanderbilt Univ Med Ctr, Dept Urology, A-1302 Medical Center North, Nashville, TN 37232-2765; **Phone:** 615-343-0234; **Board Cert:** Urology 2000; **Med School:** Univ Tenn Coll Med 1974; **Resid:** Surgery, Parkland Meml Hosp 1976; Urology, Univ Utah 1979; **Fellow:** Urologic Oncology, Meml Sloan Kettering Cancer Ctr 1980; **Fac Appt:** Prof U, Vanderbilt Univ

Soloway, Mark S MD [U] - **Spec Exp:** Bladder Cancer; Kidney Cancer; Prostate Cancer; Urologic Pathology; **Hospital:** Jackson Meml Hosp (page 82), Univ of Miami Hosp & Clins/Sylvester Comp Canc Ctr (page 82); **Address:** 1150 NW 14th St, Ste 309, Miami, FL 33136; **Phone:** 305-243-6596; **Board Cert:** Urology 1977; **Med School:** Case West Res Univ 1968; **Resid:** Surgery, Univ Hosps 1970; Urology, Univ Hosps 1975; **Fellow:** Surgery, Natl Cancer Inst 1972; **Fac Appt:** Prof U, Univ Miami Sch Med

Strup, Stephen E MD [U] - **Spec Exp:** Urologic Cancer; Minimally Invasive Urologic Surgery; Robotic Surgery; **Hospital:** Univ of Kentucky Albert B. Chandler Hosp; **Address:** MS-283 Chandler Med Ctr, 800 Rose St, Lexington, KY 40536; **Phone:** 859-323-6679; **Board Cert:** Urology 2007; **Med School:** Indiana Univ 1988; **Resid:** Urology, Thomas Jefferson Univ Hosp 1994; **Fellow:** Urologic Oncology, National Cancer Inst 1996; **Fac Appt:** Prof S, Univ KY Coll Med

Su, Li-Ming MD [U] - **Spec Exp:** Prostate Cancer; Bladder Cancer; Testicular Cancer; **Hospital:** Shands at Univ of FL; **Address:** Shands at Univ Florida, Dept Urology, 1600 SW Archer St, Gainesville, FL 32610; **Phone:** 352-265-8282; **Board Cert:** Urology 2003; **Med School:** Cornell Univ-Weill Med Coll 1994; **Resid:** Surgery, NY Presby-Cornell Med Ctr 1996; Urology, NY Presby-Cornell Med Ctr 2000; **Fellow:** Robotic Surgery, Johns Hopkins Hosp 2001; **Fac Appt:** Prof U, Univ Fla Coll Med

Teigland, Chris M MD [U] - **Spec Exp:** Prostate Cancer/Robotic Surgery; Kidney Cancer; **Hospital:** Carolinas Med Ctr; **Address:** Mckay Urology, 1023 Edgehill Rd S, Charlotte, NC 28207; **Phone:** 704-355-8686; **Board Cert:** Urology 2007; **Med School:** Duke Univ 1980; **Resid:** Surgery, Univ Utah Affil Hosps 1982; Urology, Univ Texas SW Med Ctr 1987; **Fac Appt:** Clin Prof S, Univ NC Sch Med

Terris, Martha K MD [U] - **Spec Exp:** Prostate Cancer; Brachytherapy; Urologic Cancer; Bladder Cancer; **Hospital:** Charlie Norwood VA Med Ctr - Augusta, Med Coll of GA Hosp and Clin (MCG Health Inc); **Address:** Charlie Norwood VA Medical Center, 1 Freedom Way, Augusta, GA 30904; **Phone:** 706-733-0188; **Board Cert:** Urology 2007; **Med School:** Univ Miss 1986; **Resid:** Surgery, Duke Univ Med Ctr 1988; Urology, Stanford Univ Med Ctr 1995; **Fellow:** Ultrasound, Stanford Univ 1991; **Fac Appt:** Prof S, Med Coll GA

Wallen, Eric M MD [U] - **Spec Exp:** Laparoscopic Surgery; Prostate Cancer; Urologic Cancer; Robotic Surgery; **Hospital:** NC Memorial Hosp - UNC; **Address:** Div of Urologic Surgery, CB 7235, 2113 Physicians Office Bldg, 170 Manning Drive, Chapel Hill, NC 27599-7235; **Phone:** 919-966-8802; **Board Cert:** Urology 2002; **Med School:** UCLA 1994; **Resid:** Surgery, Stanford Univ Med Ctr 1996; Urology, Stanford Univ Med Ctr 2000; **Fac Appt:** Assoc Prof S, Univ NC Sch Med

Midwest

Andriole, Gerald L MD [U] - **Spec Exp:** Urologic Cancer; Prostate Cancer; Laparoscopic Surgery; **Hospital:** Barnes-Jewish Hosp; **Address:** 4960 Children's Place, Campus Box 8242, St Louis, MO 63110; **Phone:** 314-362-8212; **Board Cert:** Urology 2003; **Med School:** Jefferson Med Coll 1978; **Resid:** Surgery, Strong Meml Hosp 1980; Urology, Brigham & Womens Hosp 1983; **Fellow:** Urologic Oncology, NCI/NIH 1985; **Fac Appt:** Prof U, Washington Univ, St Louis

Bahnson, Robert MD [U] - **Spec Exp:** Prostate Cancer; Bladder Cancer; Continent Urinary Diversions; **Hospital:** Ohio St Univ Med Ctr, Arthur G James Cancer Hosp & Research Inst; **Address:** 456 West 10th Avenue, Dept of Urology, 3142 Cramblett Med Ctr, Columbus, OH 43210-1228; **Phone:** 614-293-3646; **Board Cert:** Urology 2006; **Med School:** Tufts Univ 1979; **Resid:** Surgery, Northwestern Univ 1981; Urology, Northwestern Univ 1985; **Fellow:** Urology, Northwestern Univ 1984; Research, Univ Pittsburgh 1991; **Fac Appt:** Prof U, Ohio State Univ

Brendler, Charles B MD [U] - **Spec Exp:** Prostate Cancer; **Hospital:** Evanston/North Shore Univ Hlth Sys; **Address:** NorthShore Dept Urology, 2650 Ridge Ave Walgreen Bldg - Ste 2507, Evanston, IL 60201; **Phone:** 847-657-5730; **Board Cert:** Urology 1981; **Med School:** Univ VA Sch Med 1974; **Resid:** Surgery, Duke Univ Med Ctr 1976; Urology, Duke Univ Med Ctr 1979; **Fellow:** Urologic Oncology, Univ Hosp Wales 1980; Urologic Oncology, Johns Hopkins Hosp 1982; **Fac Appt:** Prof U, Northwestern Univ-Feinberg Sch Med

Campbell, Steven C MD/PhD [U] - **Spec Exp:** Kidney Cancer; Prostate Cancer; Bladder Cancer; **Hospital:** Cleveland Clin (page 70); **Address:** Cleveland Clinic, Glickman Urological Inst, 9500 Euclid Ave, MS Q10-1, Cleveland, OH 44195; **Phone:** 216-444-5595; **Board Cert:** Urology 2008; **Med School:** Univ Chicago-Pritzker Sch Med 1989; **Resid:** Urology, Cleveland Clinic 1995; **Fellow:** Urology, Meml Sloan Kettering Cancer Ctr 1996; **Fac Appt:** Prof S, Cleveland Cl Coll Med/Case West Res

Catalona, William J MD [U] - **Spec Exp:** Prostate Cancer; **Hospital:** Northwestern Meml Hosp; **Address:** Northwestern Med Faculty Foundation, 675 N St Clair St, Ste 20-150, Chicago, IL 60611; **Phone:** 312-695-6126; **Board Cert:** Urology 1978; **Med School:** Yale Univ 1968; **Resid:** Surgery, UCSF Med Ctr 1970; Urology, Johns Hopkins Hosp 1976; **Fellow:** Surgical Oncology, Natl Cancer Inst 1972; **Fac Appt:** Prof U, Northwestern Univ

Coplen, Douglas E MD [U] - **Spec Exp:** Pediatric Urology; Urologic Cancer-Pediatric; Testicular Cancer-Pediatric; **Hospital:** St. Louis Chldns Hosp; **Address:** St Louis Children's Hosp, 4990 Children's Pl, Northwest Tower, Ste 1120, St Louis, MO 63110; **Phone:** 314-454-6034; **Board Cert:** Urology 2005; Pediatric Urology 2008; **Med School:** Indiana Univ 1985; **Resid:** Urology, Barnes Jewish Hosp 1992; **Fellow:** Pediatric Urology, Childrens Hosp 1994; **Fac Appt:** Asst Prof S, Washington Univ, St Louis

Donovan Jr, James F MD [U] - **Spec Exp:** Prostate Cancer/Robotic Surgery; Kidney Cancer; Adrenal Tumors; Laparoscopic Surgery; **Hospital:** Univ Hosp - Cincinnati, Christ Hosp, The - Cincinnati; **Address:** Univ Cincinnati Med Ctr, Medical Arts Bldg, 222 Piedmont Ave, Ste 7000, Cincinnati, OH 45219; **Phone:** 513-475-8787; **Board Cert:** Urology 2009; **Med School:** Northwestern Univ 1978; **Resid:** Surgery, Northwestern Meml Hosp 1982; Urology, Northwestern Meml Hosp 1986; **Fellow:** Male Infertility, Baylor Coll Med 1986; **Fac Appt:** Prof U, Univ Cincinnati

Flanigan, Robert C MD [U] - **Spec Exp:** Urologic Cancer; Prostate Cancer; Kidney Cancer; Bladder Cancer; **Hospital:** Loyola Univ Med Ctr; **Address:** Loyola Univ Med-Fahey Bldg, 2160 S First Ave, rm 267, Maywood, IL 60153; **Phone:** 708-216-5100; **Board Cert:** Urology 2001; **Med School:** Case West Res Univ 1972; **Resid:** Surgery, Case West Univ Med Ctr 1978; Urology, Case West Univ Med Ctr 1978; **Fac Appt:** Prof U, Loyola Univ-Stritch Sch Med

Foster, Richard S MD [U] - **Spec Exp:** Testicular Cancer; Reconstructive Surgery; **Hospital:** IU Health Methodist Hosp; **Address:** 535 N Barnhill Drive, Ste 420, Indianapolis, IN 46202; **Phone:** 317-274-3458; **Board Cert:** Urology 2008; **Med School:** Indiana Univ 1980; **Resid:** Urology, Indiana Univ Hosp 1986; **Fac Appt:** Prof U, Indiana Univ

Gluckman, Gordon R MD [U] - **Spec Exp:** Prostate Cancer; Kidney Cancer; Minimally Invasive Urologic Surgery; Robotic Surgery; **Hospital:** Adv Luth Genl Hosp, Resurrection Med Ctr; **Address:** Northwest Suburban Urologists, 900 Rand Rd, Ste 120, Des Plaines, IL 60016; **Phone:** 847-823-3185; **Board Cert:** Urology 2006; **Med School:** Northwestern Univ 1989; **Resid:** Surgery, UCSF Med Ctr 1991; Urology, UCSF Med Ctr 1995; **Fac Appt:** Asst Clin Prof S, Ros Franklin Univ/Chicago Med Sch

Jones, J Stephen MD [U] - **Spec Exp:** Prostate Cancer; **Hospital:** Cleveland Clin (page 70); **Address:** 26900 Cedar Rd, Ste 306 South, Beachwood, OH 44122; **Phone:** 216-839-3666; **Board Cert:** Urology 2002; **Med School:** Univ Ark 1986; **Resid:** Urology, Vanderbilt Univ Med Ctr 1993; **Fac Appt:** Prof S, Cleveland Cl Coll Med/Case West Res

Kaouk, Jihad MD [U] - **Spec Exp:** Minimally Invasive Urologic Surgery; Robotic Surgery; Kidney Cancer; Bladder Cancer; **Hospital:** Cleveland Clin (page 70); **Address:** Cleveland Clinic, 9500 Euclid Ave, MC Q10, Cleveland, OH 44195; **Phone:** 216-444-2976; **Med School:** Lebanon 1993; **Resid:** Surgery, Amer Univ of Beirut Med Ctr 1996; Urology, Amer Univ of Beirut Med Ctr 1999; **Fellow:** Minimally Invasive Surgery, Cleveland Clinic 2001; Laparoscopic Surgery, Cleveland Clinic 2002; **Fac Appt:** Assoc Prof S, Cleveland Cl Coll Med/Case West Res

Kibel, Adam S MD [U] - **Spec Exp:** Prostate Cancer; Bladder Cancer; Kidney Cancer; **Hospital:** Barnes-Jewish Hosp, Barnes-Jewish West County Hosp; **Address:** 4960 Chldns Pkwy, Wohl Hosp Bldg Fl 2, Box 82, St Louis, MO 63110-1000; **Phone:** 314-362-8295; **Board Cert:** Urology 2009; **Med School:** Cornell Univ-Weill Med Coll 1991; **Resid:** Urology, Brigham & Women's Hosp 1996; **Fellow:** Urologic Oncology, Johns Hopkins Hosp 1999; **Fac Appt:** Prof U, Washington Univ, St Louis

Klein, Eric A MD [U] - **Spec Exp:** Urologic Cancer; Testicular Cancer; Kidney Cancer; Prostate Cancer; **Hospital:** Cleveland Clin (page 70); **Address:** 9500 Euclid Ave, MS Q-10, Glickman Urologic and Kidney Institute, Cleveland, OH 44195-0001; **Phone:** 216-444-5591; **Board Cert:** Urology 2008; **Med School:** Univ Pittsburgh 1981; **Resid:** Urology, Cleveland Clinic Fdn 1986; **Fellow:** Urologic Oncology, Meml Sloan Kettering Canc Ctr 1989; **Fac Appt:** Prof S, Cleveland Cl Coll Med/Case West Res

Koch, Michael O MD [U] - **Spec Exp:** Prostate Cancer; Bladder Cancer; Robotic Surgery; Reconstructive Urologic Surgery; **Hospital:** IU Health Methodist Hosp; **Address:** Indiana Cancer Pavilion, 535 N Barnhill Drive, Ste 420, Indianapolis, IN 46202; **Phone:** 317-274-7338; **Board Cert:** Urology 2007; **Med School:** Dartmouth Med Sch 1981; **Resid:** Surgery, Dartmouth-Hitchcock Med Ctr 1983; Urology, Vanderbilt Univ Med Ctr 1987; **Fellow:** Surgical Research, Dartmouth Med Sch 1984; **Fac Appt:** Prof U, Indiana Univ

Kozlowski, James M MD [U] - **Spec Exp:** Prostate Cancer; Continent Urinary Diversions; Laparoscopic Surgery; **Hospital:** Northwestern Meml Hosp, Jesse Brown VA Med Ctr; **Address:** 675 N St Clair St, Galter 20-150, Chicago, IL 60611; **Phone:** 312-695-8146; **Board Cert:** Surgery 2004; Urology 1983; **Med School:** Northwestern Univ 1975; **Resid:** Surgery, McGaw Med Ctr 1979; Urology, McGaw Med Ctr 1982; **Fellow:** Research, NCI-Frederick Cancer Rsch 1984; **Fac Appt:** Assoc Prof U, Northwestern Univ

Lee, Cheryl T MD [U] - **Spec Exp:** Urologic Cancer; Bladder Cancer; **Hospital:** Univ of Michigan Hosp; **Address:** Univ of Michigan Cancer Ctr, 1500 E Medical Ctr Drive, Reception D LB1-229, Ann Arbor, MI 48109; **Phone:** 734-647-8903; **Board Cert:** Urology 2002; **Med School:** Albany Med Coll 1991; **Resid:** Urology, Albany Med Ctr; **Fellow:** Urologic Oncology, Meml Sloan Kettering Cancer Ctr 2000; **Fac Appt:** Assoc Prof U, Univ Mich Med Sch

McVary, Kevin T MD [U] - **Spec Exp:** Prostate Cancer; Erectile Dysfunction; Minimally Invasive Surgery; **Hospital:** Northwestern Meml Hosp; **Address:** 675 N St Clair St, Galter 20-150, Chicago, IL 60611-4813; **Phone:** 312-695-8146; **Board Cert:** Urology 2010; **Med School:** Northwestern Univ 1983; **Resid:** Surgery, Northwestern Meml Hosp 1985; Urology, Northwestern Meml Hosp 1988; **Fellow:** Research, Northwestern Meml Hosp; **Fac Appt:** Prof U, Northwestern Univ

Menon, Mani MD [U] - **Spec Exp:** Prostate Cancer/Robotic Surgery; Transplant-Kidney; Urologic Cancer; **Hospital:** Henry Ford Hosp; **Address:** Henry Ford Hosp - Vattikuti Urology Inst, 2799 W Grand Bvd, Clinic Bldg - K-9, Detroit, MI 48202; **Phone:** 313-916-2066; **Board Cert:** Urology 1982; **Med School:** India 1969; **Resid:** Urology, Bryn Mawr Hosp 1974; Urology, Johns Hopkins Hosp 1980; **Fellow:** Transplant Surgery, Johns Hopkins Univ 1977; **Fac Appt:** Prof S, Univ Mass Sch Med

Montie, James MD [U] - **Spec Exp:** Bladder Cancer; Prostate Cancer; Genitourinary Cancer; **Hospital:** Univ of Michigan Hosp; **Address:** UMH Cancer Ctr, Team 3, Reception D, Level B1-229, 1500 E Med Ctr Drive, Ann Arbor, MI 48109-5913; **Phone:** 734-647-8903; **Board Cert:** Urology 1978; **Med School:** Univ Mich Med Sch 1971; **Resid:** Urology, Cleveland Clinic Fdn 1976; **Fellow:** Urologic Oncology, Meml Sloan-Kettering Cancer Ctr 1979; **Fac Appt:** Prof U, Univ Mich Med Sch

O'Donnell, Michael A MD [U] - **Spec Exp:** Bladder Cancer; Immunotherapy; Urologic Cancer; Ureter & Renal Pelvis Cancer; **Hospital:** Univ Iowa Hosp & Clinics; **Address:** 200 Hawkins Drive RCP Bldg Fl 3, Iowa City, IA 52242-1089; **Phone:** 319-384-6040; **Board Cert:** Urology 2005; **Med School:** Duke Univ 1984; **Resid:** Surgery, Brigham & Womens Hosp 1987; Urology, Brigham & Womens Hosp 1991; **Fellow:** Urology, Brigham & Womens Hosp 1993; **Fac Appt:** Prof U, Univ Iowa Coll Med

Schaeffer, Anthony MD [U] - **Spec Exp:** Incontinence after Prostate Cancer; **Hospital:** Northwestern Meml Hosp; **Address:** 675 N St Clair St, Galter 20-150, Chicago, IL 60611; **Phone:** 312-695-8146; **Board Cert:** Urology 1978; **Med School:** Northwestern Univ 1968; **Resid:** Surgery, Northwestern Meml Hosp 1970; Urology, Stanford Med Ctr 1976; **Fac Appt:** Prof U, Northwestern Univ

See, William A MD [U] - **Spec Exp:** Prostate Cancer; Bladder Cancer; Testicular Cancer; **Hospital:** Froedtert and Med Ctr of WI; **Address:** Med Coll Wisconsin, Dept Urology, 9200 W Wisconsin Ave, Milwaukee, WI 53226; **Phone:** 414-805-0805; **Board Cert:** Urology 2008; **Med School:** Univ Chicago-Pritzker Sch Med 1982; **Resid:** Urology, Univ Washington 1988; **Fellow:** Research, Natl Kidney Fdn/Univ Wash 1986; Research, Amer Fdn for Urol Dis/Univ Iowa 1990; **Fac Appt:** Prof U, Med Coll Wisc

Steinberg, Gary D MD [U] - **Spec Exp:** Bladder Cancer; Kidney Cancer; Prostate Cancer; **Hospital:** Univ of Chicago Med Ctr; **Address:** 5841 S Maryland Ave, rm J653, Chicago, IL 60637-1447; **Phone:** 773-702-3080; **Board Cert:** Urology 2003; **Med School:** Univ Chicago-Pritzker Sch Med 1985; **Resid:** Surgery, Johns Hopkins Hosp 1987; Urology, Brady Urol Inst/Johns Hopkins 1991; **Fellow:** Oncology, Johns Hopkins Hosp 1989; **Fac Appt:** Prof U, Univ Chicago-Pritzker Sch Med

Urology

Sundaram, Chandru P MD [U] - **Spec Exp:** Kidney Cancer; Prostate Cancer; Adrenal Tumors; Robotic Surgery; **Hospital:** IU Health Methodist Hosp; **Address:** Indiana Univ, Dept Urology, Indiana Cancer Pavilion, 535 N Barnhill Drive, Ste 420, Indianapolis, IN 46202; **Phone:** 317-278-3098; **Board Cert:** Urology 2009; **Med School:** India 1985; **Resid:** Urology, Univ Minn Med Ctr 1997; **Fellow:** Endourology, Beth Israel Deaconess Med Ctr/Harvard Med Sch 1998; **Fac Appt:** Prof U, Indiana Univ

Wood, David P MD [U] - **Spec Exp:** Genitourinary Cancer; Bladder Cancer; Prostate Cancer; Robotic Surgery; **Hospital:** Univ of Michigan Hosp; **Address:** UMH Cancer Ctr, Team 3, Reception D, Level B1-229, 1500 E Medical Center Drive, Ann Arbor, MI 48109-5913; **Phone:** 734-647-8903; **Board Cert:** Urology 2002; **Med School:** Univ Mich Med Sch 1983; **Resid:** Urology, Cleveland Clinic 1988; **Fellow:** Urologic Oncology, Meml Sloan-Kettering Cancer Ctr 1991; **Fac Appt:** Prof U, Univ Mich Med Sch

Zippe, Craig D MD [U] - **Spec Exp:** Prostate Cancer; Bladder Cancer; Incontinence after Prostate Cancer; **Hospital:** Univ Hosps Case Med Ctr; **Address:** 88 Center Rd, Ste 360, Bedford, OH 44146; **Phone:** 440-232-8955; **Board Cert:** Urology 2007; **Med School:** Rush Med Coll 1980; **Resid:** Urology, Columbia Presby Med Ctr 1989; **Fellow:** Brown Univ Hosp 1985; Urologic Oncology, Meml Sloan Kettering Cancer Ctr 1992

Great Plains and Mountains

Childs, Stacy J MD [U] - **Spec Exp:** Prostate Cancer; Bladder Cancer; Incontinence after Prostate Cancer; **Hospital:** Yampa Valley Med Ctr, Memorial Hosp - Craig; **Address:** 501 Anglers Drive, Ste 202, Steamboat Springs, CO 80487-8841; **Phone:** 970-871-9710; **Board Cert:** Urology 1979; **Med School:** Louisiana State U, New Orleans 1972; **Resid:** Urology, Carraway Meth Med Ctr 1977; **Fac Appt:** Clin Prof U, Univ Colorado

Crawford, E David MD [U] - **Spec Exp:** Prostate Cancer; Testicular Cancer; Bladder Cancer; **Hospital:** Univ of CO Hosp - Anschutz Inpatient Pav; **Address:** Urologic Oncology, MS F710, 1665 Aurora Ct, rm 1004, MS F-710, Aurora, CO 80045; **Phone:** 720-848-0170; **Board Cert:** Urology 1980; **Med School:** Univ Cincinnati 1973; **Resid:** Urology, Good Samaritan Hosp 1977; **Fellow:** Genitourinary Surgery, UCLA Med Ctr 1978; **Fac Appt:** Prof U, Univ Colorado

Davis, Bradley E MD [U] - **Spec Exp:** Urologic Cancer; Bladder Cancer; Reconstructive Surgery; Prostate Cancer; **Hospital:** Overland Pk Regl Med Ctr, St. Luke's Hosp of Kansas City; **Address:** Urologic Surgery Assocs, 10550 Quivira Rd, Ste 105, Overland Park, KS 66215; **Phone:** 913-438-3833; **Board Cert:** Urology 2004; **Med School:** Univ Kansas 1986; **Resid:** Surgery, St Lukes Hosp 1991; Urology, Univ Kansas Med Ctr 1991; **Fellow:** Urologic Oncology, Meml Sloan-Kettering Cancer Ctr 1993; **Fac Appt:** Asst Clin Prof U, Univ Kansas

Lugg, James A MD [U] - **Spec Exp:** Prostate Cancer; Laparoscopic Surgery; Incontinence after Prostate Cancer; **Hospital:** Cheyenne Regl Med Ctr, Univ of CO Hosp - Anschutz Inpatient Pav; **Address:** 2301 House Ave, Ste 502, Cheyenne, WY 82001; **Phone:** 307-635-4131; **Board Cert:** Urology 2008; **Med School:** Northwestern Univ 1990; **Resid:** Urology, UCLA Med Ctr 1995; **Fac Appt:** Asst Prof U, Univ Colorado

Thrasher, J Brantley MD [U] - **Spec Exp:** Prostate Cancer; Reconstructive Urologic Surgery; **Hospital:** Univ of Kansas Hosp; **Address:** 3901 Rainbow Blvd, MS 3016, Kansas City, KS 66160; **Phone:** 913-588-6146; **Board Cert:** Urology 2003; **Med School:** Med Univ SC 1986; **Resid:** Urology, Fitzsimons Army Med Ctr 1992; **Fellow:** Urologic Oncology, Duke Univ Med Ctr 1994; **Fac Appt:** Prof U, Univ Kansas

Southwest

Andrews, Paul E MD [U] - **Spec Exp:** Urologic Cancer; Minimally Invasive Urologic Surgery; Robotic Surgery; **Hospital:** Mayo Clinic - Phoenix; **Address:** Mayo Clinic-Urology, 5779 E Mayo Blvd, Phoenix, AZ 85054; **Phone:** 480-342-2951; **Board Cert:** Urology 2003; **Med School:** Texas Tech Univ 1987; **Resid:** Urology, Mayo Clinic 1993; **Fac Appt:** Prof U, Mayo Med Sch

Bans, Larry L MD [U] - **Spec Exp:** Prostate Cancer; **Hospital:** Banner Good Samaritan Regl Med Ctr - Phoenix; **Address:** Prostate Solutions of Arizona, 2525 E Arizona Biltmore Cir, Ste C236, Phoenix, AZ 85016; **Phone:** 602-426-9772; **Board Cert:** Urology 2004; **Med School:** Cornell Univ-Weill Med Coll 1978; **Resid:** Urology, Ind Univ Med Ctr 1983

Bardot, Stephen F MD [U] - **Spec Exp:** Urologic Cancer; Prostate Cancer; **Hospital:** Ochsner Med Ctr-New Orleans; **Address:** Ochsner Clinic, 1514 Jefferson Hwy Fl 4, Atrium 4 West, Dept Urology, New Orleans, LA 70121-2483; **Phone:** 504-842-4083; **Board Cert:** Urology 2002; **Med School:** Univ Kansas 1985; **Resid:** Surgery, St Luke's Hosp 1987; Urology, Kansas City Univ Med Ctr 1990; **Fellow:** Urologic Oncology, Cleveland Clinic 1991

Basler, Joseph W MD [U] - **Spec Exp:** Prostate Cancer; Urologic Cancer; **Hospital:** Audie L Murphy Meml Vets Hosp - San Antonio; **Address:** 7703 Floyd Curl Dr, MC-7845, San Antonio, TX 78229-3900; **Phone:** 210-567-5640; **Board Cert:** Urology 2001; **Med School:** Univ MO-Columbia Sch Med 1984; **Resid:** Surgery, Univ Missouri Affil Hosp 1986; Urology, Barnes Hosp/Wash Univ 1990; **Fac Appt:** Prof U, Univ Tex, San Antonio

Culkin, Daniel J MD [U] - **Spec Exp:** Urologic Cancer; Laparoscopic Surgery; **Hospital:** OU Med Ctr; **Address:** OU Medical Ctr, Dept Urology, 825 NE 10th St, Ste 5400, Oklahoma City, OK 73104; **Phone:** 405-271-6452; **Board Cert:** Urology 2006; **Med School:** Creighton Univ 1979; **Resid:** Surgery, Loyola Univ Med Ctr 1981; Urology, Loyola Univ Med Ctr 1983; **Fellow:** Neurourology, Loyola Univ Med Ctr 1984; **Fac Appt:** Prof U, Univ Okla Coll Med

Ellis, David S MD [U] - **Spec Exp:** Prostate Cancer-Cryosurgery; **Hospital:** Arlington Meml Hosp; **Address:** Urology Assocs of N Texas (UANT), Arlington-North, 1001 Waldrop Drive, Ste 708, Arlington, TX 76012; **Phone:** 817-312-8181; **Board Cert:** Urology 2000; **Med School:** Univ Tex, Houston 1982; **Resid:** Urology, Univ Texas Med Ctr 1988

Grossman, H Barton MD [U] - **Spec Exp:** Bladder Cancer; **Hospital:** UT MD Anderson Cancer Ctr; **Address:** MD Anderson Cancer Ctr, Dept Urology, 1373, 1515 Holcombe Blvd, Houston, TX 77030-4009; **Phone:** 713-792-3250; **Board Cert:** Urology 1979; **Med School:** Temple Univ 1970; **Resid:** Surgery, St Joseph Mercy Hosp 1974; Urology, Univ Michigan Med Ctr 1977; **Fellow:** Urologic Oncology, Meml Sloan Kettering Cancer Ctr 1979; **Fac Appt:** Clin Prof U, Univ Tex, Houston

Kadmon, Dov MD [U] - **Spec Exp:** Prostate Cancer; **Hospital:** St. Luke's Episcopal Hosp-Houston, Methodist Hosp - Houston; **Address:** Baylor Dept Urology, 6620 Main St, Ste 1325, Houston, TX 77030; **Phone:** 713-798-4001; **Board Cert:** Urology 1984; **Med School:** Israel 1970; **Resid:** Surgery, Barnes Jewish Hosp 1977; Urology, Barnes Jewish Hosp 1980; **Fellow:** Urology, Barnes Jewish Hosp 1982; **Fac Appt:** Prof U, Baylor Coll Med

Lerner, Seth P MD [U] - **Spec Exp:** Bladder Cancer; Testicular Cancer; Urinary Reconstruction; **Hospital:** St. Luke's Episcopal Hosp-Houston, Methodist Hosp - Houston; **Address:** 6620 Main St, Ste 1325, Houston, TX 77030; **Phone:** 713-798-6841; **Board Cert:** Urology 2002; **Med School:** Baylor Coll Med 1984; **Resid:** Surgery, Virginia Mason Hosp 1986; Urology, Baylor Coll Med 1990; **Fellow:** Urologic Oncology, LAC-USC Med Ctr 1992; **Fac Appt:** Prof U, Baylor Coll Med

Urology

Miles, Brian J MD [U] - **Spec Exp:** Prostate Cancer; Urologic Cancer; Gene Therapy; **Hospital:** Methodist Hosp - Houston, St. Luke's Episcopal Hosp-Houston; **Address:** 6560 Fannin St, Ste 2100, Houston, TX 77030; **Phone:** 713-441-6455; **Board Cert:** Urology 1984; **Med School:** Univ Mich Med Sch 1974; **Resid:** Urology, Walter Reed Army Med Ctr 1982; **Fac Appt:** Clin Prof U, Baylor Coll Med

Pisters, Louis L MD [U] - **Spec Exp:** Prostate Cancer; Bladder Cancer; Genitourinary Cancer; Prostate Cancer/Robotic Surgery; **Hospital:** UT MD Anderson Cancer Ctr; **Address:** MD Anderson Cancer Ctr, 1515 Holcombe Blvd, Unit 1373, Houston, TX 77030; **Phone:** 713-792-3250; **Board Cert:** Urology 2003; **Med School:** Univ Western Ontario 1986; **Resid:** Urology, Shands Hosp/UNIV Florida 1991; **Fellow:** Urologic Oncology, MD Anderson Cancer Ctr 1993; **Fac Appt:** Assoc Prof U, Univ Tex, Houston

Sagalowsky, Arthur I MD [U] - **Spec Exp:** Urologic Cancer; Transplant-Kidney; Testicular Cancer; Continent Urinary Diversions; **Hospital:** UT Southwestern Med Ctr at Dallas; **Address:** UT SW Med Ctr, Dept Urology, 5323 Harry Hines Blvd, J8.130, Dallas, TX 75390-9110; **Phone:** 214-648-3976; **Board Cert:** Urology 1980; **Med School:** Indiana Univ 1973; **Resid:** Surgery, Indiana Univ Hosps 1975; Urology, Indiana Univ Hosps 1978; **Fellow:** Clinical Pharmacology, Univ Tex SW Med Ctr 1980; **Fac Appt:** Prof U, Univ Tex SW, Dallas

Slawin, Kevin Mark MD [U] - **Spec Exp:** Prostate Cancer; Prostate Cancer/Robotic Surgery; **Hospital:** Meml Hermann Hosp - Texas Med Ctr, Methodist Hosp - Houston; **Address:** Vanguard Urologic Inst, Meml Hermann Med Plaza, 6400 Fannin, Ste 2300, Houston, TX 77030; **Phone:** 713-366-7847; **Board Cert:** Urology 2005; **Med School:** Columbia P&S 1986; **Resid:** Surgery, Mt Sinai Med Ctr 1988; Urology, Columbia-Presby Hosp 1992; **Fellow:** Urologic Oncology, Am Fdn Urol Dis/Baylor Coll Med 1994; **Fac Appt:** Clin Prof U, Baylor Coll Med

Swanson, David A MD [U] - **Spec Exp:** Kidney Cancer; Prostate Cancer; Testicular Cancer; **Hospital:** UT MD Anderson Cancer Ctr; **Address:** UT MD Anderson Canc Ctr, Dept Urol, 1515 Holcombe Blvd , Unit 1373, Houston, TX 77030-4009; **Phone:** 713-792-3250; **Board Cert:** Urology 1977; **Med School:** Univ Pennsylvania 1967; **Resid:** Surgery, Harbor Genl Hosp 1969; Urology, UC Davis Med Ctr 1975; **Fellow:** Urologic Oncology, Univ Tex-MD Anderson Hosp 1978

Thompson Jr, Ian M MD [U] - **Spec Exp:** Prostate Cancer; **Hospital:** Univ Hlth Syst-San Antonio; **Address:** Univ Tex Hlth Scis Ctr, Dept Urol, 8300 Floyd Curl Drive, San Antonio, TX 78229; **Phone:** 210-567-5643; **Board Cert:** Urology 2005; **Med School:** Tulane Univ 1980; **Resid:** Urology, Brooke Army Med Ctr 1985; **Fellow:** Medical Oncology, Meml Sloan-Kettering Canc Ctr 1988; **Fac Appt:** Prof S, Univ Tex, San Antonio

West Coast and Pacific

Ahlering, Thomas E MD [U] - **Spec Exp:** Prostate Cancer/Robotic Surgery; **Hospital:** UC Irvine Med Ctr, VA Long Beach Hlthcare Sys; **Address:** UC Irvine Med Ctr, 333 City Blvd W, Ste 2100, Orange, CA 92868; **Phone:** 714-456-6068; **Board Cert:** Urology 2005; **Med School:** St Louis Univ 1979; **Resid:** Urology, LAC-USC Med Ctr 1984; **Fellow:** Urologic Oncology, USC-Norris Comp Cancer Ctr 1986; **Fac Appt:** Prof U, UC Irvine

Amling, Christopher L MD [U] - **Spec Exp:** Prostate Cancer/Robotic Surgery; Kidney Cancer; Bladder Cancer; Testicular Cancer; **Hospital:** OR Hlth & Sci Univ; **Address:** 3303 SW Bond Ave, MC CH10U, Portland, OR 97239; **Phone:** 503-346-1500; **Board Cert:** Urology 2008; **Med School:** Oregon Hlth & Sci Univ 1985; **Resid:** Urology, Duke Univ Med Ctr 1996; **Fellow:** Urologic Oncology, Mayo Clinic 1997; **Fac Appt:** Prof U, Univ Alabama

Belldegrun, Arie S MD [U] - **Spec Exp:** Urologic Cancer; Gene Therapy; **Hospital:** UCLA Ronald Reagan Med Ctr; **Address:** 924 Westwood Blvd, Ste 1050, Los Angeles, CA 90024; **Phone:** 310-206-1434; **Board Cert:** Urology 1999; **Med School:** Israel 1974; **Resid:** Urology, Brigham and Women's Hosp 1985; **Fellow:** Urologic Oncology, Natl Cancer Inst, NIH 1988; **Fac Appt:** Prof U, UCLA

Boyd, Stuart D MD [U] - **Spec Exp:** Urologic Cancer; **Hospital:** USC Norris Cancer Hosp, USC Univ Hosp; **Address:** 1441 Eastlake Ave, Ste 7416, Los Angeles, CA 90089-9178; **Phone:** 323-865-3704; **Board Cert:** Urology 1984; **Med School:** UCLA 1975; **Resid:** Urology, UCLA Med Ctr 1982; **Fac Appt:** Prof U, USC Sch Med

Carroll, Peter R MD [U] - **Spec Exp:** Testicular Cancer; Prostate Cancer; Bladder Cancer; Bladder Reconstruction; **Hospital:** UCSF - Mt Zion Med Ctr; **Address:** UCSF Urologic Oncology Practice, 1600 Divisadero St Fl 3, San Francisco, CA 94115-1711; **Phone:** 415-353-7171; **Board Cert:** Urology 2006; **Med School:** Georgetown Univ 1979; **Resid:** Surgery, UCSF Med Ctr 1984; **Fellow:** Urology, Meml Sloan Kettering Cancer Ctr 1986; **Fac Appt:** Prof U, UCSF

Dalkin, Bruce MD [U] - **Spec Exp:** Urologic Cancer; Prostate Cancer; Bladder Cancer; Testicular Cancer; **Hospital:** Univ Wash Med Ctr; **Address:** Univ Washington-Dept Urology, 1959 NE Pacific St, Box 356510, Seattle, WA 98195; **Phone:** 206-598-4294; **Board Cert:** Urology 2002; **Med School:** Northwestern Univ 1985; **Resid:** Urology, Northwestern Meml Hosp 1991; **Fac Appt:** Prof U, Univ Wash

Daneshmand, Siamak MD [U] - **Spec Exp:** Bladder Cancer; Prostate Cancer; Kidney Cancer; Testicular Cancer; **Hospital:** USC Univ Hosp; **Address:** 1441 Eastlake Ave, Ste 7416, Los Angeles, CA 90089; **Phone:** 323-865-3700; **Board Cert:** Urology 2006; **Med School:** UC Davis 1996; **Resid:** Surgery, UC Med Ctr 1998; Urology, UC Med Ctr 2002; **Fellow:** Urologic Oncology, UC Med Ctr 2004; **Fac Appt:** Assoc Prof S, Oregon Hlth & Sci Univ

Danoff, Dudley S MD [U] - **Spec Exp:** Prostate Cancer; Bladder Cancer; **Hospital:** Cedars-Sinai Med Ctr; **Address:** 8635 W 3rd St, Ste 1 West, Los Angeles, CA 90048; **Phone:** 310-854-9898; **Board Cert:** Urology 1974; **Med School:** Yale Univ 1963; **Resid:** Urology, Yale-New Haven Hosp 1965; Urology, Columbia-Presby Med Ctr 1969

DeKernion, Jean B MD [U] - **Spec Exp:** Urologic Cancer; Kidney Cancer; Prostate Cancer; **Hospital:** UCLA Ronald Reagan Med Ctr; **Address:** UCLA Medical Plaza Drive, rm 140, Los Angeles, CA 90095-1738; **Phone:** 310-206-6453; **Board Cert:** Surgery 1973; Urology 1975; **Med School:** Louisiana State U, New Orleans 1965; **Resid:** Surgery, Univ Hosps-Case West Res 1967; Urology, Univ Hosps-Case West Res 1973; **Fellow:** Urologic Oncology, Natl Cancer Inst 1969; **Fac Appt:** Prof U, UCLA

Ellis, William J MD [U] - **Spec Exp:** Prostate Cancer; Kidney Cancer; **Hospital:** Univ Wash Med Ctr; **Address:** Univ Wash Med Ctr, Dept Urology, 1959 NE Pacific St, Box 356510, Seattle, WA 98195; **Phone:** 206-598-4294; **Board Cert:** Urology 2001; **Med School:** Johns Hopkins Univ 1985; **Resid:** Surgery, Northwestern Meml Hosp 1987; Urology, Northwestern Meml Hosp 1991; **Fac Appt:** Assoc Prof U, Univ Wash

Gill, Harcharan Singh MD [U] - **Spec Exp:** Urologic Cancer; Prostate Cancer; **Hospital:** Stanford Univ Hosp & Clinics; **Address:** 875 Blake Wilbur Drive, rm 2218, Stanford, CA 94305-5826; **Phone:** 650-725-5544; **Board Cert:** Urology 2004; **Med School:** Kenya 1977; **Resid:** Urology, Inst of Urology; Urology, Univ Hosp Penn 1991; **Fellow:** Urology, Univ Hosp Penn 1986; **Fac Appt:** Prof U, Stanford Univ

Urology

Gill, Inderbir Singh MD [U] - **Spec Exp:** Prostate Cancer; Kidney Cancer; Urologic Cancer; Minimally Invasive Urologic Surgery; **Hospital:** USC Norris Cancer Hosp; **Address:** USC/Norris Cancer Ctr, Dept Urology, 1441 Eastlake Ave, Ste 7416, Los Angeles, CA 90089; **Phone:** 323-865-3700; **Board Cert:** Urology 2008; **Med School:** India 1980; **Resid:** Surgery, Dayanand Med Coll & Hosp; Urology, Univ Kentucky Hosp 1993; **Fac Appt:** Prof U, Univ SC Sch Med

Holden, Stuart MD [U] - **Spec Exp:** Kidney Cancer; **Hospital:** Cedars-Sinai Med Ctr; **Address:** 8635 W 3rd St, Ste 1 W, Los Angeles, CA 90048; **Phone:** 310-854-9898; **Board Cert:** Urology 1977; **Med School:** Cornell Univ-Weill Med Coll 1968; **Resid:** Surgery, NY Hosp-Cornell 1970; Urology, Emory Univ Hosp 1975; **Fellow:** Urology, Meml Sloan Kettering Cancer Ctr 1978

Kawachi, Mark H MD [U] - **Spec Exp:** Prostate Cancer/Robotic Surgery; Minimally Invasive Urologic Surgery; **Hospital:** City of Hope Natl Med Ctr (page 69); **Address:** Div Urologic Oncology, 1500 E Duarte Rd, Duarte, CA 91010-3012; **Phone:** 626-359-8111 x62655; **Board Cert:** Urology 2004; **Med School:** USC Sch Med 1979; **Resid:** Urology, USC Med Ctr 1984

Lange, Paul H MD [U] - **Spec Exp:** Prostate Cancer; **Hospital:** Univ Wash Med Ctr; **Address:** Univ Wash Med Ctr, Dept Urology, 1959 NE Pacific St, Box 356510, Seattle, WA 98195; **Phone:** 206-598-4294; **Board Cert:** Urology 2006; **Med School:** Washington Univ, St Louis 1967; **Resid:** Surgery, Duke Univ Med Ctr 1972; Urology, Univ Minn Med Ctr 1975; **Fellow:** Immunology, Univ Minn Med Ctr 1973; Research, Natl Inst Hlth 1970; **Fac Appt:** Prof U, Univ Wash

Lieskovsky, Gary MD [U] - **Spec Exp:** Prostate Cancer; **Hospital:** USC Norris Cancer Hosp, USC Univ Hosp; **Address:** 1441 Eastlake Ave, Ste 7416, Los Angeles, CA 90089-0112; **Phone:** 323-865-3702; **Board Cert:** Urology 1980; **Med School:** Canada 1973; **Resid:** Urology, Univ Alberta Hosp 1978; **Fellow:** Urology, UCLA Med Ctr 1980; **Fac Appt:** Prof U, USC Sch Med

Lin, Daniel W MD [U] - **Spec Exp:** Bladder Cancer; **Hospital:** Univ Wash Med Ctr; **Address:** Urology Clinic at UWMC, 1959 NE Pacific St, Ste SP1266, Box 356158, Seattle, WA 98195; **Phone:** 206-598-4294; **Board Cert:** Urology 2003; **Med School:** Vanderbilt Univ 1994; **Resid:** Urology, Univ WA Med Ctr 2000; **Fellow:** Urologic Oncology, Meml Sloan-Kettering Canc Ctr 2001; **Fac Appt:** Assoc Prof U, Univ Wash

Presti Jr, Joseph C MD [U] - **Spec Exp:** Prostate Cancer; Bladder Cancer; Kidney Cancer; Testicular Cancer; **Hospital:** Stanford Univ Hosp & Clinics; **Address:** Stanford Cancer Ctr, 875 Blake Wilbur Dr MC 5826, Palo Alto, CA 94305-5826; **Phone:** 650-725-5544; **Board Cert:** Urology 2002; **Med School:** UC Irvine 1984; **Resid:** Surgery, UCSF Med Ctr 1986; Urology, UCSF Med Ctr 1989; **Fellow:** Urologic Oncology, Meml Sloan-Kettering Cancer Ctr 1992; **Fac Appt:** Prof U, Stanford Univ

Skinner, Eila C MD [U] - **Spec Exp:** Urologic Cancer; Urinary Reconstruction; **Hospital:** USC Norris Cancer Hosp, USC Univ Hosp; **Address:** USC-Keck Sch Med, Dept Urology, 1441 Eastlake Ave, Ste 7416, Los Angeles, CA 90089; **Phone:** 323-865-3707; **Board Cert:** Urology 2001; **Med School:** USC Sch Med 1983; **Resid:** Urology, LAC-USC Med Ctr 1988; **Fellow:** Urologic Oncology, LAC-USC Med Ctr 1990; **Fac Appt:** Assoc Prof U, USC Sch Med

Wilson, Timothy G MD [U] - **Spec Exp:** Prostate Cancer/Robotic Surgery; Urinary Reconstruction; **Hospital:** City of Hope Natl Med Ctr (page 69); **Address:** Div Urologic Oncology, 1500 E Duarte Rd, Duarte, CA 91010; **Phone:** 626-359-8111 x62655; **Board Cert:** Urology 2001; **Med School:** Oregon Hlth & Sci Univ 1984; **Resid:** Urology, USC Med Ctr 1990; **Fellow:** Urologic Oncology, City Hosp Natl Med Ctr 1991; **Fac Appt:** Assoc Clin Prof U, USC Sch Med

City of Hope™

Cleveland Clinic

Every life deserves world class care.

Cleveland Clinic
Taussig Cancer Institute
9500 Euclid Avenue
Cleveland, OH 44195

clevelandclinic.org/urologyTCD

State-of-the-Art Care for Urological Cancer

At Cleveland Clinic Taussig Cancer Institute, more than 250 top cancer specialists, researchers, nurses and technicians are dedicated to delivering the most effective medical treatments and offering access to the latest clinical trials for more than 13,000 new cancer patients every year. Our doctors are nationally and internationally known for their contributions to cancer breakthroughs and their ability to deliver superior outcomes for our patients. In recognition of these and other achievements, *U.S.News & World Report* has ranked Cleveland Clinic as one of the top cancer centers in the nation.

Glickman Urological & Kidney Institute

Cleveland Clinic's Taussig Cancer Institute and Glickman Urological & Kidney Institute bring together the expertise of world-renowned specialists and multidisciplinary approaches to treat urological cancers. Cleveland Clinic's urology program has been ranked #2 in the nation since 2000, by *U.S.News & World Report*.

Innovations and Experience

Cleveland Clinic urologists have been at the forefront of several surgical techniques including single-port surgery, laparoscopic radical prostatectomy and robotic urological surgery. Cleveland Clinic has the world's largest experience in partial nephrectomy, having performed more than 4,000 since the open procedure was pioneered here.

More than 3,000 patients have been treated in the brachytherapy program, jointly between radiation oncologists and urologists, at multiple locations. Cleveland Clinic pioneered the use of early chemotherapy after surgery to improve cure rates for urological cancer and was the first program to employ real-time, image-guided radiotherapy in the clinical setting.

Appointments | Information:
Call the Cancer Answer Line at
866.223.8100.

Cancer Treatment Guides

Cleveland Clinic has developed comprehensive treatment guides for many cancers. To download our free treatment guides, visit clevelandclinic.org/cancertreatmentguides.

Comprehensive Online Medical Second Opinion

Cleveland Clinic experts can review your medical records and render an opinion that includes treatment options and recommendations. Call 216.444.3223 or 800.223.2273 ext. 43223; email eclevelandclinic@ccf.org.

Special Assistance for Out-of-State Patients

Cleveland Clinic Global Patient Services offers a complimentary Medical Concierge service for patients who travel from outside of Ohio. Call 800.223.2273, ext. 55580, or email medicalconcierge@ccf.org.

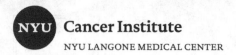

NYU Langone Medical Center
550 First Avenue , New York, NY 10016
www.NYULMC.org

NYU Clinical Cancer Center
160 East 34th Street, New York, NY 10016
www.NYUCI.org

The Stephen D. Hassenfeld Children's Center
for Cancer and Blood Disorders
160 East 32nd Street, New York, NY 10016
www.NYUMC.org/Hassenfeld

The NYU Cancer Institute is an NCI-designated cancer center and provides personalized patient care that is both compassionate and state of the art. The doctors and researchers work together to develop innovative therapies for patients. The Cancer Institute is world-renowned for excellence in cancer-focused research, personalized care, education and community outreach. Its mission is to discover the origins of human cancer and to use that knowledge to eradicate the personal and societal burden of cancer in our community, the nation and the world. For more information about our expert physicians, call 212-731-5000. *We specialize in the following areas:*

Patient-Focused Setting
The NYU Clinical Cancer Center is the principal outpatient facility of The Cancer Institute and serves as home to our patients and their caregivers. The center and its multidisciplinary team of experts provide access to the latest treatment options and clinical trials along with a variety of programs in cancer risk reduction/prevention, screening, diagnostics, genetic counseling and supportive services. In addition the NYUCI emphasizes the importance of a holistic approach to management services in complementary medicine, psychosocial support, survivorship and palliative care.

Renowned Expertise
The NYU Cancer Institute brings together experts from a variety of disciplines to create collaborative research endeavors and clinical care teams. The Cancer Institute offers a full continuum of personalized care, from prevention through diagnosis, treatment and post-treatment support. The compassion and expertise of our team members helps patients better manage the symptoms of their diseases as well as meet their special needs. Additionally, we have created special emphasis programs in diseases such as breast cancer, melanoma, GI cancer, prostate cancer, hematologic malignancies and lung cancer among others, as well as, translational programs in cancer healthcare disparities, molecularly targeted therapy, and the cell signaling pathways involved in cancer.

A Translational Approach
NYU Langone Medical Center scientists and other researchers excel in uncovering how cancer develops at the molecular level, and how we can harness that knowledge to reduce the risk of cancer and treat the disease. The Medical Center constantly seeks to create new opportunities for collaboration between investigators within our own institution, those located elsewhere in the NYU network of campuses, and researchers at other institutions.

The Stephen D. Hassenfeld Children's Center for Cancer and Blood Disorders
The center is a leading pediatric outpatient facility for the treatment of childhood cancers and blood diseases. Its unique interdisciplinary and family-centered approach combines the most advanced medical treatments with psychosocial and emotional support services for young patients and their families.

The Best in American Medicine
www.CastleConnolly.com

Other Specialties

Cardiology
(a subspecialty of INTERNAL MEDICINE)

Cardiovascular Disease: A cardiologist specializes in diseases of the heart, lungs and blood vessels and manages complex cardiac conditions such a heart attacks and life-threatening, abnormal heartbeat rhythms.

Cardiac Electrophysiology: A field of special interest within the subspecialty of cardiovascular disease which involves intricate technical procedures to evaluate heart rhythms and determine appropriate treatment for them.

Interventional Cardiology: An area of medicine within the subspecialty of cardiology which uses specialized imaging and other diagnostic techniques to evaluate blood flow and pressure in the coronary arteries and chambers of the heart, and uses technical procedures and medications to treat abnormalities that impair the function of the heart.

Training Required: Three years in internal medicine plus additional training and examination for certification in cardiovascular disease, clinical electrophysiology or interventional cardiology.

Clinical Genetics: A specialist trained in diagnostic and

therapeutic procedures for patients with genetically linked diseases. This specialist uses modern cytogenetics, radiologic and biochemical testing to assist in specialized genetic counseling, implements needed therapeutic interventions and provides prevention through prenatal diagnosis. A clinical geneticist demonstrates competence in providing comprehensive diagnostic, management and counseling services for genetic disorders. A medical geneticist plans and coordinates large scale screening programs for inborn errors of metabolism, hemoglobinopathies, chromosome abnormalities and neural tube defects.

Training Required: Two or four years

Infectious Disease:
(a subspecialty of INTERNAL MEDICINE)

An internist who deals with infectious diseases of all types and in all organs. Conditions requiring selective use of antibodies call for this special skill. This physician often diagnoses and treats AIDS patients and patients with fevers which have not been explained. Infectious disease specialists may also have expertise in preventive

medicine and conditions associated with travel.

Training Required: Three years in internal medicine plus additional training and examination for certification in infectious disease.

Internal Medicine: An internist is a personal physician who provides long-term, comprehensive care in the office and the hospital, managing both common and complex illness of adolescents, adults and the elderly. Internists are trained in the diagnosis and treatment of cancer, infections and diseases affecting the heart, blood, kidneys, joints and digestive, respiratory and vascular systems. They are also trained in the essentials of primary care internal medicine, which incorporates an understanding of disease prevention, wellness, substance abuse, mental health and effective treatment of common problems of the eyes, ears, skin, nervous system and reproductive organs.

Note: Internal Medicine normally includes many primary care physicians. However; for the purpose of this directory, no primary care physicians are included.

Training Required: Three years

Physical Medicine & Rehabilitation:

Physical medicine and rehabilitation, also referred to as rehabilitation medicine, is the medical specialty concerned with diagnosing, evaluations and treating patients with physical disabilities. these disabilities may arise from conditions affecting the musculoskeletal system such as neck and back pain, sports injuries, or other painful conditions affecting the limbs, for example carpal tunnel syndrome. Alternatively, the disabilities may result from neurological trauma or disease such as spinal cord injury, head injury or stroke.

A physician certified in physical medicine and rehabilitation is often called a physiatrist. The primary goal of the physiatrist is to achieve maximal comprehensive rehabilitation. Pain management is often an important part of the role of the physiatrist. for diagnosis and evaluation, a physiatrist may include the techniques of electromyography to supplement the standard history, physical, Xray and laboratory examinations. the physiatrist has expertise in orthotics and mechanical and electrical devices.

Training Required: Four years plus one year clinical practice.

CARDIOVASCULAR DISEASE

Mid Atlantic

Steingart, Richard MD [Cv] - **Spec Exp:** Heart Disease in Cancer Patients; Cardiac Effects of Cancer/Cancer Therapy; **Hospital:** Meml Sloan-Kettering Cancer Ctr (page 75); **Address:** 1275 York Ave, New York, NY 10065; **Phone:** 800-525-2225; **Board Cert:** Internal Medicine 1977; Cardiovascular Disease 1979; **Med School:** Mount Sinai Sch Med 1974; **Resid:** Internal Medicine, Yale-New Haven Hosp 1977; **Fellow:** Cardiovascular Disease, Mt Sinai Med Ctr 1979; **Fac Appt:** Prof Med, Cornell Univ-Weill Med Coll

CLINICAL GENETICS

New England

Bale, Allen E MD [CG] - **Spec Exp:** Cancer Genetics; **Hospital:** Yale-New Haven Hosp, Yale Med Group; **Address:** 333 Cedar St, SHM Bldg - rm I321, New Haven, CT 06519; **Phone:** 203-785-5745; **Board Cert:** Internal Medicine 1983; Clinical Genetics 1987; Clinical Molecular Genetics 2006; **Med School:** Univ Mass Sch Med 1979; **Resid:** Internal Medicine, Western Penn Hosp 1983; **Fellow:** Medical Genetics, Natl Inst of Health 1987; **Fac Appt:** Assoc Prof CG, Yale Univ

Mid Atlantic

Gilbert, Fred MD [CG] - **Spec Exp:** Cancer Genetics; **Hospital:** NY-Presby Hosp/Weill Cornell (page 78), Brooklyn Hosp Ctr-Downtown; **Address:** 1300 York Ave, Box 128, New York, NY 10065; **Phone:** 646-962-2205; **Board Cert:** Clinical Genetics 1982; Clinical Cytogenetics 1982; Clinical Molecular Genetics 2006; **Med School:** Albert Einstein Coll Med 1966; **Resid:** Internal Medicine, Barnes Hosp 1968; Internal Medicine, Natl Inst Hlth 1971; **Fellow:** Clinical Genetics, Yale-New Haven Hosp 1974; **Fac Appt:** Assoc Prof Ped, Cornell Univ-Weill Med Coll

Ostrer, Harry MD [CG] - **Spec Exp:** Genetic Disorders; Hereditary Cancer; **Hospital:** NYU Langone Med Ctr (page 79); **Address:** NYU Medical Ctr, 550 1st Ave, rm MSB136, New York, NY 10016; **Phone:** 212-263-5746; **Board Cert:** Clinical Genetics 1984; Pediatrics 1985; Clinical Cytogenetics 1990; Clinical Molecular Genetics 2010; **Med School:** Columbia P&S 1976; **Resid:** Pediatrics, Johns Hopkins Hosp 1978; Clinical Genetics, Natl Inst Health 1981; **Fellow:** Molecular Genetics, Johns Hopkins Hosp 1983; **Fac Appt:** Prof Ped, NYU Sch Med

Shapiro, Lawrence R MD [CG] - **Spec Exp:** Hereditary Cancer; **Hospital:** Westchester Med Ctr, Nyack Hosp; **Address:** Children/Women's Physicians Westchester, 503 Grasslands Ave, Ste 200, Valhalla, NY 10595; **Phone:** 914-304-5300; **Board Cert:** Pediatrics 1967; Clinical Genetics 1982; Clinical Cytogenetics 1982; **Med School:** NYU Sch Med 1962; **Resid:** Pediatrics, Chldns Hosp 1964; Pediatrics, Bellevue Hosp 1965; **Fellow:** Clinical Genetics, Mount Sinai Med Ctr 1968; **Fac Appt:** Prof Ped, NY Med Coll

Clinical Genetics

Southeast

Sutphen, Rebecca MD [CG] - **Spec Exp:** Genetic Disorders; Hereditary Cancer; Cancer Risk Assessment; **Hospital:** H Lee Moffitt Cancer Ctr & Research Inst; **Address:** 3650 Spectrum Blvd, Ste 100, Tampa, FL 33612; **Phone:** 813-396-9234; **Board Cert:** Clinical Molecular Genetics 2010; Clinical Cytogenetics 2009; Clinical Genetics 2010; **Med School:** Temple Univ 1990; **Resid:** Pediatrics, All Children's Hosp 1993; **Fellow:** Clinical Genetics, Univ S Fla Coll Med 1995; **Fac Appt:** Prof CG, Univ S Fla Coll Med

Midwest

Rubinstein, Wendy S MD/PhD [CG] - **Spec Exp:** Breast Cancer; Colon Cancer; Pancreatic Cancer; **Hospital:** Evanston/North Shore Univ Hlth Sys; **Address:** Ctr for Medical Genetics, 1000 Central St, Ste 620, Evanston, IL 60201; **Phone:** 847-570-1029; **Board Cert:** Internal Medicine 2003; Clinical Genetics 2010; Clinical Molecular Genetics 2010; **Med School:** Mount Sinai Sch Med 1989; **Resid:** Internal Medicine, Strong Meml Hosp 1992; **Fellow:** Clinical Genetics, Univ Pittsburgh 1996; Clinical Molecular Genetics, Univ Pittsburgh 1996; **Fac Appt:** Assoc Clin Prof Med, Northwestern Univ

Whelan, Alison MD [CG] - **Spec Exp:** Gynecologic Cancer Risk; Colon & Rectal Cancer Risk; Hereditary Cancer; **Hospital:** Barnes-Jewish Hosp, St. Louis Chldns Hosp; **Address:** Washington Univ Sch Med, 660 S Euclid Ave, Campus Box 8116, St Louis, MO 63110; **Phone:** 314-454-6093; **Board Cert:** Internal Medicine 1989; Clinical Genetics 2010; **Med School:** Washington Univ, St Louis 1986; **Resid:** Internal Medicine, Barnes Hosp 1989; Pediatrics, Wash Univ Sch Med 1994; **Fellow:** Research, Wash Univ Sch Med 1991; Clinical Genetics, Wash Univ Sch Med 1994; **Fac Appt:** Prof Med, Washington Univ, St Louis

Southwest

Mulvihill, John J MD [CG] - **Spec Exp:** Genetic Disorders; Fertility in Cancer Survivors; **Hospital:** Chldns Hosp OU Med Ctr; **Address:** Chldn's Hosp-OU Med Ctr, Dept Ped Genetics, Dept Pediatric Genetics, 1200 N Phillips Ave, Ste 12100, Oklahoma City, OK 73104; **Phone:** 405-271-8685; **Board Cert:** Pediatrics 1975; Clinical Genetics 1982; **Med School:** Univ Wash 1969; **Resid:** Pediatrics, Johns Hopkins Hosp 1974; **Fellow:** Research, NCI-Natl Inst Hlth 1972; **Fac Appt:** Prof CG, Univ Okla Coll Med

Plon, Sharon E MD/PhD [CG] - **Spec Exp:** Hereditary Cancer; Cancer Risk Assessment; Breast Cancer Risk Assessment; Ovarian Cancer Genetics; **Hospital:** Texas Chldns Hosp, St. Luke's Episcopal Hosp-Houston; **Address:** Texas Chldn's Hosp, 1102 Bates St, MC FC1200, Houston, TX 77030; **Phone:** 832-824-4539; **Board Cert:** Clinical Genetics 2006; **Med School:** Harvard Med Sch 1987; **Resid:** Internal Medicine, Univ Washington Affil Hosp 1988; **Fellow:** Molecular Genetics, National Cancer Inst 1990; Medical Genetics, Fred Hutchinson Cancer Research Ctr 1993; **Fac Appt:** Prof CG, Baylor Coll Med

West Coast and Pacific

Grody, Wayne W MD/PhD [CG] - **Spec Exp:** Genetic Disorders; Hereditary Cancer; **Address:** UCLA School Medicine, Div, Med Genetic & Molecular Pathology, 10833 Le Conte Ave, Los Angeles, CA 90095-1732; **Phone:** 310-825-5648; **Board Cert:** Clinical Genetics 1990; Anatomic & Clinical Pathology 1987; Clinical Biochemical Genetics 1990; Molecular Genetic Pathology 2001; **Med School:** Baylor Coll Med 1977; **Resid:** Pathology, UCLA Med Ctr 1986; **Fellow:** Clinical Genetics, UCLA Med Ctr 1987; **Fac Appt:** Prof CG, UCLA

Weitzel, Jeffrey N MD [CG] - **Spec Exp:** Breast Cancer; Ovarian Cancer; Hereditary Cancer; **Hospital:** City of Hope Natl Med Ctr (page 69); **Address:** City of Hope Cancer Ctr, 1500 E Duarte Rd, Duarte, CA 91010; **Phone:** 626-256-8662; **Board Cert:** Internal Medicine 1986; Medical Oncology 1989; Clinical Genetics 2009; **Med School:** Univ Minn 1983; **Resid:** Internal Medicine, Univ Minn Hosps 1986; Hematology, Hammersmith Hosp 1987; **Fellow:** Hematology & Oncology, Tufts-New England Med Ctr 1992; Clinical Genetics, Tufts-New England Med Ctr 1996; **Fac Appt:** Assoc Clin Prof Med, USC Sch Med

INFECTIOUS DISEASE

Mid Atlantic

Polsky, Bruce W MD [Inf] - **Spec Exp:** Infections in Cancer Patients; AIDS Related Cancers; **Hospital:** St. Luke's - Roosevelt Hosp Ctr - Roosevelt Div (page 71); **Address:** 1111 Amsterdam Ave, New York, NY 10025-1716; **Phone:** 212-523-7335; **Board Cert:** Internal Medicine 1983; Infectious Disease 1986; **Med School:** Wayne State Univ 1980; **Resid:** Internal Medicine, Montefiore Hosp 1983; **Fellow:** Infectious Disease, Meml Sloan Kettering Cancer Ctr 1986; **Fac Appt:** Prof Med, Columbia P&S

Segal, Brahm H MD [Inf] - **Spec Exp:** Infections in Cancer Patients; **Hospital:** Roswell Park Cancer Inst; **Address:** Roswell Park Cancer Inst, Elm & Carlton Streets, Buffalo, NY 14263; **Phone:** 716-845-5721; **Board Cert:** Infectious Disease 2009; **Med School:** Albert Einstein Coll Med 1992; **Resid:** Internal Medicine, New England Med Ctr 1995; **Fellow:** Infectious Disease, Natl Inst Allergy/Inf Dis 1997; **Fac Appt:** Assoc Prof Med, SUNY Buffalo

Sepkowitz, Kent MD [Inf] - **Spec Exp:** Infections in Cancer Patients; **Hospital:** Meml Sloan-Kettering Cancer Ctr (page 75); **Address:** 1275 York Ave, New York, NY 10065; **Phone:** 800-525-2225; **Board Cert:** Internal Medicine 1983; Infectious Disease 2010; **Med School:** Univ Okla Coll Med 1980; **Resid:** Internal Medicine, Roosevelt Hosp 1984; **Fellow:** Infectious Disease, Meml Sloan Kettering Cancer Ctr 1991; **Fac Appt:** Prof Med, Cornell Univ-Weill Med Coll

Great Plains and Mountains

Freifeld, Alison G MD [Inf] - **Spec Exp:** Infectious Disease during Chemotherapy; Infections in Cancer Patients; **Hospital:** Nebraska Med Ctr; **Address:** Univ Nebraska Med Ctr, 985400 Nebraska Medical Center, Omaha, NE 68198-5400; **Phone:** 402-559-8650; **Board Cert:** Internal Medicine 1985; Infectious Disease 1988; **Med School:** Johns Hopkins Univ 1982; **Resid:** Internal Medicine, Johns Hopkins Univ Med Ctr 1985

West Coast and Pacific

Palefsky, Joel M MD [Inf] - **Spec Exp:** AIDS Related Cancers; **Hospital:** UCSF - Mt Zion Med Ctr; **Address:** UCSF Med Ctr, Div Infectious Disease, 513 Parnassus Ave, Box 0654, San Francisco, CA 94143; **Phone:** 415-353-7100; **Board Cert:** Internal Medicine 1984; Infectious Disease 1988; **Med School:** McGill Univ 1980; **Resid:** Internal Medicine, Royal Victoria Hosp 1984; **Fellow:** Infectious Disease, Stanford Univ 1989

INTERNAL MEDICINE

Mid Atlantic

Quill, Timothy E MD [IM] - **Spec Exp:** Palliative Care; **Hospital:** Univ of Rochester Strong Meml Hosp; **Address:** University of Rochester Medical Ctr, 601 Elmwood Ave, Box 687, Rochester, NY 14642; **Phone:** 585-273-1154; **Board Cert:** Internal Medicine 1979; Hospice & Palliative Medicine 2008; **Med School:** Univ Rochester 1976; **Resid:** Internal Medicine, Univ Rochester/Strong Meml Hosp 1980; **Fellow:** Liaison Psychiatry, Univ Rochester Med Psych Liason Program 1981; **Fac Appt:** Prof Med, Univ Rochester

Rivlin, Richard S MD [IM] - **Spec Exp:** Nutrition & Cancer Prevention/Control; Breast Cancer; Prostate Cancer; Colon Cancer; **Hospital:** NY-Presby Hosp/Weill Cornell (page 78); **Address:** 1167 York Ave, New York, NY 10065; **Phone:** 646-898-2749; **Board Cert:** Internal Medicine 1969; **Med School:** Harvard Med Sch 1959; **Resid:** Internal Medicine, Johns Hopkins Hosp 1961; Internal Medicine, Johns Hopkins Hosp 1964; **Fellow:** Endocrinology, Diabetes & Metabolism, Natl Inst Hlth 1963; Biochemistry, Johns Hopkins Hosp 1966; **Fac Appt:** Prof Med, Cornell Univ-Weill Med Coll

Southeast

Tucker, Rodney O MD [IM] - **Spec Exp:** Palliative Care; **Hospital:** Univ of Ala Hosp at Birmingham; **Address:** UAB Ctr for Palliative Care, Ch19, Ste 219, 1530 3rd Ave S, Birmingham, AL 35294-2041; **Phone:** 205-975-8197; **Board Cert:** Internal Medicine 2002; **Med School:** Univ Alabama 1989; **Resid:** Internal Medicine, Carraway Methodist Med Ctr 1993; **Fac Appt:** Asst Prof Med, Univ Alabama

Tulsky, James A MD [IM] - **Spec Exp:** Palliative Care; **Hospital:** Duke Univ Hosp; **Address:** Ctr for Palliative Care, Hock Plaza, 2424 Erwin Rd, Ste 1105, Durham, NC 27705; **Phone:** 919-668-7215; **Board Cert:** Internal Medicine 2000; Hospice & Palliative Medicine 2006; **Med School:** Univ IL Coll Med 1987; **Resid:** Internal Medicine, UCSF Med Ctr 1990; **Fellow:** Pain & Palliative Care, UCSF Med Ctr 1993; **Fac Appt:** Prof Med, Duke Univ

Southwest

Fine, Robert L MD [IM] - **Spec Exp:** Palliative Care; **Hospital:** Baylor Univ Medical Ctr; **Address:** 3434 Swiss Ave, Ste 205, Dallas, TX 75204; **Phone:** 214-828-5090; **Board Cert:** Internal Medicine 1981; Hospice & Palliative Medicine 1993; **Med School:** Univ Tex SW, Dallas 1978; **Resid:** Internal Medicine, Baylor Univ Med Ctr 1981

West Coast and Pacific

Ferris, Frank D MD [IM] - **Spec Exp:** Palliative Care; **Hospital:** San Diego Hospice; **Address:** 4311 3rd Ave, San Diego, CA 92103-1407; **Phone:** 619-688-1600; **Board Cert:** Hospice & Palliative Medicine 1998; **Med School:** Canada 1981; **Resid:** Internal Medicine, Univ Toronto; Radiation Oncology, Univ Toronto; **Fellow:** Pain Management, Toronto-Sunnybrook Reg Cancer Ctr

Pantilat, Steven MD [IM] - **Spec Exp:** Palliative Care; **Hospital:** UCSF Med Ctr; **Address:** 521 Parnassus Ave, Box 0903, San Francisco, CA 94143-0903; **Phone:** 415-476-9019; **Board Cert:** Internal Medicine 2003; Hospice & Palliative Medicine 2001; **Med School:** UCSF 1989; **Resid:** Internal Medicine, UCSF Med Ctr 1992; **Fac Appt:** Asst Clin Prof Med, UCSF

Rabow, Michael W MD [IM] - **Spec Exp:** Palliative Care; **Hospital:** UCSF - Mt Zion Med Ctr; **Address:** 1545 Divisadero St, UCSF Gen Internal Med Practice, San Francisco, CA 94115; **Phone:** 415-353-7300; **Board Cert:** Internal Medicine 2006; Hospice & Palliative Medicine 2002; **Med School:** UCSF 1993; **Resid:** Internal Medicine, UCSF Med Ctr 1996; **Fellow:** Gastroenterology, UCSF Med Ctr 1997; **Fac Appt:** Assoc Clin Prof Med, UCSF

PHYSICAL MEDICINE & REHABILITATION

Mid Atlantic

Francis, Kathleen D MD [PMR] - **Spec Exp:** Lymphedema; **Address:** Lymphedema Physician Services, 200 S Orange Ave, Ste 111, Livingston, NJ 07039; **Phone:** 973-322-7366; **Board Cert:** Physical Medicine & Rehabilitation 2004; **Med School:** UMDNJ-NJ Med Sch, Newark 1989; **Resid:** Physical Medicine & Rehabilitation, UMDNJ-Kessler Inst Rehab 1993; **Fac Appt:** Asst Clin Prof PMR, UMDNJ-NJ Med Sch, Newark

Schwartz, L Matthew MD [PMR] - **Spec Exp:** Pain-Musculoskeletal; Cancer Rehabilitation; Lymphedema; Head & Neck Cancer; **Hospital:** Chestnut Hill Hosp; **Address:** Montgomery Rehab Assocs, 8601 Stenton Ave, Wyndmoor, PA 19038; **Phone:** 215-233-6226; **Board Cert:** Physical Medicine & Rehabilitation 1992; Pain Medicine 2003; **Med School:** UMDNJ-NJ Med Sch, Newark 1987; **Resid:** Physical Medicine & Rehabilitation, Hosp Univ Penn 1989; Physical Medicine & Rehabilitation, Thos Jefferson Univ Hosp 1991; **Fac Appt:** Asst Clin Prof PMR, Univ Pennsylvania

Stubblefield, Michael Dean MD [PMR] - **Spec Exp:** Cancer Rehabilitation; Pain-Cancer; Pain-Neuropathic; Radiation Fibrosis Syndrome; **Hospital:** Meml Sloan-Kettering Cancer Ctr (page 75); **Address:** 515 Madison Ave, Fl 5th Floor, Meml Sloan-Kettering Cancer Ctr, Outpatient Rehabilitation Ctr, New York, NY 10022; **Phone:** 646-888-1936; **Board Cert:** Internal Medicine 2001; Physical Medicine & Rehabilitation 2002; Electrodiagnostic Medicine 2003; **Med School:** Columbia P&S 1996; **Resid:** Internal Medicine, Columbia Presby Med Ctr 2001; Physical Medicine & Rehabilitation, Columbia Presby Med Ctr 2001; **Fac Appt:** Asst Prof PMR, Cornell Univ-Weill Med Coll

Southeast

King Jr, Richard W MD [PMR] - **Spec Exp:** Cancer Rehabilitation; Lymphedema; Soft Tissue Radiation Necrosis; Soft Tissue Radiation Necrosis-Breast; **Hospital:** WellStar Windy Hill Hosp, WellStar Cobb Hosp; **Address:** HyOx Medical Treatment Ctr, 2550 Windy Hill Rd, Ste 110, Marietta, GA 30067; **Phone:** 678-303-3200; **Board Cert:** Physical Medicine & Rehabilitation 1988; Undersea & Hyperbaric Medicine 2002; **Med School:** Emory Univ 1979; **Resid:** Physical Medicine & Rehabilitation, Emory Univ Hosp 1987; **Fac Appt:** Asst Clin Prof PMR, Emory Univ

Stewart, Paula JB MD [PMR] - **Spec Exp:** Lymphedema; Brain Tumors; Spinal Cord Tumors; Cancer Rehabilitation; **Hospital:** Healthsouth Lakeshore Rehab Hosp; **Address:** Healthsouth Lakeshore Rehab Hosp, 3800 Ridgeway Drive, Birmingham, AL 35209; **Phone:** 205-868-2347; **Board Cert:** Physical Medicine & Rehabilitation 2006; Spinal Cord Injury Medicine 2000; **Med School:** Univ Minn 1987; **Resid:** Physical Medicine & Rehabilitation, Mayo Clinic 1991

Physical Medicine & Rehabilitation

Midwest

Cheville, Andrea L MD [PMR] - **Spec Exp:** Lymphedema; Cancer Rehabilitation; Pain-Cancer; **Hospital:** Mayo Med Ctr & Clin - Rochester; **Address:** Mayo Clinic, Dept Physical Med & Rehab, 200 1st St SW, Rochester, MN 55905; **Phone:** 507-284-2747; **Board Cert:** Physical Medicine & Rehabilitation 2008; Pain Medicine 2004; Hospice & Palliative Medicine 2008; **Med School:** Harvard Med Sch 1993; **Resid:** Physical Medicine & Rehabilitation, UMDNJ Med Ctr 1997; **Fellow:** Pain & Palliative Care, Meml Sloan Kettering Cancer Ctr 1999; **Fac Appt:** Asst Prof PMR, Mayo Med Sch

DePompolo, Robert W MD [PMR] - **Spec Exp:** Cancer Rehabilitation; Lymphedema; **Hospital:** St. Mary's Hosp - Rochester MN (Mayo), Mayo Med Ctr & Clin - Rochester; **Address:** Mayo Clinic, Dept Phys Med & Rehab, 200 1st St SW, Rochester, MN 55905; **Phone:** 507-255-3116; **Board Cert:** Physical Medicine & Rehabilitation 1981; **Med School:** Wayne State Univ 1977; **Resid:** Physical Medicine & Rehabilitation, Univ Minnesota Affil Hosp 1980

Feldman, Joseph L MD [PMR] - **Spec Exp:** Lymphedema; **Hospital:** Evanston/North Shore Univ Hlth Sys; **Address:** 1000 Central St, Ste 800, Evanston, IL 60201; **Phone:** 847-570-2066; **Board Cert:** Physical Medicine & Rehabilitation 1971; **Med School:** Univ IL Coll Med 1965; **Resid:** Physical Medicine & Rehabilitation, Univ Ilinois Med Ctr 1969; **Fac Appt:** Asst Prof PMR, Northwestern Univ

Gamble, Gail L MD [PMR] - **Spec Exp:** Lymphedema; Cancer Rehabilitation; **Hospital:** Rehab Inst of Chicago; **Address:** Rehab Inst of Chicago, 345 E Superior St, Ste 1136, Chicago, IL 60611; **Phone:** 312-238-7670; **Board Cert:** Physical Medicine & Rehabilitation 1985; **Med School:** Mayo Med Sch 1979; **Resid:** Physical Medicine & Rehabilitation, Mayo Clinic 1983

FOX CHASE
CANCER CENTER

333 Cottman Avenue
Philadelphia, PA 19111-2497
Phone: 1-888-FOX CHASE • Fax: 215-728-2702
www.foxchase.org

RISK ASSESSMENT

The Risk Assessment Program at Fox Chase Cancer Center provides screening, education, and counseling to healthy people at increased risk for cancer. Our risk assessment team—physicians, nurses, and genetic counselors—can help you determine your chances of getting cancer and whether you and your family members are at increased risk for certain types of cancers.

The risk assessment process involves:
- A detailed review of your family history of cancer
- A look at your own medical history
- A way to learn your chance of getting a specific type of cancer
- A personal plan to reduce your cancer risk

In addition, our team will guide you through the genetic counseling and testing process along with high-risk screening, if appropriate. Participants in the program also have the option to take part in research studies that may help us learn more about cancer risk and prevention.

The Risk Assessment Program builds on Fox Chase's long and outstanding history as a leader in cancer prevention and risk assessment. In 1991, the Center established one of the first risk programs in the country for individuals with a family history of breast and/or ovarian cancer. This program served as a model for others around the country and led to risk assessment services at Fox Chase for other types of cancers.

To learn more about Fox Chase's Risk Assessment Program, call 1-877-627-9684.

CLINICAL GENETICS

Our Department of Clinical Genetics builds on Fox Chase's pioneering spirit to offer the most comprehensive risk assessment program in the Philadelphia region. It encompasses all of Fox Chase's clinical services for healthy people at risk for cancer, as well as innovative research in the areas of cancer prevention and genetics.

The department is built on the success of Fox Chase's Margaret Dyson Family Risk Assessment Program, which began in 1991. Through this program, Fox Chase developed a high-risk screening clinic for individuals with a family history of breast and/or ovarian cancer. In addition, genetic counseling was provided to both high-risk participants and breast and ovarian cancer patients.

Today, Fox Chase's comprehensive risk assessment services include examining Risk Assessment Program participants for all cancer types, including—but not limited to— breast, ovarian, uterine, gastrointestinal (including colon), prostate and thyroid cancers as well as melanoma.

The Department of Clinical Genetics is closely aligned with ongoing research initiatives in Fox Chase's Cancer Prevention and Control Program, as well as its Keystone Program in Personalized Risk and Prevention, a collaborative translational science program.

For more about Fox Chase physicians and services, visit our website, www.foxchase.org, or call 1-888-FOX CHASE.

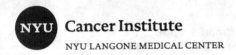

NYU Cancer Institute
NYU LANGONE MEDICAL CENTER

NYU Langone Medical Center
550 First Avenue , New York, NY 10016
www.NYULMC.org

NYU Clinical Cancer Center
160 East 34th Street, New York, NY 10016
www.NYUCI.org

**The Stephen D. Hassenfeld Children's Center
for Cancer and Blood Disorders**
160 East 32nd Street, New York, NY 10016
www.NYUMC.org/Hassenfeld

The NYU Cancer Institute is an NCI-designated cancer center and provides personalized patient care that is both compassionate and state of the art. The doctors and researchers work together to develop innovative therapies for patients. The Cancer Institute is world-renowned for excellence in cancer-focused research, personalized care, education and community outreach. Its mission is to discover the origins of human cancer and to use that knowledge to eradicate the personal and societal burden of cancer in our community, the nation and the world. For more information about our expert physicians, call 212-731-5000. *We specialize in the following areas:*

Patient-Focused Setting
The NYU Clinical Cancer Center is the principal outpatient facility of The Cancer Institute and serves as home to our patients and their caregivers. The center and its multidisciplinary team of experts provide access to the latest treatment options and clinical trials along with a variety of programs in cancer risk reduction/prevention, screening, diagnostics, genetic counseling and supportive services. In addition the NYUCI emphasizes the importance of a holistic approach to management services in complementary medicine, psychosocial support, survivorship and palliative care.

Renowned Expertise
The NYU Cancer Institute brings together experts from a variety of disciplines to create collaborative research endeavors and clinical care teams. The Cancer Institute offers a full continuum of personalized care, from prevention through diagnosis, treatment and post-treatment support. The compassion and expertise of our team members helps patients better manage the symptoms of their diseases as well as meet their special needs. Additionally, we have created special emphasis programs in diseases such as breast cancer, melanoma, GI cancer, prostate cancer, hematologic malignancies and lung cancer among others, as well as, translational programs in cancer healthcare disparities, molecularly targeted therapy, and the cell signaling pathways involved in cancer.

A Translational Approach
NYU Langone Medical Center scientists and other researchers excel in uncovering how cancer develops at the molecular level, and how we can harness that knowledge to reduce the risk of cancer and treat the disease. The Medical Center constantly seeks to create new opportunities for collaboration between investigators within our own institution, those located elsewhere in the NYU network of campuses, and researchers at other institutions.

The Stephen D. Hassenfeld Children's Center for Cancer and Blood Disorders
The center is a leading pediatric outpatient facility for the treatment of childhood cancers and blood diseases. Its unique interdisciplinary and family-centered approach combines the most advanced medical treatments with psychosocial and emotional support services for young patients and their families.

Section IV
Appendices

The Best in American Medicine
www.CastleConnolly.com

Appendix A:
Medical Boards

Intro to ABMS and Osteopathic Specialties

The following pages contain descriptions of the "official" medical specialties, approved by the American Board of Medical Specialists (for M.D.s) or by the American Osteopathic Association (for D.O.s). These are important because they are the only specialties recognized by the official governing boards. There may be physicians who call themselves one kind of specialist or another, but they may not be certified by the "official" boards. There are, in fact, over 100 such "self-designated" boards, some simply groups of physicians interested in a given area of medicine with no qualifications for membership to other groups with very specific qualifications for membership.

It is important for the medical consumer to seek out physicians certified by the ABMS or AOA to assure their doctor has had the appropriate training and passed the board certification exam.

ABMS

The ABMS is an organization of ABMS approved medical specialty boards. The mission of the ABMS is to maintain and improve the quality of medical care by assisting the Member Boards in their efforts to develop and utilize professional and educational standards for the evaluation and certification of physician specialists. The intent of certification of physicians is to provide assurance to the public that a physician specialist certified by a Member Board of the ABMS has successfully completed an approved educational program and evaluation process which includes an examination designed to assess the knowledge, skills, and experience required to provide quality patient care in that specialty. The ABMS serves to coordinate the activities of its Member Boards and to provide information to the public, the government, the profession and its Members concerning issues involving specialization and certification in medicine.

Following is a list of the addresses of the various medical specialty boards approved by the ABMS. Note that there are 24 board organizations for 25 medical specialties. Psychiatry and Neurology share the same board.

Appendix A: Medical Boards

To find out if a physician is certified, consumers can call the individual boards which may charge a fee for the information, or they can contact the ABMS at 866-275-2267 (no fee) or www.abms.org.

American Board of Allergy and Immunology
111 S. Independence Mall East, Suite 701
Philadelphia, PA 19106-3699
(215) 592-9466, (866) 264-5568

General Certification in Allergy and Immunology. Certifications awarded since 1989 are valid for 10 years. For those certified prior to 1989 there is no recertification requirement.

American Board of Anesthesiology
4208 Six Forks, Ste 900
Raleigh, NC 27609-2200
Ph: (919) 745-2200
Fax: (919) 745-2201

General Certification in Anesthesiology; with Special and Added Qualifications in Critical Care Medicine and Pain Medicine. Certifications awarded since 2000 are valid for 10 years.

American Board of Colon and Rectal Surgery
20600 Eureka Road, Suite 600
Taylor, MI 48180
(734) 282-9400

General Certification in Colon and Rectal Surgery. Certifications awarded since 1990 are valid for 10 years.

American Board of Dermatology
Henry Ford Health System
1 Ford Place
Detriot, MI 48202-3450
(313) 874-1088

General Certification in Dermatology; with Special Qualifications in Dermatopathology, and Pediatric Dermatology. Certifications awarded since 1991 are valid for 10 years.

American Board of Emergency Medicine
3000 Coolidge Road
East Lansing, MI 48823-6319
(517) 332-4800

General Certification in Emergency Medicine; with Special and Added Qualifications in Emergency Medical Services, Hospice & Palliative Medicine, Medical Toxicology, Pediatric Emergency Medicine, Sports Medicine and Undersea and Hyperbaric Medicine. Certifications awarded since 1980 are valid for 10 years.

American Board of Family Medicine
1648 McGrathiana Parkway, Ste 550
Lexington, KY 40505-4294
(859) 269-5626, (888) 995-5700

General Certification in Family Medicine; with Added Qualifications in Adolescent Medicine, Geriatric Medicine, Hospice & Palliative Care, Sleep Medicine and Sports Medicine. Certifications awarded since 1970 are valid for 7 years.

American Board of Internal Medicine
510 Walnut Street, Suite 1700
Philadelphia, PA 19106-3699
(215) 446-3500, (800) 441-2246

General Certification in Internal Medicine; with Special Qualifications in Cardiovascular Disease, Endocrinology, Diabetes and Metabolism, Gastroenterology, Hematology, Infectious Disease, Medical Oncology, Nephrology, Pulmonary Disease, and Rheumatology; and Added Qualifications in Adolescent Medicine, Advanced Heart Failure and Transplant Cardiology, Clinical Cardiac Electrophysiology, Critical Care Medicine, Geriatric Medicine, Hospice & Palliative Medicine, Interventional Cardiology, Sleep Medicine, Sports Medicine and Transplant Hepatology. Certifications awarded since 1990 are valid for 10 years.

American Board of Medical Genetics
9650 Rockville Pike
Bethesda, MD 20814-3998
(301) 634-7315

General Certification in Clinical Genetics (MD), PhD Medical Genetics, Clinical Biochemical Genetics, Clinical Cytogenetics and Clinical Molecular Genetics; with Added Qualifications in Medical Biochemical Genetics and Molecular Genetic Pathology. Certifications awarded since 2002 are valid for 2 years.

Appendix A: Medical Boards

American Board of Neurological Surgery
6550 Fannin Street, Suite 2139
Houston, TX 77030-2701
(713) 441-6015

General Certification in Neurological Surgery. Certifications awarded since 1999 are valid for 10 years.

American Board of Nuclear Medicine
4555 Forest Park Boulevard, Suite 119
St. Louis, MO 63108
(314) 367-2225

General Certification in Nuclear Medicine. Certifications awarded since 1992 are valid for 10 years.

American Board of Obstetrics and Gynecology
2915 Vine Street
Dallas, TX 75204
(214) 871-1619

General Certification in Obstetrics and Gynecology; with Special Qualifications in Gynecologic Oncology, Maternal and Fetal Medicine, Reproductive Endocrinology/Infertility; and Added Qualifications in Critical Care Medicine, Female Pelvic Medicine and Reconstructive Surgery, Hospice & Palliative Medicine. Certifications awarded since 1986 are valid for 6 years.

American Board of Ophthalmology
111 Presidential Boulevard, Suite 241
Bala Cynwyd, PA 19004-1075
(610) 664-1175

General certifications in Ophthalmology. Certifications awarded since 1992 are valid for 10 years. For those certified prior to 1992 there is no recertification requirement.

American Board of Orthopaedic Surgery
400 Silver Cedar Court
Chapel Hill, NC 27514
(919) 929-7103

General Certification in Orthopaedic Surgery; with Added Qualifications in Surgery of the Hand & Orthopaedic Sports Medicine. Certifications awarded since 1986 are valid for 10 years.

American Board of Otolaryngology
5615 Kirby Drive, Suite 600
Houston, TX 77005
(713) 850-0399

General Certification in Otolaryngology; with Added Qualifications in Neurotology, Pediatric Otolaryngology, Plastic Surgery within the Head and Neck and Sleep Medicine. Certifications awarded since 2002 are valid for 10 years.

American Board of Pathology
P.O. Box 25915
Tampa, FL 33622-5915
(813) 286-2444

General Certification in Anatomic and Clinical Pathology, Anatomic Pathology and Clinical Pathology; with Special Qualifications in Blood Banking/Transfusion Medicine, Chemical Pathology, Dermatopathology, Forensic Pathology, Hematology, Medical Microbiology, Molecular Genetic Pathology, Neuropathology and Pediatric Pathology; and Added Qualifications in Cytopathology. Certifications awarded since 1997 are valid for 10 years.

American Board of Pediatrics
111 Silver Cedar Court
Chapel Hill, NC 27514-1651
(919) 929-0461

General Certification in Pediatrics; with Special Qualifications in Adolescent Medicine, Developmental-Behavioral Pediatrics, Neonatal-Perinatal Medicine, Pediatric Cardiology, Pediatric Critical Care Medicine, Pediatric Emergency Medicine, Pediatric Endocrinology, Pediatric Gastroenterology, Pediatric Hematology-Oncology, Pediatric Infectious Diseases, Pediatric Nephrology, Pediatric Pulmonology, and Pediatric Rheumatology; and Added Qualifications in Child Abuse Pediatrics, Hospice & Palliative Medicine, Medical Toxicology, Neurodevelopmental Disabilities, Pediatric Transplant Hepatology, Sleep Medicine and Sports Medicine. Certifications awarded since 1988 valid for 7 years.

American Board of Physical Medicine and Rehabilitation
3015 Allegro Park Lane, S.W.
Rochester, MN 55902-4139
(507) 282-1776

General Certification in Physical Medicine and Rehabilitation; with Special Qualifications in Hospice & Palliative Medicine, Neuromuscular Medicine, Pain Medicine, Pediatric Rehabilitation Medicine, Spinal Cord Injury Medicine and Sports Medicine. Certifications awarded since 1993 are valid for 10 years.

Appendix A: Medical Boards

American Board of Plastic Surgery
Seven Penn Center, Suite 400
1635 Market Street
Philadelphia, PA 19103-2204
(215) 587-9322

General Certification in Plastic Surgery; with Added Qualifications in Surgery of the Hand and Plastic Surgery within the Head & Neck. Certifications awarded since 1995 are valid for 10-years.

American Board of Preventive Medicine
111 West Jackson Boulevard, Suite 1110
Chicago, IL 60604
(312) 939-2276

General Certification in Aerospace Medicine, Occupational Medicine and Public Health and General Preventive Medicine; with Added Qualifications in Undersea and Hyperbaric Medicine and Medical Toxicology. Certifications awarded since 1997 are valid for 10 years.

American Board of Psychiatry and Neurology
2150 E. Lake Cook Road, Suite 900
Buffalo Grove, IL 60089
(847) 229-6500

General Certification in Psychiatry, Neurology and Neurology with Special Qualification in Child Neurology; with Special Qualifications in Child and Adolescent Psychiatry, Pain Medicine and Sleep Medicine; and Added Qualifications in Addiction Psychiatry, Clinical Neurophysiology, Epilepsy, Forensic Psychiatry, Geriatric Psychiatry, Hospice & Palliative Medicine, Neurodevelopmental Disabilities, Neuromuscular Medicine, Psychosomatic Medicine and Vascular Neurology . Certifications awarded since 1994 are valid for 10 years.

American Board of Radiology
5441 E. Williams Boulevard, Suite 200
Tucson, AZ 85711
(520) 790-2900

General Certifications in Diagnostic Radiology, Radiation Oncology and Medical Physics; with Special Competency in Nuclear Radiology; and Added Qualifications in Hospice & Palliative Medicine, Neuroradiology, Nuclear Radiology, Pediatric Radiology and Vascular and Interventional Radiology. Radiological Physics is a non-clinical certification. Certificates are valid for 10 years.

American Board of Surgery
1617 John F. Kennedy Boulevard, Suite 860
Philadelphia, PA 19103-1847
(215) 568-4000

General Certification in Surgery and Vascular Surgery; with Special Qualifications in
Pediatric Surgery and Surgery of the Hand; and Added Qualifications in Complex
General Surgical Oncology, Hospice & Palliative Medicne, Surgical Critical Care.
Certifications awarded since 1976 are valid for 10 years.

American Board of Thoracic Surgery
633 North St. Clair Street, Suite 2320
Chicago, IL 60611
(312) 202-5900

General Certification in Thoracic Surgery with Special Qualification in Congenital
Cardiac Surgery. Certifications awarded since 1976 are valid for 10 years.

American Board of Urology
600 Peter Jefferson Parkway, Ste 150
Charlottesville, VA 22911
(434) 979-0059

General Certification in Urology with special qualifications in Pediatric Urology and
Female Pelvic Medicine and Reconstructive Surgery. Certifications awarded as of 1985
are valid for 10 years.

Osteopathic

The American Osteopathic Association (AOA) is a member association
representing more than 78,000 osteopathic physicians (D.O.s). The AOA serves as
the primary certifying body for D.O.s, and is the accrediting agency for all
osetopathic medical colleges and healthcare facilities. The AOA's mission is to
advance the philosophy and practice of osteopathic medicine by promoting
excellence in education, research, and the delivery of quality, cost-effective
healthcare within a distinct, unified profession.
American Osteopathic Association
142 E Ontario Street
Chicago, IL 60611

Consumers may call the American Osteopathic Association at (800) 621-1773 or
visit the website, www.osteopathic.org, for general certification information.

Appendix A: Medical Boards

American Osteopathic Board of Anesthesiology

General certification in Anesthesiology; with Added Qualifications in Addiction Medicine, Critical Care Medicine, and Pain Management. Certifications awarded since 2004 are valid for 10 years. For those certified prior to 2004 there is no recertification requirement.

American Osteopathic Board of Dermatology

General certification in Dermatology; with Added Qualifications in Dermatopathology and Mohs'-Micrographic Surgery. Certifications awarded since 2004 are valid for 10 years.

American Osteopathic Board of Emergency Medicine

General certification in Emergency Medicine; with Added Qualifications in Emergency Medical Services, Medical Toxicology, and Sports Medicine. Certifications awarded since 1994 are valid for 10 years.

American Osteopathic Board of Family Physicians

General certification in Family Practice and Osteopathic Manipulative Treatment (OMT); with Added Qualifications in Geriatric Medicine, Hospice & Palliative Medicine, Sleep Medicine, Sports Medicine and Undersea & Hyperbaric Medicine. Certifications awarded since March 1,1997 are valid for 8 years.

American Osteopathic Board of Internal Medicine

General certification in Internal Medicine; with Special Qualifications in Allergy/Immunology, Cardiology, Endocrinology, Gastroenterology, Hematology, Infectious Disease, Nephrology, Oncology, Pulmonary Disease, Rheumatology; with Added Qualifications in Addiction Medicine, Critical Care Medicine, Clinical Cardiac Electrophysiology, Geriatric Medicine, Hospice & Palliative Medicine, Interventional Cardiology, Sleep Medicine, Sports Medicine and Undersea & Hyperbaric Medicine. Certifications awarded since 1993 are valid for 10 years.

American Osteopathic Board of Neurology and Psychiatry

General certification in Neurology and Psychiatry; with Special Qualifications in Child/Adolescent Psychiatry and Child/Adolescent Neurology; with Added Qualifications in Addiction Medicine, Geriatric Psychiatry, Hospice & Palliative Care, Neurophysiology, Sleep Medicine. Certifications awarded since 1995 are valid for 10 years.

American Osteopathic Board of Neuromusculoskeletal Medicine

(Formerly American Osteopathic Board of Special Proficiency in Osteopathic Manipulative Medicine) General certification in Neuromusculoskeletal Medicine & Osteopathic Manipulative Medicine with added qualifications in Sports Medicine. Certifications awarded since 1995 are valid for 10 years. For those certified prior to 1995 there is no recertification requirement.

American Osteopathic Board of Nuclear Medicine

General certification in Nuclear Medicine. Certifications awarded since 1995 are valid for 10 years.

American Osteopathic Board of Obstetrics and Gynecology

General certification in Obstetrics and Gynecology; with Special Qualifications in Gynecologic Oncology; Maternal and Fetal Medicine and Reproductive Endocrinology. Certifications awarded since June 2002 are valid for 6 years.

American Osteopathic Board of Ophthalmology and Otolaryngology

General certification in Ophthalmology, Otolaryngology, and Otolaryngology/Facial Plastic Surgery; with Added Qualifications in Otolaryngic Allergy and Sleep Medicine. Certifications awarded in Ophthalmology since 2000 are valid for 10 years. For those certified prior to 2000 there is no recertification requirement. Certifications awarded in Otolaryngology and/or Otolaryngology/Facial Plastic Surgery since 2002 are valid for 10 years.

American Osteopathic Board of Orthopaedic Surgery

General certification in Orthopaedic Surgery; with Added Qualifications in Hand Surgery. Certifications awarded since 1994 are valid for 10 years.

American Osteopathic Board of Pathology

General certification in Laboratory Medicine, Anatomic Pathology and Anatomic Pathology and Laboratory Medicine; with Special Qualifications in Forensic Pathology; and with Added Qualifications in Dermatopathology. Certifications awarded since 1995 are valid for 10 years.

American Osteopathic Board of Pediatrics

General certification in Pediatrics with Special Qualifications in Adolescent and Young Adult Medicine, Neonatology, Pediatric Allergy/Immunology and Pediatric Endocrinology; with Added Qualification in Sports Medicine. Certifications awarded since 1995 are valid for 7 years.

Appendix A: Medical Boards

American Osteopathic Board of Physical Medicine and Rehabilitation Medicine

General certification in Physical Medicine and Rehabilitation; with Added Qualifications in Hospice & Palliative Medicine and Sports Medicine. Certifications awarded since 2004 are valid for 10 years.

American Osteopathic Board of Preventive Medicine

General certification in Preventive Medicine/Aerospace Medicine, Preventive Medicine/Occupational-Environmental Medicine and Preventive Medicine/Public Health; with Added Qualifications in Occupational Medicine and Undersea & Hyperbaric Medicine. Certifications awarded since 1994 are valid for 10 years.

American Osteopathic Board of Proctology

General certification in Proctology. Certifications awarded since 2004 are valid for 10 years.

American Osteopathic Board of Radiology

General certification in Diagnostic Radiology and Radiation Oncology; with Added Qualifications in Body Imaging, Diagnostic Ultrasound, Neuroradiology, Pediatric Radiology and Angiography & Interventional Radiology. Certifications awarded since 2002 are valid for 10 years.

American Osteopathic Board of Surgery

General certification in Surgery, Neurological Surgery, Plastic and Reconstructive Surgery, Thoracic Cardiovascular Surgery, Urological Surgery and General Vascular Surgery; with Added Qualifications in Surgical Critical Care. Certifications awarded since 1997 are valid for 10 years.

APPENDIX B:
Hospital Listings

The following is an alphabetical listing of all hospitals that have at least one Castle Connolly Top Doctor in this guide. Institutions listed in **Bold** are profiled in this Guide in association with Castle Connolly's Partnership for Excellence program. The abbreviations as they appear in the listings are in italics below. Due to the many changes taking place in the hospital industry, the names on this list may have changed subsequent to publication of this guide.

Abbott - Northwestern Hospital		(612) 863-4000
Abbott - Northwestern Hosp		
800 E 28th St	Minneapolis, MN 55407	MIDWEST
Advocate Christ Medical Center		(708) 684-8000
Adv Christ Med Ctr		
4440 W 95th St	Oak Lawn, IL 60453	MIDWEST
Advocate Lutheran General Hospital		(847) 723-2210
Adv Luth Genl Hosp		
1775 West Dempster St	Park Ridge, IL 60068	MIDWEST
Akron Children's Hospital		(330) 543-1000
Akron Children's Hosp		
One Perkins Square	Akron, OH 44308	MIDWEST
Albany Medical Center		(518) 262-3125
Albany Med Ctr		
43 New Scotland Ave	Albany, NY 12208	MID ATLANTIC
Albert Einstein Medical Center		(215) 456-7890
Albert Einstein Med Ctr		
5501 Old York Rd	Philadelphia, PA 19141	MID ATLANTIC
Alegent Health - Immanuel Medical Center		(402) 572-2121
Alegent Hlth - Immanuel Med Ctr		
6901 N 72nd St	Omaha, NE 68122	GREAT PLAINS AND MOUNTAINS
Alfred I duPont Hospital for Children		(302) 651-4000
Alfred I duPont Hosp for Children		
1600 Rockland Rd, Box 269	Wilmington, DE 19889	MID ATLANTIC
All Children's Hospital		(727) 898-7451
All Children's Hosp		
801 Sixth Street South	St. Petersburg, FL 33701	SOUTHEAST

Allegheny General Hospital   (412) 359-3131
Allegheny General Hosp
320 E. North Avenue   Pittsburgh, PA 15212   MID ATLANTIC

Alta Bates Summit Medical Center-Alta Bates Campus   (510) 204-4444
Alta Bates Summit Med Ctr-Alta Bates Campus
2450 Ashby Avenue   Berkeley, CA 94705   WEST COAST AND PACIFIC

Anne Arundel Medical Center   (443) 481-1000
Anne Arundel Med Ctr
64 Franklin Street   Annapolis, MD 21401   MID ATLANTIC

Arkansas Children's Hospital   (501) 364-1100
Arkansas Chldns Hosp
800 Marshall St   Little Rock, AR 72202   SOUTHWEST

Arlington Memorial Hospital   (817) 548-6100
Arlington Meml Hosp
800 W Randol Mill Rd   Arlington, TX 76012-2503   SOUTHWEST

Arthur G. James Cancer Hospital & Research Institute   (614) 293-3300
Arthur G James Cancer Hosp & Research Inst
300 West 10th Avenue   Columbus, OH 43210   MIDWEST

Atlanta VA Medical Center   (404) 321-6111
Atlanta VA Med Ctr
1670 Clairmont Rd   Decatur, GA 30033   SOUTHEAST

Audie L Murphy Memorial Veterans Hospital - San Antonio   (210) 617-5300
Audie L Murphy Meml Vets Hosp - San Antonio
7400 Merton Minter Blvd   San Antonio, TX 78229   SOUTHWEST

Aultman Hospital   (330) 452-9911
Aultman Hosp
2600 6th St SW   Canton, OH 44710-1799   MIDWEST

Banner Desert Medical Center   (480) 512-3000
Banner Desert Med Ctr
1400 S Dobson Rd   Mesa, AZ 85202   SOUTHWEST

Banner Good Samaritan Regional Medical Center - Phoenix   (602) 839-2000
Banner Good Samaritan Regl Med Ctr - Phoenix
1111 E McDowell Rd   Phoenix, AZ 85006   SOUTHWEST

Baptist Hospital - Nashville   (615) 284-5555
Baptist Hosp - Nashville
2000 Church St   Nashville, TN 37236   SOUTHEAST

Baptist Hospital of Miami (786) 596-1960
Baptist Hosp of Miami
8900 N Kendall Dr Miami, FL 33176 SOUTHEAST

Baptist Medical Center-Jackson (601) 968-1000
Baptist Med Ctr-Jackson
1225 N State St Jackson, MS 39202 SOUTHEAST

Baptist Memorial Hospital-Memphis (901) 226-5000
Baptist Memorial Hospital-Memphis
6019 Walnut Grove Rd Memphis, TN 38120 SOUTHEAST

Barbara Ann Karmanos Cancer Institute (800) 527-6266
Barbara Ann Karmanos Cancer Inst
4100 John R Detroit, MI 48201 MIDWEST

Barnes-Jewish Hospital (314) 747-3000
Barnes-Jewish Hosp
One Barnes-Jewish Hospital Plaza St. Louis, MO 63110 MIDWEST

Bascom Palmer Eye Institute (305) 326-6000
Bascom Palmer Eye Inst
900 NW 17 St Miami, FL 33136 SOUTHEAST

Baylor Clinic & Hospital (713) 798-1000
Baylor Clinic & Hosp
6620 Main St Houston, TX 77030 SOUTHWEST

Baylor University Medical Center (214) 820-0111
Baylor Univ Medical Ctr
3500 Gaston Avenue Dallas, TX 75246 SOUTHWEST

Beaumont Hospital-Royal Oak (248) 898-5000
Beaumont Hosp-Royal Oak
3601 W 13 Mile Rd Royal Oak, MI 48073 MIDWEST

Ben Taub General Hospital (713) 873-2000
Ben Taub Genl Hosp
1504 Taub Loop Houston, TX 77001 SOUTHWEST

Beth Israel Deaconess Medical Center - Boston (617) 667-7000
Beth Israel Deaconess Med Ctr - Boston
330 Brookline Ave Boston, MA 02215 NEW ENGLAND

Beth Israel Medical Center - Milton & Caroll Petrie Division (212) 420-2000
Beth Israel Med Ctr - Petrie Division
First Avenue @ 16th Street New York, NY 10003 MID ATLANTIC

Boca Raton Regional Hospital		(561) 955-7100
Boca Raton Regl Hosp		
800 Meadows Road	Boca Raton, FL 33486	SOUTHEAST

Boston Medical Center		(617) 638-8000
Boston Med Ctr		
1 Boston Medical Center Pl	Boston, MA 02118	NEW ENGLAND

Brenner Children's Hospital		(336) 716-2011
Brenner Chldrn's Hosp		
Medical Center Blvd	Winston-Salem, NC 27157-1015	SOUTHEAST

Brigham & Women's Hospital		(617) 732-5500
Brigham & Women's Hosp		
75 Francis St	Boston, MA 02115	NEW ENGLAND

Bryn Mawr Hospital		(610) 526-3000
Bryn Mawr Hosp		
130 S Bryn Mawr Ave	Bryn Mawr, PA 19010-3143	MID ATLANTIC

California Pacific Medical Center-Pacific Campus		(415) 600-6000
CA Pacific Med Ctr-Pacific Campus		
2333 Buchanan St, Box 7999	San Francisco, CA 94115	WEST COAST AND PACIFIC

Carolinas Medical Center		(704) 355-2000
Carolinas Med Ctr		
1000 Blythe Blvd, PO Box 32861	Charlotte, NC 28203-5871	SOUTHEAST

Cedars-Sinai Medical Center		(310) 423-3277
Cedars-Sinai Med Ctr		
8700 Beverly Boulevard	Los Angeles, CA 90048	WEST COAST AND PACIFIC

Centennial Medical Center		(615) 342-1000
Centennial Med Ctr		
2300 Patterson Street	Nashville, TN 37203	SOUTHEAST

Chandler Regional Medical Center		(602) 963-4561
Chandler Regional Med Ctr		
475 S Dobson Rd	Chandler, AZ 85224-5695	SOUTHWEST

Charlie Norwood VA Medical Center - Augusta		(706) 733-0188
Charlie Norwood VA Med Ctr - Augusta		
One Freedom Way	Augusta, GA 30904	SOUTHEAST

Chestnut Hill Hospital		(212) 248-8200
Chestnut Hill Hosp		
8835 Germantown Ave	Philadelphia, PA 19118	MID ATLANTIC

Cheyenne Regional Medical Center		(307) 634-2273
Cheyenne Regl Med Ctr		
214 E 23rd St	Cheyenne, WY 82001	GREAT PLAINS AND MOUNTAINS
Children's Healthcare of Atlanta at Egleston		(404) 785-6000
Chldns Hlthcare Atlanta @ Egleston		
1405 Clifton Rd NE	Atlanta, GA 30322	SOUTHEAST
Children's Hospital - Boston		(617) 355-6000
Children's Hospital - Boston		
300 Longwood Avenue	Boston, MA 02115	NEW ENGLAND
Children's Hospital - Los Angeles		(323) 660-2450
Chldns Hosp - Los Angeles		
4650 Sunset Blvd	Los Angeles, CA 90027	WEST COAST AND PACIFIC
Children's Hospital - New Orleans		(504) 899-9511
Children's Hospital - New Orleans		
200 Henry Clay Ave	New Orleans, LA 70118	SOUTHWEST
Children's Hospital - Oakland		(510) 428-3000
Chldns Hosp - Oakland		
747 52nd St	Oakland, CA 94609	WEST COAST AND PACIFIC
Children's Hospital - Omaha		(402) 955-5400
Children's Hosp - Omaha		
8200 Dodge St	Omaha, NE 68114	GREAT PLAINS AND MOUNTAINS
Children's Hospital and Clinics - Minneapolis		(612) 813-6111
Chldns Hosp and Clinics - Minneapolis		
2525 Chicago Ave S	Minneapolis, MN 55404	MIDWEST
Children's Hospital at OU Medical Center		(405) 271-5437
Chldns Hosp OU Med Ctr		
1200 N Everett Drive	Oklahoma City, OK 73104	SOUTHWEST
Children's Hospital Central California		(559) 353-3000
Chldns Hosp Central CA		
9300 Valley Children's Pl	Madera, CA 93638	WEST COAST AND PACIFIC
Children's Hospital of Michigan		(313) 745-5437
Chldns Hosp of Michigan		
3901 Beaubian Blvd	Detroit, MI 48201	MIDWEST
Children's Hospital of Orange County		(714) 997-3000
Chldns Hosp Orange Co		
455 South Main Street	Orange, CA 92868	WEST COAST AND PACIFIC

Children's Hospital of Philadelphia (215) 590-1000
Chldns Hosp of Philadelphia
34th St & Civic Center Blvd   Philadelphia, PA 19104   MID ATLANTIC

Children's Hospital of Pittsburgh - UPMC (412) 692-5325
Chldns Hosp of Pittsburgh - UPMC
4401 Penn Ave   Pittsburgh, PA 15224   MID ATLANTIC

Children's Hospital of Wisconsin (414) 266-2000
Chldns Hosp - Wisconsin
9000 W Wisconsin Ave   Milwaukee, WI 53226   MIDWEST

Children's Medical Center of Dallas (214) 456-7000
Chldns Med Ctr of Dallas
1935 Motor St   Dallas, TX 75235   SOUTHWEST

Children's Memorial Hospital- Chicago (773) 880-4000
Children's Mem Hosp -Chicago
2300 Children's Plaza   Chicago, IL 60614   MIDWEST

Children's Mercy Hospitals & Clinics (816) 234-3000
Chldns Mercy Hosps & Clinics
2401 Gilham Rd   Kansas City, MO 64108   MIDWEST

Children's National Medical Center - DC (202) 476-3000
Chldns Natl Med Ctr
111 Michigan Ave NW   Washington, DC 20010   MID ATLANTIC

Christiana Hospital (302) 733-1000
Christiana Hospital
4755 Ogletown-Stanton Rd, PO Box 6001 Newark, DE 19718-0001   MID ATLANTIC

Christus Santa Rosa Children's Hospital (512) 228-2011
Christus Santa Rosa Children's Hosp
333 N Santa Rosa St   San Antonio, TX 78207   SOUTHWEST

Christus St Vincent Regional Medical Center-Santa Fe (505) 983-3361
Christus St Vincent Reg Med Ctr-Santa Fe
455 St Michaels Dr   Santa Fe, NM 87504-2107   SOUTHWEST

Cincinnati Children's Hospital Medical Center (513) 636-4200
Cincinnati Chldns Hosp Med Ctr
3333 Burnet Ave   Cincinnati, OH 45229-3039   MIDWEST

City of Hope National Medical Center (626) 256-4673
City of Hope Natl Med Ctr
1500 E Duarte Rd   Duarte, CA 91010   WEST COAST AND PACIFIC

Cleveland Clinic   (216) 444-2200
Cleveland Clin
9500 Euclid Avenue   Cleveland, OH 44195   MIDWEST

Cleveland Clinic Florida - Weston   (954) 659-5000
Cleveland Clin - Weston
2950 Cleveland Clinic Blvd   Weston, FL 33331   SOUTHEAST

Columbus Regional Medical Center   (706) 571-1000
Columbus Regl Med Ctr
710 Center St   Columbus, GA 31902   SOUTHEAST

Community Hospital East - Indianapolis   (317) 355-5411
Commun Hosp E - Indianapolis
1500 N Ritter Ave   Indianapolis, IN 46219   MIDWEST

Community Memorial Hospital - Ventura   (805) 652-5011
Comm Meml Hosp - Ventura
147 N Brent St   Ventura, CA 93003   WEST COAST AND PACIFIC

Concord Hospital   (603) 225-2711
Concord Hospital
250 Pleasant St   Concord, NH 03301-2598   NEW ENGLAND

Connecticut Children's Medical Center   (860) 545-9000
CT Chldns Med Ctr
282 Washington St   Hartford, CT 06106   NEW ENGLAND

Cook Children's Medical Center   (682) 885-4000
Cook Chldns Med Ctr
801 7th Ave   Fort Worth, TX 76104-2796   SOUTHWEST

Cooper University Hospital   (856) 342-2000
Cooper Univ Hosp
1 Cooper Plaza   Camden, NJ 08103   MID ATLANTIC

Covenant Medical Center   (319) 272-8000
Covenant Med Ctr
3421 W 9th St   Waterloo, IA 50702-5499   MIDWEST

Crouse Hospital   (315) 470-7111
Crouse Hosp
736 Irving Ave   Syracuse, NY 13210-1607   MID ATLANTIC

CTCA at Midwestern Regional Medical Center   (847) 872-4561
CTCA at Midwestern Reg Med Ctr
2520 Elisha Ave   Zion, IL 60099   MIDWEST

Dana-Farber Cancer Institute (617) 632-3000
Dana-Farber Cancer Inst
44 Binney St Boston, MA 02115 NEW ENGLAND

Dartmouth - Hitchcock Medical Center (603) 650-5000
Dartmouth - Hitchcock Med Ctr
1 Medical Center Dr Lebanon, NH 03756-0002 NEW ENGLAND

Doctors' Hospital (305) 666-2111
Doctors' Hosp
5000 University Dr Coral Gables, FL 33146 SOUTHEAST

Doernbecher Children's Hospital/Oregon Health Science University (503) 494-8811
Doernbecher Chldns Hosp/OHSU
3181 SW Sam Jackson Park Rd Portland, OR 97201-3098 WEST COAST AND PACIFIC

Duke University Hospital (919) 684-8111
Duke Univ Hosp
2301 Erwin Rd, PO Box 3708 Durham, NC 27710 SOUTHEAST

El Camino Hospital (650) 940-7000
El Camino Hosp
2500 Grant Road Mountain View, CA 94039 WEST COAST AND PACIFIC

Elliot Hospital (603) 669-5300
Elliot Hosp
1 Elliot Way Manchester, NH 03103 NEW ENGLAND

Emory University Hospital (404) 712-2000
Emory Univ Hosp
1364 Clifton Rd NE Atlanta, GA 30322 SOUTHEAST

Englewood Hospital & Medical Center (201) 894-3000
Englewood Hosp & Med Ctr
350 Engle Street Englewood, NJ 07631 MID ATLANTIC

Evanston/North Shore University Health System (847) 570-2000
Evanston/North Shore Univ Hlth Sys
2650 Ridge Ave Evanston, IL 60201 MIDWEST

Fargo VA Medical Center (701) 239-3700
Fargo VA Med Ctr
2101 Elm St Fargo, ND 58102 GREAT PLAINS AND MOUNTAINS

Fletcher Allen Health Care-Medical Center Campus (802) 847-0000
Fletcher Allen Health Care- Med Ctr Campus
111 Colchester Ave Burlington, VT 05401 NEW ENGLAND

Florida Hospital - Celebration Health   (407) 764-4000
Florida Hosp Celebration Hlth
400 Celebration Pl   Celebration, FL 34747   SOUTHEAST

Forsyth Medical Center   (336) 718-5000
Forsyth Med Ctr
3333 Silas Creek Pkwy   Winston-Salem, NC 27103   SOUTHEAST

Four Winds Hospital   (914) 763-8151
Four Winds Hosp
800 Cross River Road   Katonah, NY 10536   MID ATLANTIC

Fox Chase Cancer Center   (215) 728-6900
Fox Chase Cancer Ctr
333 Cottman Avenue   Philadelphia, PA 19111   MID ATLANTIC

Franciscan St. Francis Health-Indianapolis   (317) 865-5000
Franciscan St. Francis Hlth-Indianapolis
8111 S Emerson Ave   Indianapolis, IN 46143   MIDWEST

Franklin Square Hospital   (443) 777-7000
Franklin Square Hosp
9000 Franklin Square Drive   Baltimore, MD 21237   MID ATLANTIC

Frazier Rehabilitation Institute   (502) 582-7400
Frazier Rehab Inst
220 Abraham Flexner Way   Louisville, KY 40202   SOUTHEAST

Froedtert and the Medical Center of Wisconsin   (414) 805-3666
Froedtert and Med Ctr of WI
9200 W Wisconsin Ave   Milwaukee, WI 53226   MIDWEST

George Washington University Hospital   (202) 715-4000
G Washington Univ Hosp
900 23rd St NW   Washington, DC 20037   MID ATLANTIC

Georgetown University Hospital   (202) 444-2000
Georgetown Univ Hosp
3800 Reservoir Rd NW   Washington, DC 20007   MID ATLANTIC

Glendale Memorial Hospital & Health Center   (818) 502-1900
Glendale Mem Hosp & Hlth Ctr
1420 S Central Ave   Glendale, CA 91204-2594   WEST COAST AND PACIFIC

Good Samaritan Medical Center - West Palm Beach   (561) 655-5511
Good Sam Med Ctr - W Palm Beach
1309 N Flagler Dr   West Palm Beach, FL 33401   SOUTHEAST

Grady Health System		(404) 616-1000
Grady Hlth Sys		
80 Jesse Hill Jr SE	Atlanta, GA 30303	SOUTHEAST

Greater Baltimore Medical Center		(443) 849-2000
Greater Baltimore Med Ctr		
6701 N Charles St	Baltimore, MD 21204	MID ATLANTIC

Greenwich Hospital		(203) 863-3000
Greenwich Hosp		
Five Perryridge Road	Greenwich, CT 06830	NEW ENGLAND

H Lee Moffitt Cancer Center & Research Institute		(813) 745-4673
H Lee Moffitt Cancer Ctr & Research Inst		
12902 Magnolia Drive	Tampa, FL 33612-9497	SOUTHEAST

Hackensack University Medical Center		(201) 996-2000
Hackensack Univ Med Ctr		
30 Prospect Avenue	Hackensack, NJ 07601	MID ATLANTIC

Hahnemann University Hospital		(215) 762-7000
Hahnemann Univ Hosp		
Broad & Vine St	Philadelphia, PA 19102	MID ATLANTIC

Harborview Medical Center		(206) 744-3000
Harborview Med Ctr		
325 9th Ave	Seattle, WA 98104	WEST COAST AND PACIFIC

Harper University Hospital		(313) 745-8040
Harper Univ Hosp		
3990 John R St	Detroit, MI 48201-2097	MIDWEST

Harrison Medical Center		(360) 377-3911
Harrison Med Ctr		
2520 Cherry Ave	Bremerton, WA 98310-4270	WEST COAST AND PACIFIC

Hartford Hospital		(860) 545-5000
Hartford Hosp		
80 Seymour St, Box 5037, PO Box 5037	Hartford, CT 06102-5037	NEW ENGLAND

Healthsouth Lakeshore Rehabilitation Hospital		(205) 868-2000
Healthsouth Lakeshore Rehab Hosp		
3800 Ridgeway	Birmingham, AL 35209	SOUTHEAST

Henry Ford Hospital		(313) 916-2600
Henry Ford Hosp		
2799 W Grand Blvd	Detroit, MI 48202	MIDWEST

Henry Ford West Bloomfield Hospital   (248) 661-4100
Henry Ford- W Bloomfield Hosp
6777 W Maple Rd   West Bloomfield, MI 48322   MIDWEST

Hilton Head Regional Medical Center   (843) 681-6122
Hilton Head Reg Med Ctr
25 Hospital Ctr Blvd, PO Box 21117   Hartsville, SC 29925-1117   SOUTHEAST

Hoag Memorial Hospital Presbyterian   (949) 645-8600
Hoag Meml Hosp Presby
One Hoag Drive   Newport Beach, CA 92663   WEST COAST AND PACIFIC

Holy Cross Hospital - Silver Spring   (301) 754-7000
Holy Cross Hospital - Silver Spring
1500 Forest Glen Road   Silver Spring, MD 20910   MID ATLANTIC

Hospital for Special Surgery   (212) 606-1000
Hosp For Special Surgery
535 East 70th Street   New York, NY 10021   MID ATLANTIC

Hospital of the University of Pennsylvania - UPHS   (215) 662-4000
Hosp Univ Penn - UPHS
3400 Spruce Street   Philadelphia, PA 19104   MID ATLANTIC

Howard University Hospital   (202) 865-6100
Howard Univ Hosp
2041 Georgia Ave NW   Washington, DC 20060   MID ATLANTIC

Huntsville Hospital, The   (256) 517-8020
Huntsville Hosp, The
101 Sivley Rd   Huntsville, AL 35801-4470   SOUTHEAST

Indiana University Health Goshen Hospital   (574) 533-2141
Indiana Univ Hlth Goshen Hosp
200 High Park Ave   Goshen, IN 46526   MIDWEST

Indiana University Health Methodist Hospital   (317) 962-2000
IU Health Methodist Hosp
I65 at 21st Street, Box 1367   Indianapolis, IN 46202   MIDWEST

Inova Fairfax Hospital   (703) 776-4001
Inova Fairfax Hosp
3300 Gallows Road   Falls Church, VA 22042   SOUTHEAST

Inova Fairfax Hospital for Children   (703) 204-6777
Inova Fairfax Hosp for Chldn
3300 Gallows Rd   Falls Church, VA 22042   SOUTHEAST

IU Health University Hospital   (317) 944-5000
IU Health University Hosp
550 N University Blvd   Indianapolis, IN 46202   MIDWEST

Jackson Memorial Hospital   (305) 585-1111
Jackson Meml Hosp
1611 NW 12th Ave   Miami, FL 33136   SOUTHEAST

Jackson North Medical Center   (305) 651-1100
Jackson N Med Ctr
160 NW 170 St   North Miami Beach, FL 33169   SOUTHEAST

Jewish Hospital - Kenwood - **Cincinnati**   **(513) 686**-3000
Jewish Hosp - Kenwood - Cincinnati
4777 E Galbraith Rd   **Cincinnati, OH 45236-2891**   MIDWEST

John M & Sally B Thornton Hospital
John M & Sally B Thornton **Hosp**
9300 Campus Point Drive   La Jolla, CA 92037   WEST COAST AND PACIFIC

Johns Hopkins Bayview Medical Center   (410) 550-0100
Johns Hopkins Bayview Med Ctr
4940 Eastern Avenue   Baltimore, MD 21224   MID ATLANTIC

Johns Hopkins Hospital   (410) 955-5000
Johns Hopkins Hosp
600 N Wolfe St   Baltimore, MD 21287   MID ATLANTIC

Kaiser Permanente South San Francisco Medical Center   (650) 742-2000
Kaiser Permanente S San Francisco Med Ctr
1200 El Camino Real   South San Francisco, CA 94080   WEST COAST AND PACIFIC

Kapiolani Medical Center for Women & Children   (808) 983-6000
Kapiolani Med Ctr for Women & Chldn
1319 Punahou St   Honolulu, HI 96826   WEST COAST AND PACIFIC

Kootenai Medical Center   (208) 666-2000
Kootenai Med Ctr
2003 Lincoln Way   Coeur d'Alene, ID 83814-2677   GREAT PLAINS AND MOUNTAINS

Kosair Children's Hospital   (502) 629-6000
Kosair Chldn's Hosp
231 E Chestnut St   Louisville, KY 40202   SOUTHEAST

LAC & USC Medical Center   (323) 266-2622
LAC & USC Med Ctr
1200 N State St   Los Angeles, CA 90033-4525   WEST COAST AND PACIFIC

LAC - Harbor - UCLA Medical Center   (310) 222-2345
LAC - Harbor - UCLA Med Ctr
1000 W Carson St,   Torrance, CA 90509-2059   WEST COAST AND PACIFIC

Lahey Clinic   (781) 744-5100
Lahey Clin
41 Mall Road   Burlington, MA 01805   NEW ENGLAND

Lakeland Regional Medical Center   (863) 687-1100
Lakeland Regl Med Ctr
1324 Lakeland Hills Blvd   Lakeland, FL 33805   SOUTHEAST

Lankenau Hospital   (610) 645-2000
Lankenau Hosp
100 Lancaster Ave   Wynnewood, PA 19096-3498   MID ATLANTIC

Lawrence & Memorial Hospital   (860) 442-0711
Lawrence & Meml Hosp
365 Montauk Ave   New London, CT 06320   NEW ENGLAND

LDS Hospital   (801) 408-1100
LDS Hosp
8th Ave & C St   Salt Lake City, UT 84143   GREAT PLAINS AND MOUNTAINS

Le Bonheur Children's Medical Center   (901) 287-5437
Le Bonheur Chldns Med Ctr
50 N Dunlap   Memphis, TN 38103-2893   SOUTHEAST

Lee Memorial Health Systems   (239) 334-5314
Lee Memorial Hlth Systems
2776 Cleveland Ave   Fort Myers, FL 33901   SOUTHEAST

Lenox Hill Hospital   (212) 434-2000
Lenox Hill Hosp
100 East 77th Street   New York, NY 10021   MID ATLANTIC

Lenox Hill Hospital (Manhattan Eye, Ear & Throat Hosp)   (212) 838-9200
Lenox Hill Hosp (Manh Eye, Ear & Throat Hosp)
210 East 64th Street   New York, NY 10021   MID ATLANTIC

Loma Linda University Medical Center   (909) 558-4000
Loma Linda Univ Med Ctr
11234 Anderson St   Loma Linda, CA 92354   WEST COAST AND PACIFIC

Long Beach Memorial Medical Center   (562) 933-2000
Long Beach Meml Med Ctr
2801 Atlantic Ave   Long Beach, CA 90801   WEST COAST AND PACIFIC

Long Island Jewish Medical Center (718) 470-7000
Long Island Jewish Med Ctr
270-05 76th Avenue   New Hyde Park, NY 11040   MID ATLANTIC

Louisiana State University Hospital (318) 675-4239
Louisiana State Univ Hosp
1501 Kings Highway P.O. Box 33932   Shreveport, LA 71130   SOUTHWEST

Loyola University Medical Center (708) 216-9000
Loyola Univ Med Ctr
2160 S 1st Ave   Maywood, IL 60153   MIDWEST

LSU Interim Public Hospital (504) 903-3000
LSU Interim Public Hosp
2021 Perdido St   New Orleans, LA 70112   SOUTHWEST

Lucile Packard Children's Hospital (650) 497-8000
Lucile Packard Chldn's Hosp
725 Welch Rd   Palo Alto, CA 94304   WEST COAST AND PACIFIC

Magee-Womens Hospital of UPMC (412) 641-1000
Magee-Womens Hosp - UPMC
300 Halket Street   Pittsburgh, PA 15213   MID ATLANTIC

Maimonides Medical Center (718) 283-6000
Maimonides Med Ctr
4802 Tenth Avenue   Brooklyn, NY 11219   MID ATLANTIC

Maine Medical Center (207) 662-0111
Maine Med Ctr
22 Bramhall St   Portland, ME 04102   NEW ENGLAND

Marin General Hospital (415) 925-7000
Marin Genl Hosp
250 Bon Air Rd   Greenbrae, CA 94904   WEST COAST AND PACIFIC

Massachusetts Eye and Ear Infirmary (617) 523-7900
Mass Eye & Ear Infirmary
243 Charles Street   Boston, MA 02114   NEW ENGLAND

Massachusetts General Hospital (617) 726-2000
Mass Genl Hosp
55 Fruit St   Boston, MA 02114   NEW ENGLAND

Mattel Children's Hospital at UCLA (310) 825-9111
Mattel Chldns Hosp at UCLA
10833 Le Conte Ave   Los Angeles, CA 90095-1752 WEST COAST AND PACIFIC

Mayo Clinic - Jacksonville, FL   (904) 953-2000
Mayo - Jacksonville
4500 San Pablo Road   Jacksonville, FL 32224   SOUTHEAST

Mayo Clinic - Phoenix   (480) 515-6296
Mayo Clinic - Phoenix
5777 E Mayo Blvd   Phoenix, AZ 85054   SOUTHWEST

Mayo Clinic - Rochester, MN   (507) 284-2511
Mayo Med Ctr & Clin - Rochester
200 First St SW   Rochester, MN 55905   MIDWEST

Mayo Clinic - Scottsdale   (480) 301-8000
Mayo Clinic - Scottsdale
13400 E Shea Blvd   Scottsdale, AZ 85259   SOUTHWEST

McLaren Regional Medical Center   (810) 342-2000
McLaren Reg Med Ctr
401 S. Ballenger Highway   Flint, MI 48532   MIDWEST

MD Anderson Cancer Center-Orlando   (407) 648-3800
MD Anderson Cancer Ctr-Orlando
1400 S Orange Ave   Orlando, FL 32806   SOUTHEAST

Medical City Dallas Hospital   (972) 566-7000
Med City Dallas Hosp
7777 Forest Ln   Dallas, TX 75230-2594   SOUTHWEST

Medical College of Georgia Hospital & Clinic (MCG Health Inc)   (706) 721-0211
Med Coll of GA Hosp and Clin (MCG Health Inc)
1120 15th Street   Augusta, GA 30912   SOUTHEAST

Medical College of Virginia Hospitals   (804) 828-9000
Med Coll of VA Hosp
1250 E Marshall St, Box 980510   Richmond, VA 23219   SOUTHEAST

Medical University of South Carolina Medical Center   (843) 792-2300
MUSC Med Ctr
171 Ashley Ave   Charleston, SC 29425   SOUTHEAST

Memorial Health University Medical Center - Savannah   (912) 350-8000
Meml Hlth Univ Med Ctr - Savannah
4700 Waters Ave   Savannah, GA 31404   SOUTHEAST

Memorial Hermann Hospital - Texas Medical Center   (713) 704-4000
Meml Hermann Hosp - Texas Med Ctr
6411 Fannin   Houston, TX 77030   SOUTHWEST

Memorial Regional Hospital (954) 987-2000
Meml Regl Hosp
3501 Johnson Street   Hollywood, FL 33021   SOUTHEAST

Memorial Sloan-Kettering Cancer Center (212) 639-2000
Meml Sloan-Kettering Cancer Ctr
1275 York Avenue   New York, NY 10021   MID ATLANTIC

Methodist Hospital System (713) 790-3311
Methodist Hosp - Houston
6565 Fannin St   Houston, TX 77030   SOUTHWEST

Methodist Hospital-Omaha (402) 354-4000
Methodist Hosp - Omaha
8303 Dodge St   Omaha, NE 68114   GREAT PLAINS AND MOUNTAINS

Methodist Hospital-San Antonio (210) 575-4000
Methodist Hosp-San Antonio
7700 Floyd Curl Dr   San Antonio, TX 78229   SOUTHWEST

Methodist University Hospital - Memphis (901) 516-7000
Methodist Univ Hosp - Memphis
1265 Union Ave   Memphis, TN 38104   SOUTHEAST

MetroHealth Medical Center (216) 778-7800
MetroHealth Med Ctr
2500 MetroHealth Drive   Cleveland, OH 44109-1998   MIDWEST

Miami Children's Hospital (305) 666-6511
Miami Children's Hosp
3100 SW 62nd Ave   Miami, FL 33155   SOUTHEAST

Miriam Hospital (401) 793-2500
Miriam Hosp
164 Summit Avenue   Providence, RI 02906-2894   NEW ENGLAND

Mobile Infirmary Medical Center (334) 431-2400
Mobile Infirmary Med Ctr
5 Mobile Infirmary Circle   Mobile, AL 36607-3513   SOUTHEAST

Montefiore Medical Center - Henry and Lucy Moses Division (718) 920-4321
Montefiore Med Ctr - Div. Moses
111 East 210 Street   Bronx, NY 10467   MID ATLANTIC

Montefiore Medical Center - Jack D. Weiler Division (718) 904-2000
Montefiore Med Ctr - Div. Weiler
1825 Eastchester Road   Bronx, NY 10461   MID ATLANTIC

Morristown Medical Center		(973) 971-5000
Morristown Med Ctr		
100 Madison Avenue	Morristown, NJ 07960-6095	MID ATLANTIC
Mott Children's Hospital		(734) 936-4000
Mott Chldns Hosp		
1500 E Medical Center Dr	Ann Arbor, MI 48109	MIDWEST
Mount Clemens Regional Medical Center		(586) 493-8000
Mount Clemens Regional Med Ctr		
1000 Harrington Blvd	Mount Clemens, MI 48043	MIDWEST
Mount Sinai Medical Center		(212) 241-6500
Mount Sinai Med Ctr		
One Gustave L. Levy Pl	New York, NY 10029	MID ATLANTIC
Mount Sinai Medical Center - Miami		(305) 674-2121
Mount Sinai Med Ctr - Miami		
4300 Alton Rd	Miami Beach, FL 33140	SOUTHEAST
Mountainview Hospital - Las Vegas		(702) 255-5074
Mountainview Hosp - Las Vegas		
3100 N Tenaya Way	Las Vegas, NV 89128	WEST COAST AND PACIFIC
National Institutes of Health - Clinical Center		(301) 496-4000
Natl Inst of Hlth - Clin Ctr		
10 Center Drive	Bethesda, MD 20892-0001	MID ATLANTIC
National Jewish Medical & Research Center		(303) 388-4461
Natl Jewish Med & Rsch Ctr		
1400 Jackson St	Denver, CO 80206-2762	GREAT PLAINS AND MOUNTAINS
Nationwide Children's Hospital		(614) 722-2000
Nationwide Chldn's Hosp		
700 Children's Drive	Columbus, OH 43205	MIDWEST
Nebraska Medical Center		(402) 559-2000
Nebraska Med Ctr		
4350 Dewey Ave	Omaha, NE 68198	GREAT PLAINS AND MOUNTAINS
Nebraska Methodist Hospital		(402) 354-4000
Nebraska Meth Hosp		
8303 Dodge St	Omaha, NE 68114	GREAT PLAINS AND MOUNTAINS
New York Eye & Ear Infirmary		(212) 979-4000
New York Eye & Ear Infirm		
310 East 14th Street	New York, NY 10003	MID ATLANTIC

NewYork-Presbyterian Hospital/Columbia   (212) 305-2500
NY-Presby Hosp/Columbia
622 W 168th St   New York, NY 10032   MID ATLANTIC

NewYork-Presbyterian Hospital/Weill Cornell   (212) 746-5454
NY-Presby Hosp/Weill Cornell
525 E 68th St   New York, NY 10021   MID ATLANTIC

NewYork-Presbyterian/Morgan Stanley Children's Hospital   (212) 305-2500
NYPresby-Morgan Stanley Children's Hosp
622 W 168th St   New York, NY 10032   MID ATLANTIC

North Carolina Memorial Hospital - UNC   (919) 966-4131
NC Memorial Hosp - UNC
101 Manning Drive, Box 7600   Chapel Hill, NC 27514   SOUTHEAST

North Shore University Hospital   (516) 562-0100
N Shore Univ Hosp
300 Community Dr   Manhasset, NY 11030   MID ATLANTIC

Northside Hospital - Atlanta   (404) 851-8000
Northside Hosp
1000 Johnson Ferry Rd NE   Atlanta, GA 30342   SOUTHEAST

Northwest Hospital - Seattle   (206) 364-0500
Northwest Hosp - Seattle
1550 N 115th St   Seattle, WA 98133-0806   WEST COAST AND PACIFIC

Northwestern Memorial Hospital   (312) 926-2000
Northwestern Meml Hosp
251 E Huron St   Chicago, IL 60611   MIDWEST

NYU Hospital for Joint Diseases   (212) 598-6000
NYU Hosp For Joint Diseases
301 East 17th Street   New York, NY 10003   MID ATLANTIC

NYU Langone Medical Center   (212) 263-7300
NYU Langone Med Ctr
550 First Avenue   New York, NY 10016   MID ATLANTIC

Ochsner Baptist Medical Center   (504) 899-9311
Ochsner Baptist Med Ctr
2700 Napoleon Ave   New Orleans, LA 70115   SOUTHWEST

Ochsner Medical Center-New Orleans   (504) 842-3000
Ochsner Med Ctr-New Orleans
1514 Jefferson Hwy   New Orleans, LA 70121   SOUTHWEST

Ohio State University Medical Center		(614) 293-8000
Ohio St Univ Med Ctr		
410 W 10th Avenue	Columbus, OH 43210	MIDWEST

Olathe Medical Center		(913) 791-4200
Olathe Med Ctr		
20333 W 151st St	Olathe, KS 66061-5352	GREAT PLAINS AND MOUNTAINS

Oregon Health & Science University		(503) 494-8311
OR Hlth & Sci Univ		
3181 SW Sam Jackson Park Rd	Portland, OR 97239-3098	WEST COAST AND PACIFIC

OU Medical Center		(405) 271-4700
OU Med Ctr		
1200 Everett Dr, PO Box 26307	Oklahoma City, OK 73104-5098	SOUTHWEST

Our Lady of the Lake Regional Medical Center		(225) 765-6565
Our Lady of the Lake Regl Med Ctr		
5000 Hennessy Blvd	Baton Rouge, LA 70808-4398	SOUTHWEST

Overland Park Regional Medical Center		(913) 541-5000
Overland Pk Regl Med Ctr		
10500 Quivira Rd	Overland Park, KS 66215	GREAT PLAINS AND MOUNTAINS

Palmetto Health Richland Memorial Hospital		(803) 434-7000
Palmetto Health Richland Mem Hosp		
5 Richland Medical Park Drive	Columbia, SC 29203	SOUTHEAST

Penn Presbyterian Medical Center - UPHS		(215) 662-8000
Penn Presby Med Ctr - UPHS		
51 N 39th St	Philadelphia, PA 19104	MID ATLANTIC

Penn State Children's Hospital		(717) 531-8521
Penn State Chldns Hosp		
500 University Dr	Hershey, PA 17033	MID ATLANTIC

Penn State Milton S. Hershey Medical Center		(717) 531-8521
Penn State Milton S Hershey Med Ctr		
500 University Drive	Hershey, PA 17033-0850	MID ATLANTIC

Pennsylvania Hospital		(215) 829-3000
Pennsylvania Hosp		
800 Spruce St, Ste 240	Philadelphia, PA 19107	MID ATLANTIC

Phoenix Baptist Hospital & Medical Center		(602) 249-0212
Phoenix Baptist Hosp & Med Ctr		
2000 West Bethany Home Rd	Phoenix, AZ 85015-2184	SOUTHWEST

Physicians Regional Healthcare System-Pine Ridge   (239) 348-4000
Physicians Regl Hlthcare Med Ctr-Pine Ridge
6101 Pine Ridge Rd   Naples, FL 34119   SOUTHEAST

Porter Adventist Hospital   (303) 778-1955
Porter Adventist Hosp
2525 S Downing St   Denver, CO 80210   GREAT PLAINS AND MOUNTAINS

Presbyterian - St Luke's Medical Center   (303) 839-6000
Presby - St Luke's Med Ctr
1719 E 19th Ave   Denver, CO 80218   GREAT PLAINS AND MOUNTAINS

Primary Children's Medical Center   (801) 588-2000
Primary Children's Med Ctr
100 N Medical Drive   Salt Lake City, UT 84113-1100   GREAT PLAINS AND MOUNTAINS

Providence Hospital - Southfield   (248) 424-3000
Providence Hosp - Southfield
16001 W Nine Mile Rd   Southfield, MI 48075   MIDWEST

Providence Portland Medical Center   (503) 215-1111
Providence Portland Med Ctr
4805 NE Glisan   Portland, OR 97213-2967   WEST COAST AND PACIFIC

Providence Saint Joseph Medical Center   (818) 843-5111
Providence St Joseph Med Ctr
501 S Buena Vista St   Burbank, CA 91505   WEST COAST AND PACIFIC

Queen's Medical Center - Honolulu   (808) 538-9011
Queen's Med Ctr - Honolulu
1301 Punchbowl Street   Honolulu, HI 96813   WEST COAST AND PACIFIC

Rady Children's Hospital - San Diego   (858) 576-1700
Rady Children's Hosp - San Diego
3020 Children's Way   San Diego, CA 92123   WEST COAST AND PACIFIC

Rehabilitation Institute of Chicago   (312) 238-1000
Rehab Inst of Chicago
345 E. Superior Street   Chicago, IL 60611   MIDWEST

Resurrection Health Care Saint Joseph Hospital   (773) 665-3000
Resurrection Hlth Care St Joseph Hosp
2900 N Lake Shore Dr   Chicago, IL 60657   MIDWEST

Rhode Island Hospital   (401) 444-4000
Rhode Island Hosp
593 Eddy Street   Providence, RI 02903-4923   NEW ENGLAND

Riley Hospital for Children		(317) 274-5000
Riley Hosp for Children		
702 Barnhill Drive	Indianapolis, IN 46202	MIDWEST
Riverview Medical Center		(732) 741-2700
Riverview Med Ctr		
1 Riverview Plaza	Red Bank, NJ 07701	MID ATLANTIC
Robert Wood Johnson University Hospital - New Brunswick		(732) 828-3000
Robert Wood Johnson Univ Hosp - New Brunswick		
1 Robert Wood Johnson Pl	New Brunswick, NJ 08903	MID ATLANTIC
Rochester Methodist Hospital		(507) 284-2511
Rochester Methodist Hosp		
201 W Center St	Rochester, MN 55905-3003	MIDWEST
Roper Hospital		(843) 724-2000
Roper Hosp		
316 Calhoun St	Charleston, SC 29401	SOUTHEAST
Roswell Park Cancer Institute		(716) 845-2300
Roswell Park Cancer Inst		
Elm and Carlton Streets	Buffalo, NY 14263	MID ATLANTIC
Ruby Memorial - WVU Hospital		(304) 598-4000
Ruby Memorial - WVU Hosp		
1 Medical Center Drive	Morgantown, WV 26506	MID ATLANTIC
Rush University Medical Center		(312) 942-5000
Rush Univ Med Ctr		
1653 W Congress Pkwy	Chicago, IL 60612-3833	MIDWEST
Sacred Heart Medical Center		(541) 686-7300
Sacred Heart Med Ctr		
1255 Hilyard St	Eugene, OR 97440-3700	WEST COAST AND PACIFIC
Saint Barnabas Medical Center		(973) 322-5000
Saint Barnabas Med Ctr		
94 Old Short Hills Rd	Livingston, NJ 07039-5672	MID ATLANTIC
Saint Francis Hospital - Memphis		(901) 765-1000
St. Francis Hosp - Memphis		
5959 Park Ave	Memphis, TN 38119	SOUTHEAST
Saint John's Health Center		(310) 829-5511
St. John's Hlth Ctr, Santa Monica		
1328 22nd St	Santa Monica, CA 90404	WEST COAST AND PACIFIC

Saint Joseph's Hospital - Atlanta   (404) 851-7001
St. Joseph's Hosp - Atlanta
5665 Peachtree Dunwoody Rd NE   Atlanta, GA 30342   SOUTHEAST

Salt Lake Regional Medical Center   (801) 350-4111
Salt Lake Regional Med Ctr
1050 E South Temple   Salt Lake City, UT 84102   GREAT PLAINS AND MOUNTAINS

San Diego Hospice   (619) 688-1600
San Diego Hospice
4311 3rd Ave   San Diego, CA 92103-7499   WEST COAST AND PACIFIC

San Francisco General Hospital   (415) 206-8000
San Francisco Genl Hosp
1001 Potrero Avenue   San Francisco, CA 94110   WEST COAST AND PACIFIC

Sanford Medical Center Fargo   (701) 234-2000
Sanford Med Ctr Fargo
801 Broadway Drive, PO Box MC   Fargo, ND 58122   GREAT PLAINS AND MOUNTAINS

Santa Clara Valley Medical Center   (408) 885-5000
Santa Clara Vly Med Ctr
751 S Bascom Ave   San Jose, CA 95128   WEST COAST AND PACIFIC

Santa Monica - UCLA Medical Center and Orthopaedic Hospital   (310) 319-4000
Santa Monica - UCLA Med Ctr & Ortho Hosp
1250 16th St   Santa Monica, CA 90404   WEST COAST AND PACIFIC

Sarasota Memorial Hospital   (941) 917-9000
Sarasota Meml Hosp
1700 S Tamiami Trail   Sarasota, FL 34239   SOUTHEAST

Scott & White Memorial Hospital   (254) 724-2111
Scott & White Mem Hosp
2401 S 31st St   Temple, TX 76508-0001   SOUTHWEST

Scottsdale Healthcare - Shea   (480) 860-3000
Scottsdale Hlthcare - Shea
9000 E Shea Blvd   Scottsdale, AZ 85258-4514   SOUTHWEST

Scripps Green Hospital   (858) 455-9100
Scripps Green Hosp
10666 N Torrey Pines Rd   La Jolla, CA 92037   WEST COAST AND PACIFIC

Scripps Memorial Hospital - La Jolla   (858) 457-4123
Scripps Meml Hosp - La Jolla
9888 Genesee Ave   La Jolla, CA 92037   WEST COAST AND PACIFIC

Seattle Children's Hospital		(206) 987-2000
Seattle Chldns Hosp		
4800 Sand Point Way NE	Seattle, WA 98105	WEST COAST AND PACIFIC
Shands at University of Florida		(352) 265-8000
Shands at Univ of FL		
1600 SW Archer Rd	Gainesville, FL 32610	SOUTHEAST
Shands Jacksonville		(904) 244-0411
Shands Jacksonville		
655 W 8th St	Jacksonville, FL 32209	SOUTHEAST
Sherman Hospital		(847) 742-9800
Sherman Hosp		
934 Center St	Elgin, IL 60120	MIDWEST
Sibley Memorial Hospital		(202) 537-4000
Sibley Mem Hosp		
5255 Loughboro Road NW	Washington, DC 20016	MID ATLANTIC
Sinai Hospital - Baltimore		(410) 601-9000
Sinai Hosp - Baltimore		
2401 W Belvedere Ave	Baltimore, MD 21215	MID ATLANTIC
Southern Arizona VA Health Care System - Tucson		(520) 792-1450
Southern AZ VA Health Care Sys - Tucson		
3601 S 6th Avenue	Tucson, AZ 85723	SOUTHWEST
Southern New Hampshire Medical Center		(603) 577-2000
Southern NH Med Ctr		
8 Prospect St	Nashua, NH 03061	NEW ENGLAND
Spectrum Health - Blodgett Campus		(616) 774-7444
Spectrum Hlth Blodgett Campus		
1840 Wealthy St SE	Grand Rapids, MI 49506	MIDWEST
St. Anthony Hospital - Oklahoma City		(405) 272-7000
St. Anthony Hosp -Oklahoma City		
1000 N Lee St	Oklahoma City, OK 73102	SOUTHWEST
St. Anthony's Hospital - St Petersburg		(727) 893-6814
St. Anthony's Hosp - St Petersburg		
1200 7th Avenue North	St Petersburg, FL 33705	SOUTHEAST
St. Christopher's Hospital for Children		(215) 427-5000
St. Christopher's Hosp for Chldn		
Erie Ave at Front St	Philadelphia, PA 19134	MID ATLANTIC

St. John's Hospital - Springfield (217) 544-6464
St. John's Hosp - Springfield
800 E Carpenter St — Springfield, IL 62769 — MIDWEST

St. Joseph Hospital (360) 734-5400
St. Joseph Hosp - Bellingham
2901 Squalicum Pkwy — Bellingham, WA 98225-1898 — WEST COAST AND PACIFIC

St. Joseph Hospital & Trauma Center (603) 883-3414
St. Joseph Hosp & Trauma Ctr
172 Kinsley St — Nashua, NH 03060 — NEW ENGLAND

St. Joseph Medical Center (410) 337-1000
St. Joseph Med Ctr
7601 Osler Drive — Baltimore, MD 21208 — MID ATLANTIC

St. Joseph's Children's Hospital (813) 554-8500
St. Josephs Chldns Hosp
3001 W Dr Martin Luther King Jr Blvd Tampa, FL 33607 — SOUTHEAST

St. Joseph's Hospital & Medical Center - Phoenix (602) 406-3000
St. Joseph's Hosp & Med Ctr - Phoenix
350 W Thomas Rd — Phoenix, AZ 85013-4496 — SOUTHWEST

St. Joseph's Hospital - Orange (714) 633-9111
St. Joseph's Hosp - Orange
1100 West Stewart Drive — Orange, CA 92868 — WEST COAST AND PACIFIC

St. Joseph's Hospital - Tucson (520) 296-3211
St. Joseph's Hosp - Tucson
350 N Wilmot Rd — Tucson, AZ 85711 — SOUTHWEST

St. Jude Children's Research Hospital (901) 495-3300
St. Jude Children's Research Hosp
262 Danny Thomas Pl — Memphis, TN 38105 — SOUTHEAST

St. Louis Children's Hospital (314) 454-6000
St. Louis Chldns Hosp
One Children's Pl — St Louis, MO 63110 — MIDWEST

St. Louis University Hospital (314) 577-8000
St. Louis Univ Hosp
3635 Vista at Grand Blvd — St Louis, MO 63110 — MIDWEST

St. Luke's - Roosevelt Hospital Center - Roosevelt Division (212) 523-4000
St. Luke's - Roosevelt Hosp Ctr - Roosevelt Div
1000 Tenth Avenue — New York, NY 10019 — MID ATLANTIC

St. Luke's - Roosevelt Hospital Center - St Luke's Hospital   (212) 523-4000
St. Luke's - Roosevelt Hosp Ctr - St Luke's Hosp
1111 Amsterdam Ave   New York, NY 10025   MID ATLANTIC

St. Luke's Boise Medical Center   (208) 381-2222
St. Luke's Boise Med Ctr
190 E Bannock St   Boise, ID 83712   GREAT PLAINS AND MOUNTAINS

St. Luke's Episcopal Hospital-Houston   (832) 355-1000
St. Luke's Episcopal Hosp-Houston
6720 Bertner Avenue, PO Box 20269   Houston, TX 77030   SOUTHWEST

St. Luke's Hospital - Chesterfield, MO   (314) 434-1500
St. Luke's Hosp - Chesterfield, MO
232 S Woods Mill Rd   Chesterfield, MO 63017   MIDWEST

St. Mark's Hospital - Salt Lake City   (801) 268-7111
St. Mark's Hosp - Salt Lake City
1200 E. 3900 S   Salt Lake City, UT 84124   GREAT PLAINS AND MOUNTAINS

St. Mary's Hospital - Rochester, MN (Mayo Clinic)   (507) 255-5123
St. Mary's Hosp - Rochester MN (Mayo)
1216 2nd St SW   Rochester, MN 55902   MIDWEST

St. Mary's Medical Center - Huntington   (304) 526-1234
St. Mary's Med Ctr - Huntington
2900 First Ave   Huntington, WV 25702-1272   MID ATLANTIC

St. Mary's Medical Center - West Palm Beach   (561) 844-6300
St. Mary's Med Ctr - W Palm Bch
901 45th St   West Palm Beach, FL 33407   SOUTHEAST

St. Patrick Hospital & Health Sciences Center   (406) 543-7271
St. Patrick Hospital - Missoula
500 W Broadway   Missoula, MT 59802   GREAT PLAINS AND MOUNTAINS

St. Peter's University Hospital   (732) 745-8600
St. Peter's Univ Hosp
254 Easton Ave   New Brunswick, NJ 08901-1780   MID ATLANTIC

St. Rose Dominican Hospital - San Martin Campus   (702) 492-8000
St. Rose Dom Hosp-San Martin
8280 W Warm Springs Rd   Las Vegas, NV 89113   WEST COAST AND PACIFIC

St. Vincent Carmel Hospital   (317) 573-7000
St. Vincent Carmel Hosp
13500 N Meridian St   Carmel, IN 46032-1496   MIDWEST

St. Vincent Indianapolis Hospital   (317) 338-2345
St. Vincent Indianapolis Hosp
2001 W 86th St   Indianapolis, IN 46260-1991   MIDWEST

St. Vincent's Medical Center - Jacksonville   (904) 308-7300
St. Vincent's Med Ctr - Jacksonville
1800 Barrs St   Jacksonville, FL 32204   SOUTHEAST

Stanford Universtiy Hospital & Clinics   (650) 723-4000
Stanford Univ Hosp & Clinics
300 Pasteur Dr   Stanford, CA 94305   WEST COAST AND PACIFIC

Steven and Alexandra Cohen Children's Medical Center of New York   (718) 470-3000
Steven & Alexandra Cohen Chldn's Med Ctr of NY
269-01 76th Ave   New Hyde Park, NY 11040   MID ATLANTIC

Stony Brook University Medical Center   (631) 444-4000
Stony Brook Univ Med Ctr
101 Nicolls Rd   Stony Brook, NY 11794-8410   MID ATLANTIC

Sunrise Hospital & Medical Center   (702) 731-8000
Sunrise Hosp & Med Ctr
3186 Maryland Pkwy   Las Vegas, NV 89109   WEST COAST AND PACIFIC

SUNY Downstate Medical Center (University Hospital of Brooklyn)   (718) 270-1000
SUNY Downstate Med Ctr
445 Lenox Rd   Brooklyn, NY 11203   MID ATLANTIC

SUNY Upstate Medical University Hospital   (315) 464-5540
SUNY Upstate Med Univ Hosp
750 E Adams Street   Syracuse, NY 13210   MID ATLANTIC

Swedish Medical Center-First Hill Campus - Seattle   (206) 386-6000
Swedish Med Ctr-First Hill-Seattle
747 Broadway   Seattle, WA 98122   WEST COAST AND PACIFIC

Tampa General Hospital   (813) 844-7000
Tampa Genl Hosp
1 Tampa General Cir, PO Box 1289   Tampa, FL 33601   SOUTHEAST

Temple University Hospital   (215) 707-2000
Temple Univ Hosp
3401 N Broad St   Philadelphia, PA 19140-5189   MID ATLANTIC

Tennessee Valley Healthcare System - Nashville   (615) 327-4751
TN Valley Healthcare Sys-Nashville
1310 24th Ave S   Nashville, TN 37212   SOUTHEAST

Texas Children's Hospital   (832) 824-1000
Texas Chldns Hosp
6621 Fannin St   Houston, TX 77030   SOUTHWEST

Texas Health Presbyterian Hospital Dallas   (214) 345-6789
TX Hlth Presby Hosp Dallas
8200 Walnut Hill Ln   Dallas, TX 75231   SOUTHWEST

Thomas Jefferson University Hospital   (215) 955-6000
Thomas Jefferson Univ Hosp
111 S 11th St   Philadelphia, PA 19107   MID ATLANTIC

Tucson Medical Center   (520) 327-5461
Tucson Med Ctr
5301 E Grant Rd   Tucson, AZ 85733-2195   SOUTHWEST

Tufts Medical Center   (617) 636-5000
Tufts Med Ctr
750 Washington St   Boston, MA 02111   NEW ENGLAND

UCLA Ronald Reagan Medical Center   (310) 267-8000
UCLA Ronald Reagan Med Ctr
757 Westwood Plaza   Los Angeles, CA 90095   WEST COAST AND PACIFIC

UCSD Medical Center-Hillcrest   (619) 543-6222
UCSD Med Ctr-Hillcrest
200 W Arbor   San Diego, CA 92103   WEST COAST AND PACIFIC

UCSF - Mount Zion Medical Center   (415) 567-6600
UCSF - Mt Zion Med Ctr
1600 Divisadero St   San Francisco, CA 94115   WEST COAST AND PACIFIC

UCSF Medical Center   (415) 476-1000
UCSF Med Ctr
505 Parnassus Ave   San Francisco, CA 94143   WEST COAST AND PACIFIC

UMass Memorial Medical Center   (508) 334-1000
UMass Memorial Med Ctr
55 Lake Ave N   Worcester, MA 01655   NEW ENGLAND

Union Memorial Hospital-Baltimore   (410) 554-2000
Union Meml Hosp-Baltimore
201 E University Pkwy   Baltimore, MD 21218   MID ATLANTIC

University Health System-San Antonio   (210) 358-4000
Univ Hlth Syst-San Antonio
4502 Medical Dr   San Antonio, TX 78229   SOUTHWEST

University Hospital - Cincinnati Univ Hosp - Cincinnati 234 Goodman St	Cincinnati, OH 45219	(513) 584-1000 MIDWEST
University Hospital - New Mexico Univ Hosp - New Mexico 2211 Lomas Blvd NE	Albuquerque, NM 87106	(505) 272-2111 SOUTHWEST
University Hospital of Brooklyn at Long Island College Hospital Univ Hosp of Bklyn at Long Island Coll Hosp 339 Hicks Street	Brooklyn, NY 11201	(718) 780-1000 MID ATLANTIC
University Hospital-UMDNJ-Newark Univ Hosp-UMDNJ—Newark 150 Bergen St	Newark, NJ 07103-2406	(973) 972-4300 MID ATLANTIC
University Hospitals Case Medical Center Univ Hosps Case Med Ctr 11100 Euclid Ave	Cleveland, OH 44106	(216) 844-8447 MIDWEST
University Hospitals Rainbow Babies & Children's Hospital UH Rainbow Babies & Chldns Hosp 11100 Euclid Ave	Cleveland, OH 44106	(216) 844-1000 MIDWEST
University Medical Center of Southern Nevada - Las Vegas Univ Med Ctr - Las Vegas 1800 W Charleston Blvd	Las Vegas, NV 89102	(702) 383-2000 WEST COAST AND PACIFIC
University Medical Center- Tucson Univ Med Ctr - Tucson 1501 N Campbell Ave	Tucson, AZ 85724-5128	(520) 694-0111 SOUTHWEST
University Medical Center-Lubbock Univ Med Ctr-Lubbock 602 Indiana Ave	Lubbock, TX 79408	(806) 775-8200 SOUTHWEST
University of Alabama Hospital at Birmingham Univ of Ala Hosp at Birmingham 1802 6th Ave S	Birmingham, AL 35249-6544	(205) 934-4011 SOUTHEAST
University of Arkansas for Medical Sciences Medical Center UAMS Med Ctr 4301 W Markham St	Little Rock, AR 72205	(501) 686-7000 SOUTHWEST
University of California - Davis Medical Center UC Davis Med Ctr 2315 Stockton Blvd	Sacramento, CA 95817	(916) 734-2011 WEST COAST AND PACIFIC

University of California - Irvine Medical Center
UC Irvine Med Ctr
101 The City Dr   Orange, CA 92868

(714) 456-7890

WEST COAST AND PACIFIC

University of Chicago Comer Children's Hospital
Univ Chicago-Comer Chldn's Hosp
5721 S Maryland Ave   Chicago, IL 60637

(773) 702-1000

MIDWEST

University of Chicago Medical Center
Univ of Chicago Med Ctr
5841 S Maryland Ave   Chicago, IL 60637

(773) 702-1000

MIDWEST

University of Colorado Hospital-Anschutz Inpatient Pavilion
Univ of CO Hosp - Anschutz Inpatient Pav
12605 E 16th Ave   Aurora, CO 80045

(720) 848-4011

GREAT PLAINS AND MOUNTAINS

University of Connecticut Health Center - John Dempsey Hospital
Univ of Conn Hlth Ctr, John Dempsey Hosp
263 Farmington Ave   Farmington, CT 06030

(860) 679-2000

NEW ENGLAND

University of Illinois Medical Center at Chicago
Univ of IL Med Ctr at Chicago
1740 W Taylor St, Ste 1400   Chicago, IL 60612

(312) 355-4000

MIDWEST

University of Iowa Hospitals and Clinics
Univ Iowa Hosp & Clinics
200 Hawkins Drive   Iowa City, IA 52242

(319) 356-1616

MIDWEST

University of Kansas Hospital
Univ of Kansas Hosp
3901 Rainbow Blvd   Kansas City, KS 66160

(913) 588-5000

GREAT PLAINS AND MOUNTAINS

University of Kentucky Albert B. Chandler Hospital
Univ of Kentucky Albert B. Chandler Hosp
800 Rose Street   Lexington, KY 40536

(859) 323-5000

SOUTHEAST

University of Louisville Hospital
Univ of Louisville Hosp
530 S Jackson St   Louisville, KY 40202

(502) 562-3000

SOUTHEAST

University of Maryland Medical Center
Univ of MD Med Ctr
22 S Greene St   Baltimore, MD 21201

(410) 328-8667

MID ATLANTIC

University of Miami Hosp & Clinics/Sylvester Comprehensive Cancer Cntr
Univ of Miami Hosp & Clins/Sylvester Comp Canc Ctr
1475 NW 12th Ave   Miami, FL 33136

(305) 243-1000

SOUTHEAST

University of Miami Hospital   (305) 325-5511
Univ of Miami Hosp
1400 NW 12 Ave   Miami, FL 33136   SOUTHEAST

University of Michigan Hospital   (734) 936-4000
Univ of Michigan Hosp
1500 E Medical Center Dr   Ann Arbor, MI 48109   MIDWEST

University of Mississippi Medical Center   (601) 984-1000
Univ Mississippi Med Ctr
2500 N State St   Jackson, MS 39216   SOUTHEAST

University of Missouri Hospital   (573) 882-4141
Univ of Missouri Hosp
1 Hospital Dr   Columbia, MO 65212   MIDWEST

University of Rochester Strong Memorial Hospital   (585) 275-2100
Univ of Rochester Strong Meml Hosp
601 Elmwood Ave   Rochester, NY 14642   MID ATLANTIC

University of South Alabama Medical Center   (251) 471-7000
Univ of S AL Med Ctr
2451 Fillingim St   Mobile, AL 36617   SOUTHEAST

University of Tennesee Medical Center   (865) 305-9000
Univ of Tennesee Med Ctr
1924 Alcoa Hwy   Knoxville, TN 37920   SOUTHEAST

University of Texas MD Anderson Cancer Center   (713) 792-2121
UT MD Anderson Cancer Ctr
1515 Holcombe Blvd   Houston, TX 77030-4095   SOUTHWEST

University of Utah Health Care   (801) 581-2121
Univ Utah Hlth Care
50 N Medical Dr   Salt Lake City, UT 84132   GREAT PLAINS AND MOUNTAINS

University of Virginia Health System   (434) 924-0211
Univ of Virginia Health Sys
1215 Lee Street   Charlottesville, VA 22908-0001   SOUTHEAST

University of Washington Medical Center   (206) 598-3300
Univ Wash Med Ctr
1959 NE Pacific St, PO Box 656355   Seattle, WA 98195   WEST COAST AND PACIFIC

University of Wisconsin Hospital & Clinics   (608) 263-6400
Univ WI Hosp & Clins
600 Highland Avenue   Madison, WI 53792   MIDWEST

UPMC Montefiore		(412) 647-2345
UPMC Montefiore		
200 Lothrop St	Pittsburgh, PA 15213	MID ATLANTIC
UPMC Passavant-McCandless		(412) 367-6700
UPMC Passavant-McCandless		
9100 Babcock Blvd	Pittsburgh, PA 15237	MID ATLANTIC
UPMC Presbyterian		(412) 647-2345
UPMC Presby, Pittsburgh		
200 Lothrop St	Pittsburgh, PA 15213	MID ATLANTIC
UPMC Shadyside		(412) 623-2121
UPMC Shadyside		
5230 Centre Ave	Pittsburgh, PA 15232	MID ATLANTIC
USC Norris Cancer Hospital		(323) 865-3000
USC Norris Cancer Hosp		
1441 Eastlake Ave	Los Angeles, CA 90033	WEST COAST AND PACIFIC
USC University Hospital		(323) 442-8500
USC Univ Hosp		
1500 San Pablo St	Los Angeles, CA 90033	WEST COAST AND PACIFIC
UT Southwestern Medical Center at Dallas		(214) 648-3111
UT Southwestern Med Ctr at Dallas		
5323 Harry Hines Blvd	Dallas, TX 75390	SOUTHWEST
VA Ann Arbor Healthcare System		(734) 769-7100
VA Ann Arbor Healthcare Sys		
2215 Fuller Rd	Ann Arbor, MI 48105	MIDWEST
VA Medical Center - Portland		(503) 220-8262
VA Medical Center - Portland		
3710 SW US Veteran Hospital Rd	Portland, OR 97239	WEST COAST AND PACIFIC
Vanderbilt Monroe Carrell Jr. Children's Hospital		(615) 936-1000
Vanderbilt Monroe Carrell Jr. Chldn's Hosp		
2200 Children's Way	Nashville, TN 37232	SOUTHEAST
Vanderbilt University Medical Center		(615) 322-5000
Vanderbilt Univ Med Ctr		
1211 Medical Center Drive	Nashville, TN 37232	SOUTHEAST
VCU Medical Center		(904) 828-9000
VCU Med Ctr		
1250 E Marshall St, PO Box 980510	Richmond, VA 23298	SOUTHEAST

Appendix B

Virginia Mason Medical Center (206) 223-6600
Virginia Mason Med Ctr
1100 Ninth Ave, Box 900 Seattle, WA 98111 WEST COAST AND PACIFIC

Wake Forest University Baptist Medical Center (336) 716-2255
Wake Forest Univ Baptist Med Ctr
Medical Center Blvd Winston-Salem, NC 27157-1015 SOUTHEAST

WakeMed Cary Hospital (919) 350-2300
WakeMed Cary
1900 Kildaire Farm Rd Cary, NC 27511-6616 SOUTHEAST

Washington Hospital Center (202) 877-7000
Washington Hosp Ctr
110 Irving St NW Washington, DC 20010 MID ATLANTIC

WellStar Windy Hill Hospital (770) 644-1000
WellStar Windy Hill Hosp
2540 Windy Hill Road Marietta, GA 30067 SOUTHEAST

Westchester Medical Center (914) 493-7000
Westchester Med Ctr
95 Grasslands Road Valhalla, NY 10595 MID ATLANTIC

Wills Eye Hospital (215) 928-3000
Wills Eye Hosp
840 Walnut St Philadelphia, PA 19107-5598 MID ATLANTIC

Wilmington Hospital (302) 733-1000
Wilmington Hosp
501 W 14th St Wilmington, DE 19801 MID ATLANTIC

Winthrop University Hospital (516) 663-0333
Winthrop Univ Hosp
259 1st St Mineola, NY 11501 MID ATLANTIC

Wolfson Children's Hospital (904) 202-8000
Wolfson Chldns Hosp
800 Prudential Dr Jacksonville, FL 32207 SOUTHEAST

Women & Infants Hospital of Rhode Island (401) 274-1100
Women & Infants Hosp of RI
101 Dudley Street Providence, RI 02905 NEW ENGLAND

Women's and Children's Hospital of Buffalo, The (716) 878-7000
Women's & Chldn's Hosp of Buffalo, The
219 Bryant St Buffalo, NY 14222 MID ATLANTIC

Yakima Valley Memorial Hospital   (509) 575-8000
Yakima Valley Mem Hosp
2811 Tieton Dr   Yakima, WA 98902-3799   WEST COAST AND PACIFIC

Yale-New Haven Hospital   (203) 688-4242
Yale-New Haven Hosp
20 York St   New Haven, CT 06510   NEW ENGLAND

Yampa Valley Medical Center   (970) 879-1322
Yampa Valley Med Ctr
1024 Central Park Dr   Steamboat Springs, CO 80487 GREAT PLAINS AND MOUNTAINS

The Best in American Medicine
www.CastleConnolly.com

Appendix C:
Selected Cancer Resources

AMERICAN CANCER SOCIETY
A site with many resources on types of cancer, treatments, coping, support, clinical research data, volunteering and current news articles. It also has a database which allows one to search by zip code to locate local resources, activities and news.

National Office   800-ACS-2345
1599 Clifton Road, NE   www.cancer.org
Atlanta, GA 30329

ANNIE APPLESEED PROJECT
Provides information, education, advocacy and awareness to those interested in complementary and alternative medical treatments.

7319 Serrano Terrace   www.annieappleseedproject.org
Delray Beach, FL 33446-2215   annieappleseedpr@aol.com

ASSOCIATION OF CANCER ONLINE RESOURCES (ACOR)
Maintains many support groups and cancer-specific information, treatment options, clinical trial findings and a large collection of cancer-related online communities.

173 Duane Street   212-226-5525
Suite 3A   www.acor.org
New York, NY 10013-3334

CANCER CARE
Provides free resources and support to cancer patients, caregivers and families with all cancers through counseling, education, information, referrals and direct financial assistance.

National Office   800-813-HOPE or 212-712-8400
275 7th Ave, Fl 22   www.cancercare.org
New York, NY 10001

CANCER NEWS
News and information on cancer diagnosis, treatment and prevention.

www.cancernews.com

CANCER RESEARCH & PREVENTION FOUNDATION OF AMERICA
Scientific research and cancer education with a focus on cancers that can be prevented through lifestyle changes or early detection followed by prompt treatment. Includes breast, cervical, colorectal, lung, prostate, skin, oral and testicular cancers.

1600 Duke Street   800-227-2732
Suite 500   www.preventcancer.org
Alexandria, VA 22314

CANCER TRACK

Comprehensive source for links to news, research, medications, treatments, support groups, regulatory agencies and online references.

www.cancertrack.com

CANCEREDUCATION.COM

Provides cancer-specific information and educational programming for patients, their families and physicians.

www.cancereducation.com

CANCERNETWORK.COM

Provides research findings and information on cancers, complications, therapies and insurance and payment issues.

www.cancernetwork.com

HEALTH FINDER

A service of the Department of Health and Human Services, Health Finder has many resources ranging from topics specifically related to cancer to broader health topics such as locating public clinics, nursing homes, health fraud advice, medical privacy and links to universities, medical dictionaries and journals. It also has a guide that presents information and resources to help patients and families get better quality healthcare.

P.O. Box 1133
Washington, DC 20013-1133

www.healthfinder.gov
healthfinder@nhic.org

MacMillan

Europe-based organization with over 4,500 pages of online cancer information, practical advice and support for cancer patients and their families.

www.macmillan.org.uk

NATIONAL CANCER INSTITUTE (NCI)

A branch of the US National Institutes of Health, NCI provides information about cancer, clinical trials, statistics, and research.

www.cancer.gov

The National Cancer Institute's (NCI's) Cancer Information Service (CIS) is a national information and education network. The CIS is a free public service of the NCI, the Nation's primary agency for cancer research. The CIS provides current cancer information to patients, their families, the public, and health professionals. The CIS provides personalized, confidential responses to specific questions about cancer.

NCI-Designated Cancer Centers
Cancer centers listed by state.

http://cancercenters.cancer.gov/cancer_centers/cancer-centers-list.html

NCI Dictionary of Cancer Terms

www.cancer.gov/dictionary

NCI Public Inquiries Office
6116 Executive Blvd
Suite 300
Bethesda, MD 20892-8322

1-800-4-CANCER (1-800-422-6237)
http://www.cancer.gov/aboutnci/cis

NATIONAL COMPREHENSIVE CANCER NETWORK (NCCN)

Outlines cancer treatment guidelines and offers cancer patients and their families information to help work with their physicians to make more informed decisions about care and treatments.

Treatment Guidelines for Patients   888.9009.NCCN

National Comprehensive Cancer Network   215-690-0300
275 Commerce Drive   www.nccn.org
Suite 300
Fort Washington, PA 19034

ONCOLINK

Information on specific types of cancer, updates on cancer treatments and news about research advances

OncoLink   www.oncolink.org
Abramson Cancer Center of the University of Pennsylvania
3400 Spruce Street - 2 Donner   215-349-8895
Philadelphia, PA 19104

ONCOLOGY NURSING SOCIETY (ONS)

Resources on prevention, detection, diagnosis, treatment and survivorship.

Oncology Nursing Society   866-257-4ONS
125 Enterprise Drive   www.ons.org
Pittsburgh, PA 15275   customer.service@ons.org

PEOPLE LIVING WITH CANCER

A website by the American Society of Clinical Oncology for patients that provides oncologist-approved information on more than 50 types of cancer and their treatments, side effects, coping, and clinical trials. It includes a "Find an Oncologist" database, live chats, message boards, a drug database and links to patient support organizations.

American Society of Clinical Oncology   571-483-1780
2318 Mill Road   www.cancer.net
Suite 800   contactus@cancer.net
Alexandria, VA 22314

YOUR DISEASE RISK

Provides education on cancers and focuses on prevention as the primary approach to controlling cancer and other chronic diseases.

Washington University in St. Louis   314-747-7222
Siteman Cancer Center   800-600-3606
660 S. Euclid Ave   www.yourdiseaserisk.wustl.edu
Box 8100
St. Louis, MO 63110

Appendix C

CHILDREN AND YOUNG ADULTS

BRAVE KIDS
Provides online resources for children with chronic, life-threatening illnesses and disabilities and their families. Local resources searchable by zip code.

Brave Kids: East Coast
1113 S. Marsh Wind Way
Ponte Verda Beach, FL 32082J

800-568-1008
www.bravekids.org
office@bravekids.org

CANDLELIGHTERS CHILDHOOD CANCER FOUNDATION
Offers support, education and advocacy for families of children with cancer, survivors of childhood cancer and the professionals who care for them.

National Office
P.O. Box 498
Kensington, MD 20895-0498

800-366-CCCF or 301-962-3520
www.candlelighters.org
staff@acco.org

CHILDREN'S ONCOLOGY GROUP
The Children's Oncology Group, in partnership with the National Childhood Cancer Foundation. Offers education and support resources.

Rush Operation Ctr
440 E. Hungton Dr., Ste 40
Arcadia, CA 91006

626-447-0064
www.childrensoncologygroup.org

CURESEARCH
Provides educational resources about cancer diagnoses, the different phases of treatment and support resources

CureSearch Headquarters
4600 East West Highway
Suite 600
Bethesda, MD 20814

800-458-6223
www.curesearch.org

KIDSHEALTH.ORG
Site designed for parents, kids and teens that discusses many health topics including cancer.

www.kidshealth.org

LIVESTRONG™ YOUNG ADULT ALLIANCE (THE LANCE ARMSTRONG FOUNDATION).
The mission of the LIVESTRONG™ Young Adult Alliance is to improve survival rates and quality of life for young adults living with cancer by promoting relevant research and the delivery of patient care, generating awareness of the issue, being a voice for young adults with cancer and advancing helpful community-based programs and services.

2201 E 6th St.,
Austin TX, 78702

877-236-8820
866-673-7205
www.livestrong.org/yaa

NATIONAL CHILDHOOD CANCER FOUNDATION
National Childhood Cancer Foundation 800.458.NCCF

440 E Huntington Drive
Suite 300
Arcadia, CA 91066-0012

www.curesearch.org

PEDIATRIC ONCOLOGY RESOURCE CENTER

A site with resources, Internet links, and references for parents, friends and families of children who have or had childhood cancer.

www.ped-onc.org/

PLANET CANCER

A website for young adults with cancer that provides support and other resources, including an online forum.

www.planetcancer.org

TEENS LIVING WITH CANCER

A website for teenagers with cancer with information on treatments, combating fear, testimonials from other teens who have or had cancer and support chat rooms.

Melissa's Living Legacy Foundation
1000 Elmwood Avenue
Ste 300
Rochester, NY 14620

585-334-0858
teenslivingwithcancer.org
info@teenslivingwithcancer.org

585-563-6221

CLINICAL TRIALS

AMERICAN CANCER SOCIETY

Free clinical trial matching and referral service.

www.cancer.org

CENTERWATCH

Provides information and resources used by patients, pharmaceutical, biotechnology and medical device companies, CROs and research centers involved in clinical research around the world. The web site provides an extensive list of IRB approved clinical trials being conducted internationally and also lists promising therapies newly approved by the Food and Drug Administration. CenterWatch also offers reports on specific illnesses, clinical trial information and therapies that patients and advocates can buy.

10 Winthrop Sq, Fl 5,
Boston, MA 02110

617-948-5100
www.centerwatch.com

COALITION OF NATIONAL CANCER COOPERATIVE GROUPS (CNCC)

A network of cancer clinical trials specialists including cooperative groups, cancer centers, academic medical centers, community hospitals, physician practices, and patient advocate groups, CNCC aims at improving the clinical trials experience for patients and physicians, and providing professional support services regulatory requirements, and providing professional support services. It offers a variety of programs and information for physicians, patient advocate groups, and patients designed to increase awareness of, and participation in cancer clinical trials.

1818 Market Street
#1100
Philadelphia, PA 19103

877-520-4457
www.cancertrialshelp.org

INTERNATIONAL FEDERATION OF PHARMACEUTICAL MANUFACTURERS & ASSOCIATIONS (IFPMA)

Provides a portal that allows one to search for comprehensive information on on-going clinical trials or results of completed trials conducted by the pharmaceutical industry.

www.ifpma.org/clinicaltrials

NATIONAL CANCER INSTITUTE (NCI)

A branch of the US National Institutes of Health, NCI provides information about cancer, clinical trials, statistics, and research.

www.cancer.gov/clinicaltrials

NATIONAL COMPREHENSIVE CANCER NETWORK (NCCN)

An alliance of 19 of the world's leading cancer centers, NCCN is a source of information to help patients and health professionals make informed decisions about cancer care. Through the collective expertise of its member institutions, the NCCN develops, updates, and disseminates a complete library of clinical practice guidelines.

275 Commerce Drive
Ste 300
Fort Washington PA,19034

Fax: 215-690-0280
888-909-NCCN
215.690.0300
www.nccn.org

SPECIFIC CANCERS

RARE CANCER ALLIANCE

Provides support and other resources for adults and children with rare cancers. Note: You are encouraged to explore the other websites listed in this appendix, as many also include information on rare cancers.

www.rare-cancer.org

SUPPORT

FERTILE HOPE

Provides reproductive information and support to cancer patients whose medical treatments present the risk of infertility.

Note: You are encouraged to explore the other websites listed in this appendix, as many also include resources for support including education materials, chat rooms, community groups and clinical advice.

866-965-7205
www.fertilehope.org

SURVIVORS

CANCER SURVIVORS NETWORK
(American Cancer Society) Provides a forum for cancer survivors to share their stories, join chats, post messages on discussion boards and create their own webpage about their stories.

www.acscsn.org

CANCERVIVE
Provides support, public education and advocacy to those who have had cancer.

LANCE ARMSTRONG FOUNDATION (LAF)
LAF provides advocacy, education, support and research for both cancer survivors and people who currently have cancer.

2201 E. Sixth Street   512-236-8820
Austin, TX 78702   www.livestrong.org

NATIONAL COALITION FOR CANCER SURVIVORSHIP (NCCS)
Provides education, advocacy and support to those affected by cancer and cancer survivors. Specifically addresses quality of care and minority issues.

1010 Wayne Avenue   301-650-9127 or 888-650-9127
Suite 770   www.canceradvocacy.org
Silver Spring, MD 20910   info@canceradvocacy.org

TRAVEL ASSISTANCE

NATIONAL PATIENT AIR TRANSPORT HELPLINE (NPATH)
Provides information about and referrals to charitable medical air transportation programs that provide long-distance travel for medical, low income, and financially vulnerable patients. The information is provided at no cost and the HELPLINE is available 24 hours a day.

National Patient Travel Center   1-800-296-1217
4620 Haygood Rd, Ste. 1   www.patienttravel.org
Virginia Beach, VA 23455   info@nationalpatienttravelcenter.org

TREATMENT

AMERICAN SOCIETY FOR THERAPEUTIC RADIOLOGY AND ONCOLOGY
Provides downloadable brochures and publications on treatment options for several specific cancers.

ASTRO Headquarters   800-962-7876
8280 Willowoaks Corporate Drive   703-502-1550
Suite 500   www.astro.org/patients
Fairfax, VA 22031

BLOOD AND MARROW TRANSPLANT INFORMATION NETWORK

Provides information about blood and marrow transplants, support groups, a list of transplant centers and testimonials from survivors.

BMI InfoNet
2310 Skokie Valley Road
Ste 104
Highland Park, IL 60035

1-847-433-3313
www.bmtinfonet.org

CANCERSYMPTOMS.ORG

(Oncology Nursing Society) Provides information and resources for learning about and managing symptoms often associated with cancer treatment.

www.cancersymptoms.org

WOMEN

BREASTCANCER.ORG

Offers information on breast cancer prevention, symptoms, treatment, research, recovery and support.

www.breastcancer.org

ENTRE MUJERES

Un guia sobre la recuperación física y emocional después de la mastectomía.

www.cancerlinks.com

LOOK GOOD. . . FEEL BETTER

Provides resources and links for women who are undergoing cancer treatment including cosmetic advice and support.

www.lookgoodfeelbetter.org

NATIONAL WOMEN'S HEALTH RESOURCE CENTER

Women's health site that includes information on various cancers.

NWHRC
157 Broad Street
Suite 106
Red Bank, NJ 07701

www.healthywomen.org (Note: Click on "Health Center" and select the appropriate topic.)
1-877-986-9472

NCI WOMEN OF COLOR

Provides basic data on how cancer affects women in minority populations.

www.womenshealth.gov/minority-health/

WOMEN'S CANCER CENTER

Many resources for women with carious kinds of cancer.

www.womenscancercenter.com

YWCA

"ENCOREplus", a program available at some YWCA locations that focuses on cancer prevention, nutrition and rehabilitation.

YWCA USA
2025 M Street, NW
Suite 550
Washington, DC 20036

800-YWCA-US1 or 202-467-0801
www.ywca.org (Note: click on the "I need help" link.)

The Best in American Medicine
www.CastleConnolly.com

Appendix D:
NCI Designated Cancer Centers

National Cancer Institute (NCI) designated Cancer Centers are recognized for their scientific excellence and extensive resources focused on cancer and cancer-related problems.

The Cancer Centers are a major source of discovery of the nature of cancer and of the development of more effective approaches to cancer prevention, diagnosis, and therapy. They also deliver medical advances to patients and their families, educate health-care professionals and the public, and reach out to underserved populations. They may be freestanding organizations, a center within an academic institution, or part of a consortium of institutions.

NCI-designation is voluntary and is awarded via a grant using a peer-review process. All NCI-designated cancer centers receive substantial financial support from NCI grants and are reevaluated each time their cancer center support grant comes up for renewal (generally every 3 to 5 years). The NCI recognizes two types of centers: Cancer Centers and Comprehensive Cancer Centers, based on the type of grant received. In terms of patient care, there is no difference in the quality of care they each provide.

For more information on NCI-designated Cancer Centers, go to the Cancer Centers Program on the Internet at: http://cancercenters.cancer.gov.

Below is a list of states where a NCI-designated Cancer Center is located. There are two different types of cancer centers included in this appendix:

*Comprehensive Cancer Center:

Provides patient services; conducts basic, population sciences, and clinical research; and engages in outreach and education activities.

Cancer Center:

Provides patient services; and conducts basic, population sciences, and clinical research.

Appendix D

*UNIVERSITY OF ALABAMA AT BIRMINGHAM COMPREHENSIVE CANCER CENTER (UAB)

Address:	North Pavilion 2500
	1802 Sixth Avenue South
	Birmingham, AL 35294
Telephone:	205-975-8222 (Cancer Answers)
	205-934-5077 (Administration)
	1-800-822-0933 (1-800-UAB-0933) (Cancer Answers)
	1-800-UAB-MIST (1-800-UAB-6478) (Referring Physicians)
Web site:	http://www3.ccc.uab.edu/

The University of Alabama at Birmingham Comprehensive Cancer Center is a National Cancer Institute (NCI)-designated Comprehensive Cancer Center that conducts research and provides services directly to cancer patients. Comprehensive Cancer Centers also conduct activities in outreach and education, and provide information on health care advances to both health care professionals and the public. An NCI-designated Cancer Center must meet a series of competitive requirements and demonstrate excellence in cancer research. For more general information about the Cancer Centers Program of NCI, please visit http://cancercenters.cancer.gov on the Internet.

---

*ARIZONA CANCER CENTER: UNIVERSITY OF ARIZONA

Address:	3838 North Campbell Avenue (clinic address)
	Tucson, AZ 85719
Telephone:	520-694-2873
	1-800-524-5928
Web site:	http://www.azcc.arizona.edu/

The Arizona Cancer Center is a National Cancer Institute (NCI)-designated Comprehensive Cancer Center that conducts research and provides services directly to cancer patients. Comprehensive Cancer Centers also conduct activities in outreach and education, and provide information on health care advances to both health care professionals and the public. An NCI-designated Cancer Center must meet a series of competitive requirements and demonstrate excellence in cancer research. For more general information about the Cancer Centers Program of NCI, please visit http://cancercenters.cancer.gov/ on the Internet.

CALIFORNIA

*CHAO FAMILY COMPREHENSIVE CANCER CENTER: UNIVERSITY OF CALIFORNIA, IRVINE

Address:	101 The City Drive
	Building 23, Route 81
	Orange, CA 92868
Telephone:	714-456-8000 (Cancer Center)
	714-456-7001 (Physician Referral Service)
Web site:	http://www.ucihs.uci.edu/cancer/

The Chao Family Comprehensive Cancer Center is a National Cancer Institute (NCI)-designated Comprehensive Cancer Center that conducts research and provides services directly to cancer patients. Comprehensive Cancer Centers also conduct activities in outreach and education, and provide information on health care advances to both health care professionals and the public. An NCI-designated Cancer Center must meet a series of competitive requirements and demonstrate excellence in cancer research. For more general information about the Cancer Centers Program of NCI, please visit http://cancercenters.cancer.gov/ on the Internet.

*CITY OF HOPE
CITY OF HOPE NATIONAL MEDICAL CENTER AND BECKMAN RESEARCH INSTITUTE

Address:	1500 East Duarte Road
	Duarte, CA 91010
Telephone:	626-256-4673 (626-256-HOPE)
	1-800-826-4673 (New Patient Services)
	1-866-434-4673 (General Information)
Web site:	http://www.cityofhope.org

The City of Hope is a National Cancer Institute (NCI)-designated Comprehensive Cancer Center that conducts research and provides services directly to cancer patients. Comprehensive Cancer Centers also conduct activities in outreach and education, and provide information on health care advances to both health care professionals and the public. An NCI-designated Cancer Center must meet a series of competitive requirements and demonstrate excellence in cancer research. For more general information about the Cancer Centers Program of NCI, please visit http://cancercenters.cancer.gov/ on the Internet.

*MOORES UCSD CANCER CENTER
UNIVERSITY OF CALIFORNIA, SAN DIEGO

Address:	3855 Health Sciences Drive
	La Jolla, CA 92093
Telephone:	858-822-6100
	1-866-773-2703
Web site:	http://cancer.ucsd.edu/

The Rebecca and John Moores University of California, San Diego Comprehensive Cancer Center is a National Cancer Institute (NCI)-designated Comprehensive Cancer Center that conducts research and provides services directly to cancer patients. Comprehensive Cancer Centers also conduct activities in outreach and education, and provide information on health care advances to both health care professionals and the public. An NCI-designated Cancer Center must meet a series of competitive requirements and demonstrate excellence in cancer research. For more general information about the Cancer Centers Program of NCI, please visit http://cancercenters.cancer.gov/ on the Internet.

STANFORD CANCER CENTER (SCC)

Address:	875 Blake Wilbur Drive
	Stanford, CA 94305
Telephone:	650-498-6000 (Referral Center)
	1-877-668-7535 (Referral Center)
	1-877-487-0237 (International Medical Services)
E-mail:	referral@stanfordmed.org
Web site:	http://cancer.stanford.edu/

The Stanford Cancer Center is a National Cancer Institute (NCI)-designated Cancer Center that conducts research and provides services directly to cancer patients. An NCI-designated Cancer Center must meet a series of competitive requirements and demonstrate excellence in cancer research. For more general information about the Cancer Centers Program of NCI, please visit http://cancercenters.cancer.gov/ on the Internet.

UC DAVIS CANCER CENTER
UNIVERSITY OF CALIFORNIA, DAVIS

Address:	Room 3003
	4501 X Street
	Sacramento, CA 95817
Telephone:	916-703-5210 (New Patient Referral Office)
	916-734-5959 (General Information)
	1-800-362-5566 (New Patient Referrals)
E-mail:	cancer.center@ucdmc.ucdavis.edu
Web site:	http://cancer.ucdmc.ucdavis.edu/

The UC Davis Cancer Center is a National Cancer Institute (NCI)-designated Cancer Center that conducts research and provides services directly to cancer patients. An NCI-designated Cancer Center must meet a series of competitive requirements and demonstrate excellence in cancer research. For more general information about the Cancer Centers Program of NCI, please visit http://cancercenters.cancer.gov/ on the Internet.

*UCLA'S JONSSON COMPREHENSIVE CANCER CENTER
UNIVERSITY OF CALIFORNIA, LOS ANGELES

Address:	8-684 Factor Building
	UCLA Box 951781
	Los Angeles, CA 90095
Telephone:	310-825-5268 (administrative office)
	1-888-662-8252 (UCLA Cancer Hotline)
	1-800-825-2631 (Cancer Screening or General Health Care)
E-mail:	jcccinfo@mednet.ucla.edu
Web site:	http://www.cancer.ucla.edu

UCLA's Jonsson Comprehensive Cancer Center is a National Cancer Institute (NCI)-designated Comprehensive Cancer Center that conducts research and provides services directly to cancer patients. Comprehensive Cancer Centers also conduct activities in outreach and education, and provide information on health care advances to both health care professionals and the public. An NCI-designated Cancer Center must meet a series of competitive requirements and demonstrate excellence in cancer research. For more general information about the Cancer Centers Program of NCI, please visit http://cancercenters.cancer.gov/ on the Internet.

*UCSF HELEN DILLER FAMILY COMPREHENSIVE CANCER CENTER
UNIVERSITY OF CALIFORNIA,
SAN FRANCISCO COMPREHENSIVE CANCER CENTER

Address:	UCSF Helen Diller Family Comprehensive Cancer Center
	Box 0981, UCSF
	San Francisco, CA 94143-0981
Telephone:	415-353-8489 (International Inquiries)
	888-444-2559 (Cancer Referral Line)
	1-800-353-2559 (Physician Referral Service)
E-mail:	referral.center@ucsfmedctr.org
Web site:	http://cancer.ucsf.edu

The UCSF Helen Diller Family Comprehensive Cancer Center is a National Cancer Institute (NCI)-designated Comprehensive Cancer Center that conducts research and provides services directly to cancer patients. Comprehensive Cancer Centers also conduct activities in outreach and education, and provide information on health care advances to both health care professionals and the public. An NCI-designated Cancer Center must meet a series of competitive requirements and demonstrate excellence in cancer research. For more general information about the Cancer Centers Program of NCI, please visit http://cancercenters.cancer.gov/ on the Internet.

*USC/NORRIS COMPREHENSIVE CANCER CENTER

Address:	1441 Eastlake Avenue
	Los Angeles, CA 90033
Telephone:	323-865-3000 (general information)
	Web site: http://ccnt.hsc.usc.edu/

The USC/Norris Comprehensive Cancer Center is a National Cancer Institute (NCI)-designated Comprehensive Cancer Center that conducts research and provides services directly to cancer patients. Comprehensive Cancer Centers also conduct activities in outreach and education, and provide information on health care advances to both health care professionals and the public. An NCI-designated Cancer Center must meet a series of competitive requirements and demonstrate excellence in cancer research. For more general information about the Cancer Centers Program of NCI, please visit http://cancercenters.cancer.gov/ on the Internet.

COLORADO

*UNIVERSITY OF COLORADO CANCER CENTER

Address: UCCC
               Anschtz Medical Campus
               13601 E 17th Pl
               Campus Box F434
               Aurora, CO 80045
Telephone: 720-848-0300
Web site: http://www.uccc.info

The University of Colorado Cancer Center is a National Cancer Institute (NCI)-designated Comprehensive Cancer Center that conducts research and provides services directly to cancer patients. Comprehensive Cancer Centers also conduct activities in outreach and education, and provide information on health care advances to both health care professionals and the public. An NCI-designated Cancer Center must meet a series of competitive requirements and demonstrate excellence in cancer research. For more general information about the Cancer Centers Program of NCI, please visit http://cancercenters.cancer.gov/ on the Internet.

CONNECTICUT

*YALE CANCER CENTER
YALE UNIVERSITY SCHOOL OF MEDICINE

Address: Post Office Box 208028 (mailing address)
               333 Cedar Street, WWW 205 (physical address)
               New Haven, CT 06520
Telephone: 203-785-4191
               1-866-925-3226 (1-866-YALECANCER)
Web site: http://yalecancercenter.org

The Yale Cancer Center is a National Cancer Institute (NCI)-designated Comprehensive Cancer Center that conducts research and provides services directly to cancer patients. Comprehensive Cancer Centers also conduct activities in outreach and education, and provide information on health care advances to both health care professionals and the public. An NCI-designated Cancer Center must meet a series of competitive requirements and demonstrate excellence in cancer research. For more general information about the Cancer Centers Program of NCI, please visit http://cancercenters.cancer.gov/ on the Internet.

DISTRICT OF COLUMBIA

*LOMBARDI COMPREHENSIVE CANCER CENTER
GEORGETOWN UNIVERSITY MEDICAL CENTER

Address:	3800 Reservoir Road, NW.
	Washington, DC 20007
Telephone:	202-444-2223 (Appointments)
	202-444-4000 (CancerLine)
Web site:	http://lombardi.georgetown.edu/

The Lombardi Comprehensive Cancer Center, Georgetown University Medical Center is a National Cancer Institute (NCI)-designated Comprehensive Cancer Center that conducts research and provides services directly to cancer patients. Comprehensive Cancer Centers also conduct activities in outreach and education, and provide information on health care advances to both health care professionals and the public. An NCI-designated Cancer Center must meet a series of competitive requirements and demonstrate excellence in cancer research. For more general information about the Cancer Centers Program of NCI, please visit http://cancercenters.cancer.gov on the Internet.

FLORIDA

*H. LEE MOFFITT CANCER CENTER AND RESEARCH INSTITUTE AT THE
UNIVERSITY OF SOUTH FLORIDA

Address:	12902 Magnolia Drive
	Tampa, FL 33612
Telephone:	813-745-4673 (813-745-HOPE) (Main)
	1-888-860-2778 (New Patient/Physician Referral)
	1-888-663-3488 (1-888-MOFFITT) (Main)
Web site:	http://www.moffitt.usf.edu/

The H. Lee Moffitt Cancer Center and Research Institute at the University of South Florida is a National Cancer Institute (NCI)-designated Comprehensive Cancer Center that conducts research and provides services directly to cancer patients. Comprehensive Cancer Centers also conduct activities in outreach and education, and provide information on healthcare advances to both healthcare professionals and the public. An NCI-designated Cancer Center must meet a series of competitive requirements and demonstrate excellence in cancer research. For more general information about the Cancer Centers Program of NCI please visit http://cancercenters.cancer.gov on the Internet.

GEORGIA

WINSHIP CANCER INSTITUTE
EMORY UNIVERSITY

Address: 1365C Clifton Road
              Atlanta, GA 30322
Telephone: 404-778-1900 (Main)
              1-888-946-7447 (1-888-WINSHIP)
Web site: http://cancer.emory.edu/

The Winship Cancer Institute, Emory University, is a National Cancer Institute (NCI)-designated Cancer Center that conducts research and provides services directly to cancer patients. An NCI-designated Cancer Center must meet a series of competitive requirements and demonstrate excellence in cancer research. For more general information about the Cancer Centers Program of NCI, please visit http://cancercenters.cancer.gov/ on the Internet.

HAWAII

CANCER RESEARCH CENTER OF HAWAII (CRCH)
UNIVERSITY OF HAWAII

Address: 677 Ala Moana Blvd,
              Gold Bond Bldg, Ste 901
              Honolulu, HI 96813
Telephone: 808-586-3010
Web site: http://www.crch.org

The Cancer Research Center of Hawaii (CRCH) is a National Cancer Institute (NCI)-designated Cancer Center that conducts research on the causes, prevention and treatment of cancer. Although CRCH does not treat patients at the facility, it can provide referrals to other facilities for medical care and second opinions and can refer patients to providers and institutions participating in clinical trials. An NCI-designated Cancer Center must meet a series of competitive requirements and demonstrate excellence in cancer research. For more general information about the Cancer Centers Program of NCI, please visit http://cancercenters.cancer.gov/ on the Internet.

ILLINOIS

*ROBERT H. LURIE COMPREHENSIVE CANCER CENTER
NORTHWESTERN UNIVERSITY

Address:	Galter Pavilion
	675 N. St. Clair, 21st Floor, Suite 100
	Chicago, IL 60611
Telephone:	312-908-5250
	1-866-587-4322 (1-866-LURIE-CC) appointment line
	1-800-543-7362 (1-800-KIDS-DOC) pediatric patients
E-mail:	cancer@northwestern.edu
Web site:	http://cancer.northwestern.edu/home/index.cfm

The Robert H. Lurie Comprehensive Cancer Center is a National Cancer Institute (NCI)-designated Comprehensive Cancer Center that conducts research and provides services directly to cancer patients. Comprehensive Cancer Centers also conduct activities in outreach and education, and provide information on health care advances to both health care professionals and the public. An NCI-designated Cancer Center must meet a series of competitive requirements and demonstrate excellence in cancer research. For more general information about the Cancer Centers Program of NCI, please visit http://cancercenters.cancer.gov/ on the Internet.

*UNIVERSITY OF CHICAGO CANCER RESEARCH CENTER

Address:	Mail Code 2115
	5841 South Maryland Avenue
	Chicago, IL 60637
Telephone:	773-702-6180
	773-834-7424 (adult)
	773-702-6808 (pediatric)
Web site:	http://cancer.uchicago.edu/

The University of Chicago Cancer Research Center is a National Cancer Institute (NCI)-designated Comprehensive Cancer Center that conducts research and provides services directly to cancer patients. Comprehensive Cancer Centers also conduct activities in outreach and education, and provide information on health care advances to both health care professionals and the public. An NCI-designated Cancer Center must meet a series of competitive requirements and demonstrate excellence in cancer research. For more general information about the Cancer Centers Program of NCI, please visit http://cancercenters.cancer.gov/ on the Internet.

INDIANA

INDIANA UNIVERSITY MELVIN AND BREN SIMON CANCER CENTER
IU SIMON CANCER CENTER

Address:	535 Barnhill Drive
	Indianapolis, IN 46202
Telephone:	317-944-0920
	1-888-600-4822
Web site:	www.cancer.iu.edu

The Indiana University Melvin and Bren Simon Cancer Center is a National Cancer Institute (NCI)-designated Cancer Center that conducts research and provides services directly to cancer patients. An NCI-designated Cancer Center must meet a series of competitive requirements and demonstrate excellence in cancer research. For more general information about the Cancer Centers Program of NCI, please visit http://cancercenters.cancer.gov/ on the Internet.

IOWA

*HOLDEN COMPREHENSIVE CANCER CENTER
UNIVERSITY OF IOWA

Address:	4802 JPP
	200 Hawkins Drive
	Iowa City, IA 52242
Telephone:	319-356-4200 (Referrals & Appointments)
	1-800-777-8442 (Referrals & Appointments)
	1-800-237-1225 (General Information)
E-mail:	cancer-center@uiowa.edu
Web site:	http://www.uihealthcare.org/

The Holden Comprehensive Cancer Center at the University of Iowa is a National Cancer Institute (NCI)-designated Comprehensive Cancer Center that conducts research and provides services directly to cancer patients. Comprehensive Cancer Centers also conduct activities in outreach and education, and provide information on health care advances to both health care professionals and the public. An NCI-designated Cancer Center must meet a series of competitive requirements and demonstrate excellence in cancer research. For more general information about the Cancer Centers Program of NCI, please visit http://cancercenters.cancer.gov/ on the Internet.

MARYLAND

GREENEBAUM CANCER CENTER (MARLENE AND STEWART) (UMGCC)
UNIVERSITY OF MARYLAND

Address:	22 South Greene Street
	Baltimore, MD 21201
Telephone:	410-328-7904 (Main and New Appointments)
	1-800-888-8823 (Main and New Appointments)
	1-800-373-4111 (Physician Referrals)
Web site:	http://www.umgcc.org/

The Greenebaum Cancer Center, University of Maryland, is a National Cancer Institute (NCI)-designated Cancer Center that conducts research and provides services directly to cancer patients. An NCI-designated Cancer Center must meet a series of competitive requirements and demonstrate excellence in cancer research. For more general information about the Cancer Centers Program of NCI please visit http://cancercenters.cancer.gov/ on the Internet.

*SIDNEY KIMMEL COMPREHENSIVE CANCER CENTER AT JOHNS HOPKINS UNIVERSITY

Address: The Harry and Jeanette Weinberg Building
               Suite 1100, 401 North Broadway
               Baltimore, MD 21231
Telephone: 410-955-8964 (Patient Referrals)
               410-955-8804 (Clinical Trials)
               410-955-5222 (Main# to SKCCC)
Web site: http://www.hopkinskimmelcancercenter.org/

The Sidney Kimmel Comprehensive Cancer Center at Johns Hopkins is a National Cancer Institute (NCI)-designated Comprehensive Cancer Center that conducts research and provides services directly to cancer patients. Comprehensive Cancer Centers also conduct activities in outreach and education, and provide information on health care advances to both health care professionals and the public. An NCI-designated Cancer Center must meet a series of competitive requirements and demonstrate excellence in cancer research. For more general information about the Cancer Centers Program of NCI, please visit http://cancercenters.cancer.gov/ on the Internet.

MASSACHUSETTS

*DANA FARBER/HARVARD CANCER CENTER

Address: 450 Brookline Ave, BP332A
               Boston, MA 02115
Telephone: 617-632-3673 (Spanish)
               1-866-408-3324 (1-866-408-DFCI) (Adult/General)
Web site: http://www.dana-farber.org

The Dana Farber/Harvard Cancer Center is a National Cancer Institute (NCI)-designated Comprehensive Cancer Center that conducts research and provides services directly to cancer patients. Comprehensive Cancer Centers also conduct activities in outreach and education, and provide information on health care advances to both health care professionals and the public. An NCI-designated Cancer Center must meet a series of competitive requirements and demonstrate excellence in cancer research. For more general information about the Cancer Centers Program of NCI, please visit http://cancercenters.cancer.gov/ on the Internet.

*BARBARA ANN KARMANOS CANCER INSTITUTE
MEYER L. PRENTIS COMPREHENSIVE CANCER CENTER
OF METROPOLITAN DETROIT

Address:	Karmanos Cancer Center
	4100 John R Street
	Detroit, MI 48201
Telephone:	1-800-527-6266 (1-800-KARMANOS)
E-mail:	info@karmanos.org
Web site:	http://www.karmanos.org

The Barbara Ann Karmanos Cancer Institute is a National Cancer Institute (NCI)-designated Comprehensive Cancer Center that conducts research and provides services directly to cancer patients. Comprehensive Cancer Centers also conduct activities in outreach and education, and provide information on health care advances to both health care professionals and the public. An NCI-designated Cancer Center must meet a series of competitive requirements and demonstrate excellence in cancer research. For more general information about the Cancer Centers Program of NCI, please visit http://cancercenters.cancer.gov/ on the Internet.

*UNIVERSITY OF MICHIGAN COMPREHENSIVE CANCER CENTER
UNIVERSITY OF MICHIGAN HEALTH SYSTEM

Address:	1500 East Medical Center Drive
	Ann Arbor, MI 48109
Telephone:	734-763-5005
	1-800-865-1125 (Cancer Answer Line)
Web site:	http://www.cancer.med.umich.edu/

The University of Michigan Comprehensive Cancer Center is a National Cancer Institute (NCI)-designated Comprehensive Cancer Center that conducts research and provides services directly to cancer patients. Comprehensive Cancer Centers also conduct activities in outreach and education, and provide information on health care advances to both health care professionals and the public. An NCI-designated Cancer Center must meet a series of competitive requirements and demonstrate excellence in cancer research. For more general information about the Cancer Centers Program of NCI, please visit http://cancercenters.cancer.gov/ on the Internet.

MINNESOTA

*MASONIC CANCER CENTER
UNIVERSITY OF MINNESOTA

Address:	Mayo Mail Code 806
	420 Delaware Street, SE.
	Minneapolis, MN 55455
Telephone:	612-624-8484 (administrative office)
	612-624-2620 (cancer information line)
	1-888-226-2376 (in IA, MN, ND, SD, WI)
E-mail:	ccinfo@cancer.umn.edu
Web site:	http://www.cancer.umn.edu

The Masonic Cancer Center is a National Cancer Institute (NCI)-designated Comprehensive Cancer Center that conducts research and provides services directly to cancer patients. Comprehensive Cancer Centers also conduct activities in outreach and education, and provide information on health care advances to both health care professionals and the public. An NCI-designated Cancer Center must meet a series of competitive requirements and demonstrate excellence in cancer research. For more general information about the Cancer Centers Program of NCI, please visit http://cancercenters.cancer.gov/ on the Internet.

*MAYO CLINIC CANCER CENTER

Address:	200 First Street SW.
	Rochester, MN 55905
Telephone:	507-284-4137 (Medical Oncology appt. office)
	Web site: http://cancercenter.mayo.edu/

The Mayo Clinic Cancer Center is a National Cancer Institute (NCI)-designated Comprehensive Cancer Center that conducts research and provides services directly to cancer patients. Comprehensive Cancer Centers also conduct activities in outreach and education, and provide information on health care advances to both health care professionals and the public. An NCI-designated Cancer Center must meet a series of competitive requirements and demonstrate excellence in cancer research. For more general information about the Cancer Centers Program of NCI, please visit http://cancercenters.cancer.gov/ on the Internet.

MISSOURI

*SITEMAN CANCER CENTER
BARNES-JEWISH HOSPITAL AND
WASHINGTON UNIVERSITY SCHOOL OF MEDICINE

Address:	Box 8100
	660 South Euclid Avenue
	Saint Louis, MO 63110
Telephone:	314-747-7222
	1-800-600-3606
E-mail:	info@ccadmin.wustl.edu
Web site:	http://www.siteman.wustl.edu/

The Siteman Cancer Center is a National Cancer Institute (NCI)-designated Comprehensive Cancer Center that conducts research and provides services directly to cancer patients. Comprehensive Cancer Centers also conduct activities in outreach and education, and provide information on health care advances to both health care professionals and the public. An NCI-designated Cancer Center must meet a series of competitive requirements and demonstrate excellence in cancer research. For more general information about the Cancer Centers Program of NCI, please visit http://cancercenters.cancer.gov/ on the Internet.

NEBRASKA

UNMC EPPLEY CANCER CENTER
UNIVERSITY OF NEBRASKA MEDICAL CENTER

Address:	UNMC Eppley Cancer Center
	985950 Nebraska Medical Center
	Omaha, NE 68198-5950
Telephone:	402-559-6500 (Peggy D. Cowdery Patient Care Center)
	1-800-922-0000 (Physician Referrals)
Web site:	http://www.unmc.edu/cancercenter/

The UNMC Eppley Cancer Center is a National Cancer Institute (NCI)-designated Cancer Center that conducts research and provides services directly to cancer patients. An NCI-designated Cancer Center must meet a series of competitive requirements and demonstrate excellence in cancer research. For more general information about the Cancer Centers Program of NCI, please visit http://cancercenters.cancer.gov/ on the Internet.

NEW HAMPSHIRE

---

*NORRIS COTTON CANCER CENTER
DARTMOUTH-HITCHCOCK MEDICAL CENTER

Address:	One Medical Center Drive
	Lebanon, NH 03756
Telephone:	603-653-9000 (Administration)
	1-800-639-6918 (Cancer Help Line)
E-mail:	cancerhelp@dartmouth.edu
Web site:	http://www.cancer.dartmouth.edu/index.shtml

The Norris Cotton Cancer Center is a National Cancer Institute (NCI)-designated Comprehensive Cancer Center that conducts research and provides services directly to cancer patients. Comprehensive Cancer Centers also conduct activities in outreach and education, and provide information on health care advances to both health care professionals and the public. An NCI-designated Cancer Center must meet a series of competitive requirements and demonstrate excellence in cancer research. For more general information about the Cancer Centers Program of NCI, please visit http://cancercenters.cancer.gov/ on the Internet.

NEW JERSEY

*CANCER INSTITUTE OF NEW JERSEY (CINJ)
ROBERT WOOD JOHNSON UNIVERSITY HOSPITAL

Address: 195 Little Albany Street
New Brunswick, NJ 08903
Telephone: 732-235-2465 (CINJ)
Web site: http://www.cinj.org

The Cancer Institute of New Jersey, based at Robert Wood Johnson Medical School, is a National Cancer Institute (NCI)-designated Comprehensive Cancer Center that conducts research and provides services directly to cancer patients. Comprehensive Cancer Centers also conduct activities in outreach and education, and provide information on health care advances to both health care professionals and the public. An NCI-designated Cancer Center must meet a series of competitive requirements and demonstrate excellence in cancer research. For more general information about the Cancer Centers Program of NCI, please visit http://cancercenters.cancer.gov/ on the Internet.

NEW MEXICO

UNIVERSITY OF NEW MEXICO CANCER CENTER
UNM CANCER RESEARCH AND TREATMENT CENTER

Address: 1200 Camino de Salud NE
1 University of New Mexico
Albuquerque, NM 87131
Telephone: 505-272-4946
1-800-432-6806 (in New Mexico)
Web site: http://cancer.unm.edu/

The UNM Cancer Center is a National Cancer Institute (NCI)-designated Cancer Center that conducts research and provides services directly to cancer patients. An NCI-designated Cancer Center must meet a series of competitive requirements and demonstrate excellence in cancer research. For more general information about the Cancer Centers Program of NCI, please visit http://cancercenters.cancer.gov/ on the Internet.

Appendix D

ALBERT EINSTEIN CANCER CENTER (AECC)
ALBERT EINSTEIN COLLEGE OF MEDICINE OF YESHIVA UNIVERSITY

Address: 1300 Morris Park Avenue
Bronx, NY 10461
Telephone: 718-430-2302
E-mail: aecc@aecom.yu.edu
Web site: http://www.aecom.yu.edu/cancer/new/default.htm

The Albert Einstein Cancer Center is a National Cancer Institute (NCI)-designated Cancer Center that conducts research and provides services directly to cancer patients. An NCI-designated Cancer Center must meet a series of competitive requirements and demonstrate excellence in cancer research. For more general information about the Cancer Centers Program of NCI, please visit http://cancercenters.cancer.gov/ on the Internet.

*HERBERT IRVING COMPREHENSIVE CANCER CENTER
NEW YORK PRESBYTERIAN HOSPITAL,
COLUMBIA UNIVERSITY MEDICAL CENTER

Address: PH 18, Room 200
622 West 168th Street
New York, NY 10032
Telephone: 212-305-2500 (Main number for Columbia University Medical Center)
1-877-697-9355 (24 hours) (Physician Referrals)
Web site: http://hiccc.columbia.edu/

The Herbert Irving Comprehensive Cancer Center is a National Cancer Institute (NCI)-designated Comprehensive Cancer Center that conducts research and provides services directly to cancer patients. Comprehensive Cancer Centers also conduct activities in outreach and education, and provide information on health care advances to both health care professionals and the public. An NCI-designated Cancer Center must meet a series of competitive requirements and demonstrate excellence in cancer research. For more general information about the Cancer Centers Program of NCI, please visit http://cancercenters.cancer.gov/ on the Internet.

*MEMORIAL SLOAN-KETTERING CANCER CENTER

Address: 1275 York Avenue
New York, NY 10065
Telephone: 212-639-2000 (General)
1-800-525-2225 (Physician Referral)
Web site: http://www.mskcc.org

The Memorial Sloan-Kettering Cancer Center is a National Cancer Institute (NCI)-designated Comprehensive Cancer Center that conducts research and provides services directly to cancer patients. Comprehensive Cancer Centers also conduct activities in outreach and education, and provide information on health care advances to both health care professionals and the public. An NCI-designated Cancer Center must meet a series of competitive requirements and demonstrate excellence in cancer research. For more general information about the Cancer Centers Program of NCI, please visit http://cancercenters.cancer.gov/ on the Internet.

NEW YORK UNIVERSITY CANCER INSTITUTE

Address:	NYU Clinical Cancer Center
	160 E 34th St
	New York, NY 10016
Telephone:	212-731-6000 (Main)
	1-888-769-8633 (Physician Referral)
Web site:	http://ci.med.nyu.edu/

The New York University Cancer Institute is a National Cancer Institute (NCI)-designated Cancer Center that conducts research and provides services directly to cancer patients. An NCI-designated Cancer Center must meet a series of competitive requirements and demonstrate excellence in cancer research. For more general information about the Cancer Centers Program of NCI, please visit http://cancercenters.cancer.gov/ on the Internet.

*ROSWELL PARK CANCER INSTITUTE

Address:	Elm and Carlton Streets
	Buffalo, NY 14263
Telephone:	716-845-2300 (Main)
	1-800-767-9355 (1-800-ROSWELL)
E-mail:	askrpci@roswellpark.org
Web site:	http://www.roswellpark.org/Home

The Roswell Park Cancer Institute is a National Cancer Institute (NCI)-designated Comprehensive Cancer Center that conducts research and provides services directly to cancer patients. Comprehensive Cancer Centers also conduct activities in outreach and education, and provide information on health care advances to both health care professionals and the public. An NCI-designated Cancer Center must meet a series of competitive requirements and demonstrate excellence in cancer research. For more general information about the Cancer Centers Program of NCI, please visit http://cancercenters.cancer.gov/ on the Internet.

NORTH CAROLINA

---

*DUKE COMPREHENSIVE CANCER CENTER
DUKE UNIVERSITY MEDICAL CENTER

Address:	Hock Plaza Suite 601
	2424 Erwin Road
	Durham, NC 27705
Telephone:	919-684-3377 (administrative offices)
	1-888-275-3853 (1-888-ASK-DUKE) (Consultation and Referral Service)
Web site:	http://www.cancer.duke.edu/

The Duke Comprehensive Cancer Center is a National Cancer Institute (NCI)-designated Comprehensive Cancer Center that conducts research and provides services directly to cancer patients. Comprehensive Cancer Centers also conduct activities in outreach and education, and provide information on health care advances to both health care professionals and the public. An NCI-designated Cancer Center must meet a series of competitive requirements and demonstrate excellence in cancer research. For more general information about the Cancer Centers Program of NCI, please visit http://cancercenters.cancer.gov/ on the Internet.

*UNC LINEBERGER COMPREHENSIVE CANCER CENTER
UNIVERSITY OF NORTH CAROLINA AT CHAPEL HILL

Address:	School of Medicine Campus Box #7295
	450 West Drive
	Chapel Hill, NC 27599
Telephone:	919-966-3036 (Main)
	1-866-828-0270 (Information or Appointments)
	1-877-668-0683 (Clinical Trials Information)
E-mail:	lccc@med.un.edu
Web site:	http://cancer.med.unc.edu/

The UNC Lineberger Comprehensive Cancer Center is a National Cancer Institute (NCI)-designated Comprehensive Cancer Center that conducts research and provides services directly to cancer patients. Comprehensive Cancer Centers also conduct activities in outreach and education, and provide information on health care advances to both health care professionals and the public. An NCI-designated Cancer Center must meet a series of competitive requirements and demonstrate excellence in cancer research. For more general information about the Cancer Centers Program of NCI, please visit http://cancercenters.cancer.gov/ on the Internet.

*WAKE FOREST UNIVERSITY COMPREHENSIVE CANCER CENTER
WAKE FOREST UNIVERSITY

Address:	Medical Center Boulevard
	Winston-Salem, NC 27157
Telephone:	336-716-4464
Web site:	http://www1.wfubmc.edu/cancer

The Wake Forest University Comprehensive Cancer Center is a National Cancer Institute (NCI)-designated Comprehensive Cancer Center that conducts research and provides services directly to cancer patients. Comprehensive Cancer Centers also conduct activities in outreach and education, and provide information on health care advances to both health care professionals and the public. An NCI-designated Cancer Center must meet a series of competitive requirements and demonstrate excellence in cancer research. For more general information about the Cancer Centers Program of NCI, please visit http://cancercenters.cancer.gov/ on the Internet.

OHIO

---

*CASE COMPREHENSIVE CANCER CENTER
CASE WESTERN RESERVE UNIVERSITY

Address:	11100 Euclid Avenue
	Cleveland, OH 44106
Telephone:	1-800-641-2422 (Phone greeting may say Ireland Cancer Center)
E-mail:	cancer@case.edu
Web site:	http://cancer.case.edu/

Case Comprehensive Cancer Center of the Case Western Reserve University is a National Cancer Institute (NCI)-designated Comprehensive Cancer Center that conducts research and provides services directly to cancer patients. Comprehensive Cancer Centers also conduct activities in outreach and education, and provide information on health care advances to both health care professionals and the public. An NCI-designated Cancer Center must meet a series of competitive requirements and demonstrate excellence in cancer research. For more general information about the Cancer Centers Program of NCI, please visit http://cancercenters.cancer.gov/ on the Internet.

*THE OHIO STATE UNIVERSITY COMPREHENSIVE CANCER CENTER (OSUCCC - JAMES)
JAMES CANCER HOSPITAL AND SOLOVE RESEARCH INSTITUTE

Address:	Suite 519
	300 West 10th Avenue
	Columbus, OH 43210
Telephone:	614-293-5066
	1-800-293-5066
E-mail:	jamesline@osumc.edu
Web site:	http://www.jamesline.com/

The Ohio State University Comprehensive Cancer Center at the James Cancer Hospital and Solove Research Institute is a National Cancer Institute (NCI)-designated Comprehensive Cancer Center that conducts research and provides services directly to cancer patients. Comprehensive Cancer Centers also conduct activities in outreach and education, and provide information on health care advances to both health care professionals and the public. An NCI-designated Cancer Center must meet a series of competitive requirements and demonstrate excellence in cancer research. For more general information about the Cancer Centers Program of NCI, please visit http://cancercenters.cancer.gov/ on the Internet.

OREGON

OHSU KNIGHT CANCER INSTITUTE
OREGON HEALTH AND SCIENCE UNIVERSITY

Address:	Oregon Health and Science University
	3181 SW Sam Jackson Park Road, CR145
	Portland, OR 97239
Telephone:	503-494-1617 (Cancer Institute)
	503-494-8311 (Health Care Services and OHSU switchboard)
	1-888-222-6478 (Main operator at OHSU)
E-mail:	cancer@ohsu.edu
Web site:	http://ohsucancer.com

The OHSU Knight Cancer Institute is a National Cancer Institute (NCI)-designated Cancer Center that conducts research and provides services directly to cancer patients. An NCI-designated Cancer Center must meet a series of competitive requirements and demonstrate excellence in cancer research. For more general information about the Cancer Centers Program of NCI, please visit http://cancercenters.cancer.gov/ on the Internet. The OHSU Cancer Institute Web site offers a listing of staff doctors by cancer specialty.

*ABRAMSON CANCER CENTER OF THE UNIVERSITY OF PENNSYLVANIA

Address: Penn Tower, 16th Floor
             3400 Spruce Street
             Philadelphia, PA
Telephone: 215-662-4000 (main number)
             1-800-789-7366 (medical referrals)
Web site: http://www.penncancer.org

The Abramson Cancer Center of the University of Pennsylvania is a National Cancer Institute (NCI)-designated Comprehensive Cancer Center that conducts research and provides services directly to cancer patients. Comprehensive Cancer Centers also conduct activities in outreach and education, and provide information on health care advances to both health care professionals and the public. An NCI-designated Cancer Center must meet a series of competitive requirements and demonstrate excellence in cancer research. For more general information about the Cancer Centers Program of NCI, please visit http://cancercenters.cancer.gov/ on the Internet.

*FOX CHASE CANCER CENTER

Address: 333 Cottman Avenue
             Philadelphia, PA 19111
Telephone: 215-728-2570 (Appointment scheduling)
             1-888-369-2427 (1-888-FOX-CHASE) (Cancer information)
Web site: http://www.fccc.edu/

The Fox Chase Cancer Center is a National Cancer Institute (NCI)-designated Comprehensive Cancer Center that conducts research and provides services directly to cancer patients. Comprehensive Cancer Centers also conduct activities in outreach and education, and provide information on health care advances to both health care professionals and the public. An NCI-designated Cancer Center must meet a series of competitive requirements and demonstrate excellence in cancer research. For more general information about the Cancer Centers Program of NCI, please visit http://cancercenters.cancer.gov/ on the Internet.

KIMMEL CANCER CENTER
THOMAS JEFFERSON UNIVERSITY HOSPITAL

Address: 233 South 10th Street
             Philadelphia, PA 19107
Telephone: 1-888-955-1212 (Kimmel Cancer Center)
             1-800-533-3669 (1-800-JEFF-NOW) (Physician Referral)
Web site: http://www.kimmelcancercenter.org/

The Kimmel Cancer Center, based at Thomas Jefferson University, is a National Cancer Institute (NCI)-designated Cancer Center that conducts research and provides services directly to cancer patients. Cancer Centers also conduct activities in outreach and education, and provide information on health care advances to both health care professionals and the public. An NCI-designated Cancer Center must meet a series of competitive requirements and demonstrate excellence in cancer research. For more general information about the Cancer Centers Program of NCI, please visit http://cancercenters.cancer.gov/ on the Internet.

*UNIVERSITY OF PITTSBURGH CANCER INSTITUTE
UNIVERSITY OF PITTSBURGH MEDICAL CENTER,
HILLMAN CANCER CENTER

Address:	5150 Centre Avenue
	Pittsburgh, PA 15232
Telephone:	412-647-2811
E-mail:	PCI-INFO@upmc.edu
Web site:	http://www.upci.upmc.edu/

The University of Pittsburgh Cancer Institute, based at the University of Pittsburgh Medical Center, is a National Cancer Institute (NCI)-designated Comprehensive Cancer Center that conducts research and provides services directly to cancer patients. Comprehensive Cancer Centers also conduct activities in outreach and education, and provide information on health care advances to both health care professionals and the public. An NCI-designated Cancer Center must meet a series of competitive requirements and demonstrate excellence in cancer research. For more general information about the Cancer Centers Program of NCI, please visit http://cancercenters.cancer.gov/ on the Internet.

SOUTH CAROLINA

HOLLINGS CANCER CENTER
MEDICAL UNIVERSITY OF SOUTH CAROLINA

Address:	Post Office Box 250955
	86 Jonathan Lucas Street
	Charleston, SC 29425
Telephone:	843-792-9300 (Patient Care and Appointments)
	843-792-2200 (Physician Referral)
	1-800-424-6872 (1-800-424-MUSC) (Health Care Connection)
	1-800-922-5250 (Physician Referral)
Web site:	http://hcc.musc.edu/

Hollings Cancer Center is a National Cancer Institute (NCI)-designated Cancer Center that conducts research and provides services directly to cancer patients. An NCI-designated Cancer Center must meet a series of competitive requirements and demonstrate excellence in cancer research. For more general information about the Cancer Centers Program of NCI please visit http://cancercenters.cancer.gov/ on the Internet.

Appendix D

*ST. JUDE CHILDREN'S RESEARCH HOSPITAL

Address:	262 Danny Thomas Place
	Memphis, TN 38105
Telephone:	901-595-3300 (General Information)
	1-866-278-5833 (Physician Referrals)
Web site:	http://www.stjude.org

The St. Jude Children's Research Hospital is a National Cancer Institute (NCI)-designated Comprehensive Cancer Center that conducts research and provides services directly to cancer patients. Comprehensive Cancer Centers also conduct activities in outreach and education, and provide information on healthcare advances to both healthcare professionals and the public. An NCI-designated Cancer Center must meet a series of competitive requirements and demonstrate excellence in cancer research. For more general information about the Cancer Centers Program of NCI please visit http://cancercenters.cancer.gov/ on the Internet.

*THE VANDERBILT-INGRAM CANCER CENTER
VANDERBILT UNIVERSITY MEDICAL CENTER

Address:	691 Preston Research Building
	Nashville, TN 37232
Telephone:	615-936-5847 (Clinical Trials or Treatment Options)
	615-936-1782 (Admin.)
	1-800-811-8480 (Clinical Trials or Treatment Options)
Web site:	http://www.vicc.org/

The Vanderbilt-Ingram Cancer Center is a National Cancer Institute (NCI)-designated Comprehensive Cancer Center that conducts research and provides services directly to cancer patients. Comprehensive Cancer Centers also conduct activities in outreach and education, and provide information on health care advances to both health care professionals and the public. An NCI-designated Cancer Center must meet a series of competitive requirements and demonstrate excellence in cancer research. For more general information about the Cancer Centers Program of NCI, please visit http://cancercenters.cancer.gov/ on the Internet.

CANCER THERAPY & RESEARCH CENTER (CTRC)
UNIVERSITY OF TEXAS HEALTH SCIENCE AT SAN ANTONIO

Address:	7979 Wurzbach Road
	San Antonio, TX 78229
Telephone:	210-450-5798 (Clinical Trial Referral Office)
	210-450-1000 (Main Operator)
	1-800-340-2872 (Main Operator)
Web site:	www.ctrc.net

The Cancer Therapy & Research Center at the University of Texas Health Science Center at San Antonio is a National Cancer Institute (NCI)-designated Cancer Center that conducts research and provides services directly to cancer patients. An NCI-designated Cancer Center must meet a series of competitive requirements and demonstrate excellence in cancer research. For more general information about the Cancer Centers Program of NCI, please visit http://cancercenters.cancer.gov/ on the Internet.

THE DAN L. DUNCAN CANCER CENTER
BAYLOR COLLEGE OF MEDICINE

Address:	One Baylor Plaza
	MS: BCM305
	Houston, TX 77030
Telephone:	713-798-1354
Web site:	http://www.bcm.edu/cancercenter/

The Dan L. Duncan Cancer Center at Baylor College of Medicine is a National Cancer Institute (NCI)-designated Cancer Center that conducts research and provides services directly to cancer patients. An NCI-designated Cancer Center must meet a series of competitive requirements and demonstrate excellence in cancer research. For more general information about the Cancer Centers Program of NCI, please visit http://cancercenters.cancer.gov/ on the Internet.

*THE UNIVERSITY OF TEXAS M.D. ANDERSON CANCER CENTER

Address:	1515 Holcombe Boulevard
	Houston, TX 77030
Telephone:	713-792-2121
	1-877-632-6789 (Patient Referral)
	1-800-392-1611 (Main)
	001-713-745-0450 (International)
Web site:	http://www.mdanderson.org/

The University of Texas M.D. Anderson Cancer Center is a National Cancer Institute (NCI)-designated Comprehensive Cancer Center that conducts research and provides services directly to cancer patients. Comprehensive Cancer Centers also conduct activities in outreach and education, and provide information on health care advances to both health care professionals and the public. An NCI-designated Cancer Center must meet a series of competitive requirements and demonstrate excellence in cancer research. For more general information about the Cancer Centers Program of NCI, please visit http://cancercenters.cancer.gov/ on the Internet.

UTAH

HUNTSMAN CANCER INSTITUTE
UNIVERSITY OF UTAH

Address:	2000 Circle of Hope
	Salt Lake City, UT 84112
Telephone:	801-585-0303
	1-877-585-0303 (Main)
	1-888-424-2100 (Cancer Information and Referrals)
E-mail:	patient.education@hci.utah.edu
Web site:	http://www.hci.utah.edu/

The Huntsman Cancer Institute is a National Cancer Institute (NCI)-designated Cancer Center that conducts research and provides services directly to cancer patients. An NCI-designated Cancer Center must meet a series of competitive requirements and demonstrate excellence in cancer research. For more general information about the Cancer Centers Program of NCI, please visit http://cancercenters.cancer.gov/ on the Internet.

VIRGINIA

MASSEY CANCER CENTER
VIRGINIA COMMONWEALTH UNIVERSITY

Address:	Post Office Box 980037
	401 College Street
	Richmond, VA 23298
Telephone:	804-828-0450 (General Information)
	804-828-5116 (New Patients)
	1-877-462-7739 (1-877-4-MASSEY)
E-mail:	askmassey@vcu.edu
Web site:	http://www.massey.vcu.edu/

The Massey Cancer Center is a National Cancer Institute (NCI)-designated Cancer Center that conducts research and provides services directly to cancer patients. An NCI-designated Cancer Center must meet a series of competitive requirements and demonstrate excellence in cancer research. For more general information about the Cancer Centers Program of NCI, please visit http://cancercenters.cancer.gov/ on the Internet.

UNIVERSITY OF VIRGINIA CANCER CENTER (UVA CANCER CENTER)
UNIVERSITY OF VIRGINIA HEALTH SCIENCE CENTER

Address:	1222 Jefferson Park Avenue
	PO Box 800834
	Charlottesville, VA 22908
Telephone:	434-924-9333
	1-800-223-9173
Web site:	http://www.uvacancer.com

The University of Virginia Cancer Center is a National Cancer Institute (NCI)-designated Cancer Center that conducts research and provides services directly to cancer patients. An NCI-designated Cancer Center must meet a series of competitive requirements and demonstrate excellence in cancer research. For more general information about the Cancer Centers Program of NCI, please visit http://cancercenters.cancer.gov/ on the Internet.

WASHINGTON

*FRED HUTCHINSON CANCER RESEARCH CENTER (FHCRC, SCCA)
SEATTLE CANCER CARE ALLIANCE

Address:	LA-205, Post Office Box 19024
	1100 Fairview Avenue North
	Seattle, WA 98109
Telephone:	206-288-7222 (SCCA)
E-mail:	hutchdoc@seattlecca.org
Web site:	http://www.fhcrc.org/

The Fred Hutchinson Cancer Research Center is a National Cancer Institute (NCI)-designated Comprehensive Cancer Center that conducts research and provides services directly to cancer patients. Comprehensive Cancer Centers also conduct activities in outreach and education, and provide information on health care advances to both health care professionals and the public. An NCI-designated Cancer Center must meet a series of competitive requirements and demonstrate excellence in cancer research. For more general information about the Cancer Centers Program of NCI, please visit http://cancercenters.cancer.gov/ on the Internet.

WISCONSIN

*UNIVERSITY OF WISCONSIN
PAUL P. CARBONE COMPREHENSIVE CANCER CENTER

Address:	600 Highland Avenue
	K5/601
	Madison, WI 53792
Telephone:	608-263-6400 (General information)
	800-323-8942 (Cancer Connect)
E-mail:	uwccc@uwccc.wisc.edu
Web site:	http://www.cancer.wisc.edu

Appendix D

The University of Wisconsin Paul P. Carbone Comprehensive Cancer Center is a National Cancer Institute (NCI)-designated Comprehensive Cancer Center that conducts research and provides services directly to cancer patients. Comprehensive Cancer Centers also conduct activities in outreach and education, and provide information on health care advances to both health care professionals and the public. An NCI-designated Cancer Center must meet a series of competitive requirements and demonstrate excellence in cancer research. For more general information about the Cancer Centers Program of NCI, please visit http://cancercenters.cancer.gov/ on the Internet.

Appendix E:
Sources of Quality Data on Hospitals

U.S. NEWS AND WORLD REPORT

U.S. News & World Report and Castle Connolly created a strategic collaboration that will bring the Castle Connolly Top Doctors® database to online visitors of the U.S. News website. The online database went live on www.usnews.com in mid-July 2011 and will be linked with the U.S. News database of Best Hospitals. This annual feature on Best Hospitals has become the standard in the field where rankings are concerned and is heavily anticipated and utilized by consumers and members of the healthcare professions. Consumers will be able to search the full database of Top Doctors across the nation, including all specialties and subspecialties. The detailed physician profiles, including designation of doctors affiliated with Castle Connolly's Partnership for Excellence hospital program, will be drawn from Castle Connolly's growing database of over 30,000 physicians currently accessible online at www.castleconnolly.com

WWW.WHYNOTTHEBEST.ORG

WhyNotTheBest.org was created and is maintained by The Commonwealth Fund, a private foundation working toward a high performance health system. It is a free resource for health care professionals and consumers interested in tracking performance on various measures of health care quality. It enables organizations to compare their performance against that of peer organizations, against a range of benchmarks and over a given period of time. Case studies and improvement tools spotlight successful improvement strategies of the nation's top performers. A regional map shows performance at the county, state and national levels. This site also includes process-of-care measures, patient satisfaction measures, readmission rates, mortality rates and average reimbursement rates. All of these performance measures are publicly reported on the Centers for Medicare and Medicaid Services website, Hospital Compare, and include data from nearly all U.S. hospitals.

THE LEAPFROG GROUP

The Leapfrog Group, http://www.leapfroggroup.org/cp, started in 1998 by a group of large employers. The Leapfrog Hospital Survey compares hospitals' performance on the national standards of safety, quality and efficiency - areas of healthcare that are most relevant to consumers. Hospitals that participate in The Leapfrog Hospital Survey achieve hospital-wide improvements that translate into saving millions of lives and cutting costs for hospitals and consumers. Leapfrog's survey results are later used to inform key employees on purchasing strategies.

HOSPITAL COMPARE

The Hospital Compare website was created through the efforts of the Centers for Medicare & Medicaid Services (CMS), an agency of the U.S. Department of Health and Human Services (DHHS), along with the Hospital Quality Alliance (HQA). The HQA was established to promote reporting on hospital quality of care. The HQA consists of organizations that represent consumers, hospitals, doctors and nurses, employers, accrediting organizations and Federal agencies. The information on this website can be used by patients requiring hospital care. This information helps the consumer and health care providers to compare the quality of care provided in participating hospitals. This information not only helps one to make good decisions about health care, but also encourages hospitals to improve the quality of the care that they provide to their communities. This website can be found at: http://www.hospitalcompare.hhs.gov/hospital-search.aspx or http://bit.ly/jdvCzW

Section V
Indices

The Best in American Medicine
www.CastleConnolly.com

Subject Index

A

America's Top Doctors 11, 12, 15, 53

American Board of Medical Specialties (ABMS) 19, 57, 58, 64, 65

American Cancer Society 4

American Osteopathic Association (AOA) 19

Lance Armstrong 9

B

Board Certification 10, 19, 20, 21, 22, 53, 57, 65

Jane E. Brody 4

C

Centers for Disease Control and Prevention 4

CenterWatch 39

Clinical trials 37-45, 47-50

Consultation 31, 32, 33, 35

Continuing medical education 21

D

Directory of Graduate Medical Education Programs 18

F

Faculty Appointment 24, 53

Fellowship 19, 21, 22, 25, 26, 53

Food and Drug Administration 41

Foreign Medical Graduates 17

Friends of Cancer Research 15

J

Joint Commission on Accreditation of Healthcare Organizations 23

L

Liaison Committee for Medical Education (LCME) 16

M

Malpractice insurance 23

Managed care 7

Mark O. Hatfield Clinical Research Center 46

Medical College Admissions Tests 16

Medical records 32, 33, 35, 41, 46

N

National Cancer Institute (NCI) 4, 15, 39, 43, 47, 48, 50

National Institutes of Health (NIH) 3, 37, 39, 45

The New York Times 4

North American Association of Central Cancer Registries 4

Northwestern University 26

P

Partnership for Excellence Program 67

Primary care physician 7, 8, 11, 16, 29

Professional Reputation 22

R

S

T

U

V

W

The Best in American Medicine
www.CastleConnolly.com

Special Expertise Index

This index lists the areas that the physicians listed in the Guide have identified as their "special expertise." These are not medical specialties. They are specific elements of disease, procedures, techniques and treatments for which these physicians are best known and are referred patients.

Spec	Name	St	Pg

A

Abdominal Imaging

Spec	Name	St	Pg
DR	Coakley, F	CA	411
DR	Fishman, E	MD	408
DR	Levy, A	DC	408
DR	Weinreb, J	CT	407
DR	Zagoria, R	NC	410

Abdominal Wall Reconstruction

Spec	Name	St	Pg
PlS	Stahl, R	CT	366

Adrenal Cancer

Spec	Name	St	Pg
EDM	Daniels, G	MA	110
EDM	Hammer, G	MI	111
Onc	Oh, W	NY	161
Onc	Quinn, D	CA	203
PHO	Wolfe, L	NY	340
S	Solorzano, C	TN	444

Adrenal Pathology

Spec	Name	St	Pg
Path	Weiss, L	CA	329

Adrenal Tumors

Spec	Name	St	Pg
S	Angelos, P	IL	445
S	Brunt, L	MO	446
S	Butler, J	CA	457
S	Duh, Q	CA	458
S	Grant, C	MN	447
S	Hanna, N	MD	435
S	Hodin, R	MA	429
S	Schulick, R	MD	438
S	Udelsman, R	CT	431
U	Donovan, J	OH	495
U	Libertino, J	MA	484
U	Sundaram, C	IN	498

AIDS Related Cancers

Spec	Name	St	Pg
Hem	Levine, A	CA	140
Inf	Palefsky, J	CA	513
Inf	Polsky, B	NY	513
Onc	Aboulafia, D	WA	196
Onc	Abrams, D	CA	197
Onc	Ambinder, R	MD	149
Onc	Henry, D	PA	156
Onc	Kaplan, L	CA	201
Onc	Mitsuyasu, R	CA	202
Onc	Remick, S	WV	162
Onc	Volberding, P	CA	205

Spec	Name	St	Pg
Onc	Von Roenn, J	IL	187
Psyc	Breitbart, W	NY	374

Airway Reconstruction

Spec	Name	St	Pg
Oto	Couch, M	VT	290
Oto	Genden, E	NY	291

Anaemia-Aplastic

Spec	Name	St	Pg
Hem	Dang, C	MD	128

Anal Cancer

Spec	Name	St	Pg
CRS	Dietz, D	OH	90
CRS	Fry, R	PA	87
CRS	Geisler, D	PA	88
CRS	Gorfine, S	NY	88
CRS	Nagle, D	MA	86
CRS	Welton, M	CA	94
DR	Coakley, F	CA	411
Onc	Berry, J	CA	197

Anal Disorders & Reconstruction

Spec	Name	St	Pg
CRS	Blatchford, G	NE	92
CRS	Marcet, J	FL	89
CRS	Rafferty, J	OH	92

Anal Sphincter Repair

Spec	Name	St	Pg
CRS	Wexner, S	FL	90

Anemia-Aplastic

Spec	Name	St	Pg
Hem	Maciejewski, J	OH	136
Hem	Mangan, K	PA	129
Onc	Claxton, D	PA	151
PHO	Boxer, L	MI	346
PHO	Camitta, B	WI	346
PHO	Wang, W	TN	345

Anemia-Cancer Related

Spec	Name	St	Pg
Hem	Rodgers, G	UT	137
Hem	Schiffman, F	RI	127
Hem	Wisch, N	NY	131

Anemias & Red Cell Disorders

Spec	Name	St	Pg
PHO	Boxer, L	MI	346
PHO	Finklestein, J	CA	353
PHO	Thomas, G	OR	355

Anorectal Disorders

Spec	Name	St	Pg
CRS	Church, J	OH	90
CRS	Efron, J	MD	87
CRS	Eisenstat, T	NJ	87
CRS	Fry, R	PA	87
CRS	Heppell, J	AZ	93
CRS	Read, T	MA	86
CRS	Senagore, A	CA	94
CRS	Shellito, P	MA	87
CRS	Stamos, M	CA	94
CRS	Stein, D	PA	89
CRS	Wise, P	TN	90

Appendix Cancer

Spec	Name	St	Pg
S	Bartlett, D	PA	432
S	Mansfield, P	TX	455
S	Paty, P	NY	437
S	Sugarbaker, P	DC	439

Autoimmune Disease

Spec	Name	St	Pg
Hem	Brodsky, R	MD	128

B

Barrett's Esophagus

Spec	Name	St	Pg
Ge	Estores, D	FL	119
Ge	Fleischer, D	AZ	121
Ge	Gerdes, H	NY	116
Ge	Greenwald, B	MD	117
Ge	Lightdale, C	NY	118
Ge	Ravich, W	MD	118
Ge	Savides, T	CA	122
Path	Montgomery, E	MD	319
S	Nava-Villarreal, H	NY	436
TS	Battafarano, R	MD	471
TS	Ferguson, M	IL	476

Biliary Cancer

Spec	Name	St	Pg
Onc	O'Reilly, E	NY	161
Onc	Patt, Y	NM	195
Onc	Posey, J	AL	175
Onc	Yen, Y	CA	206
S	Bouvet, M	CA	457
S	Cameron, J	MD	432
S	Chari, R	TN	441
S	Drebin, J	PA	433
S	Ellison, E	OH	447

Special Expertise Index

Special Expertise Index

America's Top Doctors® for Cancer 7th Edition

Special Expertise Index

Special Expertise Index

Spec	Name	St	Pg
GO	Siller, B	TX	263
GO	Smith, D	IL	261
GO	Soisson, A	UT	262
GO	Valea, F	NC	259
GO	Van Nagell, J	KY	259
GO	Waggoner, S	OH	261
GO	Walker, J	OK	264
ObG	Argenta, P	MN	266
ObG	Lengyel, E	IL	267
Onc	Scudder, S	CA	204
Path	Cho, K	MI	323
Path	Gupta, P	PA	318
RadRO	Eifel, P	TX	402

Chemo-Radiation Combined Therapy

RadRO	Cooper, J	NY	387
RadRO	Formenti, S	NY	388
RadRO	Rich, T	VA	396

Chemoembolization & Tumor Ablation

VIR	Weintraub, J	NY	415

Chest Wall Reconstruction

PlS	Stahl, R	CT	366
PlS	Yuen, J	AR	370

Chest Wall Tumors

TS	Cerfolio, R	AL	474
TS	Handy, J	OR	480
TS	Kiev, J	MD	472
TS	Marshall, M	DC	473
TS	Naunheim, K	MO	477
TS	Shrager, J	CA	480
TS	Whyte, R	CA	480

Children/Families with Severe Illness

Psyc	Rauch, P	MA	374

Clinical Trials

D	Bowen, G	UT	105
Ge	Gish, R	CA	121
Ge	Greenwald, B	MD	117
Ge	Okolo, P	MD	118
GO	Chan, J	CA	264
GO	Cornelison, T	MD	252
GO	Coukos, G	PA	253
GO	De Geest, K	IA	259
GO	Edwards, R	PA	253
GO	Follen, M	PA	254
GO	Ghamande, S	GA	257
GO	Odunsi, A	NY	255
GO	Stehman, F	IN	261
GO	Teng, N	CA	266
Hem	Djulbegovic, B	FL	132

Spec	Name	St	Pg
Hem	Flynn, P	MN	134
Hem	Greer, J	TN	132
Hem	Grever, M	OH	135
Hem	Komrokji, R	FL	132
Hem	Kraut, E	OH	135
Hem	Maddox, A	AR	139
Hem	Maslak, P	NY	129
Hem	Nademanee, A	CA	141
Hem	O'Donnell, M	CA	141
Hem	Slease, R	DE	130
Hem	Streiff, M	MD	131
N	Chamberlain, M	WA	245
N	Janss, A	GA	243
N	Newton, H	OH	244
NS	Brem, S	FL	228
NS	Markert, J	AL	228
NS	Sampson, J	NC	229
NS	Shaffrey, M	VA	230
NS	Yu, J	CA	238
Onc	Abbruzzese, J	TX	190
Onc	Advani, R	CA	197
Onc	Akerley, W	UT	188
Onc	Arun, B	TX	191
Onc	Berlin, J	TN	167
Onc	Bernard, S	NC	167
Onc	Birrer, M	MA	142
Onc	Blackwell, K	NC	167
Onc	Blobe, G	NC	167
Onc	Bunn, P	CO	188
Onc	Butler, W	SC	168
Onc	Carducci, M	MD	150
Onc	Chang, J	TX	192
Onc	Chapman, P	NY	151
Onc	Chu, E	PA	151
Onc	Cohen, R	PA	152
Onc	Disis, M	WA	199
Onc	Ellis, G	WA	199
Onc	Ensminger, W	MI	181
Onc	Estey, E	WA	199
Onc	Ettinger, D	MD	154
Onc	Fine, R	NY	154
Onc	Flaherty, K	MA	143
Onc	Friedberg, J	NY	155
Onc	Haas, N	PA	156
Onc	Hauke, R	NE	189
Onc	Hortobagyi, G	TX	193
Onc	Hwu, P	TX	193
Onc	Jurcic, J	NY	157
Onc	Kaminski, M	MI	183
Onc	Karp, J	MD	158
Onc	Kaufman, P	NH	145
Onc	Kraft, A	SC	171
Onc	Limentani, S	NC	172
Onc	Marcom, P	NC	173
Onc	Mortimer, J	CA	202
Onc	O'Connor, O	NY	160
Onc	O'Regan, R	GA	174
Onc	Orlowski, R	TX	194
Onc	Perez, E	FL	174
Onc	Perry, D	DC	162
Onc	Pinto, H	CA	202
Onc	Ready, N	NC	175
Onc	Remick, S	WV	162

Spec	Name	St	Pg
Onc	Robert-Vizcarrondo, F	AL	175
Onc	Schilder, R	PA	163
Onc	Schuchter, L	PA	163
Onc	Serody, J	NC	175
Onc	Shibata, S	CA	204
Onc	Sikic, B	CA	204
Onc	Sotomayor, E	FL	176
Onc	Triozzi, P	OH	187
Onc	Tripathy, D	CA	205
Onc	Wolchok, J	NY	166
Onc	Wolff, R	TX	196
Onc	Worden, F	MI	187
Oto	Weisman, R	CA	305
Path	Wilczynski, S	CA	329
PHO	Adamson, P	PA	334
PHO	Blaney, S	TX	351
PHO	Bruggers, C	UT	350
PHO	Croop, J	IN	346
PHO	Goldman, S	IL	347
PHO	Halligan, G	PA	337
PHO	Jakacki, R	PA	337
PHO	Kreissman, S	NC	343
PHO	Maris, J	PA	338
PHO	Neuberg, R	SC	343
PHO	Razzouk, B	IN	349
PHO	Rheingold, S	PA	339
PHO	Rosenthal, J	CA	354
PHO	van Hoff, J	NH	334
PHO	Vik, T	IN	350
RadRO	Blackstock, A	NC	392
RadRO	Bogart, J	NY	387
RadRO	Bradley, J	MO	397
RadRO	Koh, W	WA	405
RadRO	Le, Q	CA	405
RadRO	McGarry, R	KY	394
RadRO	Schild, S	AZ	404
RadRO	Senzer, N	TX	404
RadRO	Willett, C	NC	397
S	Averbook, B	OH	446
S	Julian, T	PA	435
S	Leeming, R	OH	448
S	Lowy, A	CA	459
S	Meric-Bernstam, F	TX	455
S	Olson, J	NC	443
S	Pockaj, B	AZ	456
S	Sauter, E	ND	453
S	Willey, S	DC	440
S	Yang, J	MD	440
TS	Pass, N	NY	473
U	Keane, T	SC	492
U	Moul, J	NC	493

Clinical Trials Only

Onc	Arlen, P	MD	149
Onc	Gulley, J	MD	156

Cognitive Rehabilitation

PHO	Lange, B	PA	338

Special Expertise Index

Special Expertise Index

Special Expertise Index

Special Expertise Index

Special Expertise Index

Special Expertise Index

Special Expertise Index

Spec	Name	St	Pg
TS	Fernando, H	MA	470
TS	Howington, J	IL	476
TS	Jones, D	VA	475
TS	Krellenstein, D	NY	473
TS	Maddaus, M	MN	477
TS	Mason, D	OH	477
TS	Nesbitt, J	TN	475
TS	Rice, T	OH	478
TS	Sonett, J	NY	474
TS	Weksler, B	PA	474

Minimally Invasive Urologic Surgery

Spec	Name	St	Pg
U	Andrews, P	AZ	499
U	Bagley, D	PA	485
U	Gill, I	CA	502
U	Gluckman, G	IL	496
U	Gomella, L	PA	486
U	Hall, S	NY	487
U	Kaouk, J	OH	496
U	Kawachi, M	CA	502
U	Lanteri, V	NJ	488
U	Miller, S	GA	493
U	Moul, J	NC	493
U	Strup, S	KY	494
U	Trabulsi, E	PA	490
U	Uzzo, R	PA	490

Mohs' Surgery

Spec	Name	St	Pg
D	Amonette, R	TN	101
D	Arpey, C	MN	103
D	Bailin, P	OH	103
D	Bennett, R	CA	106
D	Berg, D	WA	106
D	Bowen, G	UT	105
D	Braun, M	DC	100
D	Brodland, D	PA	100
D	Carney, J	AR	105
D	Cook, J	NC	102
D	Dufresne, R	RI	98
D	Dzubow, L	PA	100
D	Fewkes, J	MA	98
D	Flowers, F	FL	102
D	Fosko, S	MO	104
D	Garrett, A	VA	102
D	Geronemus, R	NY	100
D	Glogau, R	CA	106
D	Green, H	FL	102
D	Greenway, H	CA	107
D	Hanke, C	IN	104
D	Hruza, G	MO	104
D	Johnson, T	MI	104
D	Kriegel, D	NY	100
D	Kriegel, D	NY	100
D	Krunic, A	IL	104
D	Leffell, D	CT	99
D	Leshin, B	NC	103
D	Lim Quan, K	AZ	106
D	Maloney, M	MA	99
D	Miller, S	MD	101
D	Neel, V	MA	99

Spec	Name	St	Pg
D	Neuburg, M	WI	104
D	Nouri, K	FL	103
D	Olbricht, S	MA	99
D	Orengo, I	TX	106
D	Otley, C	MN	105
D	Prioleau, P	NY	101
D	Sober, A	MA	99
D	Swanson, N	OR	107
D	Taylor, R	TX	106
D	Wheeland, R	MO	105
D	Zitelli, J	PA	101

MRI

Spec	Name	St	Pg
DR	Elster, A	NC	410
DR	Zagoria, R	NC	410
NRad	Johnson, A	NC	413
NRad	Sze, G	CT	412

MRI & CT of Brain & Spine

Spec	Name	St	Pg
NRad	Hesselink, J	CA	414

MRI-Breast

Spec	Name	St	Pg
DR	Lehman, C	WA	412

MRI-Functional

Spec	Name	St	Pg
NRad	Faro, S	PA	412

Mucositis

Spec	Name	St	Pg
RadRO	Martenson, J	MN	400

Muir-Torre Syndrome

Spec	Name	St	Pg
D	Olbricht, S	MA	99

Multiple Myeloma

Spec	Name	St	Pg
Hem	Allen, S	NY	127
Hem	Anderson, K	MA	126
Hem	Barlogie, B	AR	138
Hem	Copelan, E	OH	134
Hem	Djulbegovic, B	FL	132
Hem	Emanuel, P	AR	138
Hem	Farag, S	IN	134
Hem	Fonseca, R	AZ	139
Hem	Gertz, M	MN	134
Hem	Goldberg, J	PA	128
Hem	Gregory, S	IL	135
Hem	Greipp, P	MN	135
Hem	Linenberger, M	WA	140
Hem	Lyons, R	TX	139
Hem	Marks, S	PA	129
Hem	Mears, J	NY	129
Hem	Rai, K	NY	129
Hem	Raphael, B	NY	130
Hem	Richardson, P	MA	127
Hem	Roodman, G	PA	130
Hem	Rosenblatt, J	FL	132
Hem	Savage, D	NY	130
Hem	Singhal, S	IL	137

Spec	Name	St	Pg
Hem	Solberg, L	FL	133
Hem	Strair, R	NJ	131
Hem	Williams, M	VA	133
NuM	Wiseman, G	MN	418
Onc	Aboulafia, D	WA	196
Onc	Ball, E	CA	197
Onc	Bensinger, W	WA	197
Onc	Bergsagel, P	AZ	191
Onc	Chanan-Khan, A	NY	151
Onc	Coleman, M	NY	152
Onc	Czuczman, M	NY	152
Onc	Flinn, I	TN	169
Onc	Foss, F	CT	144
Onc	Gerson, S	OH	181
Onc	Jillella, A	GA	171
Onc	Kwak, L	TX	193
Onc	Limentani, S	NC	172
Onc	O'Brien, T	OH	184
Onc	Orlowski, R	TX	194
Onc	Schiffer, C	MI	186
Onc	Silverman, L	NY	163
Onc	Smith, M	PA	163
Onc	Stadtmauer, E	PA	164
Onc	Straus, D	NY	164
Onc	Treon, S	MA	147
Onc	Vescio, R	CA	205
Onc	Wingard, J	FL	178
Onc	Yunus, F	TN	178
OrS	Biermann, J	MI	283
RadRO	Meredith, R	AL	395
RadRO	Wong, J	CA	407
RadRO	Yahalom, J	NY	391

Musculoskeletal Tumor Imaging

Spec	Name	St	Pg
DR	Panicek, D	NY	409

Musculoskeletal Tumors

Spec	Name	St	Pg
OrS	Berrey, B	FL	282
OrS	Bos, G	WA	286
OrS	Gebhardt, M	MA	280
OrS	Henshaw, R	DC	281
OrS	Kneisl, J	NC	282
OrS	Luck, J	CA	286
OrS	Mayerson, J	OH	284
OrS	Mott, M	MI	284
OrS	Schwartz, H	TN	283
OrS	Wittig, J	NY	282

Myelodysplastic Syndromes

Spec	Name	St	Pg
Hem	Baer, M	MD	127
Hem	Copelan, E	OH	134
Hem	Cortes, J	TX	138
Hem	Erba, H	MI	134
Hem	Greer, J	TN	132
Hem	Isola, L	NY	128
Hem	Komrokji, R	FL	132
Hem	Larson, R	IL	136
Hem	Lyons, R	TX	139
Hem	Maslak, P	NY	129
Hem	Miller, K	MA	127

America's Top Doctors® for Cancer 7th Edition

Special Expertise Index

Special Expertise Index

Special Expertise Index

Special Expertise Index

Special Expertise Index

Spec	Name	St	Pg
OrS	Wurtz, L	IN	285
Path	Brooks, J	PA	317
Path	Fletcher, C	MA	316
Path	Goldblum, J	OH	323
Path	Patchefsky, A	PA	319
Path	Rubin, B	OH	324
Path	Triche, T	CA	329
Path	Weiss, S	GA	322
PHO	Albritton, K	TX	351
PHO	Arndt, C	MN	345
PHO	Marina, N	CA	354
PHO	Meyer, W	OK	352
PHO	Meyers, P	NY	339
PHO	Olson, T	GA	344
PHO	Williams, J	AZ	352
PlS	Rockwell, W	UT	370
RadRO	Brizel, D	NC	392
RadRO	Constine, L	NY	387
RadRO	DeLaney, T	MA	385
RadRO	Donaldson, S	CA	404
RadRO	Hahn, S	PA	389
RadRO	Herman, T	OK	403
RadRO	Marcus, R	FL	394
RadRO	Michalski, J	MO	400
RadRO	Pollack, A	FL	395
RadRO	Prosnitz, L	NC	395
RadRO	Tepper, J	NC	396
RadRO	Wara, W	CA	407
RadRO	Wolfson, A	FL	397
S	Brennan, M	NY	432
S	Brown, C	IL	446
S	Dooley, W	OK	453
S	Eilber, F	CA	458
S	Eisenberg, B	NH	428
S	Feig, B	TX	454
S	Fraker, D	PA	434
S	Leitch, A	TX	455
S	Levine, E	NC	442
S	Li, B	LA	455
S	Lind, D	GA	442
S	Nakakura, E	CA	460
S	Nathanson, S	MI	449
S	Pollock, R	TX	456
S	Sondak, V	FL	444
S	Weber, S	WI	451
S	White, R	NC	445

Sarcoma-Soft Tissue

Spec	Name	St	Pg
Onc	Chow, W	CA	198
Onc	Forscher, C	CA	200
Onc	Maki, R	NY	159
Onc	Stockdale, F	CA	204
OrS	Benevenia, J	NJ	280
OrS	Healey, J	NY	281
OrS	Irwin, R	MI	284
OrS	Mayerson, J	OH	284
OrS	O'Donnell, R	CA	286
OrS	Randall, R	UT	285
OrS	Ready, J	MA	280
OrS	Schmidt, R	PA	282
OrS	Wittig, J	NY	282
PHO	Wexler, L	NY	340

Spec	Name	St	Pg
RadRO	Landry, J	GA	393
RadRO	Pezner, R	CA	405
RadRO	Wharam, M	MD	391
S	August, D	NJ	431
S	Hanna, N	MD	435
S	Heslin, M	AL	442
S	Hunt, K	TX	454
S	Pisters, P	TX	456
TS	Putnam, J	TN	476

Sentinel Node Surgery

Spec	Name	St	Pg
Oto	Pitman, K	MS	296
S	Essner, R	CA	458
S	Giuliano, A	CA	458
S	Hansen, N	IL	448
S	Klimberg, V	AR	454
S	Krag, D	VT	429
S	Nowak, E	NY	436
S	O'Hea, B	NY	437
S	Ross, M	TX	456
S	Saha, S	MI	450
S	Swistel, A	NY	439
S	Tartter, P	NY	439

Sex Cord-Stromal Tumors

Spec	Name	St	Pg
GO	Gershenson, D	TX	263

Shoulder Tumors

Spec	Name	St	Pg
OrS	Wittig, J	NY	282

Sinus Disorders/Surgery

Spec	Name	St	Pg
Oto	DiNardo, L	VA	295
Oto	Kennedy, D	PA	293
Oto	Lanza, D	FL	296
Oto	Rice, D	CA	304
Oto	Weymuller, E	WA	305

Sinus Tumors

Spec	Name	St	Pg
Oto	Har-El, G	NY	292
Oto	Koch, W	MD	293
Oto	O'Malley, B	PA	293
Oto	Snyderman, C	PA	294

Skin Cancer

Spec	Name	St	Pg
D	Amonette, R	TN	101
D	Arpey, C	MN	103
D	Bailin, P	OH	103
D	Bennett, R	CA	106
D	Berg, D	WA	106
D	Bickers, D	NY	99
D	Bolognia, J	CT	98
D	Braun, M	DC	100
D	Brodland, D	PA	100
D	Butler, D	TX	105
D	Carney, J	AR	105
D	Cook, J	NC	102
D	Curiel, C	AZ	106
D	Del Giudice, S	NH	98
D	Duvic, M	TX	106
D	Dzubow, L	PA	100
D	Eichler, C	FL	102
D	Elmets, C	AL	102
D	Fenske, N	FL	102
D	Fosko, S	MO	104
D	Garrett, A	VA	102
D	Geronemus, R	NY	100
D	Gilchrest, B	MA	98
D	Green, H	FL	102
D	Greenway, H	CA	107
D	Grichnik, J	FL	102
D	Halpern, A	NY	100
D	Kim, Y	CA	107
D	Krunic, A	IL	104
D	Kupper, T	MA	98
D	Lebwohl, M	NY	100
D	Leffell, D	CT	99
D	Leshin, B	NC	103
D	Lessin, S	PA	100
D	Lim, H	MI	104
D	Lim Quan, K	AZ	106
D	Lowe, L	MI	104
D	Lowitt, M	MD	100
D	Maloney, M	MA	99
D	Miller, S	MD	101
D	Neel, V	MA	99
D	Neuburg, M	WI	104
D	Nghiem, P	WA	107
D	Nigra, T	DC	101
D	Nouri, K	FL	103
D	Olbricht, S	MA	99
D	Otley, C	MN	105
D	Prioleau, P	NY	101
D	Ramsay, D	NY	101
D	Rigel, D	NY	101
D	Sobel, S	FL	103
D	Sober, A	MA	99
D	Sokoloff, D	FL	103
D	Swanson, N	OR	107
D	Swetter, S	CA	107
D	Taylor, R	TX	106
D	Thiers, B	SC	103
D	Tsao, H	MA	99
D	Wood, G	WI	105
D	Zitelli, J	PA	101
Onc	Biggs, D	DE	150
Onc	Daud, A	CA	198
Onc	Ernstoff, M	NH	143
Onc	Pavlick, A	NY	161
Onc	Pfister, D	NY	162
Onc	Sosman, J	TN	176
Oto	Weber, R	TX	303
Path	Bastian, B	NY	317
Path	Le Boit, P	CA	328
Path	Prieto, V	TX	326
PlS	Manson, P	MD	367
PlS	Miller, T	CA	371
RadRO	Cooper, J	NY	387
RadRO	Laramore, G	WA	405
RadRO	Machtay, M	OH	399
RadRO	Mittal, B	IL	400
RadRO	Wilson, J	WI	401

T

Special Expertise Index

Alphabetical Listing of Doctors

Alphabetical Listing of Doctors

Name	Specialty	Pg
Antin, Joseph (MA)	Onc	142
Antonia, Scott (FL)	Onc	166
Appelbaum, Frederick (WA)	Onc	197
Apuzzo, Michael (CA)	NS	235
Aranha, Gerard (IL)	S	446
Arber, Daniel (CA)	Path	327
Arceci, Robert (MD)	PHO	334
Argenta, Peter (MN)	ObG	266
Argiris, Athanassios (PA)	Onc	149
Arlen, Philip (MD)	Onc	149
Armitage, James (NE)	Onc	188
Arndt, Carola (MN)	PHO	345
Arpey, Christopher (MN)	D	103
Arteaga, Carlos (TN)	Onc	166
Arts, H Alexander (MI)	Oto	298
Arun, Banu (TX)	Onc	191
Asher, Anthony (NC)	NS	227
Ashley, Stanley (MA)	S	428
Aslanian, Harry (CT)	Ge	116
Astrow, Alan (NY)	Onc	149
Athanasian, Edward (NY)	HS	287
Atkins, Michael (MA)	Onc	142
Attas, Lewis (NJ)	Onc	149
Audell, Laura (CA)	PM	313
Augsburger, James (OH)	Oph	274
August, David (NJ)	S	431
Austin, John (NY)	DR	407
Averbook, Bruce (OH)	S	446
Awan, Azhar (IL)	RadRO	397
Axelrod, Deborah (NY)	S	431
Axelrod, Rita (PA)	Onc	149
Azodi, Masoud (CT)	GO	250
Azzoli, Christopher (NY)	Onc	149

B

Name	Specialty	Pg
Babiera, Gildy (TX)	S	453
Back, Anthony (WA)	Onc	197
Badie, Behnam (CA)	NS	235
Baer, Maria (MD)	Hem	127
Bagg, Adam (PA)	Path	317
Bagley, Demetrius (PA)	U	485

Name	Specialty	Pg
Bahn, Duke (CA)	DR	411
Bahnson, Robert (OH)	U	495
Baile, Walter (TX)	Psyc	375
Bailes, Julian E (WV)	NS	223
Bailey, H Randolph (TX)	CRS	93
Bailin, Philip (OH)	D	103
Bains, Manjit (NY)	TS	471
Bajorin, Dean (NY)	Onc	150
Balaji, K (NC)	U	491
Balducci, Lodovico (FL)	Onc	167
Bale, Allen (CT)	CG	511
Ball, Douglas (MD)	EDM	110
Ball, Edward (CA)	Onc	197
Balla, Andre (IL)	Path	323
Ballantyne, Garth (CT)	S	428
Ballantyne, Jane (PA)	PM	310
Ballen, Karen (MA)	Hem	126
Banerjee, Anuradha (CA)	PHO	352
Banks, Peter (NC)	Path	321
Bans, Larry (AZ)	U	499
Barakat, Richard (NY)	GO	252
Bardot, Stephen (LA)	U	499
Barger, Geoffrey (MI)	N	243
Barkin, Jamie (FL)	Ge	119
Barlogie, Bart (AR)	Hem	138
Barnes, Willard (DC)	GO	252
Barnett, Gene (OH)	NS	230
Baron, Joseph (IL)	Hem	133
Barredo, Julio (FL)	PHO	341
Barter, James (MD)	GO	252
Bartlett, David (PA)	S	432
Basch, Samuel (NY)	Psyc	374
Bashevkin, Michael (NY)	Onc	150
Basler, Joseph (TX)	U	499
Bassett, Lawrence (CA)	DR	411
Bastian, Boris (NY)	Path	317
Batchelor, Tracy (MA)	N	242
Battafarano, Richard (MD)	TS	471
Beall, Michael (VA)	U	491
Bear, Harry (VA)	S	440
Beart, Robert (CA)	CRS	94
Beatty, Patrick (MT)	Onc	188
Beauchamp, Robert (TN)	S	440

Alphabetical Listing of Doctors

Name	Specialty	Pg	Name	Specialty	Pg
Bouvet, Michael (CA)	S	457	Bubley, Glenn (MA)	Onc	142
Bowen, Glen (UT)	D	105	Buchholz, Thomas (TX)	RadRO	402
Boxer, Laurence (MI)	PHO	346	Buckner, Jan (MN)	Onc	179
Boxrud, Cynthia (CA)	Oph	276	Buckwalter, Joseph (IA)	OrS	283
Boyd, Stuart (CA)	U	501	Budd, George (OH)	Onc	179
Bradford, Carol (MI)	Oto	298	Bueno, Raphael (MA)	TS	470
Bradley, Jeffrey (MO)	RadRO	397	Bull, David (UT)	TS	478
Brandt, Keith (MO)	PlS	369	Bumpous, Jeffrey (KY)	Oto	295
Braun, Martin (DC)	D	100	Bunn, Paul (CO)	Onc	188
Brecher, Martin (NY)	PHO	335	Burger, Peter (MD)	Path	317
Breitbart, William (NY)	Psyc	374	Burke, Thomas (TX)	GO	262
Brem, Henry (MD)	NS	223	Burkey, Brian (OH)	Oto	298
Brem, Rachel (DC)	DR	407	Burman, Kenneth (DC)	EDM	110
Brem, Steven (FL)	NS	228	Burnett, Alexander (AR)	GO	262
Brems, John (IL)	S	446	Burnett, Arthur (MD)	U	486
Brendler, Charles (IL)	U	495	Burris, Howard (TN)	Onc	168
Brenin, Christiana M (VA)	Onc	168	Burstein, Harold (MA)	Onc	142
Brennan, Murray (NY)	S	432	Burt, Randall (UT)	Ge	120
Brenner, Malcolm (TX)	Hem	138	Burton, Allen (TX)	PM	312
Bresalier, Robert (TX)	Ge	121	Busby, J Erik (AL)	U	491
Brewer, Molly (CT)	GO	250	Bussel, James (NY)	PHO	335
Bricker, Leslie (MI)	Hem	134	Busuttil, Ronald (CA)	S	457
Brien, Earl (CA)	OrS	286	Butler, Charles (TX)	PlS	370
Brinckerhoff, Laurence (MA)	TS	470	Butler, David (TX)	D	105
Bristow, Robert (CA)	GO	264	Butler, John (CA)	S	457
Brizel, David (NC)	RadRO	392	Butler, William (SC)	Onc	168
Brockstein, Bruce (IL)	Onc	179	Butterly, Lynn (NH)	Ge	116
Brodland, David (PA)	D	100	Buys, Saundra (UT)	Onc	188
Brodsky, Robert (MD)	Hem	128	Buzdar, Aman (TX)	Onc	191
Brooks, Ari (PA)	S	432	Byrd, David (WA)	S	457
Brooks, John (PA)	Path	317	Byrd, John (OH)	Hem	134
Brown, Charles (IL)	S	446			
Brown, Karen (NY)	VIR	414			
Brown, Kimberly (MI)	Ge	119			
Browne, J Dale (NC)	Oto	295	# C		
Bruce, Jeffrey (NY)	NS	223	Cagle, Philip (TX)	Path	325
Bruera, Eduardo (TX)	Onc	191	Cain, Joanna (RI)	GO	250
Brufsky, Adam (PA)	Onc	150	Cairo, Mitchell (NY)	PHO	335
Bruggers, Carol (UT)	PHO	350	Califano, Joseph (MD)	Oto	291
Bruner, Janet (TX)	Path	325	Callery, Mark (MA)	S	428
Brunicardi, F Charles (TX)	S	453	Calvo, Benjamin (NC)	S	441
Brunt, L Michael (MO)	S	446	Cameron, John (MD)	S	432
Buatti, John (IA)	RadRO	397	Cameron, Robert (CA)	TS	479

Name	Specialty	Pg	Name	Specialty	Pg
Camitta, Bruce (WI)	PHO	346	Chandrasoma, Parakrama (CA)	Path	327
Camoriano, John (AZ)	Onc	192	Chang, Alfred (MI)	S	446
Campbell, Bruce (WI)	Oto	298	Chang, Helena (CA)	S	457
Campbell, Steven (OH)	U	495	Chang, Jenny (TX)	Onc	192
Cance, William (NY)	S	432	Chang, Karen (CA)	Path	327
Canellos, George (MA)	Onc	142	Chang, Sam (TN)	U	491
Cannistra, Stephen (MA)	Onc	142	Chang, Susan (CA)	Onc	198
Canto, Marcia (MD)	Ge	116	Chao, Nelson (NC)	Onc	168
Caputo, Thomas (NY)	GO	252	Chap, Linnea (CA)	Onc	198
Carabasi, Matthew (PA)	Onc	150	Chapman, Paul (NY)	Onc	151
Carbone, David (TN)	Onc	168	Chapman, Robert (MI)	Onc	180
Cardenosa, Gilda (VA)	DR	409	Chapman, William (MO)	S	446
Carducci, Michael (MD)	Onc	150	Char, Devron (CA)	Oph	276
Carey, Lisa (NC)	Onc	168	Charboneau, J William (MN)	RadRO	398
Carlson, John (NJ)	GO	252	Chari, Ravi (TN)	S	441
Carlson, Robert (CA)	Onc	198	Chen, Allen (MD)	PHO	335
Carney, John (AR)	D	105	Chen, Chun (NY)	NS	224
Carney, Michael (HI)	GO	264	Chen, David (PA)	U	486
Carpenter, John (AL)	Onc	168	Chen, Thomas (CA)	NS	236
Carrasquillo, Jorge (NY)	NuM	416	Cheng, Edward (MN)	OrS	283
Carroll, Peter (CA)	U	501	Cherny, W Bruce (ID)	NS	233
Carroll, William (NY)	PHO	335	Cherqui, Daniel (NY)	S	433
Carson, Benjamin (MD)	NS	224	Cheson, Bruce (DC)	Hem	128
Carter, H Ballentine (MD)	U	486	Cheung, Nai-Kong V (NY)	PHO	335
Carty, Sally (PA)	S	432	Cheville, Andrea (MN)	PMR	516
Cascino, Terrence (MN)	N	243	Chew, Helen (CA)	Onc	198
Castellino, Sharon (NC)	PHO	341	Childs, Stacy (CO)	U	498
Castle, Valerie (MI)	PHO	346	Chiles, Caroline (NC)	DR	409
Catalona, William (IL)	U	495	Chiocca, E Antonio (OH)	NS	231
Celano, Paul (MD)	Onc	151	Chitambar, Christopher (WI)	Onc	180
Cerfolio, Robert (AL)	TS	474	Chlebowski, Rowan (CA)	Onc	198
Cha, Soonmee (CA)	NRad	413	Cho, Kathleen (MI)	Path	323
Chabner, Bruce (MA)	Onc	143	Choi, Noah (MA)	RadRO	385
Chabot, John (NY)	S	432	Choti, Michael (MD)	S	433
Chachoua, Abraham (NY)	Onc	151	Chow, Warren (CA)	Onc	198
Chakravarthy, Anuradha (TN)	RadRO	392	Chowdhury, Khalid (CO)	Oto	301
Chalian, Ara (PA)	Oto	291	Choy, Hak (TX)	RadRO	402
Chamberlain, Marc (WA)	N	245	Chu, Edward (PA)	Onc	151
Chambers, Setsuko (AZ)	GO	262	Chung, Daniel (MA)	Ge	116
Champlin, Richard (TX)	Hem	138	Chung, Ki Young (SC)	Onc	169
Chan, John (CA)	GO	264	Church, James (OH)	CRS	90
Chanan-Khan, Asher (NY)	Onc	151	Ciezki, Jay (OH)	RadRO	398
Chandler, William (MI)	NS	230	Cioffi, William (RI)	S	428

Alphabetical Listing of Doctors

Name	Specialty	Pg	Name	Specialty	Pg
Civantos, Francisco (FL)	Oto	295	Come, Steven (MA)	Onc	143
Civin, Curt (MD)	PHO	335	Comenzo, Raymond (MA)	Hem	126
Clamon, Gerald (IA)	Onc	180	Conant, Emily (PA)	DR	408
Clark, Joseph (IL)	Onc	180	Connolly, James (MA)	Path	316
Clark, Orlo (CA)	S	458	Conrad, Ernest (WA)	OrS	286
Clarke-Pearson, Daniel (NC)	GO	256	Conry, Robert (AL)	Onc	169
Claxton, David (PA)	Onc	151	Constine, Louis (NY)	RadRO	387
Clayman, Gary (TX)	Oto	301	Cook, Jonathan (NC)	D	102
Cleary, James (WI)	Onc	180	Cookson, Michael (TN)	U	492
Cliby, William (MN)	GO	259	Cooper, Barry (TX)	Hem	138
Clinton, Steven (OH)	Onc	180	Cooper, Dan (CA)	PPul	357
Clohisy, Denis (MN)	OrS	283	Cooper, Jay (NY)	RadRO	387
Close, Lanny (NY)	Oto	291	Copelan, Edward (OH)	Hem	134
Cloughesy, Timothy (CA)	N	245	Copeland, Larry (OH)	GO	259
Clutter, William (MO)	EDM	111	Coplen, Douglas (MO)	U	495
Cmelak, Anthony (TN)	RadRO	392	Cordeiro, Peter (NY)	PlS	366
Coakley, Fergus (CA)	DR	411	Corey, Seth (IL)	PHO	346
Cobleigh, Melody (IL)	Onc	180	Cornelison, Terri (MD)	GO	252
Cobos, Everardo (TX)	Hem	138	Cornelius, Lynn (MO)	D	103
Coccia, Peter (NE)	PHO	350	Cortes, Jorge (TX)	Hem	138
Cochran, Alistair (CA)	Path	327	Cosgrove, G Rees (RI)	NS	222
Cockerham, Kimberly (CA)	Oph	276	Cosin, Jonathan (DC)	GO	253
Cohen, Alan (OH)	NS	231	Costantino, Peter (NY)	Oto	291
Cohen, Bruce (OH)	ChiN	246	Cote, Richard (FL)	Path	322
Cohen, Gary (PA)	VIR	414	Couch, Marion (VT)	Oto	290
Cohen, Gary (MD)	Onc	151	Coukos, George (PA)	GO	253
Cohen, Jeffrey (PA)	U	486	Couldwell, William (UT)	NS	233
Cohen, Kenneth (MD)	PHO	335	Courey, Mark (CA)	Oto	303
Cohen, Michael (IA)	Path	323	Coutifaris, Christos (PA)	RE	268
Cohen, Philip (DC)	Onc	151	Cowan, Kenneth (NE)	Onc	189
Cohen, Roger (PA)	Onc	152	Cowan, Morton (CA)	PA&I	355
Cohen, Seymour (NY)	Onc	152	Cox, James (TX)	RadRO	402
Cohn, Susan (IL)	PHO	346	Cramer, Daniel (MA)	ObG	266
Coit, Daniel (NY)	S	433	Crawford, E David (CO)	U	498
Colberg, John (CT)	U	484	Crawford, James (NY)	Path	317
Cole, David (SC)	S	441	Crawford, Jeffrey (NC)	Onc	169
Coleman, John (IN)	PlS	369	Creasman, William (SC)	GO	256
Coleman, Morton (NY)	Onc	152	Crippin, Jeffrey (MO)	Ge	119
Coleman, R Edward (NC)	NuM	417	Crocenzi, Todd (OR)	Onc	198
Collins, Dale (NH)	PlS	366	Crocker, Ian (GA)	RadRO	393
Colombani, Paul (MD)	PS	357	Crockett, Dennis (CA)	PO	356
Colon-Otero, Gerardo (FL)	Onc	169	Croop, James (IN)	PHO	346
Colquhoun, Steven (CA)	S	458	Crowe, Joseph (OH)	S	446

Alphabetical Listing of Doctors

Name	Specialty	Pg	Name	Specialty	Pg
Crowley, William (MA)	RE	267	De Simone, Philip (KY)	Onc	169
Culkin, Daniel (OK)	U	499	Decker, Gustav (AZ)	Ge	121
Cullen, Kevin (MD)	Onc	152	Deeg, H Joachim (WA)	Onc	199
Curcillo, Paul (PA)	S	433	DeKernion, Jean (CA)	U	501
Curiel, Clara (AZ)	D	106	Del Giudice, Stephen (NH)	D	98
Curley, Steven (TX)	S	453	Del Priore, Giuseppe (IN)	GO	259
Currie, John (GA)	GO	256	Delaney, Conor (OH)	CRS	90
Curtin, John (NY)	GO	253	Delaney, Thomas (MA)	RadRO	385
Cusack, James (MA)	S	428	DeLellis, Ronald (RI)	Path	316
Czuczman, Myron (NY)	Onc	152	DeLeon, Oscar (NY)	PM	310
			Della Rocca, Robert (NY)	Oph	272
			DeMars, Leslie (NH)	GO	250
			Demetri, George (MA)	Onc	143
D			Demmy, Todd (NY)	TS	471
			DePompolo, Robert (MN)	PMR	516
D'Amico, Anthony (MA)	RadRO	385	DePriest, Paul (KY)	GO	256
D'Amico, Thomas (NC)	TS	474	Dershaw, D David (NY)	DR	408
Dacey, Ralph (MO)	NS	231	Deschamps, Claude (MN)	TS	476
Dakhil, Shaker (KS)	Onc	189	Deschler, Daniel (MA)	Oto	290
Dalkin, Bruce (WA)	U	501	DeVita, Vincent (CT)	Onc	143
Dalmau, Josep (PA)	N	242	DeWeese, Theodore (MD)	RadRO	387
Daly, Mary (PA)	Onc	152	Di Bisceglie, Adrian (MO)	Ge	120
Damon, Lloyd (CA)	Hem	140	Di Giacinto, George (NY)	NS	224
Daneker, George (GA)	S	441	Di Persio, John (MO)	Hem	134
Daneshmand, Siamak (CA)	U	501	Di Saia, Philip (CA)	GO	265
Dang, Chi (MD)	Hem	128	Diaz, Eduardo (TX)	Oto	302
Daniels, Gilbert (MA)	EDM	110	Dicker, Adam (PA)	RadRO	388
Danoff, Dudley (CA)	U	501	Dickler, Maura (NY)	Onc	153
Daud, Adil (CA)	Onc	198	Dietz, David (OH)	CRS	90
David, Carlos (MA)	NS	222	Dillehay, Gary (IL)	NuM	417
Davidoff, Andrew (TN)	PS	358	Diller, Lisa (MA)	PHO	333
Davidson, Bruce (DC)	Oto	291	Dillon, William (CA)	NRad	414
Davidson, Nancy (PA)	Onc	152	DiNardo, Laurence (VA)	Oto	295
Davidson, Susan (CO)	GO	262	DiPaola, Robert (NJ)	Onc	153
Davies, Stella (OH)	PHO	346	Disa, Joseph (NY)	PlS	366
Davis, Bradley (KS)	U	498	Disis, Mary (WA)	Onc	199
Davis, Mellar (OH)	Onc	180	Dizon, Don (RI)	Onc	143
Dawson, Nancy (DC)	Onc	152	Djulbegovic, Benjamin (FL)	Hem	132
Day, Terrence (SC)	Oto	295	Domchek, Susan (PA)	Onc	153
De Angelis, Lisa (NY)	N	242	Donald, Paul (CA)	Oto	303
De Geest, Koen (IA)	GO	259	Donaldson, Sarah (CA)	RadRO	404
De Masters, Bette (CO)	Path	325	Donehower, Ross (MD)	Onc	153
De Meester, Tom (CA)	TS	479	Donohue, John (MN)	S	447
De Monte, Franco (TX)	NS	234			

Alphabetical Listing of Doctors

F

Name	Specialty	Pg	Name	Specialty	Pg
Fonseca, Rafael (AZ)	Hem	139	Furman, Wayne (TN)	PHO	341
Forastiere, Arlene (MD)	Onc	154	Futran, Neal (WA)	Oto	304
Ford, James (CA)	Onc	199			
Forero, Andres (AL)	Onc	169			
Forman, Jeffrey (MI)	RadRO	398			
Forman, Stephen (CA)	Hem	140	**G**		
Formenti, Silvia (NY)	RadRO	388			
Forscher, Charles (CA)	Onc	200	Gabram, Sheryl (GA)	S	441
Fosko, Scott (MO)	D	104	Gabrilove, Janice (NY)	Onc	155
Foss, Francine (CT)	Onc	144	Gaffney, David (UT)	RadRO	401
Fossella, Frank (TX)	Onc	192	Gaissert, Henning (MA)	TS	470
Foster, Richard (IN)	U	496	Gajjar, Amar (TN)	PHO	342
Foucar, M Kathryn (NM)	Path	325	Galandiuk, Susan (KY)	CRS	89
Fowble, Barbara (CA)	RadRO	404	Gamble, Gail (IL)	PMR	516
Fowler, Jeffrey (OH)	GO	260	Gandara, David (CA)	Onc	200
Fowler, Wesley (NC)	GO	257	Ganz, Patricia (CA)	Onc	200
Fox, Kevin (PA)	Onc	155	Garber, Judy (MA)	Onc	144
Fracasso, Paula (VA)	Onc	170	Garnick, Marc (MA)	Onc	144
Fraker, Douglas (PA)	S	434	Garrett, Algin (VA)	D	102
Francis, Kathleen (NJ)	PMR	515	Garst, Jennifer (NC)	Onc	170
Frangoul, Haydar (TN)	PHO	341	Garver, Robert (AL)	Pul	379
Frantz, Christopher (DE)	PHO	336	Garvin, James (NY)	PHO	336
Fraser, Lionel (MS)	U	492	Gawande, Atul (MA)	S	428
Frassica, Frank (MD)	OrS	281	Gaynor, Ellen (IL)	Onc	181
Frazier, Thomas (PA)	S	434	Gearhart, Susan (MD)	CRS	87
Freedman, Arnold (MA)	Onc	144	Gebhardt, Mark (MA)	OrS	280
Freedman, Gary (PA)	RadRO	388	Geisler, Daniel (PA)	CRS	88
Freifeld, Alison (NE)	Inf	513	Gejerman, Glen (NJ)	RadRO	388
Freimanis, Rita (NC)	DR	410	Geller, David (PA)	S	434
Friebert, Sarah (OH)	PHO	347	Geller, Kenneth (CA)	PO	357
Friedberg, Jonathan (NY)	Onc	155	Gellis, Stephen (MA)	D	98
Friedberg, Joseph (PA)	TS	472	Gelmann, Edward (NY)	Onc	155
Friedlaender, Gary (CT)	OrS	280	Genden, Eric (NY)	Oto	291
Friedman, Alan (MD)	PHO	336	George, Daniel (NC)	Onc	170
Friedman, Allan (NC)	NS	228	Georgiade, Gregory (NC)	PIS	368
Friedman, Debra (TN)	PHO	341	Gerdes, Hans (NY)	Ge	116
Friedman, Henry (NC)	Onc	170	Geronemus, Roy (NY)	D	100
Frim, David (IL)	NS	231	Gershenson, David (TX)	GO	263
Fromm, Geri-Lynn (TX)	GO	263	Gerson, Stanton (OH)	Onc	181
Fry, Robert (PA)	CRS	87	Gertz, Morie (MN)	Hem	134
Fuchs, Charles (MA)	Onc	144	Geschwind, Jean-Francois (MD)	VIR	414
Fung, John (OH)	S	447	Geyer, Charles (PA)	Onc	155
Funk, Gerry (IA)	Oto	298	Geyer, J Russell (WA)	PHO	353
			Ghamande, Sharad (GA)	GO	257

Alphabetical Listing of Doctors

Name	Specialty	Pg	Name	Specialty	Pg
Greenwald, Bruce (MD)	Ge	117	Halberg, Francine (CA)	RadRO	404
Greenway, Hubert (CA)	D	107	Haley, Barbara (TX)	Onc	192
Greer, Benjamin (WA)	GO	265	Hall, Simon (NY)	U	487
Greer, John (TN)	Hem	132	Halle, Jan (NC)	RadRO	393
Gregory, Stephanie (IL)	Hem	135	Halligan, Gregory (PA)	PHO	337
Greiner, Carl (NE)	Psyc	375	Hallisey, Michael (CT)	VIR	414
Greipp, Philip (MN)	Hem	135	Halpern, Allan (NY)	D	100
Grem, Jean (NE)	Onc	189	Halpern, Howard (IL)	RadRO	398
Grever, Michael (OH)	Hem	135	Halpern, Steven (NJ)	PHO	337
Grichnik, James (FL)	D	102	Haluszka, Oleh (PA)	Ge	117
Grigsby, Perry (MO)	RadRO	398	Halyard, Michele (AZ)	RadRO	403
Grillone, Gregory (MA)	Oto	290	Hamilton, Stanley (TX)	Path	326
Grody, Wayne (CA)	CG	512	Hammar, Samuel (WA)	Path	328
Grogan, Thomas (AZ)	Path	325	Hammer, Gary (MI)	EDM	111
Grosh, William (VA)	Onc	171	Hammond, Denis (NH)	Onc	144
Grossbard, Michael (NY)	Onc	156	Hammond, Dennis (MI)	PlS	369
Grossman, H Barton (TX)	U	499	Hancock, Steven (CA)	RadRO	404
Grossman, Stuart (MD)	Onc	156	Handa, James (MD)	Oph	272
Grossniklaus, Hans (GA)	Oph	273	Hande, Kenneth (TN)	Onc	171
Grubb, Robert (MO)	NS	231	Handy, John (OR)	TS	480
Gruber, Stephen (MI)	Onc	182	Hanke, C William (IN)	D	104
Grunberg, Steven (VT)	Onc	144	Hankinson, Hal (NM)	NS	234
Grupp, Stephan (PA)	PHO	336	Hanks, John (VA)	S	442
Guarini, Ludovico (NY)	PHO	337	Hanna, Ehab (TX)	Oto	302
Guillem, Jose (NY)	CRS	88	Hanna, Nader (MD)	S	435
Guinan, Eva (MA)	PHO	333	Hansen, Juliana (OR)	PlS	371
Gulley, James (MD)	Onc	156	Hansen, Nora (IL)	S	448
Gupta, Prabodh (PA)	Path	318	Har-El, Gady (NY)	Oto	292
Gururangan, Sridharan (NC)	PHO	342	Haraf, Daniel (IL)	RadRO	398
Guthikonda, Murali (MI)	NS	231	Harari, Paul (WI)	RadRO	398
Guthrie, Barton (AL)	NS	228	Harbour, J William (MO)	Oph	274
Gutin, Philip (NY)	NS	224	Harnsberger, Jeffrey (NH)	CRS	86
			Harpole, David (NC)	TS	475
			Harris, Jay (MA)	RadRO	385
H			Harris, Michael (NJ)	PHO	337
			Harris, Nancy (MA)	Path	316
Haas, Eric (TX)	CRS	93	Harrison, Louis (NY)	RadRO	389
Haas, Naomi (PA)	Onc	156	Harsh, Griffith (CA)	NS	236
Habermann, Thomas (MN)	Hem	135	Hartford, Alan (NH)	RadRO	385
Haffty, Bruce (NJ)	RadRO	389	Hartig, Gregory (WI)	Oto	298
Hageboutros, Alexandre (NJ)	Onc	156	Hartmann, Lynn (MN)	Onc	182
Hahn, Stephen (PA)	RadRO	389	Haskal, Ziv (MD)	VIR	414
Haik, Barrett (TN)	Oph	273	Hatch, Kenneth (AZ)	GO	263

Alphabetical Listing of Doctors

Name	Specialty	Pg	Name	Specialty	Pg
Haughey, Bruce (MO)	Oto	299	Hirsch, Barry (PA)	Oto	292
Hauke, Ralph (NE)	Onc	189	Hochberg, Ephraim (MA)	Onc	145
Haut, Paul (IN)	PHO	347	Hochster, Howard (CT)	Onc	145
Havrilesky, Laura (NC)	GO	257	Hoda, Syed (NY)	Path	318
Hawkins, Douglas (WA)	PHO	353	Hodes, Jonathan (KY)	NS	228
Hayani, Ammar (IL)	PHO	347	Hodin, Richard (MA)	S	429
Hayashi, Robert (MO)	PHO	347	Hoffman, Andrew (CA)	EDM	113
Hayes, Daniel (MI)	Onc	182	Hoffman, Brenda (SC)	Ge	119
Hayman, James (MI)	RadRO	399	Hoffman, Henry (IA)	Oto	299
Healey, John (NY)	OrS	281	Hoffman, John (PA)	S	435
Healey, Patrick (WA)	PS	360	Hoffman, Lloyd (NY)	PlS	366
Heber, David (CA)	EDM	113	Hoffman, Philip (IL)	Onc	182
Heimann, Ruth (VT)	RadRO	385	Hogan, Thomas (WV)	Onc	157
Heinrich, Michael (OR)	Hem	140	Holden, Stuart (CA)	U	502
Heitmiller, Richard (MD)	TS	472	Holland, James (NY)	Onc	157
Heller, Debra (NJ)	Path	318	Holliday, Michael (MD)	Oto	292
Helman, Lee (MD)	PHO	337	Hollister, Dickerman (CT)	Onc	145
Helvie, Mark (MI)	DR	410	Homans, Alan (VT)	PHO	333
Hemal, Ashok (NC)	U	492	Hong, Waun (TX)	Onc	192
Hemming, Alan (CA)	S	459	Hoppe, Richard (CA)	RadRO	405
Henderson, Randal (FL)	RadRO	393	Hord, Jeffrey (OH)	PHO	348
Heney, Niall (MA)	U	484	Horn, Biljana (CA)	PHO	353
Henry, David (PA)	Onc	156	Hornicek, Francis (MA)	OrS	280
Henschke, Claudia (NY)	DR	408	Horowitz, Ira (GA)	GO	257
Henshaw, Robert (DC)	OrS	281	Hortobagyi, Gabriel (TX)	Onc	193
Heppell, Jacques (AZ)	CRS	93	Horwitz, Eric (PA)	RadRO	389
Herbst, Roy (CT)	Onc	145	Horwitz, Steven (NY)	Onc	157
Herman, Terence (OK)	RadRO	403	Howe, James (IA)	S	448
Heros, Roberto (FL)	NS	228	Howington, John (IL)	TS	476
Herr, Harry (NY)	U	487	Hrebinko, Ronald (PA)	U	487
Herrmann, Virginia (SC)	S	442	Hricak, Hedvig (NY)	DR	408
Herzog, Thomas (NY)	GO	254	Hruban, Ralph (MD)	Path	318
Heslin, Martin (AL)	S	442	Hruza, George (MO)	D	104
Hesselink, John (CA)	NRad	414	Huben, Robert (NY)	U	487
Hetherington, Maxine (MO)	PHO	347	Huber, Philip (TX)	CRS	93
Hicks, Terry (LA)	CRS	93	Hudes, Gary (PA)	Onc	157
Hicks, Wesley (NY)	Oto	292	Hudis, Clifford (NY)	Onc	157
Hiesiger, Emile (NY)	N	242	Hudson, Melissa (TN)	PHO	342
Higano, Celestia (WA)	Onc	200	Hughes, Kevin (MA)	S	429
Hilden, Joanne (IN)	PHO	348	Hunt, Kelly (TX)	S	454
Himelstein, Andrew (DE)	Onc	156	Huntoon, Marc (MN)	PM	312
Hinshaw, Daniel (MI)	S	448	Hurd, David (NC)	Onc	171
Hiotis, Spiros (NY)	S	435	Husain, Amreen (CA)	GO	265

Alphabetical Listing of Doctors

Alphabetical Listing of Doctors

Name	Specialty	Pg
Konski, Andre (MI)	RadRO	399
Kopans, Daniel (MA)	DR	407
Kopp, Peter (IL)	EDM	112
Korones, David (NY)	PHO	337
Koss, Michael (CA)	Path	328
Koulos, John (NY)	GO	254
Kozlowski, James (IL)	U	496
Kraft, Andrew (SC)	Onc	171
Krag, David (VT)	S	429
Krasna, Mark (MD)	TS	473
Kraus, Dennis (NY)	Oto	293
Kraut, Eric (OH)	Hem	135
Kreissman, Susan (NC)	PHO	343
Kreitzer, Joel (NY)	PM	310
Krellenstein, Daniel (NY)	TS	473
Krespi, Yosef (NY)	Oto	293
Kriegel, David (NY)	D	100
Kris, Mark (NY)	Onc	158
Krishnamurthi, Smitha (OH)	Onc	183
Krontiras, Helen (AL)	S	442
Krouse, Robert (AZ)	S	455
Krunic, Aleksandar (IL)	D	104
Kucharczuk, John (PA)	TS	473
Kucuk, Omer (GA)	Onc	172
Kudrimoti, Mahesh (KY)	RadRO	393
Kuettel, Michael (NY)	RadRO	389
Kuhn, Joseph (TX)	S	455
Kun, Larry (TN)	RadRO	393
Kung, Faith (CA)	PHO	353
Kunkel, Elisabeth (PA)	Psyc	375
Kunschner, Lara (PA)	N	242
Kupper, Thomas (MA)	D	98
Kuriakose, Philip (MI)	Hem	136
Kurman, Robert (MD)	Path	319
Kurtin, Paul (MN)	Path	324
Kurtz, Robert (NY)	Ge	117
Kurtzberg, Joanne (NC)	PHO	343
Kushner, Brian (NY)	PHO	338
Kuske, Robert (AZ)	RadRO	403
Kuttesch, John (PA)	PHO	338
Kuzel, Timothy (IL)	Onc	183
Kvols, Larry (FL)	Onc	172
Kwak, Larry (TX)	Onc	193

Name	Specialty	Pg

L

La Quaglia, Michael (NY)	PS	358
Lackman, Richard (PA)	OrS	281
Lacy, Jill (CT)	Onc	145
Ladenson, Paul (MD)	EDM	110
Lage, Janice (SC)	Path	322
Laheru, Daniel (MD)	Onc	158
Lamonica, Dominick (NY)	NuM	416
Lancaster, Johnathan (FL)	GO	257
Landreneau, Rodney (PA)	TS	473
Landry, Jerome (GA)	RadRO	393
Lane, Joseph (NY)	OrS	281
Lang, Frederick (TX)	NS	234
Lange, Beverly (PA)	PHO	338
Lange, Paul (WA)	U	502
Langer, Corey (PA)	Onc	158
Lannin, Donald (CT)	S	429
Lanteri, Vincent (NJ)	U	488
Lanza, Donald (FL)	Oto	296
Lanza, Louis (AZ)	TS	478
Laramore, George (WA)	RadRO	405
Larner, James (VA)	RadRO	394
Larson, David (CA)	RadRO	405
Larson, Richard (IL)	Hem	136
Larson, Steven (NY)	NuM	417
Laske, Douglas (PA)	NS	225
Latchaw, Laurie (NH)	PS	357
Laterra, John (MD)	N	242
Lau, Christine (VA)	TS	475
Laughlin, Mary (VA)	Hem	132
Laver, Joseph (TN)	PHO	343
Lavertu, Pierre (OH)	Oto	299
Lavery, Ian (OH)	CRS	91
Lavyne, Michael (NY)	NS	225
Lawrence, Theodore (MI)	RadRO	399
Lawson, David (GA)	Onc	172
Lawson, William (NY)	Oto	293
Lazarus, Hillard (OH)	Hem	136
Le, Quynh-Thu Xuan (CA)	RadRO	405
Le Boit, Philip (CA)	Path	328
Leach, Steven (MD)	S	435
Lebwohl, Mark (NY)	D	100

Alphabetical Listing of Doctors

Name	Specialty	Pg	Name	Specialty	Pg
Lowe, Lori (MI)	D	104	Maloney, Mary (MA)	D	99
Lowitt, Mark (MD)	D	100	Mamelak, Adam (CA)	NS	237
Lowy, Andrew (CA)	S	459	Mamounas, Eleftherios (OH)	S	449
Lu, Karen (TX)	GO	263	Manera, Ricarchito (IL)	PHO	348
Lucas, David (MI)	Path	324	Mangan, Kenneth (PA)	Hem	129
Lucci, Joseph (FL)	GO	257	Mansfield, Paul (TX)	S	455
Luchtman-Jones, Lori (DC)	PHO	338	Manson, Paul (MD)	PlS	367
Luck, James (CA)	OrS	286	Mansur, David B (MO)	RadRO	400
Ludwig, Kirk (WI)	CRS	91	Mantyh, Christopher (NC)	CRS	89
Lueder, Gregg (MO)	Oph	274	Mapstone, Timothy (OK)	NS	234
Lugg, James (WY)	U	498	Marcet, Jorge (FL)	CRS	89
Lunsford, L Dade (PA)	NS	225	Marcom, Paul (NC)	Onc	173
Lurain, John (IL)	GO	260	Marcus, Judith (NY)	PHO	338
Lusher, Jeanne (MI)	PHO	348	Marcus, Robert (FL)	RadRO	394
Lyckholm, Laurel (VA)	Onc	173	Marentette, Lawrence (MI)	Oto	299
Lydiatt, Daniel (NE)	Oto	301	Margolin, Kim (WA)	Onc	201
Lydiatt, William (NE)	Oto	301	Marina, Neyssa (CA)	PHO	354
Lyerly, H Kim (NC)	S	443	Maris, John (PA)	PHO	338
Lyman, Gary (NC)	Onc	173	Mark, Eugene (MA)	Path	316
Lynch, James (FL)	Onc	173	Markert, James (AL)	NS	228
Lynch, Thomas (CT)	Onc	146	Markoe, Arnold (FL)	RadRO	394
Lyons, Roger (TX)	Hem	139	Markowitz, Sanford (OH)	Onc	184
			Marks, Lawrence (NC)	RadRO	394
			Marks, Peter (CT)	Hem	126
			Marks, Stanley (PA)	Hem	129

M

Name	Specialty	Pg	Name	Specialty	Pg
			Marsh, James (PA)	S	436
Machtay, Mitchell (OH)	RadRO	399	Marshall, Fray (GA)	U	492
Maciejewski, Jaroslaw (OH)	Hem	136	Marshall, John (DC)	Onc	159
Macklis, Roger (OH)	RadRO	399	Marshall, Margaret Blair (DC)	TS	473
Maddaus, Michael (MN)	TS	477	Martenson, James (MN)	RadRO	400
Maddox, Anne (AR)	Hem	139	Martins, Renato (WA)	Onc	201
Madoff, Robert (MN)	CRS	91	Martuza, Robert (MA)	NS	222
Magrina, Javier (AZ)	GO	263	Maslak, Peter (NY)	Hem	129
Mahvi, David (IL)	S	449	Mason, David (OH)	TS	477
Makhija, Sharmila (GA)	GO	258	Mason, Joel (MA)	Ge	116
Makhoul, Issam (AR)	Onc	194	Masood, Shahla (FL)	Path	322
Maki, Robert (NY)	Onc	159	Masters, Gregory (DE)	Onc	159
Malawer, Martin (MD)	OrS	282	Mathew, Paul (MA)	Onc	146
Malcolm, Arnold (TN)	RadRO	394	Mathisen, Douglas (MA)	TS	470
Maldjian, Joseph (NC)	NRad	413	Matthay, Katherine (CA)	PHO	354
Malik, Ghaus (MI)	NS	232	Matulonis, Ursula (MA)	Onc	146
Malkowicz, S Bruce (PA)	U	488	Mauch, Peter (MA)	RadRO	386
Maloney, David G (WA)	Onc	201	Mauro, Matthew (NC)	VIR	415

Alphabetical Listing of Doctors

Name	Specialty	Pg	Name	Specialty	Pg
Maxwell, G Patrick (TN)	PlS	368	Meredith, Ruby (AL)	RadRO	395
Mayberg, Marc (WA)	NS	237	Meric-Bernstam, Funda (TX)	S	455
Mayerson, Joel (OH)	OrS	284	Meropol, Neal (OH)	Onc	184
Maziarz, Richard (OR)	Hem	141	Messersmith, Wells (CO)	Onc	190
McAneny, David (MA)	S	430	Meyer, William (OK)	PHO	352
McCabe, Daniel (AZ)	S	455	Meyers, Bryan (MO)	TS	477
McCaffrey, Thomas (FL)	Oto	296	Meyers, Paul (NY)	PHO	339
McCarthy, Shirley (CT)	DR	407	Meyers, Rebecka (UT)	PS	360
McConnell, John (NC)	U	493	Meyskens, Frank (CA)	Onc	201
McCormick, Beryl (NY)	RadRO	390	Michalski, Jeff (MO)	RadRO	400
McCormick, Paul (NY)	NS	225	Michelassi, Fabrizio (NY)	S	436
McCraw, John (MS)	PlS	368	Mickey, Bruce (TX)	NS	234
McCurley, Thomas (TN)	Path	322	Mieler, William (IL)	Oph	275
McDermott, Michael (CA)	NS	237	Mies, Carolyn (PA)	Path	319
McDonald, Douglas (MO)	OrS	284	Mihm, Martin (MA)	D	99
McDougal, W Scott (MA)	U	484	Mikkelsen, Tommy (MI)	N	244
McFadden, David (VT)	S	430	Miles, Brian (TX)	U	500
McGahan, John (CA)	VIR	416	Milhem, Mohammed (IA)	Hem	136
McGarry, Ronald (KY)	RadRO	394	Millenson, Michael (PA)	Hem	129
McGill, Trevor (MA)	PO	356	Miller, Antonius (NC)	Onc	173
McGlave, Philip (MN)	Hem	136	Miller, Daniel (GA)	TS	475
McGovern, Francis (MA)	U	484	Miller, Donald (KY)	Onc	173
McGrath, Patrick (KY)	S	443	Miller, Kenneth (MA)	Hem	127
McGuire, William (MD)	Onc	159	Miller, Michael (OH)	PlS	369
McLean, Thomas (NC)	PHO	343	Miller, Scott (GA)	U	493
McMasters, Kelly (KY)	S	443	Miller, Stanley (MD)	D	101
McMenomey, Sean (OR)	Oto	304	Miller, Thomas (AZ)	Onc	194
McVary, Kevin (IL)	U	497	Miller, Timothy (CA)	PlS	371
Meacham, Lillian (GA)	PEn	356	Miller, Vincent (NY)	Onc	159
Mears, John Gregory (NY)	Hem	129	Millis, J Michael (IL)	S	449
Medbery, Clinton (OK)	RadRO	403	Mills, Stacey (VA)	Path	322
Medich, David (PA)	CRS	88	Milsom, Jeffrey (NY)	CRS	88
Medina, Jesus (OK)	Oto	302	Minsky, Bruce (IL)	RadRO	400
Meehan, Kenneth (NH)	Hem	126	Mintzer, David (PA)	Onc	160
Mehrara, Babak (NY)	PlS	367	Mischel, Paul (CA)	Path	328
Melamed, Jonathan (NY)	Path	319	Mitchell, Beverly (CA)	Hem	141
Melmed, Shlomo (CA)	EDM	113	Mitnick, Julie (NY)	DR	408
Melvin, W Scott (OH)	S	449	Mitsuyasu, Ronald (CA)	Onc	202
Mendenhall, Nancy (FL)	RadRO	395	Mittal, Bharat (IL)	RadRO	400
Mendenhall, William (FL)	RadRO	395	Modesitt, Susan (VA)	GO	258
Menick, Frederick (AZ)	PlS	370	Mohler, James (NY)	U	488
Menon, Mani (MI)	U	497	Moley, Jeffrey (MO)	S	449
Merchant, Thomas (TN)	RadRO	395	Molo, Mary (IL)	RE	268

Alphabetical Listing of Doctors

Name	Specialty	Pg	Name	Specialty	Pg
Monsees, Barbara (MO)	DR	410	Muto, Michael (MA)	GO	251
Montgomery, Elizabeth (MD)	Path	319	Myers, Jeffrey (MI)	Path	324
Montie, James (MI)	U	497	Myers, Jeffrey (TX)	Oto	302
Moore, Anne (NY)	Onc	160	Myerson, Robert (MO)	RadRO	400
Moore, David (IN)	GO	260	Myseros, John (VA)	NS	229
Moore, Francis (MA)	S	430			
Moore, Frank (NY)	NS	226			
Moore, Joseph (NC)	Onc	173			
Moossa, AR (CA)	S	459			
Moots, Paul (TN)	N	243	**N**		
Moran, Cesar (TX)	Path	326	Nabell, Lisle (AL)	Onc	174
Morcos, Jacques (FL)	NS	229	Nabors, L Burt (AL)	N	243
Morgan, David (TN)	Onc	174	Nademanee, Auayporn (CA)	Hem	141
Morgan, Elaine (IL)	PHO	348	Nadler, Lee (MA)	Onc	146
Morgan, Linda (FL)	ObG	266	Naff, Neal (MD)	NS	226
Morgan, Mark (PA)	GO	255	Nagle, Deborah (MA)	CRS	86
Morgan, Walter (TN)	PS	358	Nagorney, David (MN)	S	449
Morris, Monica (VA)	RadRO	395	Nakakura, Eric (CA)	S	460
Morrison, William (TX)	RadRO	403	Nand, Sucha (IL)	Hem	136
Morrow, Jon (CT)	Path	316	Nanus, David (NY)	Onc	160
Morrow, Monica (NY)	S	436	Naslund, Michael (MD)	U	488
Mortimer, Joanne (CA)	Onc	202	Natale, Ronald (CA)	Onc	202
Moscow, Jeffrey (KY)	PHO	343	Nathanson, S David (MI)	S	449
Moss, R Lawrence (OH)	PS	359	Nathwani, Bharat (CA)	Path	328
Mostwin, Jacek (MD)	U	488	Naunheim, Keith (MO)	TS	477
Mott, Michael (MI)	OrS	284	Nava-Villarreal, Hector (NY)	S	436
Motzer, Robert (NY)	Onc	160	Neel, Victor (MA)	D	99
Moul, Judd (NC)	U	493	Neglia, Joseph (MN)	PHO	348
Movsas, Benjamin (MI)	RadRO	400	Negrin, Robert (CA)	Hem	141
Muggia, Franco (NY)	Onc	160	Neifeld, James (VA)	S	443
Mukherji, Suresh (MI)	NRad	413	Nelson, Edward (UT)	S	452
Mullett, Timothy (KY)	TS	475	Nelson, Heidi (MN)	CRS	91
Mulvihill, John (OK)	CG	512	Nelson, Joel (PA)	U	489
Mulvihill, Sean (UT)	S	452	Nelson, Judith (NY)	Pul	378
Mundt, Arno (CA)	RadRO	405	Nerad, Jeffrey (OH)	Oph	275
Munker, Reinhold (LA)	Hem	139	Nesbitt, Jonathan (TN)	TS	475
Muntz, Howard (WA)	GO	265	Netterville, James (TN)	Oto	296
Murphree, A Linn (CA)	Oph	277	Neuberg, Ronnie (SC)	PHO	343
Murray, Timothy (FL)	Oph	273	Neuburg, Marcelle (WI)	D	104
Murtagh, F Reed (FL)	NRad	413	Neumann, Donald (OH)	NuM	417
Muss, Hyman (NC)	Onc	174	Neuwelt, Edward (OR)	NS	237
Mutch, David (MO)	GO	260	Newman, Elliot (NY)	S	436
Mutch, Matthew (MO)	CRS	91	Newman, Lisa (MI)	S	449
			Newton, Herbert (OH)	N	244

O

P

Alphabetical Listing of Doctors

Alphabetical Listing of Doctors

Name	Specialty	Pg	Name	Specialty	Pg
Ryken, Timothy (IA)	NS	233	Saven, Alan (CA)	Hem	141
			Savides, Thomas (CA)	Ge	122
			Sawaya, Raymond (TX)	NS	235
			Sawczuk, Ihor (NJ)	U	489
S			Sawin, Robert (WA)	PS	361
Saclarides, Theodore (IL)	CRS	92	Scarborough, Mark (FL)	OrS	282
Sagalowsky, Arthur (TX)	U	500	Scardino, Peter (NY)	U	489
Sagel, Stuart (MO)	DR	410	Schaeffer, Anthony (IL)	U	497
Saha, Sukamal (MI)	S	450	Schantz, Stimson (NY)	Oto	294
Sahin, Aysegul (TX)	Path	326	Scheff, Alice (CA)	NuM	418
Saiki, John (NM)	Onc	195	Scheinberg, David (NY)	Onc	163
Sailer, Scott (NC)	RadRO	396	Scheithauer, Bernd (MN)	Path	324
Sakamoto, Kathleen (CA)	PHO	354	Scher, Howard (NY)	Onc	163
Salem, Riad (IL)	VIR	415	Scherr, Douglas (NY)	U	489
Salem, Ronald (CT)	S	430	Schiff, David (VA)	N	243
Salgia, Ravi (IL)	Onc	185	Schiff, Peter (NY)	RadRO	390
Sallan, Stephen (MA)	PHO	333	Schiffer, Charles (MI)	Onc	186
Salo, Jonathan (NC)	S	444	Schiffman, Fred (RI)	Hem	127
Saltz, Leonard (NY)	Onc	162	Schiffman, Jade (TX)	Oph	276
Salvi, Sharad (IL)	PHO	349	Schild, Steven (AZ)	RadRO	404
Samadi, David (NY)	U	489	Schilder, Russell (PA)	Onc	163
Samant, Sandeep (TN)	Oto	297	Schiller, Alan (NY)	Path	320
Samlowski, Wolfram (NV)	Onc	203	Schiller, Gary (CA)	Hem	141
Sampson, John (NC)	NS	229	Schiller, Joan (TX)	Onc	195
Samuels, Brian (ID)	Onc	190	Schilsky, Richard (IL)	Onc	186
Sanchez, Miguel (NJ)	Path	320	Schink, Julian (IL)	GO	261
Sanda, Martin (MA)	U	485	Schlegel, Peter (NY)	U	489
Sandberg, David (FL)	NS	229	Schmidt, Richard (PA)	OrS	282
Sanders, William (GA)	U	494	Schnabel, Freya (NY)	S	438
Sandler, Alan (OR)	Onc	204	Schnipper, Lowell (MA)	Onc	146
Sandler, Eric (FL)	PHO	344	Schnitt, Stuart (MA)	Path	317
Sandler, Howard (CA)	RadRO	406	Schoenberg, Mark (MD)	U	489
Sandlund, John (TN)	PHO	344	Schoetz, David (MA)	CRS	87
Sanford, Robert (TN)	NS	229	Schomberg, Paula (MN)	RadRO	400
Santana, Victor (TN)	PHO	345	Schorge, John (MA)	GO	251
Santin, Alessandro (CT)	GO	251	Schraut, Wolfgang (PA)	S	438
Sarr, Michael (MN)	S	450	Schuchter, Lynn (PA)	Onc	163
Sasaki, Clarence (CT)	Oto	290	Schulick, Richard (MD)	S	438
Sasson, Aaron (NE)	S	452	Schuster, Michael (NY)	Hem	130
Sataloff, Dahlia (PA)	S	438	Schuster, Stephen (PA)	Hem	130
Saunders, John (MD)	S	438	Schusterman, Mark (TX)	PlS	370
Sauter, Edward (ND)	S	453	Schwartz, Burton (MN)	Onc	186
Savage, David (NY)	Hem	130	Schwartz, Cindy (RI)	PHO	334

Alphabetical Listing of Doctors

Name	Specialty	Pg	Name	Specialty	Pg
Schwartz, Herbert (TN)	OrS	283	Sherman, Carol (SC)	Onc	176
Schwartz, L Matthew (PA)	PMR	515	Sherman, Randolph (CA)	PlS	371
Schwartz, Michael (FL)	Onc	175	Sherman, Steven (TX)	EDM	112
Schwartz, Peter (CT)	GO	251	Shibata, Stephen (CA)	Onc	204
Schwartz, Theodore (NY)	NS	226	Shields, Carol (PA)	Oph	273
Schwartzberg, Lee (TN)	Hem	133	Shields, Jerry (PA)	Oph	273
Schwartzentruber, Douglas (IN)	S	450	Shields, Peter (DC)	Onc	163
Scott, Walter (PA)	TS	473	Shike, Moshe (NY)	Ge	118
Scott-Conner, Carol (IA)	S	450	Shin, Dong Moon (GA)	Onc	176
Scudder, Sidney (CA)	Onc	204	Shina, Donald (NM)	RadRO	404
See, William (WI)	U	497	Shindo, Maisie (OR)	Oto	304
Segal, Brahm (NY)	Inf	513	Shochat, Stephen (TN)	PS	359
Seiff, Stuart (CA)	Oph	277	Shrager, Joseph (CA)	TS	480
Sekhar, Laligam (WA)	NS	237	Shrieve, Dennis (UT)	RadRO	402
Selvaggi, Kathy (MA)	Onc	146	Shulman, Lawrence (MA)	Onc	147
Sen, Chandranath (NY)	NS	226	Shulman, Lee (IL)	ObG	267
Senagore, Anthony (CA)	CRS	94	Sibley, Richard (CA)	Path	329
Sencer, Susan (MN)	PHO	349	Sidransky, David (MD)	Onc	163
Sener, Stephen (CA)	S	460	Siegel, Barry (MO)	NuM	418
Senzer, Neil (TX)	RadRO	404	Siegel, Gordon (IL)	Oto	300
Sepkowitz, Kent (NY)	Inf	513	Siegel, Herrick (AL)	OrS	283
Serletti, Joseph (PA)	PlS	367	Siegel, Stuart (CA)	PHO	355
Serody, Jonathan (NC)	Onc	175	Siegelbaum, Marc (MD)	U	490
Seung, Steven (OR)	RadRO	406	Sielaff, Timothy (MN)	S	450
Sewell, C Whitaker (GA)	Path	322	Sigurdson, Elin (PA)	S	438
Shaffrey, Mark (VA)	NS	230	Sikic, Branimir (CA)	Onc	204
Shah, Jatin (NY)	S	438	Silbergeld, Daniel (WA)	NS	237
Shah, Nishit (RI)	CRS	87	Siller, Barry (TX)	GO	263
Shamberger, Robert (MA)	PS	357	Sills, Allen (TN)	NS	230
Shapiro, Charles (OH)	Onc	186	Silva, Elvio (TX)	Path	326
Shapiro, Lawrence (NY)	CG	511	Silver, Michael (IL)	Pul	379
Shapiro, Richard (NY)	S	438	Silver, Samuel (MI)	Onc	186
Shapiro, Scott (IN)	NS	233	Silverman, Jan (PA)	Path	320
Shapiro, William (AZ)	N	244	Silverman, Lewis (NY)	Onc	163
Shapshay, Stanley (NY)	Oto	294	Silverman, Paula (OH)	Onc	186
Shaw, Edward (NC)	RadRO	396	Silverstein, Melvin (CA)	S	460
Shea, Christopher (IL)	D	105	Sim, Franklin (MN)	OrS	285
Shea, Thomas (NC)	Onc	176	Simeone, Diane (MI)	S	450
Shearer, Patricia (FL)	PHO	345	Simmons, Rache (NY)	S	439
Sheinfeld, Joel (NY)	U	490	Simon, George (SC)	Onc	176
Shellito, Paul (MA)	CRS	87	Sinanan, Mika (WA)	S	461
Shen, Perry (NC)	S	444	Singer, Daniel (HI)	OrS	286
Shenk, Robert (OH)	S	450	Singer, Mark (CA)	Oto	305

Name	Specialty	Pg	Name	Specialty	Pg
Singh, Dinesh (CT)	U	485	Sokol, Thomas (CA)	CRS	94
Singhal, Seema (IL)	Hem	137	Sokoloff, Daniel (FL)	D	103
Sinha, Uttam (CA)	Oto	305	Solberg, Lawrence (FL)	Hem	133
Siperstein, Allan (OH)	S	451	Solin, Lawrence (PA)	RadRO	391
Sisti, Michael (NY)	NS	227	Solorzano, Carmen (TN)	S	444
Skibber, John (TX)	S	456	Soloway, Mark (FL)	U	494
Skinner, Eila (CA)	U	502	Sondak, Vernon (FL)	S	444
Skinner, Kristin (NY)	S	439	Sondel, Paul (WI)	PHO	350
Skinner, Michael (TX)	PS	360	Sonett, Joshua (NY)	TS	474
Sklar, Charles (NY)	PEn	356	Song, John (CO)	Oto	301
Slatkin, Neal (CA)	PM	313	Song, Shiyu (VA)	RadRO	396
Slawin, Kevin (TX)	U	500	Sood, Anil (TX)	GO	264
Slease, Robert (DE)	Hem	130	Soparkar, Charles (TX)	Oph	276
Sledge, George (IN)	Onc	186	Soper, John (NC)	GO	258
Slezak, Sheri (MD)	PlS	367	Sosa, Julie (CT)	S	430
Slingluff, Craig (VA)	S	444	Soslow, Robert (NY)	Path	320
Slivka, Adam (PA)	Ge	118	Sosman, Jeffrey (TN)	Onc	176
Small, Donald (MD)	PHO	339	Sotomayor, Eduardo (FL)	Onc	176
Small, Eric (CA)	Onc	204	Soulen, Michael (PA)	VIR	415
Small, William (IL)	RadRO	401	Souweidane, Mark (NY)	NS	227
Smalley, Stephen (KS)	RadRO	402	Spann, Cyril (GA)	GO	258
Smith, Barbara (MA)	S	430	Spetzler, Robert (AZ)	NS	235
Smith, David (FL)	PlS	368	Speyer, James (NY)	Onc	164
Smith, Donna (IL)	GO	261	Spiegel, David (CA)	Psyc	376
Smith, Joseph (TN)	U	494	Spigland, Nitsana (NY)	PS	358
Smith, Lloyd (CA)	GO	265	Spirtos, Nicola (NV)	GO	266
Smith, Matthew (MA)	Onc	147	Spitzer, Thomas (MA)	Hem	127
Smith, Mitchell (PA)	Onc	163	Spivak, Jerry (MD)	Hem	131
Smith, Paul (FL)	PlS	368	Spriggs, David (NY)	Onc	164
Smith, Russell (NE)	Oto	301	St Clair, William (KY)	RadRO	396
Smith, Thomas (VA)	Onc	176	Staats, Peter (NJ)	PM	311
Smoot, Duane (DC)	Ge	118	Stadelmann, Wayne (NH)	PlS	366
Smythe, W Roy (TX)	TS	479	Stadler, Walter (IL)	Onc	186
Snyder, David (CA)	Hem	141	Stadtmauer, Edward (PA)	Onc	164
Snyder, Peter (PA)	EDM	110	Stahl, Donna (OH)	S	451
Snyderman, Carl (PA)	Oto	294	Stahl, Richard (CT)	PlS	366
Sobel, Stuart (FL)	D	103	Staley, Charles (GA)	S	444
Sober, Arthur (MA)	D	99	Stamos, Michael (CA)	CRS	94
Soberman, Mark (DC)	TS	473	Staren, Edgar (IL)	S	451
Socinski, Mark (NC)	Onc	176	Stea, Baldassarre (AZ)	RadRO	404
Soiffer, Robert (MA)	Onc	147	Steen, Preston (ND)	Onc	190
Soisson, Andrew (UT)	GO	262	Stehman, Frederick (IN)	GO	261
Sokol, Lubomir (FL)	Hem	133	Stein, David (PA)	CRS	89

Alphabetical Listing of Doctors

Name	Specialty	Pg	Name	Specialty	Pg
Steinberg, Gary (IL)	U	497	Sun, Peter (CA)	NS	238
Steinberg, Harry (NY)	Pul	378	Sun, Weijing (PA)	Onc	164
Steingart, Richard (NY)	Cv	511	Sundaram, Chandru (IN)	U	498
Steinhagen, Randolph (NY)	CRS	89	Sundaram, Magesh (WV)	S	439
Steinherz, Laurel (NY)	PCd	355	Suntharalingam, Mohan (MD)	RadRO	391
Steinherz, Peter (NY)	PHO	340	Suster, Saul (WI)	Path	324
Stenson, Kerstin (IL)	Oto	300	Sutphen, Rebecca (FL)	CG	512
Stern, Jeffrey (CA)	GO	266	Sutton, John (NH)	S	430
Sternberg, Paul (TN)	Oph	273	Sutton, Leslie (PA)	NS	227
Stewart, Forrest (WA)	Onc	204	Sutton, Linda (NC)	Onc	177
Stewart, Paula (AL)	PMR	515	Swain, Sandra (DC)	Onc	164
Stieg, Philip (NY)	NS	227	Swanson, David (TX)	U	500
Stiff, Patrick (IL)	Hem	137	Swanson, Neil (OR)	D	107
Stock, Richard (NY)	RadRO	391	Swanson, Scott (MA)	TS	471
Stockdale, Frank (CA)	Onc	204	Swarm, Robert (MO)	PM	312
Stolar, Charles (NY)	PS	358	Swearingen, Brooke (MA)	NS	223
Stolier, Alan (LA)	S	456	Sweeney, Christopher (MA)	Onc	147
Stone, Joel (FL)	Onc	177	Sweetenham, John (OH)	Onc	187
Stone, Richard (MA)	Hem	127	Swensen, Stephen (MN)	DR	411
Stoopler, Mark (NY)	Onc	164	Swerdlow, Steven (PA)	Path	320
Stout, J Timothy (OR)	Oph	277	Swetter, Susan (CA)	D	107
Strair, Roger (NJ)	Hem	131	Swisher, Stephen (TX)	TS	479
Strauch, Eric (MD)	PS	358	Swistel, Alexander (NY)	S	439
Straus, David (NY)	Onc	164	Szabo, Robert (CA)	HS	287
Strauss, Gary (MA)	Onc	147	Sze, Gordon (CT)	NRad	412
Strauss, H William (NY)	NuM	417			
Strauss, James (TX)	Hem	139			
Streeter, Oscar (DC)	RadRO	391			
Streiff, Michael (MD)	Hem	131		**T**	
Strenger, Rochelle (RI)	Onc	147	Taetle, Raymond (AZ)	Onc	196
Stringer, Scott (MS)	Oto	297	Tafra, Lorraine (MD)	S	439
Strome, Marshall (NY)	Oto	294	Tagawa, Scott (NY)	Onc	164
Strome, Scott (MD)	Oto	294	Taghian, Alphonse (MA)	RadRO	386
Strouse, Thomas (CA)	Psyc	376	Talamonti, Mark (IL)	S	451
Strup, Stephen (KY)	U	494	Tallman, Martin (NY)	Hem	131
Stryker, Steven (IL)	CRS	92	Tanabe, Kenneth (MA)	S	430
Stubblefield, Michael (NY)	PMR	515	Taneja, Samir (NY)	U	490
Su, Li-Ming (FL)	U	494	Tannous, Raymond (IA)	PHO	350
Suen, James (AR)	Oto	303	Taplin, Mary-Ellen (MA)	Onc	147
Sugarbaker, David (MA)	TS	470	Tarbell, Nancy (MA)	RadRO	386
Sugarbaker, Paul (DC)	S	439	Tarraza, Hector (ME)	GO	251
Suh, John (OH)	RadRO	401	Tartter, Paul (NY)	S	439
Sultan, Mark (NY)	PlS	367	Tatter, Stephen (NC)	NS	230

Name	Specialty	Pg	Name	Specialty	Pg
Taylor, Lynne (WA)	N	245	Triozzi, Pierre (OH)	Onc	187
Taylor, Marie (MO)	RadRO	401	Tripathy, Debasish (CA)	Onc	205
Taylor, Peyton (VA)	GO	259	Tripuraneni, Prabhakar (CA)	RadRO	406
Taylor, R Stan (TX)	D	106	Trisal, Vijay (CA)	S	461
Tchou, Julia (PA)	S	439	Troner, Michael (FL)	Onc	177
Tebbi, Cameron (FL)	PHO	345	True, Lawrence (WA)	Path	329
Teigland, Chris (NC)	U	494	Trump, Donald (NY)	Onc	165
Teirstein, Alvin (NY)	Pul	378	Tsangaris, Theodore (MD)	S	440
Teknos, Theodoros (OH)	Oto	300	Tsao, Hensin (MA)	D	99
Tempero, Margaret (CA)	Onc	204	Tse, David (FL)	Oph	273
Teng, Nelson (CA)	GO	266	Tucker, Rodney (AL)	IM	514
Teperman, Lewis (NY)	S	439	Tufano, Ralph (MD)	Oto	294
Tepper, Joel (NC)	RadRO	396	Tufaro, Anthony (MD)	PlS	368
Terris, David (GA)	Oto	297	Tulsky, James (NC)	IM	514
Terris, Martha (GA)	U	494	Turtz, Alan (NJ)	NS	227
Tester, William (PA)	Onc	165	Tuttle, R Michael (NY)	EDM	111
Tewari, Ashutosh (NY)	U	490	Tuttle, Todd (MN)	S	451
Thayer, Sarah (MA)	S	431	Twardowski, Przemyslaw (CA)	Onc	205
Thiers, Bruce (SC)	D	103	Tyler, Douglas (NC)	S	445
Thigpen, James (MS)	Onc	177			
Thomas, Charles (OR)	RadRO	406			
Thomas, Gregory (OR)	PHO	355			
Thompson, B Gregory (MI)	NS	233	**U**		
Thompson, Ian (TX)	U	500	Uberti, Joseph (MI)	Hem	137
Thompson, John (WA)	Onc	205	Udelsman, Robert (CT)	S	431
Thompson, Reid (TN)	NS	230	Ulbright, Thomas (IN)	Path	324
Thor, Ann (CO)	Path	325	Ulissey, Michael (TX)	DR	411
Thorson, Alan (NE)	CRS	93	Unger, Michael (PA)	Pul	378
Thrasher, J Brantley (KS)	U	498	Urba, Susan (MI)	Onc	187
Ting, Jess (NY)	PlS	367	Urba, Walter (OR)	Onc	205
Tkaczuk, Katherine (MD)	Onc	165	Urist, Marshall (AL)	S	445
Tomaszewski, John (PA)	Path	321	Urken, Mark (NY)	Oto	294
Tomita, Tadanori (IL)	NS	233	Uzzo, Robert (PA)	U	490
Tomlinson, Gail (TX)	PHO	352			
Toonkel, Leonard (FL)	RadRO	396			
Topham, Neal (PA)	PlS	367	**V**		
Toppmeyer, Deborah (NJ)	Onc	165	Valea, Fidel (NC)	GO	259
Tornos, Carmen (NY)	Path	321	Valentine, Alan (TX)	Psyc	375
Torti, Frank (NC)	Onc	177	Valentino, Joseph (KY)	Oto	297
Trabulsi, Edouard (PA)	U	490	Valero, Vicente (TX)	Onc	196
Travis, William (NY)	Path	321	Vallieres, Eric (WA)	TS	480
Treon, Steven (MA)	Onc	147	Van Arsdalen, Keith (PA)	U	490
Triche, Timothy (CA)	Path	329			

Alphabetical Listing of Doctors

Name	Specialty	Pg	Name	Specialty	Pg
Weingart, Jon (MD)	NS	227	Willey, Shawna (DC)	S	440
Weinreb, Jeffrey (CT)	DR	407	Williams, James (AZ)	PHO	352
Weinstein, Gregory (PA)	Oto	295	Williams, Michael (VA)	Hem	133
Weinstein, Howard (MA)	PHO	334	Williams, Ronald (TX)	OrS	285
Weinstein, James (NH)	OrS	280	Willson, James (TX)	Onc	196
Weinstein, Sharon (UT)	PM	312	Wilson, David (OR)	Oph	277
Weintraub, Joshua (NY)	VIR	415	Wilson, J Frank (WI)	RadRO	401
Weisberg, Tracey (ME)	Onc	148	Wilson, Keith (OH)	Oto	300
Weisenburger, Dennis (NE)	Path	325	Wilson, Lynn (CT)	RadRO	387
Weisman, Robert (CA)	Oto	305	Wilson, Matthew (TN)	Oph	274
Weisman, Steven (WI)	PM	312	Wilson, Timothy (CA)	U	502
Weiss, Geoffrey (VA)	Onc	178	Wilson, Wyndham (MD)	Onc	166
Weiss, Lawrence (CA)	Path	329	Winer, Eric (MA)	Onc	148
Weiss, Marisa (PA)	RadRO	391	Wingard, John (FL)	Onc	178
Weiss, Robert (NJ)	U	491	Winick, Naomi (TX)	PHO	352
Weiss, Robert (CT)	U	485	Winter, Jane (IL)	Hem	137
Weiss, Sharon (GA)	Path	322	Wisch, Nathaniel (NY)	Hem	131
Weissler, Mark (NC)	Oto	297	Wise, Paul (TN)	CRS	90
Weitzel, Jeffrey (CA)	CG	513	Wiseman, Gregory (MN)	NuM	418
Weksler, Benny (PA)	TS	474	Wisoff, Jeffrey (NY)	NS	227
Welton, Mark (CA)	CRS	94	Witt, Thomas (IL)	S	452
Werner-Wasik, Maria (PA)	RadRO	391	Wittig, James (NY)	OrS	282
Wetzler, Meir (NY)	Onc	166	Wolchok, Jedd (NY)	Onc	166
Wexler, Leonard (NY)	PHO	340	Wolf, Gregory (MI)	Oto	300
Wexner, Steven (FL)	CRS	90	Wolfe, Lawrence (NY)	PHO	340
Weymuller, Ernest (WA)	Oto	305	Wolff, Antonio (MD)	Onc	166
Wharam, Moody (MD)	RadRO	391	Wolff, Bruce (MN)	CRS	92
Wharen, Robert (FL)	NS	230	Wolff, Robert (TX)	Onc	196
Wheeland, Ronald (MO)	D	105	Wolfson, Aaron (FL)	RadRO	397
Wheeler, Thomas (TX)	Path	327	Wollmann, Robert (IL)	Path	324
Whelan, Alison (MO)	CG	512	Woltering, Eugene (LA)	S	456
Whelan, Richard (NY)	CRS	89	Wong, Jeffrey (CA)	RadRO	407
White, Richard (NC)	S	445	Woo, Peak (NY)	Oto	295
Whitworth, Pat (TN)	S	445	Woo, Shiao (KY)	RadRO	397
Whyte, Richard (CA)	TS	480	Wood, Bradford (MD)	VIR	415
Wicha, Max (MI)	Onc	187	Wood, David (MI)	U	498
Wierman, Ann (NV)	Onc	205	Wood, Douglas (WA)	TS	480
Wilczynski, Sharon (CA)	Path	329	Wood, Gary (WI)	D	105
Wilding, George (WI)	Onc	187	Wood, R Patrick (TX)	S	457
Wiley, Joseph (MD)	PHO	340	Wood, William (GA)	S	445
Wilkins, Edwin (MI)	PlS	369	Worden, Francis (MI)	Onc	187
Wilkins, Ross (CO)	OrS	285	Wright, Cameron (MA)	TS	471
Willett, Christopher (NC)	RadRO	397	Wurtz, L Daniel (IN)	OrS	285

Alphabetical Listing of Doctors

Name	Specialty	Pg

Y

Yaddanapudi, Ravindranath (MI)	PHO	350
Yahalom, Joachim (NY)	RadRO	391
Yang, James (MD)	S	440
Yang, Stephen (MD)	TS	474
Yankelevitz, David (NY)	DR	409
Yanovich, Saul (MD)	Hem	131
Yarbrough, Wendell (TN)	Oto	297
Yeager, Andrew (AZ)	Hem	140
Yeatman, Timothy (FL)	S	445
Yeatts, R Patrick (NC)	Oph	274
Yee, Douglas (MN)	Onc	188
Yen, Yun (CA)	Onc	206
Yeo, Charles (PA)	S	440
Yetman, Randall (OH)	PlS	369
Yeung, Raymond (WA)	S	461
York, Teresa (MD)	PHO	340
Young, Robert (MA)	Path	317
Yousem, Samuel (PA)	Path	321
Yu, George (MD)	U	491
Yu, John (CA)	NS	238
Yueh, Bevan (MN)	Oto	300
Yuen, James (AR)	PlS	370
Yung, WK Alfred (TX)	N	245
Yunus, Furhan (TN)	Onc	178

Z

Zagoria, Ronald (NC)	DR	410
Zagzag, David (NY)	Path	321
Zannis, Victor (AZ)	S	457
Zeitels, Steven (MA)	Oto	290
Zelefsky, Michael (NY)	RadRO	392
Zelenetz, Andrew (NY)	Onc	166
Zietman, Anthony (MA)	RadRO	387
Zimmerman, Donald (IL)	PEn	356
Zinner, Michael (MA)	S	431
Zippe, Craig (OH)	U	498
Zitelli, John (PA)	D	101
Zuckerman, Kenneth (FL)	Hem	133
Zwischenberger, Joseph (KY)	TS	476

Acknowledgments

The publishers would like to thank the entire staff for their many hours and days of intense and precise work on this guide in order to further its goal of assisting consumers in making the best healthcare choices.

Castle Connolly Executive Management:

Chairman	John K. Castle
President & CEO	John J. Connolly, Ed.D.
Vice President, Chief Medical & Research Officer	Jean Morgan, M.D.
Vice President, Chief Strategy & Operations Officer	William Liss-Levinson, Ph.D.

Research Coordinators

Maryann Hynd, RN
Sara Sezer
Terysia Herbert
Jerville Weekes
Meagan Crooks
Cassandra Fevelo
Yuliya Nagdimova

Book Layout, Database Management	Russell Hodgson
Book Production Coordinator	Sara Sezer
Office Manager	Marcie Samartino
Director of Client Relations	Jennifer Mojave
Communications Manager	Nicki Hughes

We also would like to extend our gratitude to the American Board of Medical Specialties (ABMS) for allowing us to use excerpts, especially the descriptions of medical specialties and subspecialties, from the text of their publication "Which Medical Specialist for You?"

Other Publications from Castle Connolly Medical Ltd.:
America's Top Doctors®; *Top Doctors: New York Metro Area*;
Top Doctors: Chicago Metro Area; *Cancer Made Easier: New York— Metro Area*, *Eldercare* and others...
Order online at http://www.castleconnolly.com/books

The Best in American Medicine
www.CastleConnolly.com

Memberships for Corporations & Organizations

This service enables an employer to assist employees in identifying Top Doctors to care for themselves and their families. It is a low-cost, non-intrusive service that will result in better care and, ultimately, lower healthcare costs. For as low as a few dollars per year, employees can have complete access to the Castle Connolly website and database of Top Doctors who were nominated by their peers and screened by the Castle Connolly physician-led research team.

Instead of simply choosing a doctor's name from the phone book or a plan directory, the employee can compare physician names to the Castle Connolly database of 30,000 plus Top Doctors and select from among the best doctors in the country. This will result in overall better care, lower costs and improved morale. Once an employee logs on to the Castle Connolly database, valuable background information is available on every Top Doctor such as: medical school, board certifications, fellowships, hospital affiliations, residencies and much more, to allow them to make the best informed decision they can make when selecting a doctor.

Top Doctors can have an enormous impact. For patients and their families, the value of receiving first-class medical care is great but unquantifiable – it is measured in quality and even length of life. Employers, however, can see the results in their bottom line. Faulty diagnoses and improper treatment take a toll in productivity and ripple out into higher workplace costs. No company should have to "make do" for weeks or months without a key employee or executive, when a Top Doctor may have solved the patient's problem quickly and efficiently. The effort to identify the best doctors from ordinary ones is justified by the money saved on incorrect treatments, unnecessary surgery and days lost from work.

The Corporate Membership is suited for employers of varying sizes and can also be of great value to professional, social, civic, fraternal and religious associations. Castle Connolly may also be able to adapt and tailor the presentation of the database to meet the specific corporate client's needs.

New Movers Program

The Castle Connolly New Movers Program is designed to alleviate that concern, or even fear, as well as the time-consuming struggle to identify the right – and best – doctors and hospitals in one's new community or region. The service can be provided on a family basis (those living in the household) or for a single client. The service includes identifying primary care physicians, including Pediatricians, OB/GYN's, Internists and Family Practitioners as well as other specialists that may be needed: for example, Ophthalmologists, Allergists, Endocrinologists, Surgeons or others as required.

Perhaps nothing is more challenging to a family that has relocated to a new community than finding appropriate healthcare resources, especially physicians. While they can turn to recommendations from new neighbors and friends, or select names from the phone book or a plan directory, that is hardly adequate, especially if there are special healthcare needs in the family.

A Castle Connolly Health Advisor will identify two or three recommendations for up to six different medical specialties. If, for some reason the client wishes to change doctors within two months, Castle Connolly will identify new physicians in the same specialty. After the selection process occurs, the Health Advisor will make an introductory phone call to the physician's office. This typically facilitates faster appointments.

Doctor-Patient Advisor Program for Corporations & Organizations

The Doctor-Patient Advisor is a focused, highly personalized advisory service providing one-on-one phone consultations to individuals who have serious or complex medical problems, or anyone who feels they need assistance in finding the right doctor. It is designed to assist people in identifying the best doctors to meet their complex medical needs. Patients or their family members can speak with a nurse practitioner regarding their condition. To assist in finding a doctor, Castle Connolly identifies two to three top specialists, based on the medical condition, patient needs and the patient's specific preferences regarding geographic location, hospital affiliation, gender, age and other considerations. Because Castle Connolly's corporate programs are not insurance, they are not covered by the Employee Retirement Income Security Act (ERISA) and may be offered to selected employee groups.

The program is not designed to answer general medical or health insurance questions. Because of the breadth and depth of our database - and the extensive healthcare experience of our staff – the identification of doctors can be limited to a given region or the search can focus on finding the very best anywhere in the nation. This high level service is available at a low cost of $3.00 per employee - per month. Each employee will need to go on to an indicated website and download their specific access code and use our toll-free number to call and consult with a Castle Connolly Health Advisor to ensure the process of finding a Top Doctor is efficient and effective. Our Health Advisors are available during regular business hours Monday through Friday 9:00am-5:00pm EST.

For further information on the following programs: Corporate Membership Program, New Movers Program and Doctor-Patient Advisor Program, contact:

Jennifer Mojave
Corporate Services Manager
212.367.8400, ext. 35
or jmojave@castleconnolly.com

Strategic Partnerships

Castle Connolly Medical Ltd. has a number of strategic partnerships that may be of interest to consumers and physicians.

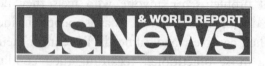

U.S. News & World Report and Castle Connolly created a strategic collaboration that will bring the Castle Connolly Top Doctors® database to online visitors to the U.S. News website. The online database went live on www.usnews.com in mid-July 2011 and will be linked with the U.S. News database of Best Hospitals. Consumers will be able to search the full database of Top Doctors across the nation, including all specialties and subspecialties. The detailed physician profiles, including designation of doctors affiliated with Castle Connolly's Partnership for Excellence hospital program, will be drawn from Castle Connolly's growing database of over 27,000 physicians currently accessible online at www.castleconnolly.com.

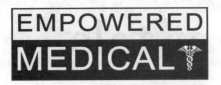

Empowered Doctor is a media, news and marketing service. Empowered Doctor produces syndicated consumer health reports. Its video and text news stories appear on major media websites, including CBS. Empowered Doctor also provides marketing services to hospitals, clinics and individual physicians by generating visibility in online search and social media. Empowered Doctor's clients benefit from the company's efficient methodologies for generating new patient referrals.

For more information call 888-333-1027 or visit www.empowereddoctor.com

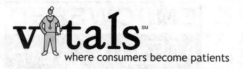
where consumers become patients

Vitals (www.vitals.com), an innovative online doctor review and comparison service from MDx Medical Inc., is the comprehensive source for vital information, peer evaluations and patient feedback on more than 700,000 doctors nationwide. Drawing upon prestigious information repositories, cutting-edge search and comparison technologies, and a robust patient feedback mechanism, Vitals has organized key information to help patients make an informed choice in their search for the right doctor. Castle Connolly and Vitals have a branding relationship in which those physicians who are Castle Connolly Top Doctors® and appear on Vitals web sites have an icon indicating their status and recognition as a Castle Connolly Top Doctor. Additional information can be found at www.vitals.com.

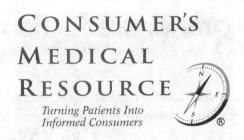

CONSUMER'S
MEDICAL
RESOURCE

*Turning Patients Into
Informed Consumers*

Consumer's Medical Resource was started in 1996 to offer high-quality, high-impact employee benefit programs to help employees and their dependents, and has been a pioneer in Medical Decision Support® services. CMR addresses all medical conditions at any point within the continuum of care, by providing personalized, evidence-based medical research, information, access to genuine, in-person second opinions and support services to employees who face serious, complicated, and chronic illness, or would like to become well-informed healthcare consumers.

Leveraging a state-of-the-art integrated model of web, phone, and print-based services, CMR enables employees to fully understand and evaluate their options so they can make the most informed medical decisions possible with their doctors. The company is privately held and currently provides services to more than 600,000 Americans, achieving extremely high levels of user and customer satisfaction, improved clinical quality outcomes, and generated excellent ROI.

Castle Connolly and CMR are working together to provide Castle Connolly's various corporate services to CMR client companies and their employees.

For more information, please visit: http://www.consumersmedical.com.

grandparents.com®
it's great to be grand.

Grandparents.com is dedicated to enhancing the lives of America's 70 million grandparents by fostering family connections, via child- and grandparent-friendly activities, travel ideas, compelling lifestyle features, expert advice, gift ideas, recipes, and more. Visitors have access to a range of tools, including groups, discussions, a homepage blog, photo sharing, and a Facebook page and Twitter feeds. Through the Grandparents.com Benefits Club, catering to America's 120 million grandparents, Boomers and seniors, members benefit from discounts and incentives they can use every day, in categories like gifts, clothes, and vitamins, plus exclusive opportunities to save on hotels, cruises, auto rentals, theme park trips, theatrical productions, and insurance. Grandparents can share their membership benefits with four extended family and household members. In 2010, Grandparents.com was ranked as the No. 3 website for seniors, boomers, and grandparents, following the U.S. Government and AARP. Castle Connolly provides access to its Top Doctors' database, its Doctor-Patient Advisor and New Movers programs for Grandparents.com members.

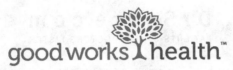

The Good Works Health government-approved platform - www.goodworkshealth.com - offers physicians the opportunity to direct donations, based on the fair market value of their time, to charities of their choice in exchange for participation in educational programs.

Participating physicians can choose from more than a million approved charities to designate as the recipients of these donations. Good Works Health's unique platform reaches a growing community of medical professionals in many specialties that are motivated by the opportunity to do good works. Castle Connolly actively works with Good Works Health to promote these opportunities to its Castle Connolly Top Doctors®

DrScore.com
PATIENTS SPEAK, DOCTORS LISTEN

Founded by Steven Feldman, M.D., DrScore.com is an interactive online survey site where patients can rate their physicians, as well as find a physician based on their service level preference.

The mission of DrScore.com is to improve medical care by giving patients a forum for rating their physician and by giving doctors an affordable, objective, non-intrusive means of documenting the quality of care that they provide. Visitors on Castle Connolly's website who are searching for "top doctors" have the option to also rate these and other physicians they have been to as patients, as well as to see if these physicians have been rated previously by other consumers on DrScore.com. Visitors to DrScore.com will be able to see if their doctors and/or other doctors are Castle Connolly "top doctors."

For more information, visit www.drscore.com.

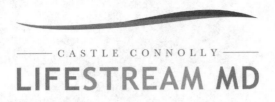

LIFESTREAM MD

Castle Connolly Medical Ltd. has a strategic relationship with Castle Connolly LifeStream MD to provide a unique health advisory service designed for families and executives, especially those who travel regularly or may have more than one residence.

Each client is assigned a Castle Connolly LifeStream MD physician who is available to them by phone 24/7/365. A client call from anywhere in the world is answered promptly and the client is connected with their Castle Connolly LifeStream MD physician advisor.

The Castle Connolly LifeStream MD physician acts as a health manager assisting in navigation of an increasingly complex health care environment. The Castle Connolly LifeStream MD physician does not replace the member's primary physician or specialists, but provides additional independent counsel and services that provide security to our members either at home or while traveling.

In the United States, the Castle Connolly LifeStream MD physician will use the Castle Connolly database of Top Doctors to assure that the client is cared for in the best medical facilities by the top doctors. Assistance in securing timely appointments with specialists and records transfers is facilitated as needed. Outside of the United States, Castle Connolly LifeStream MD has an affiliation with International SOS, the world's largest and leading provider of travel medical assistance to assure the LifeStream MD member is cared for by the best doctors and hospitals available in that region or, if necessary, is transported to a place where that care is available.

The Best in American Medicine
www.CastleConnolly.com

National Physician of the Year Awards

Castle Connolly Medical Ltd. proudly hosted its sixth annual *National Physician of the Year Awards* on March 28, 2011 at The Hudson theatre New York City. It was a spectacular evening which allowed us to recognize both the outstanding honorees and the excellence of the many thousands of physicians throughout the nation.

The Genesis of the National Physician of the Year Award.

Each year we receive thousands of nominations from physicians and the medical leadership of major medical centers, specialty hospitals, teaching hospitals and regional and community medical centers across the United States as an integral part of our research, screening and selection process to identify *America's Top Doctors®*. The selected physicians, while spread across all fifty states and involved in more than 70 medical specialties and subspecialties, all share one distinguishing professional attribute: an unwavering dedication to their patients and to medicine as a whole. Each and every one of these outstanding medical professionals is a symbol of the clinical excellence that characterizes American medicine. In honor of these exemplary physicians, Castle Connolly Medical Ltd. has created the *National Physician of the Year Awards* to recognize the thousands of excellent, dedicated physicians across the United States. Our Medical Advisory Board selected the honorees from the hundreds nominated in a special nomination process conducted months before the event.

The honorees, Drs. Armando E. Giuliano, O. Wayne Isom, and David W. Kennedy are superb examples of excellence in clinical medical practice. In addition to these awards for Clinical Excellence, Castle Connolly Medical Ltd. honored Drs. George P. Canellos, and Matthew D. Davis for their lifetime achievement in medicine. Mrs. Evelyn H. Lauder is a   tireless fundraiser for the Estee Lauder Companies' Breast Cancer Awareness Campaign and The Breast Cancer Research Foundation® organization and an exemplary recipient for the sixth National Health Leadership Award.

Each honoree received a beautiful and distinctive porcelain figurine created by the Boehm Porcelain Company exclusively for the National Physician of the Year Awards. The award features a golden caduceus, the symbol of the medical community, surrounded by a golden laurel wreath. Laurel wreaths were used by the ancients to crown and honor their leaders. The caduceus and laurel rest upon a column accented by the signature Castle Connolly logo. By combining the caduceus and the laurel wreaths, the award embodies the excellence in medical achievement that the National Physician of the Year Awards celebrates each year.

National Physician of the Year Awards

National Physician of the Year Awards Honorees:

<u>For Clinical Excellence</u>

Armando E. Giuliano, M.D., FACS, FRCSED
Chief of Science and Medicine
John Wayne Cancer Institute at Saint John's Health Center,
Santa Monica, CA

O. Wayne Isom, M.D.
Chairman of the Dept. of Cardiothoracic Surgery
New York Presbyterian-Weill Cornell Medical College

David W. Kennedy, M.D.
Otorhinolaryngology Professor at the
University of Pennsylvania

<u>For Lifetime Achievement</u>

George P. Canellos, M.D.
Served as Founding Chief of Medical Oncology at
Dana-Farber Cancer Institute;

Matthew D. Davis, M.D.
University of Wisconsin Medical Center
Chair, UW Opthalmology

<u>National Health Leadership</u>

Evelyn H. Lauder
Chairman of The Breast Cancer Research Foundation®

Previous National Physician of the Year Award Honorees

2010

Clinical Excellence
John B. Buse, M.D., Ph.D.
Director of the Diabetes Care Center, Professor, Chief of the Division of
Endocrinology and Executive Associate Dean for Clinical Research,
University of North Carolina School of Medicine, Chapel Hill

Larry Norton, M.D.
Deputy Physician-in-Chief, Memorial Hospital, Memorial Sloan-Kettering
Cancer Center, for Breast Cancer Programs
Medical Director of the MSKCC's Breast and Imaging Center, Evelyn H.
Lauder Breast Center

Ching-Hon Pui, M.D.
Department Chair of Oncology, St. Jude Children's Research Hospital
Medical Director of the St. Jude International Outreach China Program,
holder of the Fahad Nassar Al-Rashid Chair of Leukemia Research

Lifetime Achievement
Basil I Hirschowitz, M.D.
Director, Gastroenterology Division, The University of Alabama
Receipient of the Kettering Medal from the General Motors Cancer
Foundation; Friedenwald Medal of the AGA; the Schindler Medal and the
Crystal Award for lifetime contributions to Endoscopy by the ASGE;
honorary doctorate of Gothenburg University; honorary fellow of the Royal
Society of Medicine

Leonard Apt, M.D.
Professor of Ophthalmology Emeritus; Director Emeritus and Founder of
the Division of Pediatric Opthalmology and Strabismus, and Co-Director of
UCLA's Center for Child Blindness

National Health Leadership
Alexandra Reeve Givens and Matthew Reeve
Trustees, The Christopher & Dana Reeve Foundation

<u>2009</u>

Clinical Excellence
Carol R. Bradford, M.D.,
Professor and Chair
Department of Otolaryngology
University of Michigan Medical System

Diane E. Meier, M.D.,
Director, Center to Advance Palliative Care
Mount Sinai School of Medicine

Judd W. Moul, M.D.,
Chief of Urology
Duke University Medical Center

Lifetime Achievement
Emil J. Freireich, M.D., D. Sc. (Hon.),
Ruth Harriet Ainsworth Chair, Distinguished Teaching Professor
Director, Special Medical Education Programs
Director, Adult Leukemia Research Program
The University of Texas M.D. Anderson Cancer Center

Thomas E. Starzl, M.D., Ph.D.
Professor of Surgery, Emeritus
Distinguished Service Professor
University of Pittsburgh Medical Center

National Health Leadership
Page Morton Black
Chairman of the Board, Parkinson's Disease Foundation

****

2008

Clinical Excellence
Robert W. Carlson, M.D.
Medical Oncology
Stanford University Medical Center

Stanley Chang, M.D.
Ophthalmology
New York-Presbyterian Hospital

L. Dade Lunsford, M.D.
Neurological Surgery
University of Pittsburgh Medical Center

Lifetime Achievement
Jacqueline A. Noonan, M.D.
Pediatric Cardiology
University of Kentucky Medical Center

Robert W. Schrier, M.D.
Nephrology
University of Colorado Health Sciences Center

National Health Leadership
Suzanne and Robert Wright
Vice-Chair of the Board, General Electric Company
Co-founders of Autism Speaks™

****

2007

Clinical Excellence
Delos M. Cosgrove, M.D.
Chairman, Board of Governors
CEO and President
The Cleveland Clinic

Joseph G. McCarthy, M.D.
Lawrence D. Bell Professor of Plastic Surgery
Director, The Institute of Reconstructive Plastic Surgery
NYU Medical Center

Patrick C. Walsh, M.D.
University Distinguished Service Professor and Director of Urology
The James Buchanan Brady Urological Institute
The Johns Hopkins Hospital

Lifetime Achievement
Maria Delivoria-Papadopoulos, M.D.
Director, The Neonatal Intensive Care Unit
St. Christopher's Hospital for Children;
Professor of Pediatrics, Physiology and Obstetrics/Gynecology
Drexel University College of Medicine

National Health Leadership
The Honorable Nancy G. Brinker
Founder of Susan G. Komen for the Cure
Former U.S. Ambassador to Hungary

****

<u>2006</u>

Clinical Excellence
Bart Barlogie, M.D., Ph.D.
Director, Myeloma Institute for Research Therapy
University of Arkansas for Medical Services

Marilyn J. Bull, M.D.
Morris Green Professor of Pediatrics
Riley Hospital for Children

Michael J. Zinner, M.D.
Moseley Professor of Surgery
Harvard Medical School
Surgeon-in-Chief, Brigham & Women's Hospital

Lifetime Achievement
Michael E. DeBakey, M.D.
Chancellor Emeritus, Baylor College of Medicine

National Health Leadership
Princess Yasmin Aga Khan
Honorary Vice Chair
Alzheimer's Association

Castle Connolly and Social Media

Castle Connolly maintains Facebook, Twitter, LinkedIn and Sharecare accounts in an effort to keep consumers informed of the latest news not only regarding Castle Connolly Medical Ltd., its Top Doctors and Top Hospitals, but also reports on various health observances and events. A live Twitter feed can also be found on the homepage of www.castleconnolly.com.

Consumers who use our print guides, online database or refer to our regional magazine features can find up-to-date information about Castle Connolly, healthcare and medical news by logging onto these social networking sites:

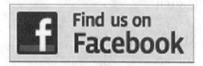

www.facebook.com/TopDoctors

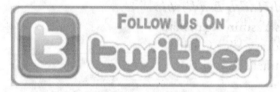

www.sharecare.com/group/castle-connolly-medical-ltd
or http://bit.ly/giuPHI

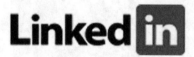

www.twitter.com/CastleConnolly

Linked in

http://linkd.in/mP4Lmb

Do you have a story about a Castle Connolly Top Doctor or Top Hospital that you want to share? If so, please email a link to the article to:

Nicki Hughes
Social Media and Research Associate
nhughes@castleconnolly.com

Castle Connolly has developed a website and database – www.AmericasTopCosmeticDoctors.com – to enable consumers to search and identify top cosmetic specialists who have been nominated by their peers through an extensive, annual survey process involving tens of thousands of American physicians. Nominated physicians' medical education, training, hospital appointments, disciplinary histories - and much more - are screened and reviewed by our physician-led research team. Those selected as top doctors may appear in a number of Castle Connolly guides/online databases, including www.topcosmeticdoctors.com. They are specially trained in cosmetic procedures and spend the majority of their time in their medical practice doing cosmetic work. The top cosmetic doctors whose profiles are included on this site are in one of only six medical specialties: Dermatology, Facial Plastic Surgery, Ophthalmology, Otolaryngology, Plastic Surgery, or Surgery. The website also includes valuable information on how to select the right cosmetic doctor for you, as well as detailed information about some of the most common procedures.

For more information visit: www.AmericasTopCosmeticDoctors.com

Doctor-Patient Advisor for Individual Consumers

Doctor-Patient Advisor is a Castle Connolly Medical Ltd. service providing one-on-one consultations with a physician or nurse practitioner to individuals who have serious or complex medical problems or to anyone who feels he/she needs assistance finding the right physician for any purpose. Each client will receive personalized assistance in identifying the appropriate specialists for his/her condition, utilizing the Castle Connolly Medical Ltd. database of physicians and hospitals, as well as individual searches, to locate the best resources to meet the client's needs.

Fee: $375. For further information call (212) 367-8400 x 16.

Premium Membership at www.CastleConnolly.com

Reap the benefits of membership with Castle Connolly. Gain access to ALL online top doctor listings and get discounts on book purchases from our extensive catalog.

• Search among more than 26,000 Castle Connolly Top Doctor listings
• Search among select hospitals and centers of excellence
• Receive a 30% discount on all book purchases
Membership Levels:
• One year - $24.95
• Two years - $34.95

For more information visit: www.CastleConnolly.com/membership

Other Products From Castle Connolly

Castle Connolly Guides

Titles Include:

- *America's Top Doctors®*
- *Top Doctors: New York Metro Area*

And Many More

To order other Castle Connolly guides at a 15% discount please visit
http://www.CastleConnolly.com/books
When ordering use discount code: **ATDC7VAN**

Castle Connolly's Top Doctors Available Online

- Free Access to 20 -25% of Castle Connolly's Top Doctors
- Purchase Access to the entire database of more than 26,000 doctor profiles

http://www.castleconnolly.com/membership

Customer Feedback

We appreciate your comments regarding our guides. Please email us at
info@castleconnolly.com

The Best in American Medicine
www.CastleConnolly.com